INTEGRATED NEUROSCIENCE AND NEUROLOGY

INTEGRATED NEUROSCIENCE AND NEUROLOGY

A CLINICAL PROBLEM SOLVING APPROACH

SECOND EDITION

Elliott M. Marcus, MD*

PROFESSOR EMERITUS OF NEUROLOGY, UNIVERSITY OF MASSACHUSETTS SCHOOL OF MEDICINE

LECTURER IN NEUROLOGY, TUFTS UNIVERSITY SCHOOL OF MEDICINE

CHAIRMAN EMERITUS DEPARTMENT OF NEUROLOGY, SAINT VINCENT HOSPITAL

AND FALLON CLINIC, WORCESTER, MA

*DECEASED.

Stanley Jacobson, PhD

PROFESSOR OF ANATOMY AND CELLULAR BIOLOGY, TUFTS UNIVERSITY

HEALTH SCIENCES CAMPUS, BOSTON, MA; AND FULBRIGHT SCHOLAR

Thomas D. Sabin, MD

PROFESSOR OF NEUROLOGY, TUFTS UNIVERSITY SCHOOL OF MEDICINE

TUFTS MEDICAL CENTER, BOSTON, MA

2014

IN MEMORIAM

Dr. Elliott Marcus, Professor of Neurology at University of Massachusetts (Emeritus). At 78, Dr. Marcus—a neurologist and educator for five decades at Tufts Medical Center, Tufts University School of Medicine, and the University of Massachusetts Medical School at Saint Vincent Hospital—died on July 25, 2011, in Massachusetts General Hospital in Boston.

Even as the end drew near, Dr. Elliott Marcus pressed on with his life's work: sharing the knowledge he had gleaned through a lifetime of dedicated study and teaching neuroscience. He received his undergraduate education at Yale University and earned an MD from Tufts University School of Medicine. He was trained in neurology at Tufts Medical Center and also served with distinction for 2 years in the US Army. He taught at Tufts University School of Medicine from 1964 to 1976, where he was the "father" of neuroscience teaching to medical students. He then moved to Saint Vincent Hospital in Worcester, Massachusetts, in 1976, where he was Chief of Neurology. He also was a Professor of Neurology at the University of Massachusetts and an active member of that department. He was a clinical neurologist and he published many papers on diagnosis and treatment of seizure disorders. He retired in 1998 and continued active teaching of neurology residents and medical students at UMass until just before his death.

Even as non-Hodgkin's lymphoma took its toll on Dr. Marcus, he pushed himself, discussing his contributions to a forthcoming book that he and Dr. Stanley Jacobson, a Professor of Anatomy and Cellular Biology at Tufts Medical School and a friend and colleague for over 40 years, were collaborating on and telling friends to make sure the work continued beyond the span of his limited days. He wanted to live and be there to teach and to be there for his grandchildren.

Friends and colleagues said he was dedicated to his work, loved his family, and inspired generations of doctors. Dr. Thomas Sabin, a Professor of Neurology at Tufts Medical School, described Dr. Marcus as a superb neurologist and someone with a brilliant intellect.

Dr. David Chad, a Professor of Neurology and Pathology at UMass Medical School, said Dr. Marcus's passion for neurology and teaching was always evident. Dr. Marcus often traveled from Florida more than a decade after his official retirement in 1998 to work with neurology students. He would talk with them, letting them learn through conversations, rather than just giving the answers. Chad said, "He had a Socratic method of teaching; he let students sort of find the truth," Chad said. "He would open the subject up. He would bring out the key issues to be discussed. He wouldn't stand up and give the answers. He'd ask questions and give feedback. He was an excellent communicator. He loved sharing what he knew. He brought scholarship to his teaching." Dr. Cynthia Brown, who first met Dr. Marcus in 1980 as a resident neurologist at UMass Medical School and Saint Vincent Hospital, described neurology as a "very intellectual specialty." "To have someone as bright and inspiring as Dr. Marcus helps to validate one's choice to be a neurologist," she said. "He's really a doctor's doctor, and it is very sad to think that the upcoming classes of medical students will not be able to have his tutorials."

Boston Globe, 2011
Melvin Mason
Stanley Jacobson

OXFORD
UNIVERSITY PRESS

Oxford University Press is a department of the University of Oxford.
It furthers the University's objective of excellence in research, scholarship,
and education by publishing worldwide.

Oxford   New York
Auckland   Cape Town   Dar es Salaam   Hong Kong   Karachi
Kuala Lumpur   Madrid   Melbourne   Mexico City   Nairobi
New Delhi   Shanghai   Taipei   Toronto

With offices in
Argentina   Austria   Brazil   Chile   Czech Republic   France   Greece
Guatemala   Hungary   Italy   Japan   Poland   Portugal   Singapore
South Korea   Switzerland   Thailand   Turkey   Ukraine   Vietnam

Oxford is a registered trademark of Oxford University Press
in the UK and certain other countries.

Published in the United States of America by
Oxford University Press
198 Madison Avenue, New York, NY 10016

© Oxford University Press 2014

All rights reserved. No part of this publication may be reproduced, stored in a
retrieval system, or transmitted, in any form or by any means, without the prior
permission in writing of Oxford University Press, or as expressly permitted by law,
by license, or under terms agreed with the appropriate reproduction rights organization.
Inquiries concerning reproduction outside the scope of the above should be sent to the
Rights Department, Oxford University Press, at the address above.

You must not circulate this work in any other form
and you must impose this same condition on any acquirer.

Library of Congress Cataloging-in-Publication Data
Marcus, Elliott M., 1932–2011, author.
Integrated neuroscience and neurology : a clinical case history problem solving approach / by Elliott M.
Marcus, Stanley Jacobson, Thomas Sabin.—Second edition.
    p. ; cm.
Includes bibliographical references and index.
ISBN 978–0–19–974443–5 (alk. paper)
I. Jacobson, Stanley, 1937– author.   II. Sabin, Thomas D., author.   III. Title.
[DNLM: 1. Nervous System Diseases—diagnosis.   2. Nervous System Diseases—therapy.
3. Nervous System—anatomy & histology.   4. Nervous System Physiological Phenomena. WL 140]
RC346
616.8—dc23
2013039951

The science of medicine is a rapidly changing field. As new research and clinical experience broaden
our knowledge, changes in treatment and drug therapy occur. The author and publisher of this work
have checked with sources believed to be reliable in their efforts to provide information that is accurate
and complete, and in accordance with the standards accepted at the time of publication. However, in
light of the possibility of human error or changes in the practice of medicine, neither the author, nor
the publisher, nor any other party who has been involved in the preparation or publication of this work
warrants that the information contained herein is in every respect accurate or complete. Readers are
encouraged to confirm the information contained herein with other reliable sources and are strongly
advised to check the product information sheet provided by the pharmaceutical company for each drug
they plan to administer.

9 8 7 6 5 4 3 2 1
Printed in China
on acid-free paper

*To our families for their infinite patience and understanding,
and to our students, teachers, and colleagues*

CONTENTS

Preface xi

SECTION ONE
INTRODUCTION TO BASIC NEUROBIOLOGY

1. Overview of the Nervous System 3
2. Overview of Localization of Function and Neurological Diagnosis 22
3. Neurocytology: Cells of the Central Nervous System 45
4. Neuroembryology and Congenital Malformations 72
5. Skeletal Muscle and Nerve-Muscle Junction 91

SECTION TWO
REGIONAL APPROACH TO NEUROANATOMY AND FUNCTIONAL LOCALIZATION

6. Spinal Cord: Structure and Function 111
7. Atlas of the Spinal Cord 133
8. A Survey of Diseases of Peripheral Nerve and Nerve Root 138
9. Spinal Cord: Clinical Considerations 162
10. Case History Problem Solving: Part I: Spinal Cord, Nerve Root, Peripheral Nerve, and Muscle 193
11. Functional Anatomy of the Brain Stem 199
12. The Cranial Nerves 221
13. Brain Stem: Clinical Considerations 252
14. Case History Problem Solving: Part II: Brain Stem and Cranial Nerves 281
15. Diencephalic Nuclei, Functional Localization, and Atlas of the Diencephalon 288

SECTION THREE
MAJOR SYSTEMS

16. Hypothalamus, Neuroendocrine System, and Autonomic Nervous System 311
17. Cerebral Cortex: Cytoarchitecture, Physiology, and Overview of Functional Localization 325
18. Motor System and Movement: Part I: Reflex Activity, Central Pattern Generators, and Cerebral Cortical Motor Functions 347
19. Motor Systems: Part II: Basal Ganglia and Movement Disorders 371
20. Motor Systems: Part III: Cerebellum and Movement and Major Fiber Pathways of the Cerebellum 395
21. Somatosensory Function and the Parietal Lobe 414
22. Limbic System 422
23. Visual System 444
24. Speech, Language, Cerebral Dominance, and the Aphasias 460
25. Case History Problem Solving: Part IV: Cortical Localization 476
26. Cerebral Hemispheres: Neuropathology and Clinical Correlation I. Vascular Syndromes 482
27. Cerebral Hemispheres: Neuropathology and Clinical Correlation II. Nonvascular Syndromes 505
28. Case History Problem Solving: Part IV: Cerebral Hemispheres 538

SECTION FOUR
COMPLEX FUNCTIONS

29. Alterations in Consciousness: Seizures, Sleep, and Coma 549
30. Learning, Memory, Amnesia, Dementia, Instinctive Behavior, and the Effects of Early Experience 575
31. Case History Problem Solving: Part V: General Cases 598
32. Case History Problem Solving: Part VI: Case History Review with Correlation to Illustrations 605
33. Atlas of the Cerebrum 614

Index 619

PREFACE

This textbook takes as a premise that, in order to make intelligent diagnosis and provide a rational treatment in disorders of the nervous system, it is necessary to develop the capacity to answer the basic questions of clinical neurology: (1) Where is the disease process located? (2) What is the nature of the disease process?

The purpose of this textbook is to enable the medical student to acquire the basic information of the neurosciences and neurology and, most important, the ability to apply that information to the solution of clinical problems. The authors also suggest that, if possible, hospital trips be a part of any Clinical Neurosciences course so that the student can put into actual practice what he or she has learned in the classroom.

We believe that this textbook will be of value to the student throughout the 4 years of the medical school curriculum.

Medical, psychiatry, and neurology residents may also find this text of value as an introduction or review.

It is truer in neurology than in any other system of medicine that a firm knowledge of basic science material, that is, the anatomy, physiology, and pathology of the nervous system, enables the student and physician to readily arrive at the diagnosis of where the disease process is located and the nature of the most likely pathology. Subsequently that knowledge may be applied to problem solving in clinical situations.

The authors have a long experience in teaching neuroscience courses at the first- or second-year medical student level in which clinical information and clinical problem solving are integral to the course. In addition, the first author has developed a case history problem-solving seminar in which all medical students at the University of Massachusetts participate during their clinical neurology clerkship rotation. This provides the students an opportunity to refresh their problem-solving skills and to review and update that basic science material essential for clinical neurology.

The second author has had extensive experience in utilizing sections of this text in neuroscience courses for advanced undergraduate college students and ancillary health profession students.

At these several levels, we have observed that this approach reinforces the subject matter learned by markedly increasing the interest of the students in both basic and clinical science material.

This text is an updated version of an earlier integrated textbook originally developed by the authors along with Dr. Brian Curtis and published by W. B. Saunders in 1972 as *An Introduction to the Neurosciences*.

Dr. Thomas Sabin reviewed all the clinical chapters and, where necessary, provided additional materials.

The present text provides an updated approach to lesion localization in neurology, utilizing the techniques of computerized axial tomography (CT scanning), magnetic resonance imaging (MRI), and magnetic resonance angiography (MRA) that were not available in 1972. In addition, the other modern clinical techniques of evoked potentials, positron emission tomography (PET), single-photon emission computerized tomography (SPECT), and functional MRI neuroimaging (fMRI) are discussed and illustrated. Multiple illustrations demonstrating the value of these techniques in clinical neurology and neuroanatomical localization have been provided. The clinical case illustrations have been utilized both in the body of the text and in special problem-solving chapters.

There are specific review and problem-solving chapters with a strong emphasis on clinical case history problem solving. These clinical problem-solving exercises are found as specific chapters with part I (Chapter 10) covering diseases of spinal cord, nerve root, peripheral nerve and muscle, part II (Chapter 14) covering disorders of the brain stem and cranial nerves, part III (Chapter 25) covering cortical localization, and part IV (Chapter 28) covering diseases of the cerebral hemispheres with an emphasis on cerebral vascular disease. Finally, parts V and VI (Chapters 31 and 32) provide case history problem solving that encompasses all regions of the brain. This final part also provides an appendix in which various clinical neuroimages are provided for identification of location of lesion and of the type pathology. A series of clinical cases is then provided in which the advanced student is requested to select the appropriate study that was utilized for the particular cases. Review questions for many of the chapters will be found at the end of the book.

The case history problem-solving exercises are designed to be utilized in weekly case history problem-solving discussion groups, with an instructor, usually a neurologist, neurosurgeon, neurology, or neurosurgical resident. Some medical school courses may provide a physical diagnosis session devoted to the neurological history and examination.

In Chapter 2 we have included an outline of a complete and abbreviated neurological history and an overview of the diagnostic studies to be utilized at each level of the neural axis.

The emphasis throughout the text, however, is on clinical diagnosis; that is, what the diagnosis is before the laboratory and imaging studies were selected. Thus, for each of the illustrative case histories, a provisional clinical diagnostic impression is provided before the results of the ancillary studies are presented. This should instill in the student the concept that the history and neurological examination must first be completed, subjected to analysis and a clinical diagnosis or differential impression established before the ancillary studies are selected.

Even in this era of modern imaging, this is the most efficient and effective approach. It has been said that 75% of neurological diagnosis is dependent on the history. The student should be aware that this stated clinical diagnostic impression does not always correspond to the final diagnosis. The case histories, in all instances, present actual patients. It is our impression that such cases are more instructive and more interesting to students than manufactured, stereotypical case histories. Because these are cases based on clinical reality, at times there are minor deviations from the classic picture, or multiple disorders are present.

In general, for the problem-solving exercises, the cases have been arranged in an increasing order of difficulty. In a number of instances within the text or within the case history problem-solving exercises, we have chosen to retain case histories from the earlier version of this text. In some instances, the history and/or findings presented were of a "classical" nature with an opportunity to study the full natural evolution of disease. In most cases, the location of disease process was clearly confirmed by surgery and/or by autopsy. This was more likely to be the case before the development of modern neuroimaging. It will also be evident that some cases were retained because those patients continued to have neurological follow-up, allowing an overview of the long-term course of particular diseases.

Chapter 27 covers, in detail, diffuse disorders of the cerebral hemispheres such as aseptic meningitis and encephalitis. Many of these topics are also covered in internal medicine courses.

It is planned that a Web page will be established by the publisher. This will provide a means for sending additional material to the reader. In addition, information regarding the solution of the clinical case history problem-solving exercises will be provided.

Most of the case histories utilized in the chapters and in the problem-solving exercises have been drawn from the files of Dr. Marcus. For a number of the cases, our associates at the New England Medical Center, Saint Vincent Hospital, Fallon Clinic, and the University of Massachusetts School of Medicine either requested our opinion or brought the case to our attention and provided information from their case files. These individual neurologists and neurosurgeons are identified in the specific case histories. We are also indebted to the many referring physicians of those institutions. Some of the cases were presented to Dr. Marcus during morning report by medical house officers at Saint Vincent Hospital. In particular, our thanks are due to our associates in Worcester: Drs. Bernard Stone, Alex Danylevich, Robin Davidson, Harold Wilkinson, and Gerry McGuillicuddy. Drs. Sandra Horowitz, Tom Mullins, Steve Donhowe, Martha Fehr, Lawrence Recht, Paula Raven, and Carl Rosenberg provided additional or follow-up clinical information from their files for some of the case histories. Our associates at the New England Medical Center, Drs. John Sullivan, Sam Brendler, Peter Carney, John Hills, Huntington Porter, Bertram Selverstone, Thomas Twitchell, C.W. Watson, and Robert Yuan and Thomas Sabin likewise provided access to some of the clinical material for the earlier version of this text. Dr. Milton Weiner at Saint Vincent Hospital was particularly helpful in providing many of the modern neuroradiological images. Dr. Sam Wolpert and Dr. Bertram Selverstone provided this material for the earlier version of the text. The normal MRIs were provided by Dr. Val Runge from the University of Texas Imaging Center. Dr. Anja Bergman (left handed) had the patience to be our normal case and the images from her brain form the normal MRIs in the basic science chapters and atlas.

Dr. Tom Smith and his associates in pathology provided much of the recent neuropathological material, particularly for the chapters on muscle, peripheral nervous system, and dementia. Drs. John Hills and Jose Segarra provided access to neuropathological material for the earlier version of the text.

Critical review of particular chapters was provided by Dr. Sandra Horowitz and Dr. David Chad.

Dr. Brian Curtis contributed material for inclusion in Chapter 6 (muscle physiology) and 7 (spinal cord physiology) and 23 (the physiology of the visual system). Dr. Curtis has contributed material included in the auditory system.

Many of the newer anatomical drawings were provided by Mary Gauthier Delaplane, now a medical student at Boston University School of Medicine, and by Dr. Sarah Cairo while a medical student at Tufts University. Dr. Marc Bard provided drawings for the earlier version of this text while a student at Tufts University School of Medicine. Dr. Mary Gauthier Delaplane and Mr. Seymour Levy provided graphic services and assisted in the layout of text and illustrations. Ms. Jane Griesbach and her associates at Saint Vincent Hospital provided photographic prints of many of the neuroimages which we had selected. Ms. Helen Johnson provided typographic assistance in the formative stages of this project.

We have continued to utilize or have modified some of the illustrations which were borrowed with permission from other published sources for the earlier version of this text.

In many of the clinical chapters, various medications are discussed. Before utilizing these medications, the reader should check dosage and indications with other sources and modify as necessary for the individual patient.

It is with great pleasure we extend our thanks to our publishers and particularly our editor, Craig Panner, who continually encouraged us and we kept our noses to the grindstone. Any faults or errors are those of the authors, and we would therefore appreciate any suggestions or comments from our colleagues.

Elliott Marcus, Stanley Jacobson, Thomas Sabin

SECTION I

INTRODUCTION TO BASIC NEUROBIOLOGY

1.

OVERVIEW OF THE NERVOUS SYSTEM

The brain is the part of the central nervous system that is housed in the cranium/skull. It consists of the brain stem, diencephalon, cerebellum, and cerebrum. At the foramen magnum the highest cervical segment of the spinal cord is continuous with the lowest level of the medulla of the brain stem. The 12 cranial nerves attached to the brain form the upper part of the peripheral nervous system and record general sensations of pain, temperature, touch, and pressure, but in addition we now find the presence of the special senses of smell, vision, hearing, balance, and taste. The blood supply to the brain originates from the first major arterial branches from the heart, ensuring that over 20% of the entire supply of oxygenated blood flows directly into the brain.

THE NERVOUS SYSTEM

One word summarizes the function of the nervous system: *reaction*. The central nervous system (brain and spinal cord) monitors and controls the entire body by its peripheral divisions, which are distributed to all the muscles, organs, and tissues. The brain has an advantageous site in the head and above the neck, which can move in about a 140-degree arc. Close to the brain are all of the specialized sense organs, which permit us to see, smell, taste, and hear our world. The central nervous system is protected by fluid-filled membranes, the meninges, and surrounded by the bony skull and vertebrae.

THE NEURON

The basic conducting element in the nervous system is the nerve cell, or neuron (Fig. 1.1). A neuron has a cell body, dendrite, and axon. The cell body contains many of the organelles vital to maintain the cell's structure and function, including the nucleus and nucleolus, and is considered the tropic center of the nerve cell. The dendrites extend from the cell body and increase the receptive surface of the neuron. The axon leaves the cell body and connects to other cells. Axons are covered by a lipoproteinaceous membrane called *myelin* that insulates the axons from the fluids in the central nervous system. The site of contact between the axon of one nerve cell and the dendrites and cell body of another neuron is the *synapse* (see Chapter 2). The cells in the nervous system are classified based on their shapes: unipolar, bipolar, and multipolar (Fig. 1.1; Table 1.1). In the central nervous system the nerve cells are supported by glia and blood vessels; in the peripheral nervous system they are supported by satellite cells, fibroblasts, Schwann cells, and blood vessels.

There are three basic categories of neurons: (1) receptors, the ganglia of the spinal dorsal roots and of the cranial nerves with general sensory components; (2) effectors, the ventral horn cells, motor cranial nerve nuclei, and motor division of the autonomic nervous system; and (3) interneurons, the vast majority of the neurons in the central nervous system. The areas in the central nervous system that contain high numbers of neuronal cell bodies are called *gray matter*, while the regions that contain primarily myelinated axons are called *white matter*. Neurons are organized into ganglia, nuclei, or layered cortices.

Ganglia

Sensory ganglia are found outside the central nervous system and contain the first-order neurons in the sensory systems, and they are the dorsal root ganglia on the 32 segments of the spinal cord and the sensory ganglia on cranial nerves (CN) V, VII, VIII, IX, and X.

Motor/autonomic ganglia are found throughout the body, and they are either sympathetic or parasympathetic ganglia.

Nuclei

Throughout the brain and spinal cord there are groupings of neurons with a common function; these are the *nuclei*. They are found throughout the spinal cord (ventral and dorsal horn), brain stem (cranial nerve nuclei, reticular formation) and diencephalon (nuclei of thalamus, hypothalamus, subthalamus, and metathalamus), basal ganglia (caudate, putamen, globus pallidus, and substantia nigra), and in the cerebral cortex (amygdaloid nuclei).

Lamina

In the cerebral cortex, cerebellar cortex, and superior colliculus, the gray matter is on the surface and organized anatomically into horizontal columns and physiologically into vertical columns, permitting a nearly infinite number of interconnections.

The Senses

Aristotle distinguished five senses: hearing, sight, smell, taste, and touch. Modern neuroscience, however, includes the *five*

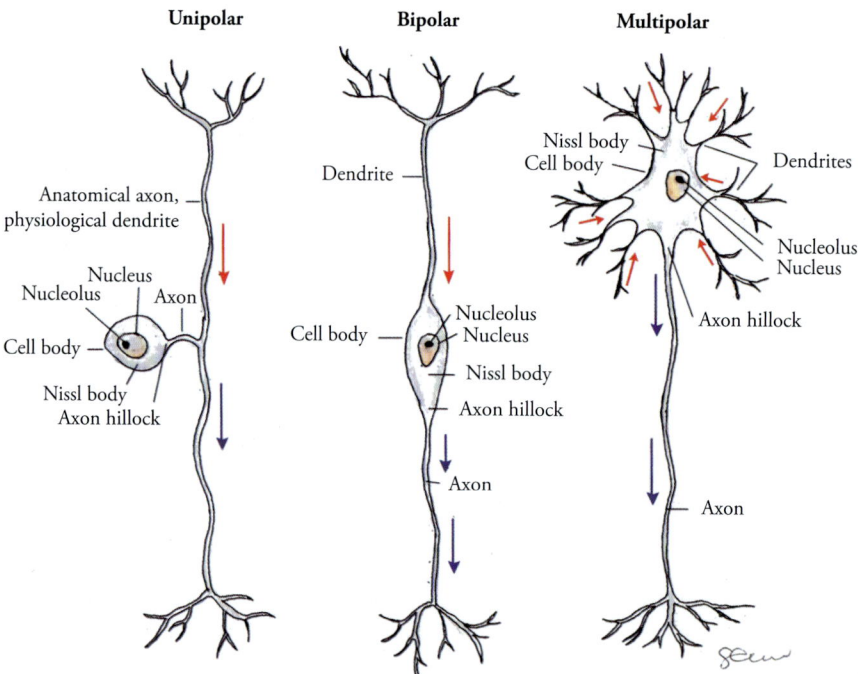

Figure 1.1 Types of Neurons in the Central Nervous System. The cells in the nervous system are classified based on their shapes: unipolar, bipolar, and multipolar. The input (red), reaches the dendrites of each cell and is then transported (blue) into the axon where it connects to the next neuron via a synaptic interruption.

special senses (balance, vision, hearing, taste, and smell) and the *four general senses* (pain, temperature, touch, and pressure). Humans have evolved a series of specialized receptors for each of these different sensory functions (Table 1.2). The special sensory apparatuses are found in the head: the eye and its protective coverings and muscles, the membranous labyrinth in the temporal bone for hearing and balance, the nose with olfactory receptors, and the tongue with taste buds. The *receptors for general sensation* (mechanicoreceptors, nociceptors, and thermoreceptors) are located primarily in the bodies largest organ, the skin (Fig. 1.2). Certain areas, such as the lips, fingers, feet, and genitalia, have a proliferation of the tactile mechanicoreceptors. Everywhere except on the soles and palms we have hair, which is an important tactile receptor but is continually being depleted by our concern for grooming. The pain receptors, or free nerve endings in the skin, are located throughout the body, but probably more receptors are in the skin over the face, lips, hands, and feet than over the rest

Table 1.1 TYPES OF NEURONS IN THE NERVOUS SYSTEM

NEURONAL TYPE	% OF NEURONS	LOCATION
Unipolar	0.05	Dorsal root ganglia of spinal cord Cranial nerve ganglia of brain stem Mesencephalic nucleus of CN V in midbrain
Bipolar	0.05	Retina, inner ear, taste buds
Multipolar		
Peripheral	0.1	Autonomic ganglia
Central	99.8	Brain and spinal cord

Table 1.2 SENSORY RECEPTORS

CLASS OF RECEPTOR	FUNCTION	LOCATION
Chemoreceptors	Taste Smell	Taste buds on tongue Olfactory mucosa in nose
Mechanicoreceptors	Balance Sound Tactile discrimination and pressure	Inner ear: semicircular canals Inner ear: cochlea Skin, muscle, tendons, joints
Nociceptor	Pain	Free nerve endings in skin and organs
Thermoreceptor	Temperature	Skin, tissues, and organs

of the body. As you review the receptors in Table 1.2, sense on your own body how the soles are especially good for feeling pressure and placing the body safely in light or darkness and the fingers and face are sensitive to touch and temperature. Remember that we have only discussed the skin receptors so far, which respond to external stimuli. However, there are also similar receptors within the respiratory, cardiovascular, endocrine, gastrointestinal, and urogenital systems that monitor our internal milieu.

Muscles

The ~640 muscles in the body form the bulk of the body and consist of three different functional and histological entities: *skeletal*, *smooth*, and *cardiac*. Skeletal muscles are found in the head, neck, arms, legs, and trunk and permit us to

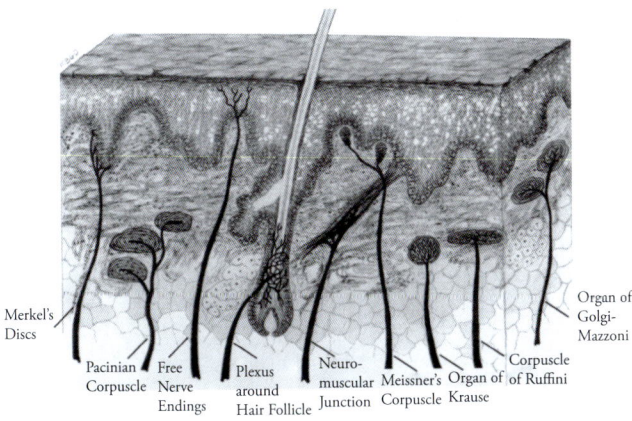

Figure 1.2 Hairy skin showing receptors.

undertake voluntary movements. Smooth, or unstriated, muscles are found in the viscera, blood vessels, and hair follicles. Cardiac muscles form auricles and ventricles of the heart.

Each muscle group has a specialized nerve ending that permits the impulse carried down the motor nerve via a peripheral nerve to stimulate the muscle through release of a specific chemical. Contraction of the three muscle groups in response to sensory information originates from the central nervous system via the efferent/motor peripheral nerves.

The general and special sensory receptors in the skin provide the *afferent* nerves that carry sensory information to the spinal cord and brain. The brain often analyzes the sensory input before the muscles, which are controlled by the efferent nerves carrying information from the brain or spinal cord, make a response. These integrative functions of the central nervous system form the bulk of the discussion in this book.

PARTS OF THE NERVOUS SYSTEM

The nervous system consists of a peripheral and central division. The central nervous system (brain and spinal cord) is surrounded by fluid-filled membranes (meninges; see Chapter 1) and housed in either the bony skull or vertebrae. In contrast, the peripheral nervous system that brings information from and to the central nervous system lacks a bony covering but is protected by the fascia, skin, muscles, and organs where it distributes. Sensory information enters the central nervous system through the afferent divisions of the peripheral nerves.

PERIPHERAL NERVOUS SYSTEM

Peripheral nerves originate from either the spinal cord or the brain. Peripheral nerves are found everywhere in the body: skin, muscles, organs, and glands. The peripheral nervous system is divided into a somatic and a visceral division. The *somatic* division innervates the skin and skeletal muscles in the body. The visceral, or *autonomic*, division innervates the cardiac muscles of the heart and the smooth muscles and receptors in the blood vessels and gastrointestinal, respiratory, urogenital, and endocrine organs. The details of the peripheral nervous system are taught as part of gross anatomy, so the student may want to review an anatomy text.

CENTRAL NERVOUS SYSTEM

The central nervous system consists of the spinal cord and brain (brain stem, cerebellum, diencephalons, and cerebrum). Attached to all of the 32 segments of the spinal cord and the brain stem are sensory ganglia that form the first link in the sensory system and bring the sensory information from the periphery into the central nervous system. The organization of the neuronal cell bodies, or the gray matter, in the central nervous system and the pathways (white matter) in each of these regions varies. In the spinal cord the gray matter is centrally placed with the white matter (tracts) located on the outside. In the brain stem and diencephalon there is an intermingling of the gray and white matter. In the cerebellum and cerebrum the gray matter is found on the surface with the white matter more centrally placed.

Motor axons exit from each of the 32 segments of the spinal cord, and all levels of the brain stem connect the central nervous system to all muscles and organs in the body. In the spinal cord, much of the brain stem, and diencephalon, the neurons are organized into nuclei, while in the superior colliculus of the brain stem, cerebellum, and cerebrum, the neurons are organized anatomically into layers and functionally into vertical columns.

SPINAL CORD

The spinal cord is that portion of the central nervous system that lies in the vertebral canal from the upper border of the atlas (first cervical vertebrae) to the lower border of the first lumbar vertebrae in the adult (or third lumbar vertebrae in the neonate). The spinal cord has 32 segments divided into five regions—cervical, thoracic, lumbar, sacral, and coccygeal—and these regions innervate specific regions in the neck and upper extremity (cervical segments), thorax and abdomen (thoracic levels), anterior leg and thigh (lumbar segments), buttock, and posterior leg and thigh (lumbar segments). This ordered relationship between the spinal cord and body produces a somatotopic organization throughout the central nervous system (Fig. 1.3).

In the spinal cord the parenchyma is organized into columns of gray and white matter with the gray matter centrally placed and surrounded by the white matter. This organization is not evident as one looks at isolated cross sections, but when these sections are reconstructed serially this columnar organization in the gray and white matter is apparent. The columns of gray matter in the spinal cord appear in the shape of a butterfly and are called horns; they are divided into a dorsal sensory horn, a ventral motor horn, intermediate zone, and commissural region. The largest neuronal cell bodies are found in the ventral horn (*ventral horn cells*), whose axons form the efferent division of the peripheral nervous system and innervate the skeletal muscles (Fig 1.4). The white matter of the spinal cord

Figure 1.3 Spinal cord cross section showing gray matter in center and white matter on the outside.

is divided into three columns: anterior, posterior, and lateral. The pathways interconnecting the spinal cord and brain are found in these columns.

The spinal cord has a tubular shape and has two regions of enlargement, the lower cervical that controls the upper extremity and the lumbosacral enlargement that controls the lower extremity.

BRAIN

The brain consists of the following regions: brain stem, cerebellum, diencephalon, and cerebrum (Fig. 1.5).

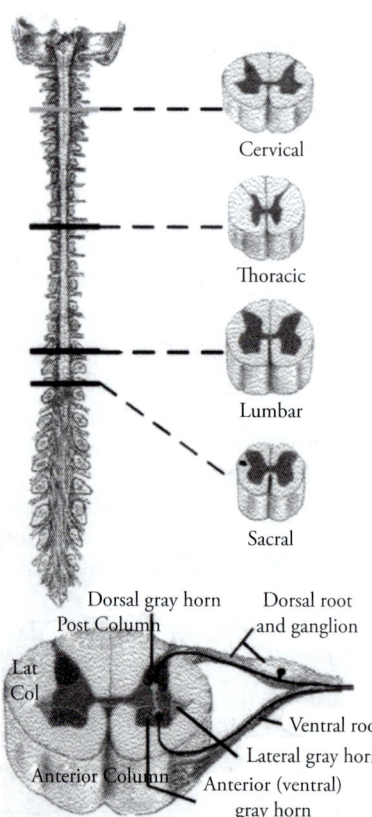

Figure 1.4 The spinal cord showing four cross section levels and the appearance of a spinal cord section with its dorsal and ventral nerves.

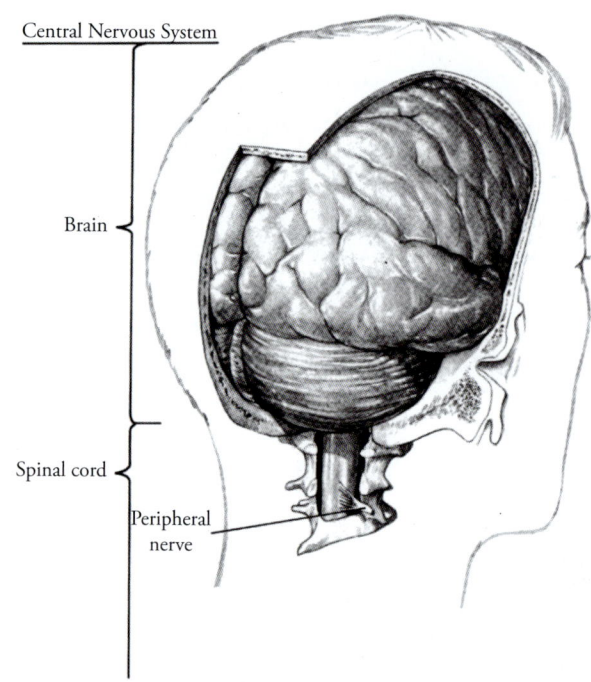

Figure 1.5 The Central Nervous System in situ. From an Introduction to Neurosciences, Curtis, Jacobson, Marcus. Saunders 1974.

The discussion of the central nervous system will start at the spinal cord and then proceed to the brain stem, to the diencephalon, and last but not least to the cerebrum.

Brain Stem

The columnar organization seen in the gray and white matter of the spinal cord is modified in the brain stem by the development of the ventricular system and the presence of the cranial nerves.

The brain stem (Fig. 1.6A) consists of three regions from inferior to superior: *medulla, pons,* and *midbrain.* The brain stem is often the most difficult region of the central nervous system for the student to learn because of the presence of the cranial nerves and associated nuclei. You may initially feel overwhelmed by its intricacy, but be patient. Approach neuroanatomy as you would a foreign language: first master the vocabulary and grammar before becoming fluent in conversation.

Reorganization of Gray and White Matter from Spinal Cord Gray to Tegmentum of Brain Stem

In the center of the brain stem, the narrow spinal canal enlarges, forming the wide fourth ventricle that divides each level of the brain stem into a region forming the floor of the ventricle of *tegmentum* and a region that forms the roof of the ventricle, the *tectum* (which consists of cerebellum, inferior and superior colliculi). The region that lies on the most anterior surface of the tegmentum is called the *basilar zone,* and it contains the descending fibers from the cerebral cortex. The columnar arrangement in the gray and white matter in the spinal cord slowly reorganizes in the lower medulla, resulting in the ventral and dorsal horn equivalent regions now lying on the floor of the ventricle with the intermediate zone forming the center of the tegmentum of the brain stem, the reticular formation.

Figure 1.6 (*A*) Location of the regions in the brain stem with the Cranial Nerve Nuclei in the brain stem on the left in blue and the sensory cranial nerve nuclei on the right in red. Only cranial nerve III-XII are found attached to the brain stem while Cranial Nerves I & II are found respectively attached to the base of the frontal lobe and diencephalon. Pure Motor Cranial Nerves—III, IV, VI, XI and XII; parasympathetic nuclei are found with CN III, VII, IX and X. Pure Sensory Cranial Nerves—II, II and VIII. Mixed Sensory and Motor Cranial Nerves—V, VII, IX and X. (*B*) Posterior surface of medulla and posterior surface of the cerebellum with the vermis, flocculonodular lobes, and cerebellar hemispheres labeled. Cerebellum.

With this reorganization the *ventral horn equivalent* contains cranial nerve motor nuclei of cranial nerves X and XII in the medulla, VI in the pons, and III and IV in the midbrain. The dorsal horn equivalent, which contains general somatic sensory and the visceral sensory nucleus of X containing general visceral sensastions and taste, lye lateral to the motor cranial nerve nuclei and are separated by the sulcus limitans. One also now finds the presence of the special sensory nucleus of cranial nerve VIII on the floor of the ventricle. The intermediate zone of the spinal cord evolves into the reticular formation in the center of the brain stem containing the motor and sensory cranial nerve nuclei innervating skin and muscles of pharyngeal arch origin and nuclei associated with the cerebellum (inferior olive), and basal ganglia (red nuclei). The medial surface of each half of the brain stem contains sensory and motor tracts, with the basilar surface containing the descending corticospinal and corticobulbar pathways. The lateral margin of the brain stem contains the anterolateral system.

Cranial Nerves (see Chapter 12)

In order to understand the functions of the brain stem, the student must first appreciate the distribution of the 12 cranial nerves with nerve I attached to the olfactory bulbs on the base of the frontal lobe, nerve II enters the diencephalon, and nerves III–XII originate in the brain stem and distribute in the head, trunk, and abdomen. Also the key to identifying dysfunction in the brain stem is to know which cranial nerve nucleus lies in each level.

The nerve rootlets of cranial nerves III and V–XII are found on the anterior surface of the brain stem, while the rootless only of cranial nerve IV exit on the posterior surface of the brain stem. Table 1.3 lists the location of the cranial nerve rootlets and nuclei in the appropriate brain stem level. Figure 1.6 demonstrates the location of the cranial nerve nuclei in the brain stem.

Chapter 6 discusses the nuclei and tracts of the brain stem in greater detail and includes many examples of the consequences of disease in the brain stem. Since the tegmentum where the cranial nerve nuclei are located is an especially important region for the student to master, we have divided this region bilaterally into five zones like an apple with the core, the center, being the reticular formation and the pulp being the surrounding four zones (Table 11.2).

Cerebellum

The cerebellum (Fig. 1.6B), similar to the cerebrum, consists of gray matter on the surface and white matter inside. It attaches to the tegmentum of the medulla and pons by three peduncles (Chapter 20). The cerebellum is divided into two lateral hemispheres and the midline vermis. From the phylogenetic (evolutionary development) standpoint there are

Table 1.3 **CRANIAL NERVE LOCALIZATION IN BRAIN STEM**

LEVEL	CRANIAL NERVE NUCLEI
Medulla: Rootlets of VII–XII	CN V spinal nucleus and tract (pain) CN VIII cochlear and vestibular CN IX, X, XI ambiguous nucleus CN IX CN X preganglionic parasympathetic CN XII tongue musculature
Pons: Rootlets of V–VII	CN V – motor nucleus (muscles of mastication) – chief sensory nucleus (tactile) – descending nucleus (pain) – mesencephalic (proprioception) CN VI lateral rectus CN VII muscles of facial expression CN VII taste and parasympathetics to face CN VIII vestibular and cochlear
Midbrain: Rootlets of III and IV	CN IV and CN III CN V mesencephalic nucleus

three regions: archicerebellum, paleocerebellum, and neocerebellum. The cerebellum functions at an unconscious level to permit voluntary motor functions to occur smoothly and accurately. Alcohol consumption and many drugs affect this region and temporarily impair, for example, gait and coordination.

In the white matter of the cerebellum are found *four deep cerebellar nuclei: fastigius*, dentatus, emboliformus, and globosus. The cerebellar cortex projects onto these nuclei, and then these nuclei project to other areas of brain stem or diencephalon. The functions of the cerebellum are detailed in Chapter 20.

Diencephalon

This region, identifiable in the gross brain after a sagittal section separates the cerebral hemispheres, lies at the upper end of the brain stem (Fig. 1.7). The third ventricle separates the right and left diencephalic masses. Their lateral margin is the posterior limb of the internal capsule, and their superior surface is the body of the lateral ventricle and the corpus callosum. The diencephalon stands as the great way station between the brain stem and cerebral cortex as all the major ascending pathways terminate here. The diencephalon consists of the following divisions: thalamus, hypothalamus, epithalamus, and subthalamus. The functional organization in the diencephalon is the basis for much of the function seen in the cerebrum and also contains the multimodal associations that make the cerebrum of the human such a potent analyzer (Table 1.4).

The *thalamus* forms the largest division of the diencephalon, and it is divided into several groupings of nuclei. All the ascending pathways terminate in thalamic nuclei and then their information is projected onto their respective region of the cerebral cortex. A detailed discussion of the thalamus is found in Chapter 15.

The *epithalamus* is a small zone on the mediodorsal portion of the diencephalon consisting of habenular nuclei, with its associative pathway, the stria medullaris, and the pineal gland; its functions are similar to the hypothalamus.

Table 1.4 **DIVISIONS OF THE DIENCEPHALON**

DIVISION	SUBNUCLEI	FUNCTIONS
Thalamus with metathalamus	Anterior, medial, lateral, and metathalamic nuclei	Termination of most ascending general and special sensory, cerebellar, and motor pathways; project onto sensory, motor, and associational areas in cerebral cortex
Epithalamus	Habenula, stria medullaris	Similar to hypothalamus but with connections to pineal gland
Hypothalamus	Anterior, medial, periventricular, and posterior	Center for homeostatic mechanisms and highest subcortical center for emotions as controls autonomics, pineal and pituitary glands
Subthalamus	Subthalamus, zona incerta	Subcortical unconscious center for movement, strong connections to basal ganglia

The *hypothalamus* is the smallest subdivision of the diencephalon and is found inferiorly in the third ventricle. However, by its controlling the pituitary gland and functioning as the "head ganglion" in the autonomic nervous system, it may well be the most important portion and emotional center of the diencephalon. The hypothalamus and the autonomic nervous system are discussed in Chapter 7.

The *subthalamus*, found below the thalamus, consists of the subthalamic nucleus and the zona incerta with its fiber pathways. It is an important subcortical region in the basal ganglia (Chapter 10).

The functions of this region are to integrate sensory and motor information and to begin to interpret this data according to the perceptions of the emotional areas in the brain.

Basal Ganglia

In a coronal section through a midpoint of the cerebral hemispheres we can identify laterally the cerebral cortex, cortical white matter, diencephalon, and basal nuclei (Fig. 1.7). Three important nuclear groups deep within the hemispheres are the corpus striatum, claustrum, and amygdala. This section focuses on the corpus striatum: the caudate nucleus, putamen, and globus pallidus. These nuclei are separated from the cerebral cortex by white matter but are functionally linked to the cerebrum. These nuclei are motor associative in function. They carry on at a subconscious level until a dysfunction, such as in Parkinson's disease or Huntington's chorea, occurs. The caudate nucleus and putamen are more laterally placed surrounding the white matter, which connects the cortex with the subcortical areas, the internal capsule. The caudate nucleus lies medial and dorsal to the thalamus. The functions of these nuclei will be discussed in further detail in Chapter 9.

Cerebrum: Cerebral Hemispheres

The cerebrum, forming the bulk of the brain and thus of the central nervous system, consists of a left and a right hemisphere containing the cortical gray matter, white matter, and

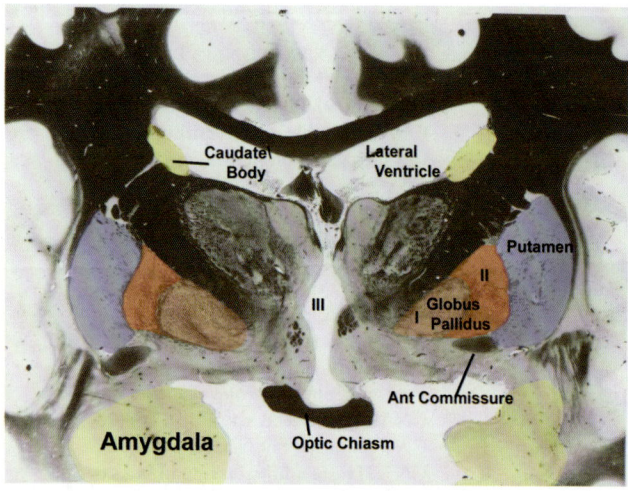

Figure 1.7 Coronal section showing basal ganglia (caudate, putamen, globus pallidus) and thalamus in relationship to the posterior limb of the internal capsule. The anterior commissure, optic chiasm and amygdala are also labeled. Myelin stain.

Figure 1.8 Gross brain with arachnoid membrane still attached.

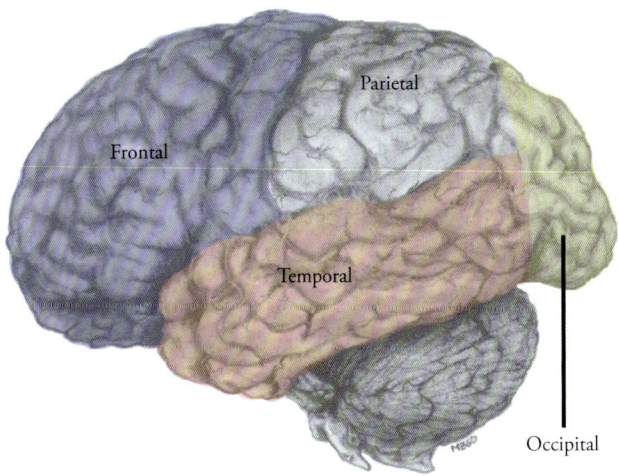

Figure 1.9 Four Lobes of the brain-Frontal, Parietal, Occipital and Temporal.

basal nuclei (Table 1.6). In each hemisphere we find four lobes: the rostral frontal lobe, the middle parietal lobe, and the posterior occipital lobe, with the inferiorly located temporal lobe (Fig. 1.9; Table 1.5).

The cerebral cortex consists of a corrugated surface, the cortical gray matter which is laminated and has six layers and is subdivided into numerous gyri, separated by narrow and deep spaces called the sulci (Fig. 1.8). The 12 to 15 billion cortical neurons are found in the cortical gray mantle. About 20% of the gray matter is found on the cortical surface while the bulk of the cortical gray mater lines the cortical sulci.

Students handling a preserved brain are often initially struck by the number of the gyri and sulci in the cerebral hemispheres and surprised by its weight (about 1500 g). If you have a series of brains to observe, note that there is a great variation in size. Remember that the size of the brain is related to the size of the skeleton, muscles, and viscera (but not adipose tissue), so a person of small stature has a proportionally smaller brain. Since women tend to be smaller than men, a woman's brain is usually smaller, although this in no way reflects intelligence or abilities. One of the first clues about the different functions in the two cerebral hemispheres was observed in stroke victims. Since the *left cerebral hemisphere* is dominant for language in right-handed people (93% of the population), strokes in that hemisphere usually affect speech. Besides language, dominant functions include initiation of movement, emotions, and artistic abilities.

Note that each hemisphere provides motor controls to the opposite side of the body. This is because the motor pathway from each cerebral cortex crosses in the transition between the spinal cord and *medulla*; consequently, the sensory fibers also cross over to the opposite side of the body. In over 90% of the human population movement initiates from the left hemisphere, making it dominant for initiation of movement.

General Features

The cerebral cortex is divided into four lobes, the frontal, parietal, occipital, and temporal lobes (Fig. 1.9). In addition, there are two other important regions in the cerebrum: the *insula* deep (Fig. 1.13) within the lateral sulcus and the *cingulate gyrus* on the medial surface of each hemisphere (Fig. 1.14). Three of the lobes also have poles: the frontal, temporal, and occipital pole. The frontal lobe (Fig 1.10) is separated from the parietal lobe by the central sulcus and from the temporal lobe by the lateral sulcus. The other lobes can be identified (Fig. 1.9) by first drawing a line from the parieto-occipital sulcus on the medial surface of the hemisphere to the preoccipital notch on the inferior lateral surface of the hemisphere. A line is then extended posteriorly from the lateral sulcus until it intersects the first line. The parietal lobe (Fig. 1.11) lies above the lateral sulcus and behind the central sulcus, anterior to the occipital lobe. The temporal lobe (Fig. 1.12) lies below the lateral sulcus anterior to the occipital lobe. The occipital lobe is most posteriorly placed (Fig. 1.12).

Functional Localization

The cerebral cortex includes frontal/motor (Fig. 1.10), parietal/sensory (Fig. 1.11), auditory (Figs. 1.12 and 1.13), and visual regions (Fig. 1.12). In addition, broad areas are involved with

Figure 1.10 Frontal Lobe and its major gyri.

Figure 1.11 Parietal lobe and its lobules.

Figure 1.13 Operculum of frontoparietal lobe removed demonstrating the insular cortex deep in the lateral sulcus and the auditory cortex in the superior temporal gyrus.

multimodal integration, which combines sensory and motor with an emotional content to determine how to respond in any situation. These emotional or limbic areas occupy much of the temporal and frontal lobes. (The *limbic* region denotes the cortical and subcortical brain areas with gray matter and tracts primarily involved with emotions, including the cingulate gyrus [Figs. 1.14 and 1.15], hippocampal formation, parahippocampal gyrus, and nuclei in the diencephalon; see Chapter 14.) Human beings also use language extensively and much of the frontal-parietal-occipital-temporal regions that abut the lateral sulcus in the left hemisphere undertake these functions. Similar areas of the right hemisphere are devoted to visual-spatial integration. You might wonder just how we have such detailed information on the organization and functions of the human nervous system. Much of it comes from research on primates or from defects observed in patients after strokes, trauma, tumors, or degenerative neurological diseases like Alzheimer's.

FUNCTIONAL LOCALIZATION IN THE LOBES OF THE CEREBRUM Besides all the functions already mentioned, the cerebral hemispheres also have the memory stores, which are the foundation for most conscious and unconscious thought, cultural activity, sexual behavior, and all of the other positive or negative traits which make the human being so distinctive. Each cortical region has a memory store that permits the function of that region (Table 1.5).

A detailed discussion of the functions of each cortical region is presented in Chapters 8 and 12–15.

Figure 1.14 Medial surface of the hemisphere with the corpus callosum and cingulate gyri identified.

Figure 1.15 Medial surface of a cerebral hemisphere with the brain stem removed revealing the inferior surface of the temporal lobe and the frontal, parietal and cuneate region of the occipital lobe labeled with an arrow pointing to the lingular gyri of the occipital lobe.

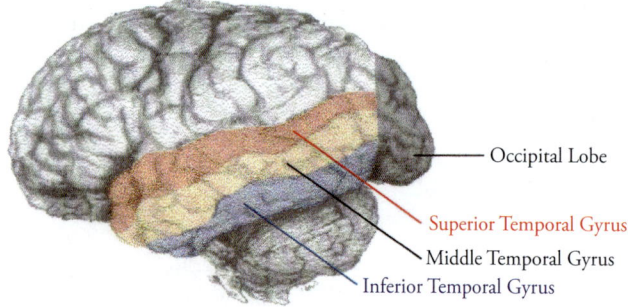

Figure 1.12 Temporal and Occipital lobes.

Cortical White Matter

The axons entering or leaving the cerebral hemispheres form three distinctive groups of fibers: associational, commissural, and subcortical (Table 1.6).

Table 1.5 OVERVIEW OF CEREBRAL FUNCTIONS

Frontal lobe Figure 1.10	Volitional movement of the muscles of the body, including limbs, face, and voice. Judgmental center
Parietal lobe Figure 1.11	Tactile discrimination from the body, body image, taste, and speech
Occipital lobe Figure 1.12	Vision (sight and interpretation)
Temporal lobe Figures 1.12 and 1.13	Emotions and new memories, hearing, language, olfaction, and visual recognition
Cingulate gyrus Figures 1.14 and 1.15	Emotions
Insular gyri Figure 1.13	Emotions and language

1. *Associational fibers.* These two types of fibers (short U and long associational) provide the integrative circuitry for movement, language, memory, and emotions. Short associational fibers, the U fibers, form the bulk of (e.g., arcuate) local connections within a hemisphere while the long associational fibers interconnect diverse areas in a hemisphere providing the multimodal (e.g., uncinate associations essential for cortical and cingulum).

2. *Commissural fibers.* Commissural fibers interconnect areas in the contralateral hemispheres and permit learning and memory in one hemisphere to be shared with the other. The bulk of the frontal, parietal, occipital, and temporal lobes is interconnected by the *corpus callosum*, best seen in the medial surface of the hemisphere. The corpus callosum consists of a rostrum, genu, body, and splenium (Fig. 1.14). The most rostral part of the temporal lobe and the olfactory cortex of the uncus are interconnected by the *anterior commissure.* The hippocampus, an important area for memory, is also connected by a commissure associated with the fornix.

3. *White matter of the cerebrum* (Table 1.6). This category of fibers includes fiber bundles reaching the cortex from subcortical areas, corticopetal (toward the cortex), and axons leaving the cortex and connecting to subcortical nuclei, corticofugal (away from the cortex).

ASSOCIATIONAL FIBERS These two types of fibers (short U and long associational) provide the integrative circuitry for movement, language, memory, and emotions.

COMMISSURAL FIBERS The bulk of the frontal, parietal, occipital, and temporal lobes is interconnected by the *corpus callosum,* best seen in the medial surface of the hemisphere. The corpus callosum consists of a rostrum, genu, body, and splenium (Fig. 1.14).

CORTICAL PROJECTION FIBERS *Corticopetal fibers* are the subcortical afferents to each cerebral hemisphere and are primarily from the thalamus of the diencephalon.

Corticofugal fibers from the cerebral hemisphere project onto subcortical structures, including the basal nuclei, diencephalon, brain stem, cerebellum, and spinal cord. The major subcortical fiber tracts leaving the cerebrum are the corticospinal, corticonuclear, corticopontine, corticomesencephalic, and the fornix.

The *internal capsule* contains the major grouping of corticofugal and corticopetal fibers of the cerebral cortex and consists of an anterior limb, genu, and posterior limb (Fig. 1.15). The anterior limb provides fibers to and from the frontal lobe. The genu provides fibers to and from the lower part of the frontal and parietal lobes (corticonuclear). The posterior limb is the largest portion of the internal capsule and includes the auditory radiations (auditory fibers to the auditory cortex), visual radiations as well as projections from the sensorimotor cortex to the spinal cord, and brain stem (corticospinal, corticonuclear, and corticopontine fibers).

Central Nervous System Pathways

Up to this point, the diverse functional gray regions in the brain and spinal cord have been identified. In order for the nervous system to work, an extensive circuitry has been established to interconnect areas throughout the central nervous system. We have just described the intrinsic white matter circuitry within the cerebrum: the associational, commissural, and subcortical fibers. The subcortical fibers consist of a multitude of axonal pathways that provide afferents to the cerebrum and efferents from the cerebrum. Many names are used for pathways within the central nervous system, including fasciculus (bundle), lemniscus (ribbon), peduncle (stalk), and tract (trail). Many of the pathways also have a name that indicates its function (e.g., the

Table 1.6 WHITE MATTER OF THE CEREBRAL HEMISPHERES

FIBER CATEGORY	FUNCTIONAL SIGNIFICANCE
ASSOCIATIONAL: short u fibers, superior longitudinal fasciculus, inferior longitudinal fasciculus, arcuate bundle, uncinate fasciculus, cingulum	Form the bulk of (e.g., arcuate) the white matter in each hemisphere and interconnect diverse areas in a hemisphere providing the multimodal associations essential for cortical control
COMMISSURAL: corpus callosum, anterior commissure, hippocampal commissure	Interconnects the left and right cerebral hemispheres (e.g., corpus callosum) and permits the learning and memory in one hemisphere to be shared with the other.
CORTICOFUGAL: corticospinal, corticobulbar/corticonuclear, corticopontines	From the cerebral cortex to subcortical gray matter > diencephalon, brain stem, cerebellum, and spinal cord; provides voluntary and involuntary controls of subcortical regions
CORTICOPETAL: thalamocorticals	Provide sensory, motor, autonomic afferents to cerebrum primarily through diencephalon

optic tract connects the eyes and visual regions, the corticospinal (Fig. 9.6) tract runs from the cortex to the spinal cord, and the corticonuclear (Fig. 9.7) tract connects the cerebral cortex to the cranial nerve nuclei). Unfortunately, the majority of the pathways have names that give no clue to function (e.g., the medial longitudinal fasciculus, lateral lemniscus, and cerebral peduncle). The major tracts and their role in the central nervous system are discussed in Chapter 6. For each pathway the student needs to learn the following:

1. Cells of origin
2. Location of the tract in the brain
3. Site of termination of pathway
4. Function

We are now going to use as an example of function within the central nervous system, a very significant region that provides volitional motor control to the muscles of the body, the motor-sensory strip.

The Motor-Sensory Cortex

This cortex is found around the central sulcus that separates the frontal from the parietal lobe and as most of the other regions in the cerebrum it has six layers. Figure 1.16, *lateral surface of the brain*, identifies the vertically oriented central sulcus which is surrounded by the precentral/motor strip and postcentral/sensory cortex. This region controls the skeletal muscles in the body that permit us to undertake so many tasks, and it is organized in a somatotopic organization (Fig. 1.16) with the head above the lateral sulcus, then comes the neck, upper extremity, thorax, abdomen, and finally the lower extremity on the medial surface of the hemisphere. The functions associated with the head occupy one-third of the motor strip, and the functions of the upper extremity and especially the hand occupy another one-third of the motor strip. The functions of the thorax and abdomen occupy 10% of the motor/sensory strip, and the many functions associated with the leg occupy 15% of the motor strip. In order to perform a skilled motor task, one is dependent on precise sensory input, so we will first describe the sensory portion of this circuit.

Sensory Information from the Foot to the Sensorimotor Cortex

In the sensory system three different neuronal groupings are traversed before the sensory information reaches the cerebral cortex from the periphery: the primary, secondary, and tertiary neurons. The sensory information of importance for precise movement originates from stretch receptors in the muscles, tendons, and joints of the hand and is encoded as electrical impulses that detail the contraction status of the muscles, tendons, and joints. The cells of origin, the primary cell bodies, are in the sensory ganglia attached to the lumbar and sacral segments of the spinal cord. The information is carried in by the dendrite of the primary sensory cell, and its axon enters the central nervous system and ascends uncrossed and ipsilaterally in the posterior column of the cord until the medullospinal junction. In the medullospinal junction *second-order nerve cells* appear in the posterior column, the gracile nucleus. The axons from the primary neurons synapse on this nucleus. The axons of the second-order axons cross the midline and ascend contralaterally in one of the major ascending white matter pathways, the medial lemniscus, into the thalamus of the diencephalon, where they synapse on the *third-order neurons in the ventral posterior lateral nucleus*, which then send fibers ipsilaterally onto the foot region on the upper end and medial surface of the postcentral gyrus.

Motor Control of the Foot from the Motor-Sensory Cortex

In the motor system two distinct neuronal groups are necessary for a movement: one in the motor cortex of the cerebrum (*the upper motor neuron*) and the other in the spinal cord or brain stem (*the lower motor neuron* [Fig. 1.16]). Motor control to the foot is carried centrifugally by the corticospinal pathway. The *corticospinal pathway* to the foot originates from layer V on the medial surface of the motor cortex of the precentral gyrus and to a lesser degree in the postcentral gyrus. The fibers before exiting the gray matter are covered with myelin and descend on the same side through the internal capsule, cerebral peduncle, pons, and medullary pyramid. The corticospinal fibers cross (decussate) to the other side of the brain in the medullospinal junction and enter the lateral column of the spinal cord. Fibers to the musculature of the leg descend to lower lumbar and sacral levels and synapse in either the intermediate region of the gray matter of the spinal cord or directly on the ventral horn cells. The axons from the ventral horn cell leave the central nervous system from the peripheral nerves that synapse on the motor endplates of the muscles in the leg which produce the contraction. The actual initiation of the movement is from the prefrontal and premotor region of the frontal lobe (see Chapter 9).

Figure 1.16 Lateral surface of the right Cerebrum. The motor (precentral) and sensory (postcentral) are marked; the somatotopic organization of this region is labeled from inferior to superior surface as follows; Head, Arm, Thorax, Abdomen and Foot. The foot region of the motor strip extends onto the medial surface of the hemisphere as the paracentral lobule.

Table 1.7 COMPARISON OF UPPER MOTOR NEURON LESION TO LOWER MOTOR NEURON LESION

Upper Motor Neuron Reflexes 2+ (normal) 3+ or 4+ are signs of upper motor neuron reflexes	Reflexes: Increase +3, +4, lesion in cortex or anywhere in corticospinal pathway. Muscles spastic, sign of corticospinal pathway, Babinski (extensor plantar response)
Lower Motor Neuron Reflexes 2+ (normal) 0>1+ are signs of lower motor neuron reflexes	Reflexes: Decrease to absent. Lesion (ventral horn cells, 0, +1, muscles flaccid and ventral roots, motor cranial atrophied, nerve nuclei and roots)

Interruption of the corticospinal pathway or destruction of the motor cortex produces *upper motor neuron paralysis* with increased reflex tone and spasticity while injury to the spinal cord ventral horn cells produces *lower motor neuron paralysis* and atrophy of the muscle and decreased reflex tone (Table 1.7).

In summary, it takes three orders of sensory neurons to provide the information to the cerebral cortex and two levels of motor neurons to produce a hand movement in response to the sensory information. Note that the sensory information ascends and crosses over, while the motor information descends and crosses so that the same side is represented in the cerebral cortex. Of course, the hand movement also needs a conscious decision to be made, which is what the cerebral cortex working as a unit does.

Demonstration of Effects of Lesions in the Brain

The following case history illustrates the effects of a tumor external to the leg region on the medial surface of the motor strip.

CASE HISTORY 1.1

This 45-year-old, right-handed, married, white mother was referred for evaluation of progressive weakness of the right lower extremity of 2 years duration. This weakness was primarily in the foot so that she would stub the toes and stumble. Because she had experienced some minor nonspecific back pain for a number of years, the question of a ruptured lumbar disc had been raised as a possible etiology. The patient labeled her back pain as "sciatica" but denied any radiation of the back pain into the leg. She had no sensory symptoms and no bladder symptoms. Six months before the consultation, the patient had transient mild weakness of the right leg that lasted a week. The patient attributed her symptoms to "menopause" and depression, and her depression had improved with replacement estrogen.

Neurological Examination

Exam revealed the patient's mental status was normal and the cranial nerves were all intact. There was a minimal drift down of the outstretched right arm, and there was significant weakness in the right lower extremity with ankle dorsiflexion and plantar flexion was less than 30% of normal. Inversion at the ankle was only 10%–20% of normal. Toe extension was 50% of normal, and there was minor weakness present in the flexors and extensors at the knee. In walking, the patient had a foot drop gait and had to overlift the foot to clear the floor. Examination of the shoes showed greater wear at the toes of the right shoe with evidence of scuffing of the toe. The patient's deep tendon stretch reflexes were increased at the patellar and Achilles tendons on

Figure 1.17 Meningioma in the left cerebral hemisphere above the leg region of the motor-sensory strip.

the right. In addition, reflexes in the right arm at the biceps, triceps, and radial periosteal were also slightly increased. The plantar response on the right was extensor (sign of Babinski), and the left was equivocal. All sensory modalities were intact. Scoliosis was present with local tenderness over the lumbar, thoracic, and cervical vertebrae, but no tenderness was present over the sciatic and femoral nerves.

Comments

It was clear that the symptoms and signs were not related to compression of the lumbar nerve roots by a ruptured disc. Such a compression (lumbar radiculopathy) would have produced a lower motor neuron lesion, a depression of deep tendon stretch reflexes, lumbar radicular pain in the distribution of the sciatic nerve and tenderness over the sciatic nerve, and no increase in reflexes in the upper or lower extremities, and no sign of Babinski. The fact that reflexes were more active in both upper and lower extremities on the right, with the sign of Babinski on the right, suggested a process involving the corticospinal tract. The fact that the weakness was greatest in the foot suggested a meningioma involving the *parasagittal motor cortex*, where the foot area is represented.

Clinical Diagnosis

With these clinical considerations in mind, a magnetic resonance image (MRI) of the patient's head was obtained and the MRI confirmed the clinical impression—of a meningioma in the right cerebral hemisphere (Fig 1.17). This tumor was successfully removed by the neurosurgeon with an essentially complete restoration of function.

Case 1.2 is an example of the effects of a lesion within the motor region in the dominant cerebral hemisphere.

CASE HISTORY 1.2

This 66-year-old, right-handed white female had the sudden onset of the feeling that the right side of her face was twisted. At the same time

Figure 1.18 Case 1-2. Glioblastoma in the face region of the left motor cortex (dominant side in this right handed individual).

she had difficulty in expressing herself. She knew what she wanted to say but had difficulty in getting the words out. These symptoms lasted for 5 minutes and then resolved completely. A similar episode had occurred 2 weeks previously and was described as a transient right-sided weakness and expressive aphasia. At that time an MRI suggested (Fig. 1.18) a possible area of early infarction in the left frontal area. Other studies of vessels in the neck and brain were negative and cardiac studies were unremarkable.

Past history of coronary artery disease for which an angioplasty had been performed with placement of a stent.

General physical exam not remarkable.

Neurological Examination

Mental status: Normal. Speech was fluent and she was able to read, name objects, and do repetitions.

Cranial nerves 2–12 were intact.

Motor system: Strength and gait were intact.

Reflexes: Deep tendon strength reflexes were symmetrical. Plantar reflexes were flexor.

Sensation: All modalities were intact.

Clinical Diagnosis

The symptoms localized to the posterior portion of the inferior frontal gyrus and the adjacent face are of the precentral gyrus. The description corresponded to a possible transient ischemic attack. However, repetitive focal seizures could not be ruled out.

Subsequent course: The patient was admitted 1 month later with a recurrence of these episodes. She had now experienced a total of 7 episodes, which were now characterized as being suddenly unable to speak; the right side of her face would contract upward and twitch. The episodes would subside over a matter of minutes except that speech deficit would now last for several hours. Examination now demonstrated problems in delayed recall. There were difficulties in repetition and speech was less fluent. The electroencephalogram (EEG) did not demonstrate any focal epileptiform discharge, and the episode was considered to represent focal seizures affecting the face and speech. Despite treatment with anticonvulsants, the episodes continue and speed problems worsened, requiring hospital readmission. Her exam now demonstrated more hesitancy with speech and less fluency. There was now flattening of the right nasolabial fold, indicating a central facial weakness.

The MRI now demonstrated an irregular rim of a contrast enhancing lesion with central necrosis located in the posterior segment of the left inferior frontal gyrus with edema of adjacent areas (Fig. 1.18). The most likely pathological diagnosis was glioblastoma-multiforme, the most malignant form of a glial tumor of the astrocytic series. The diagnosis was confirmed on subsequent biopsy of the lesion. The patient was subsequently treated with radiotherapy.

Comments

The location of the problem was apparent from the onset. The episodes of expressive aphasia localized to Broca's area in the left inferior frontal gyrus. The facial twitching suggested focal seizure originating in the adjacent area of facial representation in the precentral gyrus. Note that focal seizures involving the speech may produce transient speech arrest followed by a transient aphasia. The initial imaging studies suggested vascular damage corresponding to that localization. These studies did not include contrast enhancement. The diagnosis evolved from the transient ischemic attack (TIA) to focal seizures following an infarct to a more progressive problem of a glioblastoma. Note that because of the infarction and hemorrhage which may occur in glioblastomas, the problem may initially be incorrectly diagnosed as a stroke. There is no indication that such a delay in diagnosis alters prognosis for the glioblastoma.

THE NONNERVOUS ELEMENTS OF THE CENTRAL NERVOUS SYSTEM

ARTERIAL BLOOD SUPPLY TO THE BRAIN

The central nervous system is dependent on a continuous supply of enriched, oxygenated arterial blood. This has been accomplished by prioritizing blood supply to the brain as regards the initial branches of the major artery that leaves the heart, the aorta. Its first major branch is the common carotid, which supplies the neck, head, and brain (Fig. 1.19).

Blood flow to the brain is divided into the anterior and posterior circulation.

The *anterior circulation* (internal carotids, anterior cerebral arteries, middle cerebral arteries, and the anterior

Figure 1.19 The blood supply to the brain.

Figure 1.20 Arterial circle of Willis.

communicating arteries) supplies the basal ganglia, anterior diencephalon, the lateral surface of the cerebral hemispheres, anterior two-thirds of the medial surfaces of the cerebral hemisphere including the corpus callosum, and the orbital frontal surfaces of the cerebral hemispheres.

The *posterior circulation* (vertebral, basilar, posterior communicating and posterior cerebral arteries) supply the upper cervical spinal cord, cerebellum, brain stem, most of the diencephalon, and inferior and posterior surfaces of the temporal and occipital lobes of the cerebral hemispheres. At the base of the brain is a set of arteries called the circle of Willis (Figs. 1.20 and 1.23d) that interconnect the main portions of the anterior and posterior circulation by the formation of anterior and posterior communicating vessels.

Blood Supply to the Cerebral Hemispheres

The blood supply to the lateral surface of the brain is shown in Figure 1.21, while the arterial blood supply to the medial surface of a hemisphere is shown in Figure 1.22.

VENOUS DRAINAGE OF THE BRAIN, HEAD, AND NECK

The cerebral veins have very thin walls, no muscular layer, and no valves (Fig. 1.24). They are found on the surface of the brain or in the substance of the central nervous system.

1. *Superficial cerebral veins*. The superficial cerebral veins lie in the sulci, are thinner, and are usually external to the arteries. They consist of the superior, middle, and inferior cerebral veins.

2. *Superior cerebral veins*. A variable number of superior cerebral veins drain the superior surface of the cerebral cortex and empty into the superior sagittal sinus. The middle cerebral veins drain the bulk of the lateral and inferior surface; these veins are found in the lateral sulcus and empty into the cavernous sinus.

3. The *inferior cerebral veins* drain the lateral occipital gyrus and the temporal lobe; this vessel opens directly into the transverse sinus.

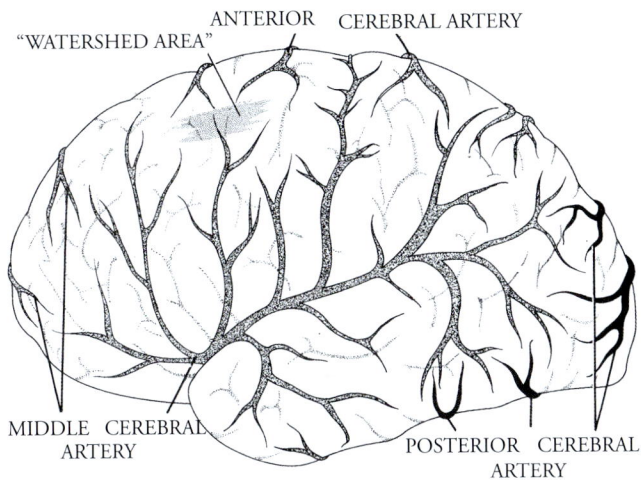

Figure 1.21 Arterial Blood supply to the Lateral surface of the brain with the distribution of the anterior, middle and posterior cerebral arteries illustrated. Note the identification of the watershed area.

Figure 1.22 Arterial blood supply to the Medial surface of a hemisphere with the distribution of the anterior, middle and posterior cerebral arteries illustrated.

Figure 1.23 MRA showing: (*A*) distribution of the common and external carotid arteries, (*B*) distribution of the vertebral and common carotid arteries, (*C*) distribution of the cerebral arteries, (*D*) arterial circle of Willis.

4. *Internal cerebral veins.* The internal and basal veins are the principal cerebral veins. They conduct blood from the center of the cerebrum and converge upon the single great cerebral vein (of Galen), which empties into the straight sinus. The vein of Galen collects venous blood from the medullary center of the cerebrum, diencephalon, basal ganglia, and midbrain.

   Each of the internal cerebral veins is formed near the interventricular foramen of Monro by the union of veins from the lenticular nuclei, caudate, septum, and chorioid plexus. The internal cerebral veins run backward in the velum interpositum in the roof of the third ventricle.

5. *Basal vein (of Rosenthal).* The paired basal veins originate near the anterior perforated substance by the union of the vessels from the corpus callosum, thalamus, insula, and anterior temporal lobe. Each vein passes posteriorly around the cerebral peduncle and unites with the internal cerebral veins behind the splenium of the corpus callosum to form the cerebral vein of Galen.

6. *Superior cerebellar veins.* The superior cerebellar veins form on the superior surface of the cerebellum and some branches join the straight sinus and great cerebral vein, while others branches run into the transverse and superior petrosal sinus.

7. *Inferior cerebellar veins.* These veins drain the inferior surface of the cerebellum and some branches end in the inferior petrosal sinus and transverse sinus, while other branches pass posteriorly into the occipital sinus.

8. *Brainstem veins.* Some of branches from the medulla and pons terminate in the superior and inferior petrosal sinuses.

9. *Sinuses.* There are six major cranial dural sinuses. The sinuses in the dura mater consist of blood vessels lined with endothelium and enwrapped between the periosteal and meningeal layers of the dura. These channels convey blood from the superficial and deep cerebral veins and from veins in the neck, orbit, meninges, and diploe ultimately back to the superior vena cava. The sinuses can be divided into median unpaired channels and lateral unpaired channel; see Table 1.8.

10. The *arachnoid granulations*, which are located in the margins of the superior sagittal sinus (Fig. 1.25), provide a mean for the cerebrospinal fluid (CSF) in the subarachnoid space to pass into the venous circulation.

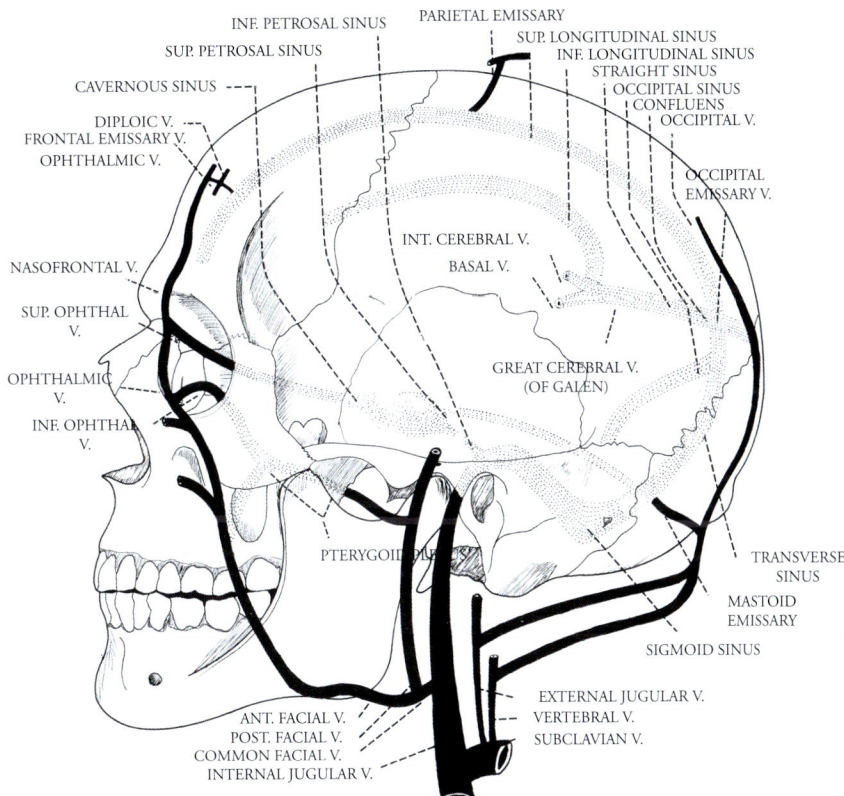

Figure 1.24 Venous drainage from the brain, head and neck.

Lateral unpaired Sinuses

a. The *superior sagittal sinus* is found in the attached margin of the falx cerebri in the inner surface of the cranium from the sagittal groove on the foramen cecum to the internal occipital protuberance. It is small anteriorly and enlarges posteriorly. At the internal occipital protuberance the superior sagittal sinus curves downward and joins the transverse sinus at the confluens. The *superior sagittal sinus* communicates with the superficial temporal veins by means of parietal emissary veins; the superior cerebral veins empty directly into it.

Paired Sinuses

a. The *inferior sagittal sinus* is found in the free margin of the falx cerebri at the junction of the falx and the cerebelli tentorium. It joins the great cerebral vein to form the straight sinus.

b. The *straight sinus* continues into the confluens sinus and then into the transverse sinus, which lies horizontally in a groove along the squamous portion of the occipital bone and the petrous portion of the temporal bone. It also lies in the attached margin of the cerebellar tentorium.

c. *Cavernous sinuses* are formed by numerous venous channels which are found in the dura around the sella turcica of the sphenoid bone (Fig. 12.7). Each continues from the medial portion of the superior orbital fissure to the apex of the petrous portion of the temporal bone. Rootlets of the III, IV, VI, and ophthalmic and maxillary branch of the trigeminal nerve are found herein. The internal carotid artery is found in the cavernous sinus with the rootlets of nerve

Table 1.8 DURAL SINUSES

PAIRED SINUSES	UNPAIRED SINUSES
Transverse	Superior sagittal
Sigmoid	Inferior sagittal
Cavernous	Straight

Figure 1.25 Layers. The scalp over the skull, and the layers of the meninges covering the brain.

Figure 1.26 Stereogram of layers of the meninges in relation to the parenchyma of the central nervous system.

VI on its lateral surface (Fig. 12.7). The cavernous sinus anteriorly receives the ophthalmic vein, middle cerebral veins, and veins from the hypophyseal (pituitary) plexus.

d. Posteriorly the superior and inferior petrosal sinuses drain the cavernous sinus and connect it respectively to the transverse sinus and the internal jugular vein.

The superior and inferior petrosal sinuses lie in grooves with the same name in the petrous portion of the temporal bone. Anteriorly the superior and inferior ophthalmic veins connect the cavernous sinus to the anterior facial vein.

e. The circular sinus surrounds the hypophyseal and connects to the cavernous sinus. The basilar plexus connects the cavernous sinus with the vertebral plexus.

f. The *sigmoid sinus* lies internal to the occipital and temporal bones. The sigmoid sinus is the continuation of the transverse sinus, and when it exits the cranial vault through the jugular foramen it becomes the internal jugular vein.

11. *Alternate pathways.* The venous blood leaves the brain principally via the internal jugular and vertebral veins and plexus.

There are additional channels by which venous blood leaves the cranial cavity:

a. One of the major pathways is provided by the following emissary veins: frontal, parietal, occipital, and mastoid.

b. In addition, the superior and inferior ophthalmic veins provide another channel by which blood leaves the cavernous sinus and enters the anterior facial vein.

c. The venous plexus around the internal carotid artery connects the cavernous sinus and the internal jugular vein.

COVERINGS OF THE BRAIN-MENINGES

The brain is enclosed by three membranes, the dura mater, arachnoid, and pia mater (Fig. 1.25). These protective fluid-filled membranes are formed by connective tissue with embedded nerves, especially in the dura. The dura mater is the most external membrane, followed by the arachnoid and finally the pia mater, which adheres to the central nervous system.

Dura Mater

The externally located dura mater (Figs. 1.25 and 1.26) consists of a tough fibrous connective tissue.

In the cranial vault the dura forms the periosteum on many of the adjacent bones and also forms an inner, or meningeal, portion that compartmentalizes the brain (Fig. 1.29):

1. *Falx cerebri* (between the cerebral hemispheres)
2. *Tentorium cerebelli* (between the cerebellum and cerebrum)
3. *Falx cerebelli* (between the cerebellar hemispheres under tentorium)

Figure 1.27 Arachnoid membrane over a gross brain.

Figure 1.28 Arachnoid granulations on the dorsal surface of brain.

18 • INTRODUCTION TO BASIC NEUROBIOLOGY

Dural Compartments in Skull

Figure 1.29 Subdivision of the cranial vault by the dura: 1-falx cerebri, 2-tentorium cerebri, 3-diaphragma sella covering over location of pituitary gland, 5-Meckel's cave containing the ganglion and nerve rootlets of CN V.

4. Diaphragma sellae covering over location of pituitary gland
5. Meckel's cave with ganglion and rootlets of CN V

The spinal dura forms a sac surrounding the spinal cord. The vertebrae have their own periosteum. The dural sac attaches at the margin of the foramen magnum to the occipital bone and to the inner surface of the second and third cervical vertebrae. It is also continuous with the perineurium on the spinal nerves and covers the filum terminale and becomes continuous with the periosteum on the coccyx as the coccygeal ligaments.

Arachnoid

This thin membrane (Fig. 1.27) is located between the dura and pia. The space between the pia and arachnoid, the subarachnoid, is filled with the CSF. The arachnoid bridges the cerebral sulci and extends from the posterior surface of the medulla to the cerebellum (cisterna magna) and below the neural ending of the spinal cord (lumbar cistern). All of these spaces contain CSF. The arachnoid is usually separated from the dura by the subdural space. The arachnoid membranes form arachnoid granulations (Fig. 1.28) (Pacchionian bodies) that permit passage of the CSF from the higher pressure in the ventricular system into the lower pressure of the venous sinuses.

Pia Mater

The pia adheres to the entire central nervous system (Figs. 1.25 and 1.26) and is continuous with the perineurium of cranial and spinal nerves. It attaches to the blood vessels entering and leaving the central nervous system and fuses with the dura. The cranial pia actually invests the cerebrum and cerebellum and extends into the sulci and fissures. It also forms the nonneural roof of the third ventricle, lateral ventricle, and fourth ventricle. The pia forms the denticulate ligaments that anchor the spinal cord to the dura between the exiting spinal nerve rootlets.

VENTRICULAR SYSTEM

The central nervous system is surrounded by CSF (Fig. 1.30). Externally, the meninges, especially the subarachnoid space,

Figure 1.30 Sagittal section through Gross Brain demonstrating location of ventricular system in brainstem (IV ventricle and cerebral aqueduct) and diencephalon (III ventricle) and opening of the interventricular foramen of Monro (white arrow) from the III ventricle into the lateral ventricle.

1 OVERVIEW OF THE NERVOUS SYSTEM • 19

Figure 1.31 3D Reconstruction of the ventricular system.

Table 1.9 COMPONENTS OF PLASMA AND CEREBROSPINAL FLUID (CSF)

	PLASMA (MG/DL)	CSF (MG/DL)
Na^+	330	310
HCO_3^-	1200	1310
Ca^{++}	10–11	5.3
K^+	17	12
HPO_4^-	3	1.8
SO_4^-	1.9	0.6
Glucose	100	70
Protein	8000	45

contain CSF. Internally, the ventricular system and cisterns contain CSF, and a specialized structure, the choroid plexus, excretes CSF. CSF also forms much of the extracellular space in the brain.

The ventricular system consists of the lateral ventricles, third ventricle, cerebral aqueduct, fourth ventricle, and spinal canal (Fig. 1.31).

1. The *lateral ventricles* are found within the cerebral hemispheres and consist of the body and the anterior, posterior, and inferior horns. A horizontal section of the brain shows the relationship between the ventricles and the central nervous system.

2. The *third ventricle* lies in the midline between the left and right diencephalon and is continuous superiorly with the frontal horn of the lateral ventricles and inferiorly with the cerebral aqueduct. Several recesses associated with the third ventricle are important radiologic landmarks: the optic recess, hypophyseal recess, and pineal recess.

3. The *cerebral aqueduct* is the narrow ventricular space in the center of the midbrain connecting the third and fourth ventricles.

4. The *fourth ventricle* forms that portion of the ventricle seen in pontine and medullary levels. The fourth ventricle is continuous laterally (foramina of Luschka) and medially (foramen Magendie) with the subarachnoid space. The *fourth ventricle* is continuous inferiorly with the narrow central canal of the spinal cord.

5. The narrow *spinal canal* is seen in the center of the gray commissure of the spinal cord.

Cerebrospinal Fluid

The ventricular system is lined by ependymal cells (see Fig. 3.27). Mostly the choroid plexus in the lateral ventricles, third ventricle, and fourth ventricle, which are supplied by the choroidal arteries, forms CSF. It is a clear, colorless, and basic fluid that resembles protein-free plasma but with many significant differences (Table 1.9).

The total volume of CSF is usually between 100 and 150 ml. The rate of formation is 20 ml/hr, or about 500 ml/day. Excess fluid is readily absorbed into the venous sinuses through the arachnoid granulations because the pressure in the CSF is higher.

Cerebrospinal Fluid Circulation

CSF flows from the lateral ventricles through the foramen of Monro into the third ventricle and then throughout the cerebral aqueduct into the fourth ventricle. In the fourth ventricle it is continuous with the subarachnoid space at the foramen Luschka (lateral) and Magendie (medial). In the subarachnoid space the fluid passes into the venous sinuses through the arachnoid granulations. An excess in CSF produces *hydrocephalus*, which is frequently a consequence of meningitis or hemorrhage (communicating hydrocephalus) or a blockage in the ventricular system (noncommunicating hydrocephalus) caused by hemorrhage, tumors, or trauma.

GLANDS ASSOCIATED WITH THE BRAIN

The brain has two glands, the pituitary and the pineal, both of which are attached to the diencephalon and associated with the hypothalamus. The pituitary or hypophysis cerebri is attached to the base of the hypothalamus. Its functions are described in the hypothalamus (Chapter 16).

The other gland, the *pineal (pine cone in shape)* or *epiphysis cerebri*, is found in the epithalamus (Figure 1.7). The pineal gland is also called the "third eye." It produces melatonin, a hormone that affects wake/sleep patterns and seasonal functions. By its location in the center of the brain above the diencephalon, its functions in relationship to light levels and diurnal cycles would not be apparent; however, fiber connections from the optic nerve and the hypothalamus reach it through the stalk of the pineal.

BIBLIOGRAPHY

Denny-Brown, D. 1957. Handbook of Neurological Examination and Case Recording. 2nd ed. Cambridge, MA: Harvard University Press.

Edelman, E. R., and Warach, S. 1993. Medical progress—Magnetic resonance imaging. N. Engl. J. Med. 328:708, 716, 785–791.

Greenberg, J. O. (Ed.). 1999. Neuroimaging: A Companion to Adams and Victor's Principles of Neurology. 2nd ed. New York, NY: McGraw Hill.

Jacobson, S, and Marcus, E. M. 2011. Neuroanatomy for the Neuroscientist. New York: Springer.

Kandel, E. R., Schwartz, J. H., and Jessell, T. M. 2011. Principles of Neurosciences. New York, NY: McGraw Hill.

Marcus, E. M., and Jacobson, S. 2003. Integrated Neuroscience. Dordrecht, The Netherlands: Kluwer Academic Press.

Martin, J. H., Brust, J. C. M., and Hilal, S. 1991. Imaging the living brain. In E. R. Kandel, J. H. Schwartz, M. S. Jessell (Eds.) Niedermeyer, E. and F. Lopes Da Silva. 1999. Electroencephalography: Basic Principles, Clinical Applications and Related Fields, pp. 155–225. Philadelphia, PA. Lippincott Williams and Wilkins

Nolte, J. 1990. The Human Brain. St. Louis, MO: Mosby.

Victor, M. and Ropper, A. 2009. Principles of Neurology. In A. H. Ropper and M. A. Samuels (Eds.) Adams and Victor's Principles of Neurology. 9th ed. New York, NY: McGraw Hill.

2.
OVERVIEW OF LOCALIZATION OF FUNCTION AND NEUROLOGICAL DIAGNOSIS

In considering the patient with neurological disease, accurate diagnosis is required for a determination of appropriate therapy and for the establishment of prognosis.

Diagnosis in neurology seeks to answer two essential questions.

1. Where is the disease (lesion) located?
   a. Central nervous system
   b. Peripheral nervous system
   c. Neuromuscular junction or muscle
2. What is the nature of the pathology?

LOCATION AND PATHOLOGY

LOCATION OF DISEASE PROCESS: SYMPTOMS AND SIGNS

Patients with neurological disease come to medical attention because of certain symptoms or complaints elicited in the history and certain signs elicited on examination. These symptoms and signs fall into several categories:

1. Disturbance of mental status (cognitive function) and language function related to disease of cerebral cortex
2. Disturbance of cranial nerve function due to direct involvement of cranial nerves or of brain stem
3. Disturbance of motor strength reflecting
   a. Disease of the lower motor neuron and the motor unit at the level of the anterior horn cell, or the nerve root or the peripheral nerve or the neuromuscular junction or muscle producing atrophy of the muscle, flaccid weakness, and a variable loss of reflex activity or
   b. Severe upper neuron disease due to involvement of motor cerebral cortex, or due to the involvement of corticospinal tracts at the level of internal capsule cerebral peduncles, basilar pons, medullary pyramids, or lateral columns of spinal cord producing spastic paralysis, increased deep tendon reflexes, and a release of the sign of Babinski.
4. Disturbance of motor control and coordination reflecting
   a. Disease of motor cortex and corticospinal tracts: loss of speed and accuracy
   b. Disease of the premotor and supplementary motor cortex/motor association cortex resulting in defects in patterns of movement and defects in the visual and tactile control of movement. Apraxia occurs and the release of automatisms may occur.
   c. Disease of cerebellum resulting in defects in coordination of limb and axial movements and of "balance"
   d. Disease of basal ganglia resulting in
      1) Slowness of movement (akinesia and bradykinesia) and/or
      2) Resting tremor and/or
      3) Other dyskinesias and/or
      4) Loss of righting reflexes and "balance" and/or alterations in tone
5. Disturbance of sensation
   a. Primary modalities (pain, touch, vibration) due to disease of peripheral nerve, nerve root, spinal cord, brain stem, or thalamus
   b. Discriminative modalities (position, sense, graphesthesia, stereognosis, tactile localization, awareness of double simultaneous stimulation) affected due to disease of posterior column system or cerebral cortex. Pain including headache—the localization of pain may reflect disease of peripheral or cranial nerve, nerve root, spinal cord, brain stem, thalamus, or cortex. Meninges and blood vessels about the head (intra and extracranial) or increased intracranial pressure, or the sinuses or orbits, or dental system, may provide the origin of headache.

DIFFERENTIATIONS OF LESION OF LOCATION

1. Disease of muscle
   a. Patients manifest lower motor neuron disease affecting limbs, trunks, and in some cases, cranial nerves. In early cases, however, deep tendon reflexes are preserved.

b. Involvement is more often proximal than distal and no sensory symptoms or signs are present.

c. No long tract motor or sensory involvement is present.

d. Cognitive function—mental status is normal but may be affected in certain hereditary types.

e. The major disorders are of two types: hereditary (muscular dystrophy or congenital myopathies) or acquired (polymyositis or dermatomyositis).

2. Disease of neuromuscular junction

   a. Patients manifest intermittent dysfunction of lower motor neuron.

   b. Involvement of cranial nerve; motor function is prominent (extraocular muscles and bulbar).

   c. When motor function is involved, the pattern is that of a lower motor neuron type lesion with atrophy, flaccid weakness, and loss of reflex function.

   d. When sensory involvement is present, some or all modalities may be involved. In the generalized type, the sensory pattern may be a glove and stocking type.

   e. Cranial nerves may be involved but without direct brain stem involvement.

f. Long tract findings are not present.

g. Cognitive function is intact.

h. If compression (entrapment) is present, localized pain may be a prominent feature.

3. Disease of peripheral nerve

   a. Motor and/or sensory and/or autonomic function are involved.

   b. The pattern of involvement indicates disease of:

      1. A specific peripheral nerve (mononeuropathy), for example, median, ulnar, radial, femoral, sciatic, peroneal, or

      2. A plexus, such as brachial, lumbar sacral (mononeuropathy), or

      3. Multiple peripheral nerves (mononeuropathy multiplex) 2-2, 2-3, 2-4.d.

   When motor function is involved; the pattern is that of a lower motor neuron type lesion as earlier.

4. Disease of nerve root or spinal nerve

   a. Motor and/or sensory function may be involved.

   b. Pain is often a prominent feature.

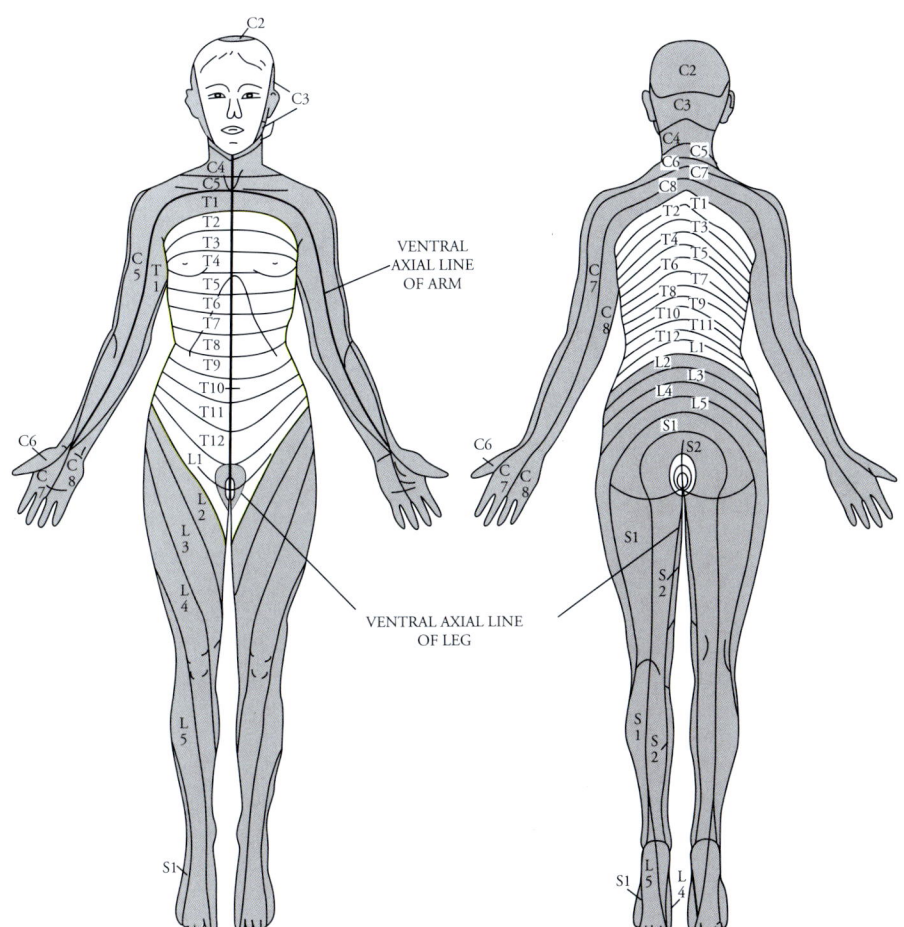

Figure 2.1 Dermatome charts of the human body determined by the pattern of hypalgesia following rupture of an intervertebral disk. (From Keegan, J.J., and Garrett, F.D.: Anat. Rec., 102:411, Wiley, 1948.)

Figure 2.2 Comparison of radicular (dermatome or segmental) and peripheral nerve innervation. (*A*) Anterior surface of the body. (*B*) Posterior surface of the body.

24 • INTRODUCTION TO BASIC NEUROBIOLOGY

Figure 2.2 Continued.

c. The symptoms and signs (pain, sensory, motor and reflex) follow a segmental (dermatomal) distribution.

If limbs are involved—proximal weakness is often greater than distal weakness.

d. Deep tendon stretch reflexes are preserved.

e. No sensory symptoms are present.

f. No long tract findings are present.

g. Cognitive function is not involved.

h. The major disorder is myasthenia gravis, an autoimmune disorder in which antibodies are produced which block and damage the acetylcholine receptor.

(Figs. 2.1 and 2.2; see also Fig. 8.18 for the upper extremity details)

5. Spinal cord: level of lesion at the spinal cord level
   a. Transverse (segmental)
   b. System involving a system of neurons or fibers over many segments
   c. Multifocal producing spotty lesions over multiple levels of the central nervous system
   d. Transverse lesions of the spinal cord: cranial nerves are not involved.
      1) Transverse lesions are usually extrinsic with the implication of compressive mass and possible surgical therapy.
      2) Four exceptions are intrinsic lesions, which involve multiple adjacent segments: syringomyelia intrinsic spinal cord tumors (astrocytomas and ependymomas), infarcts due to occlusion of the inferior spinal artery, and transverse myelitis.
      3) Generally both motor and sensory function are involved.
      4) When the motor long fiber systems are involved, the signs of an upper motor neuron lesion are produced: spastic weakness or paralysis, increased deep tendon reflexes, and the sign of Babinski.
      5) Involvement of the long fiber sensory systems may produce involvement of all modalities below the lesion in a transverse lesion or selective involvement of specific sensory modalities, for example, position and vibratory sensation when the posterior columns are involved and pain and temperature when the lateral spinothalamic tract is involved. Syringomyelia involves the decussating pain and temperature fibers in the anterior white commissure of the cervical area producing a selective dissociated pain and temperature sensory loss over the shoulders and arms, which is "cape like."
      6) Transverse lesions producing damage to the anterior horn cell or anterior root will produce signs of a lower motor neuron lesion at the segmental level of involvement. Fasciculations, twitching of muscle, will be noted in the segment involved. Fasciculations are indicative of disease of anterior horn cells (Tables 2.1–2.4).
      7) Transverse lesions producing damage to the posterior root will produce a local segmental defect at the level of involvement.
      8) Mental status, cognitive function, is not involved.

6. Brain stem. Cranial nerves findings are present with the specific lower motor neuron or sensory deficits dependent on the level of involvement.
   a. Long tract motor findings may be present which are unilateral or more often bilateral.
   b. Long tract sensory findings may be present which may be selective, that is, dissociated, for example, pain and temperature only when unilateral or bilateral and nonselective. Medial lemniscus or lateral spinothalamic may be involved.
   c. Cerebellar pathways may be involved, producing alteration in balance, stance, gait, and appendicular coordination.
   d. In general, mental status, cognitive function is well preserved, although level of consciousness may be depressed.
   e. Particular combinations of cranial nerve finding ± long tract findings are diagnostic.
      1) CN XII, XI, X, and IX due to medullary lesions
      2) CN VIII, VII, and VI due to pontomedullary involvement
      3) Trigeminal–5 midpontine with selective involvement of pain in the trigeminal distribution may be present due to involvement of the descending spinal tract and nucleus of the fifth nerve.
      4) CN III and IV, midbrain
      5) The jugular foramen syndrome (CN IX, X, XI)
      6) The cerebellar pontine angle syndrome: CN VII (facial), VIII (auditory and vestibular), and cerebellum plus or tinnitus CN V, IX, X, and XI
      7) The lateral medullary syndrome (lateral medullary tegmentum), "Wallenberg's syndrome," or syndrome of the posterior inferior cerebellar artery
      8) Ipsilateral peripheral facial weakness and contralateral hemiplegia
      9) Weber's syndrome: ipsilateral third nerve and contralateral hemiplegia
      10) Vestibular + cochlear symptoms are indicative of CN VIII disease at the level of the labyrinth or of the CN VIII. If other symptoms are present, brain stem may be involved.

7. Cerebral cortex
   a. Focal (partial) seizures are always indicative of disease involving the cerebral cortex. The specific clinical phenomena of the seizure will depend on the location of the lesion. Rapid secondary generalization of the seizure discharge may obscure the origin.
   b. Lateralized deficits in terms of upper motor neuron findings and cortical sensory deficits (somatosensory or visual) may occur based on the location of the lesion.

Table 2.1 **SEGMENTAL SENSORY PATTERNS**

THE FOLLOWING RADICULAR PATTERNS SHOULD BE COMPARED TO PERIPHERAL NERVE PATTERNS

C2	Posterior scalp versus trigeminal
C6, C7, C8	The hand
-C6	Thumb and index finger
-C7	Middle finger
-C8	Ring and little (fifth) finger
T1	Axilla
T5, T6	Xiphoid process
T10	Umbilicus
T12	Above inguinal ligament
L4	Medial calf, patella and lateral thigh
L5	Lateral calf and medial foot
S1	Posterior calf and lateral foot
S2	Posterior thigh
S3, 4, 5	Perianal areas

  c. Aphasia is always indicative of involvement of the dominant (usually left) hemisphere, in particular, involvement of the speech areas or of the fiber systems interconnecting the speech areas.

  d. Cranial nerve involvement of a lower motor neuron type does not occur. Corticobulbar involvement may produce supranuclear weakness of the lower half of the face. Bilateral corticobulbar damage may produce a pseudobulbar state involving CN V, VII, IX, X, XI, and XII. This is manifested by a hyperactive jaw jerk, spastic speech, and emotional lability.

  e. Changes in personality and behavior are indicative of disease involving the cerebral cortex, particularly the frontal and temporal lobes.

Table 2.2 **MOTOR—RADICULAR MUSCLE INNERVATIONS**

1.	Shoulder muscles	C4, C5, C6
2.	Biceps	C5, C6
3.	Triceps	C6, C7, C8
4.	Intrinsic hand muscles	C7, C8, T1
5.	Hip flexors, iliopsoas	L2, L3, L4
6.	Quadriceps	L2, L3, L4
7.	Gastrocnemius	LS, L5, S1, S2
8.	Dorsiflexors of foot (peroneal)	L4, L5, S1

Table 2.3 **DEEP TENDON STRETCH REFLEXES**

1.	Jaw	CN V—pons
2.	Biceps	C5, C6
3.	Triceps	C6, C7, C8
4.	Brachioradialis (Radial periosteal)	C5, C6, C7
5.	Fingers	C7, C8, T1
6.	Patellar	L2, L3, L4
7.	Achilles	L4, L5, S1, S2

  f. Changes in immediate (working) memory often reflect neocortical pathology, particularly involving the prefrontal areas. Changes in the ability to consolidate new learning may reflect limbic pathology (medial temporal and medial thalamus).

8. Basal ganglia

  a. There is no direct involvement of the lower motor neuron.

  b. Major upper motor neuron descending motor pathways such as the pyramidal tract are not affected.

  c. A modulating circuit is dysfunctional. This dysfunction is manifested by alterations in motor function characterized by the following findings:

   1) A lack of movement, akinesia; or slowness of movement, bradykinesia

   2) Excessive movement: tremor or dyskinesia

   3) Increased resistance to passive motor: rigidity

   4) Alteration in righting reflexes affecting gait and balance

  d. No sensory symptoms are present.

  e. No direct involvement of cranial nerve function is present, but the motor effects described earlier may alter cranial nerve function.

  f. Cognitive function is usually not directly involved, although many diseases that affect the basal ganglia also affect cerebral cortex or frontal-basal ganglia connections and thus are associated with changes in mental status.

9. The cerebellum

  a. Lower motor neuron function is not affected.

  b. Upper motor neuron function in terms of long tracts is not affected.

Table 2.4 **SUPERFICIAL REFLEXES**

1.	Upper abdomen	T7, T8, T9, T10
2.	Lower abdomen	T10, T11, T12
3.	Plantar	S1, S2

c. A modulating circuit is dysfunctional. The clinical effects of this dysfunction depend on the area of cerebellum involved.
   1) Lateral cerebellar hemisphere relates to the ipsilateral arm and leg. Deficits produce dysmetria of the arms and legs: intention tremor, finger-to-nose and heel-to-shin deficits, and an incoordination of movements.
   2) Midline cerebellum relates to the axis of the body. Deficits produce ataxia of trunk.
   3) Floccular nodular (archicerebellum) relates to the vestibular system. Deficits produce a loss of balance in sitting and standing.
d. Sensory function of a conscious nature is intact.
e. Cranial nerve function is generally intact, although speech and eye movement are altered by cerebellar dysfunction. At times vestibular function may be altered.
f. Certain aspects of cognitive function and motor learning are altered.

THE NATURE OF THE PATHOLOGY

1. The concept of extrinsic versus intrinsic:

   Extrinsic diseases are usually focal mass lesions compressing the spinal cord or brain.

   Intrinsic disorders arise within the substance of the nervous system. Disorders of muscle and neuromuscular junction are usually not due to compressive disorders.

2. The common pathological processes related to the site of lesion
   a. At the level of muscle, the common processes are (1) degenerative disorders on a genetic basis: the dystrophies primarily occurring in children, (2) genetic congenital myopathies, (3) the metabolic myopathies, often with a genetic basis, (4) the acquired inflammatory myopathies related to autoimmune disorders.
   b. At the level of the neuromuscular junction, the most common disorder is myasthenia gravis, an autoimmune disorder in which an antibody to the acetylcholine receptor blocks and damages the postsynaptic receptor. Other disorders involve a paraneoplastic related antibody to calcium channels, which alters the release of acetylcholine from the presynaptic sites. Botulinum toxin produced by an anaerobic bacterium also alters transmission at the neuromuscular junction.
   c. At the level of peripheral nerve, the most common causes of a mononeuropathy are direct trauma and the entrapment syndromes in which compression of a nerve occurs. Vascular disease may also produce a mononeuropathy. As regards polyneuropathies, the most common causes are diabetes mellitus and B vitamin nutritional deficiencies, followed by toxic and hereditary disorders. In parts of the world the infectious disorder leprosy is the most common cause of a multiple mononeuropathy or of a polyneuropathy.
   d. At the level of the nerve root, the most common disorder is compression due to ruptured disks or to the osteophytes of the degenerative disk disorder cervical spondylosis. Tumors (schwannomas) may also arise from nerve roots and peripheral nerve and in the process compress the nerves.
   e. At the level of the spinal cord, extrinsic disorders are the more common disorders. The mass may be a ruptured disc; a tumor in the epidural or intradural space; collapsed vertebrae due to metastatic disease, trauma, or infection; or an infectious process such as an epidural empyema. Intrinsic processes may be focal, system disorders, or multifocal disorders.

   Examples of focal intrinsic processes are infarcts due to anterior spinal artery occlusion, intrinsic tumors such as gliomas, or a focal enlarging cyst as in syringomyelia or transverse myelitis. Examples of system disorders are amyotrophic lateral sclerosis due to the degeneration of the motor neuron in the anterior horn or posterior lateral column disease of vitamin B12 deficiency. An example of a multifocal disorder is multiple sclera intrinsic disorders.

   f. At the level of the brain stem, most disorders are intrinsic. The most frequent disorder is vascular disease. The major type is ischemic occlusive involving the vertebral-basilar arteries producing infarcts. Other intrinsic disorders include tumors, hemorrhage, and demyelinating disease. However, the brain stem may be affected by extrinsic processes arising in cerebellum (tumors and hemorrhages) or by tumors arising from the Schwann cells in cranial nerves (primarily the vestibular nerve).
   g. At the level of the cerebellum most disorders are intrinsic. Infarcts secondary to occlusive disease are the most common. Other disorders are due to hemorrhage, neoplasms, degenerative disease, and multiple sclerosis. In infants and children, tumors are the most common disorder.
   h. At the level of the diencephalon, most disorders are intrinsic with the exception of tumors arising from the pituitary and secondarily compressing the hypothalamus. The most common intrinsic disorder is vascular disease (infarcts and hemorrhage). Other disorders are gliomas and nutritional (Wernicke's encephalopathy due to thiamine deficiency). In children, neoplasms are the most common disorder.
   i. At the level of the basal ganglia, all disorders to be considered are intrinsic, with degenerations being the most common (Parkinson's and Huntington's disease). However, the basal ganglia are also the most frequent site

of intracerebral hemorrhage related to the penetrating branches of the middle cerebral artery. These lenticulostriate branches are also subject to occlusion, producing infarct involving the internal capsule and basal ganglia.

j. At the level of cerebral cortex and subcortical white matter, the common pathological processes are intrinsic and relate to the age of the patient. In infant's hydrocephalus or congenital malformations or migration, disorders may affect cortical function. In children, adolescents, and young adults, trauma is a major consideration. In the adult, intrinsic tumors of the glial series are a major consideration. In the older patient, ischemic-occlusive vascular disease is a major neuropathologic process. In the elderly patient, the degenerative disorder Alzheimer's disease afflicts a significant proportion of the population. In all disorders involving the cerebral cortex, recurrent seizures (epilepsy) are a major consideration at all ages. Extrinsic disorders include the previously mentioned head trauma and the extrinsic tumor, the meningioma.

THE NEUROLOGICAL HISTORY AND EXAMINATION

AN OUTLINE OF THE COMPLETE NEUROLOGICAL HISTORY AND EXAMINATION

(Note that for each patient the total history and examination may be tailored so that for some cases abbreviated evaluations may be carried out in a particular area.)

The neurological examination provides a means for the systematic analysis of symptoms and signs.

The importance of the detailed history cannot be overemphasized, with 75% of neurological diagnosis dependent on the history. There are many excellent sources for the discussion and review of the Neurological Exam. We believe the following text by Drs. Morris and Jankovic is an excellent review of the Neurological Exam as it has an extensive video library which provides a practical guide to the complete exam and is a great resource for the many details of the Complete Neurological—*Neurological Clinical Examination: A Course Guide* by John Morris and Joseph Jankovic (CRC Press, 2012).

Following we have listed the basic abbreviated examination.

ABBREVIATED NEUROLOGICAL EXAMINATION

Mental Status and Language Function

1. Alertness
2. Orientation
3. Delayed recall (5/5 objects in 5 minutes)
4. Naming of five objects
5. Repetitions: "No ifs, ands or buts"

6. Cranial nerves II–XII: fundi, pupils, EOMs, facial movement and sensation, tongue move and gag, shoulder shrug, and SCM on head rotation

7. Motor system

   a. Resistance against force at shoulder abductors, biceps, triceps, wrist extensors, hand grip and finger abductors; hip flexors, quadriceps, hamstrings, ankle and toe dorsiflexors

   b. Walk a routine gait; walk a tandem gait; walk on toes and heels

   c. Stand on narrow base, eyes open, eyes closed

   d. Other cerebellar—finger to nose, alternating hand motions

   e. Any atrophy or fasciculations

   f. Any tremor or other extra movements noted

8. Reflexes

   a. Deep tendon reflexes at biceps, triceps, brachioradialis, patella, and Achilles

   b. Plantar responses

9. Sensation

   a. Pain and touch sensation—extremities, shoulders, body

   b. Vibration and position at toes

   The mini mental exam is also used in concert with the Neurological exam and it is detailed next.

Mini-Mental State Examination (MMSE)

(After Folstein, M.S., Folstein, S.E., and McHugh, P.R. "Mini-Mental State." A Practical Method for Grading the Cognitive State of Patients for the Clinician. *J. Psychiatr. Res*, 12:189–198, 1975)

1. What is today's date?

   Month___ Date___ Year___

   Day of week?___ Season___ ___ (5)

2. Where are we? City___ County___

   State___ Hospital___ Floor___ ___ (5)

3. Repeat the three words: ball—flag—tree. Record the number recited initially ___ (3).

   Repeat them up to six times for registration.

4. Subtract 7 from 100: 93–86–79–72–65.

   Spell WORLD forward and backward: D—L—R—O—W.

   (Write the greater of these two scores to the right) ___ (5)

5. Recall the three words: ball—flag—tree ___ (3).
6. Read and obey ("close your eyes") ___ (1).
7. Name these items (pen and watch) ___ (2).
8. Repeat after me ("no ifs, ands, or buts") ___ (1).
9. Take the piece of paper in your right hand, fold it in half, and put it on the floor___ (3).
10. Write a sentence:__ (1).
11. Copy this design: (1)

Total Score: ___ (30)

DIAGNOSTIC STUDIES IN NEUROLOGY

Specific laboratory studies are appropriate in providing information about disease affecting particular levels of the nervous system or about particular types of pathology.

MUSCLE AND NERVE

Electromyography

Small needles are inserted in the muscle to record the electrical activity of motor units (Fig. 2.3). Under normal circumstances,

Figure 2.3 Motor nerve conduction velocity (normal). Various points along the course of the peroneal nerve were stimulated, with recordings from extensor digitorum brevis. The differences in latencies are calculated and then divided by the distance to yield a conduction velocity of 41 meters per second. (Courtesy Neurodiagnostic Laboratory University of Massachusetts Hospital.) Edematous and acutely necrotic tissue, as infarcts and malignant tumors, usually has relatively high water content. In contrast to computerized axial tomography (CT) scan, images are obtained in the horizontal coronal and sagittal planes. As in CT scans, contrast enhancement may be utilized. Gadolinium DTPA that normally does not cross the blood–brain barrier is the agent employed. The magnetic resonance imaging (MRI) procedure may be modified to vary the appearance of cerebrospinal fluid and of tissue water content. Altering the relaxation time (the interval after the application of the radiofrequency wave) will achieve this effect. Images obtained with a short relaxation time are labeled as T1 and emphasize the normal gray-white anatomical features with the cerebrospinal fluid (CSF) appearing as black. Images produced after longer relaxation times, labeled as T2, produce increased white appearance of CSF and other water content. Demyelinating lesions in multiple sclerosis are often prominent in T2 (MRI).

at rest, with voluntary contraction, a significant number of units are recorded. These units have a range of amplitude and duration. In disease of muscle, voluntary contraction results in motor units of small amplitude and altered duration. In contrast, when the anterior horn cell or peripheral nerve has been damaged resulting in denervation, spontaneous activity is present at rest of small amplitude fibrillations (the contraction of single muscle fibers) and fasciculations corresponding to the contraction of all the fibers in a motor unit innervated by a single anterior horn cell.

Nerve Conduction Velocity

Stimulation of nerves at two points along the nerve will allow the calculation of speed of conduction over specific segments. Various points along the course of the peroneal nerve were stimulated, with recordings from extensor digitorum brevis. The differences in latencies are calculated and then divided by the distance to yield a conduction velocity of 41 meters per second (Courtesy Neurodiagnostic Laboratory University of Massachusetts Hospital). A specific site of block may be determined with normal conduction above and delayed conduction below that site, for example, median nerve at carpal tunnel or ulnar nerve at olecranon groove of the elbow. Alternatively, a general modification in conduction may be found in generalized peripheral neuropathies. Those peripheral neuropathies that involve primarily myelin produce a decrease in speed of conduction. Neuropathies that are predominantly axonal do not alter speed of conduction but may alter amplitude of the action potential. Repetitive nerve stimulation recording from appropriate muscle with measurement of the amplitude of muscle action potential may be utilized to study disorder of the neuromuscular junction. A progressive decrement occurs with myasthesia gravis and a progressive increment with Eaton Lambert syndrome. Motor nerve conduction velocity (normal).

SPINAL CORD AND NERVE ROOT

1. Simple radiological studies (Fig. 2.4). Cervical spine, thoracic spine, and lumbar sacral spine: X-rays provide information about collapse of vertebrae, narrowing of spaces, narrowing of the neural foramina, metastatic involvement of vertebrae, fractures of vertebral elements, and osteophyte (spur) formation. Neurofibromas may widen the neural foramina. Intrinsic tumors and syringomyelia may produce an increase in the diameter of the vertebral canal.

2. Computerized axial tomography scanning (CT scan) is now the most frequently employed technique in neurology, but is less frequently utilized for spinal cord.

    A computer is utilized to determine the differential attenuation of X-rays by the various tissues such as gray vs white matter versus cerebrospinal fluid (CSF) versus bone based on the differential on blood–brain barrier. When the barrier is damaged, as in tumors, brain abscesses, arteriovenous malformations (AVM) increased density will occur around or within the lesion. At barrier is also damaged in meningitis and around infarcts. For the spinal

Figure 2.4 Cervical spine X-rays. Marked enlargement of the neural foramen has occurred on the left at C5-6 extending into C6-7 consistent with a neurofibroma/schwannoma at this level. This 26-year-old female developed numbness in the left arm extending from the elbow to all of the fingers and pain in the neck and left supraclavicular area. She had absent deep tendon reflexes at left biceps and triceps. (*A*) Right neural foramina on oblique view. (*B*) Left neural foramina on oblique view. (Courtesy of Radiology Department Bay State Medical Center). See Figure 2.5 for results of magnetic resonance imaging (MRI) imaging. Previously, oil-soluble dyes (Pantopaque) were employed and had to be removed at the end of the procedure. Now water-soluble dyes are employed and these are absorbed. At times, computerized axial tomography (CT) scan is combined with myelography (Fig. 2.7). At times, the dye was terns around the brain stem.

cord, the most frequent use is in the lumbar area to image the nerve roots of the cauda equina.

3. Magnetic resonance imaging (MRI scanning) (Figs. 2.5 and 2.6) also utilizes computer-generated images. *MRI is now the study of choice for imaging spinal cord and nerve root.* Instead of utilizing X-rays, a strong magnetic field and radio frequency waves are employed. Placement of the patient's body in a magnetic field directionally orients the protons of that body. Passage of a brief radiofrequency current alters this directional orientation. When the radiofrequency current ceases, the protons realign in the

Figure 2.5 Magnetic resonance imaging (MRI) of the cervical and upper thoracic spine and spinal cord (*A*) T1-weighted and (*B*) T2-weighted from another patient: sagittal section close to midline. In both cases although degenerative disk disease is demonstrated, the spinal cord remains normal. Technique for imaging the brain stem and cerebellum (Fig. 2.11).

magnetic field. This realignment results in a signal. The signal, as in CT scans, depends on the tissue density that is the differential water content of the specific tissue. Bone has little water content; gray matter and white matter have differential water content.

4. Edematous and acutely necrotic tissue, as infarcts and malignant tumors, usually has relatively high water content. In contrast to CT scan, images are obtained in the horizontal coronal and sagittal planes. As in CT scans, contrast enhancement may be utilized. Gadolinium

Figure 2.6 Magnetic resonance imaging (MRI) of cervical spine. Same case as Figure 2.4. The cause of the enlargement of the neural foramina is now apparent. A large dumbbell tumor is present in the intraspinal bony canal and extends through the foramen to the extraspinal space. (*A*) Sagittal view; (*B*) axial/transverse view. (Courtesy Radiology Department Bay State Medical Center.)

DTPA that normally does not cross the blood–brain barrier is the agent employed. The MRI procedure may be modified to vary the appearance of CSF and of tissue water content. Altering the relaxation time (the interval after the application of the radiofrequency wave) will achieve this effect: Images obtained with a short relaxation time are labeled as T1 and emphasize the normal gray-white anatomical features with the CSF appearing as black. Images produced after longer relaxation times, labeled as T2, produce increased white appearance of CSF and other water content. Demyelinating lesions in multiple sclerosis are often prominent in T2 (MRI).

5. Other radiographic techniques utilized in the pre–CT and MRI era

Myelography: In this technique a radio contrast dye is introduced into the subarachnoid space via a lumbar puncture. The spinal cord and nerve roots are then visualized by tilt allowed to enter the fourth ventricle or the cistern.

Previously, oil-soluble dyes (Pantopaque) were employed and had to be removed at the end of the procedure. Now water-soluble dyes are employed and these are absorbed. At times, CT scan is combined with myelography (Fig. 2.7). At times, the dye was allowed to enter the lateral ventricle or the cistern around the brain stem.

6. Electrophysiological techniques for studying spinal cord function

Figure 2.7 Computerized axial tomography (CT) after metrizamide myelography: normal spinal cord. (*A*) Reference film for level of cross sections in this patient. (*B*) Scans 3, 4, 6, 7 sections through C5-C6 levels. Auditory conduction system: Wave I is associated with electrical activity generated in the cochlea at the origin of the auditory nerve. Wave II is associated with the entry of impulses from the auditory nerve into the cochlear nucleus at the medullary pontine junction. Wave III relates to signals generated at the level of the superior olivary nucleus in the lower pons. Wave IV relates to the nerve impulses generated in the lateral lemniscus. Wave V relates nerve impulses generated at the level of the inferior colliculus in the lower midbrain. Delays are noted after Wave I or between point: N12, lower cervical spine-root entry area; N14, dorsal columns and dorsal column nuclei-lower medulla; N20, thalamocortical fibers and cortex; P23, somatosensory cortex. (From Marcus, E.M. and Stone, B. In Evoked Potentials II, Ed. R.N. Nodar and C. Barber: Butterworth Publishers, Boston, 1984.)

a. H. reflex: submaximal stimulation of a mixed sensory-motor nerve at a voltage intensity which is insufficient to produce a direct orthodromic motor response (the M wave) will produce a muscle contraction after a long latency. This long latency response—the H. wave, involves the activation of the afferent fibers involved in the monosynaptic stretch reflex with activation of the anterior horn cell, anterior root motor fibers to the muscle.

b. The F response: supramaximal stimulation of a motor sensory nerve produces an even longer latency response in the muscles. This depends on antidromic activation of motor neurons, which then induces the longer latency discharge, activating the muscle fibers.

c. Evoked potentials: There are computer-averaged signals associated with peripheral and central conduction following stimulation of specific sensory systems. The specific technique relevant to spinal cord is the somatosensory evoked potential (Fig. 2.8). Stimulation of median nerve in the upper extremity or of the posterior tibial or peroneal nerves in the lower extremities produces a series of waves. These waves are related to specific points in the conduction pathway. In the case of median nerve stimulation the waves relate to brachial plexus, cervical spinal cord, and the thalamocortical system. These studies are useful in detecting whether abnormalities are present in the posterior column/medial lemniscal system in multiple sclerosis or in spinal cord compression.

Figure 2.8 Short latency somatosensory evoked potentials (SER) median nerve stimulation at wrist. Recordings from supraclavicular area (FZ-ERB), cervical spine-VII (FZ-Cervical VII), cervical spine-II (FZ-Cervical II), and somatosensory cortical projection area and scalp (F2-C3). The specific wave forms originate as follows: N10-Brachial plexus at Erb's.

Figure 2.9 Skull X-ray suprasellar tumor: craniopharyngioma. Enlarged sella turcica, and suprasellar calcification with changes in the anterior and posterior bony components (clinoids). This 23-year-old female had a 6-year history of intermittent headaches and amenorrhea and recent diplopia. She had bilateral papilledema and an elevated serum prolactin level. Refer to Figure 2.13 (*A*) for a normal comparison (see also Fig. 27.14 for a computerized tomography scan of this case).

BRAIN STEM, POSTERIOR FOSSA, AND SKULL BASE

1. Radiological studies and other imaging studies

    a. Skull X-rays have in large part been replaced by CT scan and MRI scan but are still useful in providing information about skull fractures, enlargement of the pituitary, invagination of the odontoid, and intracranial calcifications (Fig. 2.9).

    b. CT scan discussed previously may provide information regarding tumors, infarcts, and hemorrhages affecting the cerebellum and brain stem (Fig. 2.10).

    c. MRI in general has become the standard (Fig. 2.11).

2. Physiological techniques

    a. Brain stem auditory evoked potentials (Fig. 2.12): A sequence of waves occurs which have been associated with specific points in the waves I and III in patients with acoustic neuromas (vestibular schwannomas). Somatosensory evoked potentials also provide possible information about conduction delays in the medial lemniscus.

Figure 2.10 Computerized tomographic (CT) scan of the posterior fossa with contrast enhancement (C+). Cerebellar pontine angle tumor in a 65-year-old female with a 17-year history of deafness in the left ear and a minor reduction of hearing in the right ear who had additional findings of mild left peripheral facial weakness, ataxia of gait, and dysmetria of left hand. The broad base along the left petrous bone suggested a meningioma. (Courtesy of Dr. Tom Mullins.)

Figure 2.11 Magnetic resonance imaging (MRI): (*A*) T1 sagittal section in a 29-year-old woman with multiple symptoms, including headaches and depression, but with no neurological findings. MRI/MRA was obtained because sister had an aneurysm and subarachnoid hemorrhage. This study reveals an apparently benign lesion of the pineal. (*B*) T1 horizontal/axial section in a young man with multiple sclerosis. No definite demyelinating lesions are demonstrated, but the relationship of the mesial temporal areas to the mid brain is well demonstrated.

Figure 2.12 Brain stem auditory evoked potentials (BAER). This 49-year-old female had a progressive decrease in hearing in the left ear, decreased sensation on the left side of face for 2 years, and additional findings of a left peripheral facial weakness and decreased pain sensation over the face.

b. Special test of auditory and vestibular function: audiograms, caloric testing, and electronystagmograms

3. Radiological techniques no longer employed

   a. Pneumoencephalography (PEG) (Fig. 2.13): air was injected into the subarachnoid space via a lumber puncture. With the patient in the sitting position, the air would rise into the cisterns and ventricular system, allowing visualization of structures such as the fourth ventricle and aqueduct of Sylvius, as well as the lateral and third ventricle.

   b. Ventriculography: in patients with increased intracranial pressure, or with tumors mass lesions in temporal lobe or cerebellum, the PEG was dangerous with the possible complication of herniation. Instead, a needle was introduced into the frontal horn and air or

CEREBRAL HEMISPHERES

1. Imaging techniques

   a. CT scans are usually employed in cases of acute trauma, intracerebral hemorrhage, subarachnoid hemorrhage, acute infarcts, and acute brain abscess. In the case presented at the end of this chapter, an acute hemorrhage was demonstrated involving the leg and proximal arm areas (Fig. 2.29). Refer to Figure 18.12 for location of these areas on lateral surface of the cerebral hemisphere.

   b. MRI—this has become the preferred technique for imaging patients with brain tumors, malformations, seizure disorders, inflammatory disorders, and demyelinating disorders (Figs. 2.14 and 2.15).

   c. As discussed earlier, pneumoencephalograms and ventriculograms are no longer employed.

   d. Radioisotope techniques have a limited value in selected cases.

   e. Radioactive brain scans are no longer performed. Prior to the development of CT and MRI, this technique was of value in detecting lesions in which damage to the blood–brain barrier or increased metabolic activity was present. Metastatic tumors, meningiomas, glioblastomas, abscess, and acute infarcts were demonstrated but anatomical detail was poor. Several examples will be provided in the text.

2. Radioisotope flow studies are still occasionally utilized to visualize the passage of a radioisotope injected into the lumbar subarachnoid space into the ventricles, out into the cisterns, and through the subarachnoid space over the convexity to be absorbed into the venous sinuses. Normally, the isotope is no longer present in the ventricles at 48 and 72 hours. In the presence of communicating hydrocephalus (primarily normal pressure hydrocephalus),

Figure 2.13 Pneumoencephalograms: A large pituitary adenoma has ballooned out the sella turcica on the X-ray. With the injection of air, via a lumbar puncture the extrasellar extension may be seen. (A) Normal; (B) Abnormal. (Courtesy of Dr. Samuel Wolpert, New England Center Hospitals.)

Figure 2.14 Magnetic resonance imaging (MRI): multiple sclerosis. This 47-year-old female farm owner and manager had a 2-month episode of numbness ("novocaine-type sensation") over the entire right trigeminal distribution. Five years previously she had intermittent unsteadiness. Her examination demonstrated only a selective decrease in touch sensation over the entire right trigeminal distribution. The MRI studies confirmed a right midpontine tegmental lesion but also indicated multiple areas of demyelination in the white matter of the cerebral hemispheres particularly involving the corpus callosum. (*A*) T1 sagittal, (*B*) T2 horizontal views, (*C*) T2 axial of brain stem.

the isotope is still present in the cerebral ventricles at 48 and 72 hours (see Chapter 18 for an example).

3. Single-photon emission computed tomograph (SPECT) scanning remains as a modified form of the radionucleotide brain scan. Unlike the positron emission tomography scan, a cyclotronis is not necessary. Therefore, cost is less, availability is greater, but resolution is poor (Fig. 2.16).

4. Positron emission tomography (PET) scan employs positron-emitting radionucleotides combined with computer imaging of the emission to assess metabolic changes in specific areas of the brain. Resolution does yet reach the level of MRI or current high-level CT scanning but now approaches that of early CT scans. Cost is high and availability limited since a cyclotron is required to produce the short life radioisotopes required. The major clinical use is in relation to focal (partial) epilepsy (Fig. 2.17). During seizure activity, metabolic activity at the focus is increased. Between seizures the metabolic activity at the focus is decreased. The investigational use of PET scanning has provided valuable information about localization of function during the increased metabolic activity of normal cognitive activities, such as reading, motor activities, and so on. In addition, information has been provided about the localization of altered metabolic activity in patients with schizophrenia, depression, and various disorders of the basal ganglia. Functional MRI may provide a more effective technique for such metabolic correlations. Since PET scan has not been previously considered in detail, we will briefly review the technique at this point. This method combines CT with the use of positron emitting radioisotopes, which have been bound to compounds, which have significant biological function as metabolites or transmitters. In contrast to standard CT scanning (where the source of radiation is the X-ray tube), in PET the positron-emitting isotope taken up by the tissue is the source of radiation. 2-Desoxyglucose is often employed since it is taken up by the neurons and is phosphorylated

Figure 2.15 Functional magnetic resonance imaging (MRI). This 33-year-old woman had a 2-year history of focal seizures involving the right foot and arm. A large area of the left premotor and motor cortex is involved by a grade 2 astrocytoma. (*A*) The relation of the areas activated by right hand or foot movements to the intrinsic brain tumor are indicated. (*B*) Comparison of normal hemisphere to abnormal hemisphere. Note the displacement of the arm and leg areas by the tumor. (Courtesy of Drs. B.R. Buchbinder, H. Jiang, G.R. Cosgrove A Cole, D. Hoch and R. Hill at the Massachusetts General Hospital Epilepsy Center.)

Figure 2.16 Single-photon emission computed tomography (SPECT): areas of increased perfusion during seizure activity are indicated in this scan. (*A*) Ictal uptake in areas of right temporal parietal and frontal lobes. (*B*) Interictal. This 3-year-old child initially had infantile spasms with an electro-encephalographic (EEG) pattern consistent with the disorder hypsarrhythmia. Subsequently, the EEG abnormalities were right anterior quadrant or parietal. (Courtesy of Dr. Paul Marshall Pediatric Neurology University of Massachusetts.)

as is glucose but is not further metabolized. The isotope of fluorine (18F) is bonded to the desoxy glucose. The uptake of glucose or of desoxy glucose into neurons is proportional to the activity of the neurons. Thus, areas of cerebral cortex undergoing active seizure discharge will show increased activity and increased uptake. In normal individuals with activity of the visual system, for example, opening the eyes to scan a scene, activity and uptake will increase in the visual projection area of the occipital lobe. With auditory stimulation, on the other hand, activity and uptake will increase in the auditory projection area of Heschl's transverse gyrus of the temporal lobe. Areas of damage will show decreased uptake.

5. Physiological techniques

   a. Electroencephalography. This technique provides information about the electrical activity of the cerebral cortex. This activity represents primarily the summated activity of postsynaptic potentials generated in the cerebral cortex. The electroencephalogram in the normal awake adult resting with eyes closed is characterized by the alpha rhythm (Fig. 2.18). This rhythm is composed of a sequence of sinusoidal waves of 8–13 Hz (cps), which is maximal over the parietal-occipital recording. Activity faster than alpha rhythm is referred to as beta activity and may be present over frontal areas.

Figure 2.17 Positron emission tomography (PET) scans. The most prominent feature is the increased activity in visual cortex, most likely reflecting visual activity during the study. Magnetic resonance imaging (MRI) demonstrated mesial temporal sclerosis on the right, and this study did demonstrate a possible decrease in activity of the right temporal area. This 22-year-old female had complex partial seizures since puberty. She had prolonged status epilepticus as an infant related to fever. (*A*) Horizontal; (*B*) sagittal. (Courtesy of Dr. Cathy Phillips Neurology University of Massachusetts.)

Figure 2.18 (*A*) The International Federation Ten–Twenty Electrode Placement System. Frontal superior and posterior views; and a single plane projection of the head demonstrating the standard positions and the rolandic and sylvian fissures. The term *ten-twenty* is based on the placement of electrodes at particular percentages of the distance between nasion and inion. (From Jasper, H.H.: Electroenceph. Clin. NeuroPhysiol. 10: 374, 1958; Elsevier.) (*B*) The normal adult electroencephalogram. The patient is awake but in a resting state, recumbent with eyes closed. Bipolar recordings, C, central; F, frontal; O, occipital; T, temporal. (These abbreviations will be utilized in subsequent illustrations.) (*C*) Effects of eye opening and closure. Opening is associated with a blocking or suppression of the alpha rhythm of 10 cps and with the appearance of a low voltage fast-activity of 20 cps (beta rhythm). With eye closure, there is a return of the alpha rhythm.

Increased amounts of beta activity occur as an effect of various drugs such as barbiturates and benzodiazepines. Alterations occur in this normal background activity related to the following factors: (1) eye opening producing reduction of amplitude (Fig. 2.18C); (2) age: slower activity with infancy and childhood (delta 0.5–3 Hz, theta 4–7Hz) (Fig. 2.19CD ATLAS); (3) sleep (Fig. 2.20); (4) drugs and anesthesia: faster and then slower activity (Fig. 2.21).

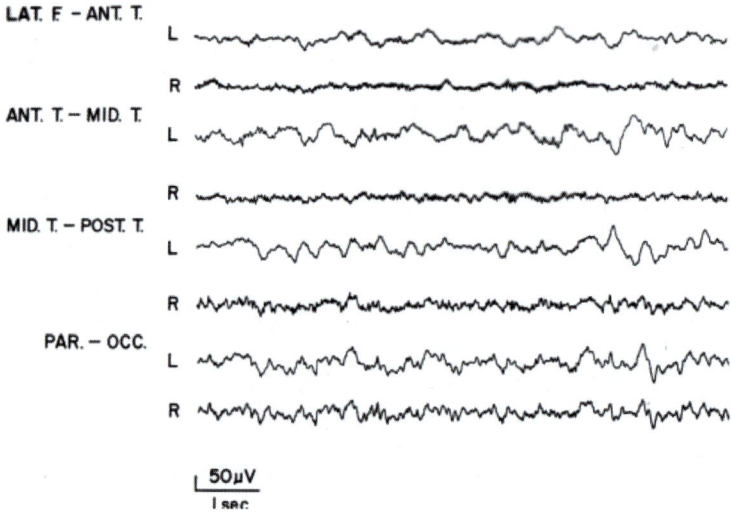

Figure 2.19 Focal 2.3 Hz slow-wave activity in the electroencephalogram: left temporal area indicating focal damage in this area. Brain abscess, left temporal lobe in a 14-year-old female secondary to an acute S aureus mastoiditis extending into the petrous ridge. Electroencephalogram. Bipolar recording. ANT- T-, anterior temporal; LAT. F., lateral frontal; MID. T., mid-temporal; OCC., occipital; PAR., parietal; POST. T-, posterior temporal.

Figure 2.20 Focal suppression of electroencephalographic (EEG) activity in right temporal area and focal slow-wave activity in right frontal. Total right middle cerebral artery occlusion in a 61-year-old female with hypertension, Case 26.4. ANT.F., anterior frontal parasagittal; ANT.T., anterior temporal; MID.T., mid-temporal; OCC., occipital; PAR., parietal; POST.F., posterior frontal (parasagittal); POST.T., posterior temporal.

Abnormalities may be (1) focal or (2) generalized. Focal abnormalities may be categorized as follows:

a. Focal spikes implying focal excessive neuronal discharge involving the cerebral cortex and associated with partial (focal) epilepsy. (See Chapter 29.)

b. Focal slow-wave activity, which implies focal cortical damage, as in infarcts, brain tumors, and brain abscess (Fig. 2.22).

c. Focal suppression of activity implies nonactive electrical tissue under the electrodes; this may be seen with a fluid collection (subdural or intracerebral hemorrhage) or with total destruction of tissue (Fig 2.23).

d. Generalized abnormalities: Generalized discharges of spike or polyspike—slow-wave complexes are associated with various types of generalized epilepsy. These will be discussed in Chapter 29.

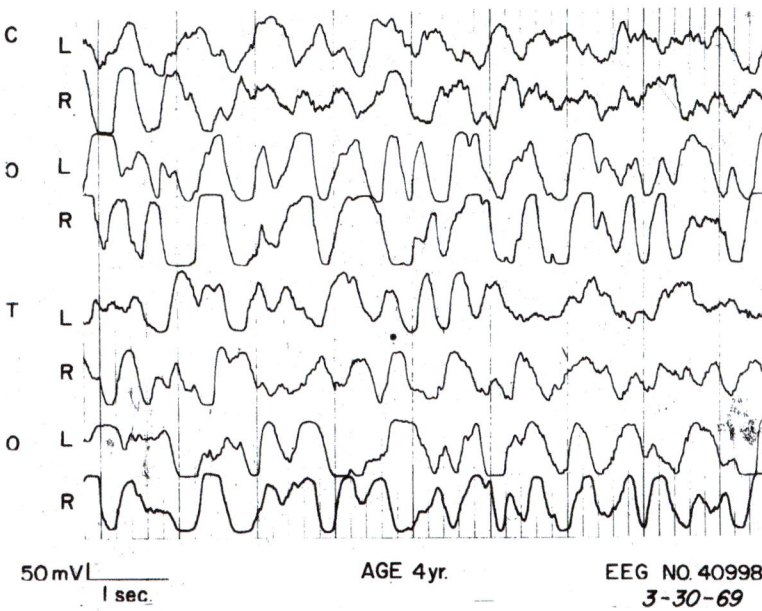

Figure 2.21 Generalized delta 1–2 Hz slow-wave activity that persisted despite attempts at arousal in this 4-year-old male who had acute viral encephalitis.

Figure 2.22 Generalized theta 5 Hz slow-wave activity. This 67-year-old female had a metabolic encephalopathy due to impaired hepatic function secondary to cirrhosis and at this point was semicomatose in a stuporous state. When the patient was more deeply comatose, the awake activity was even slower at 4 Hz. When the patient was alert during intervening periods of recovery, the dominant activity was in the alpha range.

1) Generalized bursts of 3/second spike wave complexes are associated with absence seizures previously labeled petit mal epilepsy.

2) Generalized bursts of polyspike and slow-wave complexes are associated with myoclonic seizures.

3) Generalized polyspike discharges may be found in the tonic phase of the generalized tonic clonic seizures.

d. Generalized slow waves are associated with diffuse disorders: infectious, ischemic, toxic, or metabolic encephalopathies (Figs. 2.19 and 2.20).

e. Generalized periods of suppression imply a more serious type of diffuse dysfunction, as in anoxia or a deep stage of anesthesia. It provides an example of a burst suppression pattern.

f. Total suppression of activity may be found in severe anoxic encephalopathy or the vegetative state. This total suppression of activity accompanied by an absence of brain stem reflex activity and an absence of spontaneous respiration occurs in brain death. Similar findings of total suppression of activity both electrical and reflex may also occur under condition of deep anesthesia.

g. Specialized techniques employing electroencephalography

1) Sphenoidal electrodes—these are small needle electrodes placed in the sphenoidal sinus area to record from the medial aspects of the temporal lobe.

2) Video EEG monitoring: The recording of EEG and behavior onto single videotape allows correlation of electrical activity and of clinical seizure activity. This is usually a prerequisite study prior to epilepsy surgery and is also utilized in the analysis of pseudoseizures or other unresolved "spells." Depth electrode recording: from medial temporal and other structures may be performed prior to epilepsy surgery often in combination with video monitoring.

h. Electrocorticography: recording directly from the pial surface may be utilized during epilepsy surgery.

i. Polysomnography (PSG): this technique is utilized in the evaluation of sleep disorders such as narcolepsy and sleep apnea. EEG activity from the parietal occipital or vertex areas of the scalp is correlated with:

(1) Cardiac activity (EKG) rate and rhythm

(2) Respiratory activity rate and rhythm

(3) Oxygen (O_2) saturation

(4) Extraocular movements

(5) EMG activity chins and or limb

The use of the PSG and the multiple sleep latency study will be discussed in Chapter 29.

j. Evoked potentials

k. Subdural surface grids of electrodes: may be placed on the cortical surface for better correlation of seizure discharges arising in the frontal or other neocortical areas.

(1) Visual (VER or pattern reversal visual evoked potential: PVER): the time of conduction over the entire visual pathway—to cerebral cortex is measured. Pattern reversal generates a prominent very stable wave at approximately 100 ms, the P100 wave (Fig. 2.23).

(2) Somatosensory evoked potentials: as discussed earlier, these studies may provide information regarding delays in conduction in the thalamocortical system.

6. Neuropsychological tests: a variety of tests have been developed. These include the Wechsler Adult Intelligent Score (WAIS), formerly termed the Wechsler Bellevue

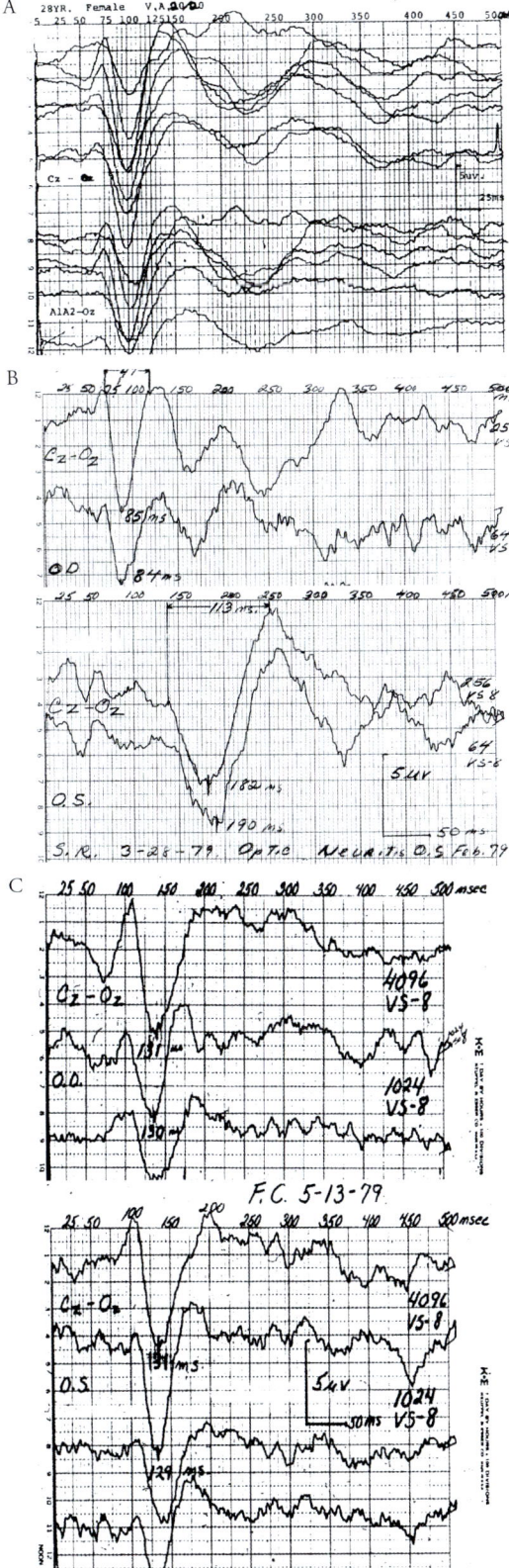

Figure 2.23 Visual evoked potentials. (*A*) Normal. Each tracing represents the summation of 256 trials at different check sizes. Note the stability of the P100 response. (*B*) Unilateral (left) optic neuritis in a young adult female 1 month previously with right eye at 85 ms and left eye at 182 ms. Normal values = 100 ms +/− 6 ms. (*C*) A patient with multiple sclerosis who had experienced several episodes of optic neuritis involving first one eye and then the other eye. Note the bilateral prolongation of the P100 responses. Spinal cord arteriovenous malformations.

Test of Adult Intelligence. This has a series of separate subtests covering multiple areas of verbal and performance functions. Total, verbal, and performance intelligence quotients are derived. A series of tests have been developed to study aphasia and frontal lobe function and are discussed in those chapters. The Wisconsin Card Sorting Test is utilized to study cognitive perseveration. The Wechsler Memory Score provides a quantitative measure of memory function. The Minnesota Multiphasic Personality index provides information regarding personality, affect, depression, and so on. Projection tests have also been developed to study personality function, such as the Rorshark and the Thematic Apperception Test. The answers to the pictures provided unless very bizarre may be difficult to score, and the results are open to several interpretations.

7. Techniques for the study of the cerebral circulation

   a. Magnetic resonance angiography (MRA)—normally in MRI scans, rapidly moving blood is not clearly imaged. However, with special software programs, a noninvasive visualization of flow through vessels can be achieved (Figs. 2.24 and 2.25). At present, resolution in the range of 2.3 mm can be achieved, allowing visualization of significant aneurysms. This procedure allows imaging of the carotid and other arteries prior to carotid-endarterectomy.

   b. In contrast, cerebral angiography (or arteriography) is invasive. A catheter must be placed in the femoral artery and advanced into the aorta and then into the carotid or vertebral arteries. Radiopaque dye is then injected to directly image the cerebral vessels. This is the best technique when detailed study of the cerebral vascular is required, for example, prior to aneurysm surgery. With the increased resolution of MRA and of CT scan angiography, direct arteriography may be replaced by these noninvasive techniques. Under special circumstances, spinal angiography employing selective catheterization of radicular arteries may be performed to visualize spinal cord AVMs.

   c. Duplex scans of the extracranial carotid and vertebral arteries: this technique combines Doppler and ultrasound techniques to image blood flow in the major extracranial arteries.

   d. Transcranial Doppler may provide gross information regarding flow in the major intracranial vessels.

CEREBROSPINAL FLUID EXAMINATION

CSF fluid is usually obtained by a lumbar puncture. The lower end of the spinal cord, the conus medullaris, does not extend below the L2 vertebra. Therefore, introduction of a needle into the subarachnoid space between the L2-L3, L3-L4, or L4-L5 spinous processes will not damage the spinal cord. CSF pressure when the patient is relaxed, but positioned on one

Figure 2.24 (A) Magnetic resonance angiography (MRA). Aortic arch and major arteries in the neck. (B1 and B2) Intracranial circulation coronal submental view demonstrated in two patients B2 labels only the differences from B1. (C) Intracranial circulation (lateral view). ACA, anterior cerebral A; ACOM, anterior communicating A; CCA, common carotid A; ECA, external carotid A; ICA, internal carotid A; MCA, middle cerebral artery; PCA, posterior cerebral artery; PCOM, posterior communicating A; SCA, superior cerebral artery; VA, vertebral artery.

Figure 2.25 Magnetic resonance angiography. Basilar vertebral (posterior) circulation. (A) AP view. (B) Lateral view. The vertebral, basilar, posterior, cerebral, and all of the circumferential cerebellar branches are evident. Lumbar puncture 2 hours after the previous puncture.

side, will be usually less than 150 mm. Values in the relaxed state greater than 200 mm are considered abnormal.

Respiration, abdominal pressure, and flexion of head on chest or thighs and knees onto abdomen will all increase the pressure.

Normally no significant red blood cells (RBCs) should be present. When the puncture is traumatic, the first tube collected will contain red cells but these should significantly decrease by the time that the fourth tube is collected. Normally, fewer than seven white blood cells (WBCs) should be present and all should be mononuclears. Any polymorphonuclears are abnormal and should raise the question of infection or inflammatory reaction. Spinal fluid glucose should be no less than 50% of the blood glucose obtained at the time of the tap or within 2 hours of prior to the lumbar puncture.

In acute bacterial meningitis the CSF glucose is low due to the interference with the transport system and/or the increased metabolic activities. Total CSF protein is usually less than 45rier as in Guillain Barré syndrome. In the latter case no cells are present. This is referred to as albumin-cytologic dissociation and may also be present in patients with diabetes mellitus or myxedema.

In patients with blocks in the lower thoracic or lumbar area, the protein level may be very high, with several grams present. The thick yellow fluid may clot in the test tube (Froin's syndrome).

The gamma globulin (IgG) percentage of the total protein may be increased under the following circumstances:

1. Production of IgG in the serum is increased.

2. IgG is selectively produced within central nervous system by plasma cells—as in multiple sclerosis or neurosyphilis. Oligoclonal bands will also be present within the gamma globulin band.

This patient in the following case history should be compared to the patient 1.1 in Chapter 1. Both began with symptoms of weakness in the leg. However, the time course for evolution of symptoms differed significantly resulting in different diagnoses.

Figure 2.26 Computerized tomography (CT) scan. Cerebral hemorrhage in a 90-year-old man with left-sided weakness primarily involving the right leg and shoulder areas of the motor cortex and the adjacent premotor cortex. See Case 2.1 at end of this chapter.

CASE HISTORY 2.1

This 90-year-old, right-handed, white male with a past history of hypertension awoke on the morning of admission with weakness of the left side, which was most marked in the leg. The initial admission examination indicated no motor function of the left leg, severe weakness of the left arm, and minimal weakness of the left side of the face. Past history indicated a previous minor "stroke" involving the left side of the body, from which he had made a full functional recovery with only minimal left-sided weakness. During year prior to admission, occasional periods of confusion had been present and progressive problems in memory had developed.

Neurological Examination

Mental status: The patient was disoriented for time and place. He was, however, cooperative and able to follow all commands. He was fluent with no disturbance of language function. His remote memory was excellent. He could repeat the name of the examiner and of his primary physician but could recall neither name after 5 minutes.

Cranial nerves: A minor left central facial weakness was present.

Motor system: He had no movement of the left leg. There was little function of the left shoulder and elbow. However, handgrip was strong and independent finger movements were present; the patient was recumbent in bed with external rotation of the left leg into a hemiplegic posture.

Reflexes: Deep tendon stretch reflexes were absent in the lower extremities and the left upper extremity. The plantar responses were extensor bilaterally (bilateral sign of Babinski).

Sensory system: No definite abnormalities within limits of testing.

Clinical diagnosis: 1. Cerebrovascular accident involving the superior parasagittal precentral gyrus either due to an anterior cerebral artery occlusion or a cerebral hemorrhage secondary to amyloid angiopathy; 2. Alzheimer's disease.

Laboratory data: A CT scan of the head demonstrated an acute hemorrhage in the right superior parasagittal Rolandic and premotor areas consistent with amyloid angiopathy. (Fig. 2.26).

Comments

This patient presents many of the neurological problems which occur in the elderly. The patient had a 1-year history of progressive memory problems, which primarily involved the formation of new memories. At age 90 such memory problems occur in more than 50% of the population. Usually, this represents the development of those degenerative changes in the neurons of the cerebral cortex seen in the process defined as Alzheimer's senile dementia. The patient had elevated blood pressure for many years and had already experienced one "stroke" affecting the left side 10–15 years previously. In the present episode, the sudden development of symptoms would suggest an additional vascular event. Compare this case to Case 1.1, in which the patient had a gradual development of weakness in the leg secondary to a meningioma. As regards the localization, the marked involvement of leg and proximal arm with relative sparing of hand and face might suggest a process involving the upper half of the motor cortex (refer to Fig. 18.12).

BIBLIOGRAPHY

Aminoff, M. J. (Ed.). 1986. Electrodiagnosis in Clinical Neurology. 2nd ed. New York, NY: Churchill Livingstone.

Atlas, S. W. (Ed.). 1991. Magnetic Resonance Imaging of the Brain and Spine. New York, NY: Raven Press.

Caplan, L. R., Dewitt, L. D., and Breen, J. C. 1999. Neuroimaging in patients with cerebrovascular disease. In Greenberg, J. O. cited here, pp 493–520.

Chiappa, K. H. 1989. Evoked Potentials in Clinical Medicine. 2nd ed. New York, NY: Raven Press.

Coughlin, W., and G. Sze. 1993. Spinal imaging. Curr. Opin. Neurol. Neurosurg. 6:571–575.

Daly, D. A., and T. A. Pedley. (Eds.). 1990. Current Practice of Clinical Eletroencephalography. 2nd ed. New York, NY: Raven Press.

Denny-Brown, D. 1957. Handbook of Neurological Examination and Case Recording. 2nd ed. Cambridge, MA: Harvard University Press.

Edelman, E. R., and Warach, S. 1993. Medical progress—Magnetic resonance imaging. N. Engl. J. Med. 328:708–716, 785–791.

Greenberg, J. O. (Ed.). 1999. Neuroimaging: A Companion to Adams and Victor's Principles of Neurology. 2nd ed. New York, NY: McGraw Hill.

Martin, J. H., Brust, J. C. M., and Hilal, S. 1991. Imaging the living brain. In E. R. Kandel, J. H. Schwartz, M. S. Jessell (Eds.) Niedermeyer, E. and F. Lopes Da Silva. 1999. Electroencephalography: Basic Principles, Clinical Applications and Related Fields. pp 135–144. Philadelphia, PA. Lippincott Williams and Wilkins.

Polachini, I., Jr. 1999. Magnetic resonance angiography. In Greenberg, J. O. cited here, pp 667–725.

Shaebitz, W., and M. Fisher. 1999. Diffusion-perfusion MRI and magnetic resonance spectroscopy in cerebrovascular disease. In Greenberg, J. O. cited here, pp 625–633.

Siewert, B., Patel, M. R., and Warach, S. 1995. Magnetic resonance angiography. The Neurologist 1:167–184.

3.

NEUROCYTOLOGY

CELLS OF THE CENTRAL NERVOUS SYSTEM

Although muscle cells can also conduct electric impulses, only neurons, when arranged in networks and provided with adequate informational input, can respond in many ways to a stimulus. Probably the neuron's most important feature is that each is unique. If one is damaged or destroyed, no other nerve cell can provide a precise or complete replacement. Fortunately the nervous system was designed with considerable redundancy; consequently, it takes a significant injury to incapacitate the individual (as in Alzheimer's or Parkinson's disease). There are two major cell types that form the nervous system: supporting cells and conducting cells. The supporting cells of the peripheral nervous system consist of Schwann cells, fibroblasts, and satellite cells, while the supporting cells in the central nervous system consist of the glia, and the lining cells of the ventricles, the ependyma, the meningeal coverings of the brain, the circulating blood cells, and the endothelial lining cells of the blood vessels. The conducting cells, or neurons, form the circuitry within the brain and spinal cord. The supporting cells are constantly being replaced, but the majority of conducting cells/neurons, once formed, remain throughout our life.

THE NEURON

The basic functional unit of the nervous system is the *neuron*. The neuron doctrine (postulated by Waldeyer in 1891, described the neuron as having one axon, which is efferent, and one or more dendrites, which are afferent. It was also noted that nerve cells are contiguous, not continuous, and all other elements of the nervous system are there to feed, protect, and support the neurons. Neurons consist of a cell body, dendrites, and an axon that terminates as a synapse. The axon is usually covered by the insulator myelin (Table 3.1).

DENDRITES

The dendrites receive input from many different sources (Figs. 3.1 and 3.2). The action potential originates at the site of origin of the axon and is transmitted down the axon in an all-or-nothing fashion to the synapse, where the impulse is transmitted to the dendritic zone of the next neuron on the chain.

Dendrites have numerous processes that increase the neuron's receptive area. The majority of synapses on a nerve cell are located on the dendrite surface. With the electron microscope the largest dendrites can be identified by the presence of parallel rows of neurotubules, which may help in the passive transport of the action potential. The dendrites in many neurons are also studded with small membrane extensions, the dendritic spines that greatly enlarge the receptive surface of the neuron.

Table 3.1 **PARTS OF A NEURON**

REGION	CONTENTS
Soma Majority of inhibitory synapses are found on its surface	The neuron's trophic center, containing the nucleus, nucleolus, and many organelles.
Dendrite	Continuation of the soma; has many branches forming large surface area; contains neurotubules and majority of synapses on its surface; Type I neurons have dendritic spines.
Axon Myelin; an insulator, covers axon	Conducts action potentials to other neurons via the synapse. Length: few millimeters to a meter.
Synapse	Site where an axon connects to the dendrites, soma or axon of another neuron. Consists of presynaptic part containing neurotransmitters, postsynaptic portion with membrane receptors separated by a narrow cleft.

SOMA

The soma (perikaryon or cell body) of the neuron varies greatly in form and size. Neuronal cell bodies are either unipolar with circular cell bodies; bipolar cells have ovoid cell bodies; and the most common cell type, the multipolar cells, have polygonal cell bodies.

GOLGI TYPE I AND II NEURONS

Neurons can also be grouped by axon length: those with long axons are called Golgi type I (or pyramidal) cells; those with short axons are called Golgi type II (or satellite) cells (Gray, 1959).

The Golgi type I cell (Fig. 3.2) has an apical and a basal dendrite, each of which has secondary, tertiary, and quaternary branches, with smaller branches arising from each of these branches that extend into all planes. They form the basic long circuitry within the central nervous system. The axons of pyramidal neurons run long distances within the cortex, but they may also exit from the cortex.

Figure 3.1 Golgi type II cells (neurons with short axons) in the motor cortex of the rat. (Golgi-Cox stain, 450×.)

The Golgi type II cell (Fig. 3.1) has a very short axon that ramifies in the gray matter; these cells have few spines on their processes. They are more numerous in the primate brain and their presence may be the basis of many of our very complex intellectual functions.

DENDRITIC SPINES

Throughout much of the central nervous system, spines are found on the dendrites. These spines were first seen in Golgi-stained sections and were considered by many as an artifact of the silver-dichromate stain, but electron micrographic studies have shown they exist and are a very important part of many neurons. In the cerebral cortex there are two basic types of neurons and a cell with a long axon, type I, and a cell with a short axon, type II. In the cerebral cortex, spines are numerous on Golgi type I pyramidal neuron/neuron with long axons and their axons form many of the long tracts within the central nervous system. The transmitter in type I cells is glutamate. Golgi type II cells (Fig 3.3) have few if any dendritic spines. The axon usually extends only a short distance within the cerebral cortex (0.3 to 5 mm).

Spines are absent from the initial segment of the apical and basal dendrite of pyramidal neurons, but they become numerous farther along the dendritic branches. Dendritic spines are bulbous, with a long neck approximately 1 to 3 microns in diameter connecting to the dendrite (Figs. 3.2, 3.3, 3.4, and 3.24).

Figure 3.2 Golgi type I cells (cells with long axons) in the motor cortex of a rat. (*A*) Entire cell: soma, axon, and dendrite, 150×. (*B*) Dendritic spines, 1100× (*A* and *B*—Golgi rapid stain). (*C* and *D*) Electron micrographs of dendritic spines with excitatory synapses, 30,000× of spiny pyramidal cell. (*D*) Dendrite with dendritic spine, which consists of a neck and a head. The spines greatly increase the surface area of the dendrite, and the neck of the spine contains the spine apparatus that is an effective capacitor. Note there are several synapses on the spine.

Figure 3.3 (*A*) Light micrograph of a 100-micron-thick parlodion section showing many pyramidal cells in the motor cortex of a monkey. Golgi rapid stain, 100×. (*B*) Light micrograph of a 100-micron-thick section showing a pyramidal cell with spines on its transverse dendrite. Golgi rapid method, 1000× (From S. Jacobson).

Figure 3.4 Molecular architecture of inhibitory and excitatory synapses. Top panels show excitatory and inhibitory synapses. Excitatory synapses target mature mushroom-shaped spines containing a prominent postsynaptic density (PSD), and inhibitory synapses are present along the dendritic shaft lacking postsynaptic thickening. Various organelles support the synapse; mitochondria provide energy, polyribosomes and RNA particles allow local protein synthesis, recycling endosomes (REs) transport internalized synaptic receptors back to the plasma membrane, and the cytoskeleton regulates spine dynamics. The abundant actin cytoskeleton is connected to the PSD and is the primary determinant of spine shape and motility. Transient invasion of dynamic microtubule into dendritic spines can regulate formation of spine head protrusions and rapid spine growth. Excitatory and inhibitory synapses contain a unique set of channels, scaffolding proteins, and other postsynaptic molecules. The microanatomy of the inhibitory and excitatory synapses and their organization of proteins and protein–protein interactions are depicted in the left and right panels, respectively. Major families of postsynaptic proteins are shown, including scaffolding proteins, adhesion molecules, and receptors. Lower panel shows major morphologic events occurring in dendritic spines upon long-term potentiation (LTP; left) or long-term depression (LTD; right). In Alzheimer's disease and mental retardation, signaling cascades are triggered similar to LTD, leading to thinner, immature spines. In contrast, cocaine addiction shows similarities to LTP, resulting in bigger, mushroom-shaped, mature spines. The molecular and morphologic changes in the synapse are hallmarks of the disease pathology and are responsible for the cognitive alterations in neuropsychiatric diseases. CamKII, Ca2+/calmodulin-dependent kinase II; AMPAR, amino-3-hydroxy-5-methyl-4-isoazolepropionate receptor; GABA, γ-aminobutyric acid; GABAR, GABA receptor; mGluR, metabotropic glutamate receptor; NMDAR, N-methyl-d-aspartate receptor; SAPAP, synapse associated protein 90/PSD-95-associated protein. (From Spronsen, Myrrhe, Hoogenraad, and Casper, 2010.)

Many spines are found on dendrites and these spines contain a spine apparatus that seems to function like a capacitor, charging and then discharging when its current load is exceeded. Immediately behind the postsynaptic membrane is an elaborate complex of interlinked proteins called the postsynaptic density (PSD), in which adhesion molecules, receptors, and their associated signaling proteins are highly concentrated (Fig. 3.4).

Dendritic spines are actin-rich protrusions from neuronal dendrites that form the postsynaptic part of most excitatory synapses. They provide compartments that locally control the signaling mechanisms at individual synapses. Many axon terminals are located on the spines. Their importance stems from the fact that they greatly expand the dendrite's receptive synaptic surface and are major sites of information processing and storage in the brain. Changes in the shape and size of dendritic spines are correlated with the strength of excitatory synaptic connections and heavily depend on remodeling of its underlying actin cytoskeleton (Hotulainen and Hoogenraad, 2010). Spine structure is regulated by molecular mechanisms that include the extrinsic factors (such as perisynaptic astroglia) and the intrinsic factors (such as organelles) that are required to build and maintain synapses. Specific mechanisms of actin regulation are also integral to the formation, maturation, and plasticity of dendritic spines and to learning and memory. Hippocampal spines show structural plasticity which may form the basis for the physiological changes in synaptic transmission that underlie learning and memory.

CYTOPLASM ORGANELLES

These structures are seen in most cells and in all neurons and glial cell types and permit each neuron to function (Table 3.2) In these eukaryotic cells the organelles tend to be compartmentalized and include the nucleus, polyribosomes, rough endoplasmic reticulum, smooth endoplasmic reticulum, mitochondria, and inclusions (Fig. 3.10). Most neuronal cytoplasm is formed in the organelles of the soma and flows into the other processes. Newly synthesized macromolecules are transported to other parts of the nerve cell, either in membrane-bound vesicles or as protein particles. As long as the soma with a majority of its organelles is intact, the nerve cell can live. Thus, it is the

Table 3.2 RATE OF AXONAL TRANSPORT OF CELLULAR STRUCTURES

TRANSPORT RATE (MM/DAY)	CELLULAR STRUCTURE
Fast 300<–>400	Vesicles, smooth endoplasmic reticulum, and granules
Intermediate 50<–>15	– Mitochondria – Filament Proteins
Slow 3<–>4	– Actin, fodrin, enolase, component CPK, calmodulin, B and clathrin
Slow 0.3<–>1	– Neurofilament protein, component tubulin, and MAPS

Data from Graftstein and Forman; McQuarrie; Wujek and Lasek.

Figure 3.5 Electron micrograph of the cerebral cortex showing the principal cell types in the central nervous system: neurons, astrocyte (astro), oligodendrocyte (oligo), and a blood vessel (BV).

trophic center of the neuron. Separation of a process from the soma produces death of that process.

NUCLEUS

The large ovoid nucleus is found in the center of the cell body (Figs. 3.5–3.9). Chromatin is dispersed as nerve cells are very

Figure 3.6 The Nissl body/rough endoplasmic reticulum in the pyramidal neurons #1 in layer v in the leg region of the motor cortex of a chimpanzee. The larger pyramidal cell is a giant cell of Betz; note the astrocyte located next to its apical dendrite. The cell stained in #2 is an astrocyte-#2. Thionin stain, 205×.

Figure 3.7 Motor neuron; ventral horn cell from a human cervical cord demonstrating the Nissl substance axon hillock and nucleolus. Nissl stain, 600×.

Figure 3.9 Ventral horn cell of a female squirrel monkey. Note the nucleus, nucleolus, and the accessory body of Barr (arrow). One micron epoxy section, 1400×.

active metabolically. Within the nucleus there is usually only a single spherical nucleolus, which stains strongly for RNA. In females, the nucleus also contains a perinuclear accessory body, called the Barr body (Fig. 3.9). The Barr body is an example of the inactivation and condensation of one of the two female sex, or X, chromosomes (Barr and Bertram, 1949). The process of inactivation of one of the X chromosomes is often called lyonization, after the cytogenetist who discovered it, Mary Lyons. Recently much progress has been made in the localization of genes associated with neurologic diseases, including trisomy's, Down's, Alzheimer's, Huntington's, and Parkinson's.

ROUGH ENDOPLASMIC RETICULUM–NISSL BODY

The rough endoplasmic reticulum or Nissl substance, which turns amino acids into proteins, is the chromodial substance found in light micrographs (Fig. 3.11). It can be demonstrated by using a light microscope and basic dyes, such as methylene blue, cresyl violet, and toluidine blue. The appearance and amount vary from cell to cell. With electron microscopy, cisterns containing parallel rows of interconnecting rough

Figure 3.8 Electron micrograph of a neuron in the rat sensory cortex demonstrating the nucleus and nucleolus (arrow). 10,000×.

Figure 3.10 Electron micrograph of a small pyramidal neuron in the rat cerebral cortex, demonstrating the following organelles: Golgi apparatus, mitochondria, lysosome, and Nissl substance (rough endoplasmic reticulum). Note the nuclear pore (arrow). 60,000×.

Figure 3.11 Electron micrograph showing inclusions: (*A*) lipofuchsin; (*B*) glycogen, lipid and Nissl substance, 30,000×.

Figure 3.12 Electron micrographs of a pyramidal neuron in the rat cerebral cortex. (*A*) Soma and nucleus. (*B*) Dendrite. Note the large amount of Nissl substance in the soma. The dendrites have less Nissl substance and many microtubules. 33,000×.

endoplasmic reticulum are revealed (Fig. 3.12). Ribosomes (clusters of ribosomal RNA) are attached to the outer surfaces of the membranes and consist of a large and a small RNA-protein subunit. The Nissl substance is most concentrated in the soma and adjacent parts of the dendrite (Fig. 3.7). It is, however, also found throughout the dendrite (Figs. 3.12B and 3.16), and even in the axon hillock.

MITOCHONDRIA

These organelles, found throughout the neuron, are the third largest organelles after the nucleus and endoplasmic reticulum and supply the energy for many activities in the eukaryotic cell. They are rod shaped and vary from 0.35 to 10 microns in length and 0.35 to 0.5 microns in diameter. The wall of a mitochondrion consists of two layers—an outer and inner membrane. The outer membrane contains pores that render the membrane soluble to proteins with molecular weights of up to 10,000. The inner membrane is less permeable and has folds called cristae that project into the center of the mitochondrial matrix. The interior of the mitochondrion is filled with a fluid denser than cytoplasm. On the inner membrane are found enzymes that provide much of the energy required for the nerve cell. These respiratory enzymes (flavoproteins and cytochromes) catalyze the addition of a phosphate group to adenosine diphosphate (ADP), forming ATP. In the cytoplasm ADP provides the energy required for cellular metabolic functions. Cations and mitochondrial DNA (mt DNA) have been demonstrated in the mitochondrial matrix. In the cytoplasm, enzymes break down glucose into pyruvic and acetoacetic acid. These substances are taken into the mitochondrial matrix and participate in the Krebs citric-acid cycle, which allows the mitochondria to metabolize amino acids and fatty acids.

Out of Africa: Lucy as the Mitochondrial Eve?

Mitochondrial DNA is derived from the mother, and an intriguing study links this mitochondrial DNA to a common human female ancestor, Lucy. *Australopithicus afarensis* is a Hominid species that lived in northeast Africa, in the Hadar region of Ethiopia. Because of the maternal inheritance of mtDNA, this work was interpreted as showing that all present mtDNA is derived from a single ancestral mtDNA belonging to a woman who lived in Africa some 2,000,000 years ago. She was nicknamed "Mitochondrial Eve," the mother of us all. Some of the implications from these data are more dramatic than is justified. One woman living 2,000,000 years ago was not the mother of us all, but was only one member of a population living then.

Until 1995, this species was the earliest known member of the Hominid family. *Australopithicus afarensis* lived from approximately 4 to 2.7 million years ago along the northern Rift valley of east Africa, and perhaps even earlier. A non-coding portion of the mitochondrial DNA (mtDNA) molecule was chosen for analysis on the assumption that it would not have been so constrained by the pressures of natural selection. The choice of mitochondrial DNA had two other advantages:

- Each cell has many (hundreds to thousands) mitochondria, so the same large number of identical mtDNA molecules, whereas it has only a single copy of each nuclear chromosome.
- We inherit our mtDNA exclusively from our mothers. The mitochondria of the sperm do not become incorporated in the fertilized egg. Unlike nuclear genes, the mitochondrial genes from two parents never get a chance to be reshuffled by crossing over before they are passed on to the next generation.

Over 600 base pairs of a noncoding region of mtDNA were sequenced in specimens collected from over 200 people. The subjects represented populations from all parts of the world, including a number of different tribal groups in Africa. The greatest diversity of sequences was found among the various African populations. Computer analysis produced many possible family trees by which the present-day sequences could be derived ultimately from a single ancestral sequence (Johanson and Edey, 1981; Johanson and Wong, 2009).

NEUROSECRETORY GRANULES

Neurons in the supraoptic and periventricular nuclei of the hypothalamus form neurosecretory material (Bodian, 1963, 1966; Palay, 1957; Scharrer, 1966). The axons of these cells form the hypothalamic-hypophyseal tract, which runs through the median eminence, down the infundibular stalk to the neurohypophysis (pars nervosa), where the axons end in close proximity to the endothelial cells. The secretory granules are 130 to 150 millimicrons in diameter and are found in the tract (see Fig. 3.13).

NEURONAL CYTOSKELETON

In silver-stained sections examined in a light microscope, a neurofibrillary network can be seen in the neurons (Fig. 3.14). Electron micrographs can distinguish microtubules, 3 to 30 μm in diameter, and neurofilaments, 1 nm in diameter. It appears that fixation produces clumping of the tubules and filaments into the fibrillar network seen in light micrographs.

Neurons in common with other eukaryotic cells contain a cytoskeleton that maintains it shape. This cytoskeleton consists of at least three types of fibers:

1. Microtubules 30 nm in diameter
2. Microfilaments 7 nm in diameter
3. Intermediate filaments 10 nm in diameter

If the plasma membrane and organelle membrane are removed, the cytoskeleton is seen to consist of actin microfilaments, tubulin-containing microtubules, and crisscrossing intermediate filaments. Neurotubules (microtubules) predominate in dendrites and in the axon hillock, whereas microfilaments are sparse in dendrites and most numerous in axons (Fig. 3.7B). Microtubules and intermediate filaments

Figure 3.13 Electron micrograph of a rat neurohypophysis. (*A*) shows neurosecretory granules in the axoplasm of filers of the hypothalamo-hypophyseal tract, 30,000×. (*B*) demonstrates a Herring body, a storage site in the terminal end of the axons from the hypothalamus, where hormones are temporarily stored prior to their release, 8000×.

are found throughout the axon. Microfilaments form much of the cytoskeleton of the entire neuron.

MICROTUBULES AND AXOPLASMIC FLOW

With the protein manufacturing apparatus present only in the soma, and to a lesser degree in the dendrites, a mechanism must exist to transport proteins and other molecules from the soma, down the axon, and into the presynaptic side. Weiss and Hisko (1948) placed a ligature on a peripheral nerve, and this produced a swelling proximal to the tie, demonstrating that material flows from the *soma*, or *trophic center*, into the axon and ultimately to the axon terminal. The development of techniques that follow this axoplasmic flow has revolutionized the study of circuitry within the central nervous system. The ability to map this circuitry accurately has given all neuroscientists a better understanding of the integrative mechanisms in the brain. There are many compounds now available to follow circuitry in the brain, and they include horseradish peroxidase, wheat germ agluttin, tetanus toxin, fluorescent molecules, and radiolabeled compounds.

Figure 3.14 Cytoskeleton of central nervous system as shown in a neurofibrillary stain (Bielschowsky) of a ventral horn cell in the cat spinal cord, showing neurofibrillary network in axons, soma, and dendrites.

Axoplasmic transport is a process responsible for movement of organelles (mitochondria), lipids, proteins, synaptic vesicles, and other parts of the cell membranes to and from the soma down the axon to the synapses and back up to the soma. Axonal transport is also responsible for moving molecules destined for degradation from the axon back to the cell body, where they are broken down by lysosomes. Microtubules provide the structural basis for transport, axoplasmic flow. This mechanism of transport is not diffusion but rather retrograde axonal transport associated with the microtubule network that exists throughout the nerve cell. The rate of flow varies depends upon the product being transported and ranges from more than 300 mm/day to less than 1 mm a day.

Direction of Axoplasmic Flow

The main direction of the flow is *anterograde*, from the cell body into the axon and synapse. There is also a very active *retrograde* flow from the synaptic region back to the cell body that is a source for recycling many of the substances found at the synaptic ending.

The particles that move the fastest, as noted in Table 3.2, consist of small vesicles of the secretory and synaptic vesicles, and the slowest group is the cytoskeletal components. Mitochondria are transported down from the cell body at an intermediate rate. The retrograde flow from the synaptic telodendria back into the soma returns any excess of material for degradation or reprocessing.

The retrograde flow permits any excess proteins or amino acids to recycle. It also permits products synthesized or released at the axonal cleft to be absorbed and then transported back to the cell. The microtubules help to transport membrane-bound vesicles, protein, and other macromolecules. This orthograde transport, or anterograde axonal transport, is the means whereby these molecules formed in the soma/trophic center are transported down the axon into the axonal telodendria. The individual microtubules in the nervous system are 10 to 35 nm in length and together form the cytoskeleton. The intermediate filaments are associated with the microtubules. The wall of the microtubule consists of a helical array of repeating tubulin subunits containing the A and B tubulin molecule. The microtubule wall consists of globular subunits 4 to 5 nm in diameter; the subunits are arranged in 13 protofilaments that encircle and run parallel to the long axis of the tubule. Each microtubule also has a defined polarity. Associated with the microtubules are protein motors, kinesins and dyneins, which when combined with cAMP are the mechanism of transport in the central nervous system. The products transported down the microtubules move similar to a humans walking rather than like an inchworm or a locomotive. During mitosis, microtubules disassemble and reassemble; however, a permanent cytoskeleton lattice of microtubules and intermediate filaments in the neuron is somehow maintained. It is not yet known how long each microtubule exists, but there is evidence of a constant turnover.

PERIPHERAL VERSUS CENTRAL NERVE STRUCTURE

Peripheral Nerve Structures

Peripheral nerves consist of many axons held together in a fascicle by connective tissue of mesodermal origin (Fig. 3.19).

Schwann Cell Cytoplasm. The peripheral nerve fiber or axon is engulfed in the Schwann cytoplasm (the neurilemmal sheath), which also forms the myelin sheath.

Epineurium. The outer layer that covers the nerve trunks and fills between the individual fascicles is called the epineurium. It consists of connective tissue cells, collagen, and some fat cells. Perineurium enwraps each of the fascicles in a dense layer of connective tissue.

Endoneurium. This region of a peripheral nerve consists of strands of collagen, fibroblasts, and other cells that run between the individual nerve fibers. The term *endoneurium* is also applied to the delicate trabeculum surrounding each nerve fiber, which is also called the sheath of Key-Retzius.

Large blood vessels are found in the epineurium and perineurium, and capillaries are seen in the endoneurium.

Peripheral axons can be classified by size and function into three major functional groups in the letter system A-B-C (Table 3.4A), or into four groups in the Roman numeral system (Table 3.4B).

Central Nervous System Structure

Axons in the central nervous system also vary in size (5 to 33 microns) and in length (0.5 mm to 1 m), but these axons cannot be readily separated into functional categories based on axonal diameter. The axons in the central nervous system run in bundles called tracts that are enwrapped by the processes of fibrous astrocytes. However, no specific coverings similar to the epineurium and perineurium and capillaries are seen in the endoneurium. Fibers can vary in diameter from less than 0.5 microns to 33 microns.

NEUROFIBRILLAR TANGLES

Neurofibrillar tangles are bundles of abnormal filaments within a neuron (Figs. 3.4-3.8). They are helical filaments that are different from normal cytoskeletal proteins (Fig. 3.14), and they contain the tau protein a microtubule binding protein (MAP) that is a normal component in neurons. In Alzheimer's disease there are accumulations of abnormally phosphorylated and aggregated forms of the microtubule binding protein tau. These large aggregates form the tangles that can be physical barriers to transport, may interfere with normal neuronal functions, and are probably toxic. Mutations in the human tau gene are found in autosomal dominant neuronal degenerative disorders isolated to chromosome 17. These familial disorders are characterized by extensive neurofibrillar pathology and are often called "taupathies" (Hutton, 2000; Lee and Trojanowski, 2013) (Fig. 3.15).

AXON AND AXON ORIGIN (AXON HILLOCK)

The axon originates at the hillock and is a slender process that usually arises from a cone-shaped region on the perikaryon (Fig. 3.16). This region includes filaments, stacks of tubules, and polyribosomes (Fig. 3.8B). The initial segment of the axon, arising from the axon hillock, is covered by dense material that functions as an insulator membrane. The axon contains some elongate mitochondria, many filaments oriented parallel to the long axis of the axon (Fig. 3.16), and some tubules. In contrast, a dendrite contains a few filaments and any tubules, all arranged parallel to the long axis of the dendrite (Fig. 3.16). Polyribosomes are present, but the highly organized, rough endoplasmic reticulum is absent.

MYELIN SHEATH: THE INSULATOR IN AN AQUEOUS MEDIA

In the nervous system axons may be myelinated or unmyelinated. Myelin is formed by a supporting cell, which in the central nervous system is the *oligodendrocyte* and in the peripheral nervous system, the *Schwann cell*. Myelin is a multilayered insulating sheath enwrapping axons of vertebrate and crustacean neurons. This increases the speed of conduction of the action potential along the axon. The breakdown of the sheath results in disruption of neuronal conduction and axoplasmic flow (as in human multiple sclerosis). The immature Schwann cells and oligodendrocyte have on their surface the myelin-associated glycoprotein that binds to the adjacent axon and may well be the trigger that leads to myelin formation. Thus, the myelin sheath is not a part of the neuron; it is only a covering for the axon.

Nodes of Ranvier

Myelin consists of segments approximately 0.5 to 3 mm in length. Between these segments are the nodes of Ranvier. The nodes of Ranvier (Fig. 3.11) permit rapid and efficient saltatory (leaping) propagation of action potentials along a myelinated axon by depolarization and rapid transfer of electric potential from node to node of Ranvier instead of a steady flow along the length of the

Figure 3.15 Electron micrograph from the rat cerebral demonstrating the differences in the density of the DNA between Neurons, Astrocytes and Oligodendrocytes, 30,000×.

Figure 3.16 Appearance of the axon hillock, axon origin. (*A*) In a Nissl stain, 400×; (*B*) in an electron micrograph, 15,000×; and (*C*) in a Golgi-rapid stain, 350×.

nerve. The axon, however, is continuous at the nodes, and axon collaterals can leave at the nodes. The myelin membrane like all membranes contains phospholipid bilayers (Fig. 3.9). In the central nervous system myelin includes the following proteins:

Proteolipid protein (51%)

Myelin basic protein (44%)

Myelin-associated glycoprotein (1%)

3,3-cyclic nucleotide (4%)

The oligodendrocytic process forms the myelin sheaths by wrapping around the axon. The space between the axonal plasma membrane and the forming myelin is reduced until most of the exoplasmic and cytoplasmic space is finally forced out. The result is a compact stack of membranes. The myelin sheath is from 3 to 100 membranes thick and acts as an insulator by preventing the transfer of ions from the axonal cytoplasm into the extracellular space.

Myelin sheaths are in contact with the axon. In light microscopy they appear as discontinuous tubes 0.5 to 3 mm in length, interrupted at the node of Ranvier (Fig. 3.29).

The axon is devoid of myelin at the site of origin (the nodes) and at the axonal telodendria. At the site of origin the axon is covered by an electron-dense membrane, and at the site of the synaptic telodendria the various axonal endings are isolated from one another by astrocytic processes. In electron micrographs each myelin lamella actually consists of two-unit membranes with the entire lamella being 130 to 180 Å thick (Fig. 3.17). Myelin is thus seen to consist of a series of light and dark lines. The dark line, called the major dense line (MDL), represents the apposition of the inner surface of the unit membranes. The less dense line, called the interperiod line (IPL), represents the approximation of the outer surfaces of adjacent myelin membranes. Only at the node of Ranvier is the axonal plasma membrane in communication with the extracellular space. The influx of Na+ at each node causes the action potential to move rapidly down the axon by jumping from node to node-saltatory conduction.

MYELINATION—SCHWANN CELL IN THE PERIPHERAL NERVOUS SYSTEM AND OLIGODENDROCYTE IN THE CENTRAL NERVOUS SYSTEM

The process of covering a naked axon with myelin is myelination. An axon starts with just a covering formed by the plasma membrane of either the *Schwann cell* or the *oligodendrocyte* (Fig. 3.18). More and more layers are added until myelination is complete. The myelin is laid down by the processes of either the Schwann cell or oligodendrocyte twisting around the axon (Geren, 1956; Robertson, 1955). In the peripheral nervous system, there is usually only one Schwann cell for each length or internode of myelin. In the central nervous system each oligodendrocyte may form and maintain myelin sheaths on 30 to 60 axons. The unmyelinated axons in the peripheral nervous system are found in the cytoplasm of the Schwann cell; in the central nervous system each oligodendrocyte enwraps many

Figure 3.17 Myelin sheath. Electron micrograph of myelin sheath from the optic nerve of the mouse demonstrating repeating units of the myelin sheath, consisting of a series of light and dark lines. The dark line, called the major dense line (MDL), represents the apposition of the inner surface of the unit membranes. The less dense line, called the interperiod line (IPL), represents the approximation of the outer surfaces of adjacent myelin membranes (67,000×). (Courtesy of Alan Peters, Department of Anatomy, Boston University School of Medicine.)

Figure 3.18 Demonstration of the cells of origin of callosal axons with the horseradish peroxidase diaminobenzidine reaction in layers II and V of the somatosensory cortex. The horseradish peroxidase was injected into the contralateral cortex 34 hours previously and transported retrogradely into this region.

axons. There can be as many as 13 unmyelinated axons in one Schwann cell (Fig. 3.19).

The *sequence of myelination* has been studied centrally in great detail (Jacobson, 1964); it begins in the spinal cord, moves into the brain stem, and finally ends up with the diencephalon and cerebrum last. A delay in myelination will produce developmental delays and may be a consequence of many factors, including genetic and nutritional ones (e.g., alcoholism-fetal alcohol syndrome), and is usually very harmful to the fetus. Breakdown of the myelin in a disease (e.g., multiple sclerosis) produces major functional deficits where they can affect the basic function of the cell—the signaling process. Fast axonal transport is associated with the microtubules. The slower components, including membrane associated proteins (MAPS), are transported inside the microtubules, but the mitochondria actually descend in the axonal cytoplasm (Table 3.3).

Scientists are investigating several different strategies for stimulating the repair of myelin:

1. Antibodies (immune proteins that attach to specific molecules) have been successfully used to stimulate myelin repair in rodents with a multiple sclerosis–like disease.

Table 3.3 **CONTENTS OF A PERIPHERAL NERVE BUNDLE**

Epineurium	Forms outer layer covering the nerve trunks and fills in between the individual fascicules; consists of connective tissue cells, collagen and some fat cells.
Perineurium	A connective tissue layer that surrounds the nerve fascicles.
Endoneurium (Sheath of Key-Retzius)	Strands of collagen and fibroblasts between individual axons. Endoneurium also refers to the delicate trabeculum surrounding each nerve fiber.
Sheath of Schwann	Engulfs each individual axon and forms myelin.

Based on the outcomes of this research, preliminary testing for safety in people with multiple sclerosis is planned.

2. Efforts are also being made to surgically replace damaged oligodendrocytes and nerve cells.

Scientists are working to identify potential sources of replacement cells for those that are damaged by multiple sclerosis. Possible sources include skin-derived cells, bone

Table 3.4 **CLASSIFICATION OF AXONS IN PERIPHERAL NERVE BY FUNCTION**

TYPE OF FIBER	DIAMETER, MICROMETERS	CONDUCTION VELOCITY, M/SEC	GENERAL FUNCTION
A. Letter System			
A-alpha	13–22	70–120	Alpha-motoneurons, muscle spindle primary endings, Golgi tendon organs, touch
A-beta	8–13	40–70	Touch, kinesthesia, muscle spindle secondary endings
A-gamma	4–8	15–40	Touch, pressure, gamma-motoneurons
A-delta	1–4	5–15	Pain, crude touch, pressure, temperature
B	1–3	3–14	Preganglionic autonomic
C	0.1–1	0.2–2	Pain, touch, pressure, temperature, postganglionic autonomic
B. Roman Numeral System			
I a	12–20	70–120	Muscle spindle primary endings
I b	11–19	66–114	Golgi tendon organs
II	5–12	20–50	Touch, kinesthesia, muscle spindle secondary endings
III	1–5	4–20	Pain, crude touch, pressure, temperature
IV	0.1–2	0.2–3	Pain, touch, pressure, temperature

Adapted from The Nervous System In Action: Michael D. Mann, Ph.D.

Figure 3.19 Peripheral nerve of a cat. (*A*) The outer wrapping of the nerve trunk, the epineurium; each nerve fascicule is surrounded by the perineurium, while each nerve is embedded in endoneurium. Bodian stain, 100×. (*B*) 1 demonstrates a large myelinated axon, and 3 points to a small myelinated and unmyelinated axon. Bodian stain, 350×.

Figure 3.20 Silver stain of a one-micron plastic embedded section showing terminal boutons on ventral horn cells, 400×.

marrow and umbilical cord blood cells, fetal cells, adult brain cells, and Schwann cells from the peripheral nervous system. The usefulness of these replacement cells will depend on finding or creating the signals needed to stimulate their transformation and growth into healthy new cells (MS Society, 2011).

CENTRAL NERVOUS SYSTEM PATHWAYS

The axons in the peripheral nervous system are organized into nerves, while in the central nervous system the axons run in groups called tracts with each axon enwrapped in myelin and groups of axons are bundled together by the processes of fibrous astrocytes. The axons vary in diameter (5 to 33 microns) and in length (0.5 mm to 1 m), but these axons cannot be separated into functional categories based on axonal diameter. These many pathways (e.g., corticospinal, spinothalamic) will be discussed within each level of the central nervous system.

SYNAPSE

Synapses can be seen at the light microscopic level (Fig. 3.20); however, to identify all the components of a synapse the electron microscope must be used. At the electron microscopic level the synapse consists of the axonal ending, which forms the presynaptic side, and the dendritic zone, which forms the postsynaptic side (Fig. 3.21). Collectively, the pre- and postsynaptic sides and the intervening synaptic cleft are called the synapse.

Synaptic Structure

The electron microscope has permitted one to reveal many new details in synaptic structure (Bodian, 1970; Colonnier, 1969; Gray, 1959; Palay, 1967). In an electron micrograph, the presynaptic or axonal side of the synapse contains mitochondria and many synaptic vesicles (Fig. 3.21). Synaptic vesicles are concentrated near the presynaptic surface with some vesicles actually seen fusing with a membrane (Fig. 3.21), illustrating that this site releases neurotransmitters. Neurofilaments

Figure 3.21 Excitatory synapses in the sensory cortex of the rat demonstrating agranular synaptic vesicles (300 to 400 Å in the presynaptic axonal side). Note the electron-dense synaptic membranes and the intersynaptic filaments in the synaptic cleft. Electron micrograph, 65,000×.

are usually absent on the presynaptic side. Pre- and postsynaptic membranes are electron dense and are separated by a 30 to 40 nm space, the synaptic cleft, which is continuous with the extracellular space of the central nervous system.

At the synapse the electrical impulse from one cell is transmitted to another. Synapses vary in size from the large endings on motor neurons (1 to 3 microns) to smaller synapses on the granule and stellate cells of the cortex and cerebellum (less than 0.5 microns). Synapses primarily occur between the axon of one cell and the dendrite of another cell. Synapses are usually located on the dendritic spins but are also seen on the soma and rarely between axons. At the synapse the axon arborizes and forms several synaptic bulbs that are attached to the plasma membrane of the opposing neuron by intersynaptic filaments (Fig. 3.12).

Synaptic Types

There are two basic types of synapses, electrical and chemical, and they differ in location and appearance.

Electrical synapses are connected by membrane bridges, gap junction connections, which permit the electric impulse to pass directly from one cell to the other. Electric synapses have almost no delay and little chance of misfiring. These synapses are seen in many fish.

Chemical synapses have a presynaptic side, containing vesicles and a gap, and the postsynaptic side with membrane receptors. The neurotransmitter released by the action potential is exocytosed and diffuses across the synaptic cleft and binds to the specific receptor on the postsynaptic membrane. Most of the synapses seen in the mammalian central nervous system are chemical.

Synaptic Transmission

Synaptic transmission in the mammalian central nervous system is primarily a chemical and not an electrically mediated phenomenon, based on the presence of:

1. A 30 to 40 nm cleft
2. Synaptic vesicles
3. Appreciable synaptic delay due to absorbance of the chemical onto the postsynaptic receptor site. In contrast, electrical synapses have cytoplasmic bridges that interconnect the pre- and postsynaptic membranes, resulting in a minimal synaptic delay as transmission is ionic rather than by release of chemical from a vesicle.

Neurotransmitters

The neurotransmitters are either amino acids or small neuropeptides. The classic neurotransmitters in the central nervous system include acetylcholine, epinephrine, norepinephrine, serotonin, glycine, glutamate, dopamine, and GABA. Acetylcholine is the best documented transmitter in the peripheral nervous system and has been isolated in synaptic vesicles in the central nervous system. Acetylcholine esterase has been found throughout the central and peripheral nervous systems and at postganglionic sympathetic endings.

Neurotransmitters fall into two broad classes:

1. Amino acids: aspartate, glutamate, its decarboxylated form g-amino-butyric acid (GABA), and glycine.
2. Biogenic amines: acetylcholine, serotonin, histamine, and the catecholamine's: epinephrine, norepinephrine, and dopamine. Except for acetylcholine, all biogenic amines are derived from aromatic amino acids tryptophan and tyrosine.

Excitatory neurotransmitters include glutamate and actylcholine.
Inhibitory neurotransmitters include GABA, histamine, neurotensin, and angiotensin.

Many other compounds have been identified as neurotransmitters. These substances are found in synaptic vesicles on the presynaptic side, and introduction of the compound into the synaptic cleft produces the same change in the resting membrane potential as stimulation of the presynaptic axon; the compound is rapidly degraded, and the membrane potential returns to the resting state.

MODULATORS OF NEUROTRANSMISSION

At certain synaptic sites the following compounds may also function as modulators (usually a slower transmitter form of neurotransmission): adenosine, histamine, octopamine, B-alanine, ATP, and taurine. Many of the neuropeptides, such as substance P, vasoactive peptide, peptide Y, and somatostatin, are also active in neurotransmission or neuromodulation. Catecholamines and 5-hydroxytryptamine are transmitters linked to synaptic transmission in the central nervous system. Noradrenaline is a transmitter at the preganglionic synapses. Many steroids and hormones have also been linked to synaptic transmission. It is still uncertain whether these compounds play a direct role in nervous transmission or if they are just related by their importance to the ongoing functions of the entire nervous system (Table 3.5).

Table 3.5 **LOCATION AND FUNCTIONS OF NEUROTRANSMITERS**

AGENT	LOCATION	FUNCTION
L-Glutamine	Excitatory neurons	Excitation
GABA	Inhibitory neurons	Inhibition (fast/slow)
Acetylcholine	Motor neurons, basal forebrain, and midbrain and pontine tegmentum.	Excitation and modulation
Monoamines – Norepinephrine – Serotonin – Histamine	Brainstem, hypothalamus – Locus ceruleus – Raphe nuclei – Hypothalamus	Modulation
Neuropeptides	Limbic system, hypothalamus, autonomics and pain pathways.	Modulation

SYNAPTIC VESICLES

The synaptic vesicles differ in size and shape and may be agranular, spherical, flattened, or round with a dense core (Figs. 3.4 and 3.21). The method of fixation for electron micrographs affects the shape of a vesicle (Table 3.6). Bodian (1970) has shown that osmium fixation produces only spheroidal vesicles. Aldehyde followed by osmium produces spheroidal and

Table 3.6 **CATEGORIES OF SYNAPTIC VESICLES**

TYPE AND DIAMETER IN NM	LOCATION
Spheroidal or flattened with a 30-40 nm. Inhibitory synapses	At neuromuscular junction and throughout clear center. Most common type in central nervous system.
Spheroidal with 38 nm 40-80 nm electron-dense granule. Excitatory	Autonomic endings in the intestines, vas deferens, and pineal body; contains catecholamines.
Spheroidal with a droplet 50 nm 80-90 nm; catecholamines present in vesicles. Excitatory	Found at preganglionic sympathetic synapses, neuromuscular junctions in smooth muscle, and in parts of the hypothalamus, basal nuclei, brain stem, and cerebellum.
Spheroidal with a large droplet that nearly fills the vesicle (Fig. 3.15). 130-300 nm. Vesicles contain vasopressin and oxytocin. Excitatory	Characteristic of nerve endings in the hypothalamus; also found in the soma, axons and presynaptic endings of nerve cells of the hypothalamic-hypophyseal tract.

Palay, 1967.

flattened vesicles. The shape of flattened vesicles may also be modified by washing the tissue in buffer or placing the tissue directly from the aldehyde into the osmium. The spheroidal vesicles retain their shape regardless of any manipulation.

SYNAPTIC TYPES

Chemical synapses consist of presynaptic axon terminals harboring synaptic vesicles and a postsynaptic region (usually on dendrites) containing neurotransmitter receptors. These neurotransmitters are made by the presynaptic neuron and are stored in synaptic vesicles at presynaptic terminals. Whether a synapse is excitatory or inhibitory determines the postsynaptic current displayed, which in turn is a function of the type of receptors and neurotransmitters operating at the synapse.

Excitatory Synapses

Excitatory synapses depolarize the membrane potential and make it more positive; they appear asymmetrical, having a prominent postsynaptic bush with presynaptic vesicles (Figs. 3.4 and 3.21). This type of synapse is most commonly seen on dendrites. Glutamate has been identified in excitatory synapses. At the excitatory synapse there is a change in permeability that leads to depolarization of the postsynaptic membrane and which can lead to the generation of an action potential.

Inhibitory Synapses

Inhibitory synapses hyperpolarize the membrane potential and make it more negative. They are symmetrical with thickened membranes on the pre- and postsynaptic side and vesicles only on the presynaptic side. GABA has been identified in the inhibitory synapses. At an inhibitory synapse the neurotransmitter binds to the receptor membrane, which changes the permeability and tends to block the formation of the action potential. Synapses on the soma are symmetrical and they are considered inhibitory.

Synaptic Architecture

Dendritic Spines

Dendritic spines are small membranous protrusions that contain the postsynaptic machinery, including glutamate receptors, the actin cytoskeleton, and a wide variety of membrane-bound organelles, such as smooth endoplasmic reticulum, mitochondria, and endosomes.

Recently it has been shown that dendritic spines in the hippocampus can be affected by stress (Chen, Dubé, Rice, and Baram, 2010) with a resultant dendritic regression and loss of dendritic spines in hippocampal neurons that is accompanied by deficits in synaptic plasticity and memory. However, the responsible mechanisms remain unresolved. In this study they found that within hours of the onset of stress, the density of dendritic spines declined in vulnerable dendritic domains. This rapid, stress-induced spine loss was abolished by blocking the receptor ($CRFR_1$) of corticotrophin-releasing hormone (CRH), a hippocampal neuropeptide released during stress. Exposure to CRH provoked spine loss and dendritic regression in hippocampal organotypic cultures, and selective blockade of the $CRFR_1$ receptor had the opposite effect. Additionally, in this study, time-lapse imaging revealed that CRH reduced spine density by altering dendritic spine dynamics, and this mechanism involved destabilization of spine F-actin. Knockout mice lacking the $CRFR_1$ receptor had augmented spine density. These findings support a mechanistic role for CRH–$CRFR_1$ signaling in stress-evoked spine loss and dendritic remodeling.

EFFECTORS AND RECEPTORS

Effectors

The motor nerves of the somatic nervous system end in skeletal muscles and form the motor end plates. Nerve endings in smooth and cardiac muscle and in glands resemble the synaptic endings in the central nervous system. Visceral motor endings are found on muscles in arterioles (vasomotor), muscles in hair follicles (pilomotor), and sweat glands (sudomotor).

Receptors

1. Cutaneous sensory. A stereogram of the skin is shown in Figure 1.3. Table 3.7 lists the mechanicoreceptors in the body.

2. Sensory endings. Sensory endings, found throughout the body, subserve pain touch, temperature, vibration, pressure, heat, and cold in the skin, muscles, and viscera as well as the specialized somatic and visceral sensations of taste, smell, vision, audition, and balance.

3. Visceral sensory. These receptors are similar to somatic sensory receptors associated with the somatic nervous system, except that they are located in the viscera and their accessory organs.

SUPPORTING CELLS OF THE CENTRAL NERVOUS SYSTEM

The central nervous system has billions of neurons, but the number of supporting cells exceeds them by a factor of five or

Table 3.7 **MECHANICORECEPTOR**

MODALITY	RECEPTOR
Sound	Cochlea in inner ear/petrous portion of temporal bone transforms mechanical into neural impulses
Light touch and vibration	Encapsulated endings—Meissner's and Pacinian corpuscles
Proprioception: Encapsulated Sensory Endings	Muscle spindles and Golgi tendon organs in joints Meissner's and Pacinian corpuscles, Merkel's tactile discs
Pain and temperature	Free nerve endings, End Bulbs of Krausse and Golgi-Mason

six. Supporting cells form a structural matrix and play a vital role in transporting gases, water, electrolytes, and metabolites from blood vessels to the neural parenchyma and in removing waste products from the neuron. In contrast to the neuron, the supporting cells in the adult central nervous system normally undergo mitotic division.

The supporting cells are divided into macroglia and microglia:

Macroglia include astrocytes, oligodendrocytes, and ependyma, and are the supporting cells or neuroglia (nerve glue) of the central nervous system (Figs. 3.5 and 3.6).

Microglia include mesodermal microglia cells (of Hortega), the perivascular cells, and any white blood cells found within the parenchyma of the central nervous system.

Schwann cells, satellite cells, and *fibroblasts* are supporting cells of the peripheral nervous system. Functions of the different supporting cells in the nervous system are summarized in Table 3.8.

ASTROCYTES

Astrocytes are of two types: fibrous (most common in white matter) or protoplasmic (most common in gray matter) (Fig. 3.20). All astrocytes are larger and less dense than the oligodendrocytes. In light micrographs, astrocytes appear as pale cells with little or no detail in the cytoplasm (Table 3.9). The nuclei are smaller than those of a neuron but larger and less dense than those of an oligodendrocyte. The astrocytes have many functions, as noted in Table 3.7. Electron micrographs demonstrate that fibrous astrocytes have many filaments, which in places appear to fill the cytoplasm. There are few microtubules, and the processes appear pale. The nuclei of these cells have some condensed chromatin adjacent to the nuclear membrane. Glycogen is also common in astrocytic processes.

Table 3.8 **FUNCTIONS OF CNS SUPPORTING CELLS**

CELL TYPE	FUNCTIONS
Astrocytes: – Fibrous type (white matter) – Protoplasmic type (gray matter)	Major supporting cells in the brain—forming microenvironment for neurons; – act as phagocyte and enwrap axons contain many filaments; – isolate synapses, enwrap blood vessels, and form membranes on brain's inner and outer surface.
Oligodendrocytes	Form and maintain myelin
Ependyma cells	Ciliated lining cells of the ventricular system
Endothelial cells	Lining cells of blood vessels in the brain that form blood-brain barrier
Microglia (pericytes)	Supporting cells and multipotential cells found in the basement membrane of blood vessels and within brain parenchyma. Can become neurons?
Mononuclear Cells	White cells from the circulation that readily enter and stay in the brain (lymphocytes, monocytes, and macrophages) and function as sentinels for the immune system

Table 3.9 **ROLE OF ASTROCYTES IN THE CENTRAL NERVOUS SYSTEM**

1) Form a complete membrane on the external surface of the brain called the external glial limiting membrane, which enwrap all entering blood vessels
2) Forms the inner glial membrane which fuses with the ependymal processes
3) Isolates neuronal processes
4) Form the skeleton of the central nervous system
5) Tend to segregate synapses and release or absorb transmitters
6) Help form the blood-brain barrier by enwrapping brain capillaries
7) Release and absorb gliotransmitters
8) If the brain is damaged by infarction, e.g., astrocytes proliferate and form scars-the scar will interfere with any successful axonal regeneration

Protoplasmic astrocytes have nuclei that are a little darker than those of a neuron. They resemble fibrous astrocytes except that they have just a few filaments. Astrocytes and adjacent neurons form the *microenvironment* of the nervous system. There are approximately 100 to 1,000 astrocytes per neuron. The central role of these cells as gliotransmitters in many neuronal functions within the central nervous system has been extensively documented, and it is summarized in Table 3.8.

Astrocytes are now thought to be involved in almost all aspects of brain function. Astrocytes generate signals that are chemical rather than electrical. Astrocytes are star-shaped glia that hold neurons in place, get nutrients to them, and digest parts of dead neurons. But because astrocytes cannot generate action potentials, they have not received a lot of attention, until recently. It has been discovered that astrocytes can indeed communicate with neurons and modify the signals they send or receive. That means astrocytes are much more involved than we thought in the processing of information and in the signaling that occurs at the synapse.

The details still need to be worked out, but astrocytes are activated when the level of calcium ions increases inside the cell. This change in concentration signals the release (typically by exocytosis) of what are now called "gliotransmitters." These small molecules travel to a neighboring cell and deliver their message in a process very similar to that used by neurotransmitters.

The role of many of these gliotransmitters is yet to be determined, but they may be able to inhibit, stimulate, or fine-tune the action potentials fired by neurons. But astrocytes may even do more. There is growing evidence that astrocytes can alter how a neuron is built by directing where to make synapses or dendritic spines. They can also attract new cells to their territory (like immune cells and perhaps even adult neural stem cells) to repair any damage. Knowing more about astrocytes will also shed light on diseases in which communication between astrocytes and neurons is altered, including Alzheimer's disease, AIDS, brain cancer, and ALS (amyotrophic lateral sclerosis, also known as Lou Gehrig's disease).

Gliotransmitters

Glia form the *internal mileu* of the central nervous system and are affected by their neighboring neurons; recently their role in neurotransmission has been documented. Gliotransmitters were first identified in 1994 and in order to be included in this category: (1) they must be synthesized and or stored in astrocytes, (2) released or triggered by physiological actions, (3) activated rapidly in neighboring cells, and (4) have a role in physiological processes (Table 3.10).

OLIGODENDROCYTES

In light micrographs the oligodendrocyte has a small darkly stained nucleus surrounded by a thin ring of cytoplasm (Figs. 3.15 and 3.13 and 3.20). In electron micrographs oligodendrocytes are dense cells with many microtubules and few neurofilaments (Fig. 3.5). Dense clumps of rough endoplasmic reticulum and clusters of polyribosomes are seen in the cytoplasm, which is denser but scantier than that in neurons. The nucleus tends to be located toward one pole of the cell, and the nuclear chromatin tends to be heavily clumped. In electron micrographs oligodendrocytes can be distinguished from astrocytes because they have a darker cytoplasm and nucleus, few if any filaments, and more heavily condensed chromatin (Fig. 3.5). The role of the oligodendrocyte is to form and maintain myelin (although they may also be responsible for breaking down myelin in multiple sclerosis). Oligodendrocytes are usually seen in close proximity to astrocytes and neurons, and all three cell types are important in forming and maintaining myelin.

ENDOTHELIAL CELLS

Endothelial cells form the lining of the capillaries in the central nervous system (Figs. 3.22 and 3.35). They are of mesodermal origin and bound together by tight junctions. Their tight junctions and a pinocytosis provide the basis of the blood–brain barrier (see later discussion).

Table 3.10 **CHEMICAL GLIOTRANSMITTERS**

GLIOTRANSMITTERS	CELLULAR STORAGE SITE	RELEASE MECHANISM	RELEASE STIMULANTS AND MODULATORS	SITE OF ACTION (RECEPTOR)	CELL TARGETS AND EFFECTS
Glutamate	SLMV, cytosol	Ca^{2+} dependent exocytosis	Glutamate, GABA, ATP, PG, TNFalpha, SDF1alpha	mGluR, AMPAR, kainite, NMDAR	Astrocyte, neurons; mostly stimulators
ATP	?DCG	Ca^2 dependent exocytosis (activation of channels and/or transporters)	ATP, glutamate, dopamine, LPA, thrombin	P2X, P2Y	Astrocytes, microglia, neurons, blood vessel cells (mostly stimulators)
Adenosine	Cytosol	Ectonucleotidase-mediated ATP dephosphorylation (activation of channels and/or transporters)	ATP, glutamate, dopamine, LPA, thrombin	A1, A2	Neurons mostly Inhibitors
d-Serine	?SLMV	Ca^2 dependent exocytosis	Glutamate	NMDAR (glycine site)	Neurons (stimulators)
Eicosanoids (PG, HETE)	Not know to be stored	Ca^{2+} dependent synthesis followed by rapid release	Glutamate, TNFalpha, SDF1alpha, noradrenaline	Eicosanoid receptors	Astrocytes, microglia, neuron, blood vessel cells (mostly stimulators)
Cytokines TNF alpha	Cell surface	Ca^{2+} dependent TACE-mediated surface proteolysis	SDF1alpha	TNFalpha receptors	Astrocytes, neurons (stimulators)
Proteins & Peptides	DCG	Ca^2 dependent exocytosis	Ach (for AchBP)	Ach binding, ANP and other peptide receptors	Neurons (AchBP; inhibitors)
Taurine and homocysteic acid?					

Key: Activation of channels and/or transporters, Ach-acetylcholine; AchBP-acetylcholine binding protein, ANP-atrial natriuretic peptide, PAR-alpha amino 3-hydorxy 5 methyl4-isoxazole propionic acid glutamate receptor, DCG-dense core granules, HETE-20-hydroxyeicosatetraenoic acid; LPA-lysophosphatidic acid; mGlur-metabotropic; glutamate receptor; NMDAR-n-methyl-d-aspartine glutamate receptor; P2X,P2Y purinergic 2X and 2Y receptors; PG-prostaglandin; SDF1alpha-stromal-derived factor; -1alpha; SLMV-synaptic like microvesicle; TNFalpha-converting enzyme; TNF–tumor necrosis factor alpha.
Eicosanoid receptors are the physiologically active substances derived from arachidonic acid, including the prostaglandins (PG), thromboxanes (TX), leukotrienes (LT) and lipoxins (LX). The PGs and TXs are collectively identified as prostanoids.
Adapted from Volterra and Meldolesi 2005. Astrocytes, from brain glue to communication elements. Modified from Volterra and Meldolesi, *Nature Review Neuroscience* 5: 626-640.

Figure 3.22 Degenerating synaptic endings in the sensory cortex of an adult rat showing dense vesicle and filaments replacing the normal-appearing axonal endings seen in Figure 3.21. Electron micrograph, 115,000×.

MONONUCLEAR CELLS: MONOCYTES AND MICROGLIA

Mononuclear Cells

Mononuclear cells—lymphocytes, monocytes, and histiocytes—are found in the central nervous system, where they act as phagocytes, breaking down myelin and neurons. Myelin destruction always triggers intense macrophage reaction within 48 hours, followed by infiltration of monocytes first and then lymphocytes. Note that astrocytes have also been shown to engulf degenerating myelin sheaths, axonal processes, and degenerating synapses (Fig. 3.23).

Microglial Cells

Microglial cells originate from monocytes that enter the brain (Fig. 3.3; Table 3.11). *Neurons, astrocytes, and oligodendrocytes are ectodermal in origin, but microglial cells are mesodermal in origin.* The ovoid microglia cells are the smallest of the supporting cells and are divided into two categories: (1) those that form perivascular cells and (2) the resting and waiting microglial cells in the parenchyma of the brain. Microglia vary in appearance, depending on developmental stage, functional state, and anatomical location; subtype terms include ramified, perivascular, amoeboid, resting, and activated. Microglia are capable of phagocytosis and play an important role in a wide spectrum of neuropathology. They have also been suggested to act in several other roles, including in secretion (e.g., of cytokines and neural growth factors), in immunological processing (e.g., antigen presentation), and in central nervous system development and remodeling have a phagocytic function as part of the reticuloendothelial system.

Pericytes are found in relation to capillaries but external to the endothelial cells and are enwrapped in the basal lamina. In electron micrographs they are not as electron dense as oligodendrocytes and lack the neurofilaments of the astrocyte and the tubules of the oligodendrocyte. The cytoplasm is denser than that of astrocytes and contains fat droplets and laminar dense bodies. The granular endoplasmic reticulum consists of long stringy cisterns. Microglia are considered multipotential cells because with the proper stimulus they can become macrophages (Vaughn and Peters, 1968). The pericyte contains actin, and this cell may well be important in controlling the channels entering the endothelial cells (Herman and Jacobson, 1988). During early development, monocytes enter the brain and, after formation of the blood–brain barrier, become trapped (Davis et al., 1994; Ling and Wong, 1993). The monocytes pass through an intermediate phase of development, the amoeboid microglia, which evolve into a down-regulated resting form, the ramified microglia. These resting microglia are found throughout the central nervous system and may well be the sentinels that alert the immune system to disease in the brain. With the appearance of any central nervous system disease (e.g., multiple sclerosis, stroke, trauma, or tumors), the resting microglia are up-regulated and become activated microglial cells. The factor or gene that up-regulates or down-regulates these cells is currently unknown.

Figure 3.23 Appearance of neurons, astrocytes (astro), and oligodendrocyte (oligo). Nissl stain, 300×.

Table 3.11 **MICROGLIAL CELLS**

CELL TYPE	FUNCTION
Monocytes	Enters brain during early development and is the stem cell of microglia
Pericyte	Found inside the brain in the (perivascular cell) basement membrane of the blood vessel; can act as a macrophage
Amoeboid Microglia	Transitional form leads to resting microglia
Resting Microglia	Down-regulated from amoeboid (ramified) microglia; probably the sentinels in the brain that raise the alarm for invasive diseases
Activated Microglia	Up regulated resting cell changes into partially activated macrophage with MHC class I and are phagocytic
Reactive Microglia	Fully activated macrophage with MHC class II and phagocytic properties. And may become Giant cells/Gitter Cells

Microglia are distributed ubiquitously throughout the brain and spinal cord, and one of their main functions is to monitor and sustain neuronal health. Microglial cells are quite sensitive to even minor disturbances in central nervous system homeostasis, and they become readily activated during most neuropathologic conditions, including peripheral nerve injury, trauma and stroke, inflammatory disease, and neurodegenerative diseases that produce neuronal injury or death. Activated microglia display changes in cell morphology, cell number, cell surface receptor expression, and production of growth factors and cytokines. The many changes occurring in activated cells reflect the altered functional states of microglia that are induced by signals arising from injured neurons. Neuronal-microglial signaling must play a fundamental role in understanding how the central nervous system responds to injury (Streit, 2010). Once the disease process has been resolved, the activated microglia can revert to resting microglial cells. The activated microglia cell is a partially activated macrophage containing the CR3 complex and class I major histocompatibility complex (MHC).

An Immunologically Privileged Site?

The central nervous system was once considered an immunologically privileged site because:

1. No specific lymph drainage from the central nervous system alerts the immune system of infection.
2. Neurons and glia do not express the major histocompatibility complex.
3. The major cell for stimulating the immune response (leukocyte dendritic cells) is not normally present in the disease-free nervous system.

However, studies have shown that there is a regular immune surveillance of the central nervous system, which is sufficient to control many viral infections (Sedgwick and Dorries, 1991). It is now known that immune cells regularly enter the brain through the capillaries and that macrophages infected with human immunodeficiency virus (HIV), for example, can infect the brain directly, the so-called Trojan-horse phenomenon (Haase, 1986; Orenstein, 2007; Price et al., 1988).

Giant Cells

Activated microglial cells can also evolve into giant multinucleated cells by the fusion of reactive cells (Fig. 3.25). They are seen in viral infections and are considered the hallmark of AIDS dementia. These cells form by fusion of reactive cells; multinucleated cells associated with viral brain infections and Creutzfeldt-Jakob disease; hallmark of AIDS dementia. reactive microglial cell, which is a fully active macrophage containing class II MHC and phagocytic activity. These cells are very active during all major disease states in the brain. They are also called Gitter cells (Fig 3.31A; Gitter cells are the eventual result of the microglial cell's phagocytosis of infectious material). In this disease with spongiform degeneration one finds the neurilemmal sheath still covered with synapses, although the neurons have degenerated. Eventually, after engulfing a certain amount of material, the phagocytic microglia becomes unable to phagocytize any further materials. The resulting cellular mass is known as a granular corpuscle, named for its "grainy" appearance, and scientists can see postinfection areas that have healed.

Prion Disease

Giant multinucleated cells are often found in patients with Creutzfeldt-Jakob disease, a transmissible spongiform degeneration caused by proteinaceous infectious particles, or prions (Fig. 3.16; Ridley and Baker, 2001).

Prion diseases or transmissible spongiform encephalopathy (TSEs) are a family of rare progressive

Figure 3.24 Dendrite with dendritic spine. The spines greatly increase the surface of many neurons. Note the many microtubules in the dendrites. The neck of the spine contains a spine apparatus. There are several excitatory synapses on the spine. 80,000×.

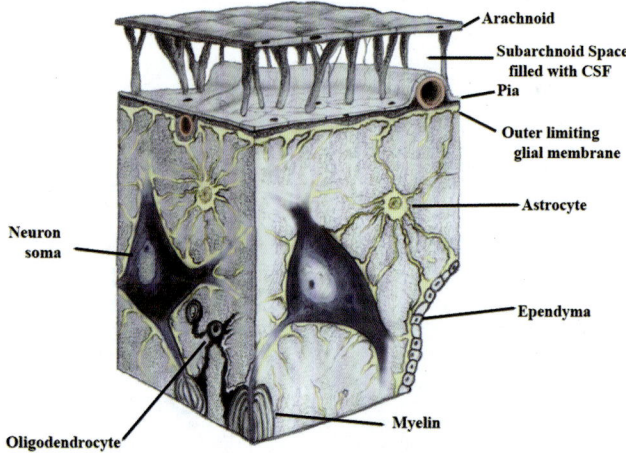

Figure 3.25 Three-dimensional reconstruction of the brain demonstrating the relationships between neurons, astrocytes, oligodendrocytes, and the covering of the pia and arachnoid of the meninges and the ependymal lining of the ventricle.

neurodegenerative disorders that affect both humans and animals. They are distinguished by long incubation periods, characteristic spongiform changes associated with neuronal loss, and a failure to induce inflammatory response. The causative agents of TSEs are believed to be prions. The term *prions* refers to abnormal, pathogenic agents that are transmissible and are able to induce abnormal folding of specific normal cellular proteins called prion proteins that are found most abundantly in the brain. The abnormal folding of the prion proteins leads to brain damage and the characteristic signs and symptoms of the disease. Prion diseases are usually rapidly progressive and always fatal. (CDC 2013)

In Figure 3.31 we have shown the appearance of Gitter cells in a patient with Creutzfeldt-Jakob disease and also the atrophic appearance of neurons with normal appearing synapses still attached to their surface (Fig. 3.36B).

EPENDYMAL CELLS

Ependymal cells line all parts of the ventricular system (lateral ventricles, third ventricle, cerebral aqueduct, fourth ventricle, and spinal canal) (Fig. 3.27). They are cuboidal, ciliated, and contain filaments and other organelles. The processes of these cells extend in the central nervous system and fuse with astrocytic processes to form the inner limiting glial membrane. Highly modified ependymal cells are found attached to the blood vessels in the roof of the body of the lateral ventricles, the inferior horn of the lateral ventricles, and the third and fourth

Figure 3.27 Ependymal lining cell in the third ventricle of a rat. Note prominent cilia extending into the ventricle (arrows) in this one-micron/μ plastic section.

ventricles. There they form the choroid plexus, which secretes much of the cerebrospinal fluid (Fig. 2.20). Ependymal cells originate from the germinal cells lining the embryonic ventricle, but they soon stop differentiating and stay at the lumen on the developing ventricles.

Supporting Cells in the Peripheral Nervous System

Satellite Cells

Satellite cells (Fig. 3.28), which are found only in the peripheral nervous system among sensory and sympathetic ganglia, originate from neural crest cells. Many satellite cells envelop a ganglion cell. Functionally, they are similar to the astrocytes, although they look more like oligodendrocytes.

Schwann Cells

Schwann cells are ectodermal in origin (neural crest) in the peripheral nervous system and function like oligodendrocytes, forming the myelin and neurilemmal sheath. In addition, the unmyelinated axons are embedded in their cytoplasm. Schwann cell cytoplasm stops before the nodes of Ranvier (Fig. 3.29), leaving spaces between the node and Schwann cells. In an injured nerve Schwann cells can form tubes that penetrate the scar and permit regeneration of the peripheral axons. Nerve growth factor is important to proliferation of the Schwann cells.

Figure 3.26 Electron micrograph of a section from the human cerebral cortex demonstrating differences in the densities of DNA in the nuclei of oligodendrocytes and microglia. 30,000×.

Figure 3.28 Cell bodies of dorsal root sensory ganglion of L1 from the a Rhesus monkeys demonstrating pseudo unipolar cells surrounded by their supportive satellite cells. 300×.

Figure 3.29 Longitudinal section of peripheral nerve fixed in osmium showing demonstrating the nodes of Ranvier (arrows, 1000×).

Figure 3.30 Ventral horn cells in the human lumbar spinal cord after injury to femoral nerve. (*A*) Normal ventral horn cell. (*B*) Chromatolytic neurons, showing a peripheral ring of Nissl substance (peripheral chromatolysis). (*C*) Chromatolytic neuron with eccentric nucleus and some dissolution of the cytoplasmic Nissl substance. Thionin/Nissl stain, 400×.

Neural Crest Cells

These cells originate embryologically as neuroectodermal cells on either side of the dorsal crest of the developing neural tube but soon drop dorsolaterally to the evolving spinal cord area (Fig. 4.2). Neural crest cells migrate out to form the following cell types in the nervous system and connective tissue: (1) Neurons formed from neural crest cells that migrated into the nervous system: dorsal root ganglion cells, cranial nerve ganglia, satellite cells, autonomic ganglion cells, Schwann cells of the peripheral nervous system, chromaffin cells of the adrenal medulla, calcitonin-secreting cells and carotid body type I cells, pigment cells of the integument, and pharyngeal arch cartilages; and (2) formation of tissues in the connective system by migration of neural crest cells: corneal endothelium and stroma, tooth papillae, dermis, smooth muscle, and adipose tissue of skin of head and neck, connective tissue of salivary, lacrimal, thymus, thyroid, and pituitary glands, connective tissue of salivary, lachrymal, thymus, thyroid, and pituitary glands, Connective tissue and smooth muscle of aortic arch origin.

RESPONSE OF NERVOUS SYSTEM TO INJURY

DEGENERATION

Neuronal death or atrophy may result from trauma, circulatory insufficiency (strokes), tumors, infections, metabolic insufficiency, developmental defects, and degenerative and heredodegenerative diseases.

1. Retrograde changes in the cell body (Fig. 3.30). Section of the axon or direct injury to the dendrites or cell body produces the following series of responses in the soma:

    a. Swelling of nucleus, nucleolus, and cytoplasm. The nucleus is displaced from the center of the cell body and may even lie adjacent to the plasma membrane of the neuron. The nucleus becomes eccentric as a direct response to injury of the axon or dendrite. Nissl substance appears to dissolve.

    b. Chromatolysis of RNA. The responses of neuronal soma to injury (chromatolysis) can be summarized in three steps.

    c. Dissolution of the Nissl substance (ribosomal RNA), called *chromatolysis* (Fig. 3.31), allows the protein-manufacturing processes to be mobilized to help the neuron survive the injury. Slow dissolution of Nissl substance starts centrally and proceeds peripherally, until only the most peripherally placed Nissl substance is left intact (which is probably essential to the protein metabolism to keep the surviving parts of the neuron alive and functional).

    d. *Proliferation* of metabolic processes in the nucleus, including mRNA, occurs. Endoplasmic reticulum and mitochondria starts manufacturing membranes and increasing the energy available in the cell. The organelles in the cell actually swell. The mRNA then begins the manufacturing of membrane that is transported down the intact tubules into the growing axonal ending (growth cone). All other organelles in the cell body and dendrites also respond to the injury. The mitochondria swell, and the smooth endoplasmic reticulum proliferates to help in the formation of new plasma membrane and new myelin. These responses represent the increased energy requirements of the nerve cell and the need to form plasma membrane during the regenerative process.

2. Recovery. If the cell survives the injury, all organelles return to normal: the nucleus returns to the center of the cell body, and the process in the nerve cell returns to its pretraumatic size. If the injury is too extensive, the neuron atrophies or dies. If seriously injured, the cell becomes atrophic or may be phagocytized.

3. Atrophic change. In atrophic change, the nerve cell is too severely damaged to repair itself. Consequently, the cell body shrinks and becomes smaller. This response is similar to the response of a nerve cell to insufficient blood supply, which produces an ischemic neuron. If necrosis occurs,

Figure 3.31 Electron micrograph of a biopsy from a 65-year-old male patient with Creutfeldt-Jakob disease. (*A*) Reactive astroglial in the cerebral cortex showing prominent digestion vacuoles, 35,000× and 8,800×. (*B*) Synapses still present on surface of atrophic neurons, in this case of spongiform neuronal degeneration, 35,000×.

the neuron cannot survive. The Nissl substance begins to disperse, and after 7 days the nucleus becomes dark and the cytoplasm eosinophilic. Within a few days, these cells are phagocytized.

4. Wallerian degeneration. When an axon is sectioned, the distal part that is separated from the trophic center (cell body) degenerates, a process called Wallerian, or anterograde, degeneration (Figs. 3.32 and 3.33). At the same time, the cell body undergoes a process called axonal, or retrograde, degeneration. If the cell body remains intact, the proximal portion begins to regenerate. The distal stump is usually viable for a few days, but its degeneration begins within 13 hours of injury. The axon starts to degenerate before the myelin sheath. In 4 to 7 days, the axon appears beaded and is beginning to be phagocytized by macrophages, which enter from the circulatory system. Fragments of degenerating axons and myelin are broken down in digestion chambers (Figs. 3.32 and 3.33), and it may take several months before all of the fragments are ingested. In the proximal portion, degenerative changes are noted back to the first unaffected node. As the myelin degenerates, it is broken up into smaller pieces that can be ingested more easily.

Figure 3.32 (*A*) Wallerian degeneration in the left medullary pyramid in the brain stem of a human several years after an infarct in the left motor-sensory strip; note the absence of myelin is on left side as this is above the decussation of the corticospinal tract. (*B*) High-powered view of the medullary pyramid; right side is normal. Weigert myelin stain, 90×.

Figure 3.33 (*A* and *B*) Electron micrograph of a degenerating axons in several fascicles of the medullary pyramid of a rat 15 days after a cortical lesion. (*A*) Arrow points to degreasing axons, 8000×. (*B*) Detail of degenerating axons, 30,000×. Note the collapsed axons and dense axoplasm and that many axons were unaffected by the cortical lesion.

REGENERATION

PERIPHERAL NERVE REGENERATION

Within a few days after section, the proximal part (attached to a functional neuronal soma) of the nerve starts regrowing. Nerve growth factor is produced after injury to the axon, and it promotes the axonal sprouting. If the wound is clean, for example, a stab sound, sewing the nerve ends together can dramatically increase the rate of recovery in the affected limb. The regenerating nerves may cross the scar within several weeks. The crossing is helped by the Schwann cells and fibroblasts, which proliferate from the proximal end of the nerve. The Schwann cells form new basement membrane and provide tubes through which the regenerating axons can grow (Fig. 3.34).

In certain peripheral nervous system diseases only segmental degeneration occurs. One example is diphtheria: the myelin sheath degenerates but the axon remains intact. Phagocytes break down the myelin, and Schwann cells rapidly reform myelin. The rate of movement of the slow component of axoplasmic flow probably accounts for the rate of axonal regrowth, which is limited to about 1 mm a day. Slow components of the axoplasmic flow (-Scb) carry actin, fodrin, calmodulin, clathrin, and glycolytic enzymes that form the network of microtubules, intermediate filaments, and the axolemma, which limit the rate of daily axonal regeneration, although functional recovery may be a little faster (Kandel,

Figure 3.34 Sciatic nerve of a rat, demonstrating the appearance of regenerating nerves 3 weeks after a crushing injury. (*A*) At the site of the crushing lesion, the nerves look normal with regenerating axons grown past the site of the injury; arrow indicates Schwann cell nucleus. (*B*) About 30 mm distal to the site of injury, note some regenerating axons and still many degenerating axon fragments. (*C*) About 35 mm distal to the crush site the transition from regenerating axons to only degenerating axons.

Schwartz, and Jesssel, 2000, 2009; McQuarrie and Grafstein, 1983; Wujek and Lasek, 1983).

As the regenerating regenerates, many axonal sprouts are seen on the axons attached to their cell bodies. If one axonal sprout penetrates the scar, the other sprouts degenerate, and the axon follows the path established by the penetrating sprout. If an axon reaches one of the tubes formed by the Schwann cells, it grows quickly and after crossing the scar descends the distal stump at a rate of approximately 1 mm/day (Guth and Jacobson, 1966; Jacobson and Guth, 1965). When the motor end plate is reached, a delay occurs while the axon reinnervates the muscle and reestablishes function. At this stage the average rate of functional regeneration is 1 to 3 mm a day.

Only a small percentage of the nerves actually reach the effectors or receptors. The basal lamina helps direct the regenerating nerve to the motor end plate. If a sensory fiber innervates a motor end plate, it remains nonfunctional and probably degenerates, and the cell body atrophies. A sensory fiber that reaches a sensory receptor may become functional, even if the receptor is the wrong one. For example, after nerve regeneration some patients complain that rubbing or pressing the skin produces pain. In these cases it would appear that fibers sensitive to pain have reached a tactile or pressure-sensitive receptor.

Motor fiber may also enervate the wrong motor end plate, as when a flexor axon innervates an extensor. In such a case, the patient has to relearn how to use the muscle. Muscle that is denervated assists the regenerating axons by expressing molecules that influence the regenerating axons. Some of the molecules are concentrated in the synaptic basal lamina of the muscle. Other molecules are up-regulated following denervation and help in attracting and reestablishing the synapse in the muscle. These up-regulated molecules include growth factors (IGF-3 and FGF-5), acetylcholinesterase (AChE), agrin, laminin, s-laminin, fibronectin, collagen, and the adhesion molecules N-CAM and N-cadherin (Hall and Patterson, 1993; Horner and Gage, 2000). Successful nerve regeneration also depends on an adequate blood supply. For example, in a large wound caused by a gun shot, nerves attempt to regenerate but may not succeed due to interruption of the blood supply.

The following is a summary of the sequence of regeneration in the peripheral nervous system:

1. Peripheral nerve interrupted.

2. The axon dies back to the first unaffected node of Ranvier, with the myelin and distal axon beginning to degenerate within 34 hours.

3. At the site of injury, the axon and myelin degenerate to form a scar.

    Phagocytosis begins within 48 hours.

4. Axons separated from the cell body degenerate. With an adequate blood supply the portion of the axon still connected to the intact cell body begins regenerating by sprouting.

5. Within 72 hours, Schwann cells begin to proliferate and form basement membranes and hollow tubes. Nerve growth factor is also formed and released, which stimulates sprouting.

6. From each of the severed axons, sprouts attempt to penetrate the scar. After one sprout successfully grows through the scar, the other sprouts die. There is a month or more delay for the axon to grow through the scar.

7. Once an axon penetrates the scar, it grows at 1 mm/day; about a third of the severed axons actually reinnervates muscle and skin.

REGENERATION IN THE CENTRAL NERVOUS SYSTEM

After an injury, axons in the central nervous system regenerate, but there seems to be no equivalent to the Schwann cell because oligodendrocytes and astrocytes do not form tubes to penetrate the scar. Instead, they form a scar that is nearly impenetrable. Even if the axons penetrate the scar, they have no means of reaching the neuron to which they were originally connected. Gage (2002) have reviewed the question of how to regenerate the damaged central nervous system in the brain that is inherently very plastic. They have noted that it is not the failure of neuronal regeneration, but it is rather a feature of the damaged environment; and it is now possible to reintroduce the factors present in the developing nervous system that produced this wonderful organ. The gene responsible for needed growth factors is probably missing or inactivated in adult tissue. Recently a brain-derived neurotropic factor has been identified, which may eventually help in finding a way to guide the axon (Goodman, 2000). Also the identification of a potent inhibitor of neurite outgrowth associated with myelin, NoGo, has focused efforts to develop agents to counteract its effects (Schwab, 2000). Animal studies have shown that neurons have considerable plasticity. That is, if some axons in a region die off, bordering unaffected axons will sprout and form new synapses over many months, filling in where the synapses were and resulting in major functional reorganization. This reorganization may eventually produce some recovery of function.

The introduction of scaffolding to assist neuronal regeneration holds great promise of successful nerve regeneration.

STEM CELLS: A SOURCE OF REPLACEMENT FOR DAMAGED NEURONS?

Neuronal stem cells have been identified in the adult brain and spinal cord. These cells under the right conditions may well be activated and help to reverse the effects of lesions in the central nervous system (Kornack and Rackic, 1999). After the implantation of immature neurons (neuroblasts) in regions affected by certain diseases (e.g., the corpus striatum of patients with Parkinson's disease), there has been some recovery (Gage et al., 1991; Sladek and Gash, 1984). In Parkinsonian patients the age of the individual receiving the transported cells seems to affect the outcome, with younger patients (less than 50 years of age) more likely to show some improvement.

NERVE GROWTH FACTORS

The first nerve growth factor (NGF) was isolated by Levi-Montalcini and Angeletti in 1968, and it is a molecule that promotes the survival and differentiation of sensory and sympathetic neurons. Recent findings point to a diversity of NGF actions and indicate that its production begins in development, extends throughout adult life and aging, and involves a variety of neurons, glia, and nonneural cells. In addition, there is a growing body of evidence that suggests that endogenous NGF signaling subserves neuroprotective and repair functions. The analysis points to many interesting unanswered questions and to the potential for continuing research on NGF to substantially enhance our understanding of the mechanisms and treatment of neurological disorders (Sofroniew, Howe, and Mobley, 2005).

REPAIR OF INJURED CENTRAL NERVOUS SYSTEM

Scaffolds

There is of course great interest in repairing the damaged central nervous system. The injured central nervous system and the resultant scar produce many molecules that inhibit successful nerve regeneration. Many attempts have been made in animal models to produce a pathway to help in nerve regeneration. These approaches have included insertion of Teflon tubes at the site of the injury; and Schwann cells, Nano fibers, and silk through the scarred portion of the spinal cord in the hope that the nerves would follow these channels. Recently scaffolds using silk or Nano fibers have been inserted to bridge the gap (Ma and Elisseeff, 2010). However, even though nerves do grow down these channels, no functional recovery occurs.

Factors to Help Regeneration

Since the pioneering work of Levi-Montalcini and Angeletti in 1968, many factors that promote neuronal survival and axon outgrowth (e.g., brain-derived neurotropic factor [BDNF], any of a group of neuropeptides as nerve growth factors that regulate the growth, differentiation, and survival of certain neurons in the peripheral and central nervous systems) have been identified and the focus is now on using these factors to stimulate growth into the injured areas and then to grow through into the uninjured area. There are many factors to test, but several seem especially promising, including the neurotropic factor (netrins 1 and 3) that produces axonal growth (Serifini et al., 1994) and also studies of programmed cell death beginning to identify genes that may be responsible for premature neuron death (Oppenheim, 2001). In addition, brain-derived ciliary neurotropic factor (CNF) that promotes the survival of various neuronal cell types may play an important role in the injury response in the nervous system. Ciliary neurotropic factor (CNTF) is a potent neuroprotective cytokine in different animal models of glutamate-induced excitotoxicity, although its action mechanisms are still poorly characterized. It also has a potential use for the clinical treatment of progressive neurodegenerative diseases involving glutamate overflow (Beurrier et al., 2009). These results suggest that we are now entering an era of brain research that offers great promise to help patients with neurodegenerative diseases, such as Huntington's, Parkinson's, and Alzheimer's.

GLIAL RESPONSE TO INJURY

Neuronal death triggers an influx of phagocytic cells from the blood stream, and the microglia proliferate and break down the dying neurons.

Necrosis

In organs with numerous fibroblasts, necrotic areas are soon filled with proliferating fibroblasts, but in the central nervous system there are few fibroblasts, and the astrocytes do not proliferate in sufficient numbers. Within a few days of an ischemic attack with infarction, neutrophils are seen at the site of injury. Shortly thereafter, microglial cells and histocytes are seen in the region of the dying cells. Microglia are distributed ubiquitously throughout the brain and spinal cord, and one of their main functions is to monitor and sustain neuronal health. Microglial cells are quite sensitive to even minor disturbances in central nervous system homeostasis, and they become readily activated during most neuropathologic conditions, including peripheral nerve injury, trauma and stroke, inflammatory disease, and neurotoxicant-induced neuronal injury. During activation, microglia display conspicuous functional plasticity, which involves changes in cell morphology, cell number, cell surface receptor expression, and production of growth factors and cytokines. The many changes occurring in activated cells reflect the altered functional states of microglia that are induced by signals arising from injured neurons. Thus, neuronal-microglial signaling plays a fundamental role in understanding how the central nervous system responds to injury. Reactive microgliosis should be viewed as a cellular effort to initiate ameliorative and reparative measures in the injured brain (Streit, 2000).

Since the blood–brain barrier is usually compromised, monocytes may now migrate into the parenchyma of the central nervous system in greater numbers and assist in phagocytosis. The time it takes for the complete removal of injured cells depends on the size of the lesion. Large infarcts may take several years before phagocytosis is complete. If the lesion is huge, such as a large infarct in the precentral gyrus, a cavity lined by astrocytic scar will form. In small lesions the neurons are phagocytized glia that proliferate, a process called replacement gliosis.

BLOOD–BRAIN BARRIER

Endothelial cells form a barrier in the central nervous system (Fig. 3.35). The endothelial cells line the capillaries and the choroids plexus are joined together by tight junctions, zonula occludens. The capillaries are not perforated, and the endothelial cells show very little pinocytosis or receptor-mediated

Figure 3.35 Schematic representation of a brain microvasculature. The blood–brain barrier is created by the tight apposition of contiguous endothelial cells. Note the endothelial cells lining blood vessels are in close contact with a variety of accessory cells such as astrocytes and pericytes which modulate the expression of blood–brain barrier characteristics. Tight junctions between contiguous endothelial cells prevent the passage of large molecules and pathogens between the blood and the brain. Tight junctions consist of rows of transmembrane proteins (major types are claudins, occludins, and junctional adhesion molecules) anchored in the membranes of two adjacent endothelial cells while the intracellular portion is anchored to cytoskeletal proteins (e.g., actin) through scaffold protein such as ZO-1. (From Cucullo, 2012, Luca Book: Mammalian Brain Development.)

endocytosis (Brightman, 1988; Pardridge, 2006). This endothelial lining is called the blood–brain barrier because it is very selective to certain large molecules and dyes and limits the entry of other substances, including amino acids, water, glucose, and electrolytes into the brain parenchyma. Making compounds lipid soluble has been on method to deliver drugs into the brain. The blood–brain barrier begins to develop in utero as the brain develops and is fully present before birth. It also may become leaky as the cerebral vasculature undergoes changes due to pathological processes, including hypertension.

In the peripheral nervous system the endothelial cells are fenestrated and very active in *pinocytosis*. *Fluid phase endocytosis in the peripheral nervous system* is relatively nonspecific; the endothelial cells engulf molecules and then internalize them by vesicular endocytosis. In *receptor-mediated endocytosis*, which is found in the central nervous system, a ligand first binds to a membrane receptor on one side of the cell. After binding to the ligand the complex is internalized into a vesicle and transported across the cell, and the ligand is usually released.

Neuwelt (2011) has developed a successful method to open the blood–brain barrier using mannitol for a short amount of time up to 2 hours and then delivering a chemotherapeutic agent directly to the area with a tumor. A catheter is threaded from the femoral artery up into the carotid on the side with the tumor and then delivers the chemotherapeutic agent methotrexate directly in to the region containing the tumor. He has successfully treated several patients with this method. Current studies are now under way using a microcatheter and magnetic resonance imaging (MRI) to improve the delivery and actually place the agent directly into the tumor site (Boockvar et al., 2012).

All vascular branches within the central nervous system are surrounded by a thin covering formed by astrocytic processes (Fig. 3.21). However, the astrocytic processes do not fuse with the endothelial lining of the blood vessel or with the processes of other cells, so they have minimal effect on limiting the entry of solutes into the brain parenchyma. Thus, the extracellular space can be entered once the materials pass through the endothelium.

The intravenous perfusion of various dye compounds (trypan blue, Evans blue, proflavin HCI, and horseradish peroxidase) demonstrate that the blood–brain barrier is leaky in certain midline regions of the third and fourth ventricle, the *circumventricular* organs (pituitary, median eminence, organum vasculosum, subfornical organ, subcommissural organ, pineal gland, and the area postrema), and in the choroid plexus and locus ceruleus (Brightman, 1989) of the fourth ventricle. These open connections between the brain and the ventricular system permit neuropeptides from the hypothalamus, midbrain, and pituitary to enter the cerebrospinal fluid and to be widely distributed in the brain and spinal cord, thus forming an alternate pathway in the neuroendocrine system. Studies have shown that the blood–brain barrier is impermeable to certain large molecules, including proteins, but substances such as small lipid-soluble compounds, including alcohol and anesthetics, gasses, water, glucose, electrolytes (NA+, K+, and CL-), and amino acids, can pass from the plasma into the intracellular space (inside neurons and glia) or into the extracellular space between neurons and glia. Acute lesions of the central nervous system, including those caused by infections, usually increase the permeability of the barrier and alter the concentrations of water, electrolytes, and protein. In viral diseases the infected leukocytes (macrophages) more easily penetrate into the brain by passing between the normally tight junctions in the endothelial cells, which is one way that HIV enters the brain directly from the blood. Tumors within the central nervous system produce growth factors that cause blood vessels to sprout. These new blood vessels have immature tight junctions that are also quite leaky. There have been many attempts with limited success to deliver chemotherapeutic agents specifically to the tumor. There have also been attempts to interfere with the formation of the blood vessel growth factors as a way to starve tumors.

Stress has been shown to open the blood–brain barrier by activating the hypothalamic-hypophyseal-adrenal axis and releasing corticotropin-releasing hormone (CRH; Esposito et al., 2001). Acute lesions of the central nervous system, including those caused by infections, usually increase the permeability of the barrier and alter the concentrations of water, electrolytes, and protein. In some viral diseases, for example, infected leukocytes (macrophages) more easily penetrate directly into the

Figure 3.36 Secretion of cerebrospinal fluid (CSF) the chorioid plexus in the fourth ventricle. Note the blood vessel (BV) in the center and the cuboidal epithelial cells that form the CSF on the outside of the vessel (300×).

brain by passing between the normally tight junctions in the endothelial cells. This is one way HIV enters the brain from the blood. Also, central nervous system tumors produce growth factors that cause blood vessels to sprout. These new capillaries have immature tight junctions that are also quite leaky and have been studied with some success as a way to deliver chemotherapeutic agents specifically to the tumor.

EXTRACELLULAR SPACE

Between the cells in the central nervous system is the extracellular space, measuring between 30 and 40 nm and filled with cerebrospinal fluid (CSF) and other solutes. The CSF is formed primarily by the chorioid plexus in the lateral ventricle, third ventricle, and fourth ventricle (Fig. 3.36). The amount of extracellular space in the brain is still a matter of controversy. Chemicals (gliotransmitters; see Table 3.7) can readily pass from the glia cells into the extracellular space and affect the neurons. Solutes from the blood plasma also readily enter through the endothelial lining into the extracellular space, and the solutes present in this space (whether deleterious or not) affect the functions of the central nervous system. A small portion of the CSF appears to be formed by the diffusion of extracellular fluid. CSF may also be reabsorbed after temporary storage in the extracellular space. Fat-soluble compounds that readily pass through the blood–brain barrier can enter the extracellular space and may be useful in resolving infections in the central nervous system or in improving the function of certain brain cells.

BIBLIOGRAPHY

Barr, M., and Bertram, R. 1949. A morphological distinction between neurons of the male and female, and the behavior of the nucleolar satellite during accelerated nucleoprotein synthesis. Nature 163: 676–678.

Bentivoglio, M. H., Kuypers, G. J. M., Catsman-Berrevoets, C. E., Loewe, H., and Dann, O. 1980. Two new fluorescent retrograde neuronal tracers which are transported over long distances. Neurosci. Lett. 18:25–30.

Bodian, D. 1970. An electron microscopic characterization of classes of synaptic vesicles by means of controlled aldehyde fixation. J. Cell Biol. 44:115.

Brightman, J. 1989. The anatomic basis of the blood-brain barrier. In E. A. Neuwelt (Ed.) Implications of the Blood- Brain Barrier and Its Manipulation. Vol. 1, p 125. New York, NY: Plenum.

Brady, S. T. 1985. A novel brain ATPase with properties expected for the fast axonal transport motor. Nature (London) 317:73–75.

Colonnier, M. 1969. Synaptic patterns on different cell types in the different laminae of the cat visual cortex. An electron microscopic study. Brain Res. 33:268–281.

Cowan, W. M., Gottlieb, D. I., Hendrickson, A. E., Price, J. L., and Woolsey, T. A. 1972. The autoradiographic demonstration of axonal connections in the central nervous system. Brain Res. 37:21–51.

Darnell, J., Lodish, H., and Baltimore, D. 1990. Molecular Cell Biology. 2nd ed. New York, NY: Scientific American Books.

Davis, E. J., Foster, T. D., and Thomas, W. E. 1994. Cellular forms and functions of brain microglia. Brain Res. Bull. 34:73–78.

De Duve, C., and Wattiaux, R. 1966. Functions of lysosomes. Ann. Rev. Physiol. 28:435.

Finger, S. 1994. Origins of Nueroscience: A History of Exploration into Brain Function. New York, NY: Oxford University Press.

Gage, F. H. 2002. Neurogenesis in the adult brain. J. Neurosci. 22:612–613.

Goodman, C. S. 1994. The likeness of being; phylogenetically conserved molecular mechanisms of growth cone guidance. Cell 78:353–356.

Graftstein, B., and Forman, D. S. 1980. Intracellular transport in neurons. Physiol. Rev. 60:1167–1183.

Gray, E. G. 1959. Axosomatic and axodendritic synapses of the cerebral cortex; an electron microscopic study. J. Anat. 93:420.

Guth, L., and Jacobson, S. 1966. The rate of regeneration of the cat vagus nerve. Exp. Neurol. 14:439.

Haase, A. 1986. Pathogenesis of lentivirus infections. Nature 2:130–136.

Hall, Z. W., and Sanes, J. R. 1993. Synaptic structure and development: the neuromuscular junction. Cell 72: 99–121.

Heimer, L. 1970. Bridging the gap between light and electron microscopy in the experimental tracing of fiber connections. In W. J. H. Nauta and S. O. E. Ebbesson (Eds.) Contemporary Research Methods in Neuroanatomy, Ann N Y Acad. Sci. 167:129–146. Springer Verlag.

Heimer, L., and Robards, M. J. 1981. Neuroanatomic Tract-Tracing Methods. New York, NY: Plenum.

Herman, I., and Jacobson, S. 1988. In situ analysis of microvascular periocytes in hypertensive rate brain. Tissue Cell 20:1–12.

Horner, P. J., and Gage, F. H. 2000. Regenerating the damaged central nervous system. Nature 407:963–970.

Hutton, M. 2000. Molecular genetics of chromosome 17 tauopathies. Ann. NY Acad. Sci. 920:63–70.

Jacobson, S., and Guth, L. 1965. An electrophysiological study of the early stages of peripheral nerve regeneration. Exp. Neurol. 11:48.

Johanson, D., and Maitland, E. 1981. Lucy, the Beginnings of Humankind. St Albans, UK: Granada.

Kernakc, D. R., and Rakic, P. 1976. Continuations of neurogenesis in the hippocampus of the adult macaque monkey. Proc. Natl. Acad. Sci. USA 96:5768–5773.

Lasek, R. J., and Joseph, B. S. 1967. Radioautography as a neuroanatomic tracing method. Anat. Rec. 157:275–276.

LaVail, J. H., and LaVail, M. M. 1972. Retrograde axonal transport in the central nervous system. Science 176:1416–1417.

Lechan, R., Nester, J., and Jacobson, S. 1981. Immunohistochemical localization of retrogradely and anterogradely transported wheat agglutinins (WGA) within the central nervous system of the rat: application to immunostaining of a second antigen within the same neuron. J. Histochem. Cytochem. 29:1255–1262.

Levi-Montalcini, R., and Angeletti, P. U. 1968. Biological aspects of the nerve growth factor. In E. E. Woolstenholme and M. O. Connor (Eds.) Growth of the Nervous System, pp. 534–565. Boston, MA: Little, Brown.

Ling, E. A., and Wong, W. 1993. The origin and nature of ramified and amoeboid microglia: a historical review and current concepts. Glia 7:9–18.

Lovgren, S. 2006. Lucy' fossil tour sparks controversy among U.S. museums. National Geographic News, November 1:55–67.

Johanson, D. C., and Wong, K. Lucy's Legacy. Crown Publishing, 2009. Washington, DC.

McQuarrie, I. G. 1988. Cytoskeleton of the regenerating nerve. In P. J. Reier, R. D. Bunge, and F. J. Seil (Eds.) Current Issues in Neural Regeneration Research, pp 23–32. New York, NY: A. R. Leiss.

Nauta, W. J. H. 1957. Silver impregnation of degeneration axons. In W. F. Windle (Ed.) New Research Techniques of Neuroanatomy, pp. 17–26. Springfield, IL: Charles C Thomas.

Neurocytology 1992. Greenfield's Neuropathology. Oxford Press.

Neuwelt, E. A., and Dahlborg, S. A. 1989. Blood-brain barrier disruption in the treatment of brain tumors: clinical implications. In E. A. Neuwelt (Ed.) Implications of the Blood-Brain Barrier and Its Manipulation. Vol. 2, pp 195–262. Springer, New York.

Newault, E., et al. 2011. Engaging neuroscience to advance transitional research in brain barrier biology. Nature Rev. Neurosci. 12:169–182.

Oppenheim, R. W. 1991. Cell death during development of the nervous system. Ann. Rev. Neurosci. 14:453–501.

Palay, S. L. 1967. Principles of cellular organization in the nervous system. In G. C. Quarton, T. Melnechuk, and F. O. Schmitt (Eds.) The Neurosciences: A Study Program. New York, NY: Rockefeller University Press.

Price, S. D., Brew, R. B., Sidtis, J., Rosenblum, M., Scheck, A., and Cleary, P. 1988. The brain in AIDS: central nervous system HIV-1 infection and AIDS dementia complex. Science 231:586–592.

Ramón y Cajal, S. 1928. Degeneration and Regeneration of the Nervous System. London, UK: Oxford University Press.

Ramón y Cajal, S. 1909. Histologie du Système Nerveux de l'Homme et des Vertèbres. Paris, France: J. A. Maloine.

Rassmussen, G. T. 1957. Selective silver impregnation of synaptic endings. In W. F. Windle (Ed.) *New Research Techniques of Neuroanatomy*. Springfield, IL: Charles C. Thomas.

Ribatti, D., Nico, B., Crivellato, E., and Artico, M. 2006. Development of the BBB: a historical point of view. Anatomical Record 289:3–8.

Reese, T. S., and Karnovsky, M. J. 1968. Fine structural localization of the blood-brain barrier to exogenous peroxidase. J. Cell Biol. 34:207.

Rio-Hortega, P del. 1919. El atercer elemento de los centros nerviosos. Boletín de la Sociedad Española del Biologica 9:69–120.

Scharrer, E. 1966. *Endocrines and the Central Nervous System*. Baltimore. MD: Williams & Wilkins.

Schwartz, J. 1980. The transport of substances in nerve cells. Sci. Am. 242:152–171.

Sedgwick, J. D., and Dorries, R. 1991. The immune system response to viral infection. Neurosciences 3:93–100.

Serafini, T., Kennedy, T. E., Galko, M. J., Mizrayan, C., Jessel, T. M., and Tessler-Lavigne, M. 1994. The netrins define a family of axon outgrowth-promoting proteins homologous to C. elegans UNC-6. Cell 78:409–424.

Sladek, J. R., Jr., and Gash, D. M. 1984. Neural Transplants: Development and Function. New York, NY: Plenum Press.

Swank, R. L., and Davenport, H. A. 1935. Chlorate-osmic formalin method for staining degenerating myelin stain. Stain. Tech. 10:87.

Vale, R. D. 1987. Intracellular transport using microtubule based molecules. Ann. Rev. Cell Biol. 3:347–378.

Vale, R. D., Reese, T. S., and Sheetz, M. P. 1985. Identification of a novel force-generating protein, kinesin, involved in microtubule based motility. Cell 42:39–50.

Vaughn, J. E., and Peters, A. E. 1968. A third neuroglial cell type. J. Comp. Neurol. 133:269–288.

Weiss, P. A., and Hiscoe, M. B. 1948. Experiments on the mechanism of nerve growth. J. Exp. Zool. 197:315–396.

Wislocki, G. B., and Leduc, E. H. 1952. Vital staining of the hematoencephalic barrier by silver nitrate and trypan blue and cytological comparisons of neurohypophysis, pineal body, area postrema, intercolumnar tubercle and supraoptic crest. J. Comp. Neurol. 96:371.

Wujek, J. R., and Lasek, R. K. 1983. Correlation of axonal regeneration and slow component B in two branches of a single axon. J. Neurosci. 3:243–251.

Young, J. Z. 1942. Functional repair of nervous tissue. Physiol. Rev. 22:318.

4.
NEUROEMBRYOLOGY AND CONGENITAL MALFORMATIONS

The brain undergoes a series of incredible changes in utero as it changes from a flat plate into a tube and then evolves into the convoluted cerebral hemisphere. This complex evolution results in several structures that start very close together (particularly the fornix, stria terminalis, corpus callosum, and anterior commissure) and move quite a distance apart.

The in utero development of the central nervous system can be divided into three periods that roughly correspond to the first, the second, and the third trimester of gestation (Table 4.1).

Newborns, through genetic inheritance, can make about 40 different sounds, and they can distinguish some sounds as being either safe or dangerous. They can also perceive certain shapes and usually have enough myelin for an organized grasp and suckling reflex.

FORMATION OF THE CENTRAL NERVOUS SYSTEM

The first evidence of the differentiation of the nervous system appears at the end of the second week of gestation. At that time a "heaping up" of ectodermal cells can be noted at the caudal end of the embryonic disk. This accumulation of cells is known as the primitive streak (Fig. 4.1A). As development continues, surface ectodermal cells involute through the primitive streak and migrate laterally, forming the intraembryonic mesoderm, interposed between the surface ectoderm and subjacent endoderm. As the intraembryonic mesoderm forms, another thickening of ectodermal cells called Hensen's node occurs at the cephalic end of the primitive streak (Fig. 4.1A). Cells migrate inward through this zone and extend between the surface ectoderm and subjacent endoderm, forming the notochord plate. The notochord is the primary "inductor" for the thickening of the ectoderm overlying and on either side of the notochord to form the neural plate, which is the origin of the central nervous system. The many factors in the notochord that underlie the formation of the neural tube and the transformation of embryonic cells into adult cells are currently being identified. The notochord ultimately degenerates as the body of the vertebrae appears and it persists as the nucleus pulposi of the intervertebral disk.

On either side of the neural plate is a thin strip of ectoderm known as the neural crest. As development proceeds, the neural plate sinks inward to form the neural groove (Figs. 4.1B and 4.2). At the beginning of the fourth week this midline groove continues to deepen until the dorsal lips of the groove meet and fuse, forming the neural tube, neurulation (Figs. 4.1C and 4.2). The adjacent neural crest separates from the overlying ectoderm and comes to lie lateral to the neural tube (Fig. 4.2). The central nervous system is derived from the neural tube; the neural crest yields many parts of the peripheral nervous system. The remaining ectoderm becomes the epidermis of the embryo (somatic ectoderm).

Before the formation of the neural tube the paraxial mesoderm begins to form the somites. Fusion of the dorsal margins of the neural groove, forming the neural tube, begins on about the twenty-second day in the region of somites 4 to 6 (Fig. 4.1C). Fusion continues in both cranial and caudal directions, and by the twenty-fifth day, only the cranial and caudal ends of the neural tube remain open (called the anterior and posterior neuropores, respectively). The lumen in the neural tube will become the ventricular system of the central nervous system.

After delineation of the neural and somatic ectoderm, the neural crest cells appear as an almost continuous column of cells along the dorsal surface, or crest, of the neural tube from the mesencephalic level through all spinal cord levels (Fig. 4.2). The neural crest cells are the primordium of the sensory ganglia, the cranial nerves and the spinal ganglia, the neurilemmal cells, satellite cells, the autonomic ganglia, and probably the pia-arachnoid membrane. Shortly after the closure of the neural tube, processes from the neural crest cells enter the spinal cord or brain stem and form the sensory roots of the spinal and cranial nerves.

Table 4.1 **IN UTERO BRAIN DEVELOPMENT**

First trimester	Establishment of basic organization of the central nervous system beginning as the neural plate, which sinks inward to form the neural groove. The neural groove continues to deepen until the dorsal lips meet and fuse, forming the neural tube, the beginning of the hollow dorsally placed central nervous system.
Second trimester	Tubular-like nervous system is changed by the massive waves of migration of neuroblasts from the germinal cell lining, producing an immature model of the adult nervous system with the beginnings of much of the circuitry in place.
Third trimester	Neuronal processes mature, and the gyri enlarge, myelination begins, and the basic circuitry continues to form, preparing the infant for functioning outside the womb.

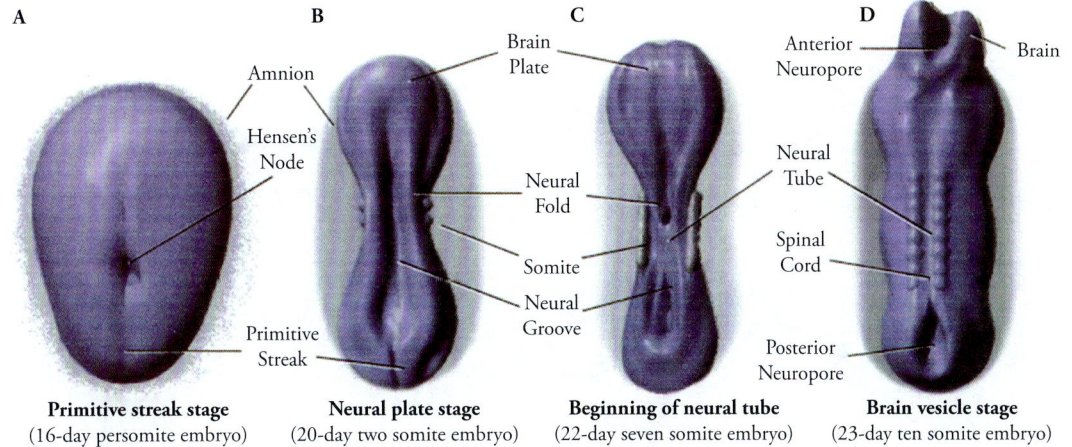

Figure 4.1 Dorsal view of human embryo. (*A*) Primitive streak stage (16-day presomite embryo). (*B*) Neural plate stage (20-day two-somite embryo). (*C*) Beginning of neural tubes (22-day seven-somite embryo). (*D*) Brain vesicles stage (23-day ten-somite embryo).

HISTOGENESIS

The walls of the neural tube throughout the nervous system consist of germinal epithelial cells that form a pseudo-stratified epithelium. After closure of the neural tube, another cell type is found external to the germinal cell layer. This new cell is the neuroblast (or immature neuron); these cells originate from the mitotic divisions of the germinal cell and form a new layer, the mantle or intermediate layer, and external to the mantle layer is a cell-free zone, the marginal layer. Subjacent to the germinal layer the subventricular region develops.

The glia are instrumental in the final formation of the central nervous system. They migrate out from the subventricular layer prior to the neuroblasts and form processes that reach the submeningeal surface and remain connected to the ventricular surface. The neurons migrate out into the region formed by the glia.

Initially the neuroblasts are connected to the lumen by an elongate process, a transient dendrite. As they migrate into the subjacent mantle layer, they lose this process and become apolar neuroblasts. Shortly thereafter two new processes appear; one becomes the axon, the other the dendrite. The axonal process elongates and more dendritic branches appear, forming a multipolar neuroblast.

Some neurons form only a single process; for example, these are the sensory ganglion of the spinal cord and cranial nerves, and the mesencephalic nucleus of cranial nerve V. Some neurons remain bipolar, for example, the olfactory receptor cells, rods, and cones of the retina, the bipolar cells in the retina, and the receptor cells in the vestibular and cochlear ganglion.

It should be noted that the germinal cells also form the supporting cells in the central system (Fig 4.3). Throughout the central nervous system neurons migrate into the intermediate (mantle) zone to become the definitive structures of the spinal cord, much of the brain stem, and the basal nuclei. He using tritiated thymidine identified this migration. In these regions the cells in the mantle layer become the gray matter, while their axons form the marginal zone or white matter. By contrast, the cerebral cortex and cerebellar cortex are formed by the migration of neuroblasts through the mantle zone into the marginal zone.

REPAIR OF DAMAGED NERVOUS SYSTEM

Since immature cells from fetuses are not as easily rejected, it has been proposed to recover neuroblasts from the brains

Figure 4.2 Coronal section showing differentiation of neural ectoderm in the neural plate stage, the neural groove stage, the neural fold stage, and the neural tube stage.

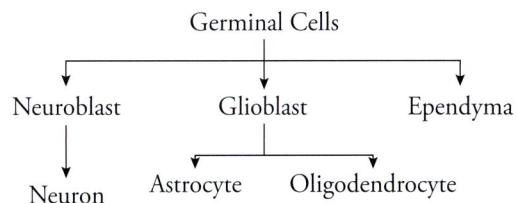

Figure 4.3 Evolution of germinal cells.

of aborted human fetuses. These fetal stem cells from human embryos would be implanted in adults replacing damaged neurons in patients with Huntington's chorea and Parkinson's disease. This line of transplant research holds great promise not only for the nervous system but also for pancreas, adrenal, and pituitary.

The implantation of fetal stem cells seems especially promising, but there is much public controversy over the use of fetal or aborted material. Recently adult stem cells have been harvested from surgical specimens and at postmortem examinations; this approach also shows much promise.

PRINCIPLES OF DIFFERENTIATION WITHIN THE CENTRAL NERVOUS SYSTEM

The following are certain rules that can be applied to the differentiation within the central nervous system (after M. Jacobson, 1978):

1. Spatial and temporal gradients of proliferation exist in the neuroepithelial germinal zone.

2. Neighboring regions have separate origins and are different cytoarchitectonically.

3. In an orderly sequence large neurons are produced first, then intermediate-sized neurons, and finally small neurons.

4. Glial cells tend to originate before neurons in any particular region of the brain.

5. Phylogenetically older parts of the brain are predisposed to arise earlier in ontogenesis.

GROWTH CONE GUIDANCE

Ramon y Cajal at the turn of the last century identified the growth cones that form connections in the developing nervous system. Since that time neurobiologists have been searching for the mechanisms that permit the formation of these synapses. Several mechanisms have been proposed, including cell adhesion, repulsion, and chemoattraction. Recently a diffusible factor that promotes outgrowth of axons in vitro has been found in the floor plate of the embryonic spinal cord (Serfanin et al., 1994). Two membrane-associated proteins were purified from the embryonic chick brain, netrin-1 and netrin-2, and each protein promotes growth cone outgrowth. Cloning cDNA encoding the netrins showed that they were homologous to UNC-6, a laminin-related protein (found in the extracellular matrix) required for migration of cells and axons in the nematode *Caenorhabditis elegans*.

This homology suggests that growth cones in the vertebrate and nematode respond to a similar molecule. Further studies with UNC-6 and the netrins have shown that these molecules may be guidance and targeting signals rather than just attractive versus repulsive molecules (Goodman, 1994). We must expect that further investigations of these molecules will lead to a better understanding of how the nervous system

Table 4.2 **THE FATE OF THE LAYERS IN THE NEURAL TUBE**

Marginal zone	At the surface covered by the presumptive pia contains pathways in the adult spinal cord and neurons in the cerebrum and cerebellum
Intermediate or mantle zone	Becomes gray matter of the adult spinal cord, brain stem and diencephalon, and contains white matter of the cerebrum and cerebellum
Subventricular zone	Forms the macroglia (astrocytes, oligodendrocytes)
Ventricular lining zone	Early on has germinal cells that form neuroblasts; in mature brain becomes ependymal lining of ventricles

actually forms and connects. An understanding of how the nervous system forms connections may ultimately lead to better methods to repair damage in the brain (see Table 4.2).

PROGRAMMED CELL DEATH

During the development of both the central and peripheral nervous system, the number of immature neurons formed is actually double that which will ultimately survive (Cowan et al., 1983). This apparent excess in formation of neurons is a mechanism whereby the size of the neuronal pool is ultimately matched to the amount of tissue actually innervated (Majno & Joris, 1995). In contrast to necrosis, which is a form of cell death that results from acute tissue injury and provokes an inflammatory response, programmed cell death (PCD) is carried out in a regulated process that generally confers advantages during an organism's life cycle:

> Programmed cell death (PCD) is a fundamental biological process, serving many important functions in animal development and homeostasis, and the pathogenesis of many diseases is attributed to its malfunctioning. Apoptosis is the most common form of PCD executed by a unique family of proteases called caspases. However, caspases are also involved in a variety of important nonapoptotic processes. Furthermore, PCD can sometimes proceed in the absence of caspases activity through alternative pathways.

NEURONAL DEATH

1. *Necrosis.* Neuronal death is necrosis, and it is unplanned cell death characterized by cellular edema and destruction of the neuronal organelles and membranes. Necrosis is commonly accompanied by the inflammatory response. This occurs usually following an injury (e.g., stroke, trauma, and tumor).

2. *Programmed cell death.* This type of degeneration is normal and planned, called *apoptosis* (a Greek term referring to the seasonal falling off of leaves); it begins with condensation and degeneration of the chromatin, blebs of the plasma membrane, and shrunken cytoplasm

with the organelles intact (Taylor, 1993). Caspases (cysteine-dependent, aspartate-specific proteases) are endoproteases that are integral to the disassembly of the cell. These enzymes exist normally in an inactive form, but once they are activated they set off a proteolytic cascade that spreads and destroys the cell. In both of these events glia and macrophages phagocytize the nerve cells, but in apoptosis the nerve cells die quietly without any inflammatory response or major activation of the phagocytes. With necrosis, there is an inflammatory response with phagocytes activated, while in apoptosis there is no injury or interruption of the blood supply and yet the cell begins to degenerate with the cell bodies appearing pyknotic.

Researchers have become more aware of this "natural" type of cell death and have also called it programmed cell death, biological/physiological cell death, or even cell suicide. Many areas in the vertebrate and invertebrate nervous system are now known to have apoptosis. It is also well established that programmed cell death occurs in most other tissues and organs and is an important means to shape the final form of the body. There have also been studies with hormones and other compounds that have decreased the number of immature neurons dying by apoptosis.

With the recognition that apoptosis is a normally occurring phenomenon, neurobiologists using molecular probes have identified genes that regulate this process. The finding of genes that control these phenomena has also permitted researches to questions whether diseases such as Huntington's chorea, Parkinson's disease, and even Alzheimer's disease are a consequence of this same gene pool being activated later in life to produce the resultant neuronal death. This promising research may well lead to gene therapy, which permits treatment of these presumed programmed cell death–caused diseases by turning off the offending genes.

DEVELOPMENT OF BLOOD VESSELS IN THE BRAIN

The blood supply to the developing brain begins by the invasion of solid cords of mesodermal endothelial cells, called Wilson's buds, which over a period of several days develop a lumen and a basement membrane. These arteries develop in the pharyngeal arches during the fourth week and are derived from the third pair of aortic arches and dorsal aortae; by 6 weeks there are well-established internal and external carotid vessels. These buds of growing endothelial cells are especially prominent as the marginal layers evolve. The blood intermediate supply evolves in direct relationship to the maturation of the central nervous system and as a consequence of the many factors released into the developing parenchyma of the central nervous system. As the astrocytes form within the central nervous system, some of their end-feet surround the basement membrane of the brain capillaries and begin to form a blood–brain barrier. The actual tight junctions between the endothelial cells that delineate the definitive blood–brain barrier are not complete until just before birth.

VENTRICULAR SYSTEM

When the neural folds fuse, a neural tube is formed. At the rostral end of the nervous system two lateral dilations appear: the primordia of the cerebral vesicles. These regions will grow rapidly, extending anteriorly, inferiorly, and posteriorly as they form the ventricles in the cerebral hemispheres.

Lateral Ventricles. The cavity in each cerebral vesicle is called a lateral ventricle. As the cerebral hemispheres grow by continued outward migration of nerve cells, the ventricles take up less and less space in the brain and are modified into a C-shaped structure with a spur extending occipitally. Each lateral ventricle in its final form is divided into an anterior horn, body, inferior horn, and posterior horn.

Foramen of Monro. Early in development, the lumen in the paired telencephalic vesicles is continuous with that of the neural tube. As the telencephalon differentiates into cerebral cortex and basal nuclei, the ventricles take up relatively less space. A narrow channel, called the interventricular foramen of Monro, persists between the cerebral ventricles and the third ventricle (Fig. 1.21).

Third Ventricle. The centrally placed cavity in the diencephalon—the third ventricle—narrows as the parenchyma of the diencephalon forms.

Cerebral Aqueduct. In the midbrain the tectum and tegmentum expand greatly and constrict the lumen so that only the narrow cerebral aqueduct remains.

Fourth Ventricle. In the metencephalon (cerebellum and pons) and myelencephalon (medulla), the tegmentum undergoes a series of flexures and expands laterally, and is overgrown by the cerebellum. As a result, the cavity in the myelencephalon and metencephalon called the fourth ventricle assumes a rhomboid shape. The fourth ventricle is continuous with the narrow cerebral aqueduct above and the constricted spinal canal below.

Spinal Canal. In the spinal cord, the expanding gray and white matter nearly obliterates the ventricular cavity so that only the small spinal canal remains.

FORMATION OF THE PERIPHERAL NERVOUS SYSTEM

Peripheral structures are innervated from nuclei in the brain stem (by the cranial nerves) and from nuclei in the spinal cord (by the spinal nerves). The twelve cranial-nerve nuclei innervate skin, glands, viscera, striated muscles, and special sense organs (eye and ear) in the head and neck. The spinal nerves innervate skin, glands, and striated muscles in the upper and lower extremities and in the thorax, abdomen, and pelvis.

SPINAL CORD DIFFERENTIATION

The origin of the spinal cord can be traced to the twentieth day. The neural plate then has two distinct regions: caudally, a single elongate cylindrical region, which will become the spinal cord; and, cranially, a shorter broader region, which will become the brain (Fig. 4.1B).

Until the third month the spinal cord fills the vertebral column. From then on the cartilage and bone grow faster than the central nervous system, and by birth the coccygeal end of the spinal cord lies at the level of the third lumbar vertebra. In an adult it is found at the level of the first lumbar vertebra.

At the end of the somite period (days 30 to 35), mitotic divisions in the spinal cord region produce thickened walls and a thin roof and floor, with almost complete obliteration of the central canal (Fig. 4.4). The ventral portion of the lateral walls develops and expands earlier than the dorsal region. The ventral portion is called the basal plate and the dorsal portion is called the alar plate. Processes from cells in the mantle layer enter the external-most region of the cord, which is called the marginal zone.

Gray matter. Four columns appear in each half of the gray matter of the spinal cord: two motors and two sensory (Table 4.3). The somatic afferent and efferent columns innervates skin and muscle related to the somites, while the visceral afferent and visceral efferent columns innervate the mucosa, glands, and smooth muscles in the visceral structures. The somatic efferent cells are the motor neurons in the ventral horn of the spinal cord; the somatic afferent cells are the neurons in the spinal ganglia. The visceral efferent cells consist of sympathetic and parasympathetic neurons.

Axons of developing motor neurons in the basal plate enter the adjoining somites, while sensory roots derived from the adjacent neural crest zone enter the dorsal or alar plate.

Table 4.3 STRUCTURE INNERVATED BY CRANIAL NERVES

STRUCTURE INNERVATED BY CRANIAL NERVES	CRANIAL NERVE
1. Muscles of somite origin	XII, VI, IV, and most of III
2. Muscles and skin of pharyngeal arches	V, VII, IX, X, and XI
3. Preganglionic parasympathetic	IX, X, VII, V, and a small part of III
4. Special sensory cranial nerves	I, II, VII, VIII, IX, and X

In the spinal cord (Fig. 4.3) the plate will become the dorsal or sensory associative horn, and the basal plate will become the ventral or motor horn. In the medulla (Fig. 4.5), pons (Fig. 3.6), and midbrain (Fig. 4.7), the alar and basal plates are restricted to the floor of the developing ventricular system. The remaining bulk of these zones consists of nuclei and tracts that are related to the head, neck, and special senses.

In the spinal cord the marginal zone also increases in width as axons that form the ascending and descending tract enter (Fig. 4.4). The formation of the dorsal and ventral horns delimits the dorsal, ventral, and lateral columns or funiculi in the marginal zone. An intermediate horn develops dorsal and lateral to the anterior horn in the thoracic and lumbar levels of the spinal cord. Cells in this horn are the preganglionic sympathetic neurons. The postganglionic visceral neurons are in the paravertebral sympathetic chain or in ganglia associated with the visceral organs. The preganglionic parasympathetic

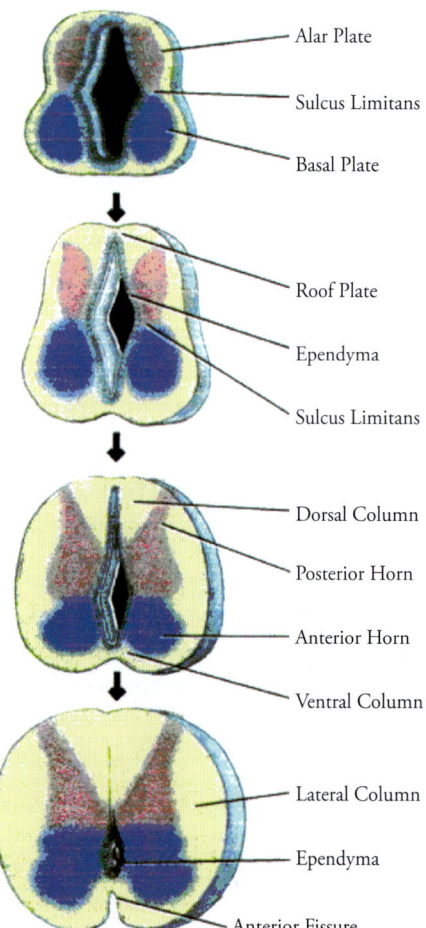

Figure 4.4 Schematic representation of the development of the spinal cord. (After Hamilton, W.J. Boyd, J.D., and Mossman, H.W.: Human Embryology. Cambridge, England, Heffer and Sons, 1964.)

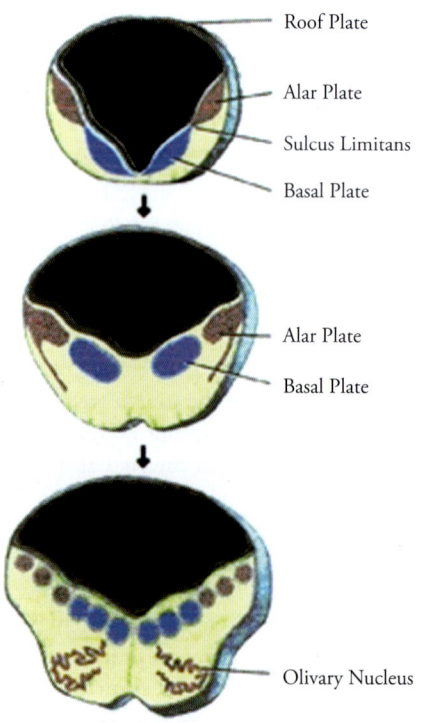

Figure 4.5 Schematic representation of the development of the medulla. (After Hamilton, W.J. Boyd, J.D., and Mossman, H.W.: Human Embryology. Cambridge, England, Heffer & Sons, 1964.)

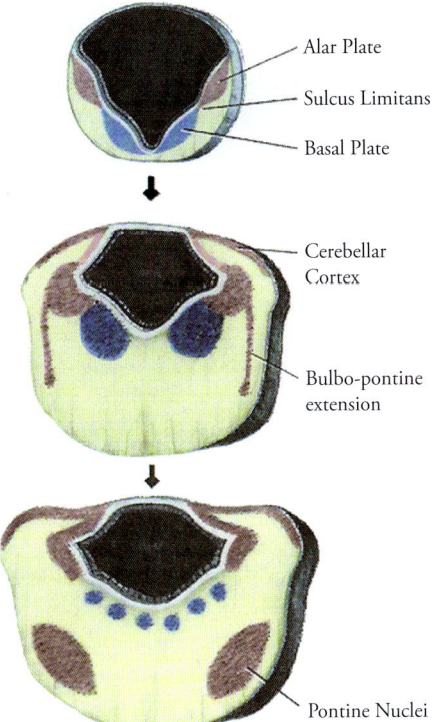

Figure 4.6 Schematic representation of the development of the pons. (After Hamilton, W.J., Boyd, J.D., and Mossman, H.W.: Human Embryology. Cambridge, England, Heffer and Sons, 1964.)

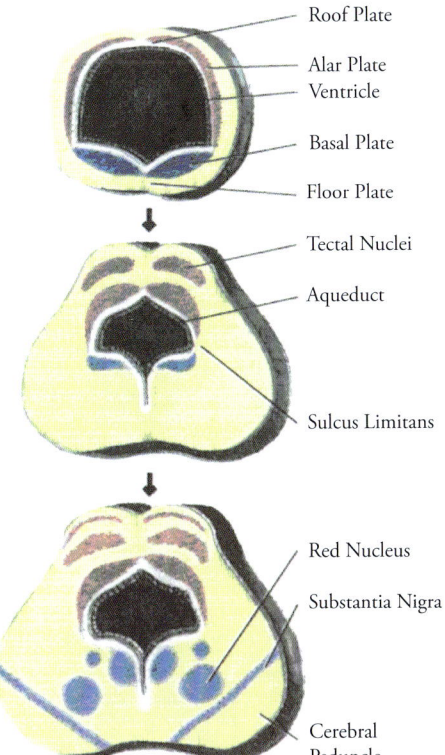

Figure 4.7 Schematic representation of the development of the midbrain. (After Hamilton, W.J., Boyd, J.D., and Mossman, H.W.: Human Embryology. Cambridge, England, Heffer and Sons, 1964.)

innervation originates from the motor neurons in cranial nerves III, VII, IX, and X and the sacral spinal cord and innervates ganglia that connect the appropriate organ or gland. Again, these ganglia differentiate very close to the appropriate structure. In the dorsal or sensory horn of the spinal cord, there are sensory neurons that provide connections throughout the spinal cord or brain stem.

The segmental arrangement of the central nervous system stops at the spinomedullary junction, which marks the site of transition from the spinal cord to the brain stem. The brain stem and cerebrum are suprasegmental with no evidence of segmentation present. These regions of the central nervous system are specialized to control structures in the head and neck as well as exerting control over the entire body.

During development the spinal cord and the somites lie close together, so the distance the axon must travel to reach its appropriate muscle is very short. Undoubtedly, chemical factors help direct the axon to the correct muscle. The sensory fibers also have only a short distance to run from the ganglia into skin or muscle and their axon into the central nervous system; again, probably by chemical mediation they establish the connection with the correct dorsal horn cells.

BRAIN DIFFERENTIATION

The brain begins development as a broad zone at the upper end of the developing central nervous system with three distinct vesicles: the prosencephalon, the mesencephalon, and the rhombencephalon.

RHOMBENCEPHALON (HIND BRAIN), FORMS THE METENCEPHALON (PONS AND CEREBELLUM) AND MYELENCEPHLON (MEDULLA)

The rhombencephalon differentiates into the metencephalon (Fig. 4.6) and myelencephalon (Fig. 4.5). This region is further divided by their relationship to the ventricular system. That portion forming the floor of the ventricle is called the tegmentum, while that forming the roof of the ventricle is called the tectum. In the spinal cord the basal plate was ventral and the alar plate dorsal. In the medulla, pons, and midbrain, both basal and alar plates are restricted to that portion of the tegmentum that forms the ventricular floor. The alar or sensory region is lateral, while the motor region is medial. The sulcus limitans, on the ventricular floor, separates the medial motor region from the lateral sensory region.

In the spinal cord the neurons are in the gray matter, in the center of the spinal cord, while the fiber tracts are on the outside. In the brain stem motor nuclei migrate to a medial position and sensory nuclei to a lateral position. The fiber tracts are on the external and medial surface; some tracts are actually in the center of the brain stem.

The dorsal portion of the alar plate in the metencephalon (pons) forms the primordium of the cerebellum. This region, the rhombic lip, thickens and the cerebellum continues to expand laterally and then medially so that a pair of lateral regions, the cerebellar hemispheres, and a medial zone, the vermis, is now formed. The ependymal lining and pia form the roof of the lower medulla, the tela choroidea.

On the anterior surface of the medulla, pons, and midbrain is the basilar region, which includes the more recently phylogenetically added descending cortical fibers. In the medulla these fibers consist of the pyramids; in the pons, they consist of the middle cerebellar peduncle and pyramids; and in the midbrain, they consist of the cerebral peduncles. Other tracts and nuclei form the bulk of the tegmentum of the pons, medulla, and midbrain (Fig. 4.8).

The ventricular lumen in pontine and medullary levels is called the fourth ventricle. The neural tube in these zones changes from a tube to a rhomboid-shaped fossa as a result of the broadening of the tegmentum and the overgrowth of the cerebellum.

The cerebellum and deep cerebellar nuclei are formed by the migration of cells. In the cerebellum there are two distinct germinal centers:

1. A region in the roof of the IV ventricle gives origin to the germinal Purkinje and Golgi II cells and glia, which migrate into the mantle layer of the cerebellum.
2. The external granule zone forms beneath the pia of the cerebellum, the external granule zone. This region gives origin to the granule cells, stellate, and basket cells and some of the glia.

The Purkinje cell layer is the first to form. A little later cells migrate inward from the more external layers to form the granular layer. In the adult the molecular layer has only a few cells, but the Purkinje layer and granule cell layer have many neurons. It appears that as the primitive neurons are migrating into their definitive place, they form many of the connections necessary for their specialized functions.

The factors that control the migration of cells into the cerebellum and cerebrum and that provide the connections that are necessary for the proper function of these structures are only now being identified. (These factors produce some of the following changes: the glia and neurons migrate and elongate at certain critical times and are supplied with an adequate blood supply that permits all this to happen.)

MESENCEPHALON FORMS THE ADULT MIDBRAIN

The mesencephalon (Fig. 4.7) begins as a wide tube with a conspicuous floor (tegmentum) and a thin roof (tectum). The addition of fibers and nuclei in the mantle zone of the tegmentum, concomitant with the formation of the superior and inferior colliculi in the tectal area, produces a narrow cerebral aqueduct with a large tegmentum and tectum.

The tectum consists of neurons that receive input from the cranial nerves that relay auditory (inferior colliculus) and visual information (superior colliculus). The cerebral

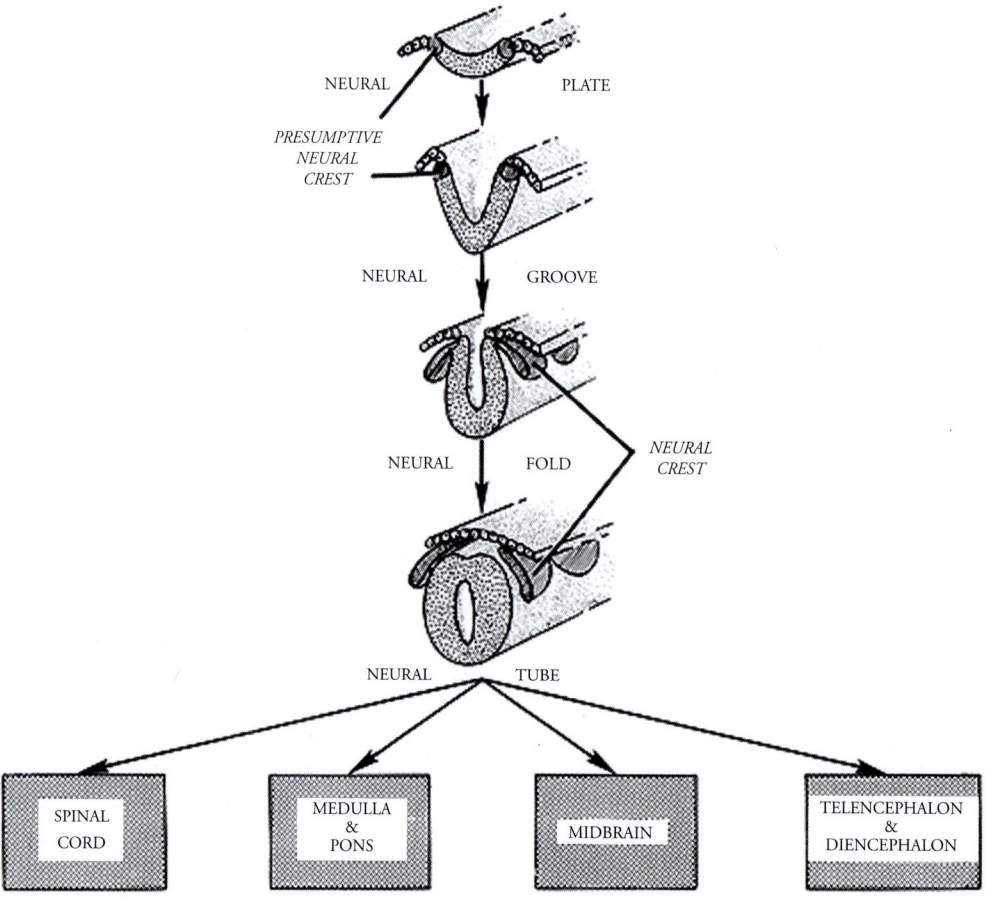

Figure 4.8 Differentiation of embryonic brain areas into adult brain regions.

peduncles form the anterior surface or basis of the midbrain, with the tegmentum located between the basis and tectum. The cerebral peduncles consist of fibers descending from the cerebrum to the brain stem and spinal cord.

PROSENCEPHALON FORMS THE CEREBRAL HEMISPHERES AND DIENCEPHALON

Three primary vesicles of brain regions are seen as the neural tube begins to close; prosencephalon (forebrain), mesencephalon (midbrain), and rhombencephalon (hindbrain). The prosencephalon (Fig. 4.9) begins to differentiate at about 30 days as a dilation of the cranial end of the neural tube (Figs. 4.2C and 4.2D); this dilation evolves into a right and left dilation. Early in development the optic vesicle, which will become the eye, appears as a lateral diverticulum of the anterior portion of the prosencephalon. In front of and above the optic stalk a pair of cerebral vesicles form. The cerebral vesicles expand superiorly, anteriorly, and posteriorly.

DIENCEPHALON

The diencephalon originates from the caudal portion of the prosencephalon (Fig. 4.1D) and represents the thickened lateral wall of the primordium of the third ventricle. The dorsal half of the diencephalon will become the thalamus and epithalamus, while the floor differentiates into the hypothalamus and neurohypophysis. The alar and basal plates are no longer found at diencephalic levels, although functionally the basal plate may well be represented as the hypothalamus. Fibers to and from the telencephalon will form the lateral limit of the diencephalon. These fibers are the internal capsule.

Pituitary Gland

The pituitary gland develops from two regions:

1. ectodermal > adenohypophysis
2. neuroectodermal from diencephalon > neurohypophysis

CRANIAL NERVES

The cranial nerves form connections to muscles, skin, glands, and blood vessels in the head and neck. A detailed discussion of the individual cranial nerves can be found in Chapter 12. In this section, the cranial nerves Table 4.3 and Figure 4.10 will be categorized on the basis of the embryonic derived structures they innervate.

Cranial Nerve Innervation for Muscles of Somite Origin

Nerve III (oculomotor) is a purely motor nerve that innervates the inferior oblique, medial, superior, inferior recti muscles and levator palpebrae superior muscles. The extrinsic eye muscles develop from mesenchyme in the orbital region.

Nerve IV (trochlear) is a purely motor nerve and innervates the superior oblique muscle of the eye. This is the only cranial with rootlets that leave the central nervous system from the posterior surface of the brain.

Nerve VI (abducens) is a purely motor nerve and innervates the lateral rectus muscle of the eye.

Nerve XII (hypoglossal) is a purely motor nerve and innervates the extrinsic and intrinsic muscles in the tongue. Occipital myotomes migrate ventrally and form the tongue musculature that is innervated by nerve XII. The epithelium and general connective tissue of the tongue arises by the fusion of pharyngeal endoderm and branchial mesoderm that are innervated by nerves VII, IX and X.

Cranial Nerves Innervating Muscles (Skeletal) and Skin in the Pharyngeal Arches

Cranial nerve innervation of the pharyngeal arches is shown in Table 4.4. After somites begin to form, five ectodermal grooves appear lateral to the embryonic pharynx and caudal to the somatoderm, or primitive mouth. The grooves are separated from one another by elevations, which gradually elongate, fuse with the opposite side, and extend laterally and anteriorly around the pharynx, forming arches. In lower vertebrates these arches form the gills, while in vertebrates without gills they are called pharyngeal arches. Many of the muscles and bones in the face and neck originate from these arches.

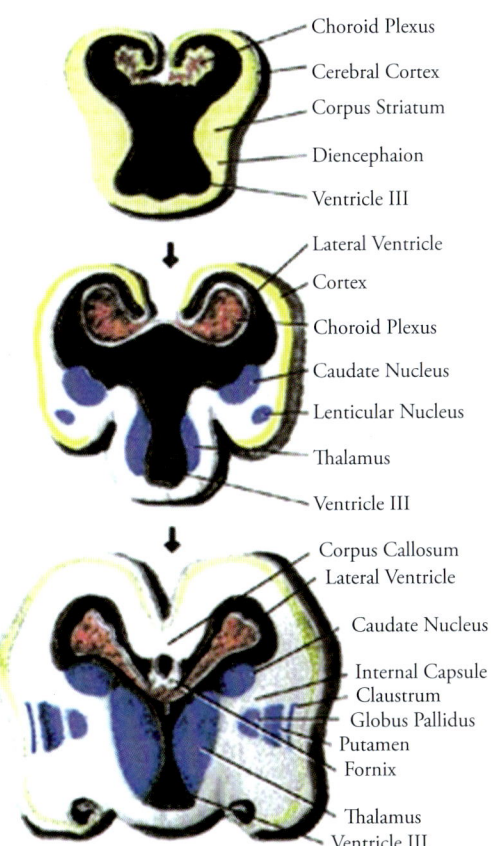

Figure 4.9 Schematic representation of the development of the telencephalon and diencephalon. (After Hamilton, W.J., Boyd, J.D., and Mossman, H.W.: Human Embryology. Cambridge, England, Heffer and Sons, 1964.)

Figure 4.10 Demonstration of origin of nerve components of the cranial nerves from the ventricular tegmentum of the brain stem. General and special somatic afferents and efferents (CN II–VI, VIII, IX–XII) and general and special visceral efferents and afferents (CN I, VII, IX, and X).

MAMMALS HAVE A TOTAL OF SIX ARCHES

1. First and second arches named, respectively, the mandibular and hyoid and the lower four unnamed (the sixth arch is rudimentary).

   a. First arch (mandibular) innervated by the trigeminal nerve—muscles of mastication form here

   b. Second arch (hyoid) innervated by the facial nerve—the muscles of facial expression form here

   c. Third arch innervated by the glossopharyngeal nerve—the stylopharyngeus forms in the third

   d. Fourth arch innervated by the superior laryngeal nerve of the vagus > cricothyroid muscles and constrictor muscles of the pharynx

   e. Fifth arch regresses

   f. Sixth arch innervated by the recurrent laryngeal nerve-vocal muscles

2. Cranial nerves associated with the pharyngeal arches: V, VII, IX, and X (Table 4.4)

   a. *Nerve V (trigeminal)* is a mixed nerve (motor and sensory) that innervates the first or mandibular arch and also contains a portion (ophthalmic) that distributes to the skin up to the vertex of the skull. The motor division of this nerve innervates the muscles of mastication derived from the first arch. The sensory division innervates the skin on the face and forehead.

   b. *Nerve VII (facial)* is a mixed nerve that distributes to the second pharyngeal or hyoid arch. The motor division of this nerve innervates the muscles of facial expression. The sensory division innervates the taste buds on the anterior two-thirds of the tongue.

   c. *Nerve IX (glossopharyngeal)* is a mixed nerve that innervates structures associated with the third arch. The motor division of this nerve innervates the stylopharyngeus muscles.

   d. *Nerve X (vagus)* is a mixed nerve that innervates structures associated with the fourth and sixth arches (the fifth arch regresses). It also provides afferent and efferent components to the heart, lungs, and much of the gastrointestinal system.

   e. *Nerve XI (accessory)* is purely motor and innervates the sternomastoid and trapezius muscles, which originate from somatic and branchial mesenchyme in the cervical region.

Preganglionic Parasympathetic Innervation to Smooth Muscle

Nerve III innervates the ciliary ganglion; postganglionic fibers then pass to the sphincter of the iris, which constricts the pupil in bright light.

Table 4.4 DERIVATIVES OF PHARYNGEAL ARCHES

PHARYNGEAL ARCH	INNERVATED BY CRANIAL NERVE	MUSCLES	SKELETON
1. Mandibular	V	Of mastication: temporal, masseter, medial and lateral pterygoid, mylohyoid, anterior belly of digastric, tensor palatine, tensor tympani	Premaxilla, maxilla, zygomatic bone, part of temporal bone, Meckel's cartilage, mandible, incus, anterior ligament of malleus, sphenomandibular ligament
2. Hyoid	VII	Of facial expression: auriculars, buccinator, frontalis, orbicularis oris and oculi, posterior belly of digastric, stylohyoid, stapedius	Stapes, styloid process, stylohoyoid ligament, lesser horn and upper part of hyoid bone
3. Unnamed	IX	Stylopharyngeus	Greater horn and lower part of body of hyoid
4. Unnamed	X-superior laryngeal branch/nerve to fourth arch	Cricothyroid, levator palatine, constrictors of pharynx	Laryngeal cartilages: thyroid, cricoid, arytenoid, corniculate, cuneiform
6. Unnamed	X-recurrent (inferior) laryngeal branch to sixth arch	Intrinsic muscles of larynx function in respiration and phonation	

Nerve VII provides innervation to the submaxillary and lacrimal ganglia associated with the following glands: submaxillary, sublingual, nasal, and lacrimal.

Nerve IX provides innervation to the parotid gland via the otic ganglion.

Nerve X provides innervation to the heart, lungs, and gastrointestinal system up to the transverse colon and the axons from the vagus synapse upon ganglia associated with these organs.

Cranial Nerves Associated with the Special Senses

Nerve I (olfactory) cell bodies are located in the nasal placode in the upper fifth of each nasal cavity. The neuroblasts in the olfactory epithelium differentiate into olfactory epithelial cells. The axons of these cells grow toward the cerebral hemisphere, pierce the roof of the nasal cavity, and enter the region of the hemisphere that will become the olfactory bulb. The primary fibers synapse in the olfactory bulb. The secondary cell bodies are located in the olfactory bulb and form the olfactory tracts.

Nerve II (optic) originates from tertiary ganglion neurons in the retina. These axons are really a tract in the central nervous system and do not constitute a peripheral nerve. The axons synapse in the lateral geniculate nucleus of the thalamus. (Students may also want to review the details of the formation of the eye from the optic vesicle and lens vesicles in a standard embryology test.)

Nerve VIII (vestibulocochlear) primary cell bodies are located in the cochlea (auditory division) and vestibule (vestibular division) of the inner ear. (Students may also want to review the details of the formation of the inner ear from the otic placode in a standard embryology textbook.)

Nerves VII, IX, and X provide innervation to the taste buds on the tongue and pharynx.

TELENCEPHALON

The telencephalon, part of the forebrain, consists of two regions: a cortical zone that becomes the cerebral hemispheres, and a deeply placed nuclear region the corpus striatum that becomes the caudate, putamen, and globus pallidus.

The telencephalon begins at 10 weeks as paired small smooth telencephalic vesicles. By birth a large, convoluted cerebral cortex is present. The first prominent features seen in the hemisphere are the formation of the primary sulci or depressions.

PRIMARY SULCI

The first of these sulci, the primary sulci, appear at about 19 weeks; they are initially the lateral or Sylvian sulcus, on the lateral surface (Fig. 4.11), and the parieto-occipital sulcus, on the medial surface (Fig. 4.12A). By 24 weeks, the Sylvian sulcus is more pronounced on the lateral surface and the calcarine

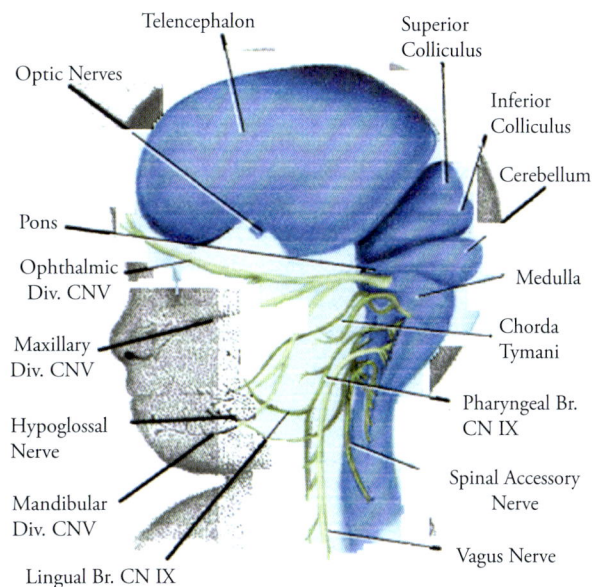

Figure 4.11 Bilateral surface of 11-week human embryo demonstrating the cranial and upper spinal nerves. (After Patten, B.M.: Human Embryology. New York, McGraw-Hill, 1953.)

Figure 4.12A Development of the lateral surface of the brain during fetal life. The lateral sulcus is first seen in the left column at 10-12, 15, 19, 22 and 24, weeks. In the middle row showing the evolution of the cortical gyri and sulci from weeks 28, 30, 32 and 34; and the right row showing development at weeks 37, 39 and 41 weeks. (From Larroche, J. CI: The Development of the Central Nervous System during Intrauterine Life. In Falkner, F. (ed.): Human Development. Philadelphia, W.B. Saunders, 1966, p. 258.)

Figure 4.12B Development of the medial surface of the brain during fetal life. The left column shows the development of the medial surface of the cerebrum at 19, 25 and 32 weeks. The right column show the development of the cerebrum at 37 and 41 weeks. (From Larroche, J. CI.: The Development of the Central Nervous System during Intrauterine Life. In Falkner, F. (ed.): Human Development. Philadelphia, W.B. Saunders, 1966, p. 259.)

sulcus is prominent on the medial surface (Fig. 4.12B). Shortly thereafter the other primary sulci—the central, callosal, and hippocampal—appear.

After about 30 weeks the primary sulci are formed, and there is a rapid increase in the secondary sulci and gyri. By term, formation of the gyri and sulci is complete. After birth the gyri increase in bulk as the neurons continue to differentiate.

The telencephalic vesicle rapidly changes shape as the frontal lobe forms and pushes anteriorly, the temporal lobe grows inferiorly, and the occipital and parietal regions expand. The olfactory bulb forms at the base of the frontal lobe by an evagination of cells that quickly obliterates any trace of the ventricle in the olfactory bulb.

The sulci begin as rather shallow depressions. However, as the neurons continue to migrate in from the ventricular surface, more and more cells are added and the gyri become larger and the sulci become deeper. In the term and adult brain more than 70% of the cortical surface is hidden from view, deep in the banks of the sulci. Therefore, when we speak of the total surface of the cerebral hemispheres, we must include not only the superficial cortex but also the hidden sulcal cortex.

The brain at birth weighs 300 to 400 g; by 1 year it weighs 1000 g. The brain continues to grow and by late childhood reaches its final weight of approximately 1500 g.

DEVELOPMENT OF CEREBRAL CORTEX

The development of certain areas is of special importance in understanding the final form of the brain. As the lateral sulcus forms, the cortex above and below the lateral fissure overgrows the cortex deep in the lateral/Sylvian fissure. This cortex, the insula, soon disappears from view and is covered over by this overgrowth of frontal, parietal, and temporal cortex.

Formation of the cerebral cortex begins around the seventh week and is completed in the first year of life. Developing from the inside to out, the first layer to form is layer VI and the last to form is layer II (tritiated thymidine studies; Berry and Rogers, 1965). The pyramidal cells in the cerebral cortex appear to mature prior to the stellate cells (Altman, 1966). Radial glial fibers form connections from the luminal surface to the pial surface that help the primitive neurons migrating later into the more superficial layers to traverse the increased cell densities in the deeper layers. The formation of the cerebrum from inside to outside permits much of the circuitry to form and also permits the columnar arrangement in the cortex to evolve.

The development of the six-layered cerebral cortex starts with the migration of neuroblasts into the deepest layer (VI–IV) first, then the cells into the external layers (I–III) last: "inside-out." Tritiated thymidine studies have been used on rodents and primates for labeling nerve cells in the germinal layer of the ventricle on their "birth days" and following them into the cerebrum and identifying their final destination (Rakic, 1972).

Commissures

Fiber bundles, called commissures (Fig. 4.13A–D) interconnect the two cerebral hemispheres. The anterior commissure

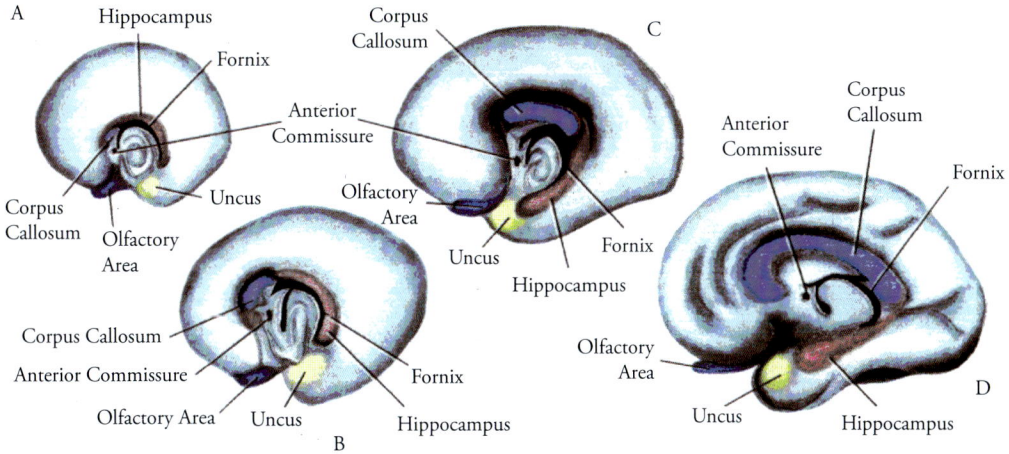

Figure 4.13 Development of the fornix and commissures of the cerebral hemispheres. (*A*) Fetus at third month. (*B*) Fetus at fourth month. (*C*) Fetus at beginning of fifth month. (*D*) Fetus at end of seventh month. (After Keibel, F., and Mall, F.P.: Manual of Human Embryology, Philadelphia, Lippincott, 1910-1912.)

interconnects the olfactory bulbs and anterior parts of the temporal lobe. The huge corpus callosum interconnects the remaining portions of the hemisphere. The hippocampal commissure interconnects the hippocampus and adjacent portions of the hippocampal gyrus. These commissures form in the lamina terminalis that marks the site of the closure of the anterior neuropore. The ventral surface of the hemispheres at this place fuse, and the fibers can then cross and interconnect the two hemispheres.

Initially, the anterior commissure, corpus callosum, and fornix (which connects the hippocampus and hypothalamus) are close to one another (Fig. 4.13A), but as the brain grows, the corpus callosum expands anteriorly, inferiorly, superiorly, and caudally with only the rostral tip remaining attached to the lamina terminalis.[1]

PRENATAL DEVELOPMENT OF CEREBRAL CORTEX

The developing cerebral hemispheres initially show the three regions common to the neural tube: the ventricular, intermediate and marginal zones. Then the subventricular zone appears. Cells of the intermediate zone migrate into the marginal zone and form the cortical layers. So that the gray matter is on the periphery and the white matter, medullary center, is located centrally.

The initial progenitor neurons first appear in the matrix/germinal area in a proliferative cell layer around the ventricle at approximately 33–42 days of development and form a structure known as the preplate (the primordial plexiform layer). Later formed neurons divide the preplate into two layers: the marginal zone (future layer 1) and the subplate (the future neurons of layer 6 and the white matter). Between the marginal zone and the subplate a transient layer the cortical plate is formed beginning approximately at embryonic day 52.

---

[1] The hippocampus anteriorly is disrupted by the formation of the corpus callosum and a small dorsal hippocampus or indusium griseum remains on the dorsal surface of the corpus callosum.

NEURONAL MIGRATION

The migration of neurons is facilitated by the presence of special primitive radial glial cells that extend between the ventricular surface and the pial surface. These glial cells essentially serve as guide wires for the migrating neurons. This radial or vertical orientation provides the basis for the columnar organization that is a characteristic of cerebral cortex. The initial migrating neurons travel through the entire marginal layer and form a temporary organizing layer in what will eventually become the relatively acellular molecular layer. This organizing layer apparently secretes an extracellular protein: Reelin. (Reelin is named after the mutant mouse—*reeler*—which has ataxic reeling movements due to the absence of this protein and in which there is total disorganization of the usual laminar pattern.) When the successive waves of migrating neurons encounter the organizing layer, the Reelin provides a signal to detach, from the glial guide wires. The initial cells to detach form the neurons of layer 6. The apical dendrites of these pyramidal cells in layers 6 and subsequently layer 5 will extend to the pial surface.

Subsequent waves of neurons detach at successively higher levels. In addition to the putative role of the protein Reelin, other factors also influence this process of migration. The radial guided migration is blocked by NMDA antagonists, suggesting a role for the transmitter glutamate. In addition, calcium ion channels may also be involved in migration. Although the previous discussion has emphasized the radial movement of neurons, it is also evident that some neurons may migrate in a direction perpendicular to the radial glial fibers. Thus, there are horizontal connections in addition to the vertical organization. The process of neurogenesis and migration is completed in the human fetus by approximately week 24. The subsequent step in the process of cortical development is a removal of those neurons in the molecular layer that served as the initial organizing layer by the process of apoptosis. The neurons in the ventricular zone, the subventricular zone, and the white matter (which have failed to reach the cortical plate forming layers 2–6) also die off by this same process. The radial glial cells lose their long fibers and differentiate into astrocytes.

The mature cerebral cortex is laminated and consists of the following six layers:

Layers 1, 2, and 3—supragranular phylogenetically newest layers and last layers to form

Layer 4—granular layer

Layers 5 and 6—infragranular layers phylogenetically are first layers to form

CHANGES IN CORTICAL ARCHITECTURE AS A FUNCTION OF POSTNATAL AGE

During postnatal development the brain increases significantly in weight from an average of 375 to 400 g at birth to 1000 g at 1 year, to a maximum of 1350 to 1410 g at age 15 years (males). This increased growth does not affect all areas of the brain to an equal extent. Thus, this growth involves a rapid expansion of the convexities of the frontal, parietal, and temporal lobes. This results in a completion of the covering of the insular lobe by the surrounding operculum and a relative displacement of the parahippocampal gyrus and occipital lobe. In addition, the cortical surface area is in a sense being increased by the deepening of sulci, with increasing complexity of the primary and secondary fissures. This process continues after the second year with the development of tertiary fissures.

Myelin formation is necessary for the functioning of the nervous system. Table 4.5 lists the chronological sequence of myelination in the brain and by implication the beginning of functions in many of these same regions.

At birth most of the intrinsic fiber systems of the spinal cord and brain stem have myelinated. The long corticospinal tracts and corpus callosum begin to myelinate during the first postnatal months. The frontopontine, temperopontine, and thalamocortical projections myelinate during the second postnatal month.

Table 4.5 MYELINATION OF BRAIN REGIONS

BRAIN REGION	WHEN MYELINATES
Spinal cord	Last trimester
Brain stem	Last trimester
Frontal, parietal, temporal, occipital-pontine fibers	First 2 months postnatal (PN)
Primordial cortical fields: motor-sensory strip	PN 1–2 months
Intermediate cortical fields: association areas adjacent to primary motor and sensory cortex—premotor and superior parietal lobule	PN 2–4 months
Terminal cortical fields: association or integration areas—prefrontal, inferior parietal, posterior temporal cortex	PN 4 months

Myelination within the cerebral hemisphere and within the cerebral cortex occurs at different rates in different areas, paralleling the changes in psychomotor development. Flechsig demonstrated that the sequence of myelination in cerebral cortex followed a logical pattern.

Although myelination of the cerebral cortex begins during the early postnatal months, it is evident that this process is not completed at this time. The initial myelination begins in the vertically oriented fibers of the infragranular layers and then extends into the supragranular layers. The myelination of horizontal plexuses occurs at a later stage. Myelination continues to increase beyond 15 years of age even until age 60 with a gradual increase in density of the myelinated fibers, particularly in the horizontal plexuses. It is important to note that even in the adult not all cortical areas will reach the same density of myelinated fibers since the underlying pattern of distribution and density of pyramidal cells and their processes will differ significantly among different cortical areas.

NEURONAL MATURATION

In addition to changes in the degree of myelination, more basic changes in the relationship between nerve cells are occurring. Thus, the neocortex has received its full complement of neurons by the end of the sixth fetal month. During postnatal development as shown in silver stains there is a progressive growth of the apical and basilar dendritic arborizations. The studies of Conel have demonstrated that the more primitive allocortex (e.g., hippocampus) attains its final structural form at an earlier stage than the neocortex. The process of maturation, however, involves more than a progressive growth and elaboration of dendrites and synapses. In addition, a remodeling of neuronal connections occurs in large part based on neuronal activity. In the early perinatal period, there may be an excessive projection of axons to their targets. Maturation in part consists of the elimination of these aberrant collateral axon branches. In the primate there are estimated to be three to four times as many axons within the corpus callosum at birth compared to the adult state. In this process the NMDA receptor may have a considerable role in both neocortex and hippocampus, with the same cascade of the events that occur in long-term potentiation also responsible for the remodeling and synaptic plasticity. Abnormalities in development or sensory/environmental deprivation may retard the structural and functional development of these processes.

ABNORMAL DEVELOPMENT

The complexity of development of the nervous system means that there is a great chance for things to go wrong. In fact, more malformations occur in the nervous system than in any other organ system. Of the 0.5% of newborn infants with a major malfunction, roughly 60% affect the nervous system.

Many defects in the brain and spinal cord are evident at birth (Table 4.6). Some defects may be limited to only the nervous system, but others may include overlying ectodermal and mesodermal structures (bone, muscle, and connective tissue).

TABLE 4.6 CONGENITAL NEUROLOGIC MALFORMATIONS

CATEGORY	RESULTANT DEFICITS
1. Abnormalities in growth and migration	Heterotopias; anencephaly; holoprosencephaly; lissencephaly; micro-, macro-, or polygyria; porencephaly; schizencephaly; agenesis; fetal alcohol syndrome
2. Chromosomal trisomy and translocation	Down's, Edward's, and Patau's syndromes
3. Defective fusion	Spina bifida, cranial bifida, Arnold-Chiari malformation
4. Abnormalities with excessive growth of ectodermal and mesodermal tissue	Tuberous sclerosis, neurofibromatosis (von Recklinghausen's disease), Sturge-Weber syndrome
5. Abnormalities in ventricular system	Syringomyelia, syringobulbia, hydrocephalus

Many of the malformations are due to genetic abnormalities. Other categories of defects can be acquired from the maternal environment: infections (syphilis, rubella, AIDS), drugs (including alcohol, cocaine, etc.), ionizing radiation, environmental toxicants, metabolic disease, and poor nutrition. The most serious defects are fatal, but even the less severe abnormalities may significantly impairment function. The following discussion covers many of the major groups of malformations of the peripheral and central nervous system. More complete lists can be found in pathology textbooks.

MALFORMATIONS RESULTING FROM ABNORMALITIES IN GROWTH AND MIGRATION WITH INCOMPLETE DEVELOPMENT OF THE BRAIN

Heterotopias

Displaced islands of gray matter appear in the ventricular walls or white matter due to incomplete migration of neurons, and this defect in neuronal migration may be seen in many of the following abnormalities. In this category of malformation, the neurons or glia have failed to migrate, and consequently the brain development is incomplete. In the normal development of the cerebrum the neurons which form the deeper cortical layers arrive first and then cells destined for outer layers appear. In this abnormality the later waves of migration stop. The axons from the first cells to arrive begin to extend throughout the brain and actually form a barrier that interferes with the next wave of migration. The newly arriving neurons, which were destined for the superficial layers, instead now form a disorganized mass of neurons deep to the cortex. The disruption of the normal pattern of cerebral cortical development results in an imbalance in the equilibrium of excitation-inhibition. Seizures often result. The routine use of magnetic resonance imaging (MRI) for the evaluation of patients with epilepsy has demonstrated the high frequency of migration disorders, particularly in the pediatric and young adult age group. Depending on the severity of the disorder, the neurological examination and intellectual development may be normal. Areas of microgyria, macrogyria, or polygyria may be encountered. For some migration disorders, a genetic basis has been established. Various seizure types are present, but neurological development, examination, and intelligence are normal. In the following malformations, neurons or glia have failed to migrate, and consequently the brain's development is incomplete. In the normal development of the cerebrum the neurons that form the deeper cortical layers arrive first and then cells destined for outer layers appear. In this abnormality the later waves of migration stop. The axons from the first cells to arrive begin to extend throughout the brain and actually form a barrier that interferes with the next wave of migration. The newly arriving neurons, which were destined for the superficial layers, instead now form a disorganized mass of neurons deep to the cortex.

GENETICALLY LINKED MIGRATION DISORDERS

1. *Type 1 X-linked dominant lissencephaly.* Most of the neurons never reach their expected destination but instead are arrested in the subcortical white matter and the subventricular proliferative zone. The cortex is smooth, since development never proceeds to the stage of development of sulci and gyri that is necessary to accommodate the large numbers of cortical neurons that would otherwise be present in a normally developed cerebral cortex. In this mutation, the cortex per se is thin with the lamination pattern consisting of a rudimentary molecular layer 1 and a thin layer 5/6. Since males have only one X chromosome, this type of lissencephaly occurs in males. Severe psychomotor retardation and seizures are the result of this process. Since females have two X chromosomes, the effects of a single mutant X chromosome are less severe. The double cortex (subcortical band heterotopia or laminar heterotopia or diffuse cortical dysplasia) syndrome is the result. There is only a partial migration defect. Some neurons arrest in the subcortical white matter, but sufficient neurons reach the intended targets so that a normal six-layered laminar pattern is present. Cognitive function fully develops but seizures are present.

2. *Miller-Dieker syndrome.* This different genetic type of lissencephaly occurs in the autosomal recessive with linkage to locus 17p13.3. Infantile spasms and mixed seizures are associated with motor and mental retardation and a characteristic facies.

3. *Bilateral nodular periventricular heterotopia* is another X-linked dominant; a relatively continuous series nodules composed of neurons is present in the ependymal layer and subventricular zone, the former proliferative zone for neurons during development. In these cases, the cortical lamination pattern is normal.

4. *Cortical microdysgenesias* is a subtle form of neuronal migration disorder. It has been described in many patients with idiopathic epilepsy: absence, juvenile myoclonic

epilepsy, and primary generalized tonic-clonic. This disorder reflects events at a late stage of prenatal cortical development. Neurological examination and psychomotor development are normal, although subtle changes in cognitive function may be present.

In the following malformations, neurons or glia have failed to migrate, and consequently the brain's development is incomplete. In the normal development of the cerebrum the neurons that form the deep cortical layers arrive first and then cells destined for the outer layers appear. In this abnormality the later waves of migration have stopped. The axons from the first cells to arrive begin to extend throughout the brain and actually form a barrier that interferes with the next wave of migration. The newly arriving neurons, which were destined for the superficial layers, instead now form a disorganized mass of neurons deep to the cortex.

The following case is an example of abnormal migration.

CASE HISTORY 4.1: BILATERAL SUBCORTICAL BAND HETEROTOPIAS: DOUBLE CORTEX

This 24-year-old, right-handed mother of two children and home health aide was admitted to the neurology service after a recurrence of seizures with a flurry of four seizures on the day of admission. Seizures had begun at age 11 and would occur every 2 months. She described the seizures as beginning with an involuntary driving of the head and eyes to the right "as though she was going to look over her right shoulder." At this point she might experience a sensation of fear. She was aware that involuntary movements of both legs would then occur as well as clonic or tonic movements of the right upper extremity. On some occasions, she would then lose consciousness and a secondarily generalized tonic-clonic seizure would then be witnessed. She had been initially treated with anticonvulsants: phenytoin and phenobarbital, without control of seizures. Carbamazepine was then utilized but produced side effects. She had discontinued all medications 14 months prior to admission.

Family history: Negative for neurological or seizure disorders.

Past history: Head trauma right frontal with short period of unconsciousness at age 9 years. She had a tubal ligation and bilateral carpal tunnel surgery 5 years prior to admission.

Neurological examination: Mental status, cranial nerves, motor system, reflexes, and sensory system were all normal.

Clinical diagnosis: Focal seizures (partial epilepsy) originating in left frontal eye field with subsequent spread to left supplementary motor cortex and amygdala (or possibly cingulate gyrus).

Laboratory Data

1. *Electroencephalogram*: normal

2. *MRI:* bilateral triangular shaped foci of heterotopic gray matter were present in the frontal white matter extending from the superolateral aspect of the frontal horns to the gray white junction superiorly.

Subsequent course: Anticonvulsant medications were readjusted. Valproic acid was added to the carbamazepine. Compliance continued to be a problem. She continued to have at least one generalized tonic-clonic and possibly several simple partial seizures per year over the next 4 years.

Comments

The description of the initial clinical phenomena and the subsequent evolution suggest initial discharge in the left frontal eye field (area 8) with subsequent spread to the (left) supplementary motor cortex (an area where there is bilateral representation of the lower extremities). In contrast to the primary motor cortex where simple clonic movements occur on stimulation, complex postures and bilateral leg movements occur on supplementary motor cortex stimulation. The tonic posture or movement of the right arm would also be consistent with such a pattern of spread. The clonic movements of the upper extremity would be consistent with additional spread to the left motor cortex. The sensation of fear could have reflected spread to the limbic system possibly by means of the adjacent cingulate gyrus eventually involving the amygdala. The actual pathology in these areas of frontal lobe consisted of heterotopias of gray matter (termed *double cortex* or *subcortical band heterotopia*), a long-standing migration disorder. With the increasing use of the MRI to investigate patients with seizure disorders, there has been increasing recognition of such migration disorders. This is an X chromosome–linked disorder. In the female with two X chromosomes, this is a relatively benign disorder. In contrast, in the male with only one X chromosome, the effects are much more severe; most neurons never reach their expected destination but instead are arrested in the subcortical white matter. The result is type 1 X-linked lissencephaly. The cortex is smooth (lissencephalic) since development never proceeds to the stage of sulci and gyri. Sulci and gyri develop normally in the process of accommodating the large number of neurons that would under normal circumstances reach the cortical layers. Such males have severe psychomotor retardation as well as seizures.

Anencephaly. Anencephaly is a lethal condition in which skull, cerebral hemisphere, diencephalon, and midbrain can be absent. The notochord does not induce the anterior neuroectoderm and the anterior neuropore does not close. The cerebral cortex and upper brainstem are represented by a tangle of meninges, glia, and vessels at the base of the skull. The amount of brain tissue absent can vary from only the cerebrum to all of the diencephalon and telencephalon. Part of the brainstem, and remnants of higher structures, are usually present. The pituitary gland and other endocrine glands are small or absent. The eyes and ears are well developed, but the optic nerves are usually absent. These children are usually born alive but do not survive the first few days. This category of almost complete absence of the brain has been used extensively for transplants of the normally formed heart, lung, or kidney into infants in need of organ donors.

In this condition the brain has failed to form two distinct cerebral hemispheres. Instead, there is a single partially differentiated hemisphere. The patient has a single ventricle, representing both lateral ventricles and the third ventricle. There are grades of severity of the malformation. In some cases of holoprosencephaly the children had trisomy 13y. In some cases these children have had only one eye, cyclopia, and a proboscis-like nose with only a single nostril.

Lissencephaly (Agyri-Pachygyri). The brain has failed to form sulci and gyri and corresponds to a 12-week embryo. There are usually also dysmorphic facial features. In some cases a few gyri do form. Neuronal migration has been arrested at this stage due to a chromosomal defect, ischemia, or infection. The studies of Reiner et al. (1993) have

Figure 4.14 Schizencephaly (*A*) 3D reconstruction with (*B*) coronal view. MRI, T2. (Courtesy of Dr Val Runge, University of Kentucky Medical Center.)

identified a specific gene deletion at chromosome 17 region p13.3, the LIS-1 gene.

Micropolygyria (Fig. 4.14). The gyri are more numerous, smaller, and more poorly developed than normal.

Macrogyria. The gyri are broader and less numerous than in the normal brain.

Microencephaly. This is another abnormal defect in which development of the brain is rudimentary and the individual has a low-grade intelligence.

Porencephaly. There are symmetrical cavities in the cortex due to the absence of cortex and white matter in these sites.

Schizencephaly (Fig. 4.15). There is an incomplete development of the cerebral hemispheres with the presence of abnormal gyri. The patient is usually retarded.

Agenesis of Corpus Callosum (Fig. 4.16). There is a complete or partial absence of the corpus callosum and septum pellucidum (see also Fig. 21.1).

The following case is an example of agenesis of the corpus callosum.

Figure 4.16 Agenesis of corpus callosum. (Courtesy of Dr. John Hills, New England Medical Center Hospitals.)

Figure 4.15 Micropolygyri. (Courtesy of Dr. John Hills, New England Medical Center.)

CASE HISTORY 4.2: AGENESIS OF CORPUS CALLOSUM (PATIENT OF DR. SANDRA HOROWITZ)

This 20-year-old female warehouse employee was referred for re-evaluation of generalized convulsive seizures that had developed at age 3 years. She had been seizure-free for 5 years. She had mild developmental delays. Full-scale Wechsler Adult Intelligence score IQ was 82, with a verbal score of 88 and a performance score of 77 (all were within low-average range). She demonstrated complete agenesis of the corpus callosum with associated alterations of gyral and sulcal patterns.

Midline sagittal section T1 weighted.

Holoprosencephaly. Only a single forebrain has formed. This deficit is also commonly accompanied by a deficit in medial facial development (Fig. 4.17). This 10-month-old white male had severe spastic diplegia (a form of "cerebral palsy") and severe developmental delays. A computerized tomography (CT) scan demonstrated a fusion of the two lateral ventricles and no frontal horns. A large cystic area extended superiorly and posteriorly.

Figure 4.17 Holoprosencephaly. (*A*) View of frontal poles. (*B*) Coronal section. Note the absence of any differentiation of the hemispheres. (Courtesy of Dr. John Hills, New England Medical Center Hospitals.)

Cerebellar Agenesis. Portions of the cerebellum, deep cerebellar nuclei, and even the pons are either absent or malformed. In some instances portions of the basal ganglia and brain stem and spinal cord may also be malformed or absent.

The cerebellar cortex forms differently than the cerebrum by migration of primitive cells from the rhombic lip of the brain stem. These cells form a layer called the external granular cell layer. From this layer, cells then migrate inward to form the internal granular cell layer.

ENVIRONMENTALLY INDUCED MIGRATION DISORDER: FETAL ALCOHOL SYNDROME

Fetal alcohol syndrome (FAS), which results when mothers drink alcohol excessively during pregnancy, causes one of the more common nongenetic causes of mental retardation (one out of 300 to 2000 live births, or up to 2%). There are other environmentally generated disorders, but FAS has the clearest etiology. The current recommendation is for pregnant women to avoid all alcohol, especially during the first trimester, or to cut back to no more than two drinks per day. Pregnant alcoholics are at high risk for premature delivery.

In FAS, pre- and postnatal growth retardation occurs along with cardiovascular, limb, and craniofacial abnormalities, such as a short palpebral fissure, thin vermillion border, and smooth philtrum. Children often have impaired fine and gross movements and developmental deficits. Microcephaly, heterotopias, and lissencephaly have been reported (Greenfield, 1992). Related to the problem of FAS is the huge rise in "cocaine babies," which have similar deficits that require lifetime care.

MALFORMATIONS RESULTING FROM CHROMOSOMAL TRISOMY AND TRANSLOCATION

Through advances in molecular biology, more and more genetic defects are being localized to specific genes. For example, in translocation syndromes like trisomy 21 (Down's syndrome), one chromosomal segment is transferred to a nonhomologous chromosome; this is called a Robertsonian translocation and most commonly affects chromosomes 13, 14, 15, 18, 21, and 22. Other defects, such as trisomy 18 (Edwards' syndrome) and trisomy 13 (Patau's syndrome), have similar neurologic findings.

Most children with Down's syndrome are moderately mentally retarded and of short stature. They have hypoplastic facies with short noses, small ears with prominent antihelices, and prominent epicanthal folds (which perhaps suggested the now outdated term *Mongolism*). Other defects include a protruding lower lip, a fissured and thickened tongue, and a simian crease on the palm. A predisposition to leukemia and congenital heart defects often proves fatal. Children with Down's syndrome constitute about 5% of children in institutions for the mentally retarded.

The brains of these children show little gross abnormality. The frontal and occipital poles are rounder than normal and the superior temporal gyrus is thinner. Conventional stains show the brain to be normal histologically, but the Golgi stain, which specifically impregnates axons and dendrites, shows sparser dendritic arborizations, fewer dendritic spines, and more anomalous spines (Becker et al., 1986; Marin-Papilla, 1972).

Patients who reach middle age may develop a degenerative disease of the nervous system called Alzheimer's disease (see Chapter 30 on dementia).

MALFORMATIONS RESULTING FROM DEFECTIVE FUSION OF DORSAL STRUCTURES

Spinal Bifida

In spinal bifida, the most common malformation in this category, the arches and dorsal spines of the vertebrae are absent. Often the bony deficit alone is present. The spinal cord, however, may be malformed either at one level or at many levels. In some instances the spinal cord, nerve root, and meninges have herniated through the midline defect in the skin and bone—meningomyelocele (Fig. 4.18). In other instances only the meninges have herniated through the midline defect; the sac is called a meningocele.

Cranial Bifida

Cranial bifida is less common the spinal bifida and usually occurs only in the suboccipital region. The cranial bones

Figure 4.18 Meningomyelocele at sacral level of the spinal cord. Arrow refers to sac, meninges, neural tissue, and overlying skin. (Courtesy of Dr. John Hills, New England Medical Center Hospitals.)

either fail to fuse or do not form. The abnormality may only be restricted to the underlying portion of the cerebrum, or it may be accompanied by a herniation of meninges (meningocele) or meninges and brain tissue (encephalocele). Cranial bifida is commonly associated with hydrocephalus and extensive brain damage.

Arnold-Chiari Malformation

In this condition there is elongation and displacement of the brain stem and a portion of the cerebellum through the foramen magnum into the cervical region of the vertebral canal. Hydrocephalus, spina bifida with meningocele, or meningomyelocele may also be associated with this abnormality, which may be fatal or produce neurological symptoms due to compression of the cervical roots and the overcrowding of the neural tissue in the posterior fossa (Fig. 9.13).

MALFORMATIONS CHARACTERIZED BY EXCESSIVE GROWTH OF ECTODERMAL AND MESODERMAL TISSUE AFFECTING SKIN, NERVOUS SYSTEM, AND OTHER TISSUES

These neurocutaneous disorders are referred to as phacomatosis (mother spot). They are all characterized by hereditary transmission, involvement of multiple organs, and a slow evolution of the disorder during the childhood and adolescent years. Due to maldevelopment, benign tumors are formed— referred to as hamartomas (body defect tumor). Moreover, there is a tendency to malignant transformation.

Tuberous Sclerosis

The triad of seizures, mental retardation, and a skin disorder called "adenoma sebaceous" characterizes this autosomal dominant disorder. The skin disorder involves the formation of nodules over the face, which are composed of angiofibromas. Within the nervous system, the nodules are usually present in a periventricular subependymal location composed of glioblast and neuroblasts. Other nodules may be present in the cerebral cortex. Giant neurons and astrocytes may be present. As these nodules (tubers) expand, the ventricular system may be blocked. Rarely malignant transformation occurs. The abnormal gene has been isolated to chromosome 9. In some manner this gene location may control an inhibitory factor. When defective, excessive growth occurs.

Neurofibromatosis (von Recklinghausen's Disease)

Two types of neurofibromatosis have been described. Type I is related to a gene locus on chromosome 17. This autosomal dominant disorder is characterized by the proliferation of cells derived from the neural crest. The cells identified in this defect include Schwann cells, melanocytes, and endoneurial fibroblasts. The presence of melanocytes produces multiple areas of skin with hyperpigmented (cafe au lait spots). Multiple tumors form in the cutaneous and subcutaneous tissues. The subcutaneous lesions may be discrete tumors and may be attached to a nerve or more diffuse—described as plexiform neuromas. The latter may produce considerable distortion of face and body. Tumors may involve peripheral, spinal, or cranial nerves. Tumors of glial and meningeal origin also occur within the central nervous system.

Type II is characterized by bilateral acoustic neuromas and has been identified with a gene locus on chromosome 22. (Case history examples and additional discussion will be found in Chapters 9, 15, and 27.)

CUTANEOUS ANGIOMATOSIS WITH ASSOCIATED MALFORMATIONS OF THE CENTRAL NERVOUS SYSTEM

Various disorders are included in this category. Often some type of vascular anomaly affecting skin (a vascular nevus) is associated with a malformation in the affected areas of the nervous system. Hemangiomas of the spinal cord may be associated with a congenital vascular nevus in the corresponding dermatome.

Sturge-Weber Syndrome

Patients with this abnormality have a large, deep port red wine nevus over much of the forehead corresponding to the distribution of the ophthalmic branch of the trigeminal nerve. The vascular malformation involves the meninges overlying the parieto-occipital cortex. In this cortical region there is calcification of the second and third layers with neuronal degeneration and proliferation of reactive glial. Atrophy occurs in the cerebrum. The specific genetic basis of this syndrome is uncertain.

MALFORMATIONS RESULTING FROM ABNORMALITIES IN THE VENTRICULAR SYSTEM

Syringomyelia

In this condition the spinal canal is abnormally large. The cavity may enlarge to destroy parts or all of the gray matter and adjacent white matter, producing a characteristic "cape-like deficit" in pain sensation (Chapter 9).

Syringobulbia

In this condition there are abnormal slit-like cavities extending from the fourth ventricle into the subjacent tegmentum of the medulla (most common) and pons, disrupting gray and white matter with accompanying cranial nerve and long tract signs (Chapter 9).

Hydrocephalus

Any abnormality in absorption of cerebrospinal fluid that produces increased cerebrospinal fluid pressure and dilation of the ventricular system is called hydrocephalus. Blockage of the flow in the ventricular system is called noncommunicating hydrocephalus, while blockage of the cerebrospinal fluid in the subarachnoid space is called communicating hydrocephalus.

Noncommunicating hydrocephalus may be caused by a cerebrospinal fluid blockage at the interventricular foramen, the cerebral aqueduct, or in the fourth ventricle, as well as by a malformation of any portion of the ventricular system. The passageways connecting the fourth ventricle to the subarachnoid space (foramina of Luschka and Magendie) may be blocked or ill formed (as in the Dandy-Walker malformation; Fig. 4.19).

Communicating hydrocephalus is caused by the inability of fluid to pass from the subarachnoid space into the venous channels (via the arachnoid granulations), or the malformation of the arachnoid villi produces excess fluid in the subarachnoid space with resultant pressure on the central nervous system. Obliteration of the subarachnoid cisterns or of the subarachnoid channels may produce this syndrome.

Figure 4.19 Noncommunicating hydrocephalus, Dandy-Walker syndrome. (Courtesy of Dr. John Hills, New England Medical Center Hospitals.)

Hydrocephalus can produce thinning out of the bones of the skull with a prominent forehead and atrophy of the cerebral cortex and white matter, compression of the basal ganglia and diencephalon, and herniation of the brain into the foramen magnum. Prior to closure of the sutures, such pressure will result in an increase in the size of the head. Depending on the severity of the brain damage, the infant may die or survive with mental retardation, spasticity, ataxia, and other defects.

BIBLIOGRAPHY

Adams, R., and Sidman, R. L. 1968. Introduction to Neuropathology. New York, NY: McGraw-Hill.

Bamberger, M. E., and Landreth, G. E. 2000. Inflammation, apopotosis and Alzheimer's disease. Neuroscientist 8:276–283.

Becker, L. E., Armstrong, D. L., and Chan, F. 1986. Dendritic atrophy in children with Down's syndrome. Ann. Neurol. 20:520.

Berry, M., and Rogers, A.W. 1966. Histogenesis of mammalian neocortex. In R. Hassler and H. Stephans (Eds.) Evolution of the Forebrain, p. 197. New York, NY: Plenum Press.

Crelin, E. S. 1974. Development of the nervous system. CIBA Clin Symp. 26(2).

Goodman, C. S.1994. The likeness of being: phylogenetically conserved molecular mechanisms of growth cone guidance. Cell 78:353–356.

Greenfield's Neuropatholgy, 5th ed. 1992. New York, NY:, Oxford University Press.

Jacobson, M. 1978. Developmental Neurobiology. 2nd ed. New York, NY: Plenum Press.

Lemire, R. J. 1975. Normal and abnormal development of the human nervous system. New York, NY: Harper & Row.

Majon, G., and Joris, I. 1995. Review. Apoptosis, oncosis, and necrosis. An overview of cell death. Amer. J. Path. 146:3–15.

Marin-Padilla, M.1972. Structural abnormalities of the cerebral cortex in human chromosomal aberrations: a Golgi study. Brain Res. 44:625.

Rakic, P. 1972. Mode of cell migration in the superficial layers of fetal monkey neocortex. J. Comp Neurol. 145:61–84.

Reiner, R., Carrazo, C. Y., Shen, Y., Weinnert, M., Fanstmetta, F., and Dubyns, W. B. 1993. Isolation of a Miller Dieker Lissencephaly gene containing G protein beta-subunit-like repeats. Nature 364:717.

Serafinin, T., Kennedy, T. E., Galko, M. J., Mirzayan, C., Jessell, T. M., and Tessler-Lavigne, M. 1994. The netrins define a family of axon outgrowth-promoting proteins homologous to C. elegans UNC-6. Cell 78:409–424.

Sonj, H. J., Ssstevesn, C. F., and Gage, F. H. 2002. Neural stem cells from adult hippocampus develop essential properties of fucnitons CNS neurons. Nature Neurosci. 5:438–445.

Taylor, R. 1993. Cell death makes for lively research. J. NIH. Res 5:59–62.

Victor, M., and Ropper, A. 2001. Principals of Neurology. 7th ed. New York, NY: McGraw Hill.

5.

SKELETAL MUSCLE AND NERVE-MUSCLE JUNCTION

Skeletal muscles are the major ending of the efferent branch of the central nervous system. We work our will upon the outside world through these muscles. Skeletal muscles occupy about 80% of the total weight of the body. They use about 6% of the resting oxygen consumption to maintain ionic gradients; after strenuous exercise they may use as much as 70% of the oxygen consumption. Each anatomic muscle is delimited by strong fascial sheets and has a characteristic origin and insertion. The basic unit of the muscle is the muscle fiber or cell that runs from one end of the muscle to the other end and has a diameter of 50 to 100 μm.

MOTOR UNITS

Anatomic muscles are subdivided into bundles of many fibers (Fig. 5.1). Each muscle fiber is innervated by only one motor nerve fiber. Groups of muscle fibers are delimited functionally by their nervous innervation. As Figure 5.1 shows, the motor nerve branches and innervates a number of muscle fibers. The muscle fibers that are innervated by a single motor neuron are called a motor unit or group. All these fibers act in the same manner since a single nerve controls them. The number of muscle fibers in a motor unit varies from 300 to 400 in the gastrocnemius (calf) muscle to 4 to 6 in the extraocular muscles. In general, the size of the muscle group is proportioned to the delicacy of the required movement. The extraocular muscles make very small, fine adjustments; the gastrocnemius muscle makes coarse, powerful movements.

When the motor nerve is stimulated, an action potential travels down the axon until it reaches the end-plate region, where it releases a chemical transmitter, acetylcholine. The acetylcholine diffuses to a specialized portion of the muscle surface, the motor end plate, and initiates a second action potential on the surface membrane of the muscle fiber. We will discuss the motor endplate in greater detail later in the chapter.

CONTRACTION

The action potential travels along the muscle surface from the end-plate region with a conduction velocity of about 1 meter/sec. The response to a single stimulus, either to the motor nerve or to the muscle surface, is called a twitch. Muscle activity usually occurs in response to a series of action potentials, a partial or complete tetanus as illustrated in Figure 5.2B–D. It can be seen that increasing the frequency of stimulation to a muscle increases the tension generated. Since motor units are in parallel, their tension is additive. The total tension a muscle produces is primarily a function of the number of motor units activated.

Sarcomeres and Filaments

When we study the structure of the muscle fiber, the mechanism of contraction becomes clearer. Figure 5.3A–D shows the structure of a 100-μm diameter muscle fiber and its component 1-μm myofibrils. The banded pattern (D) is clearly seen in the light microscope in either single living fibers or fixed and stained material. A dark A band alternates with a light I band. The I band is bisected by a thin, dark Z disk. The basic contractile unit is a length of myofibril from Z line to Z line called a sarcomere. After isolation, this unit, 1 μm in diameter and 2.5 μm long, will still contract.

At higher magnification, in the electron microscope (Fig 5.3E), it is clear that the bulk of the muscle structure is made up of two types of filaments. The larger of these filaments, the thick filament, is 10 nm in diameter and 1.5 μm long and is located entirely within the A band. Indeed, all of the properties of the A band can be attributed to these filaments. The thin filaments are 4 nm in diameter and 1.0 μm long and run from the Z line various distances into the A band. During contraction the thin filaments are pulled past the thick filaments to reduce sarcomere length.

Figure 5.1 The organization of muscle fibers into structural units, muscle bundles, and functional units, motor groups.

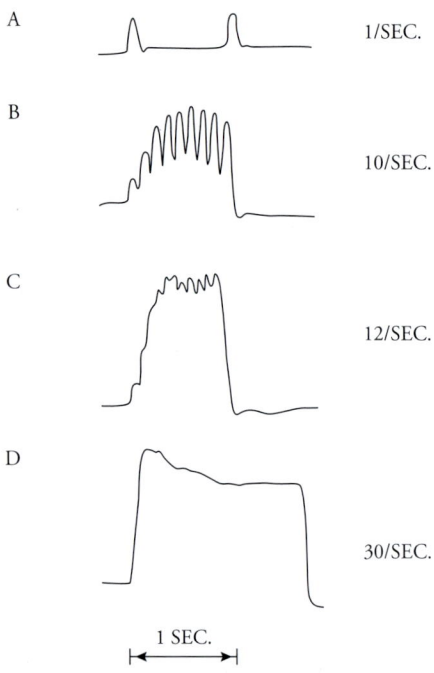

Figure 5.2 Isometric tension in response to stimuli of constant voltage and a varying frequency. Note that the total tension is greater when the frequency of stimulation is increased until a maximum (tetanus) tension is reached. Record from a human flexor carpi radialis muscle in situ. The subject's arm was held to a table with adhesive tape; stimulation was via a carbon electrode over the muscle mass in the upper forearm and a large electrocardiogram electrode at the wrist. The tension transducer was in contact with the styloid process on the wrist below the base of the thumb. Both wrist and finger flexors can be stimulated by this method.

EXCITATION CONTRACTION COUPLING

Muscle activation begins when an action potential spreads over the surface and then into the depth of each fiber. Calcium released from intracellular structures allows the thick and thin filaments to interact, produce tension, and shorten. Contraction ceases when Ca^{++} is transported into the same intracellular structures.

Reticular Structures

Skeletal muscle has an enlarged and specialized reticular network that is shown in Figure 5.4. It can be subdivided into two portions: the transverse tubules or T system and sarcoplasmic reticulum (SR). The T system is a tubular network that is continuous across the whole fiber and contains extracellular fluid. If a perfect cross section were cut across the fiber, the T system would look like a chicken-wire fence with the fibrils running through the holes in the wire. The sarcoplasmic reticulum wraps around the myofibrils like the bun around a hot dog.

The (T) system conducts the surface action potential rapidly inward to initiate contraction. When small patches of the surface membrane are stimulated to induce local contraction, the sensitivity of an area depends on its location with respect to the T system. The most sensitive location varies; it is at the Z line in the frog and at the A-I junction in the lizard and many mammals (arrows, Fig. 5.4). Inward conduction is an active, Na^+ dependent process in the tubular wall, probably much like the surface action potential. Depolarization of the transverse tubular system generates a charge equal to movement signal which precedes Ca^{++} release from the SR. This charge equal to movement signal has many similarities to the gating current of the axon.

The basic ionic mechanisms underlying the muscle action potential are quite similar to those in nerve, a regenerative increase in sodium permeability (to depolarize) which quickly inactivates, followed by an increase in potassium permeability (to repolarize). In skeletal muscle there is also a large, but unchanging, chloride permeability which participates in the repolarization phase. Chloride is in equilibrium across the membrane at a resting potential of –90 mV.

The surface area of the T system gives the "surface" action potential a slow velocity (1 m/sec). Most of the potassium channels are in the T = tubule membrane so the potassium efflux during the falling phase of the action potential is into the lumen of the T system. After several action potentials, K^+ builds up in the T lumen and begins to depolarize the fiber. In normal muscles this depolarization is not large and is buffered by the chloride conductance in the surface membrane.

Myotonia

In muscle fibers from myotonic goats the potassium buildup in the T tubules causes a significant depolarization, and action potentials continue to fire after stimulation ceases. Much the same result is obtained when normal fibers are placed in chloride-free solution.

T-SR COUPLING

The structure of the T system–terminal cisternae junction is shown in Figure 5.5A. The T tubule runs vertically in the center. The T system is ovoid and the portion adjacent to the terminal cisternae contains prominent particles.

The terminal cisternae (tc) of the sarcoplasmic reticulum shows a rich array of structures, which appear as either pits or particles depending upon the plane of fracture. At the T-tc junction are "feet," which create a distinct morphological gap. The terminal cisternae do not participate in any of the electrical events of the muscle fiber, indicating there is no ionic connection between the two. The feet are the site of Ca^{++} release from the SR that initiates contraction. After Ca^{++} is released from the terminal cisternae, the Ca^{++} concentration in the sarcoplasm rapidly builds up, as shown in Figure 5.6, well in advance of tension generation.

The ultimate result of the depolarization of the T system is Ca^{++} release from the terminal cisternae. How depolarization-induced charge movement in the T system walls induces release of Ca^{++} from the SR is far from clear. One of the authors suspects there is a chemical transmission and Ca^{++} is the first messenger. Other authors suggest a molecular rod that spans the foot process that controls calcium release from the SR.

Dantroline sodium (Dantrium) is a muscle-relaxing drug that acts directly upon the muscle fiber. One-half hour after a

SKELETAL MUSCLE

Figure 5.3 Diagram of the organization of skeletal muscle from the gross to the molecular level. A is the gross deltoid muscle, B are the muscle fascicles, C show the muscle fibers, D demonstrate the myofibrils and E show the myofilaments with F, G, H, and I are cross sections at the levels indicated. (Drawing by Sylvia Colard Keene from Bloom and Fawcett: A Textbook of Histology. Philadelphia, W.B. Saunders, 1968.)

clinical dose, the twitch tension is half its normal value; recovery occurs within 24 hours. Dantrolene sodium acts to reduce the amount of Ca^{++} released per action potential, largely by blocking release of Ca^{++} from the terminal cisternae.

The large particles elsewhere in the SR membrane are the site where Ca^{++} from the sarcoplasm is taken back into the SR, bringing about relaxation.

MOLECULAR ARCHITECTURE OF CONTRACTION

MUSCLE PROTEINS

Four major protein types have been extracted from skeletal muscle: actin, myosin, tropomyosin, and troponin. The first two are the major protein constituents; the others are a relatively small fraction of the protein. Myosin has a molecular weight of 420 kD and contains two quite different regions; a long double helical tail and a dual-headed structure containing both the ATPase and actin binding activities. Figure 5.3L–N shows the packing of the myosin molecules within the thick filaments of the band. The myosin molecule can be readily divided into two subunits—heavy and light meromyosin. The heavy meromyosin retains the adenosine triphosphatase (ATPase) and actin binding activity of the intact myosin. This fragment forms the bridges between this and the filaments. Light meromyosin rods aggregate to form a tension-bearing rod, the thick filament.

Actin has a molecular weight of 60 kD and readily forms long chains of a fibrous protein (Fig. 5.3J–K). Two chains of F-actin, wound around each other, form the thin filaments along with tropomyosin and troponin. These two regulatory

Figure 5.4 Schematic representation of the distribution of the sarcoplasmic reticulum around the myofibrils of skeletal muscle. The longitudinal sarcotubules are confluent with transverse elements called the terminal cisternae. A slender transverse tubule (T tubule) extending inward from the sarcolemma is flanked by two terminal cisternae to form the so-called triads of the reticulum. The location of these with respect to the cross-banded pattern of the myofibrils varies from species to species. In frog muscle, depicted here, the triads are at the Z line. In mammalian muscle there are two to each sarcomere, located at the A-I junctions. (Modified after L. Peachey, from Fawcett, D.W., and McNutt, S.: J. Cell Biol., 25:209, 1965. Drawn by Sylvia Colard Keene.)

proteins alter the ATPase activity of the actin-myosin complex so that calcium ions are required for ATP breakdown and consequently for muscle activity.

The immediate energy source for contraction is ATP and muscle converts chemical to mechanical energy with

Figure 5.5 (A) The T system–terminal cisternae junction. A freeze fracture study showing the T system running vertically flanked by terminal cisternae. (B) A cross sectional drawing showing the fracture planes at AA and BB. Fracture lines follow the hydrophobic (center) line of the membrane. The foot processes of the SR are stippled. (Electron micrograph courtesy of Clara Franzini-Armstrong, Ph.D., University of Pennsylvania, Philadelphia, PA.)

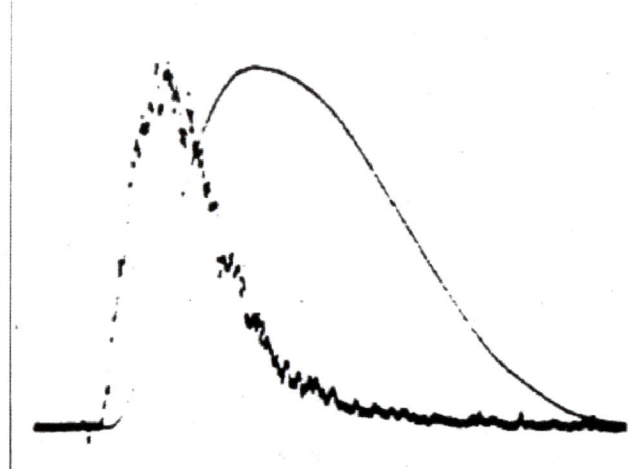

Figure 5.6 The broken line shows the average light emission from Ca^{++} sensitive protein aequorin inside a muscle fiber while the solid line is the twitch tension. Aequorin, a protein extracted from a luminescent jellyfish, emits light in proportion to Ca^{++} concentration. The light emission, hence the increasing calcium concentration within the fiber, proceeds the tension generation (solid line). (From Blinks, JR, R. Rudel, and SR Taylor, J. Physiol. 277:291–323, 1978.)

an efficiency of about 50%. Intact muscle contains relatively large quantities of creatine phosphate, an energy storage protein.

CA^{++}–TROPONIN INTERACTION

Free Ca^{++} binds to troponin on the thin filaments causing the troponin-tropomyosin to "roll-back" from the active site of actin. Actin and myosin can now interact, bridges can form, and tension is generated. The interaction continues for as long as the Ca^{++} remains elevated. In the twitch shown in Figure 5.6, Ca^{++} is rapidly taken up by the sarcoplasmic reticulum and tension declines. During tetanic stimulation, Ca^{++} remains elevated. After the surface membrane and reticulum have been removed by chemical treatment, tension generation is related to Ca^{++} concentration (Fig. 5.7). Tension is maintained for as long as Ca^{++} is present.

FILAMENT INTERACTION

A muscle fiber shortens when thin filaments slide past thick filaments. In this manner the distance between individual Z lines (sarcomere length) decreases. The decrease in muscle length is proportional to the product of the decrease per sarcomere and the number of sarcomeres per muscle.

Cross sections through the array of thick and thin filaments are shown in Figure 5.8F–I. Each set of filaments is arranged in a basically hexagonal array. In the region of overlap, section I, each of the thin filaments has three thick filaments and each neighboring thick filament has six thin filaments. Contact between the filaments is made by cross bridges (Fig. 5.8). These bridges stick out from the thick filaments and are arranged in a six-fold helix, like the treads on a spiral staircase. In this case, the stairs make a complete revolution in six steps.

Figure 5.7 A view of the central region of the band at 600,000× magnification. The projections from the thick filaments, the bridges, are the site of interaction between the thick and thin filaments. (From Huxley, H.E.: J. Biophys. Biochem. Cytol., 3:631, 1957.)

CROSS-BRIDGES

It is the interaction between the two filament arrays that produces tension; the bridges (Fig. 5.8) of the thick filaments "hook on" to and move the thin filaments. The three-dimensional structure of the heavy meromyosin (Fig. 5.3), which contains both the actin and ATP binding sites, has recently been worked out. There is a prominent cleft near the actin binding site: when it is closed (Fig. 5.9A), actin-myosin binding is strong; when it is open (Fig. 5.9B), binding is weak. A lateral pocket contains the ATP binding site; closing of the ATP binding pocket imparts a curvature to the head and a 5 nm movement of the actin binding site along the actin chain (Fig. 5.9B>C). Fig. 6.9 shows a molecular model of bridge interaction consisting of actin-myosin dissociation with ATP binding (A>B), curving of the bridge with P hydrolysis to move the myosin head 5 nm along the actin chain (B>C), head reattachment (D), and finally the power stroke as ADP dissociates (D>E).

Length–Tension Relation

Tension production, then, should be related to the number of bridges connected to thin filaments, to the degree of overlap of actin and myosin filaments, and to the sarcomere spacing. When resting muscle is fixed at various sarcomere spacing, the length of each set of filaments remains constant, as does their diameter (Fig. 5.10). The amount of overlap between the thick and thin filaments varies in direct proportion to sarcomere

Figure 5.8 The power cycle of the bridge unit of myosin. (A) The cleft between the two domains of the myosin head is closed and the myosin head is attached to an actin monomer (speckled for identification). The ATP binding pocket is open. As ATP begins binding (B), the cleft opens and the myosin head unbinds from actin. As ATP binding is completed and P hydrolysis occurs, the ATP pocket closes and the myosin head changes curvature (C) to move 5 nm along the actin chains, to bring it into alignment with the next actin monomer. As the P leaves (D), the cleft closes and the head attaches to the next actin monomer. As ADP is released (E), the pocket opens, the myosin head straightens forcing the actin chain up by 5 nm, the power stroke. (Adapted from Rayment et al., Science 261:50–65, 1993.)

length, but the A bandwidth remains constant during contraction. Experiments with contracting isolated fibrils also show the bandwidth with the I band decreases in width with decreasing sarcomere spacing. When the sarcomere spacing is just greater than the sum of the lengths of the I band filaments (3.6 μm), there should be no overlap, no bridge interaction, and consequently no tension production (Fig. 5.9B). As the sarcomere spacing decreases, the number of bridges increases and so does the tension. The number of bridges and the tension increase until all of the bridges are attached. There are no bridges in the center of the band, as can be seen in Figure 5.8.

Further shortening gives no increase in tension since there are no more bridges to interact. In fact, further shortening leads to decreased tension since one thin filament must force its way past its opposite filament, probably disturbing the bridge filament interaction. Further shortening also requires compression of the band filaments, and most of the tension that is produced goes to compress the thick filaments.

Force–Velocity Relation

We have concentrated so far on the generation of tension at constant length; to do useful work, the muscle must shorten. When a muscle shortens against a very light load, it shortens very quickly. As the load increases, the velocity decreases.

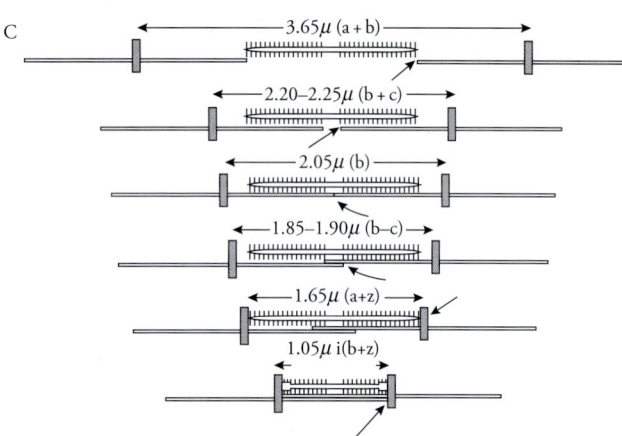

Figure 5.9 The length tension curve (*A*) and electron micrographs (*B–D*) of skeletal muscle showing the overlap of the sliding filaments. When the filaments barely overlap (*B*), tension is low. When all bridges are attached (*C*), tension is maximum. When the thin filaments overlap. (Data from AL Gordon, AF Huxley, and FJ Julian. J. Physiol. 184:170–192, 1966. Electron micrographs courtesy of Brenda Eisenberg, Ph.D., University of Illinois College of Medicine, Chicago, IL.)

A force-velocity curve is shown in Figure 5.10. A human forearm was pulling against increasingly heavy weights. The same curve can be obtained with an isolated muscle; maximum tension and maximum speed will vary, however, from muscle to muscle.

The force-velocity curve is described by the equation

$$(P + a)(V + b) = (P_o + a)b$$

where P is the force, P_o is the isometric tetanic force, V is the velocity of shortening, and a and b are constants. The constants, a and b, can be fitted uniquely and are a major goal for theoretical models of muscle function.

ACTIVE STATE

When the bridges from the thick filaments interact with the thin filaments, they develop tension 3 to 5 msec after the action potential runs along the surface. Tension cannot,

Figure 5.10 Calculated values for bridge tension, length of series elastic component, and tension. Note especially that a second stimulus can capitalize upon extension of the series elastic element and thereby increase the tension at the tendon. (F.J. Julian, Harvard Medical School, kindly supplied these records. For further details of the computation, see Julian, F.J.: Biophysical J. 9:547, 1969.)

however, be measured in the tendon for 10 to 20 msec following stimulation. What causes the delay? There is a great deal of elastic material in series with the tension-generating element, some indeed in the bridges themselves. The tension produced by the bridges must first stretch the elastic material before it can be transmitted to the tendon and the load. Consider for a moment a person pulling a stretchy nylon rope that is attached to a large rock. At first the rope stretches; only after a delay does it transmit the full force of his pull. Remember that a pull of a given force will extend the rope to a characteristic length and no further, but the stretching will take time.

Let us return to the case of the muscle. Following a single stimulus, the bridges generate their maximum tension for a very short time (Fig. 5.10). This short phase corresponds to the active state in of A.V. Hill's model. The tension is mainly expended in stretching the series elasticity; about one-half of the bridge tension appears as tendon tension. If a second stimulus follows soon after the first, the renewed bridge tension pulls on partially extended elastic elements and consequently must do less work on them to transmit tension to the tendon; more of the bridge tension is applied to the tendon. If a third stimulus follows the first two, the work the bridges do on the series elastic elements is further reduced; consequently, the work done and tension produced on the tendon is much greater during a tetanus (Fig. 5.10D) than during a twitch.

NERVE-MUSCLE JUNCTION

THE ENDPLATE

To return to the control of skeletal muscle contraction, the motor nerve enters the muscle, branches, and forms a very close junction, a synapse, with the center of each muscle fiber. The axon (presynaptic element) and muscle (postsynaptic element) remain two distinctly separate cells. The structure of the region is shown in Figure 5.11. Transmission between the axon and muscle is by means of the chemical acetylcholine (ACh).

Acetylcholine

To be considered a transmitter, a substance must meet four criteria: (a) it must be effective at the postsynaptic surface, (b) it must be liberated by the presynaptic surface in response to and in proportion to nerve stimulation, (c) there must be an enzyme system for destroying or reabsorbing liberated transmitter, and (d) there must be an enzyme system for synthesizing the transmitter.

Each of these criteria has been met by acetylcholine at the nerve-muscle junction. The idea of a chemical transmitter between nerve and muscle came from experiments by Otto Loewi in 1921 that demonstrated the slowing of the heart when the vagus nerve was stimulated. He noticed that Ringer's solution that had dripped over a slowed heart caused a second heart to slow as well. The only link between the two hearts was the Ringer's solution. Vagal stimulation liberated acetylcholine into the solution that affected the second heart. Acetylcholine can be collected from small veins in stimulated muscles.

Acetylcholine is effective in stimulating contraction if it is injected very close to the muscle. When acetylcholine is microinjected onto an excised muscle, it elicits contraction only when injected at the end-plate region. The rest of a normal muscle does not have ACh receptors. Both biochemical and histochemical studies show the presence of a cleaving enzyme, acetylcholine esterase, at the myoneuronal junction. It is present in both the postsynaptic surfaces in the subneural folds and on the presynaptic side. It is also present in fairly high concentration in the blood, which explains the general ineffectiveness of acetylcholine when injected intra-arterially.

Another enzyme, choline acetylase, reconstitutes the acetylcholine into the synaptic vesicles. The enzymes that produce the vesicles are produced in the nerve cell body; the number of vesicles decreases rapidly after section of the motor nerve. When an action potential enters the presynaptic terminal, the accompanying depolarization opens voltage-gated calcium channels. Increasing intracellular Ca^{++} is essential for neurotransmitter release, catalyzing the fusion of synaptic vesicles with the surface membrane to release ACh into the synaptic cleft (Fig. 5.12).

Acetylcholine acts on the postsynaptic membrane and destroys its selective permeability to all small ions. The membrane has an equilibrium voltage of zero millivolts. This voltage is, of course, never reached, but it would be if acetylcholine were continuously applied to the end plate. The high concentration of acetylcholine esterase prevents such an event. The depolarization brought about by the usual amount of acetylcholine causes a current to flow to the surrounding muscle fiber surface. As the current flows through the peripheral

Figure 5.11 Schematic representations of the motor end plate as seen by light and electron microscopy. (*A*) End plate as seen in histological sections in the long axis of the muscle fiber. (*B*) As seen in surface view with the light microscope. (*C*) As seen in an electron micrograph of an area such as that in the rectangle on *A*. (After R. Couteaux. From Bloom and Fawcett: A Textbook of Histology. Philadelphia, W.B. Saunders, 1968.)

Figure 5.12 A cartoon of a single acetylcholine-activated channel. Each channel has two acetylcholine binding sites—one on the cytoplasmic side of each alpha subunit. (From Miles, K. and R.L. Huganir, Molecular Neurobiology 2:91–124, 1988.)

membrane, it depolarizes that membrane and sets up a propagated action potential. The end-plate region itself is not electrically excitable; current must flow to the surrounding area, which contains classical sodium channels that must be repolarized before it can fire again.

Acetylcholine-Activated Channels

The receptor and channel are contained in a single transmembrane protein aggregate (Fig. 5.12) made up of five subunits, each of which is thought to contain three alpha helical columns with a 0.7 nm channel down the center. The receptors on the alpha subunits are some 6 nm from the gated ionic channel that is on the cytoplasmic end of the channel.

Single-Channel Recordings

Figure 5.13 shows the channel to be either open or closed. ACh concentration alters the percentage of the time the channel is open. When a microelectrode is inserted into the end-plate region, the usual resting membrane potential is recorded. When the motor nerve is stimulated, the microelectrode records an action potential, as shown in the lower traces of Figure 5.13. Careful examination of the left-hand action potential will reveal a hump on the leading edge of the action potential. This hump is the part of the end-plate potential caused by the release of acetylcholine. It is a local change in the end-plate region; no end-plate potential is seen 2 mm away (B). The end-plate potential can be seen more clearly when curarine is applied to reduce the effectiveness of the acetylcholine and to produce a subthreshold depolarization.

Small depolarizations are recorded at times when the motor nerve is quiet. They originate in the end-plate region and can be recorded only very close to it. These miniature end-plate potentials ("minis") are quantized (Fig. 5.13). They represent the release of several vesicles of ACh. The amplitude of these potentials increases as more vesicles are released. Each pocket or vesicle releases some 10^{-17} moles of acetylcholine that results in a depolarization of 0.4 mV. An action potential arriving at the presynaptic terminal causes an increase in the rate of vesicle release so that about 100 vesicles discharge their acetylcholine over a very short interval; this amount of acetylcholine is sufficient to initiate an action potential on the muscle surface.

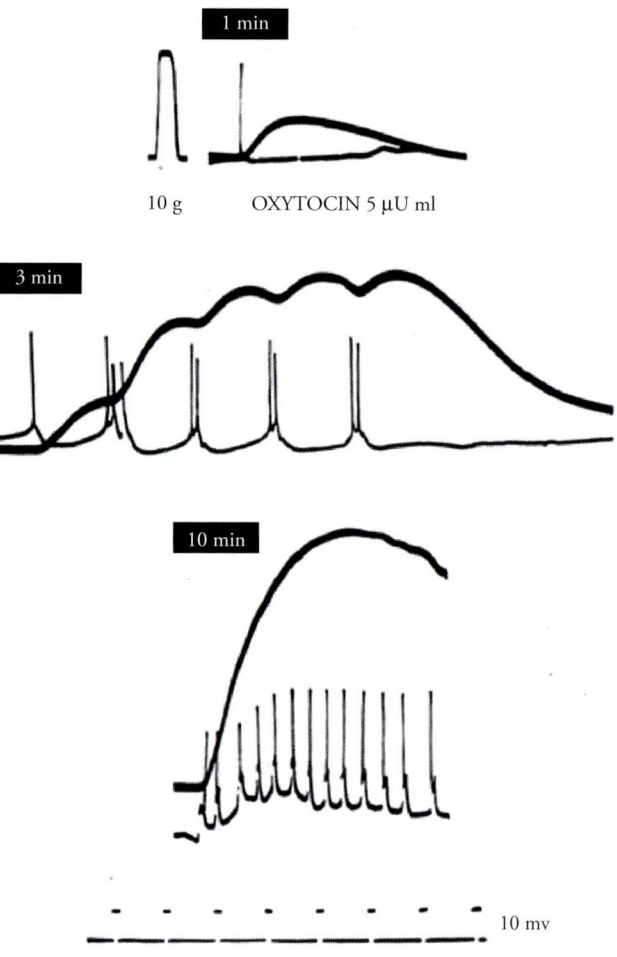

Figure 5.13 Intracellular electrical events at the end-plate regions A and B, 2 mm away. The upper traces are at high gain (3.6 mv) and slow time scale, 47 msec. In A the miniature end-plate potentials, minis, are clearly shown, whereas in B they are almost nonexistent. The two bottom traces are at low gain, 50 mv, and fast time scale, 2 msec. Note the endplate potential at the leading edge of the action potential in A. (From Fatt, P and Katz, G; J. Physiol, 117:109, 1952.)

MECHANISMS OF DRUGS ACTING ON NERVE-MUSCLE JUNCTION

DRUGS THAT COMPETE FOR RECEPTOR SITE

D-tubocurarine competes for the same postsynaptic site, as does acetylcholine; it binds more strongly to the site but does not cause a permeability change. Neuromuscular transmission is blocked because the acetylcholine cannot get to the sites. Gallamine (Flaxedil) is a synthetic d-tubocu-rarine. Several snake neurotoxins, including bungarotoxin, also bind very strongly and block the receptor. Hexamethonium and tetramethy-lammonium (TEA) also block by competitive antagonism. These drugs are slowly broken down and paralysis wears off.

Continued application of acetylcholine, and continued depolarization, does not result in continued skeletal muscle activity because the action potential mechanism must be reset after the first action potential. Any drug that produces a continual depolarization at the end plate produces a depolarization block. Nerve-muscle block and muscle relaxation should be achieved by infusing large quantities of acetylcholine, but this method is very inefficient because the acetylcholine is broken down rapidly. Succinylcholine binds to the postsynaptic surface and causes a permeability change. Since it is only slowly broken down, it produces a long-lasting depolarization. It depolarizes the muscle membrane, which contracts once and then relaxes. Decamethonium also acts in this manner.

Drugs that block the nerve-muscle junction are often used in conjunction with anesthetics to achieve muscle relaxation during surgery. It should always be borne in mind that the respiratory muscle would be blocked so that the patient must be artificially ventilated.

DRUGS THAT PROLONG THE ACTION OF ACETYLCHOLINE

Blocking the esterase activity so that the action of the released acetylcholine is prolonged can also block the end plate. The anticholinesterase, such as neostigmine, edrophonium (Tensilon), eserine, and diisopropyl fluorophosphate (DFP), all combine with acetylcholine esterase and prevent it from cleaving acetylcholine, so ACh continues to depolarize the end-plate region and to block transmission. Many insecticides block acetylcholinesterase.

Agents that block the release of acetylcholine from the presynaptic terminal will be discussed later. The various disorders affecting the neuromuscular junction are discussed in great detail later.

EFFECTS OF MOTOR NERVE ON SKELETAL MUSCLE

From the discussion so far, one might conclude that the motor nerve supplies only the stimulus to contract; this is far from the case. When the motor nerve is cut, the muscle rapidly atrophies. Its volume and strength of contraction decrease—and all of the fibers decrease in size, as does the total muscle bulk. After 3 months, the muscle bulk may have decreased to as little as 25% of its original bulk. This atrophy is not due to muscle disuse alone since disuse, such as that caused by immobilization, will cause muscle to atrophy to three-quarters of its original size in the same 3-month period. An intact motor nerve is necessary for continued survival of the muscle fiber. It would appear that the continued release of acetylcholine, or possibly some other transmitter, from the nerve is the agent responsible for this trophic influence.

DENERVATION SENSITIVITY

When the muscle is denervated, the entire surface of the muscle fiber slowly becomes sensitive to acetylcholine. After several weeks, application of acetylcholine anywhere on the surface results in an action potential and contraction. Patients who have had a motor nerve severed show great sensitivity to injected acetylcholine for this reason.

REINNERVATION

If the cut ends of a motor nerve are rejoined, sprouts from the central end will grow down the tube left by the degenerated axon. If the distance between the cut and the muscle is short and the cut ends are well aligned, the nerve will make contact with the muscle. A new end plate will form, and muscle function will be restored. Passive exercise of the muscle during regrowth is helpful to prevent disuse atrophy and contractures.

SLOW AND FAST MUSCLES

There are two sorts of skeletal muscle: red and white. The best known example of this difference is the white and dark meat of a chicken; the same qualitative differences appear in mammals.

Most muscles, particularly in mammals, are not pure red or white muscle but are made up of a mixture of fibers (Fig 5.14). The fibers in red muscles are called Type I. They are rich in mitochondria but have a relatively low myosin ATPase activity. They generate ATP from glucose as it is used. Enzymes of oxidative metabolism cause the red color. Type II fibers found in white muscles have a very active myosin ATPase activity and are relatively lacking in mitochondria. Type II fibers, which are responsive for quick, phasic contractions, depend upon an anaerobic, glycolytic metabolism; they produce large amounts of lactic acid.

Red muscle is characterized by a long twitch time, and concomitantly a low frequency of stimulation will result in tetanus. These muscles are primarily antigravity or postural muscles; their movements are characterized by long-sustained contractions. The white muscles, on the other hand, have short twitch times and are used for quick phasic movements.

The speed of contraction is determined by the pattern of activity in the motor nerve. When nerves from fast and slow muscles are crossed, the fast muscle slows down and the slow muscle speeds up (Fig. 5.14). When a limb is immobilized, the activity in motor nerves to a slow muscle, which is usually intense, decreases. After several weeks the speed of

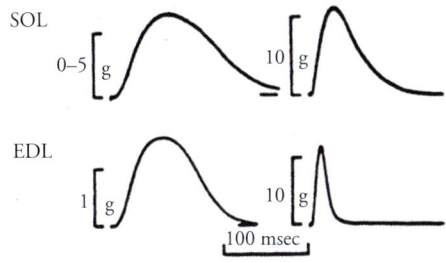

Figure 5.14 Twitch time in a fast, extensor digitorum longus (EDL) and a slow, soleus (SOL) muscle. At birth (left) the difference in twitch time is not striking, yet 5 weeks later (right) the difference is very pronounced. (From Close, R.; J. Physiol., 180:542, 1965.)

contraction has increased markedly. It is not clear how the pattern of activity alters the biochemical control mechanisms and the contractile properties of a muscle. Some authors suggest a second transmitter released in very small quantities from motor nerves is responsible for modulating which proteins are expressed from the muscle genome.

DISORDERS OF MUSCLE AND NEUROMUSCULAR JUNCTION

DISEASES OF MUSCLE

Most classifications divide these disorders into two groups: inherited and acquired (Morgan and Hughes, 1992).

Muscular Dystrophies

The major inherited diseases are the muscular dystrophies characterized by a primary degeneration of skeletal muscle. The slow but progressive destruction of muscle results in a progressive weakness initially affecting the proximal muscles.

Duchenne's Muscular Dystrophy

The most common varieties of muscular dystrophy are X linked, and almost all cases occur in males (rarely females with Turner's syndrome or X-chromosome translocation may be affected).

Duchene originally described the most common type within this group in 1868. The typical patient with Duchene's muscular dystrophy (DMD) is a boy who has delayed walking. At some point between the ages of 2 and 5 years, the patient is noted to be clumsy and slow in exercises and games. It is soon evident that proximal pelvic girdle lower extremity weakness is present. In rising from the floor the patient uses his upper extremities and hands placed on the thighs to force the body in to an erect position (Gower's sign), thus counteracting the weakness at hips and pelvis. At this point, marked enlargement of the calf muscles is present (pseudohypertrophy). With progression of the disease, increasing atrophy of muscle and increasing weakness occurs. By age 12, the patient is confined to a wheelchair. Death occurs late in the teens or early twenties from respiratory complications and/or cardiac failure (heart muscle is involved). The blood creatine kinase level while the patient is still ambulatory is at least 40 times the upper limit of normal. Levels may be 300–400 times normal. The electromyogram (EMG) demonstrates myopathic features. The muscle biopsy taken early in the course of the disease before severe atrophy is present demonstrates characteristic myopathic features including (1) widespread necrosis and phagocytosis of muscle fibers, (2) regeneration of muscle fibers, (3) marked variation in fiber size, and (4) large rounded "hypercontracted hyalinized" fibers (Fig. 5.15). In late stages replacement of muscle by proliferation of endomysial connective tissue and fat occurs.

DMD is the most common lethal, X-linked disease with an estimated incidence of 1 in 4000 live male births (see Moser, 1984). The maternal carrier can be identified based on family history and an elevated creatine kinase level in the carrier. A small percentage of carriers also have mild weakness or EMG or muscle biopsy changes. There is, however, a high frequency of isolated cases, 30%–50% suggesting a high incidence of new mutants or mutant maternal carriers. In families at risk, prenatal diagnosis is possible (Darras et al., 1987, and see later discussion).

Becker's Muscular Dystrophy

Becker's muscular dystrophy described in 1955 is a less common (1 in 20,000 male births) and less severe form of X-linked disorder. Age of onset is later; and the rate of progression is slower. The patient is still ambulatory at age 15. Life expectancy is only slightly reduced. Creatine kinase levels are markedly increased. The EMG demonstrates myopathic features. The muscle biopsy indicates features that are similar but less marked than those noted earlier.

Recent major advances have been made in our understanding of the genetics and molecular biology of these disorders (Arahata et al., 1989; Hoffman et al., 1988; see also review of Rowland, 1988). The precise locus has been identified: the short arm of the X chromosome at the region designated as Xp 21. The specific affected gene has been isolated and characterized. DNA analysis has shown that both DMD and BMD affect the same gene (allelic). Portions of the coding sequence of the gene have been used to produce polyclonal antisera directed against the normal muscle protein product of the normal gene. The specific protein, dystrophin, is a normal component of the plasma membrane, transverse tubule system of the normal muscle fiber. In patients with Duchenne's muscular dystrophy, the muscle contains less than <3% of the amounts of this protein found in control patients. In patients with Becker's muscular dystrophy, the dystrophin is normal but the size of the protein (molecular weight) is abnormal. Patients with an intermediate clinical course have results bridging these two disorders. Patients with other types of neuromuscular disorders have normal dystrophin.

Figure 5.15 Muscle histopathology I: Duchenne's muscular dystrophy. Marked variation in fiber size is present with a large dense hypercontracted hyalinized fiber (compare to Figs. 5.21 and 8.21). H&E 63×. (Courtesy of Dr. Tom Smith, University of Massachusetts Medical Center.)

Thus, a defective gene at this specific site may result in a total defect in a failure to produce this muscle protein (DMD) or the production of a muscle protein of abnormal size (BMD) or in various combinations of these deficits. Specific therapy has not yet been achieved. Corticosteroids may produce minor improvement (Brown, 1989).

The non-X-linked muscular dystrophies are less common.

Facioscapulohumeral (FSH) Dystrophy

These cases occur on an autosomal dominant basis with the gene linked to chromosome 40. The incidence is 1–2/100,000 persons. A small deletion occurs at the end of the long arm of chromosome 4q.35. The phenotypic expression is variable. Some cases begin in childhood and have a poor prognosis. Most begin in the late teens or early twenties with a slow rate of progression. Often the specific age of onset is difficult to identify. The name of the disease reflects the prominent early features of bilateral facial weakness and proximal upper extremity involvement with weakness of shoulder abduction and winging of the scapula. Subsequently, lower extremities are involved. In most cases little disability of significant degree occurs before the thirties or forties. Life span is relatively well preserved. Serum creatine kinase is borderline or only mildly elevated, reflecting the slow rate of muscle breakdown. The EMG and muscle biopsy reflect the myopathic features.

Limb Girdle Dystrophies

The limb girdle dystrophies are a heterogenous group of autosomal recessive disorders, occurring with a frequency of 1/100,000. Rarely some families follow an autosomal dominant pattern. Approximately 10% of these patients have mutations in the gene coding for sacroglycan (Duggan et al., 1997). Other mutations are also described (Dubowitz, 1997). Some begin in the upper extremities at shoulder and scapula, and some begin in the lower extremes at pelvic girdle and knees. A few mimic Duchenne's muscular dystrophy. Progression is slow and severe disability is usually not present until the thirties or even the fifties. Serum creatine kinase is moderately elevated. EMG demonstrates myopathic features; muscle biopsy demonstrates dystrophic features. From a clinical standpoint, there is considerable overlap with cases of indolent polymyositis, motor neuron disease (spinal muscular atrophy), endocrine myopathies, and carriers of the DMD gene with minor clinical manifestations.

The following case history illustrates this disorder.

CASE HISTORY 5.1

This 21-year-old white male college student was delayed in walking until age 2. During grammar school, he was the slowest runner in the class and could not keep up with his peers. In high school he first noted minor weakness in climbing stairs. By college he had trouble in climbing one flight. By his senior year, he had difficulty descending stairs.

Neurological Examination
Mental status: Intact.
Cranial nerves: Intact.

Motor system: There was proximal weakness at hips (3/5) and shoulders (4/5)[1] with intact distal strength and normal muscle bulk. Gower's sign was present in attempting to stand from a recumbent position. Gait was waddling—consistent with proximal weakness at hips.
Reflexes: Deep tendon stretch reflexes[2] were absent at triceps and radial periosteal and trace at biceps. Patellar and Achilles reflexes were normal. Plantar responses were flexor. *Sensory system:* Intact.

Clinical diagnosis: Limb girdle muscular dystrophy or a variant of motor neuron disease (Chapter 9).

Laboratory Data
Muscle enzymes: all were mildly elevated. *Motor and sensory nerve conduction velocities:* all were normal. *EMG:* demonstrated myopathic features with decreased amplitude and duration of motor units with a full interference pattern on volitional effort.

Muscle biopsy (left deltoid): reported significant dystrophic features: marked variation in muscle fiber size in a random distribution, central position of subsarcolemmal nuclei, and a significant increase in endomysial connective tissue.

Subsequent course: The patient reported at age 38 (17 years after his initial evaluation) slow progression: he was still able to walk without assistance. Climbing stairs was a problem. Face and hands were not involved.

Muscular Dystrophies with Predominant Involvement of Cranial Nerves

Cranial nerves may be affected during the course of the more common muscular dystrophies. There have, however, been several families described with adult onset with diseases beginning with predominant and relative selective involvement of cranial nerves. There is usually an autosomal dominant pattern of inheritance with a chronic progressive ophthalmoplegia or an oculopharyngeal dystrophy. Oculopharyngeal dystrophy begins in the 30s and 40s. There are geographic familial clusters: French Canadian families in Quebec and New England, and Spanish American families in the southwestern United States. A mutated gene has been located on chromosome 14q11.2-13.

Myotonic Dystrophy

This is the most common inherited form of muscular dystrophy affecting adults. It is an autosomal dominant disorder with an estimated incidence of 1/8000 in which cranial nerve and distal limb involvement are prominent. Multiple organ systems are involved with variable expression, including cataracts, baldness, mental subnormality, gonadal atrophy, other endocrine disturbances, low plasma IgG, glucose intolerance,

---

[1] The primary grading system for strength is that suggested by the Medical Research Council (MRC) during World War II:

0 = no contractions; 1 = flicker or trace of contraction; 2 = active movement with gravity eliminated; 3 = active movement against gravity; 4 = active movement against gravity and resistance; 5 = normal power. The scale is not a linear function, and because of the wide range included in grades 4 and 5 many examiners will grade 4(−), 4, 4(+), and 5(−).

[2] Deep tendon reflexes are graded as follows: 0 = absent; trace = minimally present; 1 = hyperactive; 2 = normal; 3 = hyperactive-brisk; 4 = hyperactive-unsustained clonus; 4+ sustained clonus. As above, minor gradations may be superimposed such as 2+ or 3+.

smooth muscle autonomic involvement, and cardiac conduction defects. The latter may lead to syncope and sudden death. Although cases can present in the neonatal period, the most common ages of onset are late adolescence or early adult life.

The early symptoms relate to complaints of gait difficulty and clumsiness. At this point, the more specific diagnosis may not be apparent to the nonneurological observer. (The author once saw six patients in an 8-month period at an Army basic training base with this diagnosis, referred with the more general complaints.) Examination, however, will demonstrate a distal limb weakness. Percussion of the thenar hand muscles or of the tongue will often demonstrate a myotonic reaction (prolonged contraction with delayed relaxation). Myotonia can also be demonstrated by asking the patient to squeeze the examiner's fingers and to then rapidly open the hands. Myotonia of the eyelids may be noted in the continued retraction of eyelids and a lid lag after prolonged upgaze. With progression of the disease, a significant weakness and atrophy of muscles innervated by the facial, mandibular supplied muscles, and the accessory nerve to the sternocleidomastoid muscles occurs with the development of characteristic "myopathic facies." Most patients are disabled and unable to walk by the thirties or forties. Life expectancy is reduced because of cardiac and pulmonary complications.

The creatine kinase level is usually normal. The EMG demonstrates myopathic features plus the prolonged myotonic discharges. When audio amplified, the EMG myotonic discharge sounds like a "dive bomber." The muscle biopsy shows characteristic features of chains of central nuclei, ringed fibers, and selective atrophy of type 1 fibers. The underlying molecular basis of myotonic dystrophy has recently been discovered. An unstable DNA fragment occurs on chromosome 19q 13 related to an expanded cytosine thymidine guanine (CTG) trinucleotide repeat at the end of a region encoding a protein kinase. Normally 5–30 repeats are present at this location. In myotonic dystrophy the number of repeats at this location is markedly increased by >10 fold. The greater the number of repeats, the more severe the disease (Wang et al., 1994). This protein kinase does have an effect on skeletal muscle voltage-gated sodium channels, reducing the peak sodium current. A DNA probe is available to detect the disease.

Channelopathies Affecting Skeletal Muscle

In these disorders, mutations occur in the voltage-gated channels. Table 5.1 outlines these disorders. (Modified from Neurological Channelopathies Annual Review of Neuroscience Vol. 33: 151-172 2010) Dimitri M and Kullmann and Cannon, S.C. 1998. Ion channel defects in the hereditary myotonias and periodic paralyses. Molecular Neurology. Ed. Martin, JB. New York. Scientific American, pp. 257-277.)

More recent studies, summarized by Cannon (2002), have identified mutations in the potassium channels in periodic paralysis as well as those previously described in the sodium and calcium channels.

Myotonic Congenita

In these disorders the myotonia occurs in relative isolation. An autosomal dominant form (Thomsen's disease) and an autosomal recessive form (Becker's muscular dystrophy) occur. The myotonic syndromes are characterized by an abnormal increase in membrane excitability with persistent runs of action potential in the surface membrane. Abnormal low-chloride conductance has been implicated in myotonia congenita in humans, congenital myotonia of the goat, and myotonia following ingestion of aromatic carboxylic acids.

Subsequent K^+ accumulation in the transverse tubular lumen leads to excessive depolarization and the persistent firing of action potentials. Similar results occur when normal muscle fibers are placed in a chloride-free solution.

Periodic Paralysis (Familial Periodic Paralysis)

These are relatively rare inherited (autosomal dominant) disorder of muscle that may produce acute transient weakness. These are characterized by an episodic failure of muscle membrane excitability. The attacks are often associated with marked alterations of serum potassium. There are hypokalemic and hyperkalemia forms. The hypokalemic form is the most common, occurring with a frequency of 1:100,000. As indicated in Table 5.1 some forms may be associated with myotonia. In the hyperkalemic form the basic mutation occurs in the alpha subunit of the sodium channel. This results in a disruption of fast inactivation. A minor defect in these inactivating channels (0.8%–2%) can produce myotonic runs of discharge. When >3% of inactivating channels are defective, a stabilized depolarized action potential occurs. In the hyperkalemic form attacks may be precipitated by fasting, cold, stress, or by rest after exercise. In the hypokalemic form, at the onset of the attack a significant movement of potassium and sodium ions into skeletal muscle occurs with a decrease in serum potassium. Microelectrode studies of muscle fibers from patients with

Table 5.1 CHANNELOPATHIES AFFECTING SKELETAL MUSCLE

DISORDER (EPONYM) INHERITANCE	MYOTONIA	PERIODIC WEAKNESS	LOCUS	CHANNEL
Myotonia congenita (Thomsen's) AD, (Becker's) AR	Constant	None–mild	7q35	Cl-
Potassium aggravated myotonia, AD	Variable	None	17q23-25	Na^+ (alpha)
Paramyotonia congenita (Eulenberg's), AD	Cold aggravated	Moderate–cold aggravated	17q23-25	Na^+ (alpha)
Hyperkalemic periodic paralysis (Gamstrop's), AD	Variable, K^+ aggravated	Moderate–severe, K^+ aggravated	17q23-25	Na^+ (alpha)
Hypokalemic periodic paralysis None, AD	None	Severe, decreased K^+ aggravates	1q21-31	Ca^{++} (alpha)

AD, autosomal dominant; AR, autosomal recessive.

this disorder indicate that reducing the K ion concentration in the bath solution caused the affected fibers to depolarize and become inexcitable. Normal fibers hyperpolarize under these conditions. From a molecular standpoint the missense mutation is in L-type calcium channel (alpha 1s subunit). Refer to studies of Ptacek and associates in 1994. How this channel defect relates to the microelectrode studies is unclear (Cannon, 2002). Attacks may be induced by the administration of insulin and glucose or of sodium chloride, by alcohol, stress, cold exposure, or by rest after exercise. In all types, mild persistent proximal weakness may develop later in the disease course. Muscle biopsy may demonstrate vascular changes and tubular aggregates.

In both forms the changes in serum levels of potassium are of such magnitude as to produce electrocardiogram (EKG) changes. In the hypokalemic form, serum K may be depressed to 2–3 mEq/liter. In the hyperkalemic form the level may be as high as 7–8 mEq/liter. (Normal K concentration is 5.0 mEq/liter.)

The following case presented in detail on CD-ROM illustrates many of the features of hypokalemic periodic paralysis.

CASE HISTORY 5.2: PATIENT OF DR. THOMAS TWITCHELL

This 30-year-old white housewife had experienced episodes of nighttime paralysis beginning at age 9 years. These occurred several times per month but with the administration of potassium supplementation, attacks decreased to 1–2 times per year. At age 9 years she had noted a mild persistent weakness in both proximal lower extremities which was nonprogressive but did result in difficulty in climbing steps. At age 32 episodes again became frequent, related to high carbohydrate intake, cold water exposure, or stress. Family history and a general physical examination were normal.

Neurological examination: Demonstrated only moderate weakness at hip flexors.

Neurologic diagnosis: Periodic paralysis and minor myopathic process.

Laboratory data: Erythrocyte sedimentation rate, thyroid functions, serum potassium, creatine phosphokinase, EMG, and nerve conduction studies were all normal.

Diagnostic studies: Within 15 minutes of administration of glucose and insulin the patient had increased weakness in all four extremities. By 30 minutes, the potassium level had fallen from 4.7 to 2.1 mEq/liter with the associated EKG features (flat T waves). At 60 minutes, the patient had total paralysis of all four limbs (quadriplegia) and no deep tendon reflexes could be obtained. She was flaccid and unable to lift her head from the bed. However, she was conscious, she could speak and breathe, and all cranial nerves were intact. She was given oral potassium and within 2 hours had returned to her baseline state. She was subsequently treated with potassium supplements plus acetazolamide, a drug which affects sodium potassium transport.

Congenital Myopathies

(Refer to Fardeau, 1982.) These are relatively rare disorders of muscle which primarily present with hypotonic weakness in childhood: "the floppy infant" and delay in motor developmental milestones. The specific name assigned to each of these syndromes is based on the unique features on muscle biopsy and the special histochemical stains. The first type described by Shy and Magee in 1956 is so named because type I fibers lack mitochondria in the *central core*, which instead contains disorganized tightly packed myofilaments. In *nemaline myopathy* there are peripheral collections of rod-shaped bodies—possibly derived from the Z bands. In *centronuclear myopathy*, there are chains of central muscles—surrounded by a zone devoid of myofibrillar-ATPase activity.

Metabolic Myopathies

(Refer to DiMauro, 1985; Pourmand, 2000; Rowland et al., 1986.) The metabolic myopathies are relatively rare and are inborn errors of metabolism. There are four major subcategories considered under the overall diagnosis of metabolic myopathy: (1) defects in enzymes involved in the metabolism of glucose and glycogen with the specific defect involving the lysosomal and cytosolic enzymes: *the glycogen storage diseases*; (2) abnormalities in the metabolism of lipids; (3) abnormalities of the enzymes related to the mitochondrial respiratory chain for aerobic energy production: *the mitochondrial myopathies*; and (4) abnormalities in the metabolism of adenine nucleotides. Muscle contraction utilizes ATP (adenosine triphosphate), which is converted from ADP (adenosine diphosphate) by the action of CK (creatine kinase).

Moderate exercise is fueled by aerobic conditions, with glycogen as the main fuel source. After 5–10 minutes blood glucose is utilized. Subsequently fatty acids are utilized. After 4 hours of exercise lipids and amino acids are utilized.

In high-intensity exercise anaerobic glycogen breakdown and glycolysis generate additional fuel. At rest, lipids are the predominant energy source.

The student is already aware that multiple enzymes are involved in the events of aerobic and anaerobic carbohydrate metabolism and in lipid fatty acid metabolism, which involve these enzymes. Depending on the specific deficit, (a) there may be multiple system involvement with persistent weakness, (b) selective muscle involvement with persistent weakness, or (c) exercise intolerance with easy fatigue and muscle cramps but with little persistent weakness. Note, however, that most patients with cramps or fatigue on exercise do not have a significant underlying metabolic myopathy.

The first hereditary myopathy in which a specific enzyme defect was identified was McArdle's disease. It falls into the last category (c). The enzyme muscle phosphorylase (myophosphorylase) is absent as demonstrated on special stains for this enzyme applied to the muscle biopsy. When the patient exercises, glycogen cannot be broken down to pyruvate and lactic acid and the expected rise in blood lactic acid in ischemic limb exercise fails to occur. As exercise continues, fatigue and painful cramps occur. If the patient persists, muscle breakdown will occur with a significant rise in blood and urine levels of myoglobin. Significant acute renal tubular impairment is a complication of any acute condition in which rapid breakdown of muscle occurs producing myoglobinuria. Exertional rhabdomyolysis may also occur in predisposed individuals (Greenberg and Ameson, 1966). The recent monograph edited by Pourmand (2000) provides a detailed consideration of the many other rare disorders included in this category.

In addition to the primary metabolic myopathies discussed earlier, secondary metabolic myopathies occur, for example, endocrine myopathies, thyrotoxic periodic paralysis, and drug-induced myopathies and in congestive heart failure and chronic obstructive pulmonary disease.

ACQUIRED DISORDERS OF MUSCLE

The major categories are as follows:

1. Toxic: Related to alcohol and drugs such as colchicine used in the treatment of gout or the agents employed in the treatment of elevated cholesterol levels (the statins).
2. Endocrine: Hyperthyroid (thyrotoxic myopathy), hypothyroid (myxedema myopathy), and corticosteroid myopathy. The corticosteroid myopathy occurs not only in patients with Cushing's disease but also in many patients receiving long-term corticosteroid therapy. Typically the weakness begins in the pelvic girdle and proximal muscles of the lower extremities.
3. Trauma: Closed muscle compartment compression due to trauma or a deep unconscious state produced by drugs or alcohol, etc., may produce considerable rhabdomyolysis of an acute nature (see Owen et al., 1979). Prolonged seizures or prolonged positional compression on a hard surface after a stroke may also produce this condition.
4. Inflammatory: Inflammation of muscle may occur in (a) viral disease such as influenza on Coxsackie, (b) bacterial infections by staphylococcus aureus, or (c) in parasitic infections that are of major importance in some areas of the world, such as toxoplasmosis, cysticercosis, and trichinosis. A myopathy may also occur in HIV infection. The major considerations in this section are those cases where the polymyositis occurs on autoimmune bases.

In some cases (idiopathic polymyositis and dermatomyositis), the autoimmune disease is restricted to muscle (plus skin in dermatomyositis). The cases cover a wide age range. The onset and source may be acute, subacute, or chronic. The chronic, gradually progressive pattern is the most common. Cranial nerves are usually not involved, although difficulty in swallowing may be present due to posterior pharyngeal striated muscle involvement. Proximal muscles are involved predominantly in dermatomyositis. There is more diffuse involvement in polymyositis but with a proximal predominance (limb girdle and neck flexors). In dermatomyositis there is edema and bluish (heliotrope) discoloration of the eyelids, with a scaly red rash on the face (in a butterfly pattern), shoulders, upper chest, back, and extensor surfaces of the limbs. Sedimentation rate and muscle enzymes are significantly increased. Muscle biopsy indicates segmental muscle necrosis, regeneration, and inflammatory infiltrates (Fig. 5.16). EMG indicates not only myopathic features but also the presence of fibrillations.

Figure 5.16 Muscle histopathology II: Polymyositis. Widespread necrosis of muscle fibers is present with extensive infiltration by mononuclear inflammatory cells. H&E 25×. (Compare to Fig. 5.15.) (Courtesy of Dr. Tom Smith, Neuropathology, University of Massachusetts Medical Center.)

There is an increased incidence of underlying neoplasm in adults with dermatomyositis and polymyositis (particularly in older adults). Common sites are lung and ovary. Overall incidence in all cases of dermatomyositis and polymyositis is 9% (Sigurgeirsson et al., 1992).

The term *overlap polymyositis* refers to patients who develop polymyositis within the context of already existing autoimmune connective tissue diseases: systemic lupus erythematosus (SLE), rheumatoid arthritis, periarteritis nodosa, systemic sclerosis, and Sjögren's syndrome. It has been estimated that 5%–15% of all patients with these diseases will manifest polymyositis (Isenberg, 1984).

Most patients (60%–70%) with polymyositis and dermatomyositis have a significant response to corticosteroid therapy. Nonresponders may require more definitive immunosuppressive therapy. Approximately one-third of nonresponders have another variety of myositis: *inclusion body myositis*. Such cases have a male predominance, relatively normal CPK, and greater distal involvement (see discussion in Dalakas, 1991).

The following case presented in detail on the CD-ROM demonstrates dermatomyositis complicating ovarian malignancy.

CASE HISTORY 5.3

This 69-year-old white female 2 weeks prior to admission developed difficulty swallowing and progressive weakness of all four extremities with proximal more than distal involvement. Three months prior to admission, she had partial resection of ovarian carcinoma, followed by radiotherapy and chemotherapy.

General physical examination: There was superficial redness and swelling involving the skin of both upper extremities. Liver was enlarged.

Neurologic Examination

Mental status: Intact.

Cranial nerves: The gag reflex was absent and she had difficulty handling secretions.

Motor system: Weakness was present in all four extremities proximal greater than distal.

Reflexes: Deep tendon reflexes were depressed in the upper extremities and absent in the lower extremities. Plantar responses were flexor.
Sensory system: Intact.
Clinical diagnosis: Dermatomyositis as a remote effect of ovarian carcinoma.
Laboratory data: *Erythrocyte sedimentation rate and muscle enzymes* were all significantly increased. *EMG* was consistent with polymyositis.
Subsequent course: Despite the administration of high-dosage corticosteroids (prednisone), the patient had increasing weakness. Aspiration and increasing respiratory symptoms occurred. The patient expired 7 weeks after onset of symptoms.

DISORDERS OF THE NEUROMUSCULAR JUNCTION

Diseases affecting the neuromuscular junction may be classified as to location: postsynaptic or presynaptic (see Drachman, 1986, 1994; Engel, 1984; Newsome-Davis, 1992; Richman, 1998).

POSTSYNAPTIC DISORDERS

Myasthenia Gravis

The major primary disease due to neuromuscular junction pathology in this country and western Europe is myasthenia gravis. The prevalence is 5–7.5 per 100,000. This is a disease characterized by fluctuating weakness of voluntary muscle worse on exercise, improved by rest and by administration of anticholinesterase drugs. This is primarily a disease of adults with onset between ages 10 and 70. However, neonatal and congenital cases are recognized. The peak age of onset is between ages 20 and 30. Under age 40, females are affected more often than men in a ratio of 70:30. After age 50, there is a male predominance of 60:40. Ten percent of patients have an associated tumor of the thymus gland (thymoma). These patients tend to be older with a male predominance.

The symptoms usually first appear in the muscles supplied by the cranial nerves. The extraocular muscles for control of eye and eyelid movement are first affected in 60% of cases and are affected at some stage in 90% of patients. In 15%–20% of cases with a relatively benign course, the symptoms may remain confined to the eye muscles. These cases are termed *ocular myasthenia*. In the extensive series of Grob et al. with 1487 patients (followed from 1940 to 1985), 14% of patients continued to have localized ocular myasthenia. The patient has a ptosis (closure or droop) of one or both eye lids, often most apparent on sustained upward gaze. Double vision (diplopia) results from a weakness of one or more extraocular muscles. The early occurrence of diplopia may be a reflection of the precise synchronization required between the two eyes in movement under normal conditions. A minimal weakness of one medial or lateral rectus muscle would disrupt such a precise synchronization.

Generalized myasthenia refers to progression to involve other cranial nerves and the extremity and trunk muscles. Such generalization after an ocular onset generally occurs within the first 2 years following onset. The patient will have difficulty swallowing (dysphagia), speaking (dysarthrias), and chewing (mandibular nerve–supplied muscles). In addition, a bilateral weakness of facial muscles may provide a suggestive myasthenic facies. The patient may support head or jaw with the hand to compensate for weakness. As the disease progresses, more generalized involvement of proximal limb muscles develops. In some patients there is significant involvement of the muscles of respiration. In the series of Grob et al., maximum level of weakness was reached during the first year in 55%, first 3 years in 70%, and first 5 years in 85%. After 3–5 years, the disease stabilizes.

The prognosis depends on the age of the patient, the duration of the localized form of the disease, and on the associated diseases (thymoma, thyroid disorders, other autoimmune disorders).

Myasthenia was once associated with a significant mortality due to respiratory insufficiency and infection, but this mortality rate has now been markedly reduced. In the series of Grob et al. for patients with maximum weakness in the 1940–1957 era, mortality rate was 31% and the rate of spontaneous remission was 10%. In the 1958–1966 era, the mortality rate was 15% and rate of remission was 10%. In the 1966–1985 era, mortality rate was 7% and the remission rate was 11%.

The diagnosis is readily apparent from a clinical standpoint: fluctuating weakness with no sensory findings, intact reflexes, and no long tract findings. However, there are several confirmatory diagnostic tests. Jolly in 1895 first described the electrical test that carries his name. Repetitive stimulation of a motor nerve results in a rapid decrease in the amplitude of muscle contraction "decremental response." Jolly demonstrated that the apparently fatigued muscle would still respond to direct galvanic stimulation.

In modern clinical neurophysiology the motor nerve is stimulated at a rate of 3–5 per second and the reduction in amplitude of the muscle action potential is measured. (Abnormal is greater than 10% reduction.) An agent (edrophonium or neostigmine) that blocks acetylcholine esterase is then administered. This increases the duration of available acetylcholine at the neuromuscular junction and the decremental response is reversed.

The edrophonium (Tensilon) test can be carried out in the outpatient office. This agent when administered intravenously will often transiently reverse or reduce the signs of weakness. Clinical effect occurs in 30–60 seconds and lasts 4–5 minutes. Since related cholinergic agents (anticholinesterases) play a major role in therapy the test can also be performed to determine whether the patient is receiving too little on too much of the therapeutic agent.

A very specific test is the measurement of the blood level of the acetylcholine receptor antibody positive in 85%–90% (see later).

Recently major advances have been made in our understanding of the underlying pathogenesis and pathophysiology of this disorder. This constitutes a major accomplishment for neurobiology that has been translated into improved results as regards therapy of the disease.

Adams and Victor (1989) have summarized the major historical landmarks in the study of myasthenia. Welch in 1877 and Erb in 1875 regarding electrical studies of Jolly in 1895 suggested what has come to be recognized subsequently as the location of pathology: the neuromuscular junction. The term *pseudoparalysis* as well as *myasthenia gravis* was originated by Jolly since no pathology was present at autopsy. He also recommended the use of an anticholinesterase physostigmine. Walker in 1934 noted the similarity of some of the signs to those produced by the poison curare and began the use of physostigmine. Buzzard in 1905 in a detailed clinical pathological analysis of five cases described the lesions in thymus: thymic hyperplasia, which now has been noted in over 80% of patients, and the minor lymphocytic collections in muscle. Buzzard proposed that an autotoxic agent could produce all of these findings. He also noted the association of the disease with thyrotoxic cases. Simpson in 1960 proposed an autoimmune basis for the disease because of the increased incidence of other putative autoimmune disease: thyroiditis, lupus erythematosus, and rheumatoid arthritis.

Electron microscopic studies by Zack et al. (1962), Engel and Sarta (1971), and Engel et al. (1976) had demonstrated significant changes in the postsynaptic region with shallow postsynaptic folds, a widened synaptic cleft. In contrast, the presynaptic area was normal as regards the number and size of presynaptic vesicles. Fambrough, Drachman, and Satyamuri (1973) then demonstrated a marked (three-fold) reduction in acetylcholine receptors per neuromuscular junction in motor point nerve biopsies of myasthenic patients. Compared to control subjects, there were a decreased number of binding sites for a radioactive labeled snake poison, alpha bungarotoxin, which can be purified from the venom of the cobra and krait. This toxin binds in an irreversible manner to the acetylcholine receptor. In 1973, Patrick and Lindstrom demonstrated that repeated immunization of rabbits with acetylcholine receptor protein derived from the electric organs of eels reproduced the disease. These animals develop all of the clinical and electrical features of myasthenia gravis. Antibodies to the ACh receptor protein could be identified attached to the ACh receptor. Moreover, normal animals receiving these antibodies also developed myasthenia.

Subsequently Lindstrom et al. (1976) and several other groups reported a radioimmunoassay for acetylcholine receptor antibody. This is now a standard laboratory test for myasthenia gravis with a 90% detection rate in the serum of myasthenic patients. (The serum level does not correspond to the severity of the disease.) Engel et al. (1984) were able to demonstrate immune complexes at the postsynaptic junction in biopsies from myasthenic patients. When the immunoglobulin derived from the serum of myasthenic patients is administered to mice, the characteristic myasthenic syndrome develops in the recipient animal (Toyka et al., 1974). The syndrome of neonatal myasthenia also suggests a serum or plasma transmissible factor. Fifteen percent of children born to myasthenic mothers will manifest clinical signs of weakness lasting several weeks due to passive transfer of anti-ACh receptor antibodies across the placenta. Circulating ACh receptor antibodies and electrophysiological findings can be demonstrated in these infants and even in additional neonates of myasthenic mothers who do not manifest clinical weakness.

Subsequent studies reviewed by Drachman (1986) suggest several mechanisms for antibody action: (1) there is a significant increase in the rate of degradation of ACh receptors, (2) the antibody actually blocks the binding sites of the ACh receptor, and (3) there is a complement mediated damage to and subsequent change in the geometry of the junction with a reduction in efficiency of transmission.

Cells cultured from patients with myasthenia gravis but not from control subjects can synthesize ACh receptor antibody in vitro. The highest levels of production are obtained from thymic cells of patients with medullary thymic hyperplasia. Peripheral blood lymphocyte lymph nodes and bone marrow also produce the ACh receptor antibody.

The role of the thymus appears critical from several standpoints: (1) The thymus has a central role in immunology. (2) The thymic hyperplasia involves the presence in the medulla of many germinal centers and surrounding T cell areas. Such germinal centers are rare in nonmyasthenic thymus. (3) The thymus contains muscle-like cells, and ACh receptors can be demonstrated when these cells are placed in tissue culture. Drachman (1978) has suggested that these receptor-bearing muscle cells may be particularly vulnerable to immune attack. Some alteration of these cells by lymphocytes (perhaps triggered by viral infection of thymus, etc.) could initiate any acute immune response directed against ACh receptors.

The essentials of therapy in myasthenia gravis follow from the neurobiology of the disease.

1. Initial therapy consists of anticholinesterase drugs. The main drug used is pyridostigmine (Mestinon), which has a somewhat longer duration of action than neostigmine. For some patients this will suffice, particularly if only local ocular myasthenia is present and if this responds well.

2. Generalized myasthenia will almost always require more definitive therapy directed at the immune systems.

    a. The most definitive procedure is total thymectomy. As discussed by Rowland (1987), there is now a consensus that all adults with generalized myasthenia should have this procedure relatively early in the course of the disease. In the "maximum thymectomy" series of 72 nonthymoma patients previously with moderate to severe generalized myasthenia reported by Younger et al. (1987), 46% of patients were in complete remission (on no medication), 33% were asymptomatic on 60–240 mg of pyridostigmine daily, and 10% were asymptomatic on steroids. Approximately 90% then were in complete remission or asymptomatic. An additional 6% were improved. At least 1–4 years were required to see the maximum response to therapy. There was insignificant decline in the titre of ACh receptor antibody. Although this was not a matched control series, the results are in striking contrast to the contemporary results of nonsurgical treatment of moderate to severe generalized myasthenia (see Grob, 1987). Other major centers have confirmed these results. Schumm et al. (1985) has also recommended the procedure in patients with pure ocular myasthenia, if no spontaneous remission and no satisfactory response to cholinesterase inhibitors occurs in a 6-month period. In their series, thymectomy prevented the subsequent development of generalized myasthenia; none of 18 patients progressed over two years from ocular to generalized myasthenia.

Thymectomy was originally performed primarily to remove thymomas in patients who coincidentally also had myasthenia gravis; some improvement in the myasthenia also occurred (Blalock et al., 1939). Considerable experience in subsequent years has demonstrated a poorer response of the myasthenia in such cases of thymoma to thymectomy.

b. Other types of immunosuppression may also be employed in the pre- or postoperative period or in those patients unable to tolerate thymectomy. These include corticosteroids, plasmapheresis (plasma exchange), and cytotoxic drugs (azathioprine).

The following case history, which is presented in detail on the CD-ROM, provides an example of severe generalized myasthenia gravis.

CASE HISTORY 5.4

This 44-year-old, obese (>300 lb), white, married, machine operator had noted, for several years, fatigue in his arms and legs at the end of a day. Approximately 6 to 7 weeks prior to admission, he began to have a marked intermittent weakness of the arms and legs. At the same time, he experienced significant slurring of words, difficulty in swallowing, fatigue of jaw muscles, and drooping of the lids. All of these symptoms were transient; they were not present in the morning; they were clearly precipitated by exercise. The degree of ptosis was sufficient enough to result in difficulty in driving.

Neurological Examination
Mental status: Intact.
Cranial nerves: There was significant bilateral ptosis of the eyelids and bilateral facial jaw and tongue weakness, all markedly increased by exercise. On repetitive upward gaze, a bilateral weakness of superior rectus developed.
Motor system: There was a significant weakness in shoulder abductors, elbow flexors and extensors, and handgrip, which was markedly increased by repetitive exercise.
Reflexes: Deep tendon reflexes, and plantar responses were all normal.
Sensory system: Intact.
Clinical diagnosis: Myasthenia gravis.
Diagnostic studies: An edrophonium (Tensilon) test demonstrated an almost immediate eye-opening effect with the disappearance of the bilateral ptosis. The ptosis, however, had reappeared 3 to 4 minutes after injection of 10 mg of the agent.
Subsequent course: On treatment with pyridostigmine at a dosage of 90 mg 5 times per day (approximately every 4 hours), his ocular, bulbar, and generalized weakness stabilized for 3 years. He then had additional exacerbations in part related to cholinergic crisis and in part related to progression of disease. The latter episodes responded to radiation of the thymus and subsequently prednisone therapy.

Other Postsynaptic Disorders

These are primarily toxic disorders related to pesticides (e.g., organophosphates) or neurotoxins in warfare or to bites from venomous snakes, and so on. In certain parts of the world (e.g., Sri Lanka), pesticide ingestion is a major problem.

Acetylcholinesterase Inhibitors

The usual action of acetylcholine esterase at the neuromuscular junction is to rapidly terminate the action of ACh. This allows high rates of transmission across the synapse. If acetylcholine esterase is inhibited, acetylcholine remains on the receptor and in the synaptic space.

There are two classes of acetylcholine esterase inhibitors:

a. Reversible: carbamates

b. Relatively "irreversible": organophosphates

The reversible agents include those anti-acetylcholine esterase drugs used in the treatment of myasthenia gravis. An increased availability of acetylcholine is of value in counteracting the weakness due to decreased numbers of receptors in this syndrome. Excess amounts of such drugs produce excessive amounts of acetylcholine at the receptors, as noted in the earlier case history, resulting in increased weakness referred to as "cholinergic crisis." The dose of the drug must be reduced. In the management of such patients the edrophonium ("Tensilon") test is of value.

The relatively irreversible agents (organophosphates) constitute a much more serious problem—not only does a significant acute cholinergic effect occur, but there is damage to the postsynaptic membrane and delayed effects on peripheral nerve. Senanagake and Karolliedde (1987) distinguished three syndromes. (1) The acute cholinergic syndrome is accompanied by autonomic effects, and at times central effects (coma). (2) The intermediate syndrome occurring in 10% of patients after recovery from the acute syndrome 24–96 hours after the poisoning is identical to an acute myasthenic syndrome with respiratory, cranial nerve, and proximal limb muscle involvement. If the patient survives the respiratory problems, recovery may occur in 5–18 days. (3) A delayed distal motor neuropathy occurs in some patients at 2–5 weeks after exposure.

The organophosphates are the neurotoxic agents of chemical warfare. They are also acetylcholine esterase inhibitors employed extensively as pesticides. As discussed by Davis (1987), this is a major problem in the developing countries where the sale of such chemicals is often unregulated, and the chemicals are often repackaged in unlabeled containers. The original containers are often reused. The storage and use are often unsupervised and the population is often unable to read any warning label.

The magnitude of the problem is staggering. In Sri Lanka alone between 1978 and 1980, there were 80,000 patients admitted with pesticide poisoning and 6083 of these patients died. Seventy five percent of all cases were due to organophosphorous. In Sri Lanka, the majority of complex cases were the result of ingestion with suicidal intent.

Agents That Bind to the Acetylcholine Receptor

These agents thus block access of acetylcholine to the receptor.

1. d-Tubocurarine: competes for the receptor in a reversible manner. Initially a South American Indian arrow poison, this agent is now used in anesthesia.

2. Repolarizing agents: bi-quaternary ammonium salts. These resemble acetylcholine. They are agonists that initially produce depolarization and then block the site. They are utilized to produce muscle relaxation during general anesthesia and during mechanical respiration.

3. Snake toxins: derived from the venom of the cobra and krait. These snakes are common in India, Sri Lanka, Southeast Asia, and Taiwan. The neurotoxic effect produced is often an acute myasthenic syndrome with respiratory paralysis. As discussed by Watt et al. (1986) and by Drachman (1986) for some of the toxins, such as alpha cobra toxin, the binding is reversible and can be treated with anticholinesterase. For other toxins in the group, such as alpha bungarotoxin from the Taiwan krait, the binding is less reversible and the effects of anticholinesterase less consistent. Some snake venoms also contain toxic agents that act at the presynaptic region (e.g., B. bungarotoxin of the krait).

PRESYNAPTIC DISORDERS

Eaton-Lambert (or Lambert-Eaton) Syndrome

The patient is usually an adult who has a predominantly progressive but fluctuating proximal limb weakness. In contrast to myasthenia, there are major differences: (a) bulbar ocular and respiratory muscle involvement is not common; (b) exercise improves the weakness; (c) repetitive stimulation of the motor nerve produces an incremental response in the muscle action potential, as opposed to the decremental response of myasthenia gravis.

Most patients with this disorder have an underlying malignancy, most often a small cell carcinoma of the lung. The neuromuscular syndrome, however, may precede the appearance of the tumor by months or years. In some patients (one-third) a malignancy may not be identified, but there may be other evidence of autoimmune disease.

The underlying pathophysiology relates to a decrease in the release of acetylcholine quanta from the nerve terminal (not only at the neuromuscular junction but also at cholinergic nerve endings in the autonomic nervous system). As discussed by Newsom-Davis (1992), this defect in release relates to immunoglobulin G antibody that binds to presynaptic calcium channels and prevents their voltage-gated opening. As the action potential enters the presynaptic region, fewer calcium channels open, and less Ca^{++} enters to catalyze the binding of vesicles to the surface membrane. Hence, less ACh is released.

Botulism

The toxin of the bacteria Clostridium botulinum produces an acute syndrome of paralysis involving extraocular muscles, cranial nerves muscles of respiration, and then progressively descending to involve limbs. Cholinergic autonomic junctions are also involved. Thus, the pupil, which is spared in myasthenia, often is involved (dilated). Anaerobic bacteria that may contaminate improperly canned food or preserved meat produce the neurotoxin. Clusters of cases bring this problem to the attention of public health officials. Many cases are fatal. In infants and some adults, the bacteria itself may be present in the gastrointestinal tract or in a wound producing the toxin. (see Bartlett, 1986). The toxin binds rapidly to cholinergic nerve endings and blocks the quantal release of acetylcholine. Once the toxin enters the nerve ending, the available therapeutic antitoxin, if administered, has little action. The flaccid paralysis then is often long lasting (see Chia et al., 1986).

Antibiotics

The aminoglycoside antibiotics—neomycin, streptomycin, and kanamycin—act to interfere with the quantal release of acetylcholine. In most patients this presents no significant clinical problem. However, when blood levels are high due to high dosage or renal failure and when the patient has myasthenia or a subclinical myasthenia, there may be the presentation of an acute paralysis. Most often there is an associated factor of anesthesia and the patient fails to regain normal ventilation after anesthesia has been discontinued. The effects may also be seen with other types of antibiotics.

Spider Venom: Black Widow

This toxin produces rapid release of quanta of acetylcholine storage vesicles. The clinical syndrome is characterized by severe muscle contraction followed by paralysis.

BIBLIOGRAPHY

Cannon, SC. 2002. An expanding view for the molecular basis of familial periodic paralysis. Neuromuscul Disord. 12:533–543.

SECTION II

REGIONAL APPROACH TO NEUROANATOMY AND FUNCTIONAL LOCALIZATION

6.
SPINAL CORD

STRUCTURE AND FUNCTION

Since the spinal cord is the best-understood and least complex of the major elements of the central nervous system, it is appropriate to begin the discussion of the central nervous system with it. The spinal cord has two fairly distinct functions: it conducts action potentials to and from the brain, and it relates to "its" segment.

The spinal cord is segmented, one segment per vertebra, and in the less complex nervous system of fish, the region of the body relating to each segment is a cylindrical band the width of the vertebra. Into this spinal cord segment flows all of the sensory information from the body segment: information on pain, temperature, and position of the muscles, touch, and vibration. The axons that innervate the muscles of that body segment have their nuclei in the spinal cord segment.

In the human there is only a general relationship between the sensory segments and muscles innervated by the same segment of the cord. The size and shape of the regions vary considerably, but the principle remains the same—that of relating, in sensory reception and motor control, to a delimited region of the body. At each segmental level, incoming sensory information connects, in a stereotyped manner, to motor outflow. The knee jerk reflex and the reflexive withdrawal from pain are examples of segmental spinal cord activity.

In addition to relating these functions to specific regions, the spinal cord processes incoming sensory information and sends some of it on to the brain. This is a second and basically distinct function of the spinal cord: conduction to and from the brain. These two functions are anatomically separated. Inspection of a cross section of spinal cord shows white columns surrounding a butterfly-shaped interior gray column (Fig. 6.1). The myelin sheaths of the thousands of axons running up and down in the white matter, the dorsal, lateral, and ventral funiculi, produce the white color. The thousands of cell bodies in the center give that region a gray appearance. We speak, then, of gray matter, which contains cell bodies and synapses relating to the sensory and motor activities of the segment, and of white matter, which contains axons running to and from the brain.

Each spinal cord segment has four nerve roots attached to it (Fig. 6.1). Each root is made up of many nerve bundles entering the body of the cord almost continuously. The two anterior roots, which carry axons out of the spinal cord to innervate muscles, are known as motor roots. The two posterior roots carry sensory information into the spinal cord. Since man stands vertically, we refer to posterior and anterior; in animals, dorsal and ventral. The cell bodies of all of the sensory fibers are in the posterior root ganglion. Damage to the right anterior root will paralyze motor units on the right side of the body. Damage to the left posterior root will interrupt all modalities of sensation from a small region on the left side of the body. The roots join just before they leave the spinal canal, through the intervertebral foramen, and form a single spinal nerve.

GROSS ANATOMY

The gross anatomy of the spinal cord is illustrated in Figure 6.2. The cord runs through the spinal canal of each vertebra, as is shown in Figure 6.3, and is protected by a number of layers of meninges. The pia mater is closely adherent to the cord. Cerebrospinal fluid occupies the subarachnoid space. The arachnoid lies snugly against the thick, tough dura. The spinal dura forms a protective tube beginning at the dura of the skull and tapering to a point in the region of the sacral vertebrae. Between the dura and the vertebrae lies the epidural space, usually filled with fat. The denticulate ligaments anchor the spinal cord to the dura.

The spinal cord and, more important, the spinal roots, are named in relation to the vertebral column. In humans there are 8 cervical, 12 thoracic, 5 lumbar, and 5 sacral spinal cord segments. They are shown in relation to the vertebral column in Figure 6.2. There are 7 cervical vertebrae; the C8 in Figure 6.2 is the eighth cervical spinal nerve that arises from the anterior and posterior roots of the eighth cervical spinal cord segment. The eighth cervical nerve emerges below the seventh cervical vertebrae and above the first thoracic vertebrae. The spinal nerves are always named for the spinal cord segment of origin. The intervertebral disk and foramen (Fig. 6.5) are normally named by the vertebrae above and below, that is, L4, 5 disk; L5, S1 foramen.

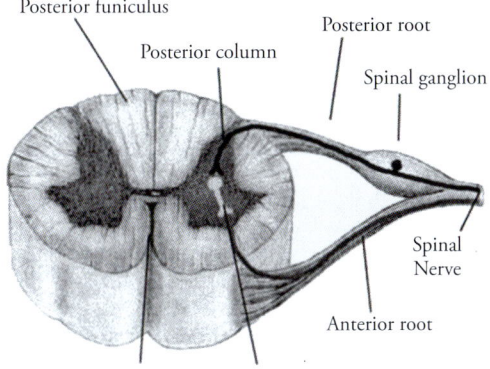

Figure 6.1 The posterior and anterior roots in relation to the gray and white matter of the spinal cord.

Figure 6.2 The lateral aspect of the spinal cord exposed within the vertebral canal. The spinous processes and the laminae of the vertebrae have been removed and the dura mater has been opened longitudinally. (From Clemente, C. (Ed.) Gray's Anatomy, Philadelphia, Lea & Febiger, 1985.)

During development and growth, particularly intrauterine growth, the vertebral column grows faster than the spinal cord it contains so that, in the adult, the spinal cord does not extend the length of the vertebral column (Fig. 6.2). As a result, the spinal roots run interiorly before they leave the spinal canal.

Figure 6.3 The relationships of the vertebral column, the meninges and spinal cord.

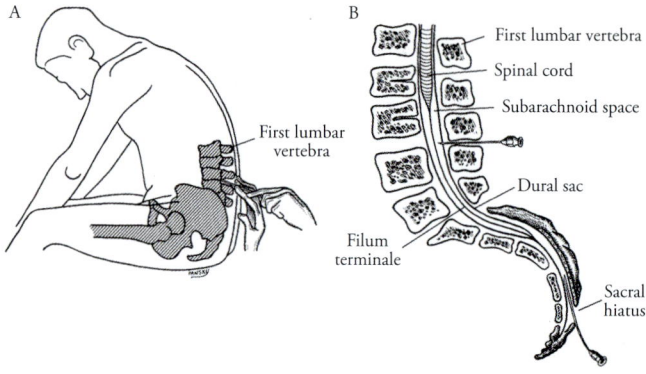

Figure 6.4 The technique of lumbar puncture. (From House and Pansky: A Functional Approach to Neuroanatomy. New York, McGraw-Hill, 1960.)

The spinal cord ends at the first or second lumbar vertebra, and below this level the spinal canal contains only spinal roots. This mass of roots reminded early anatomists of a horse's tail, so it was named cauda equina. The nerve roots run through the subarachnoid space, which is filled with cerebrospinal fluid. When a needle is inserted through the space between the fourth and fifth lumbar vertebra (Fig. 6.4), the point penetrates the dura and pushes aside the spinal roots. If the needle were inserted above L2, there would be danger of damaging the spinal cord. Samples of cerebrospinal fluid can be taken through this needle; pressure can be measured or anesthetic agents or radio-opaque dyes injected (as in Fig. 6.4).

The anterior and posterior roots join to form a spinal nerve (Fig. 6.1) just before leaving the vertebral canal through a recess in the posterior process of each vertebra as shown in Figure 6.5. The canal, the intervertebral neural foramina, is only a little larger than the nerve so that any swelling of the nerve or diminution of the diameter of the canal will pinch

Figure 6.5 A magnetic resonance image (MRI) of a normal spinal cord in the spinal canal. Sagittal section.

Figure 6.6 Typical spinal cord cross sections. (From Gross, C.M. (Ed.): Gray's Anatomy. Philadelphia, Lea and Febiger.)

the nerve. It is not uncommon for the intervertebral disk to rupture posteriorly or laterally and press on a spinal nerve as it exits. The very intense pain this pressing causes is referred to the area of the skin where the nerve began. Frequent sites where the nerve roots are pinched are the intervertebral foramina between L2 and S1, which give rise to the sciatic nerve. The pinched nerve gives the patient the impression that a hot knife is being dragged along the posterior aspect of his calf.

CROSS SECTIONS

The relative amounts of white and gray matter vary with the spinal cord level (Fig. 6.6). White matter decreases in bulk as the sections are further from the brain. Motor tracts from the brain leave the white matter to enter the gray matter and synapse with motor neurons. Sensory fibers entering the cord, section by section, also form the white matter.

A section of the cervical cord contains sensory fibers running up to the brain from the thoracic, lumbar, and sacral sections. It also contains motor fibers running down to innervate motor axons of the thoracic, lumbar, and sacral sections. The white matter of a section of the lumbar cord, however, only contains fibers to and from the lumbar segments inferior to it and the sacral segments. The white matter columns have the shape of thin pyramids with their bases at the foramen magnum and their tips at the last sacral section.

The situation in the gray matter is quite different. Since the gray matter innervates a segment, the size of the gray matter (the number of cells it contains) is related to the complexity of the segment. The hand, for example, is innervated by cervical segments 6, 7, and 8 (C6, C7, and C8) and the first thoracic segment (T1). The hand has the highest concentration of sensory receptors of any region of the body. All of these receptors send their axons into C6 to T1, where they synapse, thus increasing the girth of the posterior gray matter. The muscles of the hand can carry out very fine and intricate movements. They are innervated by nerves having their cell bodies in the gray matter of C6-T1. Such movements require many motor nerves and many cell bodies in the anterior gray matter. Consequently, the cord is enlarged at C6-T1. The situation is much the same in the lumbar region. Sensory input from and motor output to the leg is complex and the gray matter is large. The thoracic and sacral segments, on the other hand, have very small gray matter areas since they innervate only a few muscles and receive relatively uncomplicated sensory messages.

Segments can be recognized, then, by the amount of gray and white matter relative to the whole cross section. In the lower cervical segments the section is large, oval, and white matter and gray matter are nearly equal. The thoracic segments have much more white matter than gray matter and the shape of the gray matter, a thin H, is very characteristic. The lumbar segments have more gray matter than white matter, and the sacral segments are very small and have much more gray matter than white matter. The segments can also be recognized by the shapes of the gray matter. A careful review of Figure 6.6 should provide a basis for recognizing the segmental levels of spinal cord sections. The area of the body which sends sensory fibers into a given spinal cord segment is called a dermatome. These have varying shapes and sizes. Figure 6.7 may help you

Figure 6.7 Key dermatome boundaries in man. (A) Anterior surface and (B) Posterior surface. (From Zimmerman J and Jacobson S, Gross Anatomy, Little, Brown & Company, 1990.)

6 SPINAL CORD: STRUCTURE AND FUNCTION • 113

to remember the general area served by the cord segments. The muscles underlying these areas have essentially the same innervation. More detailed areas are shown in Chapter 8.

SEGMENTAL FUNCTION

ANTERIOR HORN CELLS

The final effector cell of the spinal cord, the anterior horn cell (Fig. 6.8), is probably the best place to begin a discussion of the segmental function of spinal cord segments. The extensive dendritic tree allows upward of 20–50,000 individual synaptic areas or knobs while the large cell body may have another 1–2000 synaptic knobs. Incoming axons may have more than one synaptic connection and hence exert greater control. Each anterior horn cell gives rise to one large (8 to 12 μm) axon, called an alpha motor neuron, which innervates a motor group or unit made up of 10 to 200 individual muscle fibers. There is only one motor end plate on each muscle. Therefore, for a motor group to contract, the anterior horn cell on the proximal end of the axon must fire an action potential. The muscle group is chained to its anterior horn cell. This anatomical relationship is often called the final common pathway. Activation of a specific anterior horn cell precedes activity of a motor group. There are many ways to activate this anterior horn cell; many thousand axons synapse upon it and its extensive dendritic tree.

Neurons in the anterior horn can be divided into medial and lateral groups (Fig. 6.9).

1. The medial nuclear division is divided into posterior medial and anterior medial groups. The posterior medial nucleus is most prominent in the cervical and lumbar enlargement. The medial nucleus innervates the muscles of the axial skeleton.

2. The lateral nuclear division innervates the appendicular musculature. In the thoracic region the intercostal and associated muscles are innervated by this region. In the cervical and lumbar enlargement, these nuclei become especially prominent and are divided into individual columns of nuclei (Fig. 6.9), and these nuclei columns include anterior, anterior lateral, accessory lateral, posterior lateral, and retroposterior lateral. These nuclei are represented functionally so that from medial to lateral one passes from midline spine, to trunk, upper and lower limb girdle, upper leg and arm and lower leg and arm to hand and foot. The most lateral nuclear groups innervate the muscles in the hand and foot.

3. The preganglionic autonomic nuclei lie in the intermediolateral column, a prominent lateral triangle in the gray matter (Fig. 6.6; Th.2). There are two distinct groupings. The intermediolateral nucleus from C8 to L2 is the origin of the preganglionic sympathetic neurons which synapse again either in the sympathetic trunks or in remote ganglia. The sacral nucleus in S2 to S4 is the origin of preganglionic parasympathetic fibers that run to several ganglions in the walls of the pelvic organs.

REFLEXES OF A SINGLE MUSCLE

All of the sensory axons entering the posterior roots are bipolar cells having their cell bodies in the posterior root ganglion.

Figure 6.8 A motor neuron from the cervical spinal cord of a human with prominent Nissl substance (rough endoplasmic reticulum). Thionin stain, 75×.

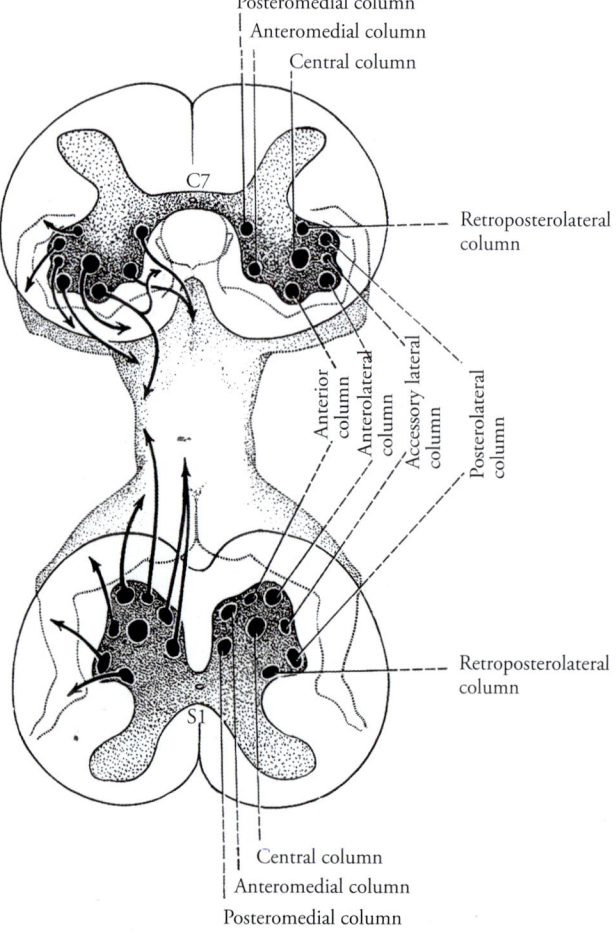

Figure 6.9 Functional localization within the anterior horns. (From Bossy, Atlas of Neuroanatomy. Philadelphia, W.B. Saunders, 1970.)

The axons can be divided into many classes by the sensory modality they carry. As far as we know, each axon carries information about only one modality, such as pain. The intensity of the pain or other sensation is coded as action potential frequency. Later in this chapter, the various modalities will be discussed in detail. For the present, two modalities will suffice for examples: muscle stretch and pain. Pain is carried by very small axons, many of them unmyelinated, which have high thresholds and slow conduction velocities. The stretching of muscles, on the other hand, leads to a barrage of action potentials in large, heavily myelinated nerve fibers. These axons have low thresholds and rapid conduction velocities.

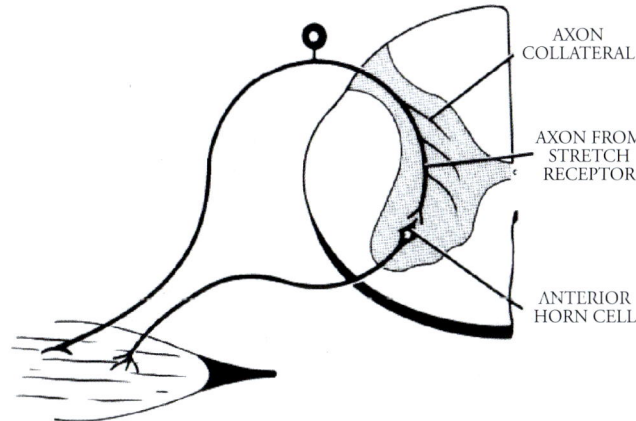

Figure 6.11 The pathway for the monosynaptic stretch reflex.

STRETCH REFLEXES

The classic stretch reflex is the knee jerk, produced by tapping the patellar tendon. This simple involuntary response is such a familiar part of the physical examination and has been used so frequently in medical humor that precise description seems unnecessary. This simple test can give the astute examiner many clues to the function and dysfunction of the nervous system.

The knee jerk is described quantitatively by Figure 6.10, which is taken from the early work of the great English physiologist Sir Charles Sherrington. As the figure indicates, after a brief stretch, the muscle contracts with a delay of about 10 msec. It can readily be shown that this is a response mediated by the spinal cord. When the nerve to the muscle is cut, the response is abolished. When the spinal cord is severed from the rest of the nervous system, the response remains.

The pathway of this response is very simple (Fig. 6.11). The axon from the stretch receptor runs into the posterior horn, and while it branches many times in the gray matter, it eventually synapses directly on the cell body of the anterior horn cells of the muscle stretched. The stretch reflex is often referred to as a monosynaptic reflex. The only muscle that contracts is the one stretched. The reflex continues for as long as the muscle is stretched (Fig. 6.12).

There are stretch reflexes in all muscles, but they are much stronger in the antigravity muscles, particularly the leg extensors. In addition to the familiar knee jerk from the quadriceps group, brisk stretch reflexes can be elicited from the ankle (the Achilles tendon), the jaw, and the biceps and triceps muscles in the arm.

Although the reflex loop is completed within a few segments of spinal cord, the magnitude of the response can be drastically altered by input from other levels. For example, grasping the hands together and pulling will greatly enhance the knee-jerk response (reinforcement). As will be discussed later, the magnitude or briskness of the response can give many clues to pathological processes.

REFLEXIVE RESPONSE TO PAIN

The majority of spinal cord responses have more flexibility than the monosynaptic response, as can be seen in the reflex withdrawal from pain. This is one of the most important of the protective reflexes of the spinal cord. The flexors are activated and the injured limb withdrawn. Figure 6.12 shows the responses of the ankle flexor muscle, the tibialis anterior, to stimulation of the nerve branches leading to the skin—branches which contain predominantly pain fibers. It can immediately be seen that the combined response is considerably greater than the sum of the two. This augmentation of response is known as facilitation and is one of the most basic integrative responses of the nervous system. The reaction is graded in response to the intensity of the stimulus and the area stimulated.

The mechanism of facilitation is shown in Figure 6.13. Stimulation of nerve A excites two anterior horn cells to threshold. Two more are excited in a subthreshold manner; they do not fire an action potential. Nerve B stimulates two totally different anterior horn cells to threshold and the same two to just below threshold. Simultaneous activation of nerves A and B brings all six cells to threshold and elicits a greater tension from the muscle.

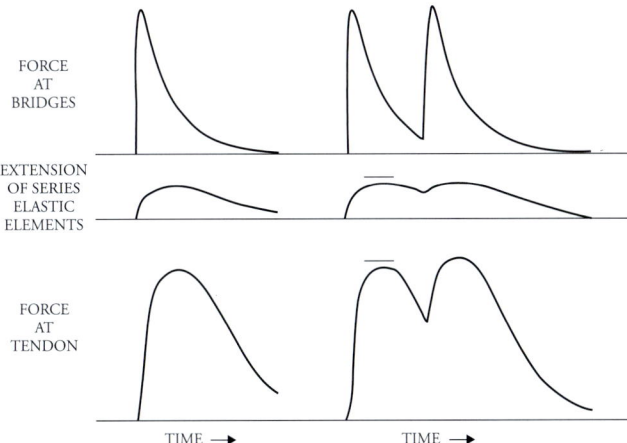

Figure 6.10 A brief stretch reflex recorded from the quadriceps tendon. The initial small, sharp response is the quick stretch which initiated the large response. The time marks are 20 msec apart. (From Ballif et al.: Proc. Roy. Soc., B98, 589, 1925.)

RECIPROCAL INNERVATION OF A JOINT

When the biceps femoralis muscle contracts, the opposing muscle, the quadriceps, is stretched because both muscles are connected to the tibia. The quadriceps group has a strong stretch

Figure 6.12 Tension response in the tibialis anterior to stimulation of the skin of (*A*) the ipsilateral foot, (*B*) ipsilateral calf, or (*C*) both. Stimulation of both sites results in a tension response greater than the sum of the individual responses: summation. Spinal rabbit. (From unpublished experiments of B.A. Curtis, M.C. Fleming, and E.M. Marcus.)

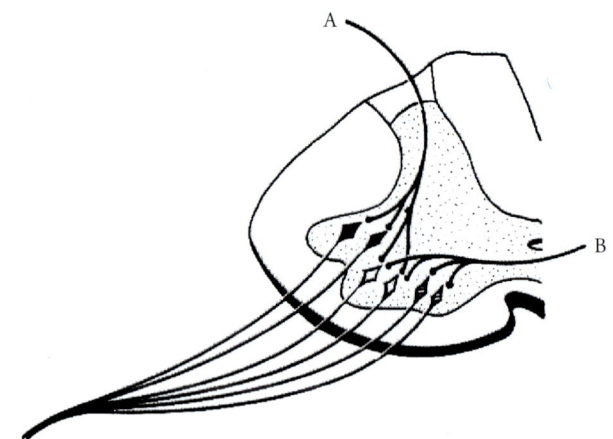

Figure 6.13 A mechanism of summation. Stimulation of nerve A fires the solid anterior horn cells and excites the clear cells. Stimulation of nerve B excites the lined cells to fire and excites the clear cells. Stimulation of both nerves fires all of the cells.

reflex which is not elicited when the biceps femoralis contracts. When the quadriceps tendon is stretched, stretch reflex tension develops (Fig. 6.14). The tension is maintained until the biceps tendon is stretched; then the tension abruptly drops. This diminution or abolition is called inhibition. Inhibition is, together with facilitation, the keystone of the integrative action of the spinal cord and probably the entire nervous system.

The pathway for the inhibitory response is shown in Figure 6.15. A collateral (branch) of the stretch receptor nerve from the biceps muscle runs to an interneuron, which in turn synapses on the anterior horn cells of the quadriceps. As far as we know, all inhibitory responses are carried out through at least one interneuron. The endings of one nerve, such as the stretch receptor nerve, all have the same effect, either facilitation or inhibition. For the nerve pathway to exhibit the other type of function, an interneuron must intercede.

The pathway for the inhibition is shown in Figure 6.14. Trains of action potentials from the stretch receptors of biceps enter the anterior root and stimulate biceps anterior horn cells and, via an interneuron, inhibit the quadriceps muscle.

MEMBRANE BASIS OF INTEGRATION

When a microelectrode is inserted into the anterior horn of the spinal cord, the tip, with luck, eventually penetrates an anterior horn cell. This penetration is signaled by the abrupt jump of voltage between the tip and the extracellular fluid from 0 to –70 mV. This intracellular work was pioneered by Sir John Eccles and his collaborators and is discussed at length in his book *The Synapse*. In this experiment the anterior roots are cut to prevent action potentials, generated by the stimulator, from traveling up the motor axons antidromically (backward). Stimulation, then, mimics only sensory input. Low-voltage stimulation activates only the larger, stretch receptor axons. The extracellular recording from the posterior root gives a signal proportional to the number of axons stimulated. After the cell is penetrated it must be identified; it is almost certain to be an anterior horn cell because of their large size. Other cell bodies and glia cells are so small that penetration is very unlikely. The destination of its axon is determined by using the stretch reflex pathway. Each muscle nerve is stimulated in turn until a short latency, all-or-nothing spike (action potential) response is obtained. This is the equivalent of a monosynaptic stretch reflex. A spike response recorded from an anterior horn cell is the counterpart of muscle tension.

EXCITATORY POSTSYNAPTIC POTENTIAL

When a flexor anterior horn cell has been located, the record in Figure 6.16 is obtained by stimulating a cutaneous nerve to mimic pain. When the nerve is stimulated at high voltage, many small pain fibers are stimulated. The response in the anterior horn cell can be the firing of an action potential, as in the lowest record. This response is the electrically recorded counterpart of the reflexive withdrawal from a painful stimulus, as shown in Figure 6.13. When the stimulus intensity is reduced, upper records; intensity is reached when no action potential is produced, yet the cell body still responds. The response is a subthreshold depolarization of the anterior horn

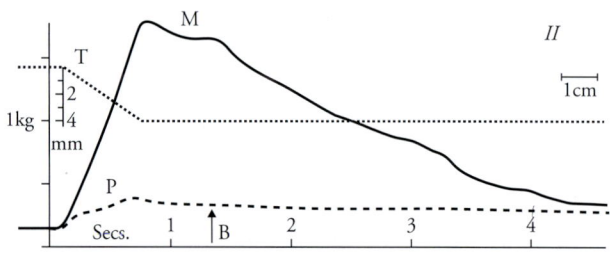

Figure 6.14 Inhibition of a stretch reflex (M) in an extensor muscle, quadriceps, by stretch, at B, of a flexor muscle, biceps. T is the applied stretch to the extensor tendon that initiated the stretch reflex. (From Liddell and Sherrington: Proc. Roy. Soc., B97, 267, 1925.)

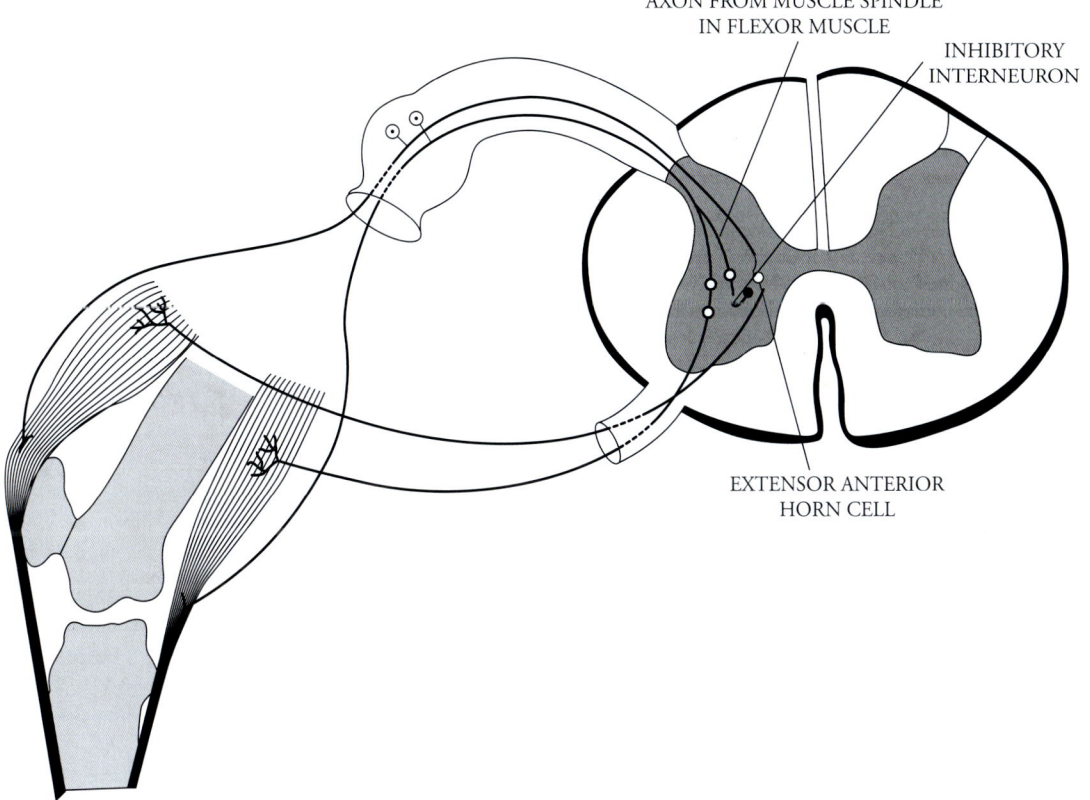

Figure 6.15 The pathway for the inhibition shown in Figure 6.14. Trains of action potentials from the stretch receptor of biceps enter the anterior root and stimulate biceps anterior horn cells and, via an interneuron, inhibit the quadriceps anterior horn cells.

cell called an excitatory postsynaptic potential (EPSP). This response brings the anterior horn cell closer to threshold, that is, closer to firing an action potential that would cause contraction of a motor group. The EPSP is localized to the cell body and dendrites. The axon is unaffected. In contrast to the action potential, it is a graded response.

The EPSPs can add up until threshold is reached and an action potential is fired as is shown in Figure 6.17. Note that the second EPSP in *A* is larger (greater depolarization) than the first. The effect of the first had not yet "worn off" and the second could add on top of it. In *B* the second EPSP follows sooner and adds up to a threshold depolarization, initiating an action potential.

This is the basic mechanism of facilitation. The two classic types of facilitation, temporal and spatial, are the same in terms of a membrane response: the EPSPs add up. Spatial response refers to the EPSPs generated as a result of the activation of two different nerves as in Figure 6.13. Temporal summation, as illustrated in Figure 6.20, means summation in time; its membrane basis depends upon the time course of the EPSP. The membrane repolarizes slowly following the initial rapid depolarization of an EPSP and a second EPSP can add upon the first. Frequently this "added boost" will bring the cell membrane to the threshold for firing an action potential in the axon.

DELAY

There is a delay of approximately 0.8 msec between the arrival of an action potential from a stretch receptor axon and response of an anterior horn cell. This delay and other features strongly support chemical transmission at the synapses on the anterior horn cell. The identity of the transmitter is still not entirely clear, although there is a great deal of evidence to suggest that L-glutamate and L-aspartate are the transmitters for many of the excitatory synapses in the spinal cord.

These transmitters destroy the selective permeability of the postsynaptic membrane, just as acetylcholine does at the myoneural junction. The equilibrium potential is then zero millivolts. The membrane never reaches zero under the influence of excitatory transmitters since they are rapidly removed. At the anterior horn cell membrane, however, unlike the myoneural junction, the amount of excitatory transmitter released is not always sufficient to depolarize the cell body to threshold.

INHIBITORY POSTSYNAPTIC POTENTIAL

When the nerve leading to the quadriceps muscle is stimulated, the membrane of a flexor (an antagonist) anterior horn cell hyperpolarizes, as shown in the recordings in Figure 6.18. This hyperpolarizing response, called an inhibitory postsynaptic potential (IPSP), moves the membrane further from threshold, making it more difficult to fire an action potential and is a postsynaptic inhibition. The IPSP is the membrane equivalent of inhibition. As noted earlier, inhibition is effected through an interneuron (Fig. 6.14).

The transmitter substances responsible for the IPSP include GABA and glycine. They specifically increase the chloride conductance of the anterior horn cell, typically for hundreds of milliseconds. The membrane potential at rest

Figure 6.16 Excitatory postsynaptic potentials (EPSPs): The upper trace of each pair is an intracellular record from a biceps anterior horn cell. The lower trace of each pair is the action current from the posterior root and is proportional to the number of sensory axons firing. As the number of axons firing increases, the depolarization (an EPSP) increases until threshold for the anterior horn cell is reached and an action potential fires. The bottom pair of records is the intracellular version of a stretch reflex. The rest of the action potential of the lower record is off the scale. The average resting potential is –70 mV. (From Brock, Coombs, and Eccles: J. Physiol., 117, 431, 1952.)

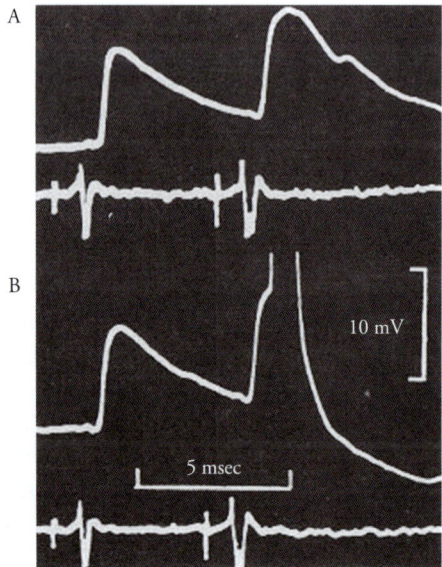

Figure 6.17 The summation of two excitatory postsynaptic potentials (EPSPs) to fire an action potential. In A the second EPSP is larger than the first. In B the second EPSP followed sooner and added upon the first to achieve a threshold depolarization, initiating an action potential. (From Brock, Coombs, and Eccles: J. Physiol., 117, 431, 1952.)

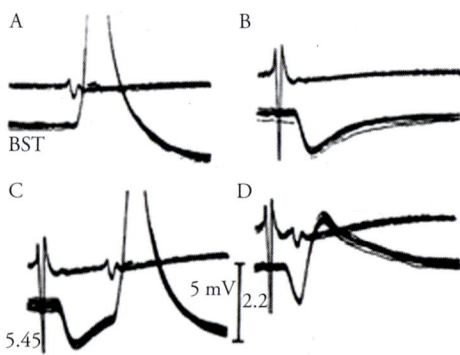

Figure 6.18 The response (an inhibitory postsynaptic potential [IPSP]) of a biceps anterior horn cell to stimulation of the quadriceps nerve. The upper trace of each pair is the action current from the posterior root; the lower is the intracellular record. The greater the number of sensory axons firing, the more negative and longer lasting is the IPSP. (From Coombs, Eccles, and Fatt: J. Physiol., 130, 396, 1955.)

is –74 mV, indicating there is considerable sodium conductance in relationship to potassium and chloride conductance. The calculated values for potassium, chloride, and sodium equilibrium voltages are VK = –90 mV, VCl = –80 mV, and VNa = +45 mV. A large increase in chloride conductance will result in a membrane potential of –80 mV, and this is the equilibrium potential at the height of the IPSP.

Summation of IPSPs and EPSPs can occur as shown in Figure 6.19. The microelectrode is recording from an anterior horn cell innervating biceps (a flexor). When the stretch receptor nerve from the biceps is stimulated (Fig. 6.19A), an action potential fires; this is the stretch reflex. When the nerve to the quadriceps (an opposing extensor) is stimulated (Fig. 6.19B), a large IPSP is recorded; this is the inhibition of a stretch reflex of an opposing muscle. When the two are stimulated 45 msec apart (Fig. 6.19C), the cell fires. When the delay was reduced, the membrane depolarizes but does not reach threshold (Fig. 6.19D).

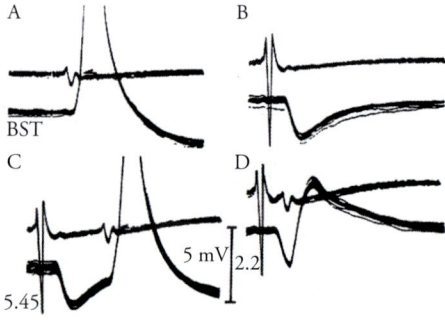

Figure 6.19 Summation of an inhibitory postsynaptic potential (IPSP) and an excitatory postsynaptic potential (EPSP). The lower trace of each pair is an intracellular recording from a biceps anterior horn cell. The upper trace is the action current in the posterior root. In A the nerve to the biceps was stimulated and an action potential evoked; this is the intracellular equivalent of a stretch reflex. In B the nerve to quadriceps was stimulated and an IPSP was evoked. In C the two were stimulated 45 msec apart and a spike resulted. In D the two were stimulated 2.2 msec apart and no action potential resulted; the IPSP generated by the quadriceps stimulus inhibited the biceps anterior horn cell. In C the hyperpolarization effect of the IPSP had declined by the time the second nerve was stimulated. (From Coombs, Eccles, and Fatt: J. Physiol., 130, 396, 1955.)

SYNAPTIC MECHANISMS

The dendritic tree and cell bodies of spinal cord neurons contain a varied collection of receptor-mediated ionic channels that are summarized in Figure 6.19 along with some of the neurotransmitters implicated in their activation. All of these ionic channels act on a time scale of milliseconds to seconds.

The fast EPSP channel (A) is very similar to the ACh channel at the myoneuronal endplate. It opens to all small ions and depolarizes rapidly and decisively. The somewhat slower IPSP Cl channel (B) is equally important. Selective increase in PK (C) usually occurs after action potential firing in the axon and is thought to be mediated by increasing Ca, possibly entering during the very positive voltages of the action potential. All of these mechanisms depend on increasing ionic permeability (decreasing cell resistance) and to rapidly changing intracellular ionic concentrations which must be restored by energy expenditure.

The next two mechanisms (D and E) rely on decreases in permeability and are more energy efficient.

The active transport of unequal numbers of ionic changes can result in changes in membrane voltage; 3Na/2K and 3Na/Ca are examples. The relative importance of this electrogenic mechanism is not clear.

Intermediate term changes in neuron baseline characteristics (more or less excitable) are produced by altering the number of active channels on the cell surface. For example, in response to noxious stimuli 5 HT is co-released from sensory a nerve which increases the C-AMP level of the interneuron causing rapid inactivation by dephosphorylation of potassium channels. Whenever an action potential enters the presynaptic region, the depolarization is prolonged because the normal increase in PK that hastens repolarization is lacking. Consequently, the voltage-gated Ca channels remain open longer, allowing greater Ca entry and hence greater transmitter release. This augmented response may last for several hours after 5 HT liberation. The key to specificity is both the type of receptor and the enzyme chain–second messenger system linked to it. Receptors for epinephrine and norepinephrine increase the number of phosphorylated, hence active, Ca channels.

Enhancement of synaptic transmission lasting one or more days occurs by increasing the amount of neurotransmitter released from each synaptic vesicle. Increase in synaptic vesicle content presumably reflects changes in gene expression that could last a very long time and might be the synaptic basis of long-term memory. This mechanism alters the importance of existing synapses. A synaptic junction that previously needed the cooperative effort of 10 other synaptic junctions to depolarize the cell body to threshold can now do so alone.

The only other major variants seen when recording from anterior horn cells are long-lasting (30 to 40 msec) responses. These are thought to involve many interneurons possibly arranged in a circular path so that an action potential "chases its tail" around the circuit for several revolutions, stimulating the anterior horn cells on each revolution. They may also be produced by long-acting neurotransmitters coreleased from the same axons that release the shorter acting neurotransmitters.

SLOW POTENTIALS

Action potentials in axons making synaptic contact with the dendrites or cell body of an anterior horn cell are expressed within the anterior horn cell as depolarizations (EPSPs, a very few of which will, by themselves, fire the cell) and hyperpolarization (IPSPs, which inhibit firing). The membrane potential of the cell is constantly changing under the influence of these two types of input. Whenever the membrane potential reaches the firing level of the axon (−55 mV), action potentials are generated with a frequency proportional to the depolarization past threshold. For the purposes of transmission, depolarization, more positive than threshold, is coded as frequency. When these action potentials bombard another cell, they are once again decoded into changes in the membrane potential of that cell body.

It is not clear why the EPSPs and IPSPs recorded from the cell body are of different amplitude. This may be due to differences in the amount of transmitter released or may be due to the location of the synapse on the cell. Since the dendrites, like the cell body, conduct potential disturbances in a decremental, cable fashion, synapses close to the cell body will have a greater influence on the membrane potential.

It is possible to show inhibition of firing of anterior horn cells without any change in the resting membrane potential; no IPSP precedes the inhibition. The inhibition is thought to take place presynaptically, either at a nearby unidentified interneuron or more probably, in the junction region between the axon and the dendrite. We will discuss this type of inhibition later in this chapter.

STRETCH RECEPTORS

THE MUSCLE SPINDLE

In the previous discussion of spinal reflexes, reference to stretch receptors was very general. The major dynamic stretch receptor is the muscle spindle. This is a bundle of modified muscle fibers that lie parallel to the rest of the muscle fibers. Its structure is shown in Figure 6.20; it is composed basically of three to five small muscle fibers, each containing a specialized, nonstriated region in their center. The striated ends of the muscle fibers can contract and are innervated by small, gamma motor neurons. These gamma motor neurons have cell bodies in the anterior horn, just as do the large alpha fibers that innervate the bulk of the muscle.

The small muscle fibers in the spindle are called intrafusal fibers, and the large muscle fibers that make up the bulk of the muscle are referred to as extrafusal fibers. The extrafusal fibers are primarily innervated by large (8–12 μm) axons. The pattern is not exclusive and there is some dual innervation—alpha motor fibers to both intra and extrafusal fibers.

There are two sensory nerves that take origin from the unstriated center region of the muscle spindle. The largest (12 μm), classified Ia, comes from the center of the sensory region. The unmyelinated ends of the nerve wrap around each of the muscle fibers and are called primary or annulospiral endings. From these endings arise the action potentials that

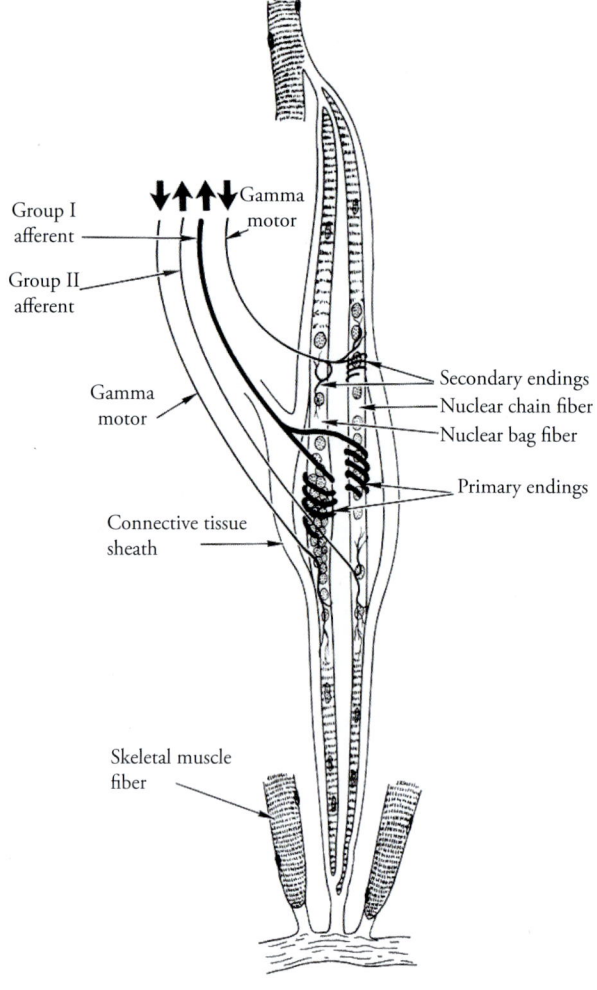

Figure 6.20 A muscle spindle. (From Gardner: Fundamentals of Neurology. Philadelphia, W.B. Saunders, 1968.)

stimulate the stretch reflexes. This axon gives off many types of collateral within the gray matter of the cord that then travel up and down the cord for several segments.

The second ending gives off a smaller nerve, classified IIa, from specialized, secondary or flower-spray endings on either side of the annulospiral ending. These axons rise to the ipsilateral cerebellum, carrying information on "unconscious position sense." They apparently play no part in the stretch reflex.

The basic function of the stretch receptor is to fire when the muscle is stretched. The response of the annulospiral ending is of short latency. The frequency of firing is at first high; it then slows down but never adapts completely.

THE GAMMA SYSTEM

The function of the intrafusal muscle fibers is more difficult to understand. The first function is to keep the muscle spindle tight as the extrafusal fibers contract; Figure 6.21 shows this. At the rest length (*A*) the spindle is tight. Any further stretch will set up a volley of action potentials in the Ia sensory nerve that will lead to a stretch reflex: contraction of the extrafusal fibers. When the extrafusal fibers contract because of firing in the alpha motor neuron alone, the spindle goes slack (*B*) and is no longer responsive to stretch. Indeed, the muscle would have to be pulled out slightly further than the rest position for the spindle to react. To rectify this situation, the gamma motor neuron fires, thus contracting the intrafusal fiber, and the spindle is tight again (*C*). Through the mechanism of the gamma motor neurons the sensitivity of the stretch reflex is maintained throughout the entire range of the limb movement. For example, the knee-jerk reflex can be elicited in many positions of the lower leg. Another function of the intrafusal fibers is to change the sensitivity of the annulospiral ending (Fig. 6.21). It can easily be seen, in the last column, that the

Figure 6.21 The effect of gamma activation of intrafusal muscle fibers upon maintenance of "tone" in the muscle spindle. In *A* the extrafusal fibers are at rest. When just the extrafusal fibers contract (*B*), the spindle becomes slack and unresponsive to small stretches. When both alpha and gamma systems are activated, the spindle is once again taut and responsive to small stretches (*C*).

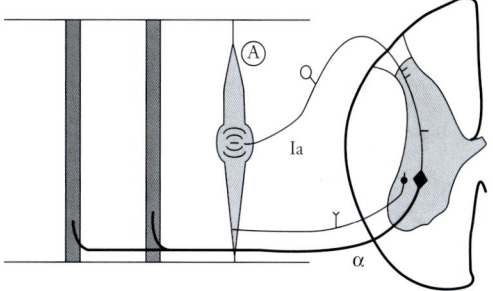

Figure 6.22 The response of an Ia fiber from an annulospiral ending to stretch and gamma activity. Notice that the number of action potentials fired increases with stretch (weight) and gamma activation. The downward deflections are stimulus artifacts of gamma stimulation. (From Kuffler, et al.: J. Neurophysiol, 14, 29, 1951.)

response to 20 g tension or an equivalent stretch can be drastically altered by activity of the intrafusal fiber. Apparently the annulospiral ending reacts to stretch or deformation whether it is from without, as in stretch, or from within, as in intrafusal muscle fiber activity.

Probably the most important function of the intrafusal fibers is to modulate contraction of the extrafusal fibers via the stretch reflex. It is clear from Figure 6.21 that activation of the gamma fibers and subsequent contraction of the intrafusal fibers set up a response in the Ia sensory fibers which is indistinguishable from the response to stretch (compare response in the upper right and lower left in Figure 6.22). This activation of the Ia sensory fiber leads to contraction of the extrafusal fibers. This is probably best shown by the accompanying sketches (Figs. 6.22 and 6.23).

The length of A is the equilibrium point for the stretch reflex when there is no gamma activity; stretch of this muscle would lead to extrafusal contraction. At A the gamma fiber is suddenly activated. During the period B, the intrafusal fibers are contracting, stretching the annulospiral ending and altering the sensitivity of the primary stretch receptor to the dashed line. The Ia ending increases its rate of firing and causes reflexive shortening of the extrafusal fibers and shortening of the muscle as a whole, as is happening in C. This process continues in D until point E is reached. At E the muscle as a whole has contracted sufficiently to decrease the stress on the center region of the muscle spindle and reduce the rate of firing of the Ia fiber to threshold for the stretch reflex.

The shortening and subsequent maintenance of muscle length and, consequently, of the joint angle was brought about by a constant gamma activation (Fig. 6.24). The rate of firing of the gamma system, initiated by the brain, has not changed during the entire time. The new position (E) is not affected by the load the muscle had to move. If the load was light, the new position was reached quickly; if the load was heavy, the new position was reached slowly. In any event, the new position was reached and maintained without further judgment from the motor centers of the brain.

This loop will provide good length control if movement is very slow. If movement is faster, this simple type of loop will begin oscillating because of nerve conduction and synaptic delays. As the muscle is contracting, its length at t = 0 is sent up the sensory nerve and arrives at the spinal cord at t + 15 msec.

γ Fibers (firing at 20/sec) activate intrafusal fibers. The annulospiral ending in deformed and discharge rate of the Ia fiber is increased.

Extrofusal fibers contract and muscle shortens. As the muscle shortens, there is less stress on the central region and the role of firing of Ia decreases.

As the rate of firing of Ia decreases, the reflexive contraction of the extrafusal fibers diminishes.

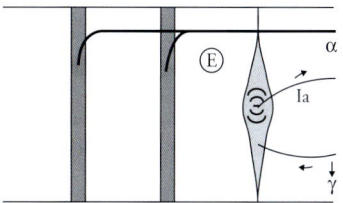

An equilibrium is reached in which the firing rate of the Ia fiber is just below threshold for reflexive contraction of the extrafusal fibers.

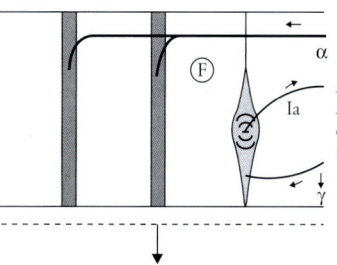

A new rest length is obtained. A slight stretch will activate the extrofusal fibers and return the muscle to its new length reflexively.

Figure 6.23 The role of the gamma system in setting a new muscle length. (Refer to text for discussion.)

6 SPINAL CORD: STRUCTURE AND FUNCTION · 121

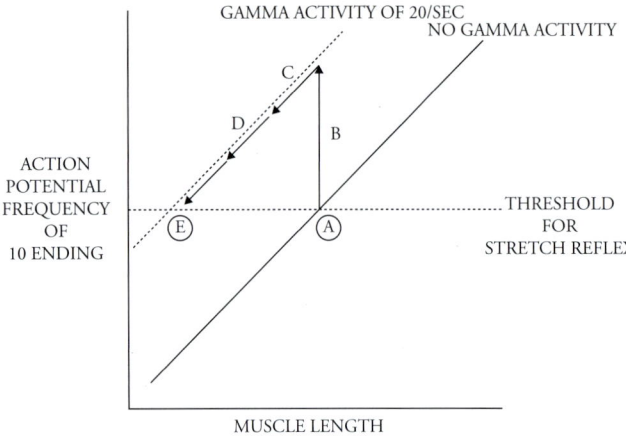

Figure 6.24 The effect of gamma activation upon maintenance of "tone" in the muscle spindle.

After a 5 msec delay the rate of firing of the anterior horn cell varies. This variation arrives via the motor nerve at the muscle in another 15 msec. Thirty-five milliseconds have elapsed, the muscle is no longer at its original length, and the "correction" is no longer correct. This will lead to a cycle of overcorrections around the intended length: oscillations.

The oscillations can be rectified if the control system is given information on the rate of change of position, velocity. With this information the control system in the spinal cord can figure out where the muscle will be at the end of the delay time and make corrections accordingly. Careful inspection of Figure 6.21, particularly the right-hand column, will show that the firing rate at the beginning of movement is faster: there is velocity information in the signal from the stretch receptor.

The difficulty with the pure gamma stimulation of muscle activity theory is that recordings such as are shown in Figure 6.21 show that the alpha fibers are activated at about the same time as the gamma fibers, not 30–40 msec later as the theory predicts. Other evidence suggests that muscle movement probably gets started by direct alpha stimulation and is later reinforced by reflexive gamma stimulation. The termination point may well be found and maintained mainly through the gamma system.

Let us digress a moment and consider the simplest type of muscle movement: opposing the thumb to the palm. Cells in the anterior horn are activated by fibers from the large descending corticospinal tract, a direct pathway, of which more will be said later. The intensity of stimulation and the number of motor groups activated are determined by the motor cortex. The motor cortex basically sets the tension that is to be developed. The distance moved is a function of the resistance to movement and the duration of the stimulus. The extent of movement is visually controlled; when the thumb reaches the desired position, the motor cortex stops stimulating the anterior horn cells.

In contrast to this type of movement, which requires constant attention if the desired position is to be achieved, many of our movements, such as walking, require little attention beyond the decision to walk along the sidewalk. Most of us can even chew gum at the same time! These movements are probably carried out through mediation of the gamma system, which allows the brain to set a desired position and then forget about it. Compare, then a corticospinal system, which produces a force, and a second system, the gamma system, which produces a new position. Although it is not completely clear at this time, it would appear that the gamma anterior horn cells are innervated by descending motor tracts other than the corticospinal. This system is controlled by neurons in the brain stem: the reticular formation, the vestibular nucleus, and the red nucleus.

GOLGI TENDON ORGANS

Golgi tendon organs are a second type of stretch receptor found in the tendinous insertion of muscles. It contains no muscle fiber system. This receptor is in series with the muscle fibers and signals tension via Ib sensory fibers. It is much more sensitive to tension generated by the muscle than to stretch of the muscle. Activation of the sensory fibers from the tendon organ causes an inhibition of the contraction of the muscle. Among the functions of the tendon organ is to protect the insertion of the muscle from too great a stress which might tear the insertion from the bone. Tension information from the tendon organ is transmitted to higher centers via both dorsal and ventral spinocerebellar tracts.

INTERNEURONS

Only a very small portions of the cells of the gray matter of the spinal cord are anterior horn cells; the vast majority are interneurons—small cells with short dendrites and axons. These cells interconnect incoming sensory axons and descending spinal cord tracts with each other and with anterior horn cells.

One such interneuron is the Renshaw cell, which must be studied in a somewhat roundabout fashion. After the posterior (sensory) roots have been cut, stimulation of a muscle nerve (for example, to the gastrocnemius) will result in action potentials traveling back up the motor nerve (antidromic) and

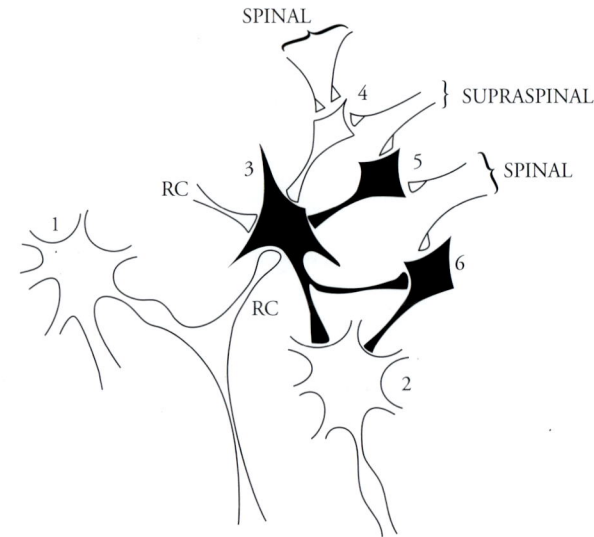

Figure 6.25 Major classes of input to Renshaw cell.

Figure 6.26 Renshaw cell activity; left-hand responses are produced by stimuli to ventral roots conducted antidromically. This activity can be inhibited (right-hand responses) by (*A*) a squeeze of the ipsilateral toe and (*B*) by stimulus to the contralateral biceps-semitendinous nerve. (From Wilson, Talbot, and Kato: J. Neurophysiol., 27, 1063, 1964.)

entering the spinal cord. An extracellular electrode records a burst of high-frequency action potentials from the Renshaw cell in response to a single volley of action potentials (Fig. 6.26). Electrophoresing dye from a recording electrode has localized these cells. After a Renshaw cell has been characterized physiologically by its response to antidromic stimulation, dye is deposited at the tip of the electrode by passing current through the microelectrode. An example of this widely used technique is shown in Figure 6.27. When many such dots are placed together on a spinal cord cross section (Fig. 6.27), they all appear in the most anterior portion of the anterior horn. This is the same region in which the axons from the anterior horn cells branch.

The firing of anterior horn cells activates the Renshaw cell with acetylcholine as the neurotransmitter. Studies of a Renshaw cell show it to remove inhibition from the anterior horn cell 2 in Figures 6.26, 6.27, and 6.28. The effect of inhibition of an inhibitory cell is called disinhibition. This does not mean that anterior horn cell 2 will fire, since that requires a facilitatory stimulus, but it be activated by antidromic stimulation of any of a great many motor nerve fibers, even from different muscles. These muscles, however, usually belong to a single functional grouping, such as knee flexors or ankle extensors. The effect of Renshaw cell activation upon other anterior horn cells is inhibitory; it depresses or totally inhibits firing. This is shown diagrammatically in Figure 6.25. Activity in anterior horn cell 1 will inhibit, via the Renshaw cell, anterior horn cell 2. This inhibition is usually to opposing muscle groups. The Renshaw cell

Figure 6.27 Localization of the Renshaw cells by the method of dye electrophoresis from the recording electrode. (*A*) The dye spot among the anterior horn cells. The dye spot, arrow, is an azure blue while the cells are purple. (*B*) The location of a number of dye spots superimposed upon a tracing of a lumbar spinal cord segment. (From Thomas and Wilson: Nature, 206:211, 1965.)

itself can be inhibited by a variety of pathways, such as squeezing the ipsilateral toes and stimulating the muscle nerve on the contralateral side (Fig. 6.26). Note that in each case the response to the antidromic stimulation is much reduced.

Since the Renshaw cell is inhibitory to anterior horn cells, inhibiting the Renshaw cell does mean that no inhibition is being applied via that particular Renshaw circuit. This phenomenon of disinhibition is quite common in the nervous system.

POSTERIOR AND VENTRAL HORN

LAMINAR ORGANIZATION

The posterior horn contains the entry of the sensory fibers and their rich synaptic connections. Many names have been proposed for the regions of the posterior and intermediate horns to

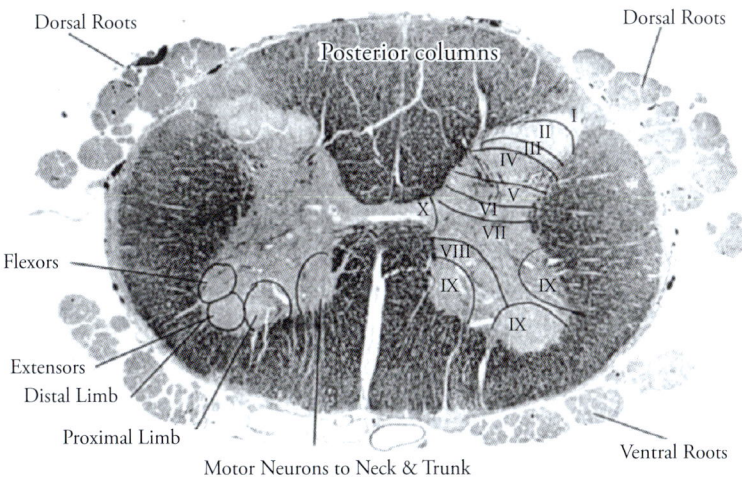

Figure 6.28 Rexed's lamination pattern of the spinal gray matter on the right and the location of ventral horn cells on the left, lumbar section. Myelin stain.

describe their anatomical and physiological variations. In order to clear up this confusion about the terminology of the organization of the gray matter of the cord, Rexed proposed a laminar organization of the cat spinal cord which has since been extended to all primates. The gray matter is divided into nine layers with a thin tenth region surrounding the central canal (Fig. 6.28).

Lamina 1 forms the cap of the dorsal horn and is penetrated by many fibers. It includes the nucleus posterior marginalis. Many intersegmental pathways arise from this layer.

Lamina 2 corresponds to the substantia gelatinosa. This nucleus extends the entire length of the cord and is most prominent in the cervical and lumbar levels. Cells in this lamina also form intersegmental connections.

Lamina 3 is the broad zone containing many myelinated axons and receives many synapses from the dorsal root fibers.

Lamina 4 is the largest zone and consists primarily of the nucleus proprius of the dorsal horn. This nucleus is conspicuous in all levels.

Lamina 5 extends across the neck of the dorsal horn and in all but the thoracic region is divided into medial and lateral portions. The lateral portion consists of the reticular nucleus that is most conspicuous in the cervical levels. Corticospinal and posterior root synapses have been identified in this lamina.

Lamina 6 is a wide zone most prominent in the cervical and lumbar enlargements. In these levels, it is divided into medial and lateral zones. Terminals from the posterior roots end in the medial region while descending fiber tracts project to the lateral zone.

Lamina 7 includes most of the intermediate region of the gray matter in the spinal cord. In this lamina are found the intermediolateral and intermediomedial nuclei. The nucleus dorsalis or nucleus spinal cerebellar of Clark is obvious in C8 through L2 levels. The axons arising from this nucleus form the posterior spinocerebellar tract. In the cervical and lumbar enlargements, this lamina includes many of the internuncials and the cell bodies of gamma efferent neurons. Axons from posterior roots, cerebral cortex, and other systems end in lamina 7. Cells in lamina 7 form tracts that project to higher levels, including cerebellum and thalamus. In the thoracic and sacral regions axons also leave this lamina to form preganglionic autonomic connections.

Lamina 8 in the cervical and lumbar enlargement is confined to the medial part of the anterior horn. Many of the axons from these nerve cells form commissural fibers in the anterior white column. Axons from descending pathways originating in the brain stem terminate here.

Lamina 9 includes the largest cell bodies in the spinal cord, the ventral horn cells. The axons of these cells (alpha motor neurons) form much of the ventral rootlets that supply the extrafusal muscle fibers. The medial group innervates the muscles of the axial skeleton while the lateral group innervates the muscles of the appendicular skeleton.

Lamina 10 includes the commissural axons.

POSTERIOR ROOT FIBERS

Sensory nerve fibers enter the spinal cord gray matter (Fig. 6.28) by a medial bundle of large, heavily myelinated fibers and a lateral bundle consisting of thinly myelinated and unmyelinated axons. The heavily myelinated medial bundles convey information from the large dorsal root ganglion cells subserving encapsulated somatic receptors (muscle spindles, pacinian corpuscles, Meissner's corpuscles), carrying information on touch, position, and vibratory senses. Upon entering the spinal cord, the axons divide into ascending and descending processes, both giving off collaterals. Many of these collaterals end in the segments above or below the level of entry. Branches from the larger fibers enter the ipsilateral posterior funiculus and ascend to the medulla. The large myelinated axons also have numerous terminals in Clark's nucleus in lamina 7. Collaterals from posterior root fibers also enter Lamina 7 and 9, ending on internuncial neurons and anterior horn cells for reflex activity.

The smaller, lateral bundle of thin axons (A delta & C fibers) conveys information from free nerve endings, tactile receptors, and other unencapsulated receptors. These fibers, conveying impulses of tissue damage, temperature, and light touch sensation, enter Lissauer's tract (fasciculus dorsal lateralis) (Figs. 6.28 and 6.34). Axons from Lissauer's tract enter laminas I, II, and III. Axons from this lamina ascend and descend in Lissauer's tract to reenter the same lamina.

NOCICEPTION AND PAIN

Any stimulus, such as heat, trauma, or pressure, which produces tissue damage or irritation, is a nociceptive stimulus. Nociceptive stimuli are the afferent arm of many reflexes; locally, a red wheal develops around a cut, withdrawal of a limb from a hot pipe is a spinal cord reflex, while tachycardia from an electric shock to the finger is a brain stem autonomic reflex. Only when this nociceptive information reaches the thalamus and cerebral cortex should we talk about pain. Pain perception by these higher centers triggers affective responses and suffering behaviors. The pain experience varies enormously from person to person and the circumstances may alter the response. Contrast the pain of your thumb being hit with a hammer when you are fixing your sailboat, doing a "chore" around the house, or holding the nail for someone else.

As a gross oversimplification, we perceive pain in two ways. The first is pricking, itching, or sharp and easily localizable, such as a razor blade cut or a mosquito bite. This type of pain is usually short lasting, up to a day or so, and is usually tolerated. In contrast, the second kind of pain may be described as dull, aching, or burning and is poorly localized. This type of pain is longer lasting (rheumatoid arthritis) or repetitive (menstrual cramps) and is often poorly tolerated, frequently coloring the person's entire view of life.

RECEPTORS

Tissue damage releases a variety of typical intracellular substances, including K^+, H^+, and bradykinin, as well as specialized compounds such as serotonin from blood platelets, substance P from nerve terminals, and histamine from mast cells. All of these substances directly stimulate the free endings of small, myelinated A delta fibers (1–5 μm diameter) and smaller, nonmyelinated C fibers (0.25–1.5 μm diameter). A second group of released substances, including prostaglandin precursors and leukotrienes, act as sensitizers. Many of these small fibers have collaterals ending in regions containing neurotransmitter vesicles that apparently amplify nociceptive stimuli by releasing substance P when the free nerve ending is stimulated.

In addition to these relatively nonspecific receptors, the upper end of the range of stimuli to temperature and pressure receptors generates nociceptive responses. For example, heating a patch of skin to 40°C with a heat lamp gives a comfortable, warm sensation. Heating to 47°C generates a painful but tolerable experience. Higher temperatures are perceived as unbearable pain.

Cold is a diverse sensation and recently a cold channel has been identified (McKeeney, Neuhauser, and Julius, 2002). Cold and warmth are sensed by thermoreceptor proteins on the free nerve endings of the somatosensory neurons; one channel, vanilloid receptor subtype 1 (VR1), is activated by temperatures above 43°C and by vanilloid compounds, including capsaicin, the component of hot chili peppers. The other vanilloid receptor type 1 (VRL-1) is sensitive to temperatures above 50°C. The cation channel that is methanol activated (cold methanol type 1 [CMR1]) is activated by temperatures of 8°C–30°C and is a member of the transient receptor potential family of ion channels with VR1 and VRL-1 also members of this family.

These nerve fibers carrying nociceptive information join peripheral nerves, segregate into spinal nerves, and once inside the spinal dura, join posterior roots. Their cell bodies are in the posterior root ganglia while the axon continues and enters the spinal cord in the lateral bundle. Nociceptive information entering on one posterior root projects for two to three segments up and down the cord in lamina I–III. From centuries-old clinical observation we know all nociceptive information reaching consciousness, hence causing pain, crosses the neuroaxis close to the segment of entry and rises in the contralateral white column.

MODULATION OF PAIN TRANSMISSION

Transmission of pain information through the chain of neurons in the posterior root is influenced by many factors, some of them originating within the segment, some from higher centers. Most of us, after cutting or bruising ourselves, rub the surrounding area and obtain relief of the pain for as long as we rub. An animal that has been hurt will lick the wound, presumably to obtain relief of pain. This subjective phenomenon is frequently spoken of as counter-irritation; stimulation of the large, myelinated touch fibers reduces the magnitude of transmission of pain sensation through the posterior horn. This modulation takes place in the substantia gelatinosa, lamina II, within the "gate" proposed by Wall and Melzak.

Several clinical observations point to the importance of large fiber inhibition of nociceptive transmission, even in the absence of apparent nociceptive stimulation. Perhaps the most painful of these condition is avulsion, traumatic tearing out, of posterior roots. Surgical severing of posterior roots, instead of giving pain relief, often results in intolerable pain. In both cases large fiber input is lost. In contrast, destruction by a laser beam of the lateral dorsal root entry zone (for small fibers) is often highly successful in blocking the flow of nociceptive information up the neuroaxis. The large fiber input is largely spared because they enter in the medial zone.

Severed peripheral nerves often generate itching or burning sensations, causalgia, which can be alleviated by stimulating the large-diameter axons central to the cut. The large-diameter axons have low thresholds so can be stimulated without stimulating the smaller, high-threshold nociceptive fibers. Activity in the large fibers suppresses background nociceptive inflow. Trans epithelial nerve stimulation (TENS) is often effective in preventing, or reducing, peripherally generated nociception from becoming pain; it is effective in closing the gate.

As mentioned earlier, branches of many incoming large axons enter the posterior column. Stimulation of the posterior column sends antidromically conducted action potentials into the posterior horn and often reduces the pain experience.

Damaged small axons are prone to developing alpha2 adrenergic receptors, so the axon becomes sensitive to norepinephrine liberated by the peripheral sympathetic nerves. Pharmacological blocking or surgically severing sympathetic outflow often reduces pain.

The major excitatory neurotransmitter in the pain system is substance P that is found in abundance in the posterior horn, particularly lamina I and II. The mechanism of postsynaptic action is a reduction in potassium permeability leading to depolarization. The major inhibitory transmitters in the pain pathway are the enkephalin/endorphin series of peptides released from cells entirely within the posterior horn, mostly lamina II. Their action is closely mimicked by the opioid peptides. At least three modes of action have been shown, although all studies are complicated by the very small size of the cell bodies in the substantia gelatinosa (lamina II). An increase in potassium permeability has been shown which hyperpolarizes the cell and acts as an IPSP. Many studies suggest these compounds also compete with the excitatory transmitters of the region, substance P and glycine, for postsynaptic sites. Other studies suggest reduction of Ca++ influx into the presynaptic terminal in response to incoming depolarization and consequent reduction of the amount of excitatory transmitter released. Other studies implicate presynaptic inhibition (see later).

Injection of opioids into the lumbar cerebrospinal fluid often reduces nociceptive transmission and reduces the pain experience. The effect is blocked by the universal narcotic blocker, naloxone. Successful acupuncture increases endorphins in the lumbar cerebrospinal fluid.

Descending axons in both the anterolateral and posterior white columns influence transmission across this chain of synapses. Supraspinal control of these enkephalin/endorphin neurons is from the brain stem, particularly from the locus ceruleus (norepinephrine) and Raphe nuclei (5HT), both in the medulla. These areas in turn are modulated by the periaqueductal gray of the midbrain that also contains an inhibitory endorphin/enkephalin system. Stimulation of these structures results in profound anesthesia (electroanesthesia).

While the descending pathways are not clear, we can suppress the flow of nociceptive information through the posterior horn by positive thinking; for example, all "pain" studies are bedeviled by a 40% placebo effect. Yes, the third, postsurgical morphine injection can be replaced with saline and still "work" half the time.

PRESYNAPTIC INHIBITION

In contrast to the cells in the anterior horn, the major mechanism of inhibition in the posterior horn is presynaptic.

After a volley of action potentials enters the posterior root, prolonged depolarization can be measured in that and adjoining posterior root axons as well as in the substantia gelatinosa. All available evidence suggests that the next cell in the transmission pathway is not depolarized. If an action potential(s) enters the endplate region of cell II, a reduced amount of excitatory transmitter is released because of the existing depolarization. The reduced amount of transmitter released by cell II causes a smaller EPSP in cell III (panel C); in this example, cell III does not reach threshold. Presynaptic inhibition appears to be particularly useful in the sensory system because specific inputs to cell III can be blocked while other inputs (such as cell IV) have not lost their influence.

Projection Fibers

After the extensive processing just described, large-diameter, myelinated axons with cell bodies in lamina I and V cross the neuroaxis near the central canal (Fig. 6.28) to join the anterior-lateral white matter. These fibers are described later in this chapter as the Spinothalamic tract as they project to the brainstem and ultimately the cerebral cortex.

VISCERAL REFERRED PAIN

Referred pain is caused by painful impulses originating in the viscera that are transmitted by the sympathetic nerves and referred to the periphery of the body. The organ in which the pain is felt belongs to the same sensory dermatome as the visceral structure where it originates as follows: lungs, C8 to T8; heart, C8 to T8; bladder, T1 to T9; testes, T10 to T12; kidneys, T11 to L1; and rectum, S2 to S4.

TRACTS

LAMINATION PATTERN

The white matter of the cord contains axons that run up and down the spinal cord connecting segment to segment (spinospinal) and to the other regions of brain to brain stem, cerebellum, diencephalon, and basal ganglia. (The white matter is divided into three regions that are delimited by the presence of the dorsal roots that separate the posterior from the lateral funiculi and the ventral roots that separate the lateral from the anterior funiculi; see Figs. 6.29 and 6.30.)

The posterior funiculus consists primarily of the posterior columns. The lateral funiculus is a solid mass of myelinated nerve fibers containing many tracts with the ascending fibers on the outside and the descending fibers closer to the gray matter. The only way that the location of individual tracts can be determined is to examine sections after an injury in the nervous system. The anterior funiculus likewise carries many ascending and descending tracts. The location of the tracts must be determined by observing any degeneration caused by discrete lesions.

In this section we will provide an overview of the pathways in the spinal cord. A detailed discussion of the individual sensory pathways are included in Chapter 11 on the brain stem and Chapter 15 on the Thalmis region with the Diencephalon. A detailed discussion of the motor pathways is found in Chapter 18, Motor system I; and Chapter 20, Motor system III, cerebellum. The discussion in this section will focus on topics relevant to only the spinal cord.

DESCENDING TRACTS IN THE SPINAL CORD

CORTICOSPINAL TRACTS

Commands for voluntary movement travel from the brain and through the spinal cord in the corticospinal tract. This tract has its origin in the cerebral cortex, most prominently

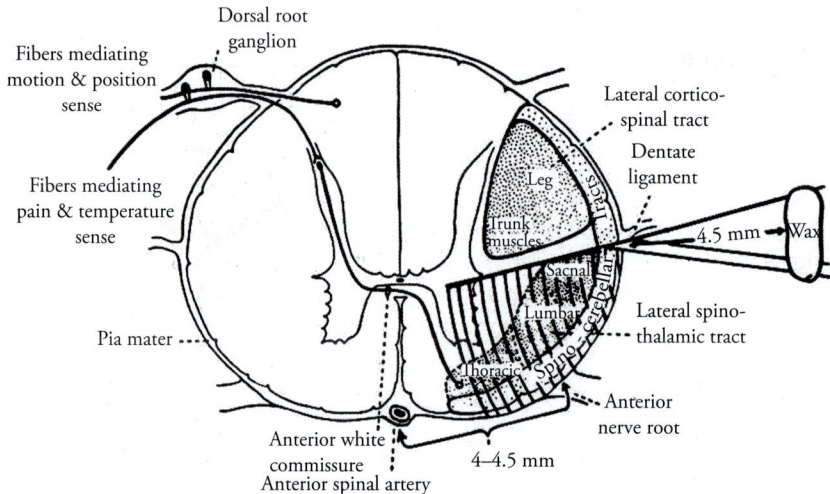

Figure 6.29 Diagram illustrating a cordotomy. The cross section of the spinal cord shows the lamination of the spinothalamic tract, the position of the pyramidal tract in relation to it, and the presence of other tracts in the lower quadrant. A piece of bone wax is mounted 4.5 mm from the tip of the knife as a depth gauge. Heavy curved lines in the ventral quadrant indicate the sweep of the knife. Note that a desire to spare the lateral corticospinal tract would result in sparing the sacral dermatomes. (From Kahn and Rand: J. Neurosurg. 9:611–619, 1952.)

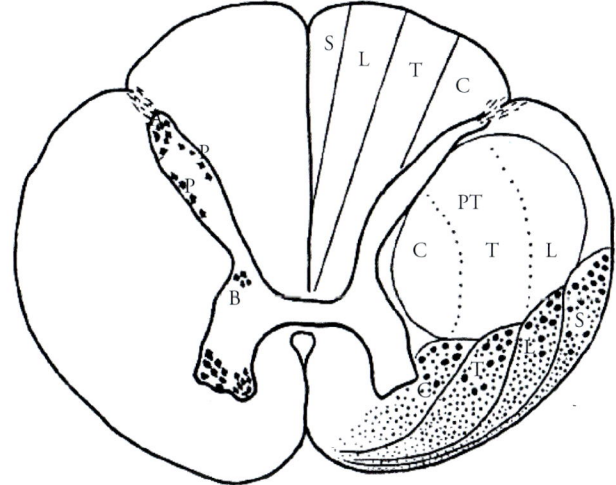

Figure 6.30 The lamination pattern of the major tracts of the spinal cord. (From Walker: Arch Neural. Psychiat. (Chicago), 43:284, 1940.)

from the motor and premotor cortex of the frontal lobe (see Chapter 17). At the junction between the medulla and the spinal cord (the level of the foramen magnum), most of the fibers cross the neuraxis, decussate, and move laterally and posteriorly to form the lateral corticospinal tract (Fig. 6.36).

The location of this pathway in the human is determined by analyzing cord sections obtained at autopsy from cases where cortical destruction has occurred in the motor areas of the precentral gyrus or in the internal capsule and axons degenerated following death of the cell body (Fig. 6.31).

The lateral corticospinal tract is the major tract for voluntary control of skeletal muscle.

Destruction of this tract leads to paralysis of skeletal muscle and the loss of voluntary movement. This paralysis is usually total distally, in the hand, and somewhat less severe in the trunk musculature. If the right tract is severed at Cl, a paralysis of both the right arm and leg will result. This is called hemiplegia, a paralysis of the arm and leg on the same side. Monoplegia is the paralysis of a single limb.

ASCENDING SENSORY TRACTS

All ascending sensory systems have three types of neurons:

1. Primary sensory neuron in dorsal root ganglion attached to each segment of the spinal cord

2. Second-order neuron in dorsal horn of spinal cord or gracile and cuneate nuclei of medulla.

   The axons of the second-order sensory neuron cross the neuroaxis, become contralateral, and form ascending pathways within the spinal cord and brain stem that terminate on third-order neurons.

3. Third-order neurons in the thalamus. Third-order neurons project to the ipsilateral sensory area of the cerebral cortex.

TACTILE DISCRIMINATION- POSTERIOR COLUMNS

Fibers in the posterior fasciculus, also known as the dorsal column (Fig. 6.32), are the major, if not exclusive, pathway for signals conveying joint position sense, tactile localization, two-point discrimination, and vibratory sensation. Fibers

Figure 6.31 The location of the corticospinal tracts as shown by degeneration caused by a lesion in the internal capsule. (From Wechsler: Clinical Neurology. Philadelphia, W.B. Saunders, 1963.)

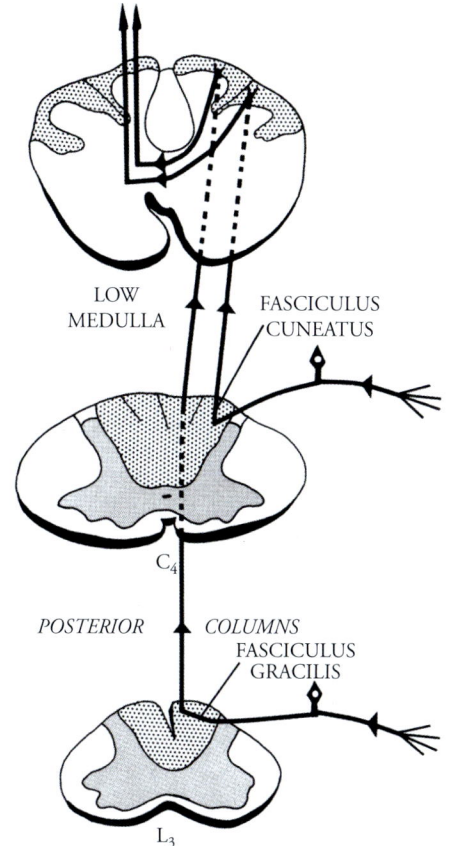

Figure 6.32 The posterior columns.

conveying touch sensation rise both in the posterior column and several other fasciculi. The fibers in this region consist primarily of heavily myelinated dorsal root ganglion fibers. Upon entering the posterior fasciculus via the medial entry root zone, these fibers divide into ascending and descending branches.

Ascending fibers from lower levels (sacral levels) lie medially while those from upper levels lie laterally. In uppermost thoracic and all cervical levels, the posterior column is divided into the medially placed fasciculus gracilis that includes fibers from the lower extremity and lower thorax and the laterally placed fasciculus cuneatus, which include fibers from the neck, upper extremity, and upper thorax. The axons in the dorsal column are primary uncrossed axons and continue without a synapse ipsilaterally up to the lower medulla where the secondary neurons begin. The axon of the secondary neuron crosses to the contralateral side and forms the medial lemniscus that ascends through pons and midbrain to the ventral posterior lateral nucleus of the thalamus. The third-order neuron in the thalamus sends its axons ipsilaterally by the posterior limb of the internal capsule onto the postcentral gyrus of the cortex.

Lesions in this pathway usually diminish tactile localization, vibratory sensation (Table 6.1). There is also loss of ability to appreciate weight differences. Position and movement sense is also affected. These deficits are most pronounced in the fingers and extremities than in the thorax or abdomen. These deficits also produce poorly coordinated movements (i.e., posterior column ataxia).

THE ANTEROLATERAL PATHWAY

Fibers carrying information on pain and temperature sense from the body all rise in the contralateral spinothalamic tract (Figs. 6.30 and 6.33). Compression, intrinsic disease, and deliberate section all result in anesthesia of the contralateral body beginning three segments below the level of disruption.

PAIN AND TEMPERATURE

Primary Cell Bodies

Cutaneous receptors for pain and temperature send axons to small and medium-sized dorsal root ganglion cells. These axons enter the spinal cord via the lateral aspects of the dorsal root entry zone. Most of these fibers enter Lissauer's tract and

Table 6.1 MAJOR PATHWAYS IN THE SPINAL CORD

PATHWAY	ORIGIN	TERMINATION	FUNCTION
Corticospinal Contralateral	Motor cortex	Lamina 7 and 9 in spinal cord	Voluntary movement of limbs
Rubrospinal Contralateral	Magnocellular portion of red nucleus in midbrain	Lamina 7 and 9	Involuntary support of movement. Facilitates flexor and inhibits extensor motor neurons, particularly arm flexors
Tectospinal Contralateral	Deep layers of superior colliculus	Lamina 7 and 9 of cervical spinal cord	Support corticospinal pathway
Vestibulospinal Uncrossed	Lateral vestibular nucleus of cranial nerve VIII	All levels of cord lamina 7 and 8	Coordination of eye and neck movements
Reticulospinal	Nucleus reticularis gigantocellularis in the medulla and from nucleus reticularis pontus caudalis and oralis of the pons	Lamina 7 and 8 of all levels of cord but especially cervical and lumbar enlargements	influence gamma motor system Facilitory to extensor motor neurons.
MLF	Cranial nerves III, V, VI, VII, & VIII, XI	Cervical cord	Coordination of eye and neck movements
Descending autonomic pathways bilateral	Hypothalamus and brain stem	Sympathetic to lamina 7 in C8-L2 Parasympathetic to Sacral nucleus of S2-S4	
Spino-spinal system	All spinal cord levels intersegmental and dorsal root fibers	Lamina	Involved in intersegmental connections or taking part in the two-neuron reflex arch
Posterior spinal cerebellar some of largest myelinated axons origin of group 1A and 1B afferent fibers. Ipsilateral	Clark's nucleus in lamina 7 from C2 to L2	Ipsilateral vermis of cerebellum	Unconscious tactile and proprioceptor information. Encapsulated (Golgi tendon organs, stretch receptors, and muscle spindles
Anterior spinocerebellar Contralateral	Lamina 5, 6, and 7 from most levels	Contralateral vermis of cerebellum	Unconscious tactile proprioception
Cuneocerebellar Ipsilateral	Accessory cuneate nucleus in low medulla	Anterior lobe and also go into the pyramis and uvula of the cerebellum	Unconscious tactile and proprioceptive information for upper extremity and neck

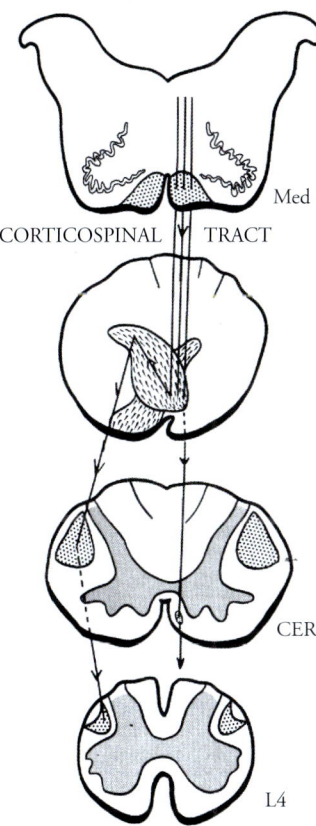

Figure 6.33 The corticospinal tracts.

branch extensively (over two or three segments on either side of the segment of entry) before entering the posterior horn, lamina I, II, and III (Fig. 6.28).

The secondary neurons arise primarily from cell bodies in lamina I and V that give origin to large axons which cross in the anterior white commissure and ascend in the contralateral anterior-lateral funiculus. As discussed earlier in the chapter (Nociception and Pain), many factors modulate information transfer across the posterior horn, between incoming nociceptive fibers and outgoing spinothalamic fibers.

There is a somatotopic arrangement in the spinothalamic tract (Figs. 6.34A and B) with the most lateral and external fibers representing sacral levels and the most intermediate and anterior fibers representing cervical levels. Pain fibers are located anteriorly to the more posteriorly placed temperature fibers. Perhaps as many as half the fibers in the tract, often called the spinoreticular tract, end in the brain stem, while many of the rest send collaterals into the brainstem on their way to the thalamus (Chapter 15). There are endings in two major nuclei of the thalamus: the ventral posterior medial nucleus and the intralaminar nuclei (see Chapter 15).

Recordings from individual spinothalamic neurons reveal four major functional categories, all contralateral.

1. Low-threshold units, activated only by gentle stimuli, for example, by stroking hairs on the arm.
2. Wide dynamic range units, activated by many types of stimuli of both high and low intensity with response graded by intensity.
3. High-threshold units, activated only by nociceptive stimuli.
4. Thermosensitive units, with high action potential frequency signaling nociception.

All of these units have small receptive fields peripherally and larger fields toward the midline. The posterior horn seems to tease apart what stimulus from what part of the body. Recording from the thalamic endings of these fibers also shows this separation of function as well as adding a wake-up function—"ouch"! A unilateral section of this tract (Fig. 6.29) for relief of pain produces a complete absence of pain and temperature from the opposite side of the body lasting for 6–9 months, but pain sensation slowly returns. Nociceptive information probably rises in Lissauer's tract until it is above the cut and then crosses.

There are several "pain" responses to nociceptive stimuli. A direct spinothalamic pathway to the contralateral ventral posterior medial nucleus of the thalamus with third order projection to the postcentral gyrus probably mediates sharp, localizable pain. Stimulation of the post central gyrus, however, rarely generates the sensation of pain. Pain is rarely reported by patients during epileptic (cortical) seizures. Apparently the thalamus tells us what (pain) and the post central gyrus tells us where. We test this pathway with the light prick of a pin and expect the patient can tell us, or point to, the location of the pin prick.

The dull throbbing quality of the pain probably ascends by a multisynaptic pathway via brain stem synapses to the midbrain and then to interlaminar thalamic nuclei with much wider cortical projection, including the limbic system. The limbic system (Chapter 22) has much to do with our outlook upon life. The thalamus alone can signal poorly localized pain to consciousness.

In addition to the spinal thalamic and spinal reticular pathways, there are other pathways that may convey pain and thermal information to the thalamus. The cervicothalamic pathway originates from the lateral cervical nucleus in the lateral column at level C1 and C2 and projects to the brain stem and thalamus. Another is the spinotectal tract running from the spinal cord to deep layers of the midbrain tegmentum to the ventral horn cells.

UNCONSCIOUS PROPRIOCEPTION FROM THE EXTREMITIES, THORAX, ABDOMEN, AND PELVIS

This information is carried up to the cerebellum by the anterior and posterior spinocerebellar tracts and the cuneocerebellar (see figures in Chapter 20). The receptors for both tracts are the neuromuscular spindles and the Golgi tendon organs.

UPPER AND LOWER MOTOR NEURONS

Causes of muscle weakness or paralysis can be grouped functionally into two categories (Table 6.2). If the difficulty is located in the corticospinal or other descending motor tract, the problem is called an upper motor neuron lesion. If the problem is in the anterior horn cell, its axon, or its motor group, the problem is called a lower motor neuron lesion. Weakness,

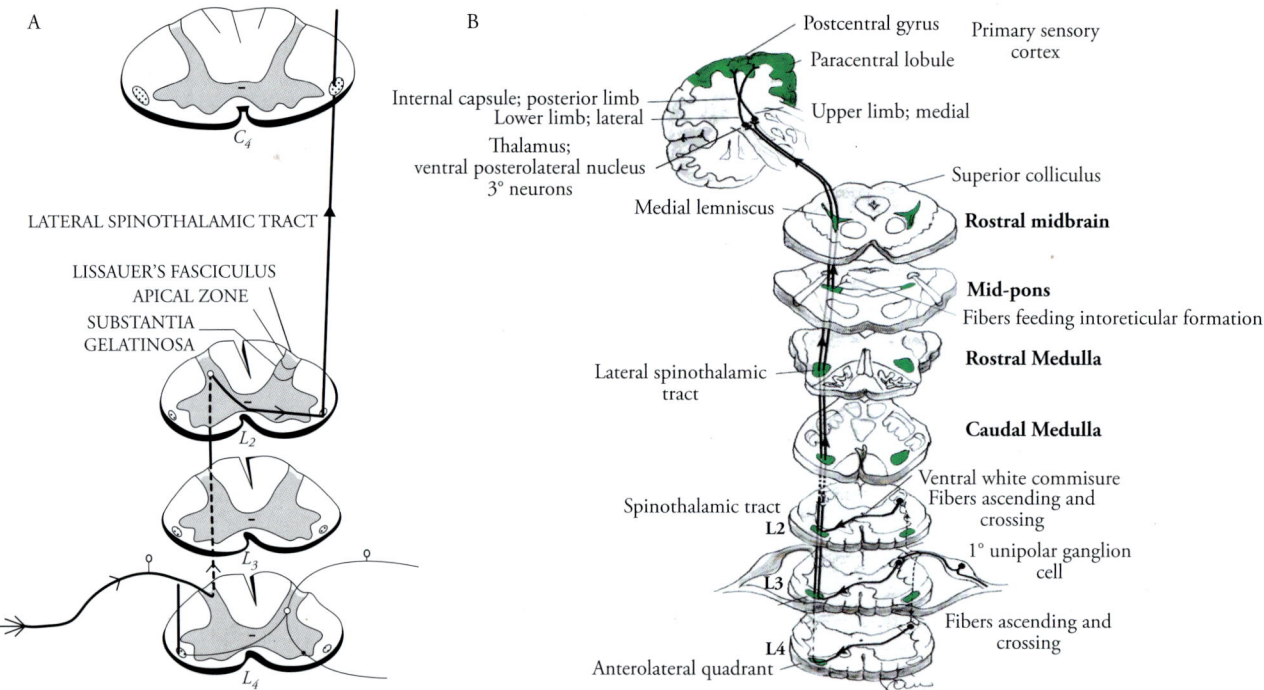

Figure 6.34 The spinothalamic tract/anterolateral system. (A) Incoming local fibers that are activated by tissue damaging stimuli may rise ipsilaterally for up to three spinal cord segments (as the fiber entering on the left) before synapsing and crossing the neuroaxis and entering the spinothalamic tract. The fiber entering on the right synapses at the level of entry, one axon crosses the neuroaxis and rises, and the other axon enters the anterior horn to participate in local reflexes, such as withdrawal from a hot surface. (B) The major projections of the spinothalamic tract are midline medulla, periaqueductal gray of the midbrain, and onto nuclei of the thalamus to reticular, ventral posterior medial, dorsomedial and intralaminar. In the thalamus, the ventral posterior lateral nucleus projects to the postcentral gyrus, the dorsomedial which projects onto frontal lobe, and the thalamic reticular and interlaminar nucleus which projects widely.

hyperreflexia, the Babinski sign, and a type of increased resistance to passive movement at a joint, spasticity, characterize the upper motor neuron syndrome. Passively moving or rotating the ankle, knee, hip, shoulder, elbow, or wrist joints easily demonstrates the increased tone. In the normal individual, the joints all move easily. When spasticity is present, the joint is easy to move for a short interval, then resistance to movement increases rapidly; upon further pressure, the resistance suddenly gives way. This latter phenomenon is often referred to as a clasp-knife reflex. In the leg, spasticity is greatest in the extensors, whereas in the arm the flexors are more affected.

Descending motor tracts normally exert an inhibitory effect on spinal cord reflexes. Hyperreflexia is a sure sign of decreased corticospinal function. Decreased function of the corticospinal tract also effects a curious reflex of the foot, Babinski's sign. If a moderately sharp object such as a key, is drawn over the lateral boundary of the sole of the foot, the toes of an adult flex (curl). In very young children and in adults with corticospinal tract destruction, the toes extend and fan out as shown in Figure 6.35.

Weaknesses, loss of reflexes, and extreme muscle loss relate to the loss of the anterior horn cell or the motor axon. The loss of reflexes and the flaccid tone of the muscles relate to the loss of the motor side of the stretch reflex pathway. Often, it

Table 6.2 UPPER MOTOR NEURON DYSFUNCTION VERSUS LOWER MOTOR NEURON DYSFUNCTION

Spasticity	Flaccidity
Hyperreflexia	Hyporeflexia
Babinski sign	Fasciculation
Very little atrophy	Severe muscle atrophy

Figure 6.35 The Babinski response. (Upper) The normal adult response to stimulation of the lateral plantar surface of the foot. (Lower) The normal infant and abnormal adult response.

ASCENDING TRACTS   **DESCENDING TRACTS**

Figure 6.36 The major ascending and descending tracts in humans.

is possible to observe spontaneous twitching of the muscle. It also conveys pain and thermal information with some synaptic interruption before reaching the thalamus.

OTHER SPINAL PATHWAYS

We have just listed the major ascending pathways (Fig. 6.36). There are also pathways from the spinal cord to: reticular formation of the brain stem to the vestibular nuclei of the medulla and pons, the inferior olive of the medulla, and to nuclei and pons and midbrain.

(See Chapter 11 on functional localization in the brain stem; for termination of the major pathways in the thalamus, see Chapter 15.)

BIBLIOGRAPHY

General

Adams, R. D., Victor, M., and Ropper, A. H. 1997. Principles of Neurology. 6th ed. New York, NY: McGraw Hill.
Brooke, M. H. 2000. Disorders of skeletal muscle. In W. G. Bradley, R. B. Daroff, G. M. Fenichel, and C. D. Marsden (Ed.) Neurology in Clinical Practice. 3rd ed., pp. 2187–2235. Boston, MA: Butterworth Heinemann.
Drachman, D. D. 1986. Pathophysiology of the neuromuscular junction. In A. K. Asbury, G. M. McKhann, and W. I. McDonald (Eds.) Diseases of the Nervous System, Clinical Neurobiology, pp. 257–268. London, UK: Wm. Heinemann.
Drachman, D. D. 1994. Medical progress—Myasthenia gravis. N. Engl. J. Med. 330:1797–1810.
Ebashi, S. 1991. Excitation-contraction coupling and the mechanism of muscular contraction. Ann. Rev. Physiology 53:1–16.
Hudson, A. J., Ebers, G. C., and Bulman, D. E. 1995. The skeletal muscle sodium and chloride channel diseases. Brain. 118:547–563.
Josephson, J. H. 1993. Contraction dynamics and power output in skeletal muscle. Ann. Rev. Physiol. 55:527–546.
Kuncl, R. W., and George, E. B. 1993. Toxic neuropathies and myopathies. Curr. Opin. Neurol. 6:695–704.
Laufer, R., and Changeux, J. P. 1989. Activity-dependent regulation of gene expression in muscle and neuronal cells. Mol. Neurobiol. 3:1–53.
Lindstrom, J., Schoepfer, R., and Whiting, P. 1987. Molecular studies of the neural nicotinic acetylcholine receptor family. Mol. Neurobiol. 1:281–338.

Lisak, R. P. (Ed.). 1994. Handbook of Myasthenia Gravis and Myasthenic Syndromes. New York, NY: Marcel Dekker.
Mastalgia, F. L., and Ojeda, V. J. 1985. Inflammatory myopathies. Ann. Neurol. 17:215–227.
Newsome-Davis, J. 1992. Diseases of the neuromuscular junction. In A. S. Asbury, G. H. McKhann, and W. I. McDonald (Eds.) Diseases of the Nervous System: Clinical Neurobiology. 2nd ed. London, UK: W. O. Heinemann.
Peachy, L. D., and Adrian, R. H. 1983. Skeletal Muscle: Handbook of Physiology. Bethesda, MD: American Physiological Society.
Penn, A. S., Richman, D. P., Ruff, R. I., and Lennon, V. A. (Eds.) 1993. Myasthenia gravis and related syndromes. Ann. NY Acad. Sci. 681:1–622.
Richman, D. P. (Ed.). 1998. Myasthenia gravis and related diseases. Ann. NY Acad. Sci. 841:1–838.
Sanders, D. C. (Ed.). 1994. Myasthenia gravis and myasthenic syndromes. Neurol. Clin. 12:229–442.
Sigurgeirsson, B., et al. 1993. Risk of cancer in patient with dermatomyositis or polymyositis. N. Engl. J. Med. 326:363–367.
Simmons, R. M. 1992. Muscular Contraction. Cambridge, MA: Cambridge University Press.
Walton, J. (Ed.). 1988. Disorders of Voluntary Muscle. 5th ed. Edinburgh, UK: Churchill Livingstone.

Specific References and Citations

Arahata, K., Ishihara, K., Kana Kura, F., et al. 1989. Mosaic expression of dystrophin in symptomatic carriers of Duchenne's muscular dystrophy. N. Engl. J. Med. 320:135–142.
Barohn, R. J. 1993. Distal myopathies and dystrophies. Sem. Neurol. 13:247–255.
Bartlett, J. C. 1986. Infant botulism in adults. N. Engl. J. Med. 315: 254–255.
Blalock, A., Mason, M. F., Morgan, H. J., et al. 1939. Myasthenia myositis. N. Engl. J. Med. 292:344–348, 403–407.
Brock, J. D., McCurroch, M. E., Horley, H. G., Buckler, A. J., et al. 1992. Molecular basis of myotonic dystrophy: expansion of a trinucleotide (CTG) repeat at the 3' end of a transcript encoding a protein kinase family member. Cell 68:799–808.
Brown, R. H., Jr. 1989. Prednisone therapy for Duchenne's muscular dystrophy. N. Engl. J. Med. 320:1592–1597.
Chia, J. K., Clark, J. B., Ryan, C. A., et al. 1986. Botulism in an adult associated with food-borne intestinal infection with Clostridium botulinum. N. Engl. J. Med. 315:239–241.
Dalakas, M. C. 1991. Polymyositis, dermatomyositis and inclusion body myositis. N. Engl. J. Med. 325:1487–1498.
Darras, B. P., Harper, J. F., and Francke, V. 1987. Prenatal diagnosis and detection of carrier with DNA probes in Duchenne's muscular dystrophy. N. Engl. J. Med. 316:985–992.

Davis, J. E. 1987. Changing profile of pesticide poisoning. N. Engl. J. Med. 316:807–808.

DiMauro, S., Monillo, E., Zevian, M., et al. 1985. Mitochondrial myopathies. Ann. Neurol. 17:521–538.

Drachman, D. B. 1978. Medical progress: Myasthenia gravis. N. Engl. J. Med. 298:136–142, 186–193.

Drachman, D. B. 1987. Present and future treatment of myasthenia gravis. N. Engl. J. Med. 316:743–745.

Dubowitz, V. 1997. The muscular dystrophies-clarity or chaos? N. Engl. J. Med. 336:650–651.

Duggan, D. J., Gorspe, J. R., Fanin, M., et al. 1997. Mutations in the sacroglycan genes in patients with myopathy. N. Eng. J. Med. 336:618–624.

Engel, A. G. 1984. Myasthenia gravis and myasthenic syndromes. Ann. Neurol. 16:519–534.

Engel, A. G., Tsujihata, M., Lambert, E. H., Lindstrom, J. M., and Lennon, V. A. 1976. Experimental autoimmune myasthenia gravis: a sequential and quantitative study of the neuromuscular junction ultrastructure and electrophysiologic correlations. J. Neuropath. Exper. Neur. 35:569–587.

Engel, A. G., and Sartai, T. 1971. Histometric analysis of the ultra structure of the neuromuscular junction in myasthenia gravis and in the myasthenic syndrome. Ann. NY Acad. Sci. 183:46–83.

Fambrough, D. M., Drachman, D. B., and Satyamari, S. 1973. Neuromuscular junction in myasthenia gravis: decreased acetylcholine receptors. Science 182:293–295.

Fardeau, M. 1982. Congenital myopathies in skeletal muscle pathology. In F. L. Mastalgia and J. Walton (Eds.), pp. 161–203. Edinburgh, UK: Churchill & Livingston.

Grob, D., Arsura, E. L., Brunner, G., et al. 1987. The course of myasthenia gravis and therapies affecting outcome. Ann. NY Acad. Sci. 505:472–499.

Hoffman, E. P., Kunkel, L. M. C., Angelini, C., et al. 1989. Improved diagnosis of Becker's muscular dystrophy by dystrophin testing. Neurol. 39:1011–1017.

Isenberg, D. 1984. Myositis in other connective tissue disorders. Clin. Rheum. Dis. 10:151–174.

Korf, B. 1995. Molecular medicine—molecular diagnosis. N. Engl. J. Med. 332:1218–1220.

Lang, B., Waterman, S., Pinto, A., et al. 1998. The role of autoantibodies in Lambert-Eatom myasthenic syndrome. Ann. NY Acad. Med. 841:596–605.

Lindstrom, J. M., Seybold, M. F., Lennon, V. A., et al. 1976. Antibody to acetylcholine receptor in myasthenia gravis: prevalence, clinical correlates and diagnostic value. Neurol. 26:1054–1059.

Mastalgia, F.C. (Ed.). 1988. Inflammatory Disease of Muscle. Oxford, UK: Blackwell.

Moser, H. 1984. Duchennes muscular dystrophy: pathogenetic aspects and genetic prevention. Hum. Gent. 66:17-40.

Owen, C. A., Mubasek, S. J., Haggers, A. R., and Rutherford, L. 1979. Intramuscular pressures with limb compression: clarification of the pathogenesis of the drug-induced muscle compartment syndrome. N. Engl. J. Med. 300:1169–1172.

Padberg, G.W. 1993. The muscular dystrophies and dystrophin. Curr. Opin. Neurol. 6:688–694.

Patrick, J., and Lindstrom, J. 1973. Autoimmune response to acetylcholine receptor. Science 180:1871–1872.

Pourmand, R. (Ed.). 2000. Metabolic myopathies. Neurol. Clin. 18:181–271.

Ptacek, L. J., Tawil, R., Griggs, R. C. et al. 1994. Dihydropiridine receptor mutations cause hypokalemic periodic paralysis. Cell 77:863–868.

Ptacek, L. J., Johnson, K. J., and Griggs, R. C. 1993. Mechanisms of disease: genetics and physiology of the myotonic muscle disorders. N. Engl. J. Med. 328:482–489.

Rowland, L. P. 1988. Clinical concepts of Duchennes muscular dystrophy: the impact of molecular genetics. Brain 111:479–496.

Rowland, L. P. 1987. Therapy in myasthenia gravis. Ann. NY Acad. Sci. 505:566–567.

Rowland, L. N., Layzer, R. B., and DiMauro, S. 1986. Pathophysiology of metabolic muscle disorders. In A. K. Asbury, G. M. McKhann, and W. T. McDonald (Eds.) Diseases of the Nervous System: Clinical Neurobiology. 2nd ed., pp.197–207. London, UK: Wm. Heinemann.

Schumm, F., Wietholter, H., Fateh-Moghadown, A., et al. 1985. Thymectomy in myasthenia with pure ocular symptoms. J. Neurol. Neurosurg. Psychiat. 48:332–337.

Sekul, E. A., and Dalakas, M. C. 1993. Inclusion body myositis: new concepts. Sem. Neurol. 13:256–263.

Senanoyake, N., and Kalliede, L. 1987. Neurotoxic effects of organophosphorous: an intermediate syndrome. N. Engl. J. Med. 316:761–763.

Sher, E., Codignola, A., Passafaro, M., et al. 1998. Nicotinic receptors and calcium channels in small cell lung carcinoma: functional role, modulation, and autoimmunity. Ann. NY Acad. Sci. 841:606–624.

Shelbourne, P., et al. 1993. Direct diagnosis of myotonic dystrophy with a disease specific DNA marker. N. Engl. J. Med. 328:471–475.

Toyka, K. V., Drachman, D. B., Griffin, D. E., et al. 1977. Myasthenia gravis: study of humoral mechanisms by passive transfer to mice. N. Engl. J. Med. 296:125–131.

Wang, Y. H., Amirhaeri, S., Kang, S., et al. 1994. Preferential nucleosome assembly at DNA triplet repeats from the myotonic dystrophy gene. Science 265:669–671.

Watt, G., Theakston, R. D. G., Hayes, C. G., et al. 1986. Positive response to edrophonium in patients with neurotoxic envenoming by cobras (Naja philippinensis). N. Engl. J. Med. 315:1444.

Weinberg, D., and Mark, E. J. 1994. Case records of the Massachusetts General Hospital—A 61-year-old man with muscular weakness. N. Engl. J. Med. 331:528–536.

Younger, D. S., Jasetzki, A., III, Penn, A. S., et al. 1987. Maximum thymectomy for myasthenia gravis. Ann. N Y Acad. Sci. 505:832–835.

Zacks, S. I., Bauer, U. C., Blumberg, J. M. 1962. The fine structure of the myasthenic neuromuscular apparatus. J. Neuropath. Exper. Neurol. 21:335.

7.
ATLAS OF THE SPINAL CORD

Figure 7.1 The entire central nervous system of a human with the cerebrum, central sulcus identified. The location of the cervical (C), thoracic (T), lumbar (L), and sacral (S) levels of the cord are noted as well as the terminal fibers from the lumbar and sacral regions of the spinal cord to the lower extremity which form the cauda equina.

ATLAS OF SPINAL CORD LEVELS with four stained section A and diagrammatic labeled section B. Sacral levels can be identified by the large amount of gray matter in comparison to white matter.

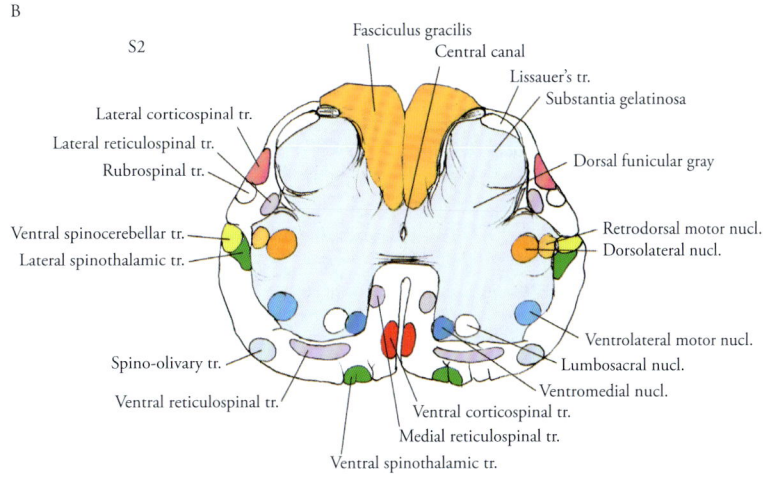

Figure 7.2 LEVEL = CERVICAL 7

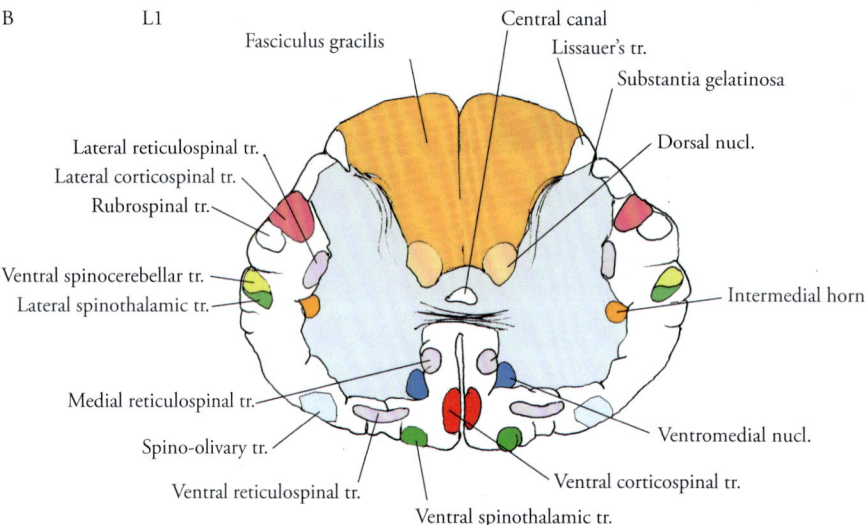

Figure 7.3 LEVEL = THORACIC 7

Gray matter. In this section there are two horns: one sensory (dorsal) and one motor (ventral). In the ventral horn the retrodorsal, dorsolateral, and ventrolateral nuclei innervate the lower extremity.

White matter. Most of the fibers forming descending tracts have ended and the bulk of the white matter consists of ascending axon and intersegmental fibers. The dorsal columns at this level contain only fibers from regions innervated by the sacral cord; these form the fasciculus gracilis.

Lumbar levels can be identified by the nearly equal amount of gray and white matter.

Gray matter. In this level two horns are present: the dorsal sensory and ventral motor.

White matter. The increase in the amount of white matter reflects first the increase in the fibers joining the posterior column from the ascending fasciculus gracilis and the presence of a large lateral column containing the corticospinal tract (crossed) above its innervations of the ventral horn to the muscles in the thigh, leg, and foot.

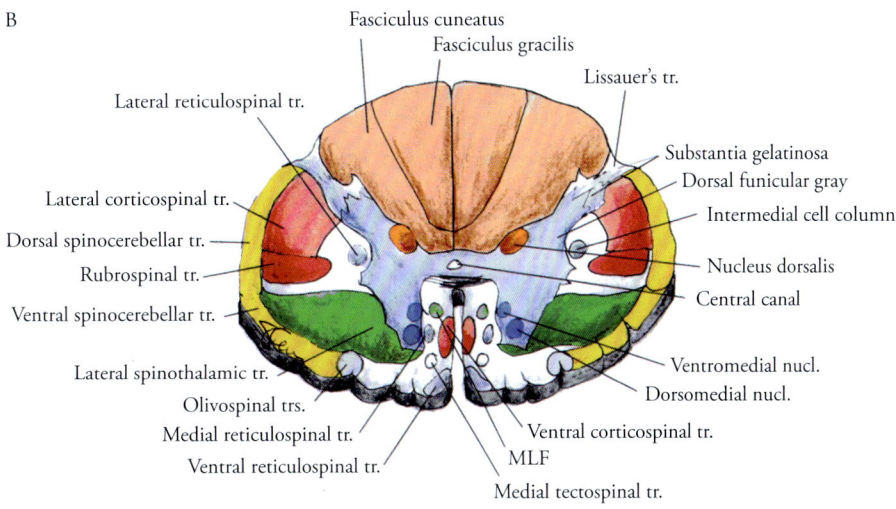

Figure 7.4 LEVEL = LUMBAR 2

Thoracic levels can always be identified by the presence of a small amount of gray matter versus a large amount of white matter, and the presence of the intermediolateral cell column, which contains preganglionic sympathetic neurons.

White matter. The ascending and descending fibers to the lower limbs, abdomen, trunk, and pelvis provide the bulk of the white matter in the lateral and posterior column.

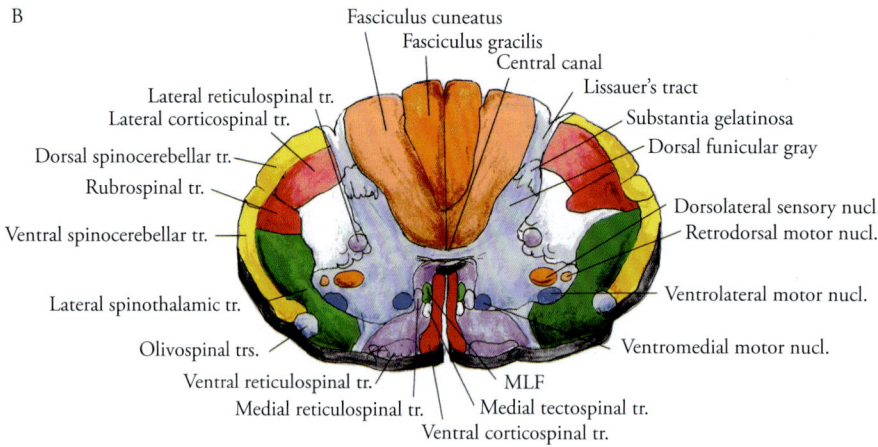

Figure 7.5 ATLAS LEVEL = SACRAL 2

This cervical level is at the cervical enlargement and can be identified as they are the largest level in the spinal cord and are ovoid in shape, with the gray matter found in the shape of a butterfly.

White matter. The bulk of this section consists of ascending and descending fibers to the extremities, thorax, abdomen, trunk, and pelvis. Note how the dorsal columns increase in size as one ascends the spinal cord due to the accumulation of the ascending general sensory fibers. The lateral column is still large as some of the corticospinal tract to the hand is still present. Re-examine the lower sections of the cord and note the decrease in bulk of the spinal cord white matter which results from the innervations from the cervical enlargement to the upper extremity. Note the decrease in bulk of the cord as one descends.

Gray matter. In this cervical level, one finds in the ventral horn the retrodorsal, dorsolateral, and ventrolateral nuclei which innervate the hand and forearm region of the upper extremity.

Figure 7.6 (*A*) Cross sections through all levels of the spinal cord in a patient with amyotrophic lateral sclerosis (ALS). Each section is stained with Luxol Fast blue and cresyl violet, the Kluver-Barra stain. (*B*) Four levels from the patient in 7.6A with cervical thoracic levels in the top row and lumbar and sacral in the bottom row. (From Kluver, H., and Barrera, E. A method for the combined staining of cells and fibers in the nervous system. J. Neuropath. Exp. Neurol. 12:400-403, 1953.)

BIBLIOGRAPHY

Abel Majuid, T., and Bowsher, D. 1985. The gray matter of the dorsal horn of the adult human spinal cord. J. Anat. 142:33–58.

Asanuma, H. 1981. The pyramidal tract. In V. B. Brooks (Ed.) Handbook of Physiology. Section I. The Nervous System. Vol II. Motor Control, pp. 703–733. Bethesda, MD: American Physiological Society.

Becksted, R., Morse, J., and Norgeren, R. 1980. The nucleus of the solitray tract in the monkey. J. Comp. Neurol. 198:259–282.

Brodal, A. 1965. The Cranial Nerves. Anatomy and Anatomical Clinical Correlation. London, UK: Oxford Blackwell.

Brodal, A. 1957. The reticular formation of the brain stem. Springfield, IL: Charles C. Thomas.

Burton, H., and Craig, A. 1979. Distribution of trigeminothalamic neurons in cat and monkey. Brain Res. 161:515–521.

Carpenter, M. B. 1991. Core Text of Neuroanatomy. 4th ed. Baltimore, MD: Williams and Wilkins.

Everts, E. Role of motor cortex in voluntary movement in primates. In V. B. Brooks (Ed.) Handbook of Physiology. Section I. The Nervous System. Vol II. Motor Control, pp. 1083–1120. Bethesda MD. American Physiological Society.

Finger, T., and Silver, W. 1987. Neurobiology of Taste and Smell. New York, NY: Wiley.

Foote, S., Bloom, F., and Aston-Jones, G. 1983. Nucleus locus cereuleus. New evidence of anatomical and physiological specificity. Physiol. Rev. 63:844–914.

Hobson, J., and Brazier, M. (Eds.). 1983. The reticular formation revisited. Brain Res. 6:1–564.

Moore, B., and Bloom, F. 1978. Central catecholamine neuron systems; anatomy and physiology of thenoreephinephrine and epinephrine systems. Ann. Rev. Neurosci. 2:113–168.

Norgren, R. 1984. Central mechansims of taste. In Darian-Smith (Ed.) Handbook of Physiology. Section I. The Nervous System. Vol 3, pp. 1087–1128. Sensory Processes. Bethesda, MD. American Physiological Society.

Riley, H. A. 1960. Brain Stem and Spinal Cord. New York, NY: Hafner.

Sinclair, D. 1982. Touch in primates. Ann. Rev. Neurosci. 5:155–194.

Wall, P and R. Melzak. Textbook of Pain. Edinburgh, Churchill Livingston. 1989.

Willis, W. 1985. Nocioceptive pathways. Anatomy and physiology of nociceptive ascending pathways. Phil Trans. Roy. Soc. London (Biol.) 308:252–268.

8.

A SURVEY OF DISEASES OF PERIPHERAL NERVE AND NERVE ROOT

In Chapter 2, we considered the differential features of disease of muscle compared to disease of peripheral nerve, disease of the nerve root, and central nervous system disease. Diseases of peripheral nerve and nerve root both represent lower motor neuron disorders. In contrast to disorders of muscle, both involve motor and sensory features. As we will discuss in greater degree, peripheral nerve disorders may involve specific nerves in a local manner (mononeuropathies) or peripheral nerve in a more generalized manner (polyneuropathies) (Table 8.1). Mononeuropathies must be distinguished from radiculopathies. This distinction can be made based on the pattern of motor deficit, the pattern of deep tendon stretch reflex deficit, the pattern of sensory deficit, and the distribution of pain. Figure 8.1A and 8.1B compares radicular (dermatomal or segmental) sensory innervations to the superficial sensory innervations of peripheral nerve.

PERIPHERAL NERVE DISEASE

Diseases involving the peripheral nerves have a combination of motor sensory and autonomic symptoms and signs. Lower motor neuron findings are present with a flaccid type weakness and atrophy. Sensory symptoms and findings (involving to a variable degree all modalities of sensation) are present within the same distribution as the motor findings. The degree of motor, sensory, or autonomic involvement will vary. These patients, however, do not show evidence of damage to the long fiber systems involved in transmitting sensory and motor information within the central nervous system.

In general, mental status is intact. Deep tendon reflexes and superficial reflexes (response to plantar stimulation) are absent within the distribution of the involved peripheral nerves. Fasciculations may be present within the distribution of the involved peripheral nerves. Damage to the sympathetic fibers, traversing the peripheral nerves, may result in alterations in sweating and skin temperatures. Nerve conduction studies demonstrate reduction in velocity (if the basic process involves loss of myelin, demyelination) or in the amplitude of the motor or sensory action potential (if the basic process involves predominately a loss of axons). In mononeuropathies the specific site of damage (conduction block) may be demonstrated. The electromyogram (EMG) will demonstrate abnormal spontaneous activity: fibrillations (onset 10–25 days after the axonal damage), positive sharp waves, and fasciculations.

As will be discussed later in greater detail, diseases of peripheral nerves are essentially of two types: (a) localized mononeuropathies involving a single peripheral nerve, often due to trauma or compression, or less often, occlusion of blood supply; and (b) symmetrical polyneuropathies—usually distal and usually due to a metabolic disturbance involving many nerves. The polyneuropathies reflect many of the systemic, toxic, and metabolic disease considered in pathology. As a general rule, any patient with a diabetes mellitus, with chronic alcoholism, or receiving chemotherapy is likely to present symptoms or signs (often subclinical) of a polyneuropathy. In many cases we are not able to establish a specific cause for the polyneuropathy. We may not have sufficient information about environmental or industrial exposure. In some cases we have insufficient information regarding the family history.

In a *mononeuropathy*, the weakness and sensory signs and symptoms are clearly within the distribution of a specific plexus peripheral nerve, for example, sciatic, radial, median, or ulnar. Common sites of compression include the radial nerve at the radial (or spiral) groove of the humerus, the ulnar nerve at the olecranon process of the elbow, the median nerve in the carpal tunnel, the brachial plexus at the thoracic outlet, and the peroneal nerve as it leaves the popliteal fossa and curves around the head of the fibula.

A specialized form of mononeuropathy, *mononeuropathy multiplex*, reflects multifocal involvement of peripheral nerve, for example, in inflammatory diseases of blood vessels.

In addition, in Von Recklinghausen's disease, multiple peripheral nerves and nerve roots may be involved by tumors arising from the Schwann cell and mesodermal components. This disorder will be discussed in relation to the spinal cord.

MONONEUROPATHIES: UPPER EXTREMITY BRACHIAL PLEXUS (C5, 6, 7, 8 T1)

Patients frequently present with a complaint of transient distal sensory symptoms and weakness involving the upper extremity occurring in relationship to sleeping posture or position of the arm. The symptoms are often bilateral. Rarely the symptoms are persistent rather than intermittent. These symptoms are referred to as the thoracic outlet syndrome or the neurovascular syndrome of the thoracic outlet. Both the brachial plexus and the subclavian artery pass through a relatively narrow area with clavicle anteriorly and the first rib posteriorly (Fig. 8.2). Alterations in posture may produce compression of the brachial artery—producing a tingling pins and needles sensations ("paresthesias") involving all fingers and a distal weakness. Often specific maneuvers will demonstrate the intermittent

Figure 8.1A and 8.1B Comparison of radicular (dermatome or segmental) and peripheral nerve innervation on the anterior versus posterior view of the body. (From Curtis BA, S Jacobson, and EM Marcus, An Introduction to the Neurosciences, WB Saunders, 1974 Philadelphia.)

B

SPINAL (RADICULAR PERIPHERAL NERVES
DERMATOMES

POSTERIOR RAMI OF CERVICAL NERVES
CERVICAL CUTANEOUS N.
POST. SUPRACLAVICULAR N.
POST. THORACIC RAMI
AXILLARY N.
INTERCOSTOBRACHIAL CUT.
LATERAL THORACIC RAMI
MED. BRACHIAL CUT.
POST. BRACHIAL CUT.
(BR. OF RADIAL)
POST. LUMBAR RAMI
ILIOHYPOGASTRIC
MED. ANTEBRACHIAL CUT.
POST. ANTEBRACHIAL CUT.
(BR. OF RADIAL)
MUSCULOCUTANEOUS
(LAT. ANTEBRACHIAL CUT.)
POST. SACRAL RAMI
SUPERFICIAL RADIAL
ULNAR MEDIAN
POST. FEMORAL CUT N.
ANT. FEMORAL CUT. N.
OBTURATOR
COMMON PERONEAL N.
SURAL N.
SUPERFICIAL PERONEAL N.
SAPHENOUS N.
DEEP PERONEAL N.

Figure 8.1B Continued

compression of the brachial artery. Neural syndromes of the outlet tend to involve primarily the ulnar nerve, or the lower roots (C8–T1). At times a cervical rib or tight band may further compress the narrow outlet.

UPPER PLEXUS

In addition to the relatively benign thoracic outlet syndrome, often trauma, traction downward as in birth injuries (Erb's), or brachial neuritis may involve the upper plexus roots C5-6 (Fig. 8.2), resulting in weakness of muscles about shoulder and flexors at elbow.

Another entity, *brachial neuritis*, presumably has a postinfectious, immunologic, or familial etiology. The specifics are often unclear. Brachial neuritis is often associated with considerable pain in the arm. Radiotherapy to the axilla for breast carcinoma may also involve the upper plexus in a relatively nonpainful syndrome.

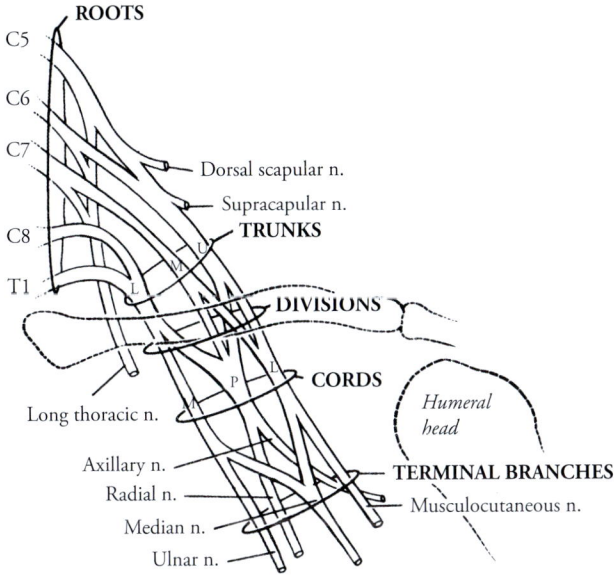

Figure 8.2 Plan of the brachial plexus: diagram of the major components in terms of roots, divisions, cords, and terminal branches. (From Mendell JR et al: Diagnosis and Management of Peripheral Nerve Disorders. Oxford, New York, 2001.)

LOWER PLEXUS

Malignant infiltration of the plexus from tumors at the apex or upper lobe of the lung ("Pancoast tumor") often involves the lower (C7, 8, T1) half of the plexus, producing severe pain. The related sympathetic plexus is often involved, producing a Horner's syndrome. Upward traction on the plexus may occur at birth (Klumpke's) or in children who suddenly are pulled up by the arm, producing damage to the lower half of the plexus (Fig. 8.2).

Case 8.1 provides an example of a brachial plexopathy and Horner's syndrome in a patient subsequently found to have an apical carcinoma of the lung.

CASE HISTORY 8.1

This 57-year-old, right-handed white male with a 30-year history of heavy cigarette smoking (two packs per day) had a 2-year history of progressive pain in the left upper extremity beginning with mild pain at the left elbow, then a lack of sensation in the left ulnar distribution. Eight months prior to admission, the left hand had become swollen and painful. Severe pain on motion at the shoulder also developed. Six months prior to evaluation, drooping of the left eyelid was first noted followed by a decrease in sweating on the left side of face and body. Three months prior to admission the patient had the onset of weakness of the left arm. The patient soon noted a decrease in sweating on the left side of face and body. The rheumatology consultant Dr. Gary Wolf noted additionally a smaller pupil on the left and referred the patient for neurological evaluation.

Physical examination demonstrated swelling, redness, change in temperature, and sweating and limitation of motion of the left arm, plus distension and firmness of the left supraclavicular space. Orthostatic hypotension was present, with a blood pressure drop on rapid stand from 170/90 flat to 100/80 standing.

Neurological Examination

Sympathetic system: A full Horner's syndrome was present on the left: mild drooping of the left eyelid (ptosis), a smaller pupil on the left, and moderate recession of the left eyeball (the right eye appeared therefore slightly more prominent).

Motor system:

a. Atrophy was present in the median (thenar eminence) and ulnar (first interosseus) distribution.

b. Weakness was present in the left arm, most marked in the median and radial distribution.

c. Minor weakness of the great toe was present bilaterally (extensor hallicus longus).

Reflexes: deep tendon reflexes were decrease in the left arm.

Sensory system:

a. Pain sensation was decreased in the left C7, C8 dermatomes.

b. Pain was decreased in the lower extremities over the feet to the level of the ankles.

c. Vibration sensation was decreased at toes and ankles.

Clinical diagnosis: Brachial plexopathy and Horner's syndrome due to apical lung tumor (Pancoast tumor). Note that the motor and sensory finding in the feet suggested an additional problem of distal peripheral neuropathy.

Laboratory Data

1. A review of previous chest X-rays indicated not only calcifications in the left upper lobe at the apex but also pleural thickness at the apex.

2. Computerized tomography (CT) of the lower neck and upper chest after venous injection of the contrast material into the left arm indicated near occlusion of the left subclavian vein at the level of the first rib and a necrotic mass in the left lower neck posterior to the thymus and carotid sheath and invading the muscular structures of the prevertebral region and arising from or extending to the left apex of the lung.

3. Nerve conduction and EMG studies indicated a severe axonal lesion of the lower half of the brachial plexus with a marked involvement of median and ulnar nerves and less of the radial nerve.

4. Biopsy of the left supraclavicular mass revealed adenocarcinoma presumably of pulmonary origin.

Subsequent Course

The patient received radiotherapy (3000 rads) to the left lung apex and the left supraclavicular area with a decrease of pain and of swelling in the arm. The patient expired 1.5 years after radiotherapy and 3.5 years after onset of symptoms.

Comments

This patient clearly presented as a major problem a neuropathy of the lower half of brachial plexus due to infiltration by an invasive adenocarcinoma of the apex of lung. Malignant tumors of the apex of the lung that involve the brachial plexus and the sympathetic ganglia in this location often carry the name of Pancoast. The swelling of the arm reflected the occlusion of the venous system draining the arm. The sympathetic changes in the arm and the Horner's syndrome reflected involvement of the chain of sympathetic ganglia. The distal peripheral neuropathy in the lower extremities may have reflected the previous excessive intake of alcohol (nutritional) or may have represented a remote effect of malignancy.

Often a brachial neuritis involves only a limited portion of the brachial plexus. Limited involvement of the long thoracic nerve (C5, 6, 7) is relatively frequent.

Case 8.2 provides an example of a neuropathy of the long thoracic nerve.

CASE HISTORY 8.2

This 29-year-old, right-handed white housewife was evaluated with a chief complaint of "my right shoulder blade is sticking out." Right shoulder pain began one day after the uncomplicated delivery of her fourth child (without general or local anesthesia). Her arm had not been secured to any arm board. Within 2 weeks she noted transient tingling of the index, middle, and ring fingers of the right hand. Within 3 weeks she first noted prominence of the scapular (winging of the scapula). Any pain had resolved by 6 weeks after onset, but the painless winging of the scapular persisted.

Neurological examination: Findings were limited to the following: tenderness was present over the right supraclavicular area and in the right axilla (palpation of brachial plexus). In pressing forward against a wall with the outstretched extended right arm, there was winging of the medial border of the scapula. The serratus anterior muscle supplied by the lesser thoracic nerve failed to fixate the scapula to the chest wall. The actions of the trapezius muscle were intact (lesions of the accessory nerve supplying the trapezius muscle may also produce winging of the scapula, but this occurs on lateral abduction of the arm). Note that cranial nerves, reflexes, and sensory system were intact.

Clinical diagnosis: Long thoracic nerve neuropathy.

Laboratory data: EMG studies 10 months after the onset indicated changes of acute and chronic denervation with reinnervation of the involved muscle.

Subsequent course: Follow-up several months later indicated no change in her clinical status.

Comments

In many cases involvement of the long thoracic nerve relates to pressure from a knapsack or backpack. However, in other cases, the involvement reflects a limited aspect of a brachial neuritis, presumably on an immunological basis. In some cases of brachial neuritis there is an autosomal dominant familial predisposition with events such as fever or pregnancy acting as triggers.

Median nerve (C5, C6, C7, C8, T1): The major syndrome of the median nerve relates to compression at the carpal tunnel by the overlying transverse carpal connective tissue (Fig. 8.3A and 8.3B). Pain and paresthesia extend into the median nerve supplied fingers per dominantly index and middle, less of thumb and median side ring finger when severe (Fig. 8.6). There is significant weakness and atrophy involving the median supplied thenar muscles of the hand -abductor pollices brevis, opponens, and the finger flexors. A positive Tinel's sign is present on percussion over the carpal tunnel. Carpal

Figure 8.3A Anatomy of the median nerve in the right upper extremity. (From Mendell JR, Kissel JT, Cornblath DR (eds): Diagnosis and Management of Peripheral Nerve Disorders. Oxford University Press, New York, 2001.)

tunnel syndrome may complicate any process where edema or swelling occurs at wrist or hand: rheumatoid arthritis (as in Case 8.3), trauma, myxedema (hypothyroid state), or acromegaly (a state associated with excessive production of pituitary growth hormone; see Chapter 16).

CASE HISTORY 8.3

This 83-year-old, right-handed white widow and retired shoe factory worker with a 20- to 30-year history of rheumatoid arthritis, in relationship to an exacerbation of her joint symptoms, had the onset of tingling paresthesia in the left median distribution of hand and fingers, most prominent in the middle finger, less in index and ring, and minor in thumb. There was pain in the hand particularly or making a fist.

Physical examination demonstrated mild inflammatory synovitis in the hands, with mild soft tissue swelling in the wrists, ankles, proximal interphalangeal joints, and metacarpal phalangeal joints.

Neurological examination demonstrated a minor weakness in left hand grip and left thumb opponens and a marked tenderness over the left carpal tunnel area with a positive Tinel's sign on palpation or

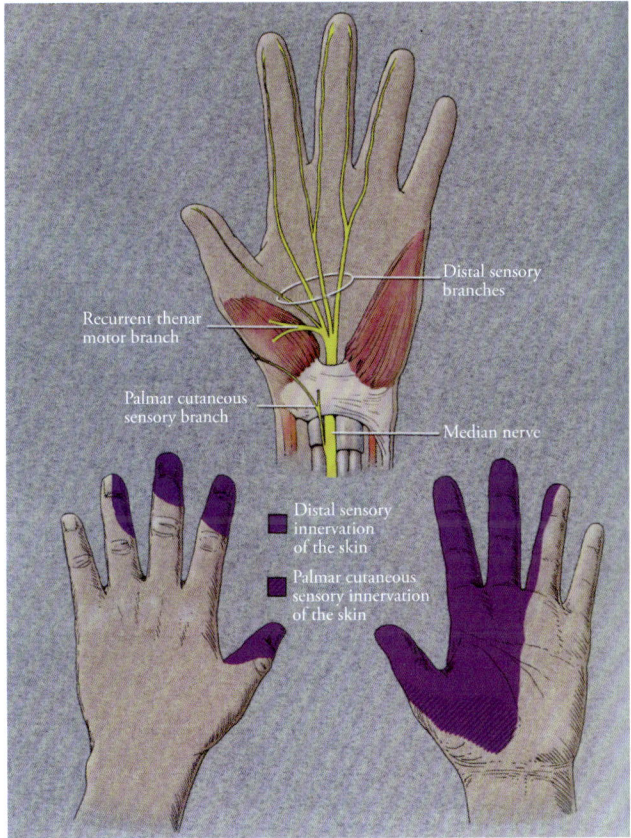

Figure 8.3B Anatomy of the right median nerve in the wrist and hand. (From Mendell JR, Kissel JT, Cornblath DR (eds): Diagnosis and Management of Peripheral Nerve Disorders. Oxford University Press, New York, 2001.)

Figure 8.4A The ulnar nerve dissected. Note exposed position of the ulnar nerve in the olecranon groove at the elbow. (From Mendell JR, Kissel JT, Cornblath DR (eds): Diagnosis and Management of Peripheral Nerve Disorders. Oxford University Press, New York, 2001.)

percussion of the median nerve in the carpal tunnel (tingling paresthesias extending from the carpal tunnel into the median nerve supplied fingers).

Clinical diagnosis: Compression of median nerve at carpal tunnel.

Laboratory data: Nerve conduction studies indicated severe delays in both sensory and motor conduction for median nerve at carpal tunnel on the left with mild findings on the right.

Subsequent course: Despite the use of nonsteroidal anti-inflammatory agents, re-evaluation 2 weeks later indicated additional progression: greater weakness of in grip and pain and touch sensation now decreased bilaterally in the median nerve distribution. Despite the use of local steroid injections, reevaluation 1 month later indicated persistence of symptoms, with atrophy present in the thenar eminence on the left. Carpal tunnel surgery on the left hand was performed with improvement of symptoms. When symptoms developed in the right hand, similar surgery was performed with relief.

Ulnar nerve (C8, T1): This nerve is often exposed to trauma as it passes through the groove behind the medial epicondyle at the elbow (Fig. 8.4). Each of us has struck our "funny bone" at some time, and we are all acquainted with the ulnar distribution of positive sensory symptoms, ring and fifth finger (Fig 8.4). Repeated trauma to the nerve or fractures at the elbow may produce more persistent symptoms, including atrophy of the hypothenar and interossei muscle and weakness of digiti quinti abductor, ring and fifth finger flexors, the interossei, and the thumb adductor.

Figure 8.4B Ulnar nerve dissection of nerves and muscles of the palm of the left hand. (From Mendell JR, Kissel JT, Cornblath DR (eds): Diagnosis and Management of Peripheral Nerve Disorders. Oxford University Press, New York, 2001.)

Figure 8.4C Cutaneous branches of the ulnar nerve. (From Mendell JR, Kissel JT, Cornblath DR (eds): Diagnosis and Management of Peripheral Nerve Disorders. Oxford University Press, New York, 2001.)

Radial nerve (C6, 7, 8): The major syndrome of this nerve relates to injury at the spiral groove of the humerus (Fig.8.5) related to fractures or to so-called Saturday night palsy (pressure effects on arm draped over a hard surface are noted due to excessive alcohol intake so that the paresthesias fail to awaken the patient and the compression therefore continues). The characteristic weakness involves the wrist and finger extensors as well as the long abductor of the thumb.

The brachioradialis muscle is usually involved. Lesions at this level, however, usually spare the triceps muscle also supplied by radial nerve. A wrist drop is characteristic. A cock up wrist splint is utilized to maintain the hand in a physiological position. With time recovery will occur.

MONONEUROPATHIES: LOWER EXTREMITY LUMBAR SACRAL PLEXUS (L1-S3)

The lumbar plexus is composed of nerve roots L1–L4 (Fig. 8.6), and the sacral plexus of nerve roots L4-S3 (Fig. 8.7). Both plexuses may be involved by malignancies within the pelvis. Both may also be commonly involved in the painful diabetic mononeuropathy that occurs on a vascular basis.

Neuropathies may commonly involve the following branches of the lumbar plexus.

1. Lateral femoral cutaneous nerve of the thigh (L2, L3). This nerve supplies the anterior-lateral aspect of the thigh. It enters the thigh by passing between the two points of attachment of the lateral aspect of the inguinal ligament to the anterior superior iliac spine (Figs. 8.6 and 8.8). There is sensitivity of the supplied cutaneous area to contact from any clothing or repetitive tactile stimulation. Tingling paresthesias are present. At times burning painful paresthesias are present; thus, the name "meralgia paresthesia."

The common causes are weight gain or weight loss. The following underlying diseases are frequent as predisposing conditions: obesity, pregnancy, diabetes, and infrequently pelvic malignancy.

2. Obturator nerve (L3, L4) (Figs. 8.6 and 8.8). This nerve supplies the adductors of the thigh. The major causes of injury relate to difficult deliveries: pressure from fetal head or forceps.

3. Femoral nerve (L2, 3, 4) (Figs. 8.6 and 8.8). This nerve supplies the quadriceps, muscle necessary for extension at the knee; and the iliacus and psoas, muscles necessary for hip flexion. Diabetic mononeuropathy on a vascular basis is the most common cause of this neuropathy. Hematomas into the iliac muscle may compress the nerve. Pelvic malignancies and pelvic surgery may injure the nerve (Fig. 8.9).

SCIATIC NERVE

Neuropathies may commonly involve the sciatic nerve (the major trunk originating from the sacral plexus) or the two major divisions of the sciatic nerve: the common peroneal and the posterior tibial nerves (Fig. 8.7). The two divisions are bound together from the plexus to just above the popliteal fossa. They are separate nerves below that point. The other branches of the sacral plexus are (a) the gluteal nerves to the gluteus medius and gluteus maximus; and (b) the pudendal nerve (S2, S3, S4) to the perineal muscle (anal sphincter).

SCIATIC NERVE (L4, L5, S1, S2)

This nerve supplies the hamstring muscles and all muscles below the knee. Common causes of injury are (a) fractures of pelvis or femur; (b) gunshot wounds of the buttock; (c) injections of medications into the buttock, for example, penicillin; and (d) diabetes mellitus mononeuropathy.

Figure 8.5 Dissection of the nerves of the right upper extremity—from posteriorly. Note the radial course of the radial nerve providing innervation to the triceps muscle, and to the extensors of wrist and finger. (From Mendell JR, Kissel JT, Cornblath DR (eds): Diagnosis and Management of Peripheral Nerve Disorders. Oxford University Press, New York, 2001.)

PERONEAL NERVE (L4, L5, S1)

This nerve has (a) superficial branch: cutaneous and muscular supply to the everter of the foot (peroneal muscles) and (b) deep peroneal or anterior tibial branch supplying the muscle or ankle and toe dorsi flexor and sensation to the dorsum of foot and lateral aspect of the calf (Fig. 8.10). This nerve passes around the head of the tibula from the popliteal fossa to the anterior aspect of the leg. In this location, the nerve is relatively superficial and very subject to pressure from leg crossing when seated in tight coats or tight boots or operating or obstetrical room stirrups. The major manifestation of compression is a foot drop or unstable ankle (due to weakness of ankle dorsiflexors and everter).

TIBIAL NERVE (L4, L5, S1, S2)

This nerve supplies the posterior calf muscles and then the gastrocnemius and soleus muscles (the plantar flexor) and then continues as the posterior tibial nerve to supply intrinsic foot muscles. It also supplies sensation to the plantar surface. The posterior tibial nerve passes behind the medial malleolus in a relatively superficial location and enters the tarsal tunnel. In this location, the nerve may be palpated and is subject to compression. Entrapment also occurs due to disease in the tendon sheaths that accompany the nerve in the tunnel.

The following case provides an example of a diabetic mononeuropathy involving the lumbar-sacral plexus in a diabetic patient who also had a symmetrical distal peripheral neuropathy (Fig. 8.11).

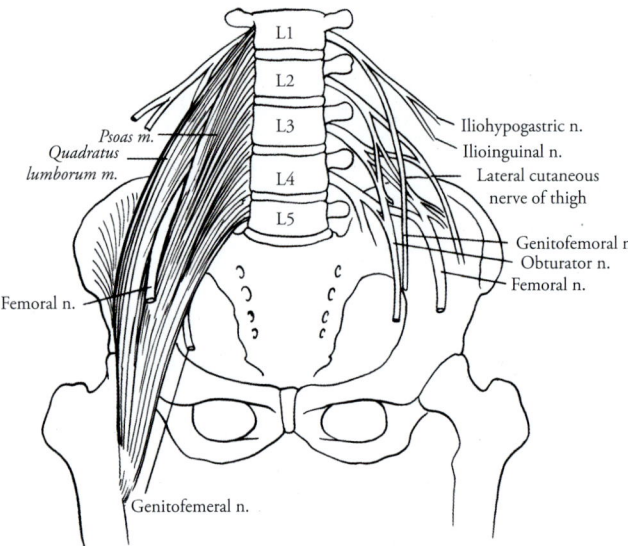

Figure 8.6 Plan of the lumbar plexus. The anterior divisions of L2, L3, and L4 unite to form the obturator nerve. The posterior divisions of L2, L3, and L4 unite to form the femoral nerve. Twigs from L2, and L3 forms the lateral femoral cutaneous nerve. (From Mendell JR et al., Diagnosis and Management of Peripheral Nerve Disorders. Oxford, 2001.)

CASE HISTORY 8.4

This 75-year-old, right-handed white widow with a 1-year history of non-insulin-dependent diabetes mellitus had the sudden onset of weakness in the right leg, most prominent at hip and knee, 3 weeks prior to evaluation. Shortly thereafter, she had the onset of a severe toothache-like pain in the lateral and anterior surface of the right leg from hip to knee. No other symptoms were present.

Neurological Examination
Mental status and cranial nerves: Intact.
Motor system: Weakness was present in the proximal muscles of the right lower extremity.
Reflexes: The deep tendon stretch reflex was absent at the right Achilles and patellar compared to left.
Sensory system: Pain sensation was decreased in a symmetrical manner over the toes and feet and two-thirds of the distance up the calves. However, there was also a focal deficit in pain sensation over the right third lumbar dermatome. Vibration was decreased at toes compared to ankles and knees in a bilateral manner.
Palpation of nerves: Significant tenderness was present over both the sciatic nerve at the sciatic notch and the femoral nerve in the femoral canal of the anterior thigh.
Clinical diagnosis: 1. Acute diabetic mononeuropathy: lumbar and to a lesser degree sacral plexopathy; 2. Diabetic distal peripheral neuropathy.
Laboratory Data
Nerve conduction studies indicated slowed conduction over the left sural nerve, absence of conduction right sural nerve and both peroneal nerves—leg to ankle. The *EMG studies* demonstrated acute denervation in sampled muscles supplied by the right femoral nerve: rectus femoris, vastus medial and iliopsoas plus muscles supplied by major components of the sciatic nerve gastrocnemius and peroneus longus. *Myelogram and CT scan of the pelvis* were normal.
Subsequent course: The patient improved but then 9 months later has an acute exacerbation in the right leg and 1 year later had a similar process involving the left leg. Over the subsequent 9 months significant improvement occurred so that she was able to ambulate with a cane.

POLYNEUROPATHIES

Polyneuropathies may be classified from several standpoints:

1. Predominantly motor versus predominantly sensory versus predominantly autonomic versus mixed

2. Acute versus subacute versus chronic

3. The site of pathology: (a) axonal—"dying back phenomena"—distal degeneration as in metabolic diseases or arsenic intoxication. (b) Segmental demyelination with the preservation of axons—as in the immunological postinfectious polyneuropathy or some connective tissue disorders or chronic lead poisoning or diphtheria.

   Note that some nutritional deficiencies affect heavily myelinated fibers in both the spinal cord and peripheral nerve. The best example is vitamin B12 deficiency. The copper deficiency seen with excessive amounts of zinc as in the recently described excessive use of dental adhesives can also be considered in this same category.

4. Etiology: Major categories represent the gamut of pathology.

   a. Infection—leprosy and HIV

   b. Inflammation: vasculitis—periarteritis

   c. Immune disorders affecting immunoglobulins and related compounds. Note that HIV may be associated with several varieties of peripheral neuropathies, the

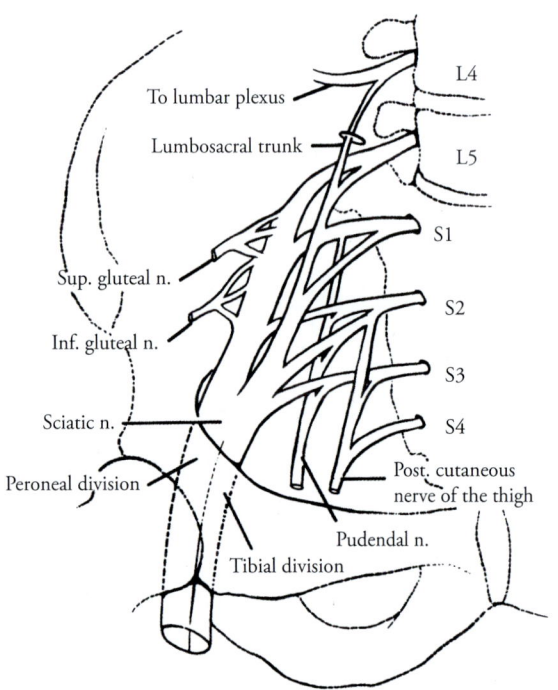

Figure 8.7 Plan of the sacral plexus. Note origin of common peroneal nerve from posterior divisions L4-S2 and of tibial nerve from anterior divisions L4-S3. The two nerves are joined together to form the sciatic nerve. (From Mendell JR, Kissel JT, Cornblath DR (eds): Diagnosis and Management of Peripheral Nerve Disorders. Oxford University Press, New York, 2001.)

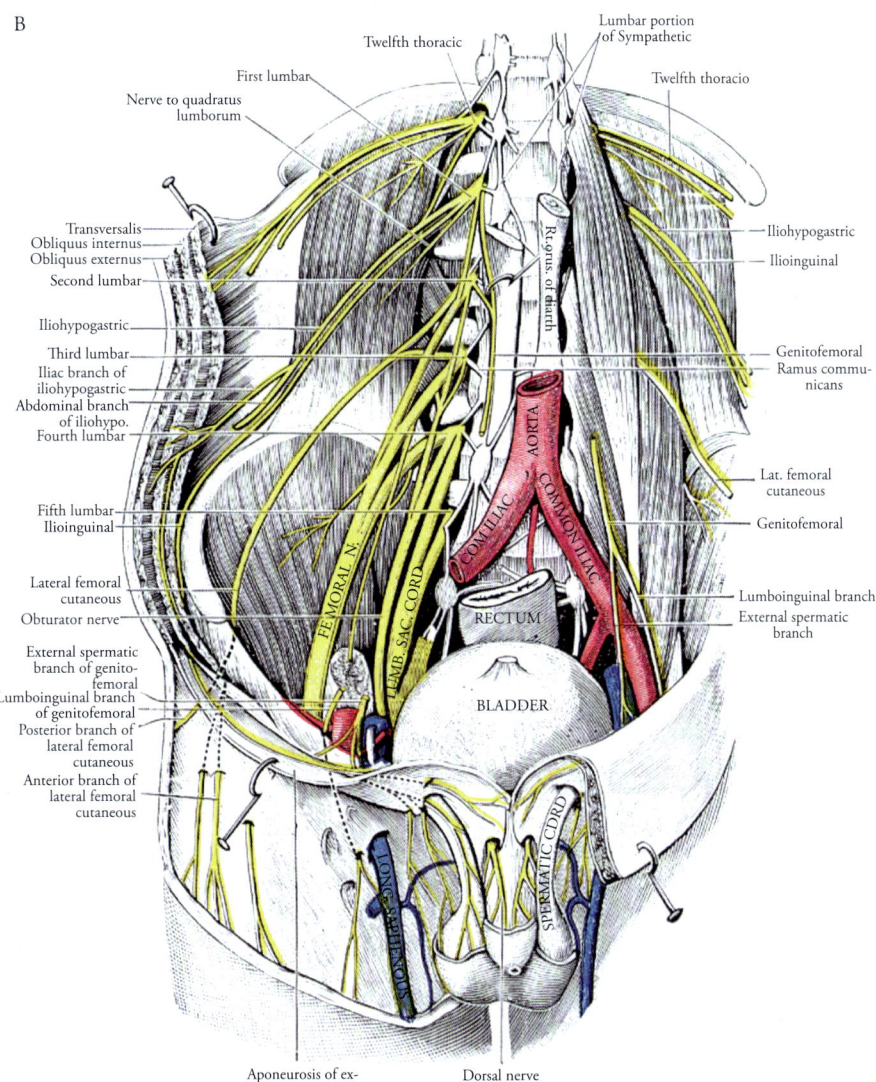

Figure 8.8 (A) Dissection of the lumbar and sacral plexuses, demonstrating their relationship to the vertebral foramina and the inguinal ligament and the sciatic notch. (From Zimmerman, J and Jacobson, S.) (B) Dissection of the Lumbar Plexus. Note relationship oof the plexus to the psoas muscle, iliacus muscle and pelvic structures. Note the course of the lateral femoral cutaneous, femoral and obturator nerves and possible sites of compression. (From Clement, Grays' Anatomy 30rth Ed., 1985, p. 1238.)

Figure 8.9 Dissection of the Sacral and Pudendal Plexuse. Sagittal View. Note the relationship of the plexus to the visceral structures. Note also the course of the obturator nerve, from the lumbar plexus, as it passes to enter the obturator canal and foramen. (With permission from Clemente, C.: Gray's Anatomy, 30th Ed. 1985, p. 1238.)

most common of which is a distal sensory peripheral neuropathy (see Gonzalez-Duarte, 2008 for additional discussion).

d. Intoxications: arsenic, lead, antineoplastic agents, and industrial chemical exposures

e. Metabolic disorders: nutritional deficiencies of B vitamins, diabetes mellitus, uremia, and critical care unit neuropathies. Note that too much of a good thing may also be bad for you. Thus, excessive amounts of pyridoxine as well as a deficiency of pyridoxine may both cause a peripheral neuropathy. In some cases a deficiency may reflect the excessive use of another agent, for example, excessive intake of zinc producing a copper deficiency as mentioned earlier.

f. Degenerations: hereditary

g. Tumors: neurofibrobromas, schwannomas

Such a classification is a simplification. Often multiple causes are present. The most obvious example is diabetes mellitus. In the United States, there are approximately 20.8 million patients with this diagnosis. Worldwide approximately 280 million people are affected. Type I diabetes is an autoimmune disorder with genetic and environmental factors that produces a severe insulin deficiency and occurs in younger age groups. In contrast, Type II diabetes, which is the larger group, occurs predominately but not exclusively in the older age groups. This is a nonimmune disorder associated with insulin resistance and impaired insulin resistance and with a strong relationship to obesity. Overall the incidence of objective neuropathy in Type I diabetes is 66% and in Type II diabetes, 59%.

The older age group also has an increased incidence of hypothyroidism, vitamin B12 deficiency, and possibly poor nutrition. Studies by indicate a significant increase in the incidence of chronic inflammatory demyelinating polyneuropathy in the 70- to 79-year-old male population to a prevalence of 6.7 to 9.5 per 100,000 population compared to a baseline of 0.81 to 1.9 per 100,000. All of these factors raise the possible coincidence of two relatively common diseases as affecting peripheral nerve occurring in the same individual. More important, in the study of 55% of 103 consecutive patients with diabetes and a distal sensory neuropathy had apparent additional causes for a peripheral neuropathy. These included alcohol use, neurotoxic medications, low vitamin B12 and B6, hypertriglyceridemia, monoclonal proteins, and paraproteinemia. Thus, a common disease such as diabetes mellitus may have a high coincidence with other diseases occurring in particular age groups and populations.

Other examples of more complex interactions are the following: (1) the use of nitrous oxide may trigger a B12 deficiency in predisposed individuals; and (2) the use of the antineoplastic agent vincristine may unmask subclinical hereditary neuropathies at low dosage exposure.

From a practical standpoint, the usual approach is to combine the several types of classification.

1. First classify as to acute, subacute, or chronic.

2. Then classify as to predominantly motor, sensory, or autonomic. The majority are mixed.

3. If possible, classify as to axonal or demyelinating based on EMG/nerve studies and in some cases on nerve biopsy. (A survey of peripheral nerve histopathology is presented in Figs. 8.12 to 8.14.)

4. Then classify as to etiology.

ACUTE PROGRESSIVE MOTOR NEUROPATHY WITH VARIABLE SENSORY FEATURES

The Guillain Barré syndrome provides the most common example of an acute rapidly progressive polyneuropathy. (Other terms used include acute idiopathic polyneuritis, acute inflammatory demyelinating polyinfectious polyneuropathy, Landry-Guillain-Barré disease).

The predominant form of Guillain Barré syndrome in North America and in Europe is *acute inflammatory demyelinating polyneuropathy* (AIDP).

This is a rapidly progressive predominantly motor peripheral neuropathy that evolves over 10–14 days and affects legs, arms, and in many cases cranial nerves. In some cases there is progression to involve the muscles of respiration. Sensory symptoms are present but in most cases sensory findings are minor compared to the motor findings. In severe cases, tracheotomy and mechanical respiratory assistance may be required.

Figure 8.10 Nerves of the right lower extremity: anatomy of the common deep and superficial peroneal nerves. The relatively superficial course of the common peroneal nerve as it passes around the head of the fibula from posterior (popliteal) location to anterior calf is best seen in this illustration. (From Mendell JR, Kissel JT, Cornblath DR (eds): Diagnosis and Management of Peripheral Nerve Disorders. Oxford University Press, New York, 2001.)

Prior to the era of modern respiratory assistance, the death rate was as high as 25%.

The essential pathology consists of perivascular inflammatory infiltrates consisting of lymphocytes and macrophages, and perivenous segmental demyelination. CD4 and CD8 T cell lymphocytes are present. Nerve roots as well as peripheral and cranial nerves are involved. In more severe cases, axons as well as myelin are involved with secondary Wallerian degeneration. The cerebrospinal fluid is usually without a cellular reaction but does show an increase in protein that peaks 1–2 weeks after onset. In most cases, slowing of motor nerve conduction will eventually be demonstrated, consistent with a demyelinating peripheral neuropathy. By week 3, 85% of patients will meet these criteria, but early in the disease conductions are often normal. Prolonged F waves or absent H waves discussed in Chapter 2 may occur within days of onset.

The underlying pathogenesis of the syndrome is now apparent. In 60%–70% of patients, a viral respiratory or gastrointestinal infection has occurred 1–2 weeks prior to the onset of the neurological symptoms. Other patients have experienced infectious mononucleosis, viral hepatitis, other viral illnesses, surgical procedures, or immunizations—(old type of serum antibodies vaccine, swine influenza vaccine of 1976).

The pathological and clinical manifestations of the disease reflect an immunological reaction directed at peripheral nerves. A similar syndrome—experimental allergic neuritis (EAN)—has been produced in rabbits and other laboratory animals 2 weeks after immunization with homogenized peripheral nerve (Waksman and Adams, 1955). More recent studies have been more specific. Rats or rabbits injected with adjuvant and bovine peripheral nerve myelin or specific myelin proteins develop the clinical paralysis syndrome plus the pathologic changes of the

Figure 8.11 Posterior tibial nerve and right medial ankle. (From Mendell JR, Kissel JT, Cornblath DR (eds): Diagnosis and Management of Peripheral Nerve Disorders. Oxford University Press, New York, 2001.)

Table 8.1 NEUROPATHOLOGICAL DIAGNOSIS AT DISCHARGE

Diabetes mellitus	22.8%
Alcohol (overlap with thiamine deficiency)	17.5%
Vitamin deficiency (B12, B6)	10.5%
Guillain Barré (acute inflammatory demyelinating polyneuropathy)	7.9%
Gammopathy	5.3%
Lyme disease	5.3%
Hypothyroidism	4.4%
Chronic inflammatory demyelinating polyneuropathy	4.4%
Paraneoplastic	3.5%
Hereditary	2.6%
Vasculitis	2.6%
Hyperthyroidism	2.6%
Critical illness	1.8%
Medication	1.8%
Misc: solvents, sarcoid, Refsum, Crohn's, polyarthritis, etc.	Each of 0.9%

human AIDP. This includes lymphocyte T cell and macrophage infiltrates, as well as demyelination. Sera from patients with the syndrome react with multiple antigens in peripheral nerve. In some studies, IgG and IgM antibodies to GM1 ganglioside from patients with the syndrome when injected into rat nerve have produced conduction block. Sera from some patients with Guillain Barré syndrome will produce demyelination in tissue culture. Overall these antibodies to GM11 are positive in a minority of all patients with the AIDP syndrome (no more than possibly 9%–25% of all patients). Even those studies with the higher percentages have probably included Fisher syndrome, AMAN, and AMSAN in the total number of patients. (See later for the much higher percentage of positive titers in these other variants.)

Differential Diagnosis

The onset of the disease has no changes in mental status, little or no early cranial nerve symptoms (these may subsequently develop), sensory symptoms but minimal sensory findings but with major motor symptoms and findings, areflexia with normal flexor or no plantar responses, and an albumin-cytologic dissociation and eventually slowing of the motor nerve conduction velocities will distinguish this syndrome from entities such as (1) spinal cord compression; (2) acute poliomyelitis; (3) botulism; (4) the acute polyneuropathy of porphyria, diphtheria, and arsenic; and (5) tick paralysis.

Treatment

As regards treatment, mild cases require only supportive treatment. Early cases should if at all possible be admitted to an intensive care unit to monitor respiration and autonomic function. Autonomic instability is often present with significant

Figure 8.12 Histopathology of peripheral nerve I: Wallerian degeneration. Considerable necrosis and degeneration of axons, myelin, and Schwann cells has occurred. The field is dominated by large macrophages containing remnant of axons, myelin, fat globules, and so on ("Digestion Chambers"). Toluidine blue, 100× (approx.). (Courtesy of Dr. Tom Smith, Neuropathology, University of Massachusetts Medical School.)

Figure 8.13 Histopathology of peripheral nerve II: chronic axonal neuropathy. A marked loss of myelinated fibers has occurred. However, these are clusters of axons surrounded by a thin myelin sheath, suggesting that degeneration of axons has occurred. Toluidine blue, 100×. (Courtesy of Dr. Tom Smith.)

orthostatic hypotension. In severe cases with progressing paralysis or respiratory muscle or pharyngeal involvement, plasmapheresis is now employed. In the cases treated by the within 2 weeks of onset, there was a definite reduction in the length of time for hospitalization, for mechanical respiration, and for resumption of walking. More recent studies have suggested that intravenous immunoglobulin G may be somewhat more effective (for a review of current concepts, see Ropper, 1992). Both therapies have their side effects. Some cases will also require respiratory assistance and or airway assistance. Glucocorticoid steroids usually have no significant effect, although massive intravenous therapy (1000 mg/day of methylprednisolone) in uncontrolled trials has been reported to have a possible effect.

The following case history provides an example of a mild case of this syndrome.

CASE HISTORY 8.5

Approximately 2 weeks after influenza infection, this 71-year-old, right-handed male awoke with tingling of the plantar surfaces of his feet, unsteadiness, and weakness at the knees. Over the next 10 days, he experienced a gradual decrease in lower extremity power but no progression of the sensory symptoms. He denied low back pain, bowel symptoms, or bladder symptoms.

Neurological Examination

Mental status and cranial nerves: All intact.

Motor system: Weakness was present in the lower extremities both proximal and distal slightly greater on right than left. A minimal dysmetria was present in the upper extremities.

Figure 8.14 Histopathology of peripheral nerve III: segmental demyelination, teased nerve fiber preparation. This 74-year-old man had a peripheral neuropathy associated with abnormality of plasma protein. (monoclonal cryoglobulinemia). (Courtesy of the authors, Lippa, C.F., Chad, D.A., Smith, T.W., Kaplan, M., Hammor, K.: Muscle and Nerve: 626–631, 1986.)

Reflexes: All deep tendon stretch reflexes were absent in upper and lower limbs except for a trace triceps. Plantars demonstrated no response to stimulation.

Sensory system: There was a mild decrease in pain and temperature sensation over toes. Perianal sensation was normal. To a greater degree, position and vibratory sensation were decreased in the toes.

Clinical diagnosis: Guillain Barré syndrome: acute postinfectious polyneuropathy.

Laboratory Data

Basic lab data: CBC, glucose, renal functions, liver functions, electrolytes, protein immunoelectrophoresis and ESR (40 mm/hr), and magnetic resonance imaging (MRI) of the spine were all normal. *CSF:* protein was increased to 206mg%, with 0 white blood cells and a glucose of 76mg%. Serological tests and cultures were negative.

EMG/nerve conduction studies demonstrated slowing of motor nerve conduction velocity—consistent with a demyelinating neuropathy.

Course: the patient's condition stabilized and he was transferred to a rehabilitation facility.

Variants

Acute motor sensory axonal neuropathy (AMSAN) and acute motor axonal neuropathy (AMAN) are variants in which motor and sensory axonal degeneration or motor axonal degeneration occurs with only minimal demyelination and inflammation. AMSAN involves both sensory and motor roots, is the more severe, and has a more prolonged recovery. These variants occur in children and young adults. The preceding infection is usually gastrointestinal caused by *campylobacter jejuni*. Epidemics have occurred in rural northern China. There may be a predilection for the Chinese and Japanese population. The clinical characteristics are a rapidly ascending quadriparesis plus respiratory failure. As in AIDP deep tendon reflexes are absent or reduced and there is an albumino-cytologic dissociation and the axon degeneration is evident on EMG/NCV studies and on pathologic examination. Nerve conduction studies indicate no responses or responses of low amplitude. Although there is macrophage infiltration in the periaxonal space, there is minimal infiltration by lymphocytes. Elevated titers of antibodies to ganglioside GM1 occur in 24%–60% of patients. The association with the antecedent campylobacter jejuni infection raises the question of molecular mimicry between a component of the infectious agent and a component of the axon. A similar question may be raised as regards AIDP and other antecedent infections.

Overall, the disease is more severe than the usual case of AIDP with more severe involvement of the cranial motor nerves (extraocular muscles are usually spared). The differential diagnosis is similar to AIDP discussed earlier. The role of immunosuppression in treatment is unclear; otherwise the supportive management is similar to AIDP.

Fisher syndrome: In this variant, there is a triad of ophthalmoplegia, ataxia, and areflexia. In general, involvement of the extraocular muscles is rare in the classical case of AIDP. There is an albuminocytologic dissociation and electrophysiological evidence of a demyelinating polyneuropathy. Other symptoms of classical AIDP are less common. What distinguishes this particular syndrome from the other variants is the presence in 89% of these patients of an elevated level of the ganglioside antibody GQ1b. These antibodies bind to antibodies in the neuromuscular junction of cranial nerves and to neurons in the molecular layer of the cerebellum. These pathologic features explain most of the main symptoms.

The disorder is relatively mild with a good prognosis for recovery.

This syndrome must be distinguished from two other syndromes: (1) Bickerstaff's brain stem encephalitis in which ophthalmoplegia, areflexia, ataxia, and paralysis are combined with drowsiness and the MRI demonstrates an actual brain stem abnormality. And (2) Wernicke's encephalopathy in which ophthalmoplegia and ataxia are combined in a rapidly progressive manner with drowsiness and impairment of recent memory. This latter syndrome is due to a thiamine deficiency and often is accompanied by an areflexia. The MRI demonstrates brain stem and diencephalic lesions.

Acute brachial neuritis is also considered a variant since in some cases electrical studies suggest involvement not only of the affected limb but also of the opposite clinically unaffected limb.

Other causes of the syndrome of acute progressive motor neuropathy:

1. The exotoxin produced by the bacillus, c. Diphtheria: pharyngeal and laryngeal muscles are affected 1–2 weeks after the pharyngeal infection followed by a general polyneuropathy: arms then legs after 4–5 weeks.

2. Acute intermittent porphyria is inherited as an autosomal dominant trait. A metabolic defect in the liver results in increased production of and high urine levels of porphobilinogen and its precursor delta aminolevulinic acid (involved in hemoglobin metabolism). The severe motor neuropathy may be accompanied by abdominal pain or psychosis or convulsions. Anticonvulsants, barbiturates, sulfa drugs, and estrogens may trigger attacks.

3. Toxic polyneuropathies:

    a. Triorthocresylphosphate: the so-called Jamaican Ginger polyneuropathy seen during the prohibition era reflected contamination of bootleg alcohol by this agent.

    b. Thallium salts

All of these acute polyneuropathies as well as many subacute and chronic polyneuropathies are characterized by an acellular cerebrospinal fluid that often has an increased protein content.

Acute polyneuropathies are distinguished from subacute and chronic polyneuropathies. There is no clear-cut distinction; subacute may evolve into chronic over years. In addition, subacute disorders may appear to have a relatively acute onset because the history may be incomplete. In addition, acute massive exposure to several toxins may produce an acute syndrome that mimics AIDP, for example, arsenic and N hexane.

Subacute Polyneuropathies

The common causes are toxic and metabolic, producing a distal symmetrical sensory, motor neuropathy often with painful feet (dysesthesia and hyperesthesia).

1. *Nutritional deficiencies* of B vitamins: thiamine, B12 pyridoxal phosphate, and folic acid, often multiple are frequently encountered. (a) In association with alcoholism, (b) in chronic elderly intensive care patients –"critical illness polyneuropathy), in the "dry" or neuropathic form of beri-beri seen in prisoner of war camps, in famine, or in underdeveloped parts of the world. A neuropathy is also seen in the "wet form" of beri-beri in association with congestive heart failure. The nutritional neuropathies are reviewed in detail. A more detailed consideration of B12 and the nervous system will be found in Chapter 9 of this book on the spinal cord. A more detailed consideration of thiamine and the nervous system will be found in Chapter 30 of this book on the problem of memory disorders (Wernicke-Korsakoff syndrome).

2. *Heavy metal intoxication*. Arsenic—distal sensory motor. A more acute form associated with acute arsenic intoxication also occurs. Lead—predominantly motor with greater involvement of the upper extremities (wrist drops due to radial nerve involvement).

3. *Hexacarbon industrial solvents* used in glues and plastic production n-hexane and methyl-n-butyl ketone (see Spenser et al., 1975).

4. *Other industrial agents*: acrylamide, trichloroethylene.

5. *Medication induced*: (a) isoniazid (INH) for treatment of tuberculosis—produces a pyridoxine deficiency; (b) nitrofuradontins used for the treatment of bladder infection; (c) antineoplastic agents, including cis-platinum and vincristine; (d) thalidomide no longer available once marketed as a tranquilizer; (e) drugs used to prevent seizures (anticonvulsants)—phenytoin is the most prominent in this group—usually the syndrome is subclinical.

6. *Uremic polyneuropathy* occurs in 60%–70% patients with chronic renal failure. The syndrome clears slowly with renal transplantation.

Chronic polyneuropathy: Common causes are as follows:

1. *Diabetes mellitus*: distal symmetrical predominantly sensory—axonal—peripheral neuropathy (see case 4 earlier); etiology is not clear but may involve accumulation of glucose, fructose, and sorbitol in nerves. In addition, a vascular etiology is also postulated due to accumulation of substances in the wall of small blood vessels with swelling of basement membranes and endothelial cells. Autonomic neuropathies or painful distal neuropathies may occur. In the laboratory study for overall diagnosis in all patients with a sensory neuropathy, the positive yield for blood tests is 11% for fasting glucose, 26% for A1C and for glucose tolerance test. (Presumably the 2 hr postprandial blood sugar would yield results between the fasting and glucose tolerance blood sugar levels.) Successful pancreatic transplantation may halt progression of the disease. See earlier discussion of epidemiology.

2. *Remote effects of malignancy*: carcinoma of lung, ovary, and breast. Mixed sensory motor, motor, or selective sensory.

3. *Complications of connective tissue disorder*: periarteritis, rheumatoid arthritis. In some cases this is a complication of HIV infection.

4. *Leprosy*: the most common worldwide infectious cause of peripheral neuropathy

5. *Chronic inflammatory demyelinating polyneuropathies* (CIDP) subacute-chronic. In contrast to Guillain Barré syndrome (AIDP and its variants) which usually reaches an end point in a matter of days or less than 4 weeks, these disorders present a progressive or relapsing remitting form of the more common acute idiopathic polyneuropathy. The clinical course is progression with or without remissions over 2 months. The clinical findings are in many ways similar. An immunologic basis is presumed although not always

demonstrated. There is a crossover with peripheral neuropathies seen with the para-proteinemias.

As with the acute disorders, three variants may be specified:

a. Chronic inflammatory peripheral neuropathy: the most common and the chronic analog of AIDP: a predominantly motor neuropathy with no clear cut antibody. There is an good response to steroids, plasmapheresis, and immunoglobulin G.

b. Multifocal motor neuropathy, the chronic analog of AMAN in which IgM anti-GM1 is demonstrated. Despite this immunologic basis, there is a poor response to immune therapy. This disorder was initially confused with long-term motor neuron disease of amyotrophic lateral sclerosis.

c. Lewis-Sumner syndrome, the chronic analog of AMSAN syndrome. No anti-GM1 antibody is demonstrated. There is a good response to steroids.

For additional discussion:

6. Abnormalities of plasma proteins usually a monoclonal abnormality of immunoglobulins (multiple myeloma, macroglobulinemia, cryoglobulinemia, and benign monoclonal gammopathy).

7. Hereditary peripheral neuropathies. Mixed sensory motor inherited polyneuropathies without a clearly defined metabolic abnormality. In the series of 205 patients referred to the Mayo Clinic (Dyck et al., 1981) with chronic polyneuropathies of unknown cause, 86 or 42% were found to have an inherited disorder of this type.

The classification of hereditary neuropathies has been markedly reorganized by genetic testing. Most have been now grouped into the overall diagnosis of Charcot Marie Tooth disease (CMT), also known as hereditary motor and sensory neuropathy (HMSN). (The classification will be employed later.) The classical description of CMT (the old original term was peroneal muscular atrophy) includes distal atrophy, sensory loss, and foot deformity of various type, including the classical pes cavus (high-arched foot due to uncompensated action of the plantar flexors and failed contraction of the peroneal ankle and toe dorsiflexors). The course is variable and there are in specific families additional different features and different ages of onset.

The following recent classification covers multiple disorders within major groups: CMT 1: Autosomal dominant demyelinating is characterized by demyelination with the hypertrophic onion bulb changes that are seen when demyelination and remyelination has occurred (Fig. 8.15). Note that onion bulb formation may also occur with repeated episodes of CIDP. The nerves may also be grossly enlarged. A marked reduction occurs in nerve conduction velocity on nerve conduction studies. Multiple subtypes have been identified: CMT 1A,1B 1C,1D,1E 1F/2E (in which cerebellar tremor and ataxia also occurs). Other variants will undoubtedly be discovered. All of these subtypes are transmitted as an autosomal dominant and have slow conduction, implying a demyelinating disorder. Type CMT 1A accounts for 60% of all hereditary peripheral neuropathies and is linked to a point mutation occurring on chromosome 17 at the PMP 22 gene segment. This gene encodes myelin protein and appears to be duplicated. Note that myelin protein also means the Schwann cell of origin whose extensions surround the axons.

Figure 8.15 Histopathology of peripheral nerve IV: hypertrophic "onion bulb" neuropathy. Repeated episodes of segmental demyelination and remyelination may result in finely myelinated axons surrounded by whorls of overlapping intertwined processes of Schwann cells. In addition, this microscopic field demonstrates a significant decrease in total numbers of fibers and a significant increase in connective tissue. Toluidine blue, 63× (approx.). (Courtesy of Dr. Tom Smith.)

CMT 2: Autosomal dominant: axonal has a somewhat variable age of onset. Nerve conduction velocity is normal; there is no histologic evidence of demyelination. The underlying pathology is considered neuronal. Multiple subtypes (CMT2A1—CMT-2 Po) have so far been described. Pupillary and hearing abnormalities may be described in some of the variants.

CMT 2: Autosomal recessive; axonal. Six varieties have so far been described, including infantile and childhood onset

CMT 3: Dejerine Sotta's syndrome is a less common but more severe recessive or autosomal dominant disorder beginning in the first decade of life with both sensory and motor features. There is severe weakness and areflexia. The disorder may map to PMP-22 as above or 8q23 or reg21q or 17 p or to other sites. The essential pathologic change is demyelination with subsequent remyelination to produce the hypertrophic onion bulb formations (Fig 8.15). Nerves are grossly enlarged to palpation; progression is more rapid and disability greater.

CMT 4: Autosomal recessive; demyelinating. So far 11 varieties have been described. Early onset: congenital, infantile, or childhood is the usual pattern.

CMT: X linked. Both dominant and recessive forms have been described. Central nervous system involvement is usually present, including optic atrophy, hearing loss, possible mental retardation, and MRI changes.

Other CMT groups:

Autosomal dominant: with intermediate varieties

dHMN: Autosomal dominant motor predominant

dHMN: Autosomal recessive motor predominant

HSAN (hereditary sensory and autonomic neuropathy): Within this group of eight disorders is the HSAN III familial dysautonomia (Riley-Day disease). A deficiency of serum dopamine B hydroxylase, the enzyme that converts dopamine to norepinephrine, results in severe abnormalities of the sympathetic autonomic nervous system. In addition, small myelinated and unmyelinated fibers are involved, producing a selective loss of pain and temperature sensibilities.

HMSN (hereditary motor and sensory neuropathy): Among the now nine subgroup members of this group is a previously described entity now listed as HMSNIV: Refsum disease. Hereditary ataxic polyneuritis (autosomal recessive). Phytanic acid (a fatty acid) accumulates in blood and nerves. The symptoms begin in late childhood or adolescence. In addition to a peripheral neuropathy, cerebellar ataxia, a degeneration of the retina (retinitis pigmentosa), neurogenic deafness, and a degeneration of cardiac muscle (cardiomyopathy) are present in most patients.

Miscellaneous group: A variety of cases are included in this group, including Andermann syndrome in which hypotonia and areflexia occur in infants.

Case 8.6 provides an example of a patient with autosomal dominant Charcot Marie Tooth disease and slow nerve conduction consistent with CMT 1 of demyelinating type as indicated the most common variant of the CMT classification.

CASE HISTORY 8.6

This 50-year-old, single, white male was referred for evaluation of progressive weakness of the legs. The patient had a deformity of both feet all of his life which produced difficulty when walking for much of his life. He related this to weakness in feet and difficulty with balance of feet. The patient had developed at some time in the early grade school years difficulty in hands, primarily a weakness in movements of fingers and grip. He felt that he had some atrophy of hand muscles all of his life. Approximately 10–12 years prior to admission, the patient began to note a progression in weakness of his hands. During the last year or two prior to admission, the patient had noted increased difficulty in movements of feet and difficulty in lifting toes and feet. He denied any specific numbness in hands and legs.

Family history was significant. The patient's brother had a similar deformity of the feet (pes cavus). In addition, the brother had weakness and lack of control of the feet. The patient's mother and grandmother had similar difficulty with foot deformity and weakness in lower extremities. In a collateral line involving many cousins for four generations, multiple family members had developed difficulty in their feet as children, and somewhat later in life had developed weakness in feet and occasionally had developed at age 35 or 40 difficulty with weakness and atrophy of hands. In most of these family members, some progression of disability began to occur between the ages of 35 and 50. This was confirmed by the evaluation of a first cousin who developed numbness in foot, foot drop, and imbalance in walking at age 30 and weakness and atrophy in the hands at age 35. His examination was similar to the patient in this case.

Neurological Examination

Mental status and cranial nerves: Intact.
Motor system:

1. Strength was intact at hip and knee but markedly decreased at ankle dorsiflexors and everter. In upper extremities, shoulders, elbows, and wrists were intact as regards strength; however, all movements in hands were weak without any selectivity as to ulnar, radial, or median. Thus, finger abductors, thumb abductors, opponens and thumb adductor were all weak.

2. There was atrophy of intrinsic muscles of hands with marked atrophy in the first interosseous space. There was flattening of thenar and hypothenar eminences. Bilateral pes cavus, deformity of the feet (high arches), was present with slight in-turning of both feet at ankles.

Reflexes: Deep tendon reflexes were everywhere absent and there was no response to plantar stimulation.

Sensory system: Pain sensation and touch were decreased in lower extremities to just below the ankles, but intact in the upper extremities. Vibratory sensation was absent at toes and ankles but present at knees and slightly decreased at fingers compared to wrists. Rare errors were made in position sense at toes.

Clinical diagnosis: Charcot Marie Tooth disease most likely autosomal dominant demyelinating.

Laboratory Data

Nerve conduction studies: There was indicated marked slowing of motor nerve conduction velocity in the upper extremities (median and ulnar nerves were studied) consistent with a demyelinating process. Sensory evoked potentials were absent.

No responses were obtained on stimulation of the peroneal and posterior tibial nerves in the lower extremities.

EMG studies: There were neuropathic changes of denervation: fibrillations.

Muscle biopsy of calf muscle (gastrocnemius): This was consistent with a neuropathic process: grouped muscle atrophy (similar to Fig. 8.16).

Sural nerve biopsy: Large fiber axons were reduced in number and occasionally fragmented. There was an apparent marked increase in small fiber axons.

Subsequent Course

Over the next 16 years the patient had a very slow progression. At the time of his death in 1984 at age 66 (apparent cardiac arrest during a minor surgical procedure), he was still able to walk slowly without assistance or the use of a walker or cane. He occasionally did need assistance in rising from a chair. He was able to live by himself and to prepare his own meals.

Figure 8.16 Histopathology of muscle III: neurogenic atrophy in a patient with Charcot Marie Tooth disease. Grouped atrophy is evident. H&E, 63× (approx.) (Courtesy of Dr. Tom Smith.)

Comments

This patient presented a slowly progressive peripheral neuropathy that was predominantly motor. The extensive family history suggested an autosomal dominant disorder. The nerve conduction studies in the upper extremities were consistent with a demyelinating disorder. In the lower extremities where longer lengths of demyelinated nerves were studied, the delay in conduction was so severe that no responses could be obtained. As a demyelinating peripheral neuropathy progresses, there are changes in the proteins in myelin and axonal structure and axonal transport. As discussed by the disruption of the interaction between Schwann cells (involved in myelin formation) and the axon results in dysfunction of the axon physiology. Eventually axonal atrophy and fiber degeneration occurs. This would then explain the findings of the muscle and sural nerve biopsy. Final classification would be CMT 1A.

OTHER INHERITED PERIPHERAL NEUROPATHIES

Bassen Kornsweig syndrome—a rare autosomal recessive syndrome which begins in infancy; the metabolic defect is a deficiency of beta lipoprotein and of cholesterol. As earlier, peripheral nerve, cerebellum, heart, and retina are all affected. In addition—fatty stools, (steatorrhea) retarded growth, and an abnormal appearance of red blood cells (acanthocytosis) is present.

Porphyria, in contrast to the previous processes, produces an acute syndrome. There is a combination of peripheral neuropathy, abdominal symptoms, and alterations in mental function: think of the "madness of King George III."

Familial amyloid polyneuropathy autosomal dominant (Andrade type). Amyloid accumulates in blood vessel walls and in the endoneurium. An often painful syndrome occurs that begins in the adult with sensory and autonomic symptoms and slowly progress to a full polyneuropathy over 10–15 years.

Spino cerebellar degenerations: Many of these disorders including many of the autosomal dominant disorders (SCA) and the autosomal recessive Friedreich's (FRDA) have evidence of a peripheral neuropathy. In many of the autosomal dominant disorders, to be discussed in the cerebellar Chapter 20, there is an excessive number of trinucleotide repeats (CAG or CTG). In FRDA, the most common of the hereditary ataxias discussed in the spinal cord chapter, there is a GAA triplet expansion in the fraxtin gene on chromosome 9.

Hereditary peripheral nerve channelopathies: These are relatively rare disorders/mutations of the sodium or potassium channels which result in episodes of axonal hyperexcitability or of in excitability. At the present time three are known to involve the Na v 1.7 form which is encoded by the SCN 9A gene which is highly expressed in the dorsal root ganglion nociceptive and in sympathetic neurons. Two of the autosomal dominant syndromes are characterized by paroxysmal attacks of pain and dysautonomia. An autosomal recessive syndrome of this sodium channel results in a syndrome of isolated loss of pain sensation.

The potassium channel abnormalities may involve the KCNQ2 gene with episodic muscle cramps and contractions or the KCNA1 gene with attacks of cerebellar ataxia and myokymia (muscle contraction). Both are autosomal dominant and rare with an overlap with neonatal seizures. (See cerebellar Chapter 20 for additional information.)

Unknown cause in chronic peripheral neuropathy: Even when the patient had been fully investigated in a specialized center, a specific etiology may still not be found. In the Mayo Clinic series (Dyck et al., 1981) previously cited, 24% of patients remained in the unknown etiology; today this percentage would undoubtedly be lower, due to the more specific recognition of varieties of CIDP and of additional categories of hereditary peripheral neuropathy.

DISORDERS OF THE NERVE ROOT: RADICULOPATHY

The major problem affecting the nerve root is compression by a ruptured disk or by osteophytes projecting into the neural foramen from the degenerative process affecting the disks (spondylosis).

These processes primarily involve the cervical and lumbar areas. These problems are among the most frequently encountered in the neurological office. In the cervical area the C5-C6 and the C6-C7 interspaces are most frequently involved with compression of the C6 or C7 nerve roots. Less often the C5 or C8 nerve roots are involved. The relationship of the disk space to the nerve root and to the spinal cord is demonstrated in Figure 8.17.

In the lumbar area the L4-L5 (L5 nerve root) and L5-S1 (S1 or L5 nerve root) interspaces are most frequently involved. Less often the L3-L4 or L2-L3 disk interspaces are involved with involvement of the L4 or L3 nerve roots.

In the diagnostic analysis of a radiculopathy, the following features should be considered:

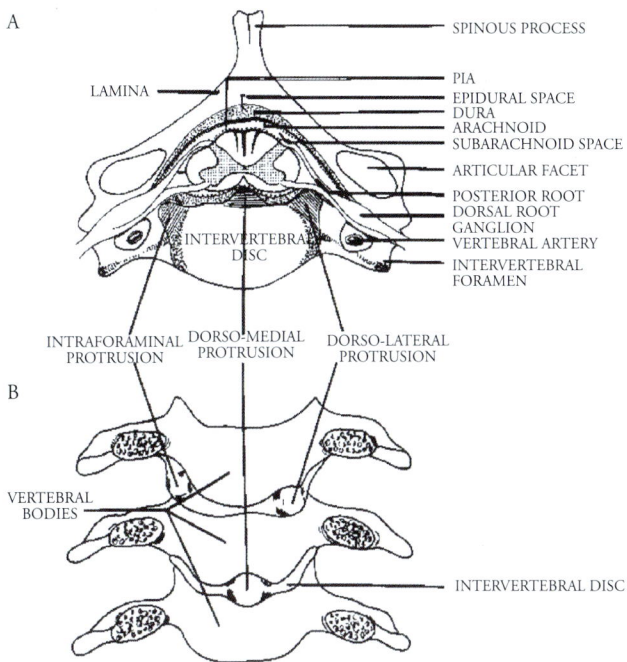

Figure 8.17 Anatomic relationships of the cervical spinal cord and the cervical intervertebral disks. Lateral and midline disk protrusions are indicated. (Modified after Frykholm, Acta. Chir. Scand. 101:345, 1951.)

1. The acute onset of pain in the limb in a radicular distribution (Fig. 8.1) with associated pain in the neck or lumbar spine
2. In general the radicular pain is out of the proportion to the neck or back pain.
3. The radicular pain is described as a sharp, shooting, burning, or electric shock-like or toothache-like pain. The pain is exacerbated by maneuvers that suddenly increase pressure within the cerebrospinal fluid space, for example, coughing, sneezing, or straining at stool.
4. Radicular sensory symptoms plus or minus radicular sensory findings may be present
5. Selective weakness of muscles supplied by a specific cervical or lumbar nerve root may be present.
6. Selective depression of a deep tendon stretch reflex supplied by a specific cervical or lumbar nerve root may be present.
7. In restricted lateral disk herniations in the cervical area, no long tract sensory, motor, or reflex findings should be present; that is, there should be no evidence for an upper motor neuron lesion. In restricted lateral disk herniations in the lumbar area, no bladder symptoms should be present.
8. With midline herniations in the cervical area, signs of spinal cord compression may be present and are considered in Chapter 9.
9. With midline herniations in the lumbar area, urinary retention and a disturbance of sexual functions may be present due to involvement of the cauda equina.

OVERVIEW OF SENSORY SYMPTOMS AND FINDINGS

The usual distribution of hypalgesia and of radicular pain in the upper extremity is demonstrated in Figure 8.18. See also Figure 2.1 for the lower extremity.

In considering sensory symptoms as compared to sensory findings, when there is involvement of a single nerve root, it is important to note that sensory symptoms (radicular pain and paresthesias) may be present, although the examination demonstrates no actual sensory deficit as regard pain or touch sensation. This is a reflection of the fact that there is an overlap of radicular sensory fields. Thus, one-half of the dermatome of C7 is also supplied by C6 and the other one half by -8 (Fig. 8.21a). The total sensory field then for a single nerve root is therefore more extensive than demonstrated in the standard sensory diagrams (Fig. 8.19b).

The following case history provides an example of cervical root compression secondary to a herniated disk.

CASE HISTORY 8.7

This 45-year-old, right-handed married white female educational coordinator 2 weeks prior to evaluation had acute onset pain in

Figure 8.18 Dermatome charts of the upper extremity in man outlined by the pattern of hypalgesia, following rupture of an intervertebral disk. (From Keegan, J.J., and Garrett, F.D., Anat. Rec. 102:417, 1948.)

the neck radiating into left arm with pain and tingling in the index and middle finger of the left hand. The pain would shoot into the arm if she coughed or sneezed or strained to move her bowels. Four months previously the patient had experienced pain in the neck extending to the left shoulder area but that symptom had cleared. In the last several days prior to consultation the patient had developed twitching of biceps and triceps muscles. She had no leg or bladder symptoms.

Neurological Examination
Mental status and cranial nerves: Intact.
Motor system: Intact
Reflexes: The left triceps deep tendon stretch reflex was absent or reversed. Plantar responses were flexor;
Sensory system: Pain sensation was decreased over the left index and middle fingers.
Neck: Neck motion was limited for extension and rotation and there was tenderness over the spinous processes of C7 and T1 and over the left supraclavicular area.

Clinical diagnosis: Cervical 7 radiculopathy secondary to lateral rupture of disk.

Subsequent course: The use of cervical traction, cervical collar, nonsteroidal anti-inflammatory agents, various pain and anti-muscle spasm agents, epidural injection, and various measures in physical

Figure 8.19A The method of remaining sensibility to demonstrate the sensory skin field of a nerve root. Sherrington sectioned three roots above and three below the intact root to be studied. In this diagram the overlap of the third and fifth thoracic spinal roots is demonstrated. (From Ransom, S., and Clark, S.: The Anatomy of the Nervous System, 10th Edition. Philadelphia, W. B. Saunders, 1959, p. 129.)

Figure 8.19B Dermatomes in man demonstrated by the method of remaining sensibility. (From Lewis, T.: Pain. New York, Macmillan, 1942, p. 20, after Foerster.)

therapy for 4 weeks failed to produce any relief. Pain was now predominantly in the arm and her examination now demonstrated additionally significant weakness at the left triceps muscle. Magnetic resonance imaging (Fig. 8. 20) demonstrated a lateral disk rupture at the C6-C7 interspace. The patient underwent a left-sided laminectomy at that level with removal of ruptured disk material. She had a resolution of symptoms except for a minor residual tingling, a decrease in pain sensation over the index finger, and a mild decrease of the left triceps deep tendon stretch reflex.

Comments

For cervical radiculopathy, at-home cervical traction, a cervical collar, cervical pillow, and nonsteroidal anti-inflammatory agents are usually effective. Most (75% and possibly as high as 90%) patients will usually respond to these measures. When these measures fail and radicular symptoms and findings persist, surgical therapy may be considered. At such a time MRI scan is appropriate. However, these considerations relate to lateral rupture of the disk without signs of long tract spinal cord involvement. If there is any evidence of midline spinal cord involvement, then an immediate MRI should be obtained.

Cervical spondylosis: This diagnostic term refers to the process in which degeneration of the nucleus pulposus of the disk space occurs

Figure 8.20 Lateral protrusion of a cervical disk: Case 8.7: Cervical radiculopathy magnetic resonance imaging: (*A*) sagittal section; (*B*) transverse section.

(often at multiple levels). This results in narrowing of the disk space, bulging of the annulus fibrosis and the formation of osteophytes (bony spurs). Depending on the diameter of the bony canal, when these events occur in the midline, spinal cord compression may occur. This topic is discussed in Chapter 9 on the spinal cord. When these events occur in the lateral position, nerve root compression may occur from projection of bony spurs into the neural foramina with the symptoms of a radiculopathy.

The following case reviews a more complex example of a lumbar radiculopathy in which diagnosis and management had been delayed.

CASE HISTORY 8.8

This 37-year-old, right-handed white female day care worker in relationship to heavy lifting had the acute onset of persistent pain in the lumbosacral area shooting as a sharp pain into the left buttock. One month later, she developed numbness in the left posterior thigh and left posterior calf to the ankle. Three months later she had the acute onset of severe pain in the lumbar area now extending to the posterior thigh and subsequently to the posterior calf as a shooting pain and tingling paresthesias now extended into the small toes. The pain in the leg was triggered by coughing or straining at stool. Despite a prolonged period of bed rest, pain medication, and nonsteroidal anti-inflammatory agents, no improvement occurred.

Neurological Examination (6 months after onset of symptoms)
Mental status and cranial nerves: Intact.
Motor system: Significant weakness was present on the left at toe extensors, ankle dorsiflexors, everter and inverter's with minor atrophy in the calf.
Reflexes: The Achilles deep tendon stretch reflex was absent on the left compared to active (3) right Achilles. Both patellar deep tendon reflexes were active (3).
Sensation: Pain sensation was markedly decreased on the left side over the L5 and S1 dermatomes and to a considerable degree over S2-S5.
Straight leg raising, palpation of nerves, and back: On straight leg rising, pain was present in both leg and back at 45–50 degrees on the left. On palpation, there was marked tenderness over the left sacroiliac area and over the left sciatic nerve at the sciatic notch and over the left posterior tibial nerve behind the medial malleolus of the ankle. The patient was in severe pain sitting, standing, or recumbent.
Clinical diagnosis: Rupture of disk with involvement of L5, S1, and probably cauda equine (based on the sensory findings).
Laboratory data: MRI (Fig. 8.21) demonstrated a massive rupture of the disk at the L4-L5 level with inferior extension and marked compression of the cauda equina.
Subsequent course: The patient eventually agreed to surgical removal of the ruptured disk, 5 weeks after the initial neurological evaluation. She had some relief of pain but over the next 3 years she continued to have a foot drop with significant weakness at left ankle and toes, an absent left Achilles reflex, and sensory deficits over the left L5 distribution.

Comments

The major consideration in the diagnosis of herniated disk was the historical information regarding the nature and distribution of the pain and tingling paresthesias. The findings of tenderness over the sciatic nerve and its branches and the findings on straight leg raising were consistent with a radiculopathy. The severe degree of weakness, the depression of the Achilles deep tendon reflex, and the widespread sensory deficit suggested that several roots of the cauda equina had been involved by this massive rupture at the L4-L5 interspace. Most patients with restricted lateral disk herniation at this level will have more limited findings usually involving only the L5 nerve root. In patients with long-standing severe deficits, surgical therapy is often not successful in reversing all of the neurological deficits. Most patients (75% and possibly as high as 90%) with a more limited lumbar radiculopathy respond to a period of strict bed rest for 3 to 5 days on a firm mattress and bed board, nonsteroidal anti-inflammatory agents, heat or cold, and possibly the temporary use subsequently of a back support. Those who fail this therapy may require local steroid

Figure 8.21 Lateral protrusion of a lumbar disk: Case 8.8: lumbar radiculopathy magnetic resonance imaging: (*A*) sagittal section; (*B*) transverse section.

injection or surgical therapy. Only if surgical therapy is a consideration should MRI studies be obtained.

BACK PAIN

Benign nonmalignant back pain alone, either acute or chronic, is an extremely common complaint. Usually it is benign in nature. However, a complete history and general physical examination is indicated to identify immediate precipitating events. In addition, a survey of any past history of malignancy, or change in bowel habits, or urinary pattern or in menses, etc. must be obtained. A rectal and or pelvic examination is indicated particularly when there is no clear-cut history of trauma. In the middle-aged or older male patient, appropriate laboratory studies to rule out prostatic malignancy are indicated (prostatic specific antigen [PSA]). If such a survey is negative and no neurological symptoms or signs are present, then lumbar MRI scan is not indicated. Plain films of the lumbar spine will usually suffice to rule out orthopedic disease. Such benign back pain does not require a course of bed rest. Nonsteroidal anti-inflammatory agents, modification of posture, heat or cold, and weight loss if indicated are appropriate measures. Activities at work may have to be temporarily modified and a support garment may be utilized.

Schwannoma Arising from the Nerve Root

These tumors arise from Schwann cells of the peripheral nerve or nerve root. When the nerve root is involved, the tumor may be present within the bony canal and/or external to the bony canal. The tumor may enlarge the neural foramen. Depending on the size and location of the tumor, the nerve root alone may be involved (Fig. 8.22) or the spinal cord may also be involved (refer to Chapter 9). When the tumor arises from a nerve root within the cauda equina, multiple nerve roots may be involved. Tumors of the lumbar roots may also be visualized by CT scan (Fig. 8.23).

Tabes Dorsalis

This late complication of syphilis involving the nervous system is a result of the infectious agent, the spirochete involving

Figure 8.23 This 23-year-old female had multiple neurofibromas/schwannomas. In this computerized tomography (CT) scan, a schwannoma at the lumbar level is demonstrated.

Figure 8.22 Schwannoma of nerve root at L2 level. Magnetic resonance imaging (MRI). This 53-year-old female had an 18-month history of progressive low back pain that began to radiate to the right foot with numbness of the lateral aspect of the right foot and numbness of left thigh. Examination demonstrated only decreased pain sensation of the left anterior thigh and lateral aspect of the right foot. An MRI of the lumbar spine demonstrated a circumscribed Schwannoma at the lumbar-2 level, subsequently removed by Dr. Alex Danylevich.

the posterior (dorsal) root and to some extent the dorsal root ganglion producing secondary degeneration in the posterior columns. The topic is discussed in greater detail in Chapter 9 on the spinal cord.

Disease of the Dorsal Root Ganglion

The major disease involving the dorsal root ganglia is infection by the herpes zoster/varicella virus. In actuality this is a reactivation of a virus remaining dormant in the dorsal root ganglion after previous varicella (chickenpox) infection. Diseases that alter the immune system such as infection, for example, HIV, or lymphomas may activate the virus and in some cases generalized zoster may occur. Ten to twenty-five percent of patients with generalized lymphoma will develop H. zoster. (This complication may be reduced by the prophylactic administration of the antiviral agent acyclovir.)

In addition, local irritation of a nerve root or a primary neoplastic process arising in organs closely related to the dermatome may activate the virus.

The clinical disorder begins with sharp lancinating pain in a radicular distribution. Within 3 or 4 days, the involved dermatome demonstrates a vesicular eruption. The thoracic dermatomes are most frequently involved. In approximately 20% of cases, cranial nerve root sensory ganglion are involved, most often cranial nerves 5 (primarily the ophthalmic division) and 7. Although the dorsal root ganglion is primarily involved, occasionally the anterior root or horns are involved, producing atrophy and weakness. Rarely, the spinal cord is involved, producing a clinical myelitis. The antiviral agent acyclovir is effective in reducing the duration of disease. *Postherpetic neuralgia* is the term applied to the persistent severe pain occurring in 20% of patients 1 month after the rash has healed. The occurrence of this chronic pain syndrome is more frequent in elderly patients: 75% of patients with H. zoster who are over the age of 70 years continue to have severe pain 1 month after healing of the cutaneous lesions. Treatment with lidocaine skin patches, the tricyclic antidepressant nortriptyline, the anticonvulsant gabapentin, or oral opioids may produce a moderate reduction in pain in some of these patients. A recent study has demonstrated the effect of intrathecal methylprednisolone in patients who were still refractory at 1 year (Kotani et al., 2000).

For additional review of varicella zoster infection.

The herpes simplex virus may also remain dormant in the sensory root ganglion and may be activated to produce radicular pain. With the type 2 virus (vaginalis), the sacral segments are often involved, and urinary retention may occur.

Complications of Lumbar Puncture and of the Intrathecal Administration of Medications

Although the lumbar puncture with access to the subarachnoid space is a very safe procedure, rare complications may occur under specific circumstances.

In patients with low platelet counts (<40,000 per cubic mm) hemorrhage may occur around the nerve roots of the cauda equina, producing paralysis of both lower extremities and of bladder function. In rare patients, persistent bleeding may occur from a lacerated subarachnoid vein.

The administration of materials into the subarachnoid space may result in the development of arachnoiditis. This is a process of inflammation about the nerve roots primarily of the cauda equine with radicular pain, weakness, sensory symptoms, and bladder symptoms. This was one of the complications of pantopaque myelography, which employed an oil-soluble dye which had to be removed at the end of the procedure. This procedure is no longer employed. In the treatment of certain lymphomas and leukemias, intrathecal administration of metrotrexamide or less often of ARA-C may be employed to reduce any incidence of central nervous system involvement by these disorders. Although not frequent, arachnoiditis is a possible complication.

BIBLIOGRAPHY

Suggested Readings

Adamsh, R. D., Victor, M., and Ropper, A. H. 1997. Principles of Neurology. 6th ed. New York, NY: McGraw Hill.

Asbury, A. K. 1992. Disorders of peripheral nerve. In A. K. Asbury, G. M. McKhann, and W. I. McDonald (Eds.) Diseases of the Nervous System: Clinical Neurobiology. 2nd ed., Vol. 1, pp.252–269. London, UK: Wm. Heinemann.

Bosch, E. P., and Smith, B. E. 2000. Disorders of peripheral nerves. In W. G. Bradley, R. B. Daroff, G. M. Fenichel, and C. D. Marsden (Eds.) Neurology in Clinical Practice. 3rd ed., pp. 2045–2130. Boston, MA: Butterworth Heinemann.

Chad, D. A. 2000. Disorders of nerve roots and plexuses. In W. G. Bradley, R. B. Daroff, G. M. Fenichel, and C. D. Marsden (Eds.) Neurology in Clinical Practice. 3rd ed., pp. 2019–2044. Boston, MA: Butterworth Heinemann.

Dawson, D. M., Hallet, M., and Millender, L. H. 1990. Entrapment neuropathies. 2nd ed. Boston, MA: Little, Brown and Co.

Dyck, P. J., Thomas, T. K., Griffin, J. W., et al. 1993. Peripheral Neuropathy. 3rd ed. Philadelphia, PA: W. B. Saunders.

Logigian, E. L. (Ed.). 1999. Entrapment and Other Focal Neuropathies. Neurol. Clin. 17:407–673.

Medical Research Council. 1943. Aids to the investigation of peripheral nerve injuries. 2nd ed. London, UK: Her Majesty's Stationary Office.

Mitchell, S. W. 1872. Injuries of Nerves and Their Consequences. Philadelphia, PA: Lippincott. Reprinted 1983, Birmingham, AL, The Classics of Neurology and Neurosurgery Library.

Rowland, L. P. (Ed.). 1989. Merritt's Textbook of Neurology. 8th ed. Philadelphia, PA: Lea & Febiger.

Specific Citations

Asbury, A. K. 1981. Diagnostic considerations in Guillain-Barré syndrome. Ann. Neurol. (Suppl.) 1–5.

Asbury, A. K. 1988. Understanding diabetic neuropathy. N. Engl. J. Med. 319:577–578.

Asbury, A. K., and Gibbs, C. J. 1990. Autoimmune neuropathies: Guillain-Barré syndrome. Ann. Neurol. (Suppl.) 27:S1–S79.

Arcasoy, S. M., and Jett, J. R. 1997. Superior pulmonary sulcus tumors and Pancoast syndrome. N. Engl. J. Med. 337:1370–1359.

Bolton, C. F., Young, G. B., and Zochodne, D. W. 1993. The neurological complications of sepsis. Ann. Neurol. 33:94–100.

Caputo, G. M., Cavanagh, P. R., Ulbrecht, J. S., et al. 1994. Current concepts—assessment and management of foot disease in patients with diabetes. N. Engl. J. Med. 331:854–860.

Clark, C. M., and Lee, D. A. 1995. Drug-therapy: prevention and treatment of the complications of diabetes mellitus. N. Engl. J. Med. 332:1210–1217.

Cornblatt, D. R., McArthur, J. C., Kennedy, G. E., et al. 1987. Inflammatory demyelinating peripheral neuropathies associated with human T-cell lymphocytic virus Type III infection. Ann. Neurol. 21:32–40.

Dalakas, M. C., and Engel, W. K. 1981. Chronic relapsing (dysimmune) polyneuropathy: pathogenesis and treatment. Ann. Neurol. 9:S134–S145.

Dawson, D. M. 1993. Entrapment neuropathies of the upper extremities. N. Engl. J. Med. 329:2013–2018.

Deyo, R. A., Diehl, A. K., and Rosenthal, M. 1986. How many days of bed rest for acute low back pain? N. Engl. J. Med. 315:1064–1070.

Downie, A. 1982. Peripheral nerve compression syndromes. In U. B. Matthews and G. H. Glaser (Ed.) Recent Advances in Neurology 3:47–66. Edinburgh, UK: Churchill Livingstone.

Dyck, P. J. 1982. Current concepts in neurology: the causes, classification and treatment of peripheral neuropathy. N. Engl. J. Med. 307:283–286.

Dyck, P. J. 1992. New understanding and treatment of diabetic neuropathy. N. Engl. J. Med. 326:1287–1288.

Dyck, P. J., Thomas, P. K., Asbury, A. K., et al. (Eds.). 1987. Diabetic Neuropathy. Philadelphia, PA: W. B. Saunders.

Dyck, P. J., Karnes, J. L., Daube, J., et al. 1985. Clinical neuropathological criteria for the diagnosis and staging of diabetic neuropathy. Brain. 108:861–880.

Dyck, P. J., Lais, A. G., Ohta, M., et al. 1975. Chronic inflammatory polyradiculoneuropathy. Proc. Mayo Clinic. 50:621–637.

Dyck, P. J., Oviatl, K. F., and Lambert, E. H. 1981. Intensive evaluation of referred unclassified neuropathies yields improved diagnosis. Ann. Neurol. 10:222–226.

Feasby, T. E. 1992. Inflammatory demyelinating polyneuropathies. Neurol. Clin. 10:651–670.

Frymoyer, J. W. 1988. Back pain and sciatica. N. Engl. J. Med. 318:291–300.

Giannini, C., and Dyck, P. J. 1995. Basement membrane reduplication and pericyte degeneration precede development of diabetic polyneuropathy and are associated with its severity. Ann. Neurol. 37:498–504.

Guillain-Barré Syndrome Study Group. 1985. Plasmapheresis and acute Guillain-Barré syndrome. Neurology 35:1096–1104.

Harding, A. E., and Thomas, P. K. 1980. The clinical features of hereditary motor and sensory neuropathy Types I and II. Brain 103:259–280.

Hay, J., and Arvin, A. M. (Ed.). 1994. Varicella zoster virus infection: new insights into pathogenesis and post herpetic neuralgia. Ann. Neurol. 35(Suppl.):S1–S72.

Hayes, M., and Hedley-Whyte, E. T. 1994. Case records of the Massachusetts General Hospital—A 77-year-old woman with fever, sweats, and pain in the head and legs. N. Engl. J. Med. 331:1293–1300.

Jackle, K. A., Young, D. F., Foley, K. M. 1985. The natural history of lumbosacral plexopathy in cancer. Neurology 35:8–15.

Kopell, H. P., and Thompson, W. A. L. 1960. Peripheral entrapment neuropathies of the lower extremities. N. Engl. J. Med. 262:56–60.

Kotani, N., Kushikata, T., Kimura, F., et al. 2000. Intrathecal methylprednisolone for intractable post herpetic neuralgia. N. Engl. J. Med. 343:1514–1519.

Kennedy, W. R., Navarro, X., Goetz, F. C., et al. 1993. Effects of pancreatic transplantation on diabetic neuropathy. N. Engl. J. Med. 322:1031–1038.

Kissel, J. T., and Mendell, J. R. 1992. Vasculitic neuropathy. Neurol. Clin. 10:761–781.

Kyle, R. A. 1992. Monoclonal proteins in neuropathy. Neurol. Clin. 10:713–734.

Leffert, R. D. 1972. Brachial plexus injuries. N. Engl. J. Med. 291:1059–1067.

McCombe, P. A., McLeod, J. G., and Pollard, T. D. 1987. Peripheral sensorimotor neuropathy associated with systemic lupus erythematosis. Brain 110:533–549.

McCombe, P. A., Pollard, T. D., and McLeod, J. G. 1987. Chronic inflammatory demyelinating polyneuropathy: a clinical and electrophysiological study of 92 cases. Brain 110:1617–1630.

McKhann, G. M., and Griffin, J. W. 1987. Plasamapheresis and the Guillain-Barré syndrome. Ann. Neurol. 22:762–763.

McLeod, J. G., Tuck, R. R., Pollard, J. D., et al. 1984. Chronic polneuropathy of undetermined cause. J. Neurol. Neurosurg. Psychiatry 47:530–535.

Miralles, G. D., O'Fallon, J. R., and Talley, N. J. 1992. Plasma- cell dyscrasia with poly neuropathy: the spectrum of POEMS syndrome. N. Engl. J. Med. 327:1919–1923.

Roa, B. B., Garcia, C. A., Suter, V., et al. 1993. Charcot-Marie-Tooth disease type IA: association with a spontaneous point mutation in the PMP22 gene. N. Engl. J. Med. 329:96–101.

Rogers, L. R., Borkowski, G. P., Albers, J. W., et al. 1993. Obturator mononeuropathy caused by pelvic cancer: six cases. Neurology 43:1489–1492.

Ropper, A. H. 1986. Severe acute Guillain Barré syndrome. Neurology 6:429–432.

Ropper, A. S. 1992. The Guillain Barré syndrome. N. Engl. J. Med. 326:1130–1136.

Rosenfeld, M. R., and Dalnava, J. 1993. Paraneoplastic syndromes and progressive motor dysfunction. Semin. Neurol. 13:281–298.

Simpson, D. M., and Olney, R. K. 1992. Peripheral neuropathies associated with human immunodeficiency virus infection. Neurol. Clin. 10:685–711.

Shy, M. E., Kamholz, J., and Lovelace, R. E. (Ed.). 1999. Charcot-Marie-Tooth disorders. Ann. NY Acad. Sci. 883:xiii–544.

So, Y. T., and Olney, R. K. 1994. Acute lumbosacral polyradiculopathy in acquired immunodeficiency syndrome: experiences in 23 patients. Ann. Neurol. 35:53–58.

Small, G. A., and Lovelace, R. E. 1993. Chronic inflammatory demyelinating polyneuropathy. Semin. Neurol. 13:305–312.

Spencer, P. S., Schaumberg, H., Raliegh, R. L., et al. 1975. Nervous system degeneration produced by the industrial solvent methyl-n-butyl ketone. Arch. Neurol. 32:219–222.

Sterman, A. B., Schaumburg, H. H., and Asbury, A. K. 1980. The acute sensory neuropathy syndrome: a distinct clinical entity. Trans. Am. Neurol. Assoc. 104:22–25.

Takigawa, T., Yasuda, H., Kikkawa, R., et al. 1995. Antibodies against GM1 ganglioside affect K+ and Na+ currents in isolated rat myelinated nerve fibers. Ann. Neurol. 37:436–442.

Vandermeche, F. G. A., Schmitz, P. I. M., and The Dutch Guillain-Barré Study Group. 1992. A randomized trial exchange in Guillain-Barré syndrome. N. Engl. J. Med. 326:1123–1129.

Waksman, B. H., and Adams, R. D. 1955. Allergic neuritis: an experimental disease of rabbits induced by injection of peripheral nerve and adjuvant. J. Exp. Med. 102:213–255.

Watkins, P. J. 1990. Diabetic autonomic neuropathy. N. Engl. J. Med. 322:1078–1079.

9.

SPINAL CORD

CLINICAL CONSIDERATIONS

Disease affecting the spinal cord is a frequent cause of chronic neurological disability. Often young adults are involved in injuries due to war, motor vehicle accidents, motorcycle accidents, and diving and skiing accidents. Special units have been developed for the care and rehabilitation of the unfortunate victims of these injuries. Early recognition and management of a potential spinal cord compromise are essential.

It is important to differentiate extrinsic (compressive) and intrinsic diseases of the spinal cord. Continued spinal cord compression will produce irreversible damage. For extrinsic diseases, surgical therapy is then indicated as early as possible. In general, extrinsic compressive lesions (Table 9.1) manifest a number of local segmental features at the level of the lesion as well as long tract findings below the level of the lesion.

ACUTE SPINAL CORD COMPRESSIONS OR TRANSECTIONS

THE PHENOMENA OF SPINAL SHOCK AND THE PATTERN OF REFLEX RECOVERY

After the acute and sudden loss of supra segmental control, a temporary depression of segmental reflex activities occurs. Deep tendon stretch reflexes are depressed. Cutaneous and autonomic reflexes may also be affected. The excitability of alpha and gamma motor neurons and of interneurons is depressed. This is more prominent in humans than in species such as the cat or dog related to the progressive encephalization of function that has occurred in the primates. In the frog, the duration is fleeting; in the cat, spinal shock lasts a matter of minutes or hours. In the monkey, duration is a matter of days or weeks. In humans, the duration is usually of several weeks. In the cat or dog, spinal shock follows damage to the vestibulospinal and ventral reticular spinal tracts. In primates, spinal shock depends more on damage to the corticospinal tracts. It is important to note that the depth and duration of spinal shock depends on the rapidity (acuity) and completeness of spinal cord section. Slowly evolving chronic spinal cord compressions are not characterized by spinal shock. Fever or infection will prolong the duration of spinal shock or may result in a recurrence of spinal shock once recovery has occurred.

Immediately after an acute transection, the patient will demonstrate a depression of all the deep tendon stretch reflexes and to a lesser degree the flexion reflexes. The limbs will be flaccid and paralyzed. The bladder will be flaccid, that is, hypotonic or atonic due to depression of the bladder stretch reflex.

Within a short period of time (1–5 weeks), the flexion reflexes, including the sign of Babinski, will recover and remain prepotent. The flexion reflex (the withdrawal of the foot and leg on painful stimulation) is a polysynaptic reflex. The afferent component of the reflex arc is mediated by group II and III myelinated fibers and group IV unmyelinated fibers, from a variety of receptors in skin, muscle, and joints. Initially in the human, the flexion reflex may be manifested as a *mass reflex*. When fully developed, this mass reflex may consist of generalized reflex flexor spasms of the muscles of the trunk and lower extremities accompanied by sweating, emptying of the bladder, and in males penile erection and ejaculation. Initially, the receptive field for triggering this response is quite extensive, involving any tactile or nociceptive stimulus to the foot, leg, abdomen, or thorax. With the passage of time, the mass reflex becomes less prominent and local sign develops. The more specific reflex movement then depends on the more specific location of the stimulus. For example, a painful stimulus to the outer border results in flexion, inversion, and adduction as opposed to a similar stimulus to the inner border of the foot that results in flexion, eversion, and abduction. The mass reflex may return if fever or infection occurs.

Over a number of weeks to months, depending on the completeness of transection (longer if complete), the monosynaptic stretch reflexes with other extensor reflexes and postures will return. The monosynaptic stretch reflex is a segmental reflex. The afferent component consists of heavily myelinated Ia fibers that originate in the stretch receptors of the muscle spindle. The efferent limb is composed of fibers from the alpha motor neuron of the anterior horn. The deep tendon stretch reflexes will then become hyperactive. There will be a spastic rather than a flaccid weakness. Bladder emptying and bowel evacuations return 3 to 4 weeks after injury. The bladder will subsequently become hypertonic, that is, spastic with small capacity. The extensor capabilities may consist of crossed extension (the contralateral lower limb extends when the ipsilateral lower limb is responding to a painful stimulus by flexion). Sweating below the level of transection may not return for 3–4 months. In the cat and dog, alternate flexion/extension, alternate stepping, and in high cervical preparations interlimb reflexes may occur (the upper limb movements are appropriately triggered by lower limb responses). With marked extensor tone, a partial capacity for brief periods of standing may return. Clearly

Table 9.1 CONSEQUENCES OF EXTRINSIC COMPRESSION OF SPINAL CORD

SYMPTOMS AND SIGNS	ANATOMICAL CORRELATION
1. Radicular pain at level of compression	Posterior root and ganglion
2. Radicular sensory symptoms at level of compression	Posterior root and/or posterior horn
3. Segmental atrophy, weakness, and fasciculations at level of compression	Segmental lower motor neuron findings due to involvement of the anterior horn cells and anterior roots.
4. Segmental depression of deep tendon stretch reflexes	Involvement of the anterior root and anterior horn or of posterior root and or horn. The monosynaptic reflex arc has been interrupted as regards its afferent or efferent component
5. Long tract findings below the level of the lesion	a. Spastic (UMN) weakness, increased deep tendon reflexes, and Babinski sign (extensor plantar response) due to damage to descending pyramidal tracts b. Spastic neurogenic bladder due to bilateral involvement of UMN control with release of the segmental bladder stretch reflexes c. Deficits in position, vibration, and other proprioceptive and light touch sensation due to posterior column damage d. Deficits in pain and temperature sensation due to lateral spinothalamic pathway damage

there is a phylogenetic factor; such extensor capabilities are more limited in the spinal human. In comparison the capabilities of the frog or chicken with a high cervical transection are well described in common terminology.

THE BROWN-SEQUARD HEMISECTION SYNDROME

Transactions of the lateral one-half of the spinal cord or lateral compressions of the spinal cord, for example, by tumors such as schwannomas, meningiomas, or metastases, will produce a classical syndrome which reflects the anatomy of the spinal cord and of the spinal cord pathways (Table 9.2). Ipsilateral corticospinal signs are combined with ipsilateral posterior column findings affecting vibration and position sensation (plus other proprioceptive sensation), with contralateral deficits in pain and temperature. *In general, unless the spinal cord has been hemisected by a knife, it is rare in clinical practice to have the pure classical picture. Instead, variations on the classical picture may be seen with lateral compressions, at times with bilateral findings, and so on.*

THE PROGRESSIVE SUBACUTE OR CHRONIC ANTERIOR MIDLINE COMPRESSION SYNDROME

The spinal cord is gradually compressed backwards against the bony canal elements. Based on the clinical and experimental studies of Tarlov, the following sequence is often noted.

Initially the bilateral symptoms and signs will be relevant to posterior columns followed by symptoms and signs of lateral column involvement and finally by symptoms and signs relevant to the lateral spinothalamic system. From a clinical standpoint, the initial symptoms may consist of a numbness of the lower extremities and a sensory ataxia. An ascending spastic weakness of the lower extremities will then develop followed by an ascending deficit in pain and temperature sensation. Such a pain and temperature deficit will initially involve the sacral segments, then lumbar segments, followed by the thoracic segments, and finally the lower cervical segments. This sequence reflects the lamination pattern of the lateral spinal thalamic system in which sacral segments are most extrinsic and cervical segments most intrinsic. As a general rule then, extrinsic lesions do not have sacral sparing. The earlier involvement of posterior and lateral columns may reflect the sequence of structural compression or the greater vulnerability of the heavily myelinated fibers. *It is important then to realize that the apparent upper level of sensory level for pain and*

Table 9.2 CLINICAL SIGNS IN BROWN-SEQUARD SYNDROME

DEFICIT	CAUSE OF CLINICAL DEFICIT
A spastic weakness below and ipsilateral to the side of transection/damage	Injury to the lateral column/cortical spinal system
Deep tendon reflexes increased below and ipsilateral to the side of transection/damage	Injury to lateral column/cortical spinal system
The sign of Babinski will also be present ipsilateral to the side of transection/damage	Injury to pyramidal tract in the lateral column
Ipsilateral loss of vibration, position sense, and all other proprioceptive sensory modalities below the level of transection/compression	Injury to posterior column
A contralateral loss of pain and temperature sensation present beginning one or two segments below the level of the transection/compression	Involvement of the lateral spinothalamic tract
An ipsilateral band of weakness atrophy and fasciculations may be present at the level of transection	Damage to the anterior root and or the anterior horn
Ipsilateral depression of deep tendon stretch reflexes at the level of transection/compression	Damage to the afferent or efferent components involved in the monosynaptic stretch reflex arc

temperature may not be the actual level of compression. When the patient is seen early in the course of spinal cord compression, the apparent level of sensory deficit will be considerably lower than the actual level of compression. It is important to recognize that slowly evolving extrinsic lesions (such as intradural meningiomas and neurofibromas) despite considerable distortion of spinal cord may produce only minimal symptoms and have a good response to surgical therapy. In contrast, rapidly evolving lesions such as metastatic epidural tumors, more often present a relatively acute or subacute course and often have a poor response to therapy. At times such metastatic lesions are complicated by vascular compromise or compression by involved vertebrae.

SPECIFIC EXTRINSIC LESIONS OF THE SPINAL CORD

FRACTURE DISLOCATIONS

In civilian life, most injuries to the cord do not represent actual lacerations of the spinal cord but are a result of crush injuries caused by fracture dislocations in the cervical or thoracic area (Fig. 9.1). Vascular effects often complicate such crush injuries. Infarction (related to compression of anterior spinal artery and of veins) and hemorrhage may occur often in a central cord location (the latter is referred to as hematomyelia). After resorption of a hemorrhage, a cystic cavity may remain. Falls transmit force to the thoracic vertebrae; the resulting compression fractures may collapse the vertebrae and caused a sharp angulation of the axis of bony support. A similar compression and collapse may also occur from other nontraumatic causes such a tuberculosis of the spine (Pott's disease),
metastatic carcinoma, and osteoporosis. Injuries to the cervical spine resulting from fracture dislocation are common in auto accidents and in diving accidents. In rheumatoid arthritis, the odontoid is commonly fractured and dislocated. It is important to note that fractures of the vertebrae may occur without a marked degree of dislocation. In such cases great care must be taken in moving these patients. Thus, in fractures of the cervical spine, the patient should remain supine with the neck immobilized to avoid flexion and extension during transportation. (Utilize a makeshift collar or sandbags.) Once the patient arrives at a treatment center, additional measures such as traction or spinal fusion must be considered so that no compromise of the spinal cord occurs. The use of very high-dosage corticosteroids may have some value in reducing the edema of the spinal cord.

CERVICAL DISK DISEASE

This is probably the most common cause of cervical spinal cord compression. Acute lateral or midline rupture of disk material may occur in the cervical area related to trauma or sudden coughing or straining. The term *cervical spondylosis* refers to a more chronic process. The disk degenerates with increasing age, the disk material then begins to bulge, the disk space narrows, and the secondary formation of osteophytes (bony spurs) occurs. The osteophytes may project laterally into the neural foramina, producing spurs. The osteophytes may project laterally into the neural foramina, producing nerve root compression and/or may be located in a midline location, producing spinal cord compression (Fig. 8.19). Not all bulging disks and osteophytes compress the spinal cord. In some patients, the vertebral canal is sufficiently wide so that

Figure 9.1 Traumatic lesions of the spinal cord. (*A*) Fracture dislocation of thoracic vertebra has crushed and almost transected the thoracic spinal cord. (*B*) A fracture dislocation of the cervical spine (due to an auto accident 2 weeks prior to death) has produced an almost complete transection of the spinal cord at the C7 level. (From Blackwood, W., Dodds, T.C., and Somerville, J.C.: Atlas of Neuropathology, 2nd Edition, Baltimore, Williams and Wilkins, 1964, p. 147.)

Figure 9.2 Ascending and descending degeneration: cervical spondylosis with spinal cord compression myelin stains. Upper cervical spinal cord above level of compression: ascending degeneration predominantly in posterior columns.

no compromise of the spinal cord occurs. In other patients the bony canal is relatively narrow (spinal stenosis) and compromise occurs. The pattern of ascending and descending degeneration found at autopsy following cervical spinal cord compression in a patient with cervical spondylosis is demonstrated in Figure 9.2 from a case in which a 64-year-old male had a 6-year history of progressive spastic paraparesis with atrophy and fasciculations of C4-C8 supplied muscles, bilateral corticospinal and posterior column findings in the lower extremities, and a deficit in pain sensation below the T10 level. Softening of the spinal cord was present at the C7 level.

The following case illustrates a relatively acute syndrome of spinal cord compression secondary to rupture of the cervical disk.

CASE HISTORY 9.1

This 34-year-old female after 2 weeks of prolonged hyperextension of her neck while painting walls and ceilings developed a transient 6-hour period of weakness in both her legs. She then developed pain in the right side of her neck, her right shoulder and right upper arm, followed by weakness in the right leg. Shortly thereafter she noted intermittent prickly sensations (paresthesias) in both lower extremities and she was unable to walk.

Neurologic Exam

Mental status and cranial nerves: Intact.

Motor: Weakness was present in the right upper extremity most prominent at the triceps and wrist extensors (4/5) with a lesser degree of weakness at deltoid, pectorals, wrist flexors, and finger abductors plus a minor degree of weakness at right ankle dorsiflexion (4.5/5). Gait was ataxic.

Reflexes: Bilateral ankle clonus was present with bilateral Babinski signs.

Sensation: Vibratory sensation was decreased in the right lower extremity at toes ankle and knee with associated proprioceptive deficits. Pain sensation was decreased in the left lower extremity from the toes to the groin. The entire buttock and the perianal area were also involved in this deficit.

Clinical diagnosis: Partial Brown-Sequard syndrome due to acute ruptured cervical disk involving the right side of cervical cord.

Laboratory data: *Computerized tomography (CT) myelogram* demonstrated a probable extruded disk at the C5-C6 level to the right of the midline displacing the spinal cord posteriorly and to the left (Fig. 9.3).

Cerebral spinal fluid protein was significantly elevated to 141mg % (normal is less than 45mg %), consistent with a spinal cord cerebrospinal fluid (CSF) block.

Subsequent course: She was unwilling to have a magnetic resonance image (MRI) or any neurosurgical procedure undertaken to remove the disk. With the use of a cervical collar, she had rapid resolution of her symptoms and continued to do well over the next 8 years.

The MRI scan remains the study of choice in patients with cervical spine pathology as demonstrated in Figure 9.4 in the case of the following patient.

This 31-year-old male jumped off a truck carrying an 80-pound bag on his shoulder. The following morning, he awoke with severe pain throughout the spine on coughing, and intermittent tingling of both hands for approximately 4 months. Nine months later, he still had an equivocal plantar response and the MRI demonstrated a ruptured disk at the C5-6 interspace.

Metastatic carcinoma: Metastatic malignancy may involve the vertebrae without producing spinal cord or nerve root compression. However, continued growth of the tumor or vertebral collapse may lead to spinal cord compression. The tumor may spread to the epidural space from the vertebral involvement, producing spinal cord compression. Vertebral collapse may also produce spinal cord compression from bony elements of the vertebrae. A metastatic tumor may also appear in the epidural space without direct involvement of the vertebrae. In such cases, tumor within the thoracic or abdominal cavity may have spread through the neural foramina directly or through the lymphatics into the epidural space. Lymphomas in the thoracic or abdominal cavity in a paravertebral location often spread in this manner. Spread

Figure 9.3 Cervical disk rupture: Brown-Sequard syndrome, case history 9.1: computerized tomography (CT) scan of cervical cord post metrizamide myelography.

Figure 9.4 Acute rupture of cervical disk midline and right lateral at C5-C6. (*A*) Magnetic resonance imaging (MRI) T1-weighted sagittal section of cervical spinal cord slightly to right of midline demonstrating a ruptured intervertebral disk at C5-C6 interspace. (*B*) Transverse sections at C5-C6 interspace. Cross-section at approximately C5, C6 demonstrating an extra dural mass to the right of the midline displacing the spinal cord posteriorly and to the left.

of metastatic tumor may also occur via the venous plexus or via other hematogenous routes. The majority of metastatic tumors involve the thoracic and lumbar areas. The majority of cases originate from primary disease in the lung, breast, prostate, and kidney. Based on the autopsy studies of Barron in 1959, 5% of all systemic cancers will eventually develop spinal epidural spread. A significant proportion of patents presenting with epidural spinal cord compression secondary to metastatic disease may not have been previously known to have a malignancy. In a series collected by Stark et al. (1982) from a large general hospital (The London Hospital), 47% of the patients were in this category; 14% of patients never had the primary location determined.

The following case demonstrates the consequences of metastatic carcinoma producing spinal cord compression.

CASE HISTORY 9.2

This 55-year-old white housewife first noted pain in the thoracic-right scapular area, 5 months prior to admission. Three months prior to admission, a progressive weakness in both lower extremities developed, resulting in a bed-ridden state in which she was unable to move her legs or even to wiggle her toe. She had also noted a progressive pins-and-needles sensation involving both lower extremities. At the same time she developed difficulty with the control of bowel movements and urination. At age 40, 15 years prior to this admission, she had undergone a left radical mastectomy for an infiltrating carcinoma of the breast with regional lymph node involvement.

Neurological Examination

Mental status and cranial nerves: Intact.

Motor system: A marked flaccid weakness was present in both lower extremities with retention of only a flicker of flexion at the left hip.

Reflexes: Plantar responses were extensor bilaterally (bilateral sign of Babinski).

Sensory system: Position sense was absent at toes, ankles, and knees and impaired at the hip bilaterally. Vibratory sensation was absent below the iliac crests bilaterally.

Pain sensation was absent from the toes through the T6-T7-dermatome with no evidence of sacral sparing. Tenderness to percussion was present over the midthoracic vertebrae (T4 and T5 spinous processes).

Clinical diagnosis: Spinal cord compression at T4-T5 vertebral level most likely secondary to metastatic epidural tumor.

Laboratory data:

X-ray studies: The patient had multiple metastatic lesions in lungs, T4, T5 vertebrae, and head of femur.

Emergency myelogram: a complete block to the flow of contrast agent at the T5 level due to an extradural lesion displacing the spinal cord to the left was demonstrated.

Subsequent course: An emergency thoracic T3-T4 laminectomy demonstrated adenocarcinoma, presumably metastatic from breast in the vertebral processes, laminae and epidural space. Following removal of the tumor and subsequent radiotherapy, movement had returned to the lower extremities to a moderate degree.

Comments

In this case, a myelogram was performed. At this time the most appropriate diagnostic procedure would be an MRI scan. However, in circumstances where that study cannot be performed on an emergency basis, then an emergency myelogram or myelogram CT is appropriate. The presence of persistent mid thoracic-scapular back pain in a patient with a past history of breast malignancy should always prompts a search for metastatic lesions in the vertebrae. In any case the earliest development of motor or sensory symptoms in a patient with a history of malignancy should lead to a prompt neurological evaluation and investigation. (The present standard of investigation would include appropriate MRI study of the spine, which has the advantage of allowing studies not only of the specific area of compression but also of the spinal cord above and below the area of compression. Thus, other epidural lesions may be identified.) The best treatment of metastatic spinal cord compression is a high index of suspicion and early recognition to prevent the result seen in this case.

Note the presence of a severe flaccid paralysis of the lower extremities with a dense sensory level implies a poor prognosis for recovery.

Acute epidural abscess: The dura mater of the spinal cord is separated from the periosteum of the surrounding bony canal by a narrow space containing fatty tissue, the epidural space. This space may be infected by an infection in adjacent tissues, for example, skin (furuncles) or bone (osteomyelitis) involving the vertebrae. Alternatively, hematogenous spread of infection from distant sources may occur. The usual organism is staphylococcus aureus. The usual site is midthoracic. The epidural abscess is rare compared to meningitis and brain abscess. Nevertheless, early recognition is necessary. Prompt drainage, decompressive laminectomy, and antibiotic therapy are essential to avoid the poor prognosis of continued spinal cord compression.

The early symptoms of severe back pain and fever are followed by radicular pain or weakness and the acute or subacute development of the signs of spinal cord compression. Approximately half the cases evolve over a period of greater than 2 weeks. The latter cases are usually secondary to vertebral osteomyelitis. If treatment is delayed, functional transaction of the spinal cord is the usual outcome related both to the direct effects of compression and the indirect effect of compression of the blood supply and the involvement of the blood vessel walls by the infectious process. The diagnosis is established by the appropriate clinical history, MRI study demonstrating blockage of the subarchnoid space by an epidural mass, and subsequent aspiration of pus from the epidural space.

Tuberculous involvement of the vertebrae with secondary spinal cord compression: Tuberculosis was once a common disease in urban centers of the United States and Europe. In other parts of the world, for example, India, tuberculosis remains a common disease. Tuberculous involvement of joints, tuberculous arthritis, is a complication of untreated tuberculosis in children. A very common site of involvement is the dorsal spine. The process often appears to begin in the disk space and then involves the adjacent vertebrae. The disease process, tuberculous spondylitis (Pott's disease), results in destruction of the body of the vertebrae and of the intervertebral disk. Collapse of the vertebrae and severe angulation of the bony canal occurs. In addition, the chronic infection may spread into the epidural space as a local mass of infection or may accumulate as a mass under the ligament posterior to the vertebral bodies. All of these factors may contribute to spinal cord compression.

Diagnosis can now be established by MRI scan. Treatment consists of drainage of any mass pockets of infection compressing the spinal cord, antituberculous chemotherapy, immobilization, and possibly fusion of the spine.

INTRADURAL-EXTRAMEDULLARY SPINAL CORD TUMORS (MENINGIOMAS AND SCHWANNOMAS)

In many earlier operative series this category of extrinsic tumor internal to the dura but external to the substance of the spinal cord, accounted for the largest percentage of spinal cord tumors. Such series accumulated prior to the advent of the MRI tended to underestimate epidural metastatic tumors because such patients were usually not admitted to specialized neurological-neurosurgical units. For example, among 567 cases of spinal cord tumors collected from the literature by Merritt, in 1967, 59% were intradural extramedullary, 25% were extradural, and 11% were intramedullary. The extradural tumors have already been considered in relationship to metastatic spread of carcinoma and lymphoma.

The intramedullary tumors (essentially gliomas) will be considered later when intrinsic lesions are discussed: astrocytomas and ependymomas.

Essentially, two types of tumor constitute in a relatively equal proportion all of the intradural lesions: meningiomas and schwannomas (neuromas or neurofibromas). Both types are benign in the sense that they are not locally invasive and do not spread to distant sites.

Meningiomas

These tumors arise from the arachnoidal cell clusters. Since the more common location is the cerebral hemisphere, a more complete discussion of histologic types will be found in a later chapter. The typical gross appearance of this tumor in relation to the spinal cord is shown in Figure 9.5.

These tumors occur most frequently in middle-aged females (many meningiomas have estrogen receptors and to a lesser degree progesterone receptors). The ratio of female to male at the spinal cord level is 8:1. (Among cerebral meningiomas, the ratio is closer to 2:1.) The most frequent location

Figure 9.5 Gross appearance of meningioma compressing the ventrolateral aspect of thoracic spinal cord. (From Russell, D.S., and Rubinstein, L.J.: Pathology of Tumors of the Nervous System, 2nd Edition. Baltimore, Williams and Wilkins, 1963, p. 45.)

is the thoracic portion of the spinal cord, in part, because the thoracic segments constitute the longest extent of the spinal cord. Other areas, however, are not immune. In the upper cervical area these tumors may arise in relation to the foramen magnum, producing both lower brain stem and upper cervical cord symptoms.

The symptomatology of a typical meningioma arising in the thoracic spinal cord area might include thoracic back pain that radiated around to the interior chest in coughing and straining at stool. Ascending sensory upper motor neurological symptoms in the lower extremities might evolve slowly over 6 to 12 months. Examination might demonstrate the findings of the bilateral transverse or Brown-Sequard hemisection discussed earlier. In addition, local tenderness would be present over the spinous processes at the level of involvement.

Note that local tenderness over the spinous processes is common in extradural and intradural extramedullary tumors. MRI scan (or CT-myelogram if MRI is not available) would reveal an intradural extramedullary tumor with partial or complete block to the flow of CSF. CSF protein would be increased. These tumors require early neurosurgical intervention to avoid progression to a chronic paraplegic state. With the slow growth of the tumor, the capacity for recovery of function despite considerable distortion of the spinal cord is usually quite surprising once the compression has been relieved.

Schwannomas

These benign tumors arise from the cells of the nerve sheath. These tumors, as noted earlier, may arise in relationship to peripheral nerve, cranial nerves, or nerve root. As discussed earlier, those that arise in relation to nerve root within the bony canal may compress nerve root and/or the spinal cord depending on location and size of the tumor. The symptoms and signs may be very similar to those of a meningioma. Because these tumors arise from the nerve root, radicular pain is often more common than in meningiomas.

The use of MRI to image schwannomas is demonstrated in Figure 9.6. The clinical summary is as follows:

> This 43-year-old male had several months of pain in the cervical area that radiated into the anterior chest on coughing plus tingling from this area to the sacral area on sneezing. He had a marked decrease in all deep tendon reflexes in the right upper extremity. and percussion tenderness over the C6-7 spinous processes. All symptoms resolve following removal of the tumor. Note that the tumors may attain considerable size and produce only minimal spinal cord symptoms. As with all spinal cord lesions, the preferred neuroimaging technique is the MRI scan.

The following case history demonstrates in greater detail the course of a schwannoma compressing spinal cord.

Figure 9.6 Schwannoma with compression of spinal cord. Magnetic resonance imaging (MRI) with contrast enhancement. (*A*) Sagittal section-midline. (*B*) Coronal section between posterior arches and dorsal surface of spinal cord. (*C*) Transverse section-T1-vertebral level.

CASE HISTORY 9.3

This 65-year-old, right-handed female first noted weakness in her legs and pain in the lower thoracic spine 18 months prior to admission. Coughing would cause the pain to radiate around into the left flank and left lower quadrant. Two months prior to admission, she developed numbness, "diminished feeling to the skin," which began in the toes and now extended to the waist. Weakness had also progressed. For the last week the patient had difficulty in urination, unable to completely empty her bladder.

Neurological Examination
Mental status: Intact.
Cranial nerves: Intact.
Motor system: Mild weakness was present in both legs distal more prominent than proximal.
Reflexes: The patellar and Achilles deep tendon stretch reflexes were increased bilaterally. The plantar responses were equivocal bilaterally.
Sensory system:

a. Pain and touch sensation was decreased bilaterally from the L1 dermatome down to the toes without sacral sparing and with more marked involvement on the left.
b. Position sense was decreased bilaterally at toes but somewhat more markedly on the right. Vibratory sensation was decreased bilaterally below L1-D12.

Spine: Percussion over the D10 spinous process produced pain radiating around into the left lower quadrant and inguinal area. Coughing produced a similar phenomena.
Clinical diagnosis: Extrinsic probable intradural tumor compressing spinal cord at the D (T)-10 vertebral level, possibly a schwannoma.
Laboratory data: Neuroimaging studies demonstrated an intradural extramedullary tumor arising from the left D11 nerve root and compressing the spinal cord.
Subsequent course: Resection of the tumor, a schwannoma, by the neurosurgeon, Dr. Michael Scott, produced a significant resolution of symptoms.
Comments

The progressive 18-month course of motor and sensory findings in the lower extremities extending to the waist all suggested a benign intradural extramedullary tumor. The possibility of a tumor arising from the D (T) 10, 11 nerve root was suggested by the history and findings of coughing reducing pain radiating in to the left lower quadrant of the abdomen. In addition, the examination demonstrated clear-cut tenderness and reproduction of symptoms by percussion over the T10 vertebral spinous process.

Neurofibromatosis Type I (von Recklinghausen's disease): This is an autosomal dominant inherited disease characterized by multiple peripheral neurofibromas (tumors composed of Schwann cells, collagen, and reticulin fibers). There are also various anomalies of the skin (multiple >6 café au lait spots and cutaneous neurofibromas), iris (Lisch nodules-pigmented hamartomas), and skeletal system. Large plexiform neurofibromas may produce marked facial deformities. Patients may also manifest meningiomas or intrinsic gliomas involving the optic nerve, brain, or spinal cord, but such central lesions are less common than in type II neurofibromatosis considered next. This form of neurofibromatosis is also referred to as peripheral neurofibromatosis; and occurs once in 3000 live births. The mutated NF1gene has been localized to chromosome 17q. The CT scan and MRI appearance of schwannomas involving nerve roots has been presented in Chapter 8.

Neurofibromatosis Type II: This type also known as central neurofibromatosis is also an autosomal dominant but is rare compared to neurofibromatosis type 1 occurring 1 in 50,000 births. The mutated NF2 gene has been localized to chromosome 22. In contrast to type 1, peripheral manifestations are uncommon. Skin and bone lesions do not occur. Instead, the patients have multiple types of tumors of the central nervous system. Most patients eventually develop bilateral vestibular schwannomas. (This problem will be discussed in greater detail in the brain stem chapter.)

INTRINSIC DISORDERS OF THE SPINAL CORD

Three general categories of intrinsic disease must be distinguished:

1. Local disease affecting one or more adjacent segments:

    a. Infarcts produced by occlusion of the anterior spinal artery

    b. Transverse myelitis

    c. Intramedullary spinal cord tumors: gliomas (astrocytomas and ependymomas)

    d. Syringomyelia

2. System diseases affecting one or more neuronal or fiber systems:

    a. Motor neuron disease

    b. Tabes dorsalis (a form of tertiary neurosyphilis)

    c. Combined system disease (a result of vitamin B12 deficiency)

    d. Spinal cerebellar degeneration (usually familial or paraneoplastic or alcohol related)

3. Multifocal disorders: various levels of the nervous system are affected. At any given level, a specific lesion is not restricted to a specific neuronal or fiber system:

    a. Multiple sclerosis

    b. Other demyelinating disorders

    c. Collagen vascular disease, lupus erythematosus, and vasculitis

SPECIFIC INTRINSIC SYNDROMES: LOCAL DISORDERS

VASCULAR DISEASE: ANTERIOR SPINAL ARTERY OCCLUSION

Primary vascular disease affecting the spinal cord is not common, although a secondary vascular component may be present in many of the spinal cord compression syndromes discussed earlier. Any understanding of the clinical syndrome found in vascular disease of the spinal cord is dependent on knowledge of the anatomy of the arterial supply of the spinal cord (Fig. 9.7). The major artery of the spinal cord is the anterior spinal artery that is located in a midline position at the anterior median fissure. This single thin midline vessel has a bilateral origin from the intracranial portions of each vertebral artery. The arterial flow as this vessel descends is dependent on additional supply from the radicular arteries. These radicular arteries are derived from the cervical portion of the vertebral artery, particularly at C3 and C5 levels and the inferior thyroid artery at the C6 level. Additional radicular arteries originate from the aorta as the intercostal thoracic lumbar and sacral arteries. Most of the radicular arteries of the thoracic area do not contribute a significant supply. However, the middle thoracic artery usually at T7 and the artery of the lumbar enlargement, (the artery of Adamkiewicz), which usually arises between T10 and L2, are of particular importance. There are then border zones of blood supply in the rostral-caudal axis between the cervical and lumbar segments of major supply. The actual border zones of circulation are at segments T4 and L1. When the transverse anatomy is considered, the following arterial supply exists:

1. *Anterior spinal artery.* This midline vessel supplies the anterior and lateral columns and almost all of the gray matter except for the posterior horns.

2. *Posterior spinal arteries.* These paired vessels supply the posterior horns and the posterior columns. Each is derived from the intracranial segment of a vertebral artery. These posterior spinal arteries also receive contributions from the posterior branches of the radicular arteries.

3. *Anastomotic vessels.* At each level, coronal arteries at the periphery of the spinal cord connect the anterior spinal artery and the posterior spinal arteries. These anastomotic vessels at the periphery also serve to interconnect the blood supply of adjacent segments. A transverse border zone or watershed must also exist in the central gray matter where penetrating branches of the anterior spinal artery meet the penetrating branches of the posterior spinal artery. Since the largest area of the spinal cord is supplied by a single anterior spinal artery, it is not surprising that most vascular disease involving the spinal cord presents as the syndrome of the anterior spinal artery, that is, infarction of the territory supplied by this vessel (Fig. 9.8). In the case illustrated, a 71-year-old male had the acute onset of a flaccid paraplegia with an absence of deep tendon reflexes in the lower extremities and a pain sensory level at T7-T8. No recovery occurred.

Actual primary occlusion of this vessel is rare. The usual cause of the syndrome relates to diseases of the aorta or to surgical procedures involving the heart, aorta, or related vessels. Clamping of the upper aorta for the surgical treatment of an aneurysm of the aorta may result in a decrease in blood flow in the critical intercostal branches supplying the spinal

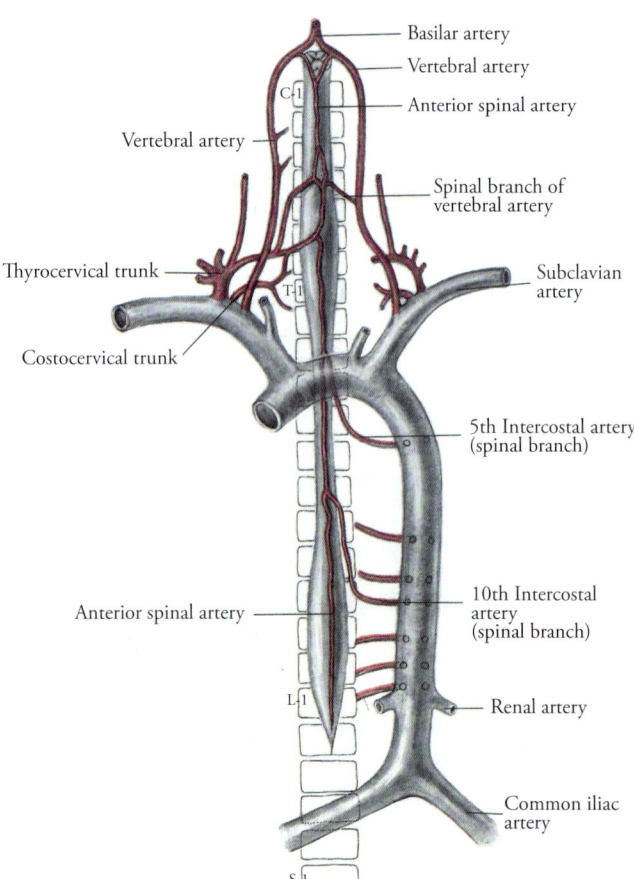

Figure 9.7 Vascular anatomy of the spinal cord. Anterior spinal artery: the major radicular (segmental) blood supply is diagrammed. (From Clemente, C., Gray's Anatomy, 30th Ed, Philadelphia, Lea and Febiger, 1988.)

Figure 9.8 Infarction of spinal cord in distribution of anterior spinal artery secondary to occlusion of radicular artery at T6. (Courtesy of Dr. Jose Segarra.)

cord. A dissecting aneurysm of the aorta (a tear within the wall of the vessel with blood under high pressure dissecting down the media of the wall of the blood vessel) often results in the occlusion of intercostal and other vessels arising from the aorta. Other arteries arising from the arch of aorta such as vertebral and carotids may also be occluded depending on the site of the dissection. In other instances, the occlusion of intercostal branches, particularly at T10, may occur during surgical procedures on the kidney or lumbar sympathetic ganglia. The resultant neurological syndrome is manifested by the acute onset of a paraplegia which is usually flaccid due to spinal shock and a bilateral deficit in pain and temperature below the level of lesion *with preservation of vibratory and position sense*. If the area of infarction involves the lumbar sacral area, the anterior horn cells will also be destroyed. The legs will then remain flaccid, muscle atrophy will develop, deep tendon stretch reflexes will never recover, and spasticity will never develop. The prognosis then for a significant degree of recovery is usually poor. Theoretically, if the thoracic spinal cord were infarcted, with preservation of the lumbar and sacral segments, deep tendon reflexes could recover and spasticity without atrophy in the lower extremities could develop after several days.

In distinguishing other acute processes producing paraplegia, the rapidity of onset and the anatomical pattern of infarction seen in occlusion of the anterior spinal artery should be considered. Other processes such as trauma or hemorrhage into the spinal cord (*hematomyelia*) from rupture of a malformed blood vessel (*as in an arteriovenous malformation*) may produce an acute syndrome. The history and findings as well as the MRI scan and the CSF examination would be distinguishing factors. Spinal arteriovenous malformations may also produce a progressive syndrome with episodes of acute exacerbation related to infarction and hemorrhage, but the anatomical pattern will differ from the acute anterior spinal artery syndrome. Multiple sclerosis may also produce a subacute or occasionally a relatively acute sputtering onset of symptoms, but the anatomical pattern will differ and lesions will usually be present elsewhere in the nervous system. Acute transverse myelitis to be discussed subsequently and the spinal cord compressions discussed earlier do not produce the anatomical pattern of the anterior spinal artery syndrome.

THE SYNDROME OF ACUTE OR SUBACUTE TRANSVERSE MYELITIS

When all other causes of an acute or subacute myelopathy have been excluded, there remain a group of patients without evidence of an extrinsic compressive or intrinsic vascular lesion. Usually the upper or mid thoracic spinal cord is involved. In the 1978 series of Ropper and Poskanzer (in which all patients had myelography, since this was prior to the modern era of neuroimaging), 138 patients presented from 1955 to 1975 with an acute myelopathy or myelitis. *In this overall group, 82 (59%) had an anatomical mass lesion, usually an epidural metastatic tumor; four (3%) had a dissecting aortic aneurysm and presumably an anterior spinal artery syndrome; and 52 (38%) remained in the transverse myelitis category.*

Of the 52 patients in this residual transverse myelitis category, 33% had a prior viral illness and presumably could have had a postinfectious myelitis. Six percent had cancer of the lung, ovary, or prostate but without spinal cord compression and presumably had a remote effect of malignancy. Thirteen percent of patients eventually developed multiple sclerosis with the transverse myelitis as the presenting syndrome.

The remaining 48% of this group of 52 patients had no specific possible etiology and could be labeled as idiopathic. (The more recent studies of Jacob and Weinshenker [2008] have suggested other etiologic factors to be excluded from this idiopathic group: prior vaccinations, infections such as herpes zoster and herpes simplex, and inflammatory conditions such as lupus erythematosus, vasculitis, and neurosarcoidosis. In addition, the demyelination group has been broadened to include not only multiple sclerosis but also the entity of neuromyelitis optica (NMO). (This will be discussed later in the chapter.)

In 21% of these patients with transverse myelitis, the appearance of symptoms was acute with mid thoracic back pain, weakness of legs, sensory deficit below the level of lesion, and urinary retention evolving over less than 1 to 12 hours. In 69% of patients the symptoms progressed in an ascending manner over 14 days and then stabilized with the findings of a spastic paralysis and spastic bladder. In 10% of patients, the course was a stuttering progression over 10–28 days. The progressive patients had a better prognosis than those with the acute onset. In the era prior to MRI scans, myelograms were usually normal but occasional patients were found to have mild swelling of the spinal cord. In cases of transverse myelitis, pathological examination of the spinal cord reveals an acute or subacute necrotic process involving a number of segments. In other cases, areas of demyelination are present. The MRI is able in most cases to image these pathologic changes. In mild cases or early in the evolution of the disease, the MRI may be normal.

The following case illustrates the diagnostic dilemma provided by such cases of transverse myelitis.

CASE HISTORY 9.4: PATIENT OF DR. THOMAS MULLINS AND DR. BERNARD STONE

This previously healthy 42-year-old white female awoke 3 days prior to admission with sudden onset of a dull aching midthoracic back pain and tingling of her lower extremities. Over the next 12 hours her T6–T8 back pain became severe and she developed mild weakness of the lower extremities and urinary retention. An emergency myelogram revealed a widened spinal cord at T8. Over the next 24-hour period back pain decreased in intensity, and sensation and strength improved, but she continued to have urinary retention. At that time bilateral Babinski signs were found. She was treated with high-dosage corticosteroids (dexamethasone). The patient had experienced two previous episodes of back pain in the T6–T8 distribution but without any neurological symptoms.

Neurological Examination
Mental status: Intact.
Cranial nerves: Intact.

Figure 9.9 Transverse myelitis: (A) Case 9.4, magnetic resonance imaging (MRI) T1-weighted. This 42-year-old female had the sudden onset of back pain at T6-8, followed by tingling and weakness in the lower extremities plus urinary retention evolving over 12 hours and then improving. (B) This 54-year-old female with a prior history of non-Hodgkin's lymphoma developed a progressive quadriparesis over 6 days, and then rapidly improved, possibly related to treatment with high-dosage corticosteroids.

The following abnormal findings were present:
Motor system:

a. Strength in hip flexion and extension was moderately weak bilaterally (4/5).
b. Gait was ataxic with occasional side steps; she was unable to perform tandem gait.

Reflexes: Patellar deep tendon stretch reflexes were hyperactive bilaterally, but plantar responses were now flexor.

Sensory system:

a. There was decreased sensation for pinprick in the S-3 distribution.
b. There was asymmetric loss of vibration sense in both lower extremities, more so on the right than left.

Clinical diagnosis: Transverse myelitis, etiology uncertain.
Laboratory Data

a. *Myelogram-CT scan of the dorsal spine* indicated a widened spinal cord at the T7 level.
b. *MRI scan of the spine* confirmed the enlargement of the spinal cord at T7-T8 (Fig. 9.9A).
c. *CSF*: protein was elevated to 55 mg%; no significant cells were present.
d. *Spinal angiography with catheterization of T6 through T11 radicular arteries on left and right* revealed no vascular malformation.

Subsequent course: Significant improvement occurred. Neurological examination, 2 months after onset of symptoms, indicated only bilateral Babinski signs and decreased pinprick over the right perineum. Repeat CT/myelography at that time indicated widening of the spinal cord at T7-8 with a possible small cavity at the T6 level. Repeat MRI scan 7 months after onset of symptoms demonstrated considerable resolution of the thoracic lesion. Neurological follow-up after 7 years detected no additional symptoms or signs.

Comments

In the era before MRI and spinal CT/myelography, this patient would have been placed in the general category of transverse myelitis. How many cases of transverse myelitis reported in that era would have that general diagnosis today is unclear. In this case, initially, a possible hemorrhage or hemorrhagic component was suspected but was never confirmed, in terms of CSF studies, and no malformation was identified. Nevertheless, the previous episodes of back pain in the same thoracic area might raise the question of a very minor vascular malformation which had been destroyed in the process of a small intrinsic hemorrhage. The absence of additional symptoms over the next 7 years would make multiple sclerosis unlikely. Cranial MRI scan could have answered the question of additional lesions in nervous system but was not performed in this case. The patient was very reluctant to undergo a cranial MRI. A number of postinfectious viral and inflammatory diseases are associated with a myelitis, but these generally produce an increased cellular response in the CSF.

Devic's syndrome neuro myelitis optica (NMO) as originally described was a syndrome consisting of a relatively acute onset transverse myelitis and a bilateral optic neuritis. Relapses were said not to occur and the brain was said to be spared. It was classically stated to extend over three or more contiguous vertebral levels. This syndrome was considered a variant of multiple sclerosis, which occurred with increased frequency in Asian and non-Caucasian populations. In Japan 20%–30% of all multiple sclerosis cases were described as the optic nerve and spinal cord combination. As discussed by Pittock (2008), the new criteria for diagnosis include a spinal cord lesion on T2 MRI that involves three or more contiguous vertebral segments. There are recurrent attacks of optic neuritis which are more often unilateral. In 80% of cases, relapses occur. Initially the brain MRI is normal but eventually lesions will be present in 60% of cases. As with multiple sclerosis, relapsing cases are much more common in women 5–10/1 versus males. This is a severe inflammatory demyelinating disorder. In contrast to multiple sclerosis, a significant number of acute inflammatory cells are present in the CSF, including neutrophils and eosinophils. In contrast to classical multiple sclerosis, the oligoclonal bands of intrathecal Ig synthesis are not present in the CSF.

The actual spinal cord lesions demonstrate changes that are in contrast to classical multiple sclerosis. While there is extensive contiguous demyelination, there is also extensive cavitation and necrosis involving gray as well as white matter. Moreover, there is in the serum a specific autoantibody, NMO IgG. This antibody is directed against a protein of the water channel complex AQP4. This NMO antibody binds to the membranes of the aquaporin 4 channel. AQP4 is a protein found in the plasma membranes of the foot processes of astrocytes abutting microvessels and pia. As such it is critical for the function of the blood–brain barrier and the CSF–brain barrier. Since this protein is present in other tissues outside the CNS as well, other organs are also affected. Other autoimmune disorders such as myasthenia gravis, hypothyroidism, and pernicious anemia may also occur in one-third of relapsing NMO patients. Treatment consists of high-dosage intravenous methyl prednisolone (1000 mg per day x 5 days). In resistant cases plasma pheresis may be employed. Because of the necrotic nature of the lesion, residual disability is common.

Subacute-chronic HTLV associated progressive myelopathy HAM/ tropical spastic paraparesis: This is a myelopathy produced by the retrovirus HTLV that causes human T cell leukemia. A chronic meningo-encephalomyelitis is associated with demyelinating lesions in posterior and lateral columns. A sensory level may be present in the thoracic area. In tropical areas, the incidence of infected individuals may be as high as 128/100,000. The risk factors for transmission of the disease include many of the factors found with HIV infection: sexual transmission, intravenous drug use, blood transfusions, and mother to child via breast milk. *However, most infected individuals remain asymptomatic.* Less than 0.25%–3.8% develop tropical spastic paraparesis. Another 2%–3% develop T cell leukemia. The CSF and MRI findings are similar to multiple sclerosis (which actually has a lower incidence in tropical as opposed to temperate areas). Differentiation may be made by a determination of antibody levels in serum and CSF. A more detailed discussion will be found in Oh and Jacobson (2008).

Intrinsic spinal cord tumors: Rarely, metastatic tumors may be found within the substance of the spinal cord. However, most intramedullary tumors are intrinsic, arising from the glial (astrocytic or ependymal) components. The glioma arising from the astrocytic series of cells is the most frequent intrinsic tumor of the spinal cord found in the cervical thoracic spinal cord. Most spinal cord ependymomas arise at the lower end of the spinal cord in the filum terminale but may also occur in the cervical spinal cord. In general, astrocytomas are more common in children and adolescents, and ependymomas are more common in young adults. Intrinsic tumors of the spinal cord are rare compared to intrinsic tumors of the cerebral hemispheres and compared to extrinsic tumors of the spinal cord.

Ependymomas are often relatively localized and are to some extent discrete tumors. Astrocytomas, on the other hand, often tend to infiltrate the surrounding tissue without any particular limiting border. Several or many adjacent segments may be thus involved by the tumor. *In children, however, the astrocytoma has a long extent and does appear to have limiting borders and thus may be shelled out at surgery with excellent results.* These gliomas often have a cystic component and the cyst may be drained at surgery. The overall diameter of the spinal cord is increased and this may be visualized on MRI scans or with myelography. The increased mass of the spinal cord produces pressure on the pedicles of the vertebrae. Plain X-ray films of the spine may demonstrate the resultant increased interpeduncular distance. From a histological standpoint the spinal cord astrocytoma is usually of a uniform appearance with a relatively low to moderate grade of malignancy (grade 1–2). This is reflected in the usual clinical course that extends over a period of several years with a 5-year survival after surgery of up to 90% of patients. Contrast this to the astrocytoma that infiltrates the cerebral hemispheres which has a much more malignant histological grade of 3–4, and a much shorter survival.

A typical case is that of a young adult or child who presents with a several-year history of a slowly progressive lower motor neuron weakness and atrophy of one extremity involving multiple segments. Sensory symptoms in that extremity might develop at the same time or subsequently with or without radicular pain. As the process continues, upper motor neuron weakness of the ipsilateral leg might be followed by a similar involvement of the opposite leg. Subsequently a slowly progressive lower motor neuron weakness might develop in the ipsilateral or opposite upper extremity. Depending on the pattern of infiltration, long tract sensory findings might be present or absent. Bladder function would usually be well preserved. Very little local tenderness would be present over the vertebrae in contrast to extrinsic tumors. The changes in plain spine X-rays, MRI, or myelography/CT have been noted earlier. The patient would improve following an extensive laminectomy, drainage of any cystic component, and in some cases removal of tumor. In these cases, usually pediatric, it may be possible to discretely separate the tumor which may have a long longitudinal extent from the surrounding tissue. Radiotherapy will also produce considerable improvement.

Syringomyelia: this disease usually affects the cervical portion of the spinal cord but may extend into thoracic and lumbar segments. The basic pathology involves the formation of an irregular cavity (syrinx) in a central or paracentral location (Fig. 9.10). The cavity is surrounded by a border of gliosis (an area of proliferation of astrocytes with the production of glial fibers). Initially the cavity is usually ventral to and distinct from the central canal that is lined normally by ependymal cells. As the disease progresses, the syrinx may, however, extend into the central canal. The location of the syrinx is critical for understanding the early symptoms and signs that develop. The syrinx initially involves those pain and temperature fibers crossing the midline in the anterior white commissure. Thus, the initial symptoms and signs relate to a selective loss of pain and temperature sensation in the cervical segments, producing a cape-like deficit (Fig. 9.11). Since initially, touch, vibratory, and proprioceptive sensation are preserved, this is referred to as a dissociated sensory deficit. The patient often reports painless burns and painless trauma to the hands and arms. Although these symptoms and findings are usually bilateral, occasionally because of the irregular shape of the syrinx the symptoms and signs may be predominantly unilateral. The subsequent course of syringomyelia is variable since the syrinx often varies in its shape and pattern of expansion. The anterior horns, however,

Figure 9.10 Syringomyelia producing enlargement of the cervical spinal cord, destroying the anterior white commissure and the anterior horn. A dense border of gliosis is evident around the cavity. (Holzer stain for glia.) (Courtesy of Dr. E. Ross.)

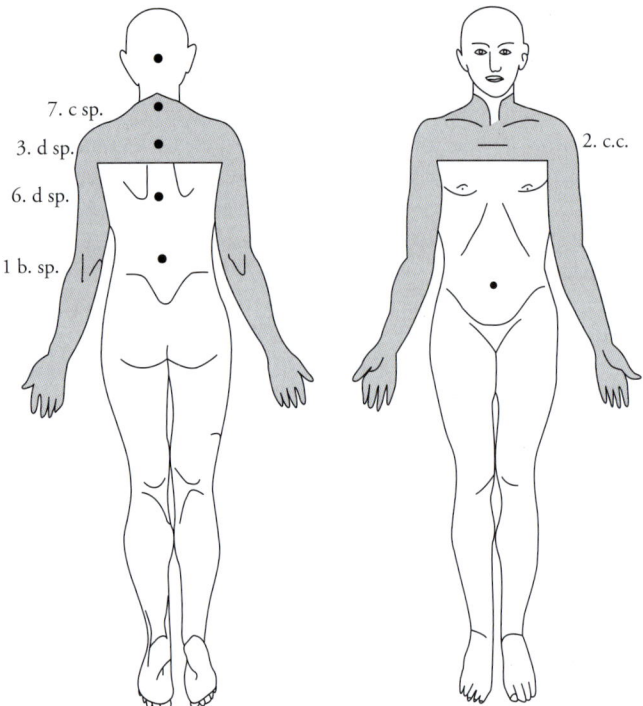

Figure 9.11 Syringomyelia with dissociated sensory loss. The cape-like distribution of a selective pain and temperature deficit with intact touch sensation over the upper extremities is demonstrated.

are often subsequently involved, resulting in local atrophy, fasciculations, and local flaccid paralysis of hand or upper extremity muscles with a segmental loss of deep tendon stretch reflexes. As the syrinx continues to expand, lateral and at times posterior columns may be involved with resultant long tract motor and sensory findings. Although the process is most prominent in the cervical spinal cord, the syrinx may extend into the thoracic and lumbar spinal cord. In addition, the process may extend into the medulla as *syringobulbia*. In such cases, the syrinx is usually present as a slit-like cavity extending in a ventral lateral direction from the floor of the fourth ventricle (the continuation of the central canal) into the dorsal lateral medullary tegmentum. In this location, many of the symptoms and signs relevant to the medulla will be similar to those of the lateral medullary infarct to be discussed in the brain stem Chapter 13. The symptoms and signs of syringobulbia may be unilateral, although bilateral lesions may occur with involvement of the nucleus ambiguous. The slit-like cavity may be difficult to visualize on MRI scans of the brain. The precise etiology of syringomyelia is variable, and the underlying pathophysiology is often not clear.

In type I syringomyelia, there is an abnormality, usually developmental at the cervicomedullary junction.

The Chiari or Arnold Chiari malformation is a frequent association.
Two types of the Chiari malformation are recognized: type I and type II.

In type I Chiari malformations, the cerebellar tonsils extend down through the foramen magnum, compressing the cervical medullary junction.

In type II Chiari malformations, there is caudal displacement of the lower end of the medulla and fourth ventricle as well as of the cerebellar tonsils through the foramen magnum. As a result, the brain stem is elongated and distorted with an abnormal bend. Other abnormalities at this junction may include the *Dandy-Walker malformation* in which the fourth ventricle is markedly dilated due to a closure or failure of development of the foramina of Magendie and Luschka. In other cases a meningioma may be present at the junction, or inflammation of the meninges (arachnoiditis) may have occurred. In all of these abnormalities a dilatation of the central canal (hydromyelia) usually occurs, and the syrinx appears to develop from this dilated central canal. In some of these cases hydrocephalus is also present.

In type II syringomyelia, no specific etiology is present. These cases referred to as idiopathic constitute approximately 60% of all cases of syringomyelia.

In type III syringomyelia, the syrinx appears to relate to other disease of the cervical spinal cord. In approximately 8%–16% of patients with syringomyelia, there is an associated intramedullary tumor. Note that the border of the syrinx is composed of proliferating astrocytes. Syringomyelia may also follow severe spinal cord trauma or following spinal cord compression, developing late after the event from areas of necrosis (myelomalacia).

Diagnosis can be made based on the clinical findings with confirmation by MRI studies of the spine and brain.

The following case provides an example of syringomyelia.

CASE HISTORY 9.5

This 33-year-old female had a 3-year history of intermittent pain and paresthesias extending from the left cervical area to the left arm and hand predominantly involving the middle finger. In the last 3 months, weakness of the left arm had developed and paresthesias of the left arm had become more continuous.

Neurological Examination
Mental status: Intact.
Cranial nerves: Intact.
Motor system: A mild weakness was present at the left triceps muscle.
Reflexes: There was depression of all deep tendon stretch reflexes in the left upper extremity.

Figure 9.12 Syringomyelia. Case 9.5 magnetic resonance imaging (MRI) scan. Cervical 6-thoracic 9: Sagittal section 10 mm right of the midline. The point of widest enlargement of the spinal cord is opposite the T4 vertebral body.

Figure 9.13 Arnold Chiari malformation associated with syringomyelia. Case 9.5 magnetic resonance imaging (MRI).

Sensory system: There was a selective cape-like decrease of pain and temperature sensation in the left upper extremity (shoulder and arm). In addition, there was a selective decrease in pain sensation over the T3-T5 dermatomes on the right.

Clinical diagnosis: Syringomyelia.

Laboratory Data

MRI scan of the spinal cord demonstrated an extensive irregular cavity extending from C2 to T9 with a major enlargement of the spinal cord at the T4 vertebral level (Fig. 9.12).

MRI scan of the head demonstrated a type I Arnold Chiari malformation with displacement of the cerebellum below the foramen magnum (Fig. 9.13).

Subsequent course: Dr. Alex Danylevich performed a laminectomy at T4 and shunted the large cavity into the subarachnoid space.

Figure 9.14 and he following case history represent a more complex and more advanced example of syringomyelia and syringobulbia.

CASE HISTORY 9.6

This 60-year-old white male maintenance worker 5 years prior to admission had the relatively sudden onset of a novocaine-like sensation behind the right ear and transient numbness of the right arm and leg. Three years prior to admission he began to drop objects from the right hand and developed decreased sensation in the right arm. On several occasions he was unaware that he burned his right arm and hand. The patient had sustained lumbar trauma at age 20 requiring lumbar spine fusion. A sister had died of a brain tumor.

Neurological Examination

General observations: There were numerous scars over the right hand and arm and to a lesser degree of the left hand.

Mental status: Intact.

Cranial nerves: The following abnormalities were present:

a. A dysconjugate rotary nystagmus was present, most marked on gaze to the right and greatest in the abducting eye. At a later point in time downbeat nystagmus was present.

b. There was decreased pain and temperature over all three divisions of the right trigeminal nerve with decreased corneal sensation. Touch sensation was intact.

c. Head was tilted to the left.

Motor system: The following findings were present:

a. Strength was intact.
b. Gait was broad based and ataxic; the patient was unable to do tandem walking. Eye closure did not change these findings, suggesting a cerebellar basis for these abnormalities.
c. Minimal incoordination was present on finger-to-nose testing and heel-to-shin testing of the right arm and leg.

Reflexes:

a. All upper extremity deep tendon stretch reflexes were 0 to 1. The lower extremities were 2+.
b. Plantar responses were flexor.

Sensory system:

a. There was a marked selective decrease in pain and temperature sensation over the C2-T4 dermatomes on the right and to a lesser degree in the same distribution on the left.
b. In contrast, position, vibration, and light touch sensation were intact.

Clinical diagnosis:

1. Syringomyelia
2. Syringobulbia
3. Possible Arnold Chiari malformation

Laboratory Data

A *myelogram* showed a diffuse expansion of the cervical spinal cord from T2 to C1. CT scan at 4–5 hours, after this study confirmed the diffuse expansion of the spinal cord and also showed a small syrinx at the C2 level.

MRI Scan (Fig 9.14). Midline sagittal section demonstrated a central cavity beginning at the cervical two segment and extending well into the upper thoracic segments. There was also noted a Chiari type 1 malformation.

Transverse sections demonstrated the irregular nature of the central cavity. (1) C1 level, no definite cavity was present. (2) At the C2 level, the cavity was predominately right sided, extending into right posterior column. (3) At the C4 level, bilateral cavities were present.

Subsequent course: The neurosurgeon Dr. Bernard Stone performed an extensive laminectomy in the upper dorsal-cervical spine area. The posterior spinal cord was thinned out "almost paper thin," particularly on the right side corresponding to the transverse images of the MRI scan. A cystic cavity was found at a depth of less than 1 mm. Using microsurgical technique, a small 1 mm incision was made with the laser into the spinal cord on the right, just posterior to the root entry zone. A thin silastic tube was inserted into the cavity, allowing continuous drainage into the subarachnoid space. Following surgery, the patient demonstrated a moderate improvement in his gait and minor subjective sensory improvement. He no longer sustained burns of the arm. However, 1 year after surgery, progression resumed. At 2 years following surgery he had weakness of the right arm and a severe ataxia. Pain and temperature sensation were now deficient over the entire right side of the body as well as the right arm and right foot. In addition, position and vibratory sensation were now impaired in both lower extremities at the foot. Repeat MRI scan demonstrated a slightly larger syrinx. His condition stabilized

Figure 9.14 Syringomyelia. Case history 9.6 magnetic resonance imaging (MRI). This 60-year-old male had clinical findings of syringomyelia and syringobulbia. (*A*) Midline sagittal section demonstrating a central cavity beginning at the cervical 2 segment and extending well into the upper thoracic segments. Note also the Chiari type 1 malformation. (*B*) Transverse sections demonstrating the irregular nature of the central cavity. (1) Cervical 1 level, no definite cavity. (2) Cervical 2 level cavity is predominately right sided, extending into right posterior column. (3) Cervical 4 level bilateral cavities.

over the next 3 months and then began to progress with increased rotatory and downbeat nystagmus, suggesting increased brain stem involvement.

Comments

Although the relatively sudden onset of symptoms at 55 years of age may be somewhat confusing, the anatomical localization should provide no problems. The initial symptom of the tingling behind the right ear, plus sensory symptoms in the right arm and leg, suggested that the cervical spinal cord was involved as high as the C2 and possibly the C1 segment. The more specific diagnosis is also very clear.

The clues to the more specific diagnosis as regard the spinal cord are the following findings:

1. The painless burns and trauma to the hands were greater in the right than the left.
2. The dissociated sensory loss in a cape-like distribution of pain sensation on the neurological examination with preservation of other sensory modalities.

All suggested involvement of the decussating pain and temperature fibers in the anterior white commissure just anterior to the central canal of the spinal cord.

The selective decrease in pain and temperature sensation over all three divisions of the trigeminal nerve on the right indicated involvement of the descending spinal tract of the fifth cranial nerve either at a lateral medullary level or at the level of the upper cervical spinal cord.

However, the occurrence of nystagmus, which was greater in the abducting eye, can only indicate involvement of the medial longitudinal fasciculus (MLF) at a low pontine level. Nystagmus in the setting of syringomyelia must mean that an associated syringobulbia is also present, with involvement of the vestibular nuclei and the MLF. The cerebellar findings in this case may indicate involvement of the inferior cerebellar peduncle in the lateral medulla. It is to be noted that the usual lesion of syringobulbia is often a slit-like lesion extending in a diagonal manner from the floor of the fourth ventricle into the lateral medulla. Therefore, the findings in syringobulbia are reminiscent of the lateral medullary syndrome to be discussed in the brain stem Chapter 13. In some cases the nucleus ambiguous is also involved to such a degree that laryngeal and pharyngeal function are significantly affected.

Downbeat nystagmus and cerebellar findings are frequently seen in the Arnold-Chiari malformation. It is important to realize that syringomyelia and syringobulbia are progressive diseases, as demonstrated in this case. This case suggests that it is not always possible to demonstrate a continuous appearance of the syrinx. The cavity, particularly at a brain stem level, may be a narrow slit which may not be imaged by the MRI, particularly by the earlier generation of MRI scanners (the study was performed in 1987). The improvement with drainage and decompression suggests that the cystic cavity is under pressure, adding an additional factor as regards the development of symptoms.

SYSTEM DISEASES OF THE SPINAL CORD

These are diseases in which there is a relatively selective involvement of particular neuronal cell groups and/or their fibers. At times, several related cell or fiber systems are involved.

System diseases are not of a uniform etiology. Nutritional deficiencies, infections, and familial/hereditary degenerative disorders are found in this category. Note that some system diseases are also systemic diseases but some are limited to specific systems of the central/and or peripheral nervous system with no systemic nonneurological involvement.

SPECIFIC SYSTEM DISEASES

DISORDERS OF THE ANTERIOR HORN CELL

Acute Anterior Poliomyelitis

This disease is caused by a filterable virus that invades the central nervous system. The virus spreads from the gastrointestinal tract by means of a viremia or by spreading up the axis cylinders of the autonomic nerve fibers. On reaching the central nervous system, the virus then involves preferentially the large motor neuron of the spinal cord and brain stem, resulting in damage, degeneration, or death of these neurons and inflammatory changes in the surrounding tissue (Fig. 9.15). Neurons in the posterior horn and interneurons of the spinal cord are to a lesser degree often involved in the acute stage. The correlated clinical phenomena consist of a prodromal period of fever, malaise, headache, plus gastrointestinal and upper respiratory symptoms. This is followed in some patients, by a stage of meningeal irritation and then in some patients, by the development of a flaccid paralysis. This involves, in an irregular manner, many of the muscles of the extremities and trunk (the spinal form) or the muscles supplied by the bulbar motor

Figure 9.15 Acute anterior poliomyelitis. Lumbar spinal cord, with a loss of large anterior horn motor neurons and replacement by clusters of mononuclear cells. Cresyl violet stain, 100×. (Courtesy of Dr. Jose Segarra.)

nuclei (the bulbar form). Muscles affected in the bulbar form include the facial, palatal, pharyngeal, and tongue. In the acute phase, cramps are often a significant symptom. Respiratory paralysis may occur in severe cases because of the involvement of the motor nuclei of the diaphragm and intercostal muscles or from damage to the respiratory centers in the medulla.

The spinal fluid findings are typical of aseptic meningitis with a predominantly lymphocytic response; however, very early in the disease polymorphonuclear cells may predominate. The majority of patients with anterior poliomyelitis viral infection make a complete or significant recovery. A significant proportion may actually be labeled as nonparalytic cases because a paralysis fails to develop even in the acute state. However, an estimated 20%–30% of all cases have a significant residual deficit or disability: a flaccid paralysis with atrophy, fasciculations, and loss of deep tendon stretch reflexes. In many cases, one limb, often a lower extremity, is predominantly involved. In bulbar cases, many patients remain respirator dependent. We may presume that in the majority of cases many neurons invaded by the virus manifest a transient dysfunction but are not destroyed. Recent interest has centered on the development of additional weakness and atrophy many years after the acute episode called the *post polio syndrome*. The underlying pathological basis for this progression is not entirely clear. The muscles involved, however, appear to be those previously affected in a clinical or subclinical manner with or without residual paralysis. Electromyography in many patients after the acute phase of poliomyelitis demonstrates changes in many muscles that were not clinically affected by the acute disease. Presumably this is a reflection of the subclinical involvement of the anterior horn cell motor neurons supplying those muscles.

With the development of the Salk vaccine (formalin inactivated virulent strains) and the Sabin (attenuated live virus) vaccine, infections with the poliomyelitis virus are now extremely rare in the United States and other developed countries. Worldwide eradication is now possible but economic factors, warfare, and misinformation regarding the effects of the vaccines have prevented such eradication in many parts of Africa and Asia. In countries where the natural disease (due to the "wild," naturally occurring virus) has been eliminated, rare cases are still encountered as a result of infection from immunization with the live attenuated virus. In addition, adults who have not been immunized may be infected by exposure to infants or children who have just been immunized with the live attenuated virus.

The following case history presents an example of poliomyelitis in an adult who had not been immunized and who was evaluated on June 14, 1968.

CASE HISTORY 9.7

This 54-year-old white housewife developed on June 4, 1968, a poorly defined illness characterized by fever, malaise, headache, nausea, and loss of appetite. Approximately 5 days later she noted an aching sensation in her right leg and then rapidly developed a weakness and then a paralysis of the right lower extremity. The following day, the left leg also became weak. She was unable to get out of bed to stand or to walk. No sensory symptoms or radicular pains were present. She had to compress her abdomen in order to void. Her temperature rose to 101°F.

Past history: The patient had never received any type of poliomyelitis immunization.

Neurological Examination (10 days after onset)
Mental status and cranial nerves: Intact.
Motor system:

a. Fasciculations were present in the thigh muscles bilaterally.
b. Strength was decreased as follows: right biceps: 4+/5(80%), right triceps: 2/5(20%), right lower extremity 0/5 except minimal wiggle of toes, unable to lift left leg off of bed, (1/5) with marked weakness of proximal thigh muscles: 1/5 (10%) but with intact distal strength.

Reflexes:

a. Deep tendon stretch reflexes were 2/4 except for the right triceps, patellar, and Achilles, which were absent bilaterally.
b. Plantar responses: The left was flexor. There was no response on the right.
3. *Sensory system*: Intact.

Clinical diagnosis: Acute anterior poliomyelitis.
Laboratory Data

1. *CSF:* Initial studies on June 9, 1968 (5 days after onset): 15 cells/cu mm (9 lymphocytes, 6 polymorphonuclears), protein increased to 85mg%, glucose normal at 60mg%. Repeat studies on the sixth day after onset of symptoms now indicated an increase in cells to 26 lymphocytes per cu mm.
2. *Viral studies* following transfer to the infectious disease service indicated isolation of poliomyelitis virus type I from the stool. When acute and convalescent serum were compared, a rise in antibody titers to poliomyelitis virus was apparent.

Subsequent course: The severe leg cramps were relieved by warm wet packs. Over a period of several days following the above evaluation, the right triceps deep tendon reflex returned and within an additional period of several days, strength in the right upper extremity had returned to normal. After several additional weeks, strength in the left lower extremity improved, but the right lower extremity remained unchanged despite intensive physiotherapy. At the time of rehabilitation hospital discharge on September 27, 1968, the patient had been fitted with long leg braces and trained in the use of crutches, with which at the time of discharge she was able to ambulate and to accomplish the activities of daily living.

Comments

Acute anterior poliomyelitis was formerly primarily a disease of children and young adults, since this was the population with the lowest previous exposure and therefore the lowest level of immunity. Occasional cases did occur in middle-aged or older adults (one of the most notable being that of President Franklin D. Roosevelt). As discussed earlier, with the development of immunization to the common strains of the virus, there has been an almost total elimination of the disease in modern industrial societies, where the rare cases that occur are primarily in nonimmunized individuals.

From the neurological standpoint, the neurological findings in this case were restricted to a lower motor neuron syndrome manifested by flaccid weakness, a loss of deep tendon reflexes, and fasciculations. Fasciculations represent apparent spontaneous contractions of motor units: the group of muscle fibers supplied by a single anterior horn cell. Although occasional fasciculations may occur in the majority of normal individuals as a benign phenomenon, the occurrence of frequent fasciculations usually represents the dysfunction of a diseased anterior horn cell. At times in other diseases with fasciculations, the basic pathological process is actually present in the anterior root or the proximal peripheral nerve. Although actual atrophy was not found in this patient during the acute phase of her illness, an examination in later years would demonstrate a significant degree of atrophy in those muscles still affected by a flaccid weakness.

The spinal fluid findings in this case were typical of a mild aseptic meningitis, that is, a nonbacterial meningitis. This type of CSF formula is often found in viral infections of the central nervous system. The occurrence of cramps as a prominent feature may reflect involvement of the posterior horn interneurons (found in acute cases which come to autopsy) or perhaps may be due to involvement of the gamma motor neurons. The major impact of the disease, however, is on alpha motor neurons and brain stem motor neurons.

SPINAL MUSCULAR ATROPHIES

This is a group of genetic disorders that involve the anterior horn cell, without involvement of the corticospinal or sensory systems. All are autosomal recessive. Four types are identified based on age of onset. The later the age of onset, the slower the progression. The earlier the age of onset, the more likely that bulbar motor neuron involvement and respiratory failure will be present in addition to the findings of anterior horn cell involvement. The incidence of the infantile and juvenile forms of the disease is estimated as 1 in 6000–20,000 births. The major disease to be differentiated is usually a disease of muscle, that is, a myopathic process. Electromyographic (EMG) studies, muscle biopsy, and genetic studies are useful in establishing the diagnosis.

Types are based on age of onset.

Type I, infantile form (Werdnig-Hoffman disease): onset: last trimester of pregnancy to 6 months: floppy infant.

Type II (intermediate/arrested form of spinal muscular atrophy): onset <18 months: delayed motor dates.

Type III, juvenile form (Kugelberg-Welander disease): onset 5–15 years: proximal limb weakness.

Type IV, adult-onset spinal muscular atrophy: onset >20 years: very slowly progressing proximal limb weakness. Note overlap with the progressive muscular atrophy form of amyotrophic lateral sclerosis discussed next.

Underlying molecular basis: types I, II, III have all been mapped to chromosome 5 at region 5q11.2–5q13.3, where a survival motor neuron (SMN) gene is located. Deletions in exons on this gene occur in these patients. The genetic defect responsible for the type IV, adult-onset cases is unknown.

X-Linked Recessive Bulbospinal Neuronopathy (Kennedy's disease): This adult-onset disease affects males over the age of 30 years. Degeneration of motor neurons in spinal cord and brain stem occurs. There are minor sensory findings. The disease is rare compared to the progressive muscle atrophy form of amyotrophic lateral sclerosis to be considered next but somewhat more common than the adult-onset type of spinal muscular atrophy. *The importance of this disorder relates to the underlying molecular basis: an abnormal increase in the trinucleotide cytosine-adenine-guanine (CAG) repeats in the region of the androgen receptor gene on the X chromosome.* Many of these patients will have gynecomastia; some will have testicular atrophy. In normal individuals, there are 17–26 CAG repeats. In the affected patients, there are 40–65 repeats. A similar expansion in the number of CAG trinucleotide repeats occurs in other diseases involving different aspects of motor function but affecting different chromosomes: Huntington's disease and the adult-onset autosomal dominant spinocerebellar degenerations. The CAG trinucleotide repeats encode polyglutamine. With excessive function, protein aggregation occurs in the motor neuron nucleus, resulting in degeneration. As in these other disorders, the higher the number of repeats, the earlier the age of onset.

DISORDERS OF THE MOTOR SYSTEM AFFECTING BOTH THE LOWER MOTOR NEURON AND THE UPPER MOTOR NEURON

Amyotrophic Lateral Sclerosis (Motor Neuron or Motor System Disease)

This is a progressive degenerative disorder of the motor neurons of the anterior horn cells, the bulbar motor neurons, and the neurons of the motor cortex. This is a relatively common degenerative disease of unknown etiology affecting predominantly adults of 40 to 60 years of age. Prevalence is estimated at 4–6 per 100,000. Approximately 10% of cases are inherited, usually as an autosomal dominant and rarely as an autosomal recessive. A variety of genetic mutations have been described. However, in 15%–20% of the autosomal dominant families a mutation has been mapped to the gene locus for superoxide dismutase on chromosome 21. Although this is the most common genetic mutation, overall this has been implicated in only 1%–2% of all amyotrophic lateral sclerosis (ALS) cases. This enzyme is involved in the detoxification of the free radical superoxide to hydrogen peroxide. Whether injury from free generation of free radicals is responsible for the neuronal degeneration in sporadic cases is uncertain. There is an overlap of some familial cases with a subset of patients with frontotemporal lobar degeneration.

Clustering of cases of ALS has been noted among the Chamorros on Guam, on the Kii peninsula of Japan, and in western New Guinea. In these clusters, there is an overlap with cases of the Parkinson's dementia complex. In these areas, the prevalence of ALS was formerly 100 times that of sporadic cases in other parts of the world when studied in the 1950s. With improvement in nutrition and in water supplies, the incidence in these areas has decreased. Thus, possible toxic factors have been suggested, although a possible predisposition may have also been present in theses populations.

As regards the etiology in most sporadic cases of ALS, the hypothesis of glutamate excitotoxicity has gained prominence in recent years. Glutamate serves as the major excitatory transmitter in the central nervous system. Excessive long-term ingestion of the chickpea (Lathyrus sativus), which contains a neurotoxin, a glutamate receptor agonist, may produce a neurological syndrome (lathyrism) in which selective damage to the motor cortex occurs. As we will discuss later in relation to dementia, an epidemic of food poisoning related to contaminated mussels occurred in the Canadian Maritime Provinces in the early 1980s with manifestations of motor neuron disease and dementia. Domoic acid, a potent glutamate receptor agonist, was found to be the specific neurotoxin. Related to glutamate excitotoxicity is the role of subsequent influx of excessive amounts of intracellular calcium. Intracellular calcium binding proteins protect against the effects of excessive intracellular calcium. The neurons that degenerate in ALS such as the large cortical pyramidal cells, the bulbar motor neurons, and the alpha motor neurons of the spinal cord have a low activity of these calcium binding proteins. In contrast, those neurons that are not affected in ALS such as the oculomotor neurons, the sensory neurons, the cerebellar Purkinje cells, and the nucleus relevant for the bladder (Onuf's nucleus) have a high level of immune-reactivity for calcium binding proteins.

An additional hypothesis as to etiology concerns the possible failure of nerve growth factor. However, administration of nerve growth factor has been ineffective in reversing the effect of the disease.

As regards the glutamate excitotoxicity hypothesis, a mild glutamate antagonist is available as riluzole. The effects on progression of the disease are minor. Life may be prolonged through the use of respiratory assistance and parenteral feeding methods. But such measures must consider the advanced directives of the patient regarding quality of life.

The majority of cases referred to as *classical ALS eventually* have involvement of all of the systems listed in Table 9.3. However, the disease may begin with involvement of the bulbar motor neuron or of the spinal cord lower motor neuron or of the upper motor neuron. The onset may be asymmetrical and limited to one limb. The terms applied to only one of the systems involved are presented in Table 9.3.

The diagnosis in those cases with a classical ALS syndrome can be established on the basis of the clinical signs and symptoms.

LABORATORY STUDIES AND DIFFERENTIAL DIAGNOSIS

Those cases with a progressive bulbar symptomatology may require MRI studies to exclude other brain stem pathology such as a brain stem glioma. Those cases with a progressive corticospinal syndrome will require an MRI study of brain and cervical spinal cord to exclude other treatable conditions such as parasagittal or foramen magnum meningioma. Those cases with a progressive spinal muscular atrophy syndrome will require nerve conduction studies to exclude motor neuropathies. These latter patients will also require studies for immunologic and toxic causes.

Electromyography in anterior horn cell disease will show evidence of both denervation and reinnervation. Some of the muscle fibers of a motor unit that have lost their innervations may be reinnervated by axonal sprouting from surviving anterior horn cells. Muscle biopsy will demonstrate grouped motor unit atrophy (as in Fig. 9.16). Thus, a group of muscle fibers all innervated by the same anterior horn cells will be atrophic, whereas a neighboring group of muscle fibers innervated by an intact anterior horn cell will be well preserved.

MRI studies of the brain, particularly in patients with prominent upper motor symptoms and signs, will demonstrate atrophy in the motor and premotor areas.

Table 9.3 CORRELATION OF CLINICAL SIGNS AND NEUROPATHOLOGY IN AMYOTROPHIC LATERAL SCLEROSIS AND RELATED DISORDERS

CLINICAL SIGN	LOCATION OF NEUROPATHOLOGY	IF THIS SYSTEM ONLY IS INVOLVED
1. Atrophy, fasciculations, flaccid weakness, and loss of deep tendon stretch reflexes (DTRs)	Alpha motor neurons of anterior horn	Progressive muscular atrophy
2. Bulbar palsy (CN V, VII, IX, X, XI, XII)	Bulbar motor neurons of medulla and pons	Progressive bulbar palsy
3. Upper motor neuron findings of spastic weakness, increased DTRs, and sign of Babinski	Degeneration of corticospinal tracts secondary to loss of large/giant pyramidal cells in motor cortex (Fig. 9.16)	Primary lateral sclerosis
4. Pseudobulbar findings of increased jaw jerk and gag plus pseudobulbar speech	Bilateral degeneration of corticobulbar tracts secondary to loss of large/giant pyramidal cells in motor cortex	Progressive pseudobulbar palsy

Figure 9.16 Amyotrophic lateral sclerosis. Degeneration of the corticospinal tracts is demonstrated in this myelin stain. (*A*) Degeneration of motor pathways in cervical and thoracic (top row), and lumbar and sacral levels (bottom row). (*B*) Cervical level showing degeneration of lateral corticospinal tract bilaterally and medial corticospinal tract on left side. (Courtesy of Dr. Emanuel R. Ross.)

COURSE OF THE DISEASE

Overall median duration of disease ranges from 23 to 52 months. Twenty to twenty-five percent of all patients live longer than 5 years and 8%–16% of patients survive beyond 10 years. *The prognosis of patients with ALS depends on the type of disease and on the initial manifestations as indicated in Table 9.4.*

Note that questions have been raised as to whether cases of primary lateral sclerosis (PLS) and progressive muscular atrophy (PMA) represent diseases that are distinct from classical ALS. Cases that remain as pure anterior horn cell longer than 36 months are usually classified as PMA. The age of onset is usually younger as well. Overall, younger patients have a better prognosis. Cases that remain as pure corticospinal longer than 36 months are usually classified as PLS. The following case history demonstrates the full clinical extent of a classical case of ALS.

CASE HISTORY 9.8

This 66-year-old married white male merchant, 9 months prior to evaluation, had the insidious onset of a progressive weakness and atrophy involving the lower extremities and subsequently a similar but lesser involvement of the upper extremities. Three months prior to evaluation, the patient had the onset of thickness of speech, a difficulty in swallowing solids, and to a lesser degree a difficulty in swallowing liquids. At the same time, stiffness in both lower extremities developed.

There had been no sensory symptoms, no urinary symptoms, and no change in mental status. There had been a weight loss of 30 lb.

Neurological Examination
Mental status: Intact.
Cranial nerves:

V: the jaw jerk was hyperactive (deep tendon stretch reflex).
VII: A bilateral peripheral paralysis was present involving the upper and lower face with a paucity of facial expression.
IX, X: Although a gag reflex was present, elevation of the uvula was poor. The voice was hoarse and speech was of low volume.
XII: Ridges of atrophy and fasciculations were present along the lateral borders of the tongue.

Motor system: Widespread muscular atrophy, fasciculations, and weakness were present in all four extremities.
Reflexes:

a. The deep tendon stretch reflexes at the biceps, triceps, and patellar were hyperactive at 3 +. However, the right Achilles reflex was 2 + and left was decreased at 0 to 1.
b. The plantar responses were both extensor (bilateral sign of Babinski).

Sensory system: Intact.
Clinical diagnosis: Amyotrophic lateral sclerosis (fully developed classical type).

Table 9.4 SURVIVAL RELATED TO ONSET OR TYPE

CLASSICAL AMYOTROPHIC LATERAL SCLEROSIS	DURATION (MEAN)	RELATIVELY PURE FORMS	DURATION
Overall	36 months		
Bulbar onset	17 months*	Progressive bulbar palsy	17 months
Corticobulbar onset	24 months		
Spinal motor neuron onset	33 months	Progressive muscular atrophy (PMA)	159 months (13 years)
Corticospinal onset	36 months	Primary lateral sclerosis (PLS)	224 months (19 years)**

*Worst prognosis.
**Best prognosis.
Source: From Matsumoto et al. (1998) and Mackay (1963).

Laboratory data: The EMG studies and muscle biopsy were consistent with the diagnosis of ALS.

Subsequent course: The patient experienced additional difficulty in swallowing. He expired 3 months after the above evaluation, approximately 1 year after the onset of his disease.

Table 9.4 outlines the clinical features and the neuropathologic correlation in ALS.

Other diseases with selective involvement of the cortical spinal tracts: In addition to primary lateral sclerosis, another very slowly progressive disorder has been identified: hereditary (or familial) spastic paraplegia. The prevalence of this disease may be as high as 3–10 per 100,000. In 70%–85% of cases the transmission of the disease occurs as an autosomal dominant. Genetic studies have indicated linkage to different chromosomes for different families: 14q or 15q or 2 p. Less often an autosomal recessive pattern is present. Various mutations have been identified, and a review is provided by Dion et al. (2009). A dysfunction of axonal transport has been suggested as the mechanism for the effects of the mutation.

In most cases, onset of disease occurs in childhood or adolescence, less often, after age 35. Initially the lower extremities are primarily involved, with delays in motor development or clumsiness in walking or athletic activity. As the disease progresses, the spastic paraparesis becomes evident. As in many of these degenerative disorders, a deformity of the feet, pes cavus may occur. Later in the disease, the upper extremities may be involved. In addition, a minor decrease in vibratory sensation in the lower extremities may be noted, and pathological examination of the nervous system demonstrates a minor degeneration of the posterior columns in addition to the marked degeneration of the corticospinal tracts.

Degeneration of the posterior columns secondary to disease of the posterior root: Tabes dorsalis (Fig. 9.17): This is a late complication of the sexually transmitted disease syphilis caused by the spirochete Treponema pallidum. Three stages of the disease are recognized: primary, secondary, and tertiary. A lesion of abraded skin and/or mucous membranes that begin as a painless papule, which then subsequently ulcerates to form the chancre, characterizes the *primary stage*. This chancre may involve the genitalia or lips or oral cavity or anus. The primary lesion develops after an incubation period of approximately 20 days and may persist for an additional 14–40 days. There is an associated painless lymphadenopathy. Primary lesions involving the vagina, cervix, or anus may go unrecognized and in other locations may be mistaken for other transient diseases.

In approximately one-third of these patients, asymptomatic spread to the nervous system may be documented by a CSF examination. The *secondary stage* of disease begins at a variable interval of 2–12 weeks after contact. It is characterized by a generalized maculopapular rash, which may be confused with other infectious exanthemas and constitutional symptoms such as fever fatigue and generalized lymphadenopathy. The symptoms may be so mild that the patient has little awareness of this stage of the disease. Again approximately one-third of patients would demonstrate a meningeal infection if spinal fluid examination were to be performed at this point. However, only 1% to 2% of patients in the secondary stage actually have symptoms of meningitis.

After a variable period following infection of months to 30 years, the late or tertiary manifestations involving the nervous system and the cardiovascular system appeared in 28% of all patients in the pre-antibiotic era. Symptomatic neurosyphilis developed in 7%–9% of all patients in that era. Prior to the antibiotic era, tertiary neurosyphilis constituted a major neurological problem. A resurgence of the disease may occur in the future.

The various types of tertiary neurosyphilis are listed in Table 9.5. Note that the primary process in almost all these syndromes relates to the late effects of meningeal infection and inflammation. The essential lesion in tabes dorsalis relates to involvement of the posterior roots with secondary degeneration of the posterior columns. In contrast, the papillary changes that occur in tabes dorsalis reflect involvement of the pretectal area of the midbrain and will be discussed in Chapter 13, which concerns the brain stem.

The clinical symptoms and signs of tabes dorsalis are listed in Table 9.6.

CASE HISTORY 9.9

This 40-year-old male had a 4-year history of severe lancinating-type pains in either leg, which were worsened by exposure to cold weather or hot water. This was accompanied by a progressive deterioration of gait, which was particularly impaired in the dark. He could not determine where his feet were placed. He would often go 18–20 hours without voiding.

Neurological Examination
Mental status: Intact.
Cranial nerves: The pupils were small, did not respond to light, but did respond to accommodation (Argyll-Robertson pupil).
Motor system: A gross ataxia of gait and stance was present, worse with eyes closed (positive Romberg sign).
Reflexes: Deep tendon reflexes were absent in the lower extremities.
Sensory system:

a. Position and vibratory sensations were absent at toes and ankles.
b. Pain sensation was decreased over the nose and nipples.

Clinical diagnosis: Tabes dorsalis.
Laboratory data: The diagnosis was confirmed by positive serological tests for syphilis in serum and CSF.
Comments
The diagnosis of tabes dorsalis is dependent on the recognition of the clinical pattern of disease. It may not be possible to obtain a reliable

Figure 9.17 Tabes dorsalis. Ascending degeneration of the posterior columns in a 67-year-old white male with tabes dorsalis, abdominal crises, luetic aortitis, and luetic optic neuritis. Myelin stain. (Courtesy of Dr. Jose Segarra.)

Table 9.5 **THE SYNDROMES OF TERTIARY NEUROSYPHILIS**

TYPE AND % OF ALL TERTIARY NEUROSYPHILIS (PREDOMINANT SYNDROME)	LOCATION OF PATHOLOGY	DELAY IN ONSET AFTER INFECTION
Acute meningitis	Meninges plus cranial neuropathies	2 months to 26 years usually < 1 year
Meningovascular (16%)	Meninges and arteries in subarachnoid space (arteritis with infarcts in brain and spinal cord)	Several months to 20 years, average of 7 years
General paresis (12%)	Invasion of cerebral cortex by the spirochete with dementia and personality changes (see Chapter 30)	20 years
Tabes dorsalis (30%)	Inflammation and infection of posterior roots and secondary degeneration of posterior columns plus (see Table 9.6)	10–25 years
Mixed usually general paresis and tabes	Combined cerebral cortex and posterior roots plus (see Table 9.6)	10–25 years
Chronic granulomas (gummas)	Skin, bones, central nervous system	Rare
Asymptomatic (31%)	Asymptomatic meningitis	Usually 1 year

Source: From Merritt, Adams, and Solomon (1946).

history of the primary or secondary lesions. The clinical diagnosis is confirmed by serological tests of the serum and by CSF examination demonstrating a positive serological test, some mild increase in mononuclear cells, a mild elevation of protein, and an increase in gamma globulin. The serological test are of two types: (1) the nonspecific reagin antibody tests such as the RPR and the VDRL; and (2) the specific treponemal antibody test such as the fluorescent treponema antibody absorption test (FTA ABS). As regards the nonspecific antibody tests, a positive serum test alone indicates only previous infection without necessarily indicating neurosyphilis. Moreover, a false-positive test may occur in other febrile illnesses and other immunological disorders. A false-negative nonspecific test in the serum may occur in up to 30% of patients with chronic neurosyphilis. The specific antibody tests on serum are positive in almost all cases of neurosyphilis. The positive nonspecific test of the spinal fluid when contamination of the spinal fluid by blood has been ruled out is diagnostic of neurosyphilis.

Table 9.6 **TABES DORSALIS: CORRELATION OF CLINICAL FINDINGS AND LOCATION OF NEUROPATHOLOGY**

CLINICAL SIGN	LOCATION OF PATHOLOGY
1. Loss of conscious proprioception: involving the lower extremities	Degeneration of heavily myelinated fibers entering the posterior columns
2. Loss of unconscious proprioceptive information	Loss of medium-diameter fibers from the posterior horn on their way to neurons in the nucleus dorsalis (Clarke's column)
3. Unsteadiness of stance and gait: sensory ataxia. Positive Romberg sign	Loss of proprioceptive information in posterior columns from lower extremities to cerebellum and cerebrum
4. Loss of the deep tendon stretch reflexes manifested as an absence of the patellar and Achilles reflexes.	Loss of the heavily myelinated Ia fibers in the posterior root
5. Bladder dysfunction—hypotonic flaccid dilated bladder occurs, atonic neurogenic bladder	Loss of the afferent fibers in the posterior roots of S2, S3, and S4 conveying stretch information from detrusor muscle of the bladder (interferes with reflex contractions of the detrusor muscle and subsequent emptying of the bladder)
6. Fleeting sharp pains in the legs, the back, the body, or face: so-called lightening pains. At times the viscera may also be involved.	Damage to small-diameter fibers conveying pain sensation
7. Loss of sensation in the feet and subsequent trauma may result in trophic ulcers	Damage to sensory fibers from the leg with degenerative changes in at joints (Charcot's joints)
8. Abnormalities of the pupillary response to light (the ArgyllArgyll Robertson pupil). Pupil is small (miotic), irregular, fails to respond to light and to sympathetic stimulation. Pupil does accommodate.	Lesion in pretectal region of upper midbrain or possibly in ciliary ganglion

Case 9.9 provides an example of tabes dorsalis.

Penicillin is the treatment of choice of neurosyphilis. The current recommendations of the US public health service are that the patient receive 24,000,000 units a day intravenously for at least 14 days. In patients who are sensitive to penicillin, other antibiotics such as erythromycin and tetracycline may be used. This should eliminate the activity of the organism. However, many of these symptoms and signs will persist since the chronic damage to nerve roots and nervous system from the meningeal or the meningoencephalitic inflammation or vascular components has already occurred. A reexamination of the spinal fluid at 6 months may continue to show a weakly positive serological test for syphilis, but all other abnormalities (such as cellular activity or increased gamma globulin) should clear. The serum nonspecific serological tests may continue to remain weakly positive, but if all other tests are negative, it is not necessary to retreat with antibiotics.

Combined degeneration of the posterior and lateral columns

Subacute combined degeneration: Combined system disease due to vitamin B12 deficiency: The combination of posterior and lateral column degeneration may be seen in several diseases involving the spinal cord. Of these various causes, the most important characteristic syndrome is that of *subacute combined degeneration secondary to vitamin B12 (cyanocobalamine) deficiency*.

In most cases the basic defect is a lack of intrinsic factor, the enzyme produced by the parietal cells of the gastric mucosa, the same cells that produce gastric acid. In most cases, this occurs on a genetic or immunological basis or as a result of a previous gastrectomy. Intrinsic factor is necessary for the absorption of vitamin B12. That absorption of vitamin B12 occurs in the distal ileum.

In a few cases, the deficiency of vitamin B12 does not indicate a deficiency of intrinsic factor but rather reflects an overall severe nutritional deficiency (e.g., a diet deficient in this vitamin) or represents a failure of the absorption of vitamin B12. Such a malabsorption syndrome may occur with any inflammatory condition involving the distal ileum such as regional ileitis or a tropical or nontropical sprue. In other instances a blind loop has occurred and bacterial growth has resulted in consumption of vitamin B12.

In rare instances, the presence in the small intestine of the fish tapeworm *D. latum* may also result in the consumption of vitamin B12 by the parasite. Two active forms of cobalamine have been identified in humans. Methylcobalamin functions as the cofactor for the conversion of homocysteine to methionine. When the reaction fails to occur, folate metabolism is impaired, and as a result there is a defect in DNA synthesis. As a result, megaloblastic maturation fails to occur and the characteristic *megaloblastic picture of pernicious anemia results*. The methionine that results from this conversion is also utilized for the production of choline and choline-containing phospholipids. When defective, the formation and maintenance of myelin may be impaired. The second form of cobalamine, adenosylcobalamin, is necessary for the conversion of methylmalonyl coenzyme A to succinyl coenzyme A. As a result, abnormal fatty acids may be synthesized and incorporated into neuronal lipids. Although the precise metabolic defect responsible for the neurological syndromes is not entirely clear, the first reaction is considered to be the more likely explanation.

Note that when conversion of homocysteine to methionine fails to occur, high serum concentration of cobalamine metabolites, methylmalonic acid, and homocysteine will be found. The usual level of B12 in the serum is greater than 200pc/ml. A level between 200 and 250 or 300 pc/ml has been considered borderline in some studies. In general most patients who develop neurologic symptoms will

Figure 9.18 Combined systems disease. Degeneration of posterior and lateral columns is demonstrated in this myelin stain of cervical spinal cord. (Courtesy of Dr. Emanuel R. Ross.)

have levels of B12 less than 100 pc/ml. For patients with borderline level, methylmalonic acid and homocysteine levels may be obtained. Approximately 30% to 70% of all patients with pernicious anemia develop neurological symptoms and signs. Even when severe anemia is present, the neurological state may be relatively normal and the explanation for sparing of neurological function is unclear.

On the other hand, severe signs of neurological involvement may be present in the absence of anemia. In some instances folic acid may been present in the absence of vitamin B12. *Folic acid will correct the anemia but will not affect the progression of the neurological syndromes.*

The neurological syndromes relate to the degeneration of myelin and subsequently of axons.

1. The major site of involvement is the spinal cord (Fig. 9.18). Initially the process is most severe in the heavily myelinated fibers of the posterior columns. This results in paresthesias in the extremities and a sensory ataxia accompanied by a positive Romberg sign.
2. At the same time, the same process affecting the heavily myelinated sensory fibers also affects peripheral nerves, resulting in paresthesias and a loss of deep tendon reflexes.
3. Subsequently the heavily myelinated fibers of the lateral columns are involved, predominantly affecting the lateral cortical spinal tracts. Bilateral Babinski signs will be found.
4. Hyperactive deep tendon reflexes are not likely in the early stages because of the effects of the peripheral neuropathy. However, after treatment with vitamin B12, hyperactive deep tendon reflexes may emerge. Less often the cerebral hemisphere white matter may be involved. Rarely for unknown reasons this site predominates, producing a progressive dementia.
5. Occasionally the optic nerve is involved, producing an optic neuropathy.

The following case history provides an example of combined system disease.

CASE HISTORY 9.10

This 48-year-old house painter had a 16-week history of progressive impairment of gait, mainly unsteadiness and imbalance worse in the dark than in the light and tingling paresthesias of all his toes. Twelve weeks prior to admission, tingling began in his fingers. Weakness had not been a major complaint, although he had noted shortly before admission some sense of heaviness in his legs on climbing steps.

Neurological examination: The following features were present.

Mental status: Intact.

Cranial nerves: Intact.

Motor system: The patient had minor difficulty walking a tandem gait with eyes open. His gait was worse with eye closure. The Romberg test was positive.

Reflexes:

a. Deep tendon stretch reflexes were 2 + excepting Achilles, which were 0.
b. Plantar responses were extensor (bilateral sign of Babinski).

Sensory system:

a. Vibratory sensation was absent at toes, ankles, and knees. Position sense was decreased at toes.
b. There was a minimal decrease in pain and touch sensation over the toes.

Clinical diagnoses: Combined system disease (subacute degeneration).

Laboratory Data

1. Hematocrit was slightly low at 34%. Blood smear indicated macrocytosis of red blood cells and hypersegmentation of the polymorphonuclear leukocytes.
2. No vitamin B12 was detected in the serum (normal values are 200–900 pg/ml). The Schilling test without intrinsic factor indicated 1% urinary excretion of the orally administered radioactive vitamin B12. Normally at least 8%–10% of administered radioactive B12 appears in the urine over 24 hours. When the Schilling test was repeated with the addition of orally administered intrinsic factor, the urinary excretion of radioactive vitamin B12 increased to 12% (normal values are 8%–22% excretion). There was a good reticulocyte response to the administration of the vitamin B12.
3. Bone marrow aspiration indicated megaloblastic changes in the erythroid series.
4. There was no gastric acid; on gastric analysis even with histamine stimulation. Gastric cytology was negative for cancer cells. Upper GI series was normal.

Subsequent course: The patient was treated with intramuscular injections of 100 mcg of vitamin B12 daily for 14 days and then was switched to 1000 mcg once a month. (The current recommendations are 1000 mcg of vitamin B12 [cyanocobalamin] daily for 5 days than weekly for an additional 3 weeks and then monthly for the lifetime of the patient.) When seen in follow-up at 5 months following his hospitalization, the patient reported exhibited improvement in gait. He was now able to walk a tandem gait with eyes open.

His Romberg test, however, remained positive. Deep tendon stretch reflexes and plantar responses were unchanged. Sensory examination now indicated that position sense was intact, although vibration was still absent at the toes and ankles and the minimal deficit in pain and touch over the toes was unchanged.

Comments

The findings in this case suggested predominant involvement of the posterior columns of the spinal cord with a sensory ataxia, with distal paresthesias of the extremities and an absence of position and vibration at toes and ankles. The deficit in position and vibration was far out of proportion to the minimal involvement of pain and touch sensation.

These symptoms could not then have been related simply to a peripheral neuropathy. Nevertheless, some peripheral nerve involvement was undoubtedly present since the Achilles deep tendon reflexes were absent and there was a minimal distal decrease in pain sensation. There was also clear-cut involvement of the corticospinal system since bilateral Babinski's signs were present. The administration of vitamin B12 would be expected to readily reverse the hematological changes, and this was already evident in the reticulocyte response to the early vitamin B12 administration.

As regards the neurological disease, at an early stage, some of these symptoms may represent a dysfunction of myelin and axons without actual structural damage. When patients are treated early, at a stage when axonal damage has not yet occurred and damage to myelin is minor, a significant improvement may occur although some neurological signs may still be present on examination. The objective is always to prevent progression and disability in this treatable disease. When treatment is delayed so that severe damage to myelin and subsequently to axons has occurred, significant disability may remain, although progression should be prevented. Patients with gastric carcinoma may also have a deficiency of intrinsic factor and for that reason gastroenterology studies were performed.

Spinal forms of spinal cerebellar degeneration: Spinal cerebellar degenerations represent overlapping groups of degenerative diseases that occur on a familial basis. As will be discussed in Chapter 20 on the cerebellum, the mutations and molecular basis for many of these disorders have now been established.

Friedreich's ataxia: In most series of hereditary ataxia, this type accounts for 50% of all cases. It is the most common of the autosomal recessive type and is certainly the most common of the early-onset ataxias. The prevalence of this disease in Europe and the United States is 1–2 cases per 100,000. The initial symptom: an ataxia of gait appears in childhood or adolescence, although rarely symptoms may appear in the young adult years. Subsequently, pyramidal tract findings and dysarthria may appear. Approximately 50% of the patients have a distal wasting, suggesting peripheral nerve involvement. Most patients have a distal loss of deep tendon reflexes and a *distal* sensory neuropathy involving large-diameter fibers. Deformities of the feet, including pes cavus (Fig. 9.19), are common. Deformities of the vertebral spine such as scoliosis (curvature) or kyphoscoliosis are also common. In some cases blindness due to optic nerve involvement and deafness due to eighth cranial nerve involvement are prominent. The majority of patients have abnormal electrocardiograms. Cardiac arrhythmias and ventricular enlargement are common due to myocardial muscle and conduction system involvement. Ten percent of patients have overt diabetes mellitus. The disease is slowly progressive with a mean age of death in the 30s due to cardiac involvement and the bed-ridden state.

Pathological examination (Fig. 9.20) demonstrates a loss or degeneration of axons that is most severe in the posterior columns of the cervical spinal cord and is accompanied by a significant loss of cells in the posterior root ganglion. The corticospinal, spinocerebellar (lower extremities), and cuneocerebellar pathways (upper extremities) also demonstrate a degeneration of axons. There is also a loss of neurons in Clark's column, the cells of origin of the spinocerebellar pathway. In some cases, there is a minor loss of Purkinje cells in the superior vermis of the cerebellum, the termination of the spinocerebellar pathway. There is usually a mild loss of neurons in the dentate nuclei of the cerebellum and of the inferior olivary nuclei of the medulla which project to the cerebellum. A more significant loss of neurons is found

Figure 9.19 Friedreich's ataxia: pes cavus. A similar abnormality of the foot may occur in other disease states. (From Wechsler, I.: Clinical Neurology, 9th Edition. Philadelphia, W.B. Saunders, 1963, p. 123.)

in the nuclei for cranial nerves 8, 10, and 12. Mild degenerative changes may be noted in the optic nerves. In contrast, the peripheral nerves demonstrate a more significant loss of large myelinated axons.

From the standpoint of clinical pathological correlation, the ataxia is primarily a sensory ataxia due to involvement of posterior columns, dorsal root ganglia, peripheral nerve, and to a lesser degree, the spinocerebellar pathway. However, some cerebellar component is also present. The dysarthria reflects involvement of cranial nerves 10 and 12 in addition to a possible cerebellar component.

The underlying genetic basis of the disease: There is an unstable expansion of a trinucleotide repeat GAA (guanine adenine adenine), which maps to the chromosome locus 9q 13. On normal chromosomes,

Figure 9.20 Friedreich's ataxia. Degeneration of posterior columns and, to a lesser extent, of lateral columns is demonstrated in this myelin stain of cervical spinal cord. (From Wechsler, I.: Clinical Neurology, 9th Edition, Philadelphia, W.B. Saunders, 1963, p. 28.)

the number of GAA repeats ranges from 7 to 22. In contrast, 96% of patients with Friedreich's ataxia have both alleles expanded to 100–2000 repeats. Patients with a larger number of repeats have an earlier age of onset and a more severe form of the disease. They are also more likely to have a cardiomyopathy. The trinucleotide expansion results in a decrease in a protein which has been labeled *frataxin* and which may function as a mitochondrial iron transport. The buildup of untransported iron could then result in defects of free radical regulation and oxidative metabolism. Other disorders of trinucleotide repeats are discussed with regard to Huntington's disease in Chapter 19 and autosomal dominant cerebellar degenerations in Chapter 20.

The following case history demonstrates the typical history and findings in a case of Friedreich's ataxia followed over many years.

CASE HISTORY 9.11

This part-time college student was initially seen for evaluation of a progressive ataxia at age 22 years. At age 9 years, the patient had noted the onset of a progressive change in handwriting and then an impairment of hand coordination. Difficulty in walking and balance had been initially noted at age 12. An evaluation at the Children's Hospital Medical Center in Boston at age 15 indicated a positive Romberg test and an absence of deep tendon stretch reflexes.

Up until age 18 years, the patient had been able to walk by holding on to the walls. Subsequently he required the assistance of one person. By age 21 he required the assistance of two people. At age 18 years, a progressive change in voice began. At the same time, the patient noted a weakness in both lower extremities with "a collapsing at the knees." In recent years, a change in vision had occurred requiring frequent changes of glasses. Despite these symptoms, the patient continued to do relatively well as a part-time college student. The patient had been adopted at an early age and no information concerning parents or siblings was available.

General physical examination: The heart rate was irregular.
Neurological examination: The following features were present:
Mental status: Intact.
Cranial nerves: The following abnormal findings were present:

a. Extraocular pursuit movements were jerk-like rather than smooth
b. There was frequent facial grimacing.
c. Dysarthria was present with slurring of speech.

Motor system: multiple abnormalities were present:

a. There was minor atrophy of the hand muscles and a more marked atrophy in the muscles of the lower legs and feet.
b. There was mild weakness in the distal portions of the upper extremities and in the hands with a more significant weakness in the lower extremities, most marked distally.
c. Hypotonia was present in all four extremities with excessive rebound on passive motion and release.
d. There was a marked bilateral intention tremor on finger-to-nose testing and a marked impairment of alternating movements of the hands and fingers. (An intention tremor is a movement perpendicular to the line of movement and usually implies disease of the cerebellar hemisphere or of pathways related to the lateral cerebellum.) A significant tremor of the head was also present.
e. The patient was unable to stand or walk except with the support of two individuals. Attempts to have him stand on a broad base

indicated a marked truncal ataxia, which usually implies disease of the midline cerebellum or of fiber systems related to the midline cerebellum.

Reflexes:

a. Deep tendon stretch reflexes were everywhere absent.
b. Plantar responses were equivocally extensor bilaterally.

Sensory system: The following abnormalities were present:

a. There was a distal decrease in pain sensation in the lower extremities up to the ankles.
b. Vibratory sensation was totally absent at toes and ankles and decreased at knees. This modality was also absent at the fingertips and markedly decreased at wrists.
c. Joint position sense was markedly defective at the toes and defective to a lesser degree at the fingertips.

Clinical diagnosis: Friedreich's ataxia.

Laboratory data: The *electrocardiogram* demonstrated the following features: a marked sinus arrhythmia, occasional nodal beats, and premature atrial contractions. In addition, abnormal T-wave inversions occurred.

Subsequent course: The patient was able to complete college. Using a motorized wheelchair and other aids, he was able to function as an accountant and as the town auditor. Follow-up visits over the next 20 years indicated continued progression with the development of bilateral optic atrophy, bilateral sensory-neural hearing loss, bilateral cortical bulbar findings, increasing dysarthria, and increasing motor and sensory deficits in all four extremities. After increasing cardiac difficulties he expired at age 41. Throughout the course of his disease, mental status and motivation were extremely well preserved.

Comments

The early symptoms and findings based upon the neurological examination when the patient was 15 years of age clearly indicated predominant involvement of posterior columns and an absence of the deep tendon stretch reflexes. The history at that time also indicated a problem in coordination of hand movements, suggesting the possibility of some cerebellar involvement at that time. His subsequent evaluation at age 22 indicated that progression of the posterior column disorder had occurred. In addition, there was now evidence of severe disease of the cerebellum or cerebellar pathways: intention tremor, impairment of alternating hand movements, ataxia of the trunk, and a dysmetria of eye movements. Moreover, there was also evidence of a distal sensory motor peripheral neuropathy. Equivocal plantar responses were also now present. Dysarthria was also very apparent. With time the involvement of all these systems progressed. In addition, involvement of the optic nerves and the eighth cranial nerve for hearing added to the severe disabilities. At the time that this patient was initially seen and followed, a genetic test for this disorder was not available. Today, a specific diagnosis could be established through the use of genetic tests for the expansion of the GAA trinucleotide repeats on chromosome 9.

MULTIFOCAL DISORDERS AFFECTING THE SPINAL CORD

Two categories of pathology produce multifocal symptoms and signs affecting the central nervous system disease: demyelinating disease and vascular disease, particularly small vessel disease such as vasculitis. When the spinal cord is considered, the first variety occurs frequently; the second is encountered less frequently.

DEMYELINATING DISEASES

In this category of disease we mean a pathological process in which there is a primary destruction of normally formed myelin. We have already indicated other disorders in which damage to myelin is but one step in the destruction of the axon. In other disorders destruction of myelin is secondary to infarction. There is moreover another group of disorders, *the leukodystrophies*, occurring in childhood, adolescence, or early adult life in which an extensive loss of myelin occurs. This loss, however, involves the destruction of defectively formed myelin. Such disorders usually occur on a genetic basis due to mutations.

MULTIPLE SCLEROSIS

(Note additional discussion of multiple sclerosis will be found in Chapter 27.) *Among the primary demyelinating diseases, the most common variety is multiple sclerosis.* This is a relatively common disorder whose etiology, although still considered as uncertain, suggests an immunological basis. Young and middle-aged adults are primarily affected with most patients first demonstrating symptoms between the age of 18 and 50 years. *Multiple sclerosis is the most common neurological disorder of young adults.* The frequency of disease varies based on geographic origin. Those who reside in the northern United States, Canada, and northern Europe have an incidence of disease and prevalence of disease far beyond those in the southern United States and southern Europe. The prevalence of disease in equatorial areas is less than 1 per 100,000. In contrast, the prevalence in the southern United States and southern Europe is 6–14 per 100,000. In northern Europe and northern United States the prevalence has been reported as 30–80 per 100,000. In Olmstead County, Minnesota, where the detailed epidemiologic studies of the Mayo Clinic have been performed, the annual incidence of new cases was 8 per 100,000 with a prevalence of 177 cases per 100,000 population. Additional studies have demonstrated that those who reside in the northern temperate zone for the first 15 years of their lives are at greatest risk as opposed to those who spent those years in a more tropical climate. Within a given geographic area whites are at higher risk than blacks. Women are at increased risk compared to men in all geographic areas. Overall, women constitute 70%–75% of all cases. Note that a predominance of females is found in all autoimmune disorders.

As discussed by Noseworthy et al. (2000), while it is unlikely that viral invasion of the nervous system directly causes the disease, it is possible that molecular mimicry— the antigenic similarity between viral organisms and neural tissue—may trigger the autoimmune response. Viral infections may also trigger exacerbations of the disease. We have earlier discussed this concept with regard to Guillain-Barré syndrome. As with that disorder, an acute experimental model of postinfectious encephalomyelitis was developed, demonstrating an acute allergic response to myelin when the myelin is accompanied by an adjuvant immune stimulus. The diseases, however, differ as discussed next. Sera from patients with multiple sclerosis when added to cultures of cerebellar neurons from newborn mice under some circumstances can damage myelin, inhibit remyelination, and block axonal conduction. The current hypothesis is that multiple sclerosis is mediated by T-cell sensitization to myelin. Genetic and familial clustering has been noted. *The disease is characterized by the dissemination of the disease in time and space.* Thus, there is the diagnostic criterion that various lesions be acquired at different times. Thus, the model of experimental allergic encephalomyelitis does not meet this criteria. At any given moment in multiple sclerosis, the various lesions will be at a different stage of development. It is also a diagnostic criterion that multiple levels of the neural axis are affected. At a given level, the lesion cuts across various fiber systems. It is not a system disease. The pathologic picture varies with the stage of the disease. The initial areas of involvement are perivenous with infiltration of mononuclear cells, plasma cells, and lymphocytes (usually T cells). A slight degeneration of oligodendrocytes may be noted. There is destruction of myelin. There is then a stage of infiltration by macrophages in which destroyed myelin is removed. There is then a stage of astrocytic proliferation with the production of glial fibers. The areas of gliosis result in the firm sclerotic gray appearance of old lesions and thus the name *multiple sclerosis* (Fig. 9.21). In some early cases remyelination by oligodendrocytes has been reported. As the disease progresses, actual destruction of axons may occur as demonstrated at pathologic exam and by MRI scans. Perivascular infiltration by plasma cells and lymphocytes is the probable source for the production of increased amounts of immunoglobulin G in the CSF of most patients with active multiple sclerosis. Among all patients with multiple sclerosis, 40%–60% will have such an elevation. Immunoelectrophoresis of the CSF will demonstrate a more specific abnormal population of oligoclonal bands within the IgG in 75%–85% of patients. These findings, however, are not specific for multiple sclerosis; similar findings are also present in neurosyphilis and postinfectious encephalomyelitis.

Cases may be classified according to the anatomical involved in the initial acute stage: spinal, cerebellar-brain stem, optic nerve, or cerebral hemisphere. A more important classification takes into account the pattern of evolution of the disease. For example:

1. Relapsing/remitting: these cases are younger and demonstrate the significant predominance of females.

2. Primary progressive: these cases constitute an older middle-aged group and there is no predominance of females.

3. Secondary progressive.

Some patients have a benign disease with only one or two episodes with a relatively complete remission. Overall 85% of patients begin with a relapsing/remitting course and 15% with a primary progressive course.

Figure 9.21 Multiple sclerosis affecting the spinal cord. (*A*) A 58-year-old male with a long history of progressive multiple sclerosis. At postmortem examination multiple plaques of variable age were present in the nervous system. (Courtesy of Dr. Jose Segarra.) (*B*) This 44-year-old male 20 years previously had experienced a single acute episode of possible multiple sclerosis involving spinal cord and was asymptomatic in the interim until his acute death from an unrelated cause. (Courtesy of Dr. Jose Segarra.)

Diagnosis of multiple sclerosis is based on the clinical history and examination. When patients have clear-cut evidence of lesions disseminated in time and space, they are referred to as manifesting definite multiple sclerosis. When dissemination in time or in space is present, the label of probable multiple sclerosis has been employed. When patients of appropriate age present with the initial findings of syndromes that are seen commonly in multiple sclerosis such as transverse myelitis, or optic neuritis, or the brain stem syndrome of internuclear ophthalmoplegia (discussed in the brain stem Chapter 13), or an acute cerebellar syndrome, they are labeled as possible multiple sclerosis. The main ancillary technique for diagnosis is the MRI scan. The MRI scan has simplified the diagnosis since many cases of possible or probable now have been shifted into the definite category at first presentation. The visual evoked potential may also be of value in providing evidence of an optic nerve lesion in patients with involvement of other areas of the nervous system.

The following case is an example of multiple sclerosis beginning with an episode affecting spinal cord but in which the MRI scans demonstrated not only the suspected spinal cord lesion but also cerebral lesions.

CASE HISTORY 9.12

This 32-year-old female registered nurse had a 6-month history of tingling paresthesias in the lower extremities beginning in the toes on the right foot and then the left and gradually spreading to the rib margin on the right and slightly lower on the left. Three months later she developed tingling of the ring and fifth fingers bilaterally. Six weeks prior to evaluation, a positive *Lhermitte's sign developed: flexion of the neck produced electric shock sensations that extended down from the buttocks into lower extremities.*

Neurological Examination
Mental status: Intact.
Cranial nerves: Intact.
Motor system: Intact.
Reflexes: The left plantar response was extensor; the right equivocal.
Sensory system:

a. Pain and cold were decreased up to the L1-L2 vertebrae posteriorly (but possibly at times to the rib margin on the right) and anteriorly up to D7 dermatome on the right and to D9 dermatome on the left.
b. Vibratory sensation was bilaterally decreased at toes, ankles, and knees with a greater defect on left than right.

Neck: Examination demonstrated no local tenderness, but flexion of the neck confirmed the positive Lhermitte's sign.
Clinical diagnosis: Cervical myelopathy.
Comments
While the Lhermitte's sign could be seen in multiple sclerosis, this sign also could be produced by compression of posterior columns from an extrinsic cause. (The original description was encountered in soldiers of World War I related to concussion of the cervical spinal cord.)
Laboratory Data

1. *MRI of the cervical spine* (Fig. 9.22) demonstrated a large area of demyelination at C2 involving the right lateral column and to the lesser degree the left posterior column.
2. *MRI of the brain* (Fig. 9.23) demonstrated multiple demyelinating lesions in both cerebral hemispheres (not all are seen in the illustration).
3. CSF studies were consistent with the diagnosis in terms of an increased cell count of 18 lymphocytes plus a markedly elevated immunoglobulin G index. Two oligoclonal bands were present (normal 0-1).

Subsequent course: The patient received a 5-day course of high-dosage intravenous methyl prednisolone with some improvement in the sensory symptoms in her leg. She had subsequent episodes affecting spinal cord and brain stem and was treated with beta interferon.

The following includes several episodes indicating clear-cut clinical involvement of the spinal cord in a patient followed over a number of years. In addition, several episodes relevant to brain stem are also documented. The history of the patient's brother with a single episode of transverse myelitis is also presented. The patient was seen and followed prior to the era of MRI scans. The student may wish to review this case after the study of the brain stem (Chapter 13).

Figure 9.22 Multiple sclerosis involving the spinal cord. Case 9.12: (*A*) sagittal section; (*B*) transverse section.

Figure 9.23 Multiple sclerosis involving brain. Case 9.12, multiple sclerosis involving the brain.

CASE HISTORY 9.13

At age 29 years, this white, married, male real estate broker and flyer awoke one morning with tingling paresthesias involving the left hand, which slowly spread to involve the left half of the trunk and left leg. Symptoms improved that morning; then they recurred and also involved the right arm. Shortly thereafter, incoordination and weakness of the left arm developed.

Neurological examination at that time demonstrated decreased touch pain and temperature sensation over the entire left arm, trunk, thigh, and plantar surface of the foot. A cervical spinal cord lesion was suspected, but the cervical myelogram, CSF fluid, and immunological studies were all normal. Over the next several weeks the patient made a complete recovery.

At age 31, the patient developed, over a period of 7–10 days, a progressive flaccid weakness and tingling of the left hand accompanied by a weakness of the distal left leg. Deep tendon reflexes were increased on the left and a left Babinski sign was present. When numbness and weakness of the left side of the face then developed, a right cerebral hemisphere lesion was suspected. However, all diagnostic studies available at that time, including a right carotid arteriogram, an electroencephalogram, and radioactive brain scan, were normal. Within 4 days, a significant improvement had occurred with only the reflex findings remaining.

At age 32, in association with a minor viral infection and fever, the patient developed progressive weakness of the right arm and leg followed by a disturbance of speech, a dysarthria. A lesion of the left internal capsule was suspected.

One month later, as these symptoms were beginning to clear, the patient developed a bilateral impairment of central vision, urinary retention, and left-sided weakness.

Neurological examination now revealed a central and paracentral scotoma (a defect in vision suggesting a lesion of the optic nerve). An independent scotoma was also present in the nasal field of the left eye. A mild distal right hemiparesis was present with increased deep tendon reflexes and a Babinski sign on the right. Within 2 days a significant degree of improvement had occurred in all symptoms and signs. Based on the urinary retention, a possible lumbosacral spinal cord lesion was suspected. In addition, a cervical spinal cord and bilateral optic nerve lesions were also presumed to be present.

Two weeks later, the patient developed burning pains over the right side of the face involving the eye, tongue, and upper teeth. These symptoms suggested involvement of the trigeminal system at a pontine or medullary level. These symptoms resolved over several days and the patient was then asymptomatic for the next 10 months.

At age 33, the patient awakened with a numbness and tingling paresthesias below the knees which gradually ascended that day to involve primarily the buttocks and perianal areas. Later that evening, the patient began to have difficulty in voiding and required catheterization by his local physician. In addition, a general sensation of weakness of the lower extremities was noted.

Neurological examination: The following findings were present:
Mental status: Intact.
Cranial nerves: Intact.
Motor system:

a. A minor decrease in strength was present bilaterally at hip flexors and ankle dorsiflexors.
b. Gait was broad based with ataxia present on attempts to walk heel to toe. A positive Romberg test was present.

Sensory system:

a. A dense bilateral deficit in pain sensation was present over the lower sacral segments (S3, S4, and S5) with a circular distribution about the anus. Temperature sensation was relatively well preserved.
b. A marked bilateral decrease in vibratory sensation was present at the toes and ankles with a lesser decrease at the knees. Position sense was relatively well preserved.

Clinical diagnosis: Relapsing/remitting type of multiple sclerosis. "Benign type of multiple sclerosis." This most recent episode represented an acute lesion at the level of sacral spinal cord.

Laboratory Data

a. Cystometrogram indicated a defect in reflex voiding in response to distension of the bladder. The patient had no sensation of distension up to 450 cc of saline but as distension of the bladder was increased he had a progressive increase in discomfort. No spontaneous voiding occurred even after a total of 750 cc had been instilled. Normally the sensation of distension and desire to void begins to occur at 200 cc and spontaneous voiding occurs at 450 cc.

Subsequent course: Significant improvement again occurred without specific therapy. On the second day in the hospital the ability to void had returned. By the fifth day the neurological examination was normal except for the broad-based gait.

Ten days later, an exacerbation occurred with difficulty in voiding and weakness and numbness in the right lower extremity requiring readmission to the hospital.

Neurological examination now revealed that deep tendon stretch reflexes in the lower extremities were now hyperactive with bilateral Babinski signs and absent abdominal reflexes. Pain sensation was now decreased below the level of the umbilicus bilaterally but more marked on the left. Vibratory sensation was markedly decreased below the level of the T12 spinous process bilaterally but more marked on the right. Position sense was markedly defective at the toes on the right, with a minor defect on the left. After a week of bed rest in the hospital, almost all of the symptoms resolved. This episode was attributed to a lesion at the level of a thoracic spinal cord, essentially a transverse myelitis. While a bilateral involvement had occurred, it was evident that many components of a right-sided Brown-Sequard spinal cord syndrome were present.

Three months later the patient developed tingling paresthesias of the left side of the face, accompanied by a paralysis of all facial muscles on the left side and a decrease in hearing in the left ear.

These brain stem symptoms suggested a lesion at the left pontomedullary junction. (Refer to brain stem Chapter 13) and soon cleared. Periodic examinations over the next 8 years indicated no significant exacerbations of the disease process and no significant disability. He did have a minor tremor. In the interim the patient continued to pursue his usual business activities and continued to pilot his own airplane. He gave up flying at age 46 and purchased a 37-foot sailboat, which he often sailed solo to Florida and the Bahamas. He experienced occasional bladder and balance problems and a minor tremor, but these did not interfere with his activities. He expired at age 50 of a massive myocardial infarct.

Comments

This patient expired in 1984, just before the availability of the MRI scan. From a clinical standpoint, there would be little doubt concerning the diagnosis of multiple sclerosis of a relatively benign relapsing/remitting type. This patient clearly had dissemination of lesions in time and space which involved the spinal cord at multiple levels, the brain stem, the cerebral hemispheres, and the optic nerves. From the standpoint of the spinal cord as delineated earlier, this patient had various types of syndrome. He did not manifest a phenomenon frequently encountered in patients with involvement of the posterior columns in the cervical area: Lhermitte's sign. Sudden flexion of the neck induces a tingling electric shock sensation down the spine into the buttocks and at times into the legs. From a diagnostic standpoint other causes of lesions disseminated in time and space such as vasculitis, lupus erythematosus, and neurosyphilis were essentially eliminated by the negative findings of arteriography, sedimentation rate, immunological studies, and CSF serology.

This patient was extremely fortunate in the sense that over the 21 years of his symptomatic disease, he did not develop secondary progression. The majority of patients with this history would sooner or later experience symptoms or demonstrate signs which did not resolve and which might provide a disability of minor or major degree. The studies of Percy published in 1971 covering all cases seen in Rochester, Minnesota, 25 years after onset of multiple sclerosis indicated than one-third of the patient's were still working and two-thirds were still ambulatory. The earlier studies of McAlpine published in 1961 indicated that among patients followed for a minimum of 10 years, approximately one-third were dead, one-third were disabled, and one-third had no physical restrictions or disabilities that affected work or home life. It is evident that this earlier study underestimated benign or mild cases of the type that were probably lost to follow-up. Moreover, these earlier studies were performed prior to the introduction of significant immunosuppression therapy.

Why did this patient have such a benign course? Did he have a genetic background which might have predisposed him to a benign type of multiple sclerosis? In this case, there is additional information that suggests such a predisposition. The patient's older brother, a naval flyer, had been hospitalized at age 33 with a diagnosis of para-infectious myelitis. Over 3 days, the brother developed a Brown-Sequard syndrome with weakness of left arm and leg accompanied by increased left-sided deep tendon stretch reflexes and left Babinski sign in addition to a deficit in pain and temperature sensation below the C4 segment. CSF examination indicated an increased number of cells (50 lymphocytes) with a minor increase in protein (53 mg/100 m l) and a probable increase in the percentage of gamma globulin. This patient (the naval aviator) recovered completely over a period of 3 weeks. He returned to his duties as a naval flier and experienced no additional episodes during the succeeding 27 years. The brother's case would be labeled as an acute postinfectious myelitis and would be included as a type of transverse myelitis discussed earlier in this chapter.

Present clinical and MRI studies indicate that most patients with relapsing/remitting multiple sclerosis do have an increasing lesion load, resulting eventually in symptoms or signs that do not resolve. The present approach then is to utilize early in the disease course agents that modify the immune system. Agents such as the beta interferons decrease relapses and secondary progression. The effects are evident from both a clinical and MRI standpoint. Acute exacerbations are usually treated with high-dose intravenous corticosteroids with the patient receiving 1000 mg a day of methylprednisolone for 5–7 days. This shortens the course of the exacerbation with the possibility of less residual disability. There is no clear-cut therapy for primary progressive multiple sclerosis, although various major immunological therapies have been investigated.

BIBLIOGRAPHY

Suggested Readings

Adams, R. D., Victor, M., and Ropper, A. H. 1997. Principles of Neurology. 6th ed. New York, NY: McGraw Hill.

Burke, D., and Lance, J. W. 1992. The myotatic unit and its disorders. In A. K. Asbury, G. M. McKhann and W. I. McDonald (Eds.). Diseases of the Nervous System, pp. 270–284. Philadelphia, PA: W. B. Saunders.

Byrne, T. N., and Waxman, S. G. 1990. Spinal Cord Compression: Diagnosis and Principles of Management. Philadelphia, PA: F. A. Davis.

Ditunno, J. F., Jr., and Formal, C. S. 1994. Current concepts: chronic spinal cord injury. N. Engl. J. Med. 330:550–556.

Greenberg, J. 1993. Handbook of Head and Spine Trauma. New York, NY: Marcel Dekker.

Hughes, J. T. 1978. Pathology of the Spinal Cord. 2nd ed. Philadelphia, PA: W. B. Saunders.

Mitsumoto, H. 2000. Disorders of upper and lower motor neurons. In W. G. Bradley, R. B. Daroff, G. M. Fenichel, and C. D. Marsden (Eds.). Neurology in Clinical Practice. 3rd ed., pp. 1985–2015. Boston, MA: Butterworth Heinemann.

Noseworthy, J. H., Lucchinetti, C., Rodriquez, M., and Weinshenker, B. C. 2000. Medical progress: multiple sclerosis. N. Engl. J. Med. 343:938–952.

Rosenblum, R. B. 2000. Disorders of bones, joints, ligaments and meninges. In W. G. Bradley, R. B. Daroff, G. M. Fenichel, and C. D. Marsden (Eds.). Neurology in Clinical Practice. 3rd ed., pp. 1953–1984. Boston, MA: Butterworth Heinemann.

Rowland, L. P. (Ed.). 1989. Merritt's Textbook of Neurology. 8th ed. Philadelphia, PA: Lea & Febiger.

Tarlov, I. M. 1957. Spinal cord compression: mechanisms of paralysis and treatment. Springfield, IL: Charles C. Thomas.

Young, R. R., and Woolsey, R. M. 1995. Diagnosis and Management of Disorders of the Spinal Cord. Philadelphia, PA: W. B. Saunders.

Citations

Baker, A. S., Ojemann, R. O., Swartz, M. N., et al. 1975. Spinal epidural abscess. N. Engl. J. Med. 293:463–468.

Barnes, C. D., and Schadt, J. C. 1979. Release of function in the spinal cord. Prog. Neurobiol. 12:1–13.

Barron, K. D., Hirano, A., Asaki, S., et al. 1959. Experiences with metastatic neoplasms involving the spinal cord. Neurology 9:91–106.

Bauer, H. J. 1978. Problems of symptomatic therapy in multiple sclerosis. Neurology 28:8–20.

Bensimon, G., Lacomblez, L., Meiininger, V., et al. 1994. A controlled-trial of Riluzole in amyotrophic lateral sclerosis. N. Engl. J. Med. 330:385–391.

Bracken, M. B., Shepard, M. J., Collins, W. F., et al. 1990. A randomized controlled trial of methylprednisolone or naloxone in the treat-ment of acute spinal cord injury. N. Engl. J. Med. 322:1406–1411.

Bresnan, M. J., Shoukumas, G. M., and Hedley-White, E. T. 1978. Case records of the Massachusetts General Hospital: a 17-year-old girl with numbness of the right leg, recent onset of vertigo and right-sided weakness. N. Engl. J. Med. 316:150–157.

Brew, B. J., and Price, R. W. 1988. Another retroviral disease of the nervous system: chronic progressive myelopathy due to HTLVI. N. Engl. J. Med. 318:1195–1197.

Brice, J., and McKissock, W. 1978. Surgical treatment of malignant extradural spinal tumors. BMJ. 1:1341–1344.

Brody, I. A., and Wilkins, R. H. 1968. Neurological classics X: Brown-Sequard syndrome. Arch. Neurol. 19:347–348.

Brown, R. H. 1994. Clinical implications of basic research: a transgenic-mouse model of amyotrophic lateral sclerosis. N. Engl. J. Med. 331:1091–1092.

Brown, R. H., Jr. 1993. Inherited motor neuron diseases: recent progress. Semin. Neurol. 13:365–368.

Bryne, T. N. 1992. Current concepts—spinal cord compression from epidural metastases. N. Engl. J. Med. 327:614–619.

Buchan, A. M., and Barnett, H. J. M. 1992. Infarction of the spinal cord. In H. J. M. Barnette, J. P. Mohr, B. M. Stein, and F. M. Yatsu (Eds.). Stroke [Pathophysiology, Diagnosis and Management]. Vol. 2., pp. 707–720. New York, NY: Churchill Livingstone.

Buchan, A. M., and Barnett, H. J. M. 1992. Vascular malformations and hemorrhage of the spinal cord. In H. J. M. Barnett, J. P. Morh, B. M. Stein, and F. M. Yatsu (Eds.). Stroke [Pathophysiology, Diagnosis and Management]. Vol. 2, pp. 721–729. New York, NY: Churchill Livingstone.

Bucy, P., and Perot, P. 1975. Injury to the spinal cord. In D. B. Tower (Ed.). The Nervous System, pp. 421–431. New York, NY: Raven Press.

Calabresi, P. A., Giang, D. W., and Goodman, R. D. 1993. Progressive spinal multiple sclerosis. Semin. Neurol. 13:322–332.

Chad, D., and Richardson, E. P., Jr. 1985. Transverse myelopathy and later development of multiple intracerebral lesions in a 64-year-old man: case records of the Massachusetts General Hospital, #52–1985. N. Engl. J. Med. 13:1646–1656.

Chamberlain, S., Shaw, J., Rowland, S., et al. 1988. Mapping of the mutation causing Friedreich's ataxia to human chromosome. Nature 334:248–250.

Choi, D. W. 1992. Amyotrophic lateral sclerosis and glutamate—too much of a good thing? (Editorial) N. Engl. J. Med. 326:1493–1495.

Collins, W. F., and Chehzazi, B. 1982. Concepts of the acute management of spinal cord injury. In W. B. Matthews and G. H. Glaser (Eds.). Recent Advances in Clinical Neurology, 326: pp. 1494-1496. Edinburgh, UK: Churchill-Livingstone.

Cooper, P. R., and Epstein, F. 1985. Radical dissection of intra-medullary spinal cord tumors in adults: recent experience in 29 patients. J. Neurosurg. 63:492–499.

Corboy, J. R., and Price, R. W. 1993. Myelitis and toxic inflammatory and infectious disorders. Curr. Opin. Neurol. Neurosurg. 6:564–570.

Cruickshank, J. K., Rudge, R., Dalgleish, A. G., et al. 1989. Tropical spastic paraparesis and human T cell lymphotrophic virus Type I in the United Kingdom. Brain 112:1057–1090.

Deng, H. X., Hentati, A., Tainer, J. A., et al. 1993. Amyotrohic lateral sclerosis and structural defects in Cu, Zn superoxide dismutase. Science 261:1047–1050.

Durr, A., Cossee, M., Agig, Y., et al. 1996. Clinical and genetic abnormalities in patients with Friedreichs ataxia. N. Engl. J. Med. 335:1169–1175.

Drucker, T. B. 1990 Treatment of spinal cord injury. (Editorial) N. Engl. J. Med. 322:1459–1461.

Epstein, F. J., Farmer, J. P., and Freed, D. 1992. Adult intramedullary astrocytomas of the spinal cord. J. Neurosurg. 77:355–359.

Epstein, F., and Epstein, N. 1982. Surgical treatment of spinal cord astrocytomas of childhood. J. Neurosurg. 57:685–689.

Foster, J. B. 1975. Syringomyelia. In W. B. Matthews (Ed.). Recent Advances in Clinical Neurology, pp. 234–251. Edinburgh, UK: Churchill Livingstone.

Geisler, F. H., Dorsey, F. C., and Coleman, W. P. 1991. Recovery of motor function after spinal cord injury: a randomized placebo control-led trial with GM-1 ganglioside. N. Engl. J. Med. 324:1829–1838.

Gessian, A., and Gout, O. 1992. Chronic myelopathy associated with human T—lymphocytic virus Type I. (HTLV-I). Ann. Intern. Med. 117:933–946.

Greenberg, H. S., Kim, J. H., and Posner, J. B. 1980. Epidural spinal cord compression from metastatic tumor: results with a new treatment protocol. Ann. Neurol. 8:361–366.

Harding, A. E. 1993. Hereditary spastic paraplegias. Semin. Neurol. 13:333–336.

Harding, A. E. 1981. Friedreich's ataxia: a clinical and genetic study of 90 families with an analysis of early diagnostic criteria and intrafamily clustering of familial features. Brain 104:589–620.

Harding, A. E. 1992. Hereditary ataxias and related disorders. In A. K. Asbury, G. M. McKhann, and W. I. McDonald (Eds.). Diseases of the Nervous System. 2nd ed., pp. 1169–1178. Philadelphia, PA: W. B. Saunders.

Hay, J., and Arvin, A. M. 1994. Varicella zoster virus infection: new insights into pathogenesis and post herpetic neuralgia. Ann. Neurol. 35(Suppl.):S1–S72.

Hollsberg, P., and Lafler, D. A. 1995. What is the pathogenesis of human T cell lymphotrophic virus type I—associated myelo-pathy/ tropical spastic paraparesis. (Editorial) Ann. Neurol. 37:143–145.

Johnson, R. T., and McArthur, J. C. 1987. Myelopathies and retroviral infections. Ann. Neurol. 21:113–116.

Jubelt, B., and Drucker, J. 1993. Post polio syndrome: an update. Semin. Neurol. 13:283–290.

Kiernan, J. A., and Hudson, A. J. 1994. Frontal lobe atrophy in motor neuron disease. Brain 117:747–757.

Kleyn, P. W., and Gillian, T. C. 1993. Progress toward cloning of the gene responsible for childhood spinal muscular atrophy. Semin. Neurol. 13:276–282.

Krauss, W. E., and McCormick, P. C. 1993. Cervical spondylotic myelo-pathy. Semin. Neurol. 13:343–348.

Lindenbaum, S., Heatton, F. B., Savage, D. G., et al. 1988. Neuropsychiatric dis-orders caused by cobalamin deficiency in the absence of anemia or macrocytosis. N. Engl. J. Med. 318:1720–1728.

Logigian, E. L., and Murray, M. B. 1994. Case records of the Massachusetts General Hospital—a 19-year-old man with rapidly progressive lower extremity weakness and dysesthesias after a respiratory tract infection—Case 42–1994. N. Engl. J. Med. 331:1437–1444.

Long, D. M. 1993. Lumbar and cervical spondylosis and spondylotic myelopathy. Curr. Opin. Neurol. Neurosurg. 6:576–580.

Logue, V., and Edwards, M. R. 1986. Syringomyelia and its surgical treatment. J. Neurol. Neurosurg. Psychiat. 44:273.

Mackay, R. P. 1963. Course and prognosis in amyotrophic lateral sclerosis. Arch. Neurol. 8:117–127.

Mandell, G. L., Douglas, R. G., and Bennett, J. E. 1985. Principles and Practice of Infectious Disease. 2nd ed. New York, NY: Wiley.

Marra, C. M. 1995. Neurosyphilis: a guide for clinicians. The Neurologist 1:157–166.

Matthews, W. B. (Ed.). 1991. McAlpine's Multiple Sclerosis. 2nd ed. Edinburgh, UK: Churchill Livingstone.

McAlpine, D. 1961. The benign form of multiple sclerosis. Brain 84:186.

McCormick, P. C. 1993. Spinal vascular malformations. Semin. Neurol. 13:349–358.

Melki, J., Lefebvre, S., Burglen, L., et al. 1994. De novo and inherited deletions of the 5q13 region in spinal muscular atrophies. Science 264:1474–1477.

Mendell, L. M. 1984. Modifiability of spinal synapses. Physio. Rev. 64:260–324.

Mitsumoto, H., Chad, D. D., and Pioro, E. P. 1998. *Amyotrophic Lateral Sclerosis*. Philadelphia, PA: F. A. Davis.

Morier, D. R., Baldelli, P., Delbono, O., et al. 1995. Amyotrophic lateral sclerosis immunoglobulins increase Ca2+currents in a motor neuron line. Ann. Neurol. 37:102–109.

Munsat, T. L., and Bradley, W. C. 1979. In H. R. Tyler and D. M. Dawson (Eds.). Neuromuscular Disease in Current Neurology. 2:79–103. Boston, MA: Houghton Mifflin.

Munsat, T. L., and Golden, J. A. 1992. Case records of the Massachusetts General Hospital—a 70-year-old man with progressive muscle weakness and agitated depression: motor neuron disease. N. Engl. J. Med. 327:1298–1305.

Palav, F., DeMichele, G., Vilcaez, J. J., et al. 1995. Early onset ataxia with cardiomyopathy and retained tendon reflexes—maps to the Friedreich ataxia locus on chromosome 9q. Ann. Neurol. 37:359–362.

Percy, A. K., Nobrega, F. T., and Okazak, H. 1971. Multiple sclerosis in Rochester, Minnesota: a 60 year appraisal. Arch. Neurol. 25:105–111.

Pringle, C. E., Hudson, A. J., Munoz, D. G., et al. 1992. Primary lateral sclerosis: clinical features, neuropathology and diagnostic criteria. Brain 115:495–520.

Rodichok, L. N., Ruickdeschel, J. C., Harper, G. R., et al. 1986. Early detection and treatment of spinal epidural metastases. Ann. Neurol. 20:696–702.

Roman, G. C., Spencer, P. S., and Schoenberg, B. S. 1985. Tropical myelo-neuropathies: the hidden endemics. Neurol. 35:1158–1170.

Ropper, A. H., and Poskanzer, D. C. 1978. The prognosis of acute and subacute transverse myelopathy based on early signs and symptoms. Ann. Neurol. 4:51–59.

Rossier, A. B., Foo, D., Shillito, J., et al. 1985. Post traumatic cervical syringomyelia. Brain 108:439–461.

Rowland, L. P. 1984. Looking for the cause of amyotrophic lateral sclerosis. N. Engl. J. Med. 311:979–981.

Rowland, L. P. 1994a. Amyotrophic lateral sclerosis: theories and therapies. (Editorial) Ann. Neurol. 35:129–130.

Rowland, L. P. 1994b. Riluzole for the treatment of amyotrophic lateral sclerosis—too soon to tell. (Editorial) N. Engl. J. Med. 330:636–637.

Rowland, L. P., Santoro, M., Lange, D. J., et al. 1991. Diagnosis of ALS. Ann. Neurol. 30:225–227.

Rowland, L. P., and Schneier, N. A. 2001. Medical progress: amyotrophic lateral sclerosis. N. Engl. J. Med. 344:1688–1700.

Rubenstein, A. F., Bunge, R. P., and Housman, D. E., et al. (Eds.). 1986. Neurofibromatosis. Ann. NY Acad. Sci. 485:1–414.

Sabin, A. B. 1981. Paralytic poliomyelitis: old dogmas and new perspectives. Rev. Inf. Dis. 3:543–564.

Smith, R. A. (Ed.). 1992. Handbook of Amyotrophic Lateral Sclerosis. New York, NY: Marcel Dekker.

Sorensen, S. V., Mulvihill, J. J., Nielsen, A. 1986. Long term follow-up of Von Recklinghausen neurofibromatosis. N. Engl. J. Med. 314:1010–1015.

Stark, R. J., Henson, R. A., and Evans, J. W. 1982. Spinal metastases: a retrospective study from a general hospital. Brain 105:189–213.

Tandan, R., and Bradley, W. G. 1985. Amyotrophic lateral sclerosis. Ann. Neurol. 18:172–280.

Tramont, E. C. 1991. Syphilis of the central nervous system. In H. P. Lambert (Ed.). Infections of the Central Nervous System, pp. 207–217. Philadelphia, PA: B. C. Decker.

Victor, M., and Rothstein, J. D. 1992. Neurologic manifestations of hepatic and gastrointestinal diseases. In A. K. Asbury, G. M. McKhann, and W. I. McDonald (Eds.). Diseases of the Nervous System. 2nd ed., pp. 1442–1455. Philadelphia, PA: W. B. Saunders.

Walker, M. D. 1991. Acute spinal cord injury. N. Engl. J. Med. 324:1885–1887.

Werteleck, W., Rouleau, G. A., and Superneau, D. W., et al. 1988. Neurofib-romatosis 2: clinical and DNA linkage studies of a large kindred. N. Engl. J. Med. 319:278–283.

Wilkins, R. H., and Brody. I. A. 1967. Neurological classics II: Babinski's sign. Arch. Neurol. 17:441–446.

Wilkins, R. H., and Brody, I. A. 1968. Neurological classics VIII: Romberg's sign. Arch. Neurol. 19:443–447.

Williams, B. 1980. On the pathogenesis of syringomyelia: a review. J. Roy. Soc. Med. 73:798–806.

Williams, D. B., and Windebank, A. J. 1991. Subject review-motor neuron disease (amyotrophic lateral sclerosis). Mayo Clinic Proc. 66:54–82.

Wright, P. F., Kim-Farley, R. J., DeQuadroe, C. A., et al. 1991. Strategies for the global eradication of poliomyelitis by the year 2000. N. Engl. J. Med. 325:1774–1779.

Zervas, N. T., and Pile-Spellman, J. 1992. A 64-year-old woman with the abrupt onset of paraparesis after 10 months of increasing episodic leg weakness: (AVM of spinal cord). N. Engl. J. Med. 326:816–824.

10.
CASE HISTORY PROBLEM SOLVING

PART I: SPINAL CORD, NERVE ROOT, PERIPHERAL NERVE, AND MUSCLE

LESION DIAGRAMS: For each of the following diagrams, indicate the spinal cord structures involved, the clinical symptoms and signs that would be present, and the most likely pathology. That is, name the disease or syndrome (Fig. 10.1 to 10.9).

CASE HISTORIES SPINAL CORD. PART I

Each of the following case histories deals with disease at the level of muscle peripheral nerve root and spinal cord. For each case relevant to spinal cord, be prepared to draw a diagram of the lesion indicating the appropriate spinal cord level, the location of the lesion, and the nature of the pathologic process. If disease of the spinal cord is present, decide whether the process is intrinsic or extrinsic and whether it involves a single-level lesion or is a system disease.

CASE HISTORY 10.1

A 48-year-old white male, while lifting a heavy object, approximately 2 months prior to neurological consultation, had the sudden onset of pain in the posterior cervical area and radiating into the right shoulder, down the posterior aspect of the right arm into the elbow. Coughing or straining at stool resulted in a shooting, burning electric shock–type pain in the above distribution, also extending at times

Figure 10.1

Figure 10.2

Figure 10.3

Figure 10.4

193

Figure 10.5

Figure 10.8

Figure 10.6

Figure 10.9

Figure 10.7

into the index and middle fingers. In association with the pain, he experienced tingling "pins-and-needles" parenthesis in the right upper extremity in a distribution similar to that noted earlier. During this period the patient also noted minor weakness of the right hand. The lower extremities and bladder were not involved. When symptoms persisted, neurological consultation was obtained.

Neurological Examination
Mental status: Intact.
Cranial nerves: II–XII intact.

Motor system:
a. There was significant weakness of the right triceps (50% of normal) with minimal weakness of the right wrist extensor and the finger abductors of the right hand. There was no weakness of the lower extremities.
b. Gait was intact.
c. No definite atrophy was present.
d. Rare fasciculations were noted in the right triceps muscles.

Biceps:	right, 2+; left, 2+
Triceps:	right, 0; left, 2+
Brachioradialis:	right, 1 to 2+; left, 2+
Patellar:	right, 2+; left, 2+
Achilles:	right, 2+; left, 2+

Reflexes:
a. Deep tendon reflexes
b. Plantar responses: right flexor, left flexor.

Sensory system: A minor decrease in pain sensation was present over the right middle finger. Pain, touch, position, and vibratory sensation were otherwise intact.

Neck: There was limitation of neck motion in all directions due to pain. Pressure over the lower cervical spinous processes produced a radiation of pain onto the right upper extremity. There was also local tenderness on pressure over the right supraclavicular area.

QUESTIONS

1. Is the spinal cord directly involved by this lesion? If so, indicate the level. If not, cite evidence against such involvement. Are the anterior roots involved? If so, indicate the level. If not, cite evidence against such involvement. Are the dorsal roots involved? If so, indicate the level. If not, cite evidence against such involvement.
2. What is the localizing significance of the relatively selective weakness of the right triceps muscle?
3. What is the explanation for the occasional fasciculations noted in the right triceps muscle?
4. What is the localizing significance of the selective depression of the triceps deep tendon reflex? Review also the segmental levels involved in the biceps, radial, patellar, and Achilles deep tendon reflexes.
5. What is the localizing significance of the distribution of pain and numbness experienced by the patient?
6. What is the localizing significance of the restricted pain deficit in the right hand?
7. Taking into account the history and the general rule that common problems occur most commonly, indicate the most likely pathology.
8. Why did coughing and straining at stool produce an exacerbation of the pain?
9. How would you manage this problem from the standpoint of treatment, at this point, assuming that no treatment had been rendered previously?
10. Which imaging studies should be obtained and when should these studies be obtained?

Subsequent course: The patient had a reduction in pain and sensory symptoms following the use of cervical traction. Strength improved and the triceps deep tendon reflex returned.

CASE HISTORY 10.2

This 58-year-old white housewife presented with a 7-month history of throbbing mid-thoracic back pain, which at time would radiate to the anterior chest and was aggravated by coughing or by straining at stool. Two months prior to admission, numbness of the right foot was noted, which gradually spread up the leg so that within a 6-week period, a level just below the breast anteriorly and just below the scapula posteriorly was involved. Six weeks prior to admission, a similar ascending numbness of the left foot developed. One month prior to admission, weakness of both lower extremities was noted, the right being weaker than the left. For 2 months, difficulty in control of urination had been present.

General physical examination: Normal.
Neurological Examination
Mental status: Intact,
Cranial nerves: Intact.
Motor system:

a. A bilateral decrease in strength was present at hip, knees, and ankles.
b. Gait was shuffling, possibly spastic.

Reflexes:

a. Deep tendon reflexes were active in the upper extremities, possibly related to a significant degree of anxiety. The patellar reflexes were markedly hyperactive (4+).

b. The plantar response was markedly extensor on the left and borderline on the right.

Sensory system:

a. Pain and temperature sensation were decreased bilaterally below the xiphoid-sternum anteriorly and the T6 spinous process posteriorly. The degree of impairment was greater on the right than the left side.
b. Position sensation was absent at the left toes.
c. Vibratory sensation was absent at the left toes and decreased at the left ankle and knee.

Vertebral percussion tenderness was present over the T3-T5 spinous processes.

Laboratory Data

X-rays: Thoracic spine X-ray was negative.

Chest X-ray was negative.

QUESTIONS

1. This patient has an incomplete example of a more classical syndrome. In your analysis consider the significance of this selective combination of signs and symptoms:

   a. The degree of impairment of pain and temperature sensation was greater on the right side than the left.

   b. Position and vibratory sensation was absent at left toes but intact on the right.

   c. The plantar response was markedly extensor on the left but borderline on the right.

   What is the name of the syndrome?

2. Where is the lesion located? Be specific and indicate basis for your conclusions.
3. Is the pathology intrinsic or extrinsic?
4. Provide a differential diagnosis as to the nature of the pathology and defend your conclusions.
5. What diagnostic studies would you request? When would you obtain those studies?
6. What therapy would you recommend?
7. What type of consultation would you request? When would you obtain this consultation?
8. What results would you expect from therapy?

CASE HISTORY 10.3

This 16-year-old right-handed white female high school student, 7 days prior to admission, awoke with a bilateral sensation of numbness and tingling of teeth and gums. Three days prior to admission, she awoke with numbness of the hands and the plantar surfaces of the feet. On the day prior to admission, she began to experience diffuse weakness of all four limbs and of her face. This worsened over 24 hours.

Past history: This was unremarkable; she did smoke 5-10 cigarettes per day.

General physical examination: Blood pressure was significantly elevated for age (140/90), and with elevated pulse of 116. Temperature was 97.6°F (oral) and respiration, 20. There was mild erythema of the pharynx but no lymphadenopathy.

Neurologic Examination

1. *Mental status and cranial nerves*: normal.
2. *Motor system*: there was diffuse weakness: right upper extremity 3+-4+/5, left upper 5-/5.
   Symmetric weakness was present in lower extremities in the following muscles: iliopsoas 3/5, hamstrings 4/5, gastrocnemius 4/5, anterior tibials 4/5, and extensor hallucis longus 4/5.
3. *Reflexes*: Deep tendon stretch reflexes were everywhere absent. Plantar responses were flexor.
4. *Sensory system*: this intact except for a minimal decrease in pinprick over the soles of the feet.

Laboratory Data

1. *Cerebrospinal fluid (CSF): day of admission*: tube #1; 1800 red blood cells (RBCs), 5 lymphocytes; tube #4: 3 RBCs, 1 lymphocyte. Protein normal: 36 mg%, glucose normal: 70.
   CSF: 1 week after admission: protein: elevated to 92 mg%, no significant cells were present.
2. White blood cells (WBCs): slightly elevated: 12,600.
3. Erythrocyte sedimentation rate (ESR) and antinuclear antibody (ANA) were normal.
4. Monospot and hepatitis A IgM antibody were positive.

Questions

1. Localize the lesion. Is this a problem of spinal cord, peripheral nerve, or muscle?
2. How do you interpret the absence of deep tendon reflexes?
3. How do you interpret the CSF findings?
4. Now be more specific as to the type of pathology: assign a clinical diagnosis. What eponym is assigned to this diagnosis?
5. What would electromyographic (EMG)/nerve conduction studies demonstrate?
6. What would a nerve biopsy demonstrate?
7. How would you manage this case in terms of treatment if clinical findings improved? Note that findings may already have been improving: the bilateral facial weakness of which she had complained was no longer present.
8. What measures should be undertaken if weakness was progressing and respiration was compromised?

CASE HISTORY 10.4

This 47-year-old white male, inspector of small parts, entered the hospital complaining of weakness and numbness in both legs. Five months prior to admission, the patient had noted a burning-type pain extending over the right forearm. Soon thereafter, he became aware of a gradually increasing numbness, pins-and-needles sensation involving his legs; first the right and then the left. This was followed by a weakness of both lower extremities, which increased in severity. Urgency of urination, occasional bowel incontinence, and increasing impotence were also noted.

Neurological Examination
Mental status: Intact.
Cranial nerves: Intact.
Motor system:

a. Strength was intact in the upper extremities but decreased in the lower extremities to 50% of normal. The involvement of the right leg was greater than that of the left leg.

b. A mild degree of spasticity was present at the knees and ankles, with a spastic gait.
c. No atrophy or fasciculations were present.

Reflexes:

a. Deep tendon stretch reflexes at triceps were decreased bilaterally (0 to 1+) compared to biceps and radial periosteal (brachioradialis), which were active (2 to 3+). The patellar and Achilles deep tendon reflexes were all hyperactive (3+ to 4+).
b. Superficial reflexes: bilateral extensor plantar responses were present (bilateral Babinski signs). Abdominal reflexes were decreased bilaterally.

Sensory system:

a. Position sense was defective for gross movements of the great toes bilaterally.
b. Vibratory sensation was markedly decreased below the level of the T7 spinous process.
c. Pain and light-touch sensation were markedly decreased below the level of the umbilicus. Sacral segments were involved. There was also a poorly defined band of decreased pain sensation over the upper thorax. Pain sensation was somewhat greater on the left than on the right.

Laboratory Data

1. *Glucose tolerance test* revealed a diabetic-type curve, with a fasting blood sugar of 122, 30-minute sample of 205, 60-minute sample of 218, and 150-minute sample of 142 mg/100 ml.
2. *Lumbar puncture* revealed a partial dynamic block with the head in extension. CSF protein was elevated to 80 mg/100 ml (normal 45 mg/100 ml).

Questions

1. Indicate the level of the lesion in this case and the structures involved in the pathology.
2. Assuming that the pain in the upper extremities early in the course of the disease had some localizing significance, why was the sensory level for pain present only up to the level of the umbilicus (T10) (that is, pain sensation was absent or decreased below the umbilicus)?
3. Was the pathology in this case intrinsic or extrinsic (compressive) to the spinal cord? Cite the evidence for your conclusions.
4. What diagnostic procedures would you undertake prior to surgery? When should these studies be obtained?
5. Granted that the patient had, among other findings, posterior and lateral column signs, why is the diagnosis of combined system disease unlikely in this case?

Hospital course: Surgery was performed by Dr. Samuel Brendler. Examination two weeks after surgery revealed some return of pain sensation over the thorax, abdomen, and lower extremities. Walking had improved. Evaluation 2 months after surgery indicated continued improvement as regards gait. Position sense had returned to the lower extremities, but vibration sense was still absent.

CASE HISTORY 10.5

This 73-year-old retired executive was referred for evaluation of paresthesias (pins-and-needles sensation and numbness) involving all four extremities. Approximately 8 months previously, while hospitalized for gallbladder surgery, the patient developed a glove-and-stocking distribution of paresthesias involving all four extremities in a symmetric manner. The level of sensory symptoms gradually ascended over the ensuing weeks and months; in the lower extremities, as far as the perineum; in the upper extremities, to the level of the elbows. In the several months prior to admission, the patient had also noted increasing unsteadiness of gait, primarily when attempting to walk in the dark.

Family history: There were several relatives with pernicious anemia but no relatives with neurological disease.

Neurological Examination
Mental status: Intact.
Cranial nerves: Intact.
Motor system:
a. Strength was intact.
b. Gait was broad-based, with unsteadiness on the turns. The degree of ataxia was increased by eye closure.
c. The patient with eyes open and standing on a narrow base was relatively steady. When his eyes were closed, a significant swaying was apparent (Romberg test positive).
d. Cerebellar tests, such as bringing the finger to the nose, when performed with eyes open, were not remarkable.

Reflexes:
a. Deep tendon reflexes were everywhere absent.
b. Plantar responses were extensor bilaterally (bilateral Babinski signs).

Sensory system:
a. Vibratory sensation was absent at the toes and ankles and markedly decreased at the knees and iliac crests in a symmetric manner. There was also a significant decrease at the fingers, with a lesser decrease at the wrists and elbows.
b. Joint position sense was defective for fine-amplitude movements at the toes but elsewhere was intact.
c. Pain and light-touch sensation were intact.

Questions

1. This patient presents a common neurologic syndrome. Indicate the anatomical site or sites of pathology. Present a differential diagnosis and indicate the most likely pathology.
2. Does this patient have a single-level lesion or a system disease?
3. Discuss the diagnostic significance of the sensory symptoms and findings.
4. Explain the absence of deep tendon reflexes.
5. What is the significance of a "positive Romberg sign?"
6. Indicate the significance of bilateral extensor plantar responses (sign of Babinski).
7. Outline what additional tests you would perform to confirm the diagnosis. Indicate the normal values for those tests.
8. What treatment would you undertake? (Be specific.)
9. Consider the apparent paradox; the relatives had pernicious anemia but no neurological findings. This patient had neurological findings but no definite anemia. What is your explanation?
10. Which diagram corresponds to this case?

CASE HISTORY 10.6

This 39-year-old white married airplane mechanic had the gradual onset of muscle weakness approximately 18 months prior to admission. This involved both arms and legs, with greater involvement of the proximal muscles than of the distal muscles. Gradual progression occurred so that 14 months before admission, significant difficulty in walking was experienced. Shortly thereafter, the patient experienced difficulty in swallowing, but this problem improved following his hospitalization the previous year. Weakness of extremity musculature also improved following the use of cortisone. The patient at no time had difficulty in voiding. He had no sensory symptoms; he had had no actual pain or tenderness in the muscles.

Neurologic Examination
Mental status: Intact.
Cranial nerves: Intact.
Motor system: The patient had severe weakness and atrophy of muscles (both proximal and distal) of all four extremities but with clearly more marked involvement of the proximal musculature. The patient was unable to lift his arms above the shoulder and unable to lift his legs off the bed. No fasciculations were present.

Reflexes:
a. Deep tendon stretch reflexes were everywhere absent except at the ankle where normal 2+ reflexes were found.
b. Plantar responses were flexor.

Sensory system: No abnormalities were present.

Laboratory Data

1. Erythrocyte sedimentation rate was elevated to 45 mm/hr.
2. Electromyogram and muscle biopsy were consistent with the clinical diagnosis.

Subsequent course: Following treatment with prednisone in high dosage, the patient had a gradual improvement in strength.

Questions

1. Does this patient have a problem localized to spinal cord, nerve root, peripheral nerve, or muscle?
2. Present a differential diagnosis of this problem and indicate the most likely diagnosis.
3. Outline the expected findings on electromyography and muscle biopsy.
4. Would any other laboratory data be of help in establishing the diagnosis?

ADVANCED CASES

CASE HISTORY 10.7

This 21-year-old single white female was admitted to the hospital because of progressive difficulty in walking. Nearly 4 years before admission, the patient first noted a relatively rapid onset of weakness in the left hand. Three months later, she noted a throbbing pain in the neck that radiated into the left arm and left hand and was accompanied by some numbness (paresthesias) of the fingers of the left hand. Weakness of the left upper extremity slowly progressed and was accompanied by atrophy. Four months before admission, a more rapid progression of left arm symptoms was noted, and weakness of both lower extremities began, initially on the left and to a greater extent than the right. Just before admission, weakness of the right upper extremity was noted. Bladder symptoms were not present.

Neurological Examination
Mental status: Intact.
Cranial nerves: Intact.
Motor system:

a. Severe atrophy of all muscles of the left upper extremity was present, with flexion (claw-hand deformity) contracture.

Fasciculations were present in almost all of the left upper extremity muscle groups. Mild atrophy of the intrinsic muscles of the right hand was also noted.

b. There was weakness of the muscles of the left upper extremity, most marked distally but also involving the shoulder girdle, with a lesser weakness of the muscles of the right upper extremity. Both lower extremities were weak, the left more so than the right.

c. Spasticity was present bilaterally on passive movement at the knees and ankles.

Reflexes:

a. Deep tendon reflexes were depressed in the left upper extremity. The biceps reflex was absent: the triceps and brachial radialis (radial periosteal) reflexes were hypoactive (1+). In the right upper extremity, the biceps reflex was depressed (1+), whereas the triceps was 2+.

In both lower extremities, the patellar and Achilles were hyperactive to a marked degree (4+).

b. Superficial reflexes: Plantar responses were extensor bilaterally. Abdominal reflexes were absent.

Sensory system:

a. Pain and temperature sensation were intact.
b. There was a slight distal decrease in vibratory sensation at the toes, but position sense was intact

Cranium and vertebral column: No local tenderness or abnormalities were present.

Laboratory Data

1. *Cervical spine X-rays* showed bony changes: widening of the spinal canal in anteroposterior and lateral diameters was noted.
2. *Thoracic spine X-rays* showed that kyphoscoliosis was present.
3. *Cerebrospinal fluid* protein was increased to 150 mg/100 ml, but no cells were present.

QUESTIONS

1. Where is the pathology located (be specific)?
2. Present a differential diagnosis. In this case you will need to consider the radiology findings.
3. What is the most likely pathology?
4. What is your diagnostic approach to this patient?
5. Outline your therapeutic approach to this patient.
6. What therapeutic results are expected?

CASE HISTORY 10.8

This 37-year-old white male was evaluated by Dr. Sandra Horowitz for a diagnosis of upper extremity disability. His neurologic history had begun 20 years previously with weakness in both upper extremities. An extensive laminectomy had been performed 19 years earlier by Dr. Bernard Stone.

Neurological Examination
Mental status and cranial nerves: Intact.
Motor system:

a. Severe flaccid weakness was present for voluntary movement in the upper extremities, particularly at the shoulders.
b. Spasticity was present on passive motion of the lower extremities.
c. The gait was also ataxic.

Reflexes:

a. The deep tendon reflexes were absent in the upper extremities but hyperactive in the lower extremities at patella and Achilles.
b. The plantar responses were extensor bilaterally.

Sensation:

a. Pain and temperature were selectively decreased over the shoulder and arms.
b. Other modalities were intact.

Laboratory Data

A magnetic resonance imaging (MRI) scan of the cervical spine was performed.

QUESTIONS

1. What is the significance of the selective decrease in pain and temperature over the shoulders and arms?
2. What would you expect the MRI to demonstrate?
3. Select the appropriate MRI from the group of illustrations below that best corresponds to this case, taking into account both the history and neurological findings.
4. What therapeutic approaches are possible?

11.

FUNCTIONAL ANATOMY OF THE BRAIN STEM

This chapter presents an overview of the anatomy of the brain stem and its relationship to the cerebellum, diencephalon, and cerebrum and describes certain functional centers. Figures 9.1 and 9.2 demonstrate the appearance of the gross brain stem. Examine Atlas Figure 33.9 for a coronal section showing the relationship between the tegmentum and tectum of the brain stem and the ventricular system. The brain stem consists of the medulla, pons, and midbrain (Figs. 11.1 and 11.2). Figure 11.1 is an illustration of the main features of the gross brain, while Figure 11.2 compares the appearance of the gross brain to that of the brain in situ in a magnetic resonance image (MRI) from a living patient. We will first start at the medullospinal junction and then discuss several levels of the medulla, pons, and midbrain. The discussion of each level will include the important functions, nuclei, and tracts found in that level. The medulla, pons, and midbrain are subdivided by their relationship to the ventricular system. One division, the tectum, forms the roof and walls or the posterior surface; the other division, the tegmentum, forms the floor or anterior surface. The basis forms the anterior surface of the tegmentum.

The tectum in medullary, pontine, and midbrain levels consists of regions that have highly specialized functions related to the special senses and movement. The tegmentum contains cranial nerve nuclei, the reticular formation, and tracts that interconnect higher and lower centers, as well as tracts that interconnect the brain stem with other portions of the central nervous system. The basis consists of the descending fibers from the cerebral cortex to the brain stem, cerebellum, and spinal cord. Table 11.1 lists the general contents of each region of the brain stem.

TEGMENTUM

The tegmentum of the brain stem (medulla, pons, and midbrain), where the sensory and motor nuclei of Cranial Nerves III–XII are located, is continuous (Figs. 11.1 and 11.2), and it can be divided functionally into five zones: ventricular, lateral, medial, central, and basilar. This is done to help the student understand the basic plan of the brain stem. Each half of the brain stem can be visualized as an apple, with the core being the reticular formation and the pulp formed by the four surrounding zones (Figs. 11.3A–C; Table 11.2).

FUNCTIONAL LOCALIZATION IN CORONAL SECTIONS OF THE BRAIN STEM

The previous chapters on the brain stem have discussed gross anatomy and cranial nerves. In this section, we will discuss the functional anatomy of the brain stem by examining coronal sections at representative levels through the medulla, pons, and midbrain. Each level will contain the following illustrations:

A—a myelinated section with the nuclei and tracts labeled on the outline that follows.

B—an MRI at a similar level. (Please remember that the MRI is from a living patient, whereas the brain sections were obtained from postmortem examination.)

Although the discussion in this chapter of each level is confined to the coronal section under examination, it should be noted that most nuclei and all tracts extend through more than just one level. Therefore, when reading this section, the student should keep in mind the origin and destination of structures identified in each of these sections. It is especially important that the student understand the function and clinical importance of the anatomical structures.

The cranial nerve nuclei and many pathways (e.g., corticospinal, corticonuclear, and spinothalamic) in the brain stem are clinically important because any functional abnormality in these systems helps to identify where the disease process is occurring in the central nervous system.

DIFFERENCES BETWEEN THE SPINAL CORD AND BRAIN STEM

The interior gray matter and exterior white matter of the spinal cord gradually change to a mixture of gray and white matter in the brain stem. Table 11.3 identifies the nuclei and tracts in the spinal cord and lists their functional equivalents in the brain stem. The student should be aware that the development of the cerebellum, midbrain, and cerebrum has greatly affected the neural contents of the many nuclei and tracts (for example, the following nuclei—inferior olive of the medulla, pontine gray of the pons, red nucleus and substantia nigra of the midbrain, and the corticonuclear and corticopontine tracts).

Table 11.1 **REGIONS IN THE BRAIN STEM**

REGION	CONTENTS
Tectum (roof) posterior surface of brain stem	Cerebellum for medulla and pons over IV ventricle; superior and inferior colliculi for midbrain
Tegmentum (floor) floor of IV ventricle and cerebral aqueduct	Cranial nerve nuclei and all ascending and descending tracts except for tracts in basis
Basis—anterior surface of brain stem	Corticospinal, corticonuclear, and corticopontine tracts

Figure 11.1 Gross appearance of the brain stem, diencephalon, and basal ganglia. (*A*) Ventral surface of brain stem and diencephalon demonstrating prominent medulla, pons and the midbrain with the cerebral peduncle, and the rootlets of cranial nerves II-XII. (*B*) Dorsal/posterior surface of the brain stem, diencephalon, third ventricle with pineal gland and basal ganglia. Note the prominent funiculi of the trigeminal, gracile and cuneate systems, in the medulla, and the cerebellar peduncles in the pons, and the open IV ventricle. Note the rootlets of the only cranial nerve seen on the posterior surface of the brain stem, Cranial nerve IV.

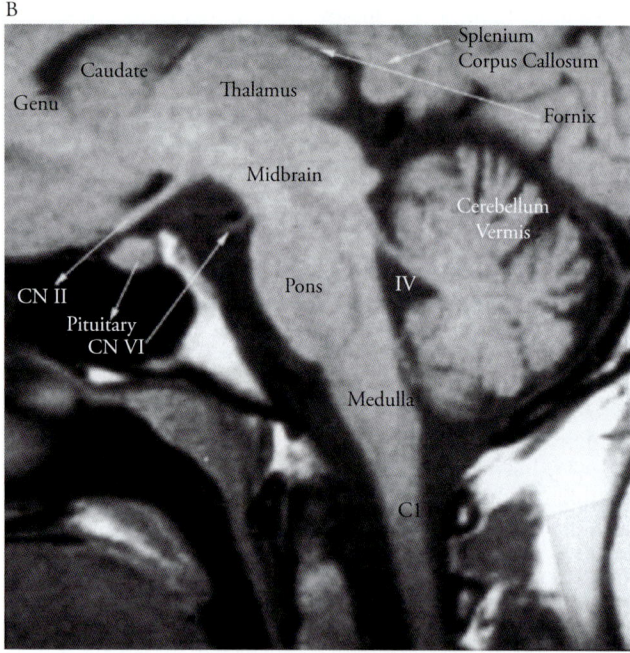

Figure 11.2 The regions of the brain stem. Sagittal magnetic resonance imaging, T1 weighted. (*A*) Gross view of the brain stem in sagittal section of the brain demonstrating medial surface of hemisphere, corpus callosum, diencephalon, brain stem, and cerebellum. (*B*) Magnetic resonance imaging. Sagittal section of brain stem with thalamus, cerebellum and IV ventricle, cerebral aqueduct and cranial nerves II and VI, and pituitary in sellae.

MEDULLA

Blood Supply: Vertebral Arteries and Their Branches

The first level we have included is at the sensory and motor decussation (Fig. 11.4). This section has mostly spinal cord elements, the ventral horns, and the three white matter columns; however, one can also note brain stem elements—the gracile and cuneate nuclei. This region is the transitional zone and the region is the size and shape of the spinal cord. As we move up the brain stem, we come to the widened medulla with the opening of the fourth ventricle.

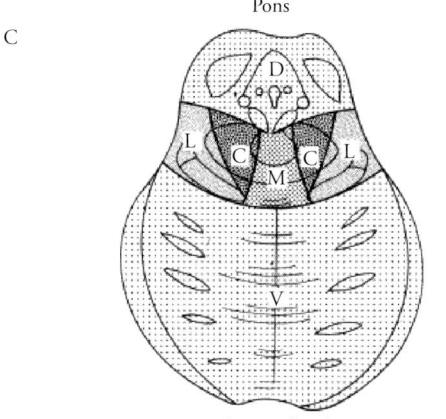

Figure 11.3 Regions in the brain stem, coronal sections; (*A*) medulla; (*B*) pons; and (*C*) midbrain.

The brain stem tegmentum and the gray and white matter appear intermingled; however, there is a basic organization of the tracts in the brain stem zones, as shown in Table 11.4.

Gross Landmarks in the Medulla

The tegmentum of the medulla has two distinct levels, a narrow lower portion, which is similar to the spinal cord, and a broader upper portion, which includes the landmarks that are a hallmark of this level: the medullary pyramids and the inferior olivary prominence.

Level: Spinomedullary Junction with Motor Decussation

Gross Features

This level resembles the spinal cord as the dorsal columns are conspicuous; the trigeminal funiculus is more laterally placed. On the anterior surface of the spinal cord, the medullary pyramids containing the corticospinal tracts are evident (Fig. 11.4A). Note that the descending pathway on the right side has first crossed (decussated) with the fibers, shifting from the anterior surface of the medulla, then entered the lateral funiculus of the spinal cord. The narrow spinal canal is present in the gray matter above the pyramidal decussation. (It has been reported that the corticospinal tract from the dominant hemisphere for movement, the left hemisphere, in over 90% of us, crosses as a unit, as evident here, while the corticospinal tract from the nondominant hemisphere trickles over slowly. The photograph in the medullary spinal junction seems to suggest that is what is going on here, but we had no data to confirm the handedness of this patient.)

Motor Cranial Nerve Nuclei

Only the cranial portion of nerve XI is present at the lateral margin of the reticular formation (Fig. 11.4A). It innervates the sternocleidomastoids and reached their maximum bulk with the addition of the last of the fibers from the uppermost cervical levels. The somatotopic arrangement of the tactile fibers in the posterior column is as follows: the most medial fibers are sacral, then come the lumbar, thoracic, and most laterally, cervical fibers.

Spinothalamics/Anterolateral Column

Pain and temperature from the extremities, abdomen, thorax, pelvis, and neck are carried by the lateral spinothalamic tract located at the lateral surface of the medulla. Light touch from the extremities, thorax, abdomen, pelvis, and neck is carried via the anterior spinothalamic tract, which is seen on the surface of the medulla just posterior to the corticospinal tract. In the spinothalamic pathways sacral fibers are on the outside while cervical fibers are on the inside. The dorsal and ventral spinocerebellar tracts are found in the lateral funiculus. The rubrospinal and tectospinal tracts, which are important in supporting voluntary trapezius muscles that rotate the head and elevate the shoulders, respectively.

Sensory Cranial Nerve Nuclei

The primary axons convey pain and temperature from the head and neck and are located in the spinal tract of the fifth cranial nerve; these fibers have descended from the pons (Fig. 11.4A). The second-order axons originate from the underlying descending nucleus and their axons cross and then ascend contralaterally to the ventral posterior medial nucleus of the thalamus. The nucleus lateral to the pyramidal tract is the inferior reticular nucleus, a portion of the reticular formation.

White Matter

At this level the tracts are still in the same positions as in the spinal cord. Tactile discrimination (fine touch, pressure, vibration sensation, and two-point discrimination) and proprioception from the extremities, thorax, abdomen, pelvis, and neck are carried via the dorsal columns. The nuclei can now be seen that are the 2° neurons in this pathway, the gracile and cuneate nuclei. The gracile and cuneate tracts (fasciculi) have motor movements and are found in the lateral funiculus and near the midline in the medullary and pontine levels.

Table 11.2 **THE FIVE ZONES IN THE TEGMENTUM**

ZONE	GRAY MATTER	WHITE MATTER
Ventricular	Medulla: nuclei of CN XII and vagal (X) trigones, IX, V, solitary nucleus, vestibular and cochlear nerves of VIII and nuclei Pons: nuclei of CN V, VI, and VII median eminence with facial colliculus Midbrain: nuclei of CN III and IV, V, red nucleus	All levels: descending autonomics. Medulla: solitary tract
Lateral	Inferior olive—medulla Descending nucleus of V—medulla, pons C1-C3	All levels: spinothalamic and rubrospinal Medulla: spinocerebellars, trigeminal afferents, inferior cerebellar peduncle Pons: lateral lemniscus Midbrain: lateral lemniscus and medial lemniscus
Medial	Reticular formation, raphe nuclei	All levels: medial longitudinal fasciculus and raphe nuclei tectospinal Medulla: medial lemniscus
Central/core	Reticular formation central and lateral nuclei Medulla: ambiguous nucleus of IX, X–XII; descending pons: motor nucleus of V, facial nucleus, parapontine nucleus. Midbrain: red nucleus and substantia nigra	Ascending and descending reticular tracts; descending autonomics from hypothalamus
Basilar	Medulla: arcuate Pons: pontine nuclei	Medulla: pyramid. Pons: inferior and middle cerebellar peduncle Midbrain: cerebral peduncle

Level: Lower Medulla at Sensory Decussation

Gross Features

At this level the fourth ventricle narrows. The funiculus gracilis and the funiculus cuneatus are conspicuous on the posterior surface of the spinal canal, while the medullary pyramids are prominent on the anterior surface (Fig. 11.5A and B).

Ventricular Zone

Motor Cranial Nerve Nuclei

This section contains the inferior extent of the hypoglossal nerve (XII) and the dorsal motor nucleus of the vagus nerve (X, Fig. 11.5A). The hypoglossal nucleus innervates the intrinsic and extrinsic musculature of the tongue, while the dorsal motor nucleus of the vagus nerve provides parasympathetic preganglionic innervation of the viscera. This level marks the superior extent of the cranial portion of the eleventh cranial nerve in the ambiguus nucleus.

Sensory Cranial Nerve Nuclei

Pain and temperature from the head are conveyed by the descending nucleus and tract of nerve V that is prominent anterior to the cuneate nucleus. Note that myelinated ipsilateral primary axons are on the outside of the second-order neurons, while the second-order neurons are leaving the inner surface of the nucleus, crossing and entering the medial lemniscus, forming the trigeminothalamic (quintothalamic) tract.

Table 11.3 **GRAY AND WHITE MATTER EQUIVALENTS IN SPINAL AND BRAIN STEM STRUCTURES**

REGION OF SPINAL CORD	EQUIVALENT REGION OF BRAIN STEM
Dorsal (sensory) horn	Ventricular zone, lateral region with sensory cranial nerves VII, IX, X; lateral zone cranial nerve V
Ventral (motor) horn	Ventricular zone, medial Motor cranial nerves—III–VI, X–XII Reticular formation with motor nuclei of cranial nerves V, VII, IX, and X
Intermediate zone	Reticular formation and associated nuclei
Sympathetic intermediolateral cell column T1–T11, L1 and L2 parasympathetic cell column S2–S4	Parasympathetic nuclei of cranial nerves III, VII, IX, and X
Lateral column = corticospinal/crossed, rubrospinal, spinothalamic	Basilar zone = corticospinal/not crossed Lateral zone = spinothalamic and rubrospinal
Posterior column = uncrossed gracile and cuneate fasciculi	Medial lemniscus = crossed tactile information
Anterior column = medial longitudinal fasciculus, vestibulospinal, reticulospinal, spinothalamic	Medial zone = medial longitudinal fasciculus, lateral zone vestibulospinal, tectospinal, reticular formation, reticulospinal, lateral zone vestibulospinal

Table 11.4 MAJOR TRACTS IN TEGMENTAL ZONES

Ventricular zone	Solitary tract and autonomic tracts
Medial zone	Medial longitudinal fasciculus, tectospinal, medial lemniscus
Lateral zone	Spinothalamic, rubrospinal, cerebellar peduncles, and lateral lemniscus. Medial lemniscus enters this zone in pons and midbrain.
Central core	Descending autonomics and central tegmental tract
Basilar zone	Corticospinal and corticonuclear

Figure 11.4 Brain stem at transition level between cervical spinal cord and medullar-sensory decussation. Coronal lateral zone.

White Matter

Pain and temperature from the extremities, thorax, abdomen, pelvis, and neck are carried via the lateral spinothalamic tract. The spinothalamic are located in the lateral funiculus throughout the spinal cord and brain stem.

The anterior spinothalamic tract is adjacent to the lateral spinothalamic tract. The tract carrying unconscious proprioception from the upper extremity originates from the external cuneate nucleus and its fibers enter the cerebellum through the posterior spinocerebellar tract. The function of this nucleus is similar to that of Clark's column in the spinal cord. The vestibulospinal tract is found internal to the spinothalamic tracts. The dorsal and ventral spinocerebellar tracts are seen on the surface of the medulla covering the spinal tract of nerve V and the spinothalamic tracts. The rubrospinal tract is an important afferent relay to the alpha and gamma neurons in the spinal cord. It originates from the red nucleus in the tegmentum of the midbrain, crosses the midline, and descends. It is found in the lateral funiculus of the medulla internal to the spinocerebellar tract and anterior to spinal portion of nerve V throughout the pons and medulla. It is important in postural reflexes. The tectospinal tract is phylogenetically an old tract, being the equivalent of the corticospinal tract in nonmammalian vertebrates. It originates from the deep layers of the superior colliculus and to some extent from the inferior colliculus. It is seen anterior to the medial longitudinal fasciculus throughout the medulla, pons, and midbrain and is important in coordinating eye movements and body position.

Medial Zone

The medial lemniscus is the largest pathway in the medial zone. However, as we progress superiorly in the brain stem, these fibers migrate laterally to finally enter the lateral zone in the midbrain. This migration is necessary for the medial lemniscus to be correctly positioned as it enters the thalamus.

Tactile discrimination and proprioception are conveyed from the extremities, thorax, abdomen, pelvis, and neck by the axons in the fasciculus gracilis and cuneatus. The nucleus gracilis and the nucleus cuneatus form the second-order neurons in this pathway and are conspicuous in this section.

Internal arcuate fibers are seen leaving the inner surface of the gracile and cuneate nuclei, curving around the ventricular gray, crossing the midline (sensory decussation), and accumulating behind the pyramid and beginning the formation of one of the major ascending highways, the medial lemniscus. The serotonin-containing raphe nucleus of the reticular formation is found in this zone throughout the brain stem. The medial longitudinal fasciculus is located in the midline of the tegmentum just below the hypoglossal nucleus and above the tectospinal and medial lemniscal pathways. In all levels of the brain stem it will be in this subventricular position.

Central Zone

The central core of the medulla, pons, and midbrain consists of the reticular formation, which is important for many vital reflex activities and for the level of attentiveness.

Basilar Zone

This level contains the corticospinal fibers just before they cross in the medullospinal junction. Note that the pyramidal system is named for the passage of the corticospinal fibers through this pyramidal-shaped region, respectively (Fig. 11.5 A,B). One of the important concepts from this section is that axons that form the volitional motor pathway, pyramidal system, originate in the cerebral cortex. These tracts are located in the basis of the brain stem and include the corticospinal and corticonuclear fibers that run in the medullary pyramid. Motor system fibers that do not run in the medullary pyramid are considered extrapyramidal (e.g., cerebellar peduncles, rubrospinal tectospinal, etc.) The location of the major structures in the tegmentum of the medulla is listed in Table 11.5.

Figure 11.5 Brain stem at lower medullary level. Coronal section. (*A*) Mylein and diagrammatic labels. (*B*) MRI.

Table 11.5 **MAJOR TRACTS AND NUCLEI IN MEDULLARY TEGMENTAL ZONES**

Ventricular zone: Cranial nerve nuclei of VIII, X, and XII (motor nuclei medial; sensory lateral) solitary nucleus and tract

Lateral zone: Cranial nerve rootlets exit in relation to the inferior olive with the XII nerve anterior to the olive and the rootlets of IX, X, and XI posterior to the olive. Rootlets for VIII exit in the cerebellopontine angle.
Tracts: Inferior cerebellar peduncle, spinothalamic, rubrospinal; nuclei: external cuneate, descending nuclei and tract of V

Medial zone: Nuclei—raphe or medial reticular
Tracts = medial longitudinal fasciculus, tectospinal, medial lemniscus

Central zone: Nuclei of reticular formation, ambiguous nuclei of IX–XI, inferior olivary complex
Tracts: central tegmental tract, the major ascending reticular pathway

Medullary basis: Tracts contains corticospinal and corticonuclear tracts in medullary pyramid

Level: Inferior Olive of the Medulla

Gross Features

At this level the medullary tegmentum expands laterally with the prominent inferior olive located behind the pyramids. The floor of the fourth ventricle contains the median eminence and the vestibular and cochlear tubercles. The median eminence consists of aqueductal gray, while the vestibular tubercle is formed by the medial vestibular nucleus and the descending root and nucleus of cranial nerve VIII. The dorsal cochlear nucleus forms the cochlear tubercle. The ventricle at this level is at its widest extent (Figs. 11.6A and 11.6B). The sulcus limitans in the ventricular floor separates the medially placed motor cranial nuclei from the laterally placed sensory cranial nuclei.

Ventricular Zone

Motor Cranial Nerve Nuclei

This level marks the superior extent of nerve XII and the dorsal motor nucleus of nerve X. The ambiguous nucleus in the lateral margin of the reticular formation contains cell bodies innervating the pharynx and larynx (nerve X, Fig. 11.6A).

Lateral Zone

Sensory Cranial Nerve Nuclei

a. Trigeminal. Pain and temperature are conveyed from the face by nerve V. The descending nucleus and tract of cranial nerve V are nearly obliterated by the olivocerebellar fibers.

b. Solitary tract and nucleus. Taste and visceral sensations are found in the solitary nucleus and tract in the tegmental gray below the medial vestibular nucleus. Fibers from cranial nerves VII, IX, and X ascend and descend in this tract, carrying general sensations from the viscera (nerve X) and gustatory sensations from the taste buds in the tongue (nerves VII and IX) and epiglottis (nerve X).

c. Vestibular. The medial and descending vestibular nuclei are present with first-order axons (Fig. 11.6B) found in the

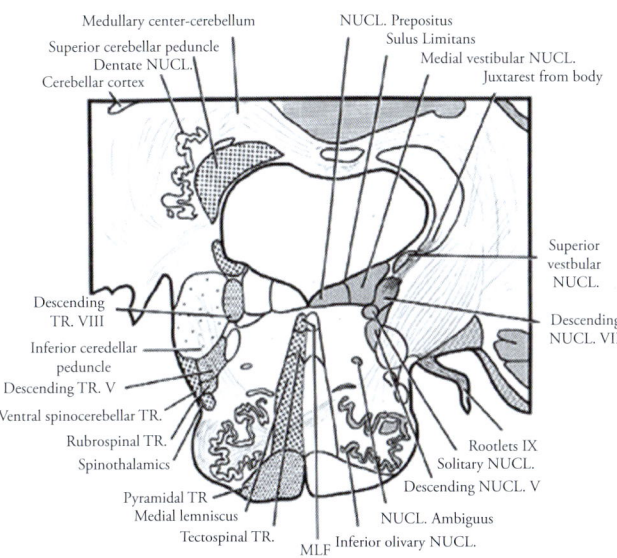

descending root of cranial nerve VIII, interstitial to the descending nucleus. Fibers may be seen running from the vestibular nuclei into the medial longitudinal fasciculus.

d. Auditory. The dorsal and ventral cochlear nuclei are second-order nuclei in the auditory pathway and receive many terminals from the cochlear portion of nerve VIII seen within its borders.

Cerebellar

The conspicuous inferior olivary nucleus in the anterior portion of the medullary tegmentum consists of the large main nucleus and the medial and dorsal accessory nuclei. The entire complex is important in supplying information to the cerebellum. Removal of the olive in animals produces contralateral increase in tone and rigidity in the extremities, with concomitant uncoordinated movements. The olive connects to the contralateral cerebellar hemispheres via the inferior cerebellar peduncle. The climbing fibers found on the dendrites of Purkinje's cells in the cerebellum originate in the inferior olive. The olive also has strong connections with the red nucleus and receives input from the spinal cord, cerebellum, red nucleus, intralaminar nuclei, and basal ganglia. The central core of this section, as in other levels, consists of neurons of the reticular formation.

Medial Zone

The serotonergic raphe nuclei of the reticular formation are found in this zone. The position of the MLF, tectospinal and medial lemniscus corresponds to that in the previous level (Fig. 11.6A).

Basilar Zone

The medullary pyramids are prominent at this level. The rootlets of cranial nerve XII exit lateral to the pyramid (Figs. 11.6A and B).

LEVEL: LOWER PONS AT LEVEL OF FACIAL NERVE AND FACIAL COLLICULUS

Ventricle Equivalent Level MRI

PONS

Figure 11.6 Brain stem at mid-medullary level. Coronal section.

Blood Supply—Basilar Artery and Its Branches Cross Landmarks

The hallmark of pontine levels is the prominent basis ponti that is present on the anterior surface. The cerebellum forms the posterior surface. The tegmentum takes up much less of these levels due to the massive enlargement of the pontine basis. With the cerebellum removed the posterior surface of the tegmentum demonstrates the three cerebellar peduncles (see Fig. 1.15): inferior cerebellar peduncle, middle cerebellar peduncle, and superior cerebellar peduncle—posterior surface and the fourth ventricle is now opened.

Gross Features

The bulk of this section consists of the middle cerebellar peduncle brachium pontis and the cerebellum. In Figure 11.7 the bulk of the cerebellum has been removed. The fourth

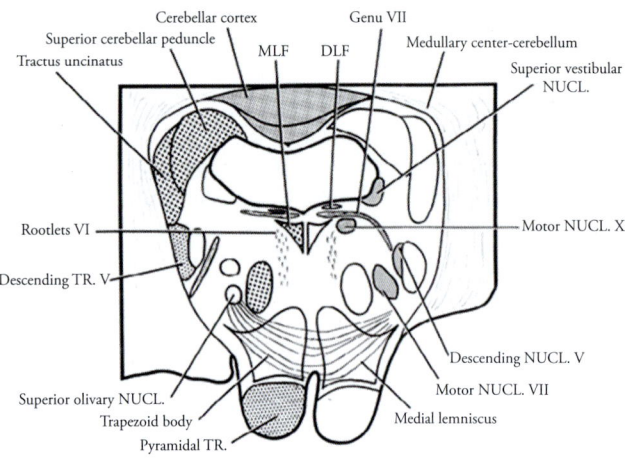

Figure 11.7 Brain stem at pontine level of cranial nerve VII. Coronal section.

ventricle narrows as it nears the cerebral aqueduct. The medullary pyramids are present at the anterior surface. Note that the inferior olive is no longer present.

VENTRICULAR ZONE

MOTOR CRANIAL NERVE NUCLEI

1. The nucleus of nerve VII is conspicuous at the lateral margin of the tegmentum. This nucleus innervates the muscles of facial expression. In the pons, in close proximity to the ventricular floor, the rootlet of this nucleus swings around the medial side of the nucleus of nerve VI, forming the internal genu of nerve VII. These fibers then pass lateral to the nucleus of nerve VII and exit from the substance of the pons on the anterior surface in the cerebellopontine angle (Fig. 11.7B).

2. The nucleus of nerve VI innervates the lateral rectus muscle of the eye. The rootlet leaves the anterior surface of the nucleus and has the longest intracerebral path of any nerve root. The fibers finally exit on the anterior surface of the brain stem near the midline at the pontomedullary junction. The close proximity of the nucleus of nerve VI to the rootlets of nerve VII demonstrates why any involvement of the nucleus of nerve VI usually produces a concomitant alteration in function of nerve VII. The nucleus of nerve VI and the internal genu of the rootlets of nerve VII form the prominent facial colliculus on the floor of the fourth ventricle.

Cerebellar Pathways

At this level the middle and inferior cerebellar peduncles form the lateral walls of the ventricle as well as the bulk of the cerebellar medullary center (Fig. 11.7B). The ventral spinocerebellar tract is seen lateral to the superior cerebellar peduncle that it enters and then follows back into the cerebellum. The superior cerebellar peduncle consists primarily of axons carrying impulses from the dentate nucleus of the cerebellum to the red nucleus and the ventral lateral nucleus in the thalamus. This tract is also called the dentatorubrothalamic tract. The tractus uncinatus connects the deep cerebellar nuclei with the vestibular nuclei and reticular formation bilaterally.

LATERAL ZONE

Sensory Cranial Nerve Nuclei

Pain and temperature are conveyed from the head (Fig. 11.7B). At pontine levels the descending nucleus of nerve V is small, while the tract is large. The superior vestibular nucleus is seen at the lateral margin of the ventricle with primary vestibular fibers present in its substance.

Auditory sensation at this level is related to the superior olive that is seen inferior to the motor nucleus of nerve VII. The superior olive is one of the secondary nuclei in the auditory pathway. The auditory fibers are seen accumulating inferior to the superior olive and cutting through the medial lemniscus to form the lateral lemniscus.

White Matter

At this pontine level, some of the ascending tracts are starting to move more laterally (Fig. 11.7B). The medial lemniscus will shift laterally and approach the rubrospinal and spinothalamic tracts.

Tactile discrimination and proprioception from the limbs, thorax, pelvis, abdomen, and neck are conveyed by fibers in the medial lemniscus, which is seen posterior to the corticospinal tract. Pain and temperature from the head are conveyed by the secondary trigeminothalamic tracts, which are found in the medial lemniscus and ascend to the nucleus ventralis posteromedialis in the thalamus.

Pain and temperature from the extremities, thorax, abdomen, pelvis, and neck are carried in the lateral spinothalamic tract, which is near the anterior surface of the pons, close to the medial lemniscus.

The anterior spinothalamic tract that is mixed in with the lateral spinothalamic tract carries light touch.

The gustatory fibers from the tongue are found in the solitary tract. The secondary fibers ascend bilaterally in the medial lemniscus. Fibers carrying visceral sensations also synapse in the solitary nucleus.

MEDIAL ZONE

The raphe or the medial reticular nuclei are present in this level. The medial lemniscus at this level contains secondary fibers from the dorsal columns and the spinothalamic, trigeminothalamic, and solitary tracts. The medial longitudinal fasciculus and tectospinal tracts are still present near the midline in the floor of the fourth ventricle with the medial longitudinal fasciculus conspicuous under the floor and the tectospinal tract below it.

CENTRAL ZONE

In the center of the pontine tegmentum, the main efferent ascending tract of the reticular system, the central tegmental tract, occupies the bulk of the reticular formation (Figs. 11.7A and 11.7B). The rootlet of cranial nerve V and motor nucleus of nerve internal to the nucleus of VI is the parapontine reticular nucleus that coordinates eye movements.

Cranial nerve V is conspicuous bilaterally near the entering rootlet of nerve V. Each of these nuclei provides innervation to the ipsilateral muscles of mastication.

BASILAR ZONE

The descending corticospinal and corticonuclear pathways are nearly obscured by the fibers of the middle cerebellar peduncle and the pontine gray (Fig. 11.7B). Table 11.6 reviews the contents of the pontine tegmentum.

LEVEL: UPPER PONS AT THE MOTOR AND MAIN SENSORY NUCLEI OF NERVE V

GROSS LANDMARKS

The bulk of this section consists of the middle cerebellar peduncle and cerebellar cortex. The fourth ventricle begins to narrow as it nears the cerebral aqueduct (Fig. 11.8).

VENTRICULAR ZONE

In this level there are no somatic motor cranial nerve nuclei on the floor of the ventricle. With the nuclei in the ventricular floor being for visceral functions.

Table 11.6 **MAJOR CONTENTS OF TEGMENTAL ZONES OF THE PONS**

Ventricular zone: Nuclei = Median eminence with facial colliculus (nucleus of VI), superior vestibular nucleus of VIII

Lateral zone: Nuclei = main sensory of V, descending of V; tracts—spinal of V and spinothalamic and rubrospinal

Central zone: Nuclei reticular formation, facial nucleus, parapontine reticular nucleus, superior olive and lateral lemniscus
Tracts crossing of lateral lemniscal nucleus of cochlea

Medial zone: Nuclei = Raphe nuclei of the reticular formation.
Tracts = medial longitudinal fasciculus, tectospinal, crossing auditory fibers, medial lemniscus

Basilar zone: Middle cerebellar peduncle with pontine gray that forms the bulk of the pons at these levels.
Tracts: Corticobulbar from frontal eye fields, synapse here and then connect via the medial longitudinal fasciculus to the nuclei of IV and III.

LATERAL ZONE

Motor Cranial Nerve Nuclei

Muscles of mastication (Fig. 11.8A).

Sensory Cranial Nerve Nuclei

Tactile discrimination from the face is carried by the trigeminal root into the main sensory nucleus of nerve V, seen lateral to the intrapontine root of nerve V (Fig. 11.8A). The secondary fibers originate from this nucleus and ascend crossed and uncrossed. The crossed fibers run adjacent to the medial lemniscus (ventral trigeminothalamic), while the uncrossed fibers run in the dorsal margin of the reticular formation (dorsal trigeminothalamic). Both fiber pathways terminate in the ventral posterior medial nucleus of the thalamus.

Proprioception from the majority of the muscles of mastication, facial expression, and those that innervate the motor nuclei of III, IV, and VI in the head is carried in by the mesencephalic root and ends in the mesencephalic nucleus of nerve V, located lateral to the walls of the fourth ventricle in the upper pontine and midbrain levels. Note cranial nerves V and VII in the MRI in Figure 11.8B. These neurons are the only primary cell bodies (dorsal root ganglion equivalent) in the central nervous system. These axons synapse on the chief nucleus of V. The jaw jerk is a monosynaptic stretch reflex. The sensory receptor is in the mesencephalic nucleus of nerve V and the effector is the motor nucleus of nerve V. The superior olive is one of the nuclei in the auditory system. Auditory fibers are seen running through the superior olive or inferior to it, cutting through the medial lemniscus and crossing the midline, forming the trapezoid body. The fibers are then found lateral to the medial lemniscus and are known as the lateral lemniscus. The pontine nuclei are conspicuous in the basilar portion of the pons.

White Matter

At this level the medial lemniscus has moved from the midline to a more lateral position, and many of the ascending sensory systems are now either in the medial lemniscus or adjacent to it (Fig. 11.8A).

MEDIAL ZONE

The raphe nuclei of the reticular formation are evident in this level. In this section the midbrain forms the roof and floor of the narrow cerebral aqueduct, while the pons makes up the basilar portion. The roof is the inferior colliculus, an important nucleus in the auditory pathway.

TECTUM

INFERIOR COLLICULUS

The gray matter of the inferior colliculus forms the tectum at this level (Figs. 11.9A and 11.9B). The inferior colliculus is divided into three nuclei, a large central nucleus, and a thin dorsal nucleus, the paracentral or cortical nucleus, and an external nucleus. The central and cortical nucleus functions as a relay.

Central Zone

In the reticular formation the central tegmental tract is conspicuous. The external cochlear nucleus functions for the acusticomotor reflexes through the tectospinal pathway. The brachium of the inferior colliculus carries auditory information onto the medial geniculate nucleus of the diencephalon. The tectospinal pathway descends from this region and terminates on motor nuclei of the lower cranial nerves and upper cervical ventral horn cells.

Basilar Zone

The corticospinal tract is found in the pontine gray and white matter.

MIDBRAIN

BLOOD SUPPLY: BASILAR ARTERY AND POSTERIOR CEREBRAL ARTERIES

Gross Landmarks

On the anterior surface of the midbrain we find the principal landmark of this level, the cerebral peduncles with the third cranial nerve exiting from the medial surface of the cerebral peduncles in the interpeduncular fossa. On the posterior surface of the midbrain we find the corpora quadragemini and the superior and inferior colliculi. The fourth cranial nerve exits from the posterior surface of the midbrain and the junction with the pons. In a coronal section through the midbrain one finds the red nucleus in the tegmentum of the midbrain (Fig. 11.9B). Also in the inferior levels in the tegmentum just before the red nucleus one finds the crossing of the superior cerebellar peduncle.

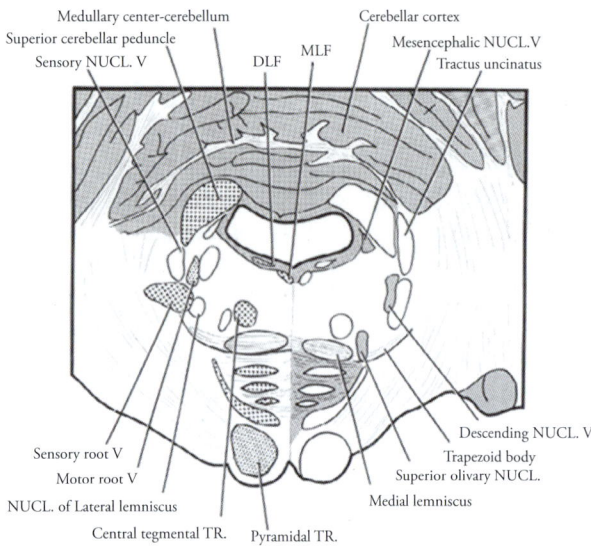

LEVEL: INFERIOR COLLICULUS AND PONTINE BASIS TEGMENTUM

VENTRICULAR ZONE

The periaqueductal gray is conspicuous in midbrain levels (Figs. 11.9A and 11.9B). Descending and ascending tracts associated with the visceral brain are found here. In the midbrain, the lower half of the periaqueductal gray and some other nuclei in the tegmentum are part of the midbrain limbic area. This zone is important in our level of attentiveness. Bilateral lesions to the periaqueductal gray and midbrain tegmentum usually produce comatose patients.

Motor Cranial Nerve Nuclei

The nucleus of cranial nerve IV is seen indenting the medial longitudinal fasciculus in lower regions of the midbrain (Fig. 11.9A). The axons of this nucleus pass posteriorly (unique for a cranial nerve) and exit the brain at the midbrain-pontine junction, where the fibers then proceed anteriorly to reach the superior oblique muscle through the superior orbital fissure.

Figure 11.8 Brain stem at pontine level of cranial nerve V. Coronal medial longitudinal fasciculus is larger in this section between the motor nuclei of cranial nerves III and VI because it contains many vestibular and cerebellar fibers necessary for accurate eye movements. The tectospinal fibers always lie below the medial longitudinal fasciculus.

Sensory Cranial Nerve Nuclei

Proprioception is conveyed from the muscles in the head and neck (Fig. 11.9A). The mesencephalic nucleus of nerve V is located at the lateral margin of the periaqueductal gray. Remember these are the only primary sensory neurons in the central nervous system; their axons join the medial lemniscus and ascend to the ventral posterior medial nucleus in the thalamus. This nucleus controls the superior oblique muscle of the eye.

LATERAL ZONE

At this level the medial lemniscus and the other major ascending tracts are stretched over the lateral surface of the tegmentum of the midbrain (Fig. 11.9A). The spinothalamic and trigeminothalamic fibers are found lateral to the medial lemniscus, while the auditory fibers are located above them. Thus, the following sensory modalities for the entire body are located here: tactile discrimination, proprioception, pain and temperature, and gustatory and visceral sensations.

Auditory Fibers

The lateral lemniscus is seen superior to the medial lemniscus (Fig. 11.9A). These secondary auditory fibers are now entering the inferior colliculus. Many of these fibers synapse and then continue up into the medial geniculate as the brachium of the inferior colliculus.

MEDIAL ZONE

The raphe nuclei of the reticular formation are very conspicuous in these levels (Fig. 11.9A). The medial longitudinal fasciculus is prominent in the floor of the ventricle as it nears cranial nerve III; the fibers located within it are important in coordinating ocular movements.

CENTRAL ZONE

This zone in the lower tegmentum of the midbrain is nearly completely filled with the crossing fibers of the superior cerebellar peduncle (Fig. 11.9A). Ultimately, all these fibers decussate and continue up to the red nucleus, where some fibers synapse, but the majority of these axons bypass the red nucleus and terminate on the ventral lateral thalamic nuclei.

BASILAR ZONE

The bulk of this region is taken up by the pontine gray and descending fibers from the cerebrum to the pontine gray, the corticopontine system. The corticospinal and corticobulbar fibers are also present here (Fig. 11.9A).

LEVEL: SUPERIOR COLLICULUS AND PONTINE BASIS

TECTUM

Superior Colliculus

The superior colliculi form the rostral portion of the midbrain tectum (Fig. 11.10). The parenchyma of the superior colliculus is organized in layers. There are four layers containing gray and white matter from inside out: stratum zonale, stratum cinereum,

Figure 11.9 Brain stem at inferior collicular level. Coronal section.

Figure 11.10 Brain stem at superior collicular level. Coronal section.

stratum opticum, and stratum lemnisci. The superficial layers of the superior colliculus receive their input from the retina and visual cortex with the contralateral upper quadrant medially and the contralateral lower quadrants laterally. In contrast, the deeper layers receive their input from polysensory sources, including the cerebellum, inferior colliculus, spinal cord, reticular formation gracile, cuneate, trigeminal nuclei, and visual regions.

A portion of the tectospinal pathway originates at this level and descends in the lower brain stem to terminate on the lower cranial nerves and ventral horn cells of the spinal cord. (Remember the tectospinal and tectobulbar fibers terminate on the same motor nuclei as the corticonuclear and corticospinal pathways.) The zone of the tectum just above the superior colliculus, the pretectal zone, is important in light reflexes.

TEGMENTUM

GROSS FEATURES

In this section the roof and floor are formed by the midbrain, while the basilar portion is made up of peduncles and the pons. The fibers of the frontopontine tract are seen entering the rostral end of the pons. The roof is the superior colliculus, an important station in the visual pathway. The cerebral aqueduct forms the narrow ventricular lumen. (Fig. 11.10B). The superior colliculus is a laminated structure important in relating eye movements and body position; the fibers from the tectum of the superior collus projects onto the inferior pulvinar nuclei of the thalamus which then projects onto V2 and V3. The tectospinal tract originates from its deepest layer and provides connections onto certain cranial and spinal neurons.

VENTRICULAR ZONE

Sensory Cranial Nerve Nuclei

Proprioception is conveyed from the muscles in the head and neck by the mesencephalic nucleus of nerve V, located at the lateral margin of the periaqueductal gray in the superior collicular levels as well as in the upper pontine and inferior collicular levels (Fig. 11.10A).

Motor Cranial Nerve Nuclei

Cranial nerve III is visible in the floor of the cerebral aqueduct, adjacent to the medial longitudinal fasciculus (Fig. 11.10A). This nerve supplies the medial, inferior, and superior rectus muscles and the inferior oblique and superior levator muscles of the eyelid. The Edinger-Westphal nucleus of nerve III is also present; it provides preganglionic parasympathetic innervation to the constrictor muscle of the pupil via the ciliary ganglion.

LATERAL ZONE

White Matter

Medial Lemniscus
At this level in close proximity to the medial lemniscus includes most of the ascending sensory fibers (Table 11.7). This

Table 11.7 **MAJOR CONTENTS OF TEGMENTAL ZONES IN MIDBRAIN**

Ventricular zone: Cranial nuclei IV (inferior colliculus), CN III (superior colliculus).
Parasympathetic: Edinger-Westphal nucleus, associated with CN III to the pupillary constrictor.
Interstitial nucleus of Cajal and nucleus of Darkschewitsch important in pupillary reflexes.
Tracts: medial longitudinal fasciculus and descending autonomics and ascending reticular fibers.

Lateral zone: Tracts: medial lemniscus, lateral lemniscus, spinothalamic and brachium of inferior colliculus, with a confluens of the major ascending tracts

Central zone: Nuclei reticular nuclei with red nucleus and origin of rubrospinal tract. Substantia nigra present just posterior to cerebral peduncle.

Medial zone: Nuclei of raphe which forms serotonergic pathway. Tracts: Medial longitudinal fasciculus with tectospinal and decussation of superior cerebellar peduncle and rubrospinal tract. The tectospinal and rubrospinal tracts originate in midbrain

Basilar zone (cerebral peduncle): Descending tracts containing from medial to lateral frontotemporal, corticobulbar/nuclear, corticospinal, parietopontine, temperopontine, occipitopontine. Nerve rootlets of CN III on medial surface of peduncle.

tract is stretched out over the inferior and lateral surface of the tegmentum, with the fibers that mediate pain and temperature from the extremities, thorax, abdomen, and pelvis located at its superior extent. The trigeminal fibers form its middle portion, and the fibers that mediate tactile, proprioceptive, and visceral sensations are placed medially (Fig. 11.10A).

ANTEROLATERAL COLUMN

Lateral Spinothalamic

Pain and temperature from the limbs, thorax, and pelvis are found in this pathway.

Anterior Spinothalamic

Light touch fibers from the limbs, abdomen, and neck are seen in close proximity to the lateral spinothalamic pathway.

Auditory Pathway

The fibers from the inferior colliculus (called at this level the brachium of the inferior colliculus) are seen at the inferior surface of the superior colliculus. On the left side they enter the medial geniculate nucleus of the metathalamus, at which point they reach their final subcortical center.

Cerebellar Fibers

The superior cerebellar peduncle continues to cross in the tegmentum of the midbrain; just above this level many of these fibers synapse in the red nucleus, while others will continue to the ventral lateral nucleus in the thalamus.

CENTRAL ZONE

The central tegmental tract is conspicuous in the midbrain tegmentum in the reticular formation (Fig. 11.10A). The red nucleus is found in the medial edge of the reticular formation. In the human it consists of a small magnocellular region and a large parvocellular region. Fibers from all cerebellar nuclei, but especially the dentate, synapse here.

Corticorubral fibers run bilaterally from the motor cortex synapse and also terminate here in a somatotopic relationship. Fibers from the red nucleus terminate directly or indirectly in the cerebellum and on many of the motor nuclei in the brain stem and spinal cord, which also receive input from the corticospinal and corticonuclear pathways. The red nucleus receives many inputs from the contralateral cerebellum (interposed nucleus and the lateral cerebellar nucleus) and an input from the ipsilateral motor cortex. It has minimal if any direct projections in the human onto the thalamus, although it most likely influences the cerebellar input onto the thalamus and basal ganglia. The substantia nigra is also located in this level, just behind the cerebral peduncle. Its functions are discussed in the relationship between the basal ganglia and movement (see Chapter 18).

MEDIAL ZONE

The serotonergic raphe nuclei of the reticular formation are present in this level. The medial longitudinal fasciculus in the floor of the cerebral aqueduct is conspicuous and connected across the midline. The oculomotor complex indents the MLF and receives ascending fibers from cranial nerves VI and VIII through the MLF (Fig. 11.10A).

The tectospinal fibers at this level are primarily from the superior colliculus.

BASILAR ZONE

Cerebral Peduncles

This is at the level of the red nucleus, CN III, and the cerebral peduncles. Figure 11.11 is a stained section through the cerebral peduncles demonstrating the relationship between

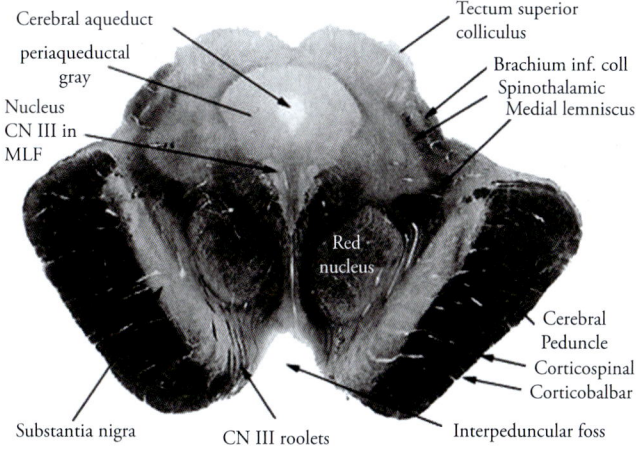

Figure 11.11 Brain stem at level of cerebral peduncles and cranial nerve III. Weil stain. Coronal section.

the peduncles, and cranial nerve III. The corticospinal fibers and many of the corticobulbar fibers are still in the peduncle. In Figure 11.10B, a coronal section through the brain, the relationship of the cerebral peduncle to the medial temporal lobe demonstrates that the cerebral peduncles are adjacent to the medial temporal lobe. This may be significant if herniation of the temporal lobe produces compression of the cerebral peduncle and cranial nerve III with the accompanying cranial nerve and upper motor neuron signs. Table 11.7 lists the significant structures in the tegmental zones of the midbrain.

VENTRICULAR ZONE

Cranial Nerve Nuclei: The Nucleus of Nuclei IV (Inferior Collicular Level) and III (Superior Collicular Level)

The parasympathetic nucleus of Edinger-Westphal, associated with cranial nerve III, to the pupillary constrictor is also present. The interstitial nucleus of Cajal (NIC) is the largest and most prominent of the cell groups of the medial longitudinal fasciculus (MLF). It contains two distinct cell classes, a group of large pyramidal-shaped neurons and small to fusiform, or round cells (Zuk et al., 1982). The NIC is probably involved in oculomotor control and in particular in the process of velocity to position integration in the vertical plane. The nucleus of Darkschewitsch is found here and it is important in pupillary reflexes.

- Tracts = MLF, with tectospinal and decussation of superior cerebellar peduncle and rubrospinal tract. The tectospinal and rubrospinal tracts originate in the midbrain.
- Lateral Zone: Tracts = Medial lemniscus, lateral lemniscus, spinothalamic and brachium of inferior colliculus, with a confluens of the major ascending tracts.
- Central Zone: Nuclei = Reticular formation with red nucleus and origin of rubrospinal tract. Substantia nigra present just posterior to the cerebral peduncle. Tracts = central tegmental and origin of rubrospinal.
- Medial Zone: Nuclei = Raphe nuclei which forms the serotonergic pathway.
- Basilar Zone: Tracts = Cerebral peduncle containing from medial to lateral frontopontine, corticonuclear, corticospinal, parietopontine, temperopontine, and occipitopontines.

FUNCTIONAL CENTERS IN THE BRAIN STEM

Now that the main anatomical features of the brain stem have been discussed, it is appropriate to identify some important functional centers located in the brain stem and diencephalon. During this discussion, it will become evident that the cranial nerves are the pivotal point for many of these activities.

RETICULAR FORMATION

The central core of the medulla, pons, and midbrain tegmentum consists of the reticular formation. Upon microscopic examination, this region is seen to consist of groupings of neurons separated by a meshwork of medullated fibers, a reticulum. With a Golgi neuronal stain, the Golgi type I cells with long axons are shown with their dendrites extending transversely and the axons bifurcating into ascending and descending branches, which run throughout the system. Each neuron receives input from at least 1000 neurons, and each neuron connects to as many as 10,000 neurons in the reticular formation.

The reticular formation of the brain stem blends inferiorly into lamina VII of the cord while superiorly it is continuous with the hypothalamus and dorsal thalamus of the diencephalon. Many nuclei have been identified in the reticular formation.

Functionally, the nuclei can be divided into cerebellar and noncerebellar nuclei (Table 11.8). The cerebellar portion of the reticular formation includes primarily the lateral and paramedian nuclei of the medulla, and the tegmental nucleus of the pons.

The noncerebellar portion nuclei are divided anatomically into three columns: the raphe, central, and lateral groupings.

Most of the nuclei in the reticular formation consist of large cells with ascending and descending axons. Functionally, the reticular formation in the medulla is especially important since the descending reticulospinal fibers and much of the ascending reticular system originate there.

Descending Reticulospinal System

The nucleus reticularis gigantocellularis is found in the rostral medullary levels, dorsal and medial to the inferior olive. This nucleus gives origin to much of the lateral reticulospinal tract, which is primarily an ipsilateral tract, running in the lateral funiculus of the spinal cord in all levels and terminating on internuncial neurons. The axons from the nucleus reticularis pontis oralis and caudalis form much of the medial reticulospinal tract, which runs in the anterior funiculus in all levels and terminates on internuncial neurons.

The lateral reticular nucleus is located in the lateral margin of the reticular formation dorsal to the inferior olive, while the ventral reticular nucleus is found in the caudal end of the medulla, dorsal to the inferior olive. These two nuclei, in conjunction with the nuclei in the pons and midbrain, form much of the ascending reticular fibers in the central tegmental tract distributing to neurons in the thalamus (intralaminar and

Table 11.8 **FUNCTIONAL GROUPINGS OF NUCLEI IN THE RETICULAR FORMATION**

NONCEREBELLAR	CEREBELLAR RELATED
Raphe, central, and lateral in tegmentum of brain stem	Lateral and paramedian l nuclei of medulla and tegmental nucleus of the pons

reticular), hypothalamus, and corpus striatum. The paramedian reticular nucleus is found near the midline at mid-olivary levels, dorsal to the inferior olive, and provides direct input into the anterior lobe of the cerebellar vermis.

Input to Reticular Formation

The reticular formation receives information via the ascending spinal tracts (spinotectal, spinoreticular, spinothalamic, and spinocerebellar), from the brain stem itself (olivoreticular, cerebelloreticular, and vestibulospinal), from the cerebral hemispheres (corticoreticular), from the basal ganglia, and from the hypothalamus. The cranial nerves are another important source, especially nerves I, II, V, VII, VIII, and X for sensory information that appears to project most heavily onto the central nuclei. The hypothalamus and striatum also project to the reticular system via the dorsal longitudinal fasciculus on the floor of the cerebral aqueduct and fourth ventricle and the more diffuse descending fiber systems in the core of the reticular formation.

Output

The medial lemniscus is a specific point-to-point relay system with few synapses (a closed system), while the fiber tracts of the reticular system are a multisynaptic nonspecific system (an open system) (Table 11.9).

The central tegmental tract is the principal fiber tract of the reticular formation. Its descending portions are located in the medial tegmentum, and its ascending portions are located in the lateral tegmentum. The ascending system projects to the thalamic intralaminar and reticular nuclei, hypothalamus, basal ganglia, substantia nigra, and red nucleus. The reticular system is functionally important in controlling our "posture" by its reflex relationship to the position of our body in space and in controlling our internal milieu by maintaining the stability of our viscera. The descending system synapses via the reticulospinal tract onto interneurons that mediate their effects through alpha and gamma motor neurons in the spinal cord and via autonomic pathways and cranial nerves onto visceral neurons.

Ascending Reticular System

This fiber system is the structural and functional substrate for maintaining consciousness. It also receives proprioceptive, tactile, thermal, visual, auditory, and nociceptive information via the spinal and cranial nerves. Many sensations (cutaneous, nociceptive, and erotic) activate the system. The sensory information ascends via the central tegmental tract into the limbic-midbrain area from which information can be more directly passed into the thalamus and hypothalamus. This midbrain to diencephalon to telencephalon circuit seems especially important in determining our level of consciousness.

Role of Descending Systems

The reticular formation is also important in controlling posture and orientation in space. Stimulation of the nucleus reticularis and gigantocellularis of the medulla inhibits the knee jerk. Stimulation of reticularis oralis/caudalis of the pons facilitates the knee jerk. The lateral part of the reticular formation is the receptor area, while the medial portion is the effector zone and the origin of the central tegmental and reticulospinal tracts. Many of the functions vital to the maintenance of the organism are found in the medulla.

Neurochemically Defined Nuclei in the Reticular Formation Affecting Consciousness

1. Cholinergic nuclei

    a. Located in the dorsal tegmentum of the pons and midbrain, cells in the mesopontine nuclei, and in the basal forebrain region

    b. Project diffusely to the cerebral cortex through the thalamus and have a modulating influence on cerebral cortical activity and wakefulness

2. Monoamine nuclei. In the reticular formation we find cells containing norepinephrine and serotonin.

    a. The norepinephrine-containing cells are found in the locus ceruleus (blue staining) in the upper pons and midbrain, and they project widely upon nuclei in the spinal cord, brain stem, thalamus, hypothalamus, and corpus striatum, which are important for maintaining attention and wakefulness.

    b. Serotinergic nuclei. These nuclei are found in the raphe of the medial tegmental zone in the medulla, pons, and midbrain. The nuclei in the pons and medulla project onto the spinal cord and brain stem while the nuclei in the upper pons and midbrain project onto to the thalamus, hypothalamus, corpus striatum, and cerebral cortex. The serotinergic system facilitates sleep. An area outside of the reticular formation, the histamine-containing area of the posterior hypothalamus, is also important in maintaining wakefulness.

Table 11.9 **MAJOR PATHWAYS OF THE RETICULAR FORMATION**

TRACT	RETICULAR NUCLEUS OF ORIGIN	TERMINATION OF PATHWAY
Lateral reticulospinal	Gigantocellularis	Spinal cord and autonomic interneurons
Medial reticulospinal	Pontis oralis and caudalis	Spinal cord and autonomic interneurons
Central tegmental	Lateral and ventral	Thalamic nuclei—intralaminar and reticular; hypothalamus, corpus striatum, substantia nigra

RESPIRATION CENTERS

Respiration is under the control of neurons in the respiratory center in the upper medulla and pons. Sensory fibers from the lungs ascend via cranial nerve X and enter the solitary tract and proceed onto the neurons in the reticular formation in the medulla and pons. Specific regions in the medulla control inspiration or expiration. The medullary respiratory center itself is responsive to the carbon dioxide content in the blood. Increased CO_2 produces increased respiration, and decreased CO_2 produces decreased respiration. In the pons the pneumotaxic centers are related to the frequency of the respiratory response. These centers play onto the medullary respiratory center to determine the respiratory output. The axons from cells in medullary reticular center descend to the appropriate *spinal cord levels to innervate the diaphragm.* Axons from cells in the medullary reticular center descend to the appropriate spinal cord levels to innervate the diaphragm and the intercostal and associated muscles of respiration. The vagus nerve itself provides preganglionic innervation of the trachea, bronchi, and lungs.

The respiratory response is also modified by cortical and hypothalamic input; that is, emotionally stimulated individuals breathe more rapidly because of the hypothalamic influence on the brain stem and spinal cord. The actual respiration occurs with the intercostal muscles, the accessory muscles, and the lungs expanding and contracting in concert with associated vascular changes (autonomic nervous system)

CARDIOVASCULAR CENTERS

The carotid body (innervated by sensory fibers of cranial nerve IX) is found distal to the bifurcation of the common carotid artery, and the aortic body, innervated by the sensory fibers of cranial nerve X is found near the origin of the subclavian arteries. These carry information on blood pressure into the solitary tract and then into the medullary respiratory center. These sites are sensitive to oxygen-carbon dioxide pressure; when oxygen is reduced, ventilations increase; when oxygen increases, ventilations decrease. Neural control over the tone of the arterioles is exercised through vasoconstrictor fibers and sometimes vasodilator fibers. A vasomotor center in the medulla extends from the midpontine to the upper medullary levels. In the lateral reticular formation of the medulla, stimulation elicits an increase in vasoconstriction and an increase in heart rate–pressor center. In the lower medulla, stimulation of the depressor center produces a decrease in vasoconstriction and a decrease in heart rate. The carotid body (innervated by cranial nerve IX) and the aortic body (cranial nerve X) contain specialized pressure receptors stimulated by an increase in the size of these blood vessels. This information runs via nerves IX and X to the medulla and depresses activity. Most sensory nerves, cranial and spinal, contain some nerve fibers, which when stimulated, cause a rise in arterial pressure by exciting the pressor region and inhibiting the depressor centers. Higher centers also influence respiratory and vascular centers in the medulla and alter blood flow, depending on the psychic state; that is, mental activity decreases peripheral blood (constricts vessels), while emotional states can produce increased blood flow, blocking vasodilation.

DEGLUTITION

The act of swallowing starts volitionally but is completed by reflex activity.

1. The food is first masticated (motor nucleus of nerve V) and reduced to smaller particles, called the bolus, which is lubricated by saliva from the salivary glands (nerves VII and IX).
2. The bolus is propelled through the oral pharyngeal opening when the tongue is elevated against the soft palate (nerve XII), and the facial pillars are relaxed.
3. The oral pharyngeal pillars close and the superior and middle pharyngeal constrictor muscles (ambiguous nucleus of nerve X) force the bolus along into the laryngeal pharynx, where the pharyngeal walls contract, closing the opening superiorly.
4. At the same time, the tracheal opening is closed by the epiglottis and glottis, as the larynx, trachea, and pharynx move up. This movement is noted externally as the bobbing of the thyroid eminence (Adam's apple).
5. Finally the inferior constrictor muscle contracts, pushing the bolus into the esophagus, where peristaltic waves and gravity carry it through the esophagus.

Cranial nerves V, IX, X, and XII perform the motor part of the activity, while nerves V, VII, IX, and X form the sensory function.

VOMITTING

Vomiting is produced by many stimuli and is usually a reflex activity. The vomitus is composed of the gastric contents.

1. Caused commonly by irritation of the oropharynx, gastrointestinal mucosa, and genitourinary and semicircular canals. Stimulation of the vestibular system, including the semicircular canals and the nerve itself, may also produce vomiting.
2. The afferent nerves travel via the vagus and glossopharyngeal tracts into the solitary tract. After synapsing on the dorsal motor nucleus of cranial nerve X, the information is conveyed via the vagus nerve to the stomach. Impulses are also passed down to the cervical and thoracic level onto the ventral horn cells that control the simultaneous contraction of the intercostal, diaphragmatic, and abdominal musculature.
3. Nausea and excessive salivation precede the deep inspiration associated with retching. The glottis is closed and the nasal passages are sealed off. The descent of the diaphragm and the contraction of the abdominal muscles exert the pressure that causes the stomach to contract in a direction contrary to normal peristalsis and forces vomitus through the relaxed cardia of the stomach and into the esophagus.

EMETIC CENTER

The area postrema is found in the caudal end of the fourth ventricle above the obex of the medulla. This area is very vascular and contains many venous sinuses. The blood–brain barrier is lacking in this region. The vagal, glossopharyngeal, and hypoglossal nuclei are strongly interconnected with the area postrema. This region is very sensitive to changes in pressure or to drugs whose passage into this area is not inhibited by any blood–brain barrier.

COUGHING

Irritation of the lining of the larynx or trachea produces coughing. The stimulus is picked up by free nerve endings associated with the internal laryngeal branch of cranial nerve X, which carries it up into the solitary tract, following the same pathway as in vomiting, except that the muscles contract alternately rather than simultaneously with the intercostal muscle contracting suddenly.

LOCALIZATION IN THE BRAIN STEM AT BIRTH

The following Figures 11.12-11.16 are coronal sections from the brain stem of a full-term fetus, demonstrating the anatomical basis for the ability of the newborn to suckle, grasp, and also respond to painful stimuli. The following structures are myelinated: cranial nerve rootlets, spinothalamic, and medial lemniscus. As expected, the corticospinal and corticobulbar fibers are not yet myelinated and will not be myelinated until 4–6 months after birth.

LOCALIZATION OF DISEASE PROCESSES IN THE BRAIN STEM

Pathological processes affecting the brain stem can usually be well localized from an anatomical standpoint. This is a direct consequence of the fact that these disease processes in general involve a particular combination of cranial nerves (as in acoustic neuroma of the cerebellar pontine angle vestibular schwannoma [acoustic neuroma] at the cerebellar pontine angle) or produce a particular combination of extrinsic and ipsilateral cranial nerve dysfunction and contralateral long tract findings (as in the midbrain infarction of Weber's syndrome, which results in a combination of ipsilateral third nerve dysfunction and contralateral pyramidal tract findings).

Moreover, when anatomical-pathological correlation is considered, the brain stem, of all sites in the central nervous system, provides the best example of how the anatomical pattern of involvement may allow the prediction of the actual pathological processes. The student has, of course, already encountered several examples of this phenomenon at the level of the spinal cord. Thus, the clinical finding of a selective dissociated loss of pain and temperature in a cape-like distribution over the shoulders and upper extremities implies an anatomical process in a pericentral location involving the anterior commissure. One could readily deduce that an intrinsic pathological process was present and, moreover, could assume that in most cases the pathological process was that of syringomyelia.

At the level of the brain stem such examples of close correlation occur frequently. Thus, the combined progressive involvement of the ipsilateral cranial nerve VIII (auditory and vestibular), nerve VII (facial), and nerve V (trigeminal), manifested by deafness and tinnitus (vestibular), nerve VII (facial), and nerve V manifested by a buzzing or ringing sound in the ear, dizziness, peripheral facial paralysis, and unilateral facial numbness, not only indicates the location of the pathology (the cerebellar pontine angle) but also suggests the actual nature of the pathology: vestibular schwannoma (acoustic neuroma): tumor arising from Schwann cells of the sheath of nerve VIII. While other pathological lesions may occur at this site, they are much less common.

There are several possible approaches to the problem of localization of disease processes in the brain stem. We will first consider a number of guidelines for localization. We will then consider in greater detail the particular anatomical syndromes

Figure 11.12 Closed medulla at birth demonstrating myelinated nucleus cuneatus and nucleus gracilis and myelination of the medial lemniscus, medial longitudinal fasciculus (mlf), trigeminal system (descending nerve and tract of V), spinothalamics, and core of reticular formation with medullary pyramid lacking myelin. Weil myelin stain.

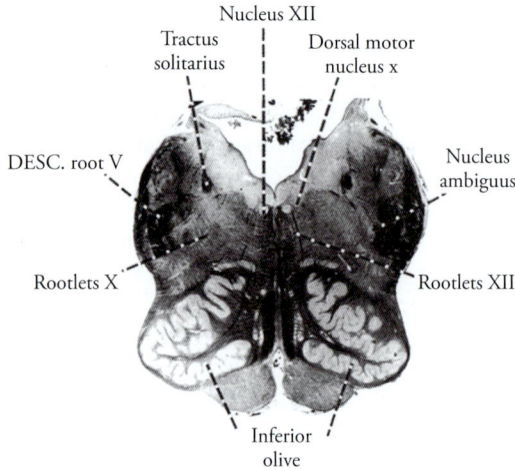

Figure 11.13 Medulla at level of inferior olive demonstrating myelinated medial lemniscus, medial longitudinal fasciculus (mlf), trigeminal system, rootlets of the vagus nerve, spinothalamics with medullary pyramid lacking myelin. Weil myelin stain.

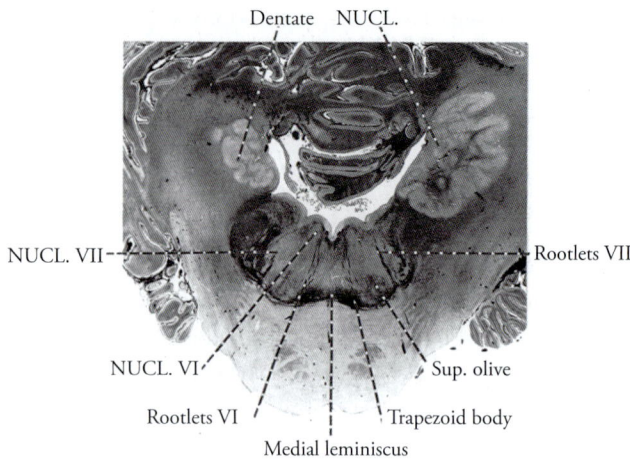

Figure 11.15 Pons at level of facial colliculus demonstrating myelinated rootlets of cranial nerves VI and VII, medial lemniscus and lateral lemniscus, and inferior cerebellar peduncle. The middle cerebellar peduncle and the corticospinal tract are showing some initial staining. Weil myelin stain.

Figure 11.14 Pons at level of vestibular nerve. Demonstrating myelinated vestibular nerve rootlets, medial lemniscus, central tegmental tract of reticular system, and beginning of myelination in the inferior cerebellar peduncle. Weil myelin stain.

Figure 11.16 Inferior colliculus of midbrain demonstrating myelination of rootlets of cranial nerve IV, medial longitudinal fasciculus (MLF), medial lemniscus, inferior colliculus, decussation of the superior cerebellar peduncle, and some in the cerebral peduncle. Weil myelin stain.

and the various types of pathology in terms of specific extrinsic and intrinsic syndromes. When speaking of the anatomical syndromes of the brain stem in clinical neurology, we will limit our considerations to the medulla oblongata, pons, and midbrain.

GUIDELINES FOR LOCALIZING BRAIN STEM DISEASE

1. Mental status is not directly involved (except that lesions involving the tegmentum of the upper brain stem—reticular formation, etc., may alter level of consciousness).

2. No muscle atrophy is presented, except that relevant to local involvement of cranial nerves.

3. Limb weakness, if present, involves central control and spasticity.

4. Deep tendon reflexes are increased in a bilateral or unilateral manner. A unilateral or bilateral sign of Babinski may be present.

EFFECTS OF INTERRUPTING LONG MOTOR PATHWAYS: CORTICOSPINAL AND CORTICOBULBAR PATHWAYS

1. The pyramidal (corticospinal) tracts:

   a. Decussate low in the medulla.

   b. Damage to the pyramidal tract above this decussation will produce contralateral upper motor neuron signs. Within the brain stem, the left and right pyramidal tracts are situated closest together at the level of the pyramidal decussation and are most widely separated at the level of the upper midbrain-internal capsule. Lesions in the medulla will often produce bilateral effects; in the midbrain, unilateral or bilateral effects. Throughout their extent in the brain stem, the corticospinal tracts are located in a ventral (or basilar) location. Lesions limited to the dorsal (tegmental or tectal) portions of the brain stem then are less likely to produce signs of pyramidal tract involvement.

2. Corticobulbar fibers

   a. Descend to the cranial nerve motor nuclei in close proximity to the corticospinal tracts.

   b. Lesions here produce a supranuclear lesion, as regards motor control of the cranial nerves, below the lesion.

   c. For each cranial nerve motor nucleus (V, VII, and XII, ambiguous) decussate, separately, somewhat above the level of that motor nucleus.

   d. In humans (compared to the cat) direct corticobulbar fibers can be traced to the trigeminal, facial, hypoglossal, and spinal accessory motor neurons.

   e. Corticobulbar control of the cranial nerve motor nuclei is bilateral to the laryngeal, pharyngeal, palatal, and upper facial musculature.

   f. The motor neurons supplying the lower half of the face and the genioglossus muscle of the tongue receive predominantly unilateral corticobulbar fibers.

   g. The effects of a unilateral corticobulbar lesion then will be limited to an upper motor neuron type weakness of the contralateral lower facial muscles (termed supranuclear or central) and a minor weakness of the tongue (with slight deviation of the tongue on attempted midline protrusion to the side contralateral to the lesion).

   h. Bilateral damage to the corticobulbar fibers will produce an upper motor neuron type weakness of the muscles of the pharynx, larynx, tongue, face (upper and lower muscles), and jaw. The resulting syndrome, termed a pseudobulbar palsy, will have the qualities which the student has come to associate with an upper motor neuron lesion: impairment of voluntary control, weakness without atrophy, and a release of segmental brain stem reflex activity from higher control. Thus, the jaw jerk, a stretch reflex, will be hyperactive. Since the muscles and brain stem motor nuclei are also involved in emotional expression (consider laughing, crying, the facial expression of rage, and so forth), bilateral corticobulbar lesions will result in a loss of higher control and a release of these motor components of emotional expression.

CEREBELLAR DYSFUNSTION

1. Cerebellar symptomatology may be noted frequently in diseases affecting the brain stem and may provide information as to localization. On the other hand, expanding lesions of the cerebellum may secondarily compress the brain stem. Diseases affecting the cerebellum will be considered later in greater detail (Chapter 19); here we will simply indicate certain general rules at this point.

2. Diseases affecting the midline cerebellum (vermis) or its fiber systems result in a disturbance of equilibrium (sense of balance) and an ataxia (unsteadiness) of the trunk. This may be evident on sitting, standing, or walking. If an ataxia in walking occurs, we speak of an ataxia of gait.

3. Diseases affecting the lateral aspects of the cerebellum or of the fiber systems related to the lateral cerebellum produce lateralized symptoms affecting the limbs. Thus, an unsteadiness (ataxia of dysmetria) of arm and leg movements will be noted. In addition, a characteristic tremor will be present—intention tremor, in which oscillations of movement perpendicular to the line of movement occur (in the finger-to-nose and heel-to-shin tests). The lateralized unsteadiness of the lower extremity will result in an impairment of gait. The ataxia of gait will have, however, a lateralized quality in the sense that the patient will tend to fall or deviate to a particular side.

4. In general, pathology affecting the cerebellar hemisphere produces symptoms ipsilateral to the side of involvement. This reflects the fact that the dorsal spinocerebellar and cuneocerebellar pathways are essentially uncrossed. Moreover, the major outflow from the cerebellar hemisphere, the dentatorubrothalamic pathway of the superior cerebellar peduncle, decussates in the upper pons before reaching the rubral and ventral lateral thalamic areas and then onto the motor cortex. The major efferent pathways from the motor cortex cross again in the pyramidal decussation. Because of this double decussation, data then from the right cerebellar hemisphere will eventually influence the anterior horn cells of the right arm and leg.

Lesions of Cerebellar Peduncles

Inferior cerebellar peduncle and the adjacent spinocerebellar and cuneocerebellar pathways in the lateral medulla will produce ipsilateral symptoms. Superior cerebellar peduncle below its decussation will produce ipsilateral symptoms; above the decussation, contralateral symptoms.

5. Whether lateralized cerebellar symptoms reflect intrinsic disease of the brain stem or disease of the cerebellum will depend on the associated signs and symptoms. Thus, the ipsilateral intention tremor and ataxia seen in the lateral medullary infarction (see Chapter 16) and due to damage of the restiform body (inferior cerebellar peduncle) and the adjacent spinocerebellar and cuneocerebellar pathways is clearly associated with the signs and symptoms referable to the involvement of the adjacent intrinsic structures: the ipsilateral descending spinal tract of the fifth nerve; the lateral spinothalamic pathway (producing contralateral deficits in pain and temperature), the ipsilateral Horner's syndrome, and the ipsilateral nucleus ambiguous or vagal

dysfunction producing hoarseness, defective gag reflex, and dysarthria. On the other hand, the ipsilateral intention tremor and ataxia due to an abscess or tumor (e.g., cystic astrocytoma) of the lateral cerebellum will not have this association but rather will be associated with the signs and symptoms of increased intracranial pressure. Common midline lesions of the cerebellum secondarily compressing the brain stem are tumors such as medulloblastomas and hemangioblastomas. The ependymoma, although arising from the floor of the fourth ventricle, is sometimes included in the midline cerebellar syndrome category.

DECEREBRATE RIGIDITY

Decerebrate rigidity is a consequence of a pathological transection of the brain stem between the vestibular nuclei and the red nuclei of the midbrain.

Pyramidal tracts and lesions of the pyramidal tracts are not involved in the phenomena. Instead, there is a marked increase in extensor tone due to the release of the extensor facilitatory area in the reticular formation in the tegmentum of the pons and midbrain and a marked increase in stretch reflexes. For further discussion of the anatomical basis of decerebraste rigidity refer to chapter 18.

INTERRUPTION OF LONG SENSORY SYSTEMS: MEDIAL LEMNISCUS AND SPINOTHALAMICS

Effects of Lesions

The spinothalamic tracts are on the lattermost margin of the brain stem; therefore, in the medulla they are separate from the medial lemniscus. An intrinsic paramedian lesion is likely to produce bilateral involvement of the medial lemniscus. Since the medial lemniscus is quite separate from the lateral spinothalamic pathway, selective involvement of contralateral position and vibratory sensation, as opposed to pain and temperature sensation, may occur.

At the level of the midbrain and thalamus, these systems are close together. Therefore, selective involvement of position and vibration as opposed to pain and temperature is less likely.

CRANIAL NERVE DYSFUNCTION

1. Motor cranial nerves

    a. The effects of a lesion involving the motor nuclei of a cranial nerve or of the motor fibers of a cranial nerve will be ipsilateral to the lesion. The effects will be those of a lower motor lesion: atrophy and weakness, and a loss of segmental reflex activity. With regard to the facial nerve, the effects are often referred to as peripheral. In a local lesion of the brain stem, it is the segmental ipsilateral motor findings, in association with the contralateral corticospinal and corticobulbar findings below the level of the lesion, which allow for localization (termed hemiplegia alternans or alternating hemiplegia).

    b. The nuclei of the somatic motor cranial nerves (III, IV, VI, and XII) are located close to the midline. These nuclei tend to be involved, then, by paramedian lesions rather than by lateral lesions. Intrinsic lesions in a paramedian location tend to produce, early in their course, a bilateral involvement of these nuclei. These nuclei are also all located in a relatively dorsal position. These nuclei would be involved early by a lesion in a dorsal or tegmental location. Except for cranial nerve IV, the fibers of these cranial nerves all exit in a relatively paramedian ventral location.

Sensory Cranial Lesions2. Cranial nerve V lesions

   a. In the main sensory root of the trigeminal nerve, in its course within or external to the midpons, will produce ipsilateral deficits in pain, temperature, and touch over the face.

   b. In the descending spinal tract of the trigeminal nerve or of its associated nucleus will produce ipsilateral deficit in pain and temperature sensation over the face with sparing of facial touch sensation. These structures are situated close to the lateral spinothalamic tract, the combination of contralateral pain and temperature deficit over the body and extremities with ipsilateral pain and temperature deficit over the face is frequently found as a consequence of lesions which involve the dorsolateral tegmental portion of the medulla, for example, infarction of the territory of the posterior inferior cerebellar artery, which supplies this sector. A similar combination may be found in the infarction of the dorsolateral tegmentum of the caudal pons: the territory of the anterior inferior cerebellar artery.

   c. The descending spinal tract (analogous to and, in a sense, the direct continuation of Lissauer's tract) and associated nucleus (analogous to the substantia gelatinosa) descend into the upper cervical spinal cord. Although there is considerable overlap, the primary trigeminal fibers synapse on the nucleus of the descending spinal nucleus at the following levels: mandibular division fibers at a lower pontine–upper medullary level; the maxillary division at a medullary level; and the ophthalmic division fibers at a lower medullary and upper cervical cord level.

   There is overlap at the upper cervical cord level between the upper cervical segment pain fibers and the ophthalmic division pain fibers. It is not surprising, then, that pain originating in the C2 and C3 roots or segments of the spinal cord may sometimes be referred to the ophthalmic division of the face (orbit and forehead), for example, the pain of cervical 2 and 3-occipital neuralgia is often referred to the orbit.

   d. The secondary pain fibers decussate and join the ventral secondary trigeminal tract (also labeled trigeminothalamic or quintothalamic tract), which, at a medullary level, is located just lateral to the medial lemniscus. At a pontine and midbrain location, the secondary trigeminal tract is just lateral to and essentially continuous with the medial lemniscus and adjacent to the lateral spinothalamic path. A lesion that involves this tract would then usually produce contralateral deficits in pain and temperature over a variable portion of the face in association with a contralateral deficit in pain and temperature and/or position and vibration over the affected arm, leg, and trunk.

CLINICAL SIGNS AFTER LESIONS IN THE TEGMENTUM OF THE BRAIN STEM

Although all nuclei and tracts in the brain stem are important to the proper function of the central nervous system, lesions in only certain tracts and nuclei produce abnormal responses detectable at the bedside and important for diagnosis and treatment of disease. Remember injury to any cranial nerve usually produces a defect that helps you to localize just where in the brain stem the lesion is located. (See also Chapters 15 and 16.) Table 11.10 provides only a brief overview of the major deficits seen after lesions in one of the five zones of the tegmentum.

1. Disease involving the brain stem does not directly affect most aspects of mental status such as memory, abstract reasoning, comprehension, and the ability to perform calculation—functions usually associated with the cerebral cortex. Brain stem lesions may interfere with the ability to test these functions in the sense that a patient with a transection of the upper pons or midbrain will usually be unable to convey information from the cerebral cortex to the cranial nerve and spinal cord motor neurons so that expression of the cortical functions cannot occur. The patient is akinetic and mute. Lesions involving the reticular formation at the diencephalic and mesencephalic junction will interfere with mental status in the sense that the alertness and arousal aspects of consciousness are defective. The patient then remains in a comatose state, either failing to arouse from this state when stimulated or arousing only for brief periods. For additional discussion refer to Chapter 29 Alterations in Consciousness.

2. Pathological processes that involve the brain stem may have effects, moreover, which are not simply limited to the brain stem. Thus, occlusion of the basilar artery may not only produce infarction (ischemic damage) of the brain stem but also may produce infarction of the territory supplied by the posterior cerebral arteries. This includes the calcarine cortex, the medial and inferior aspects of the temporal lobe, and the diencephalon. The medial aspects of the temporal lobe (the hippocampus) and the medial thalamic areas apparently provide the anatomical substrate for recent memory (the learning of new information).

3. Space-occupying lesions of the brain stem or posterior fossa may also secondarily interfere with mental status through a blockade of the ventricular system. With blockade of the fourth ventricle or aqueduct (or for that matter the third ventricle), cerebrospinal fluid pressure increases and is transmitted to the lateral ventricle. The lateral ventricles dilate and since the skull is a rigid container (after closure of the sutures), the white matter and gray matter of the cerebral hemisphere are subjected to compression with an alteration in mental status. The patient frequently presents a drowsy appearance and when roused he often manifests a diffuse defect in memory, comprehension, and abstract reasoning. With relief of the obstruction to the flow of cerebrospinal fluid, a rapid reversal in this state should occur. An increase in intracranial pressure, particularly when sudden, is often associated with headache, nausea, and vomiting.

More recent diagnostic approaches have involved earlier diagnosis by computerized tomography (CT) or MRI scan (MRI is the preferred imaging approach). The surgical approach may now include excision of the tumor utilizing the operating microscope (see Stein, 1979).

Table 11.10 **CLINICAL DEFECTS FROM LESIONS IN THE TEGMENTAL ZONES OF THE BRAIN STEM**

Ventricular zone: Interruption of motor cranial nerves III, IV, VI, X, and XII produce lower motor neuron signs. Interruption of sensory nuclei of VIII produces dizziness and deficits in hearing while injury to the solitary nucleus produces deficits in taste.

Lateral zone: Interruption of the spinothalamic tract produces contralateral decrease in pain and temperature from the body. Injury to the rootlet or chief sensory or descending nucleus of cranial nerve V produces sensory finding of ipsilateral deficits in pain, temperature, and touch from the head and ipsilateral weakness in chewing.

Medial zone: Interruption of the medial lemniscus, depending on the level of the lesion, produces loss of touch, pain, and temperature from the head or body; injury to the medial longitudinal fasciculus produces deficits in coordination of eye movements.

Central zone: Lesions here produce abnormalities in the functions associated with cranial nerve nuclei of VII, IX, X, and XI. The descending parasympathetic and sympathetic fibers can also be interrupted affecting the pupil (Horner's) and sweat glands. (See Chapter 11 on cranial nerves)

Basilar zone: Destruction of the corticospinal tract produces an upper motor neuron lesion with loss of volitional movement in the contralateral body muscles; interruption of the corticonuclear tract produces weakness of volitional movement of the muscles in the contralateral head and neck.

ANATOMICAL BASIS OF DECEREBRATE RIGIDITY

The studies of Sherrington demonstrated that the corticospinal tracts—that is, pyramidal tracts—were not involved in decerebrate rigidity since with hemisection of the brain stem at the intercollicular level the unilateral rigidity which occurred was ipsilateral to the hemisection. Sherrington also was able to indicate that deafferentation decreased rigidity in a limb. Decerebrate rigidity was conceived to be a release phenomenon.

The studies of Rhines demonstrated that stimulation of the reticular formation in a ventromedial area of the medullary tegmentum produced a decrease in decerebrate rigidity, a decrease in the quadriceps deep tendon reflex, and a decrease in the movement which could be elicited by simultaneously stimulating the motor cortex. This area was labeled the bulbar reticular inhibitory area. From an anatomical standpoint the inhibitory area of the medulla corresponds to the nucleus reticularis gigantocellularis. The neurons of this nucleus give rise to the lateral reticulospinal tract, which is found in the lateral column of the spinal cord. In contrast, stimulation of a region of the reticular formation in the pons and midbrain resulted in an increase in the degree of decerebrate rigidity. In addition, the quadriceps deep tendon reflex (the knee jerk) was increased and responses to stimulation of the motor cortex were facilitated. This facilitatory area extends into the subthalamus, the adjacent hypothalamus, and the intralaminar areas of the thalamus (e.g., centrum medianum). This area in the more lateral tegmental reticular formation in the pons and midbrain may be termed a brain stem (or bulbar reticular) facilitatory area. From an anatomical standpoint the facilitatory area of the pons corresponds to the nucleus reticularispontis oralis and caudalis.* The neurons of this nucleus give rise to that medial reticulospinal tract found in the anterior column. It is important to note that the inhibitory area of the medulla is driven from other inhibitory areas. Among these are the anterior portions of the cerebral cortex (the suppressor areas indicated as areas 4S and 8) and the caudate nucleus. The anterior lobe of the cerebellum also exerts an inhibitory driving influence, although it is uncertain whether this cerebellar influence is as significant in primates and man as in the cat. It is now recognized that flexors and extensors are not equally affected by these facilitatory and inhibitory systems. Rather, it is more proper to speak of these areas as bulbar reticular extensor inhibitory area (since actually flexor tone is increased by stimulation of these areas) and bulbar reticular extensor facilitatory area (since flexor tone is decreased by stimulation of this area). In the decerebrate animal the effects of the extensor facilitatory system predominate because the extensor inhibitory system must be driven from higher centers. These higher centers, of course, are disconnected from the inhibitory area in the brain stem by the section through the brain stem. On the other hand, the facilitatory center is driven by afferent inputs from below, that is, the collaterals of ascending sensory fibers derived from the spinothalamic tracts and the trigeminal system.

These brain stem reticular areas give rise to reticulospinal pathways which descend to the spinal cord level to influence stretch reflexes. In addition, vestibular centers give rise to facilitatory vestibulospinal pathways which may also influence to some degree stretch reflexes. As regards the effects of these brain stem reticular centers on stretch reflexes, one may postulate two possible mechanisms of action. There might well be a facilitation or inhibition of large alpha motor neurons. On the other hand, these centers might exert their effects through a facilitation or inhibition of the small gamma neurons. This latter situation would alter tension on the spindle and change the rate of discharge of the muscle spindle.

Granit and Kaada have demonstrated that stimulation of the facilitatory area did augment the spindle discharge. Stimulation of the inhibitory area reduced the spindle discharge. Both effects, then, were exerted via the gamma system. Classic decerebrate rigidity may be considered essentially "gamma rigidity." Alpha rigidity is less common and results when the cerebellum, particularly the anterior cerebellum, is destroyed in the decerebrate preparation (anemic decerebrate preparation) produced by vascular occlusion. The facilitatory effect may be exerted on the alpha motor neuron by the vestibulospinal tract. There is some evidence that although alpha rigidity may occur in the cat, this is probably not a significant form of rigidity in the primate.

BIBLIOGRAPHY

Carpenter, M. B. 1991. Core Text of Neuroanatomy, 4th ed Baltimore, Williams and Wilkins.

Gwyn, D. G., and Rutherford, J. G. 1982. Cytoarchitecture, neuronal morphology, and some efferent connections of the interstitial nucleus of cajal (INC) in the cat. J. Comp. Neurol. 212:278–292.

Riley, H. A. 1960. Brain stem and spinal cord, New York, Hafner.

---

* As discussed previously, the nucleus gigantocellularis and the nucleus reticularis pontis oralis and caudalis may be considered as a relatively continuous cell column within the reticular formation, with a major role in reticulospinal motor activities. The other major cell groupings are the paramedian cell groups (paramedian reticular nuclei and reticulotegmental nucleus) concerned with cerebellar relationships and the lateral reticular nucleus. This lateral area of reticular formation is the major relay area for afferent collateral input to the reticular formation.

12.

THE CRANIAL NERVES

The cranial nerves originate from a diverse group of nuclei and ganglia and innervate primarily the skin and muscles of the shoulder, head, and neck. The structures innervated by the cranial nerves are especially important for many of the communications skills of humans, including facial expression, language, sight, smell, taste, and hearing. Facial expression provides the motor component of the expression of our emotions. An additional function of cranial nerves (CN) III, VII, IX, and X is to provide the parasympathetic innervation to the eyes, heart, and gastrointestinal system in the body; that is one of the major survival mechanisms for our species (Fig. 12.1).

In Figure 12.1 the origins of the cranial nerves at each level of the brain stem and base of diencephalon cerebrum are noted. CN I originates from the olfactory bulbs; CN II originates in the retina and terminates in the lateral geniculate nucleus of the thalamus; CN III and CN IV originate from the midbrain with CN III exiting the midbrain between the

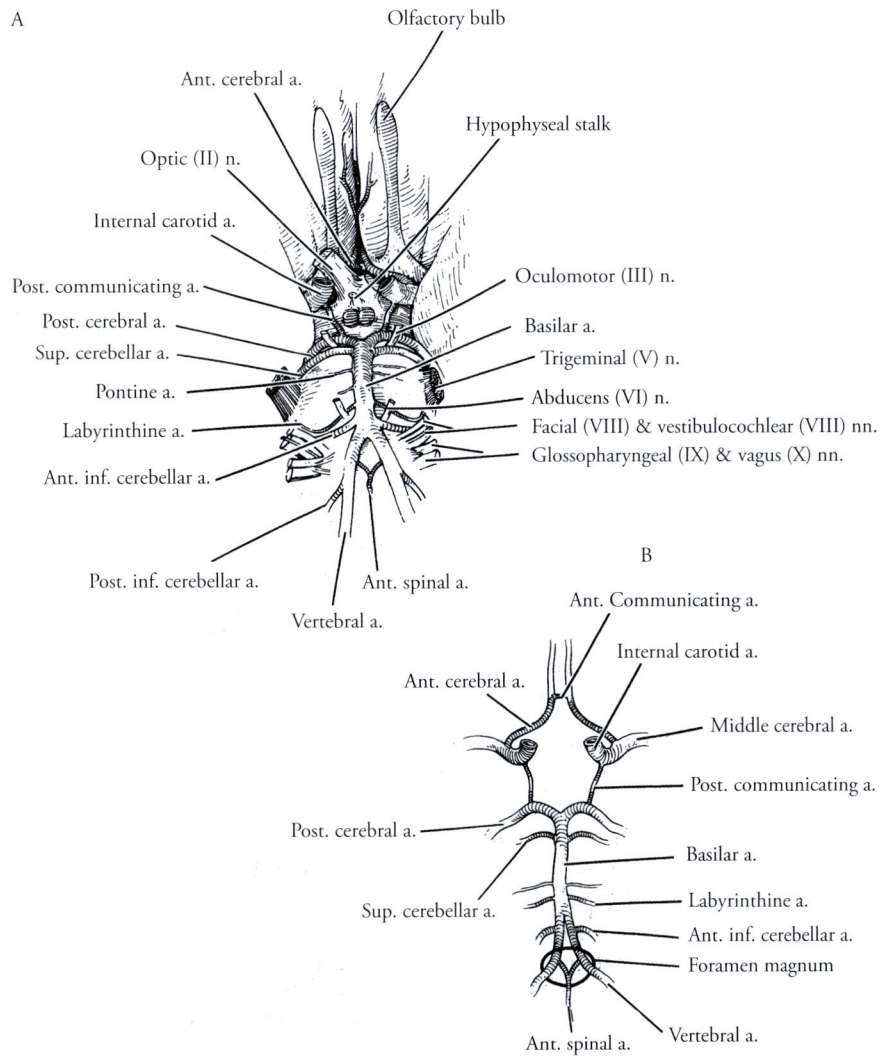

Figure 12.1 (*A*) Origins and relationship of the cranial nerve rootlets to the arterial circle of Willis. (*B*) The arteries forming the circle of Willis. (From J. Zimmerman and S. Jacobson, Anatomy, 1989, Figure 7-36, Little, Brown & Company, Boston.)

superior cerebellar and posterior cerebral arteries.; CN V–VII originate from the pons with cranial nerve VI found in a paramedian position between the labyrinthine and anterior inferior cerebellar arteries. CN VIII–X originate from the medulla in the cerebellopontine angle. CN IX originates from the lower medulla and also from the upper cervical levels, while the hypoglossal nerve (XII). originates from the medulla and its axons leave the medulla lateral to the medullary pyramid CN XI also originates from C2–C5 and descends through the foramen magnum of the spinal cord (Figs. 12.2 and 12.3).

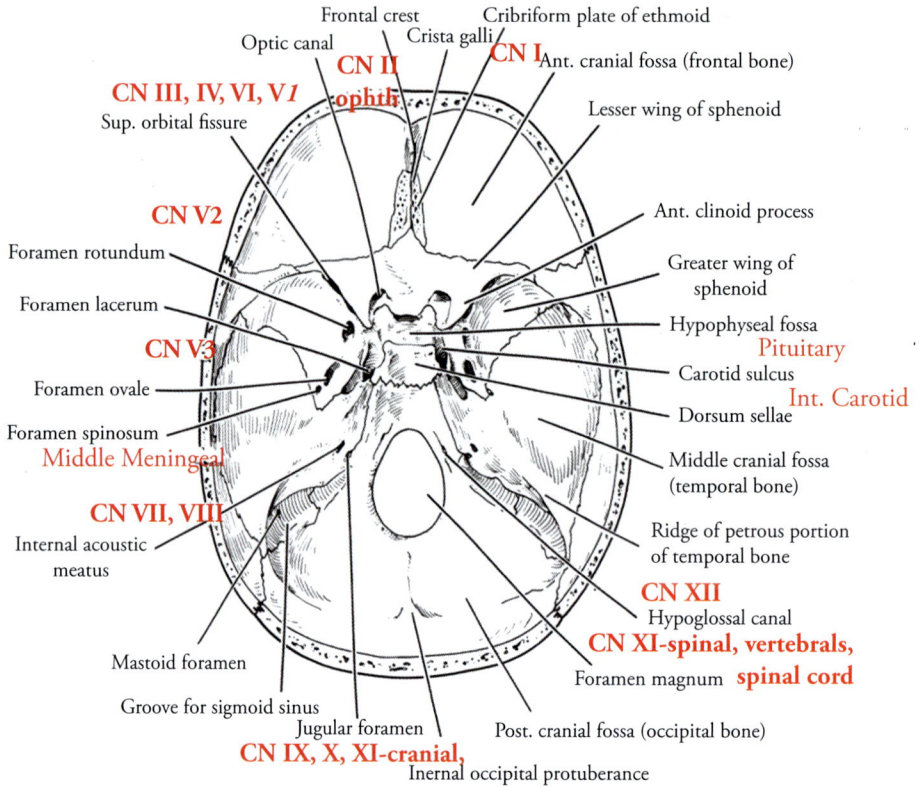

Figure 12.2 Location of cranial nerve nuclei in tegmentum of the brain stem with motor nuclei medial and sensory lateral separated by the sulcus limitans. (From Gray's Anatomy.)

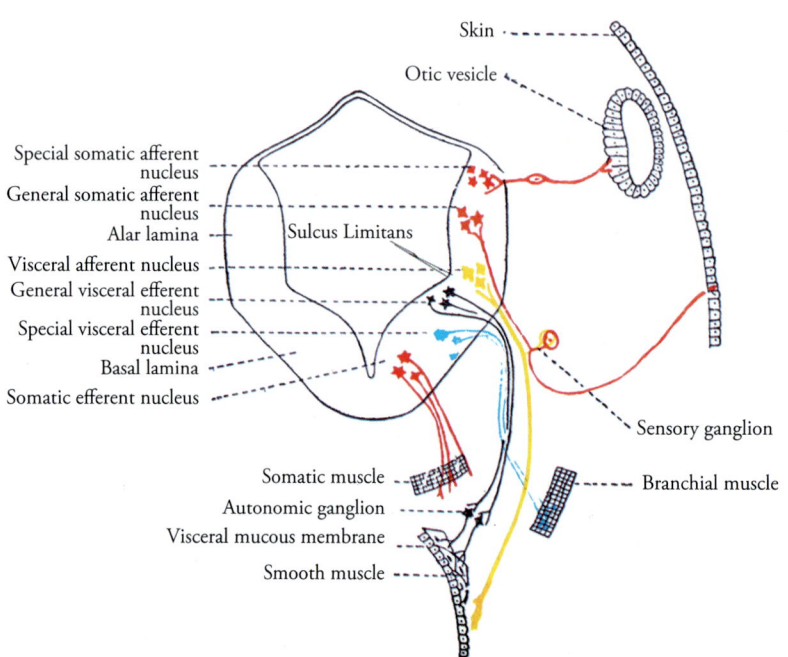

Figure 12.3 Internal surface of the base of the skull with the foramina and fissures labeled and cranial nerves passing through it identified (in red). (From J. Zimmerman and S. Jacobson, Anatomy, 1989, Figure 7-6, Little, Brown & Company, Boston.)

COMPONENTS OF THE CRANIAL NERVES

In the spinal cord, the neurons are arranged in continuous columns of cells, each of which is connected to a structure with a specific function. This grouping of neurons with similar anatomic and physiologic function is called a nerve component. In the spinal cord, the neurons innervate general structures such as skin skeletal muscles, blood vessels, glands, and viscera. They do not innervate the special sense organs: the eye, the ear, or the taste buds.

In the brain stem, cranial nerve nuclei that innervate structures of a similar embryonic origin are found in approximately the same position throughout the medulla, pons, and midbrain. These nuclei are arranged in columns, near the ventricular floor or in the reticular formation (Fig. 12.2).

All the motor and sensory nuclei in the spinal cord are of a general nature and are designated in the nerve component scheme of Herrick (1948) as follows.

MOTOR (EFFERENT)

To skeletal muscle, CN III–VII, IX–XII

– To smooth muscle and glands, CN III, IX, and X

– To cardiac muscle, CN X

SENSORY (AFFERENT)

– From cutaneous and proprioceptive receptors V, VII, IX, and X

– From viscera, CN IX, and CN X

In addition to these general categories in nerves of the spinal cord, we find in the cranial nerves, neurons innervating the special sensory receptors (ear, eye, taste buds) or muscles in the face, pharynx, and larynx, which originated from pharyngeal arches (Figs. 12.3 and 12.4). These special categories are present only in cranial nerves (see Table 12.1).

The discussion that follows will review the functions and clinical disorders associated with each of the 12 cranial nerves. At the end of this chapter we have included Table 12.2 that summarizes the cranial nerve syndromes produced by mass lesions.

GENERAL FUNCTIONS AND CLINICAL DISORDERS OF EACH CRANIAL NERVE

CRANIAL NERVE I: OLFACTORY

The olfactory nerve (Fig. 12.5) originates from receptor cells in the nasal mucosa. The unmyelinated nerve fibers combine into about 20 bundles, pierce the cribiform plate, and end in the glomerular layer of the olfactory bulb (see Chapter 22 for

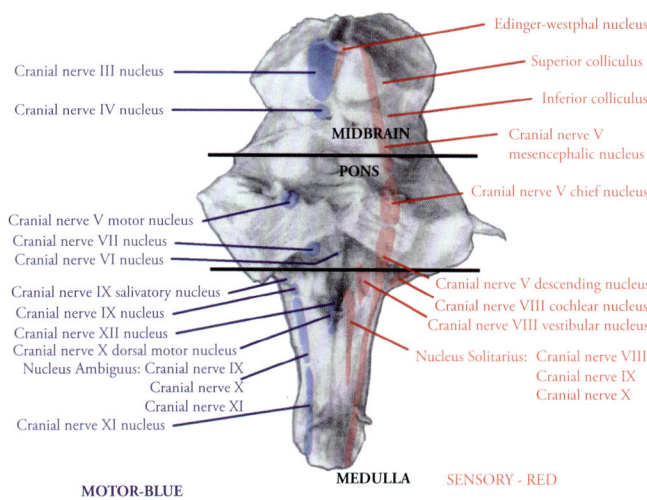

Figure 12.4 Location of cranial nerve nuclei in the brain stem with sensory nuclei on the right lateral and motor nuclei on the left. (From S. Jacobson and E. M. Marcus, Neuroanatomy for the Neuroscientist, Springer 2011.)

a discussion on chemoreception). These fibers have an especially important input to the amygdala (a cluster of nuclei deep within the anterior/medial sector of the temporal lobe). This is the only cranial nerve associated solely with the telencephalon.

CLINICAL DISORDERS: DEFECTS IN SMELL (ANOSMIA)

The most frequent causes of unilateral or bilateral anosmia are as follows:

1. Disease of nasal mucosa producing swelling and preventing olfactory stimuli from reaching the olfactory receptors.

2. Head trauma—resulting in shear effects, tearing the filaments of olfactory receptor cells passing through the cribiform plate.

3. Less common cause of unilateral anosmia is an olfactory groove meningioma compressing the olfactory bulb and tract.

4. The normal process of aging and degenerative central nervous system disorders, including Alzheimer's disease and Parkinson's disease.

CRANIAL NERVE II: OPTIC

The optic nerve (Fig. 12.6), because it is invested with glial cells not Schwann cells, is actually a tract of the central nervous system. The optic nerve originates from the axons of the ganglion cells (tertiary neurons) of the retina, which are ensheathed with myelin as they leave the neural retina. These axons form the optic nerve, which exits the orbit via the optic foramen; then pass through and are rearranged in the optic chiasm to form the optic tract; and finally terminate in the optic thalamus (lateral geniculate nucleus) and superior colliculus.

Table 12.1 **COMPONENTS OF THE CRANIAL NERVES**

FUNCTIONS	CRANIAL NERVE
1. Motor to skeletal muscles of somite origin	Nerve III (midbrain), IV (midbrain), VI (pons), and XII (medulla) *Location*: Brain stem tegmental zone = ventricular
2. Motor to the parasympathetic	Edinger-Westphal nucleus (midbrain) Superior salivatory nuclei nerve VII (see Fig. 11.13) (pons), Inferior salivatory nucleus of nerve IX (medulla), Dorsal motor nuclei of nerve X (medulla) *Location*: Brain stem tegmental zone = ventricular
3. Motor to skeletal muscles of pharyngeal and visceral origin	Motor nuclei of nerves V, VII, IX, and X (pons and medulla) *Location*: Brain stem tegmental zone = ventricular
4. Sensory visceral and gustatory sensation—general sensation from the viscera as well as taste sensation	Solitary nucleus. Primary cell bodies are located in the sensory ganglia of nerves VII, IX, and X
5. Sensory—cutaneous and proprioceptive nucleus from skin and muscles in the head and neck	Trigeminal nuclei—mesencephalic nucleus (midbrain), chief sensory (midpontine), and descending nucleus of nerve V (lower pons> cervical level spinal cord). General sensations carried in by nerves III, IV, VI, VII, XI, and XII synapse in the descending nucleus of cranial nerve V. *Location:* lateral zone medulla
6. Special sensory	Olfaction I: base of frontal lobe, olfactory bulb, Vision II: retina>lateral geniculate nucleus of thalamus>occipital lobe VIII hearing and balance: tegmentum pons and medulla

CLINICAL DISORDERS

A complete or partial unilateral loss of vision is produced by retinal or optic nerve disease. Partial lesions produce a scotoma, "a hole in the visual field."

1. Retinal disease

   a. Transient—carotid occlusive disease

   b. Central retinal artery thrombosis—sudden and persistent

   c. Central venous thrombosis

   Degeneration—retinitis pigmentosa

   Tumors—malignant melanoma

2. Optic nerve disease: Optic neuropathy

   a. Optic neuritis: demyelination as manifestation of multiple sclerosis

   b. Ischemic optic neuropathy

   c. Toxic effects, for example, methanol poisoning usually bilateral

   d. Deficiency states: for example, thiamine and B12: usually bilateral

   e. Familial degeneration: Leber's optic neuropathy

   f. Compression: by masses

      – Inner third sphenoid wing or olfactory groove:

      – Meningioma

      – Glioma of optic nerve

      – Long-standing papilledema

      – Pituitary masses (usually involve optic chiasm producing a bitemporal hemianopia)

   g. Complication of other disorders:

      – Sarcoid

      – Lymphoma

      – Immunologic

CRANIAL NERVE III: OCULOMOTOR

The oculomotor nucleus (Fig. 12.7) is a pure motor nucleus and is found in the tegmentum of the midbrain in sections containing the superior colliculus. This nucleus indents the medial longitudinal fasciculus. *The oculomotor complex can be differentiated into a somatic and visceral portion.*

The somatic portion consists of the lateral nuclear complex and a single central nucleus, the Edinger-Westphal. The individual muscles are represented in the lateral nuclear complex, but data on the exact location and extent of crossed and uncrossed innervation of the eye muscles are incomplete.

The *visceral portion of the Edinger-Westphal nucleus* in the floor of the cerebral aqueduct provides the preganglionic parasympathetic fibers to the ciliary ganglion in the orbit. The postganglionic motor fibers pass to the muscles of accommodation and pupillary constriction, permitting constriction of the pupil in response to light and an increase in the thickness

Table 12.2 SUMMARY OF THE NUCLEI AND FUNCTIONS OF EACH CRANIAL NERVE

CRANIAL NERVE	LOCATION OF CELL BODIES	FUNCTION
I. Olfactory	Neuroepithelial cells in nasal cavity	Olfaction
II. Optic-central pathways discussed in Chapter 21	Ganglion cells in retina	Vision
III. Oculomotor	Oculomotor nucleus in tegmentum of upper midbrain	Eye movements, levator palpekal supenored, superior medial and inferior rectus, inferior oblique Pupillary constriction and accommodation of lens for near vision through ciliary ganglion
	Edinger-Westphal nucleus in tegmentum of upper midbrain—preganglionic to ciliary ganglion	
IV. Trochlear	Trochlear nucleus in tegmentum of lower midbrain	Eye movements (contralateral), superior oblique muscle
V. Trigeminal	Primary trigeminal ganglion, Secondary mesencephalic (midbrain), chief sensory (pons), and descending spiral nuclei (pons, medulla, upper cervical levels)	Cutaneous and proprioceptive sensations from skin and muscles in face, orbit nose, mouth, forehead, teeth, paranasal sinuses, meninges, and anterior two-thirds of tongue
	Motor nucleus in pons	Muscles of mastication
VI. Abducens	Abducens nucleus in tegmentum of pons	Eye movements, ipsilateral, involving lateral rectus muscle
VII. Facial	Primary geniculate ganglion: -Secondary nucleus solitarius -Motor nucleus in lateral margin of pons -Superior salivatory nucleus in pons -Preganglionic parasympathetic to ganglia associated with these glands	Gustatory sensations from taste buds in anterior two-thirds of tongue Muscles of facial expression and platysma; extrinsic and intrinsic ear muscles, stapedius muscle Glands of nose and palate and the lacrimal, submaxillary and sublingual glands through pterygopalatine and submandibular ganglia
VIII. Vestibulo-acoustic (central pathways discussed in Chapter 15)	Primary vestibular and cochlear ganglion, temporal bone Secondary cochlear nuclei in medulla Secondary vestibular nuclei in medulla and pons	Audition equilibrium, coordination, orientation in space
IX. Glossopharyngeal	Primary inferior ganglion; secondary nucleus solitarius Inferior salivatory nucleus in medulla nucleus ambiguus Preganglionic to otic ganglion	Interoceptive palate and posterior one-third of tongue, carotid body Gustatory sensations from taste buds in posterior one-third of tongue Secretions from parotid gland through otic ganglion Swallowing, stylopharyngeus mm Visceral sensations
X. Vagus	Primary superior inferior ganglion; dorsal motor nucleus — preganglionic (parasympathetic innervation); nucleus ambiguus in medulla	Visceral sensations from pharynx, larynx aortic body and thorax and abdomen Gustatory sensation from taste buds in epiglottis and pharynx Skeletal muscles in pharynx and larynx Smooth muscles in heart, blood vessels, trachea, bronchi, esophagus, stomach, intestine to lower colon
XI. Spinal accessory	Cranial portion ambiguus nucleus in medulla; spinal portion: C2, C3, and C4	Innervation sternomastoid Trapezius and MM of pharynx, larynx, except cricothyroids
XII. Hypoglossal	Hypoglossal nucleus in medulla	Innervation of intrinsic and extrinsic muscles of the tongue except palatoglossal MM

of the lens for accommodation (focus on objects within 6 inches of the eye).

The somatic fibers from the nuclear complex of nerve III pass anteriorly through the tegmentum of the midbrain. Some fibers run through the red nucleus and others pass lateral or medial to it, finally entering the medial margin of the cerebral peduncle and reuniting in the interpeduncular fossa to form nerve III. Nerve III emerges from the midbrain superior to the pons between the superior cerebellar artery and the posterior cerebral artery. It then penetrates the dura, enters the cavernous sinus, where it lies lateral to the internal carotid artery, and enters the orbit via the superior orbital fissure (Fig. 12.8A) and separates into superior and inferior divisions. The *superior division* innervates the levator palpebra superioris and the superior rectus muscles, while the *inferior division* supplies the medial and inferior rectus and inferior oblique muscles and sends roots from the Edinger-Westphal nucleus to the ciliary ganglion. The superior rectus muscle elevates

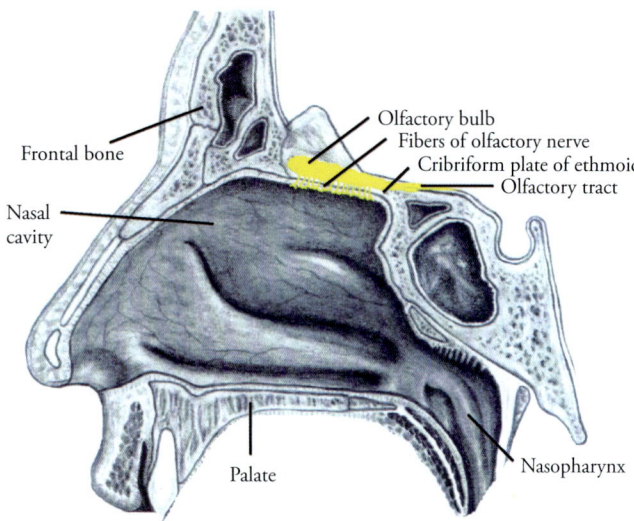

Figure 12.5 The olfactory nerve: cranial nerve I.

the eyeball and turns it upward and inward. The medial rectus muscle adducts the eyeball. The inferior rectus muscle depresses the eyeball and adducts it to some degree, turning the eye downward and inward. The major action of the inferior oblique muscle occurs when the eyeball is adducted; contraction of the inferior oblique muscle both elevates and rotates the eye. The superior levator palpebra controls the eyelid.

CLINICAL DISORDERS

1. *Complete paralysis of nerve III* produces ptosis of the lid, paralysis of the medial and upward gaze, weakness in downward gaze, and dilation of the pupil. The eyeball deviates laterally and slightly downward: the dilated pupil does not react to light or accommodation. Paralysis of the intrinsic muscles (the ciliary sphincter, or pupil) is called internal ophthalmoplegia, while paralysis of the extraocular muscles (recti and obliques) is called external ophthalmoplegia.

Figure 12.6 The optic nerve: cranial nerve II.

2. *Causes of cranial nerve III dysfunction*

   a. *Compression syndromes* involve both pupillary and extraocular muscles. Initially only the pupil may be involved. See Case 12.1.
      - Aneurysm of posterior communication internal carotid artery junction
      - Lesions within the cavernous sinus
      - Herniation of temporal lobe
      - Tumors—meningioma of tuberculum sellae or sphenoid wing

   b. Noncompression syndromes
      - Diabetic cranial neuropathy (vascular)—pupil may be spared, at time of extraocular involvement. However, diabetes mellitus may be associated with a pseudotabetic pupil
      - Ophthalmaloplegic migraine

The following case is an example of involvement of the oculomotor nerve secondary to an aneurysm.

CASE HISTORY 12.1

This 50-year-old, right-handed, white male factory foramen was referred for evaluation of ptosis and diplopia involving the left eye. Approximately 2 weeks prior to admission, the patient developed a bifrontal headache; during the week prior to his evaluation the headache had become a left-sided aching pain. It increased in intensity during the 2 days prior to admission and was present as a constant pain interfering with sleep. If the patient were to cough, he had additional pain in the left eye. On the day of admission the headache became much more severe; it was now the worst headache he had ever experienced. In retrospect, the patient reported that lights had been brighter in the left eye for approximately 1 week. At 3:00 p.m. on the day of admission the patient noted the sudden onset of diplopia, which was more marked on horizontal gaze to the right and was not present on horizontal gaze to the left. At approximately the same time he noted the rapid onset of ptosis involving the left lid.

General physical examination: There was moderate resistance to flexion of the neck.

Neurological Examination
Findings were limited to the left cranial nerve III.

1. The left pupil was fully dilated to approximately 7 mm. There was no response to light or accommodation.
2. Total ptosis of the left eyelid was present.
3. No medial movement of the left eye was present; there was no upward movement of the left eye possible. The patient had minimal downward gaze of the left eye. He had full lateral movement of the left eye. Movements of the right eye were full and the pupil was normal in size and responses.

Clinical diagnosis: Subarachnoid hemorrhage secondary to an aneurysm at the junction of the posterior communicating and internal carotid arteries.

Figure 12.7 The oculomotor, trochlear, and abducens nerves (respectively, cranial nerves III, IV, and VI), and the location of their nuclei in the pons and midbrain of the brain stem. Lateral view of right eye. (*A*) Cranial nerves III, IV, and VI in pons and midbrain. (*B*) Cavernous sinus containing internal carotid artery and cranial nerves III, IV, VI, and V1 (maxillary of trigeminal). Case 12.4. A metastatic tumor nodule was present and found to have destroyed the left abducens nucleus and part of the adjacent paramedian pontine reticular formation. (*C*) Pontine tegmental level with metastatic tumor into facial colliculus affecting ipsilateral cranial nerves VI (to lateral rectus) and VII (to muscles of facial expression). Pupil is unaffected.

Laboratory Data

1. Lumbar puncture demonstrated bloody spinal fluid with no definite clearing from Tube 1 to Tube 3 and approximately 40,000 fresh red blood cells in each tube.
2. Four-vessel angiography: The left posterior cerebral arose from the left internal carotid artery as a continuation of the posterior communicating artery. At the junction of the posterior communicating and the internal carotid arteries, a 13 mm aneurysm was present directed posteriorly. Other vessels were within normal limits.

Subsequent course: The neck of the aneurysm was clipped by the neurosurgeon, Dr. Bernard Stone. Adhesions and clots were present between the aneurysm and the third cranial nerve. The patient did well except that the third nerve paralysis was still present at the time of discharge, 3 weeks after surgery.

Comments

The occurrence on the day of admission of the worst headache ever experienced by the patient suggested the possibility of a subarachnoid hemorrhage. Most (85%) patients with an acute subarachnoid hemorrhage have an underlying saccular aneurysm.

There are three major locations for single intracranial aneurysms:

1. the junction of the posterior communicating and the internal carotid arteries,
2. the junction of the anterior communicating and anterior cerebral arteries, and
3. the bifurcation of the middle cerebral artery in the Sylvian fissure.

The posterior communicating artery is adjacent to and runs parallel to the third cranial nerve. With hemorrhage, compression of or bleeding into the nerve symptoms will develop relevant to cranial nerve III. Thus, in patients with prodromal symptoms, a third nerve syndrome allows the prediction of this specific location of the aneurysm. Because of the arrangement of the fibers within this nerve, the initial symptoms of compression often involve the pupillary fibers. In retrospect, the early symptoms of lights being brighter in the left eye, 1 week before the ptosis and diplopia developed, would be consistent with a pupil that was unable to constrict in response to light. We will discuss in greater detail in a later chapter that one can predict the middle cerebral location when symptoms and signs relevant to the middle cerebral artery occur. The anterior communicating location is often difficult to predict because weakness in both legs may occur but may be accompanied by loss of consciousness due to bilateral frontal lobe involvement. In many patients, in all locations, the bleeding may be so massive that loss of consciousness rapidly follows the sudden headache, and localization is not possible. Management of intracranial aneurysms will be discussed in Chapter 26 on vascular syndromes.

CRANIAL NERVE IV: TROCHLEAR

The trochlear nucleus (Fig. 12.7) is purely motor and located in the medio superior part of the tegmentum in the lower parts of the mesencephalon. It extends throughout the inferior collicular levels and is nearly continuous with the lateral nuclear complex of nerve III.

The nucleus of nerve IV indents the medial longitudinal fasciculis (MLF). Nerve IV is a unique cranial nerve as (1) its rootlets are on the posterior surface of the brain stem, and (2) the fibers cross as they exit the brain stem. The fibers proceed inferiorly and posteriorly in the periaqueductal gray, decussate in the anterior medullary velum, exit from the substance of the brain at the caudal end of the inferior colliculus, and then run ventrally, lateral to the nerve III rootlets. In the cavernous sinus, the nerve is lateral to the nerve III rootlets and enters the orbit through the superior orbit fissure, where it terminates in the superior oblique muscle. The major action of the superior oblique muscle occurs with the eye adducted. In that position the muscle is in line with the globe. Since the muscle is attached posteriorly, on the superior surface of the globe the globe will be tilted down. With the eyeball in the physiologic condition, contraction of this muscle results in rotation of the eyeball.

CLINICAL DISORDERS

Trauma is the primary cause of defects in CN IV movement. A nuclear lesion of nerve IV paralyzes the contralateral superior oblique muscle while a lesion in the nerve roots after decussation involves the ipsilateral muscle. A selective unilateral impairment of downgaze when the eye is adducted is usually due to a lesion of this cranial nerve. To compensate, the head may be held in a tilted position. However, a thrombosis or tumor in the cavernous sinus may also affect this nerve along with cranial nerves III, V, and VI.

CRANIAL NERVE V: TRIGEMINAL

The trigeminal nerve (Fig. 12.8A) is the largest cranial nerve and provides sensory fibers from the face (the first branchial arch)—including the posterior surface of the ear, the scalp up to the vertex, and the undersurface of the lower jaw—and motor fibers to the mastication muscles. The sensory root contains the *semilunar or gasserian ganglia,* which is larger than the motor root. Within the brain stem are one motor and three sensory nuclei. The motor nucleus of nerve V is located at the midpontine levels medial to the trigeminal root at the lateral part of the reticular formation. The three main branches of nerve V are ophthalmic, maxillary, and mandibular. Except for the mesencephalic nuclei, the primary cell bodies for the sensory fibers are located in the trigeminal (semilunar or Gasserian) ganglion in the middle cranial fossa.

PRIMARY SENSORY CELL BODIES (TRIGEMINAL GANGLION)

The primary sensory cell bodies of nerve V are found in the semilunar ganglion in Meckel's cave (cavum Trigeminal). They are unique as they are the only 1° sensory neurons found within the cranial cavity. They are located in the middle cranial fossa, in a recess in the petrous portion of the temporal

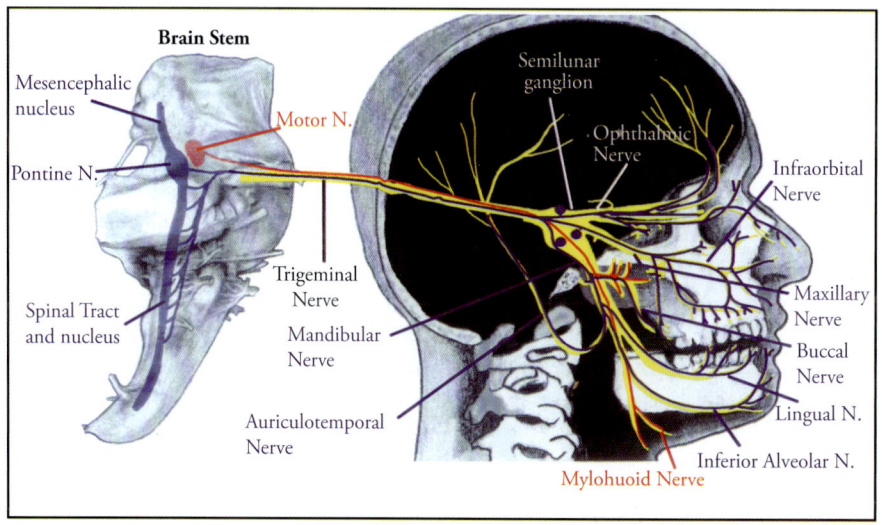

Figure 12.8A The trigeminal nerve: cranial nerve V.

Figure 12.8B Case 12.3. Distribution of lesions of H. zoster ophthalmicus in a 44-year-old physician. Note that there is no involvement of the nasociliary branch and thus there was no involvement of the cornea.

bone below the superior petrosal sinus. This is the largest sensory ganglion in the human. The centrally directed axons of the cells in the semilunar ganglion constitute the sensory root of the trigeminal nerve.

Trigeminal Peripheral Branches

1. *The ophthalmic branch of the trigeminal nerve (V1).* This nerve originates from the medial part of the semilunar ganglion, passes into the lateral wall of the cavernous sinus, and divides into its terminal branches in the superior orbital fissure. The smallest division of CN V, V1 innervates the skin of the forehead and scalp to the vertex, the upper eyelid, the skin of the anterior and bridge of the nose, the eyeballs, cornea, and ciliary body, conjunctiva, and iris, the mucosa in the frontal and nasal sinuses, and the cerebral falx and tentorium.

2. *The maxillary nerve (V2)* arises from the middle of the semilunar ganglion in the cavernous sinus. It leaves the middle cranial fossa via the foramen rotundum and enters the pterygopalatine fossa, where it becomes the infraorbital nerve. The maxillary division of nerve V (V2) supplies the skin on the temples; lateral surface of the nose, the lower eyelid, the upper cheek and the upper lip; the gums and molar, premolar, and canine teeth (superior dental plexus); and the mucous membranes of the mouth, nose, and maxillary sinus. The maxillary nerve also supplies the dura in the middle cranial fossa (middle meningeal nerve).

3. *The mandibular division of nerve V (V3),* the largest of the three divisions, is formed by the union of the sensory and motor root at the inferior border of the semilunar ganglion. The motor root exits the middle cranial fossa through the foramen ovale, where it joins the sensory root. The motor portion of the trigeminal innervates the muscle of mastication and the tensor tympani and tensor veli palatini. The sensory root supplies the skin of the chin, lower jaw, and temporal-mandibular joint, the dura in the middle and anterior cranial fossa, the lower teeth and gums, the oral mucosa, and part of the ear.

SECONDARY SENSORY NUCLEI IN THE BRAIN STEM

The sensory root enters the mid pons and divides into short ascending and long descending fibers.

The short ascending fibers terminate in two nuclei: the chief sensory nucleus and the mesencephalic nucleus.

Those fibers mediating light touch and light pressure sensation terminate in synapses on second-order neurons in the principal (chief) sensory nucleus.

The *chief sensory nucleus* of nerve V is found in the mid-pontine tegmentum, lateral to the root of nerve V. It receives cutaneous sensory information from the face and head and the nasal and oral cavities and transmits this information to the thalamus via fibers that travel with or adjacent to the medial lemniscus. This nucleus is in a sense the analog of the nuclei gracilis and cuneatus of the posterior columns.

The short ascending fibers mediating proprioceptive information from the face to the masseter and related trigeminal muscles and the ocular muscles terminate in the mesencephalic nucleus.

The *mesencephalic nucleus* is located lateral to the fourth ventricle and the cerebral aqueduct in the upper pontine and midbrain levels. This is the only primary sensory nucleus (dorsal root ganglion equivalent) located within the central nervous system. The mesencephalic and motor nuclei provide a two-neuron reflex (monosynaptic) arc for the jaw jerk.

The *descending or spinal nucleus* of nerve V is the equivalent of the substantia gelatinosa in the dorsal horn of the spinal cord. Pain and temperature fibers synapse here. External to the descending nucleus of nerve V is the descending tract of nerve V. This tract is the equivalent of Lissauer's tract of the spinal cord. Within this tract the fibers from the ophthalmic nerve descend to the third cervical level. The maxillary fibers descend to the first cervical level. The pain fibers from the mandibular and cranial nerves VII, IX, X, XI, and XII descend through the lower medullary levels.

The *secondary fibers from the spinal nucleus of CN V* are principally crossed and they ascend in the medial lemniscus to the ventral posterior medial nucleus in the thalamus.

MOTOR FUNCTIONS

The motor root originates in the motor nucleus of nerve V in the pons; joins with the mesencephalic root; and exits from the middle cranial fossa in the foramen ovale, where it then unites with the sensory root. The motor, or mandibular, nerve (V3) innervates the muscles of mastication (Table 12.3).

Function

The combined actions of the muscles associated with the mandible are listed in Table 12.4.

Table 12.3 **MUSCLES OF MASTICATION: INNERVATION BY V3: MANDIBULAR BRANCH OF CRANIAL NERVE V**

MUSCLE	MOVEMENT OF MANDIBLE
Lateral	Works in unison with the other muscles
Pterygoid	Working by itself moves the jaw laterally; protrudes and depresses mandible
Medial pterygoid	Works in unison with the other muscles to elevate the mandible; assists the external pterygoid muscle in protruding mandible
Temporal	Elevates and retracts the mandible
Masseter	Elevates and slightly protrudes the mandible
Mylohyoid	Elevates the floor of mouth and tongue
Anterior belly	Elevates and stabilizes the hyoid bone of digastric

The mandibular branch of the trigeminal nerve also innervates the tensor veil palatine and tensor tympani muscle.

1. *Tensor veli palatine* tenses the palate and draws it to one side and thus prevents food from entering the nasal pharynx.
2. *Tensor tympani muscle* located in the inner ear pulls on the malleus that tenses the tympanic membrane and diminishes the amplitude of the vibrations caused by a loud noise.

CLINICAL DISORDERS

Injury to the trigeminal nerve paralyzes the muscles of mastication, with the jaw deviating toward the side of the lesion. Injury may also block sensation of light touch, pain, and temperature in the face and results in the absence of the corneal and sneeze reflexes.

Table 12.4 **MOVEMENTS OF THE MANDIBLE**

IN MASTICATION, THE JAWS MOVE UP AND DOWN, FORWARD AND BACKWARD, AND LATERALLY

ACTION OF MANDIBLE	MUSCLE GROUP
1. Elevation	Masseter, temporal, and medial pterygoid
2. Depression and opening of the mandible	Lateral pterygoid muscle, in concert with suprahyoid muscles (mylohyoid, digastric, geniohyoid, infrahyoid)
	Depressors of the hyoid (sternohyoid and mylohyoid muscles), along with gravity
3. Protrusion	The medial and lateral pterygoid muscles of the jaw assisted by the masseter muscle
4. Retraction	The temporal and digastric of the jaw muscles
5. Side-to-side movement	The pterygoid muscles permit side-to-side movement

Localization of Motor Dysfunction of the Trigeminal Nerve

a. Lesions in the pons may affect only the motor nuclei and produce a paresis or paralysis of the ipsilateral muscles. If the lesion is destructive, atrophy and fasciculations of the affected muscles result. The jaw jerk is also absent.

b. Since the cortical innervation of the muscles of mastication is bilateral, *unilateral supranuclear lesions* may produce only a slight weakness, with a minimal increase in the jaw jerk. In contrast, a *bilateral capsular or cortical lesion* will produce marked paresis or even paralysis in the muscles of mastication, with an exaggerated jaw jerk, essentially the findings of an upper motor lesion.

c. Pontine lesions usually injure both the main sensory and motor nuclei, causing paralysis of the muscles of mastication and diminished tactile sensation ipsilaterally. Lesions of the lower lateral pontine tegmentum at the dorsal lateral medullary tegmentum may damage the descending tract and nucleus of V.

d. Tumors in the cerebellopontine angle or acoustic nerve may compress the trigeminal tubercle and cause an ipsilateral loss of the corneal reflex.

Localization of Sensory Dysfunction of the Trigeminal Nerve

Trigeminal neuralgia (tic, douloureux) is a disorder characterized by recurrent paroxysms of stabbing pains along the distribution of the involved branches. The overall incidence of the syndrome has been estimated as 4.3 per 100,000 per year.

1. Clinical signs of trigeminal neuralgia

a. Etiology: "idiopathic," with mean age of onset in the 50s. Patients with an age of onset in the 20s or 30s often have an underlying disease of brain stem, such as multiple sclerosis or arteriovenous malformation, or may have an underlying systemic disease.

b. Trigger points produce the pain on tactile stimulation. The pain is of short duration, a lancinating pain, usually occurring in clusters or paroxysms. Pain may resolve spontaneously only to recur months later.

c. Location of pain. The second (maxillary division) is most frequently involved. The third (mandibular division) is next in frequency. The first (ophthalmic division) is least common. The pain is unilateral, rarely bilateral.

d. Clinical findings. There are no sensory or motor findings on examination, although after frequent repeated episodes the patient may complain of minor numbness and a more persistent aching type pain.

e. Treatment. Though many of these cases respond to medication—such as carbamazepine, some do not and require surgical therapy. Patients with onset after age 40 may have compression of the trigeminal nerve by an anomalous loop of an artery compressing the nerve or root entry zone. Treatment in such cases that fail to respond to medications involves relocating the loop of the superior cerebellar artery or insulating the nerve from the pulsation of the vessel by inserting a soft implant between nerve and vessel. Other surgical procedures are designed to alter transmission through the Gasserian ganglion.

Other Causes of Trigeminal Symptoms

a. Compression or invasion of nerves by nasopharyngeal tumors which have infiltrated the base of the skull through the foramen rotundum (maxillary) or foramen ovale (mandibular) or other points of erosion.

b. Dental pathology or maxillary sinusitis may produce pain within the appropriate divisions of the trigeminal nerve; tingling and numbness in the mandibular or less often maxillary division may occur spontaneously or may follow dental procedures.

c. Herpes zoster involvement of the Gasserian ganglion. Acute pain almost always occurs in the ophthalmic division followed in 4–5 days by cutaneous lesions. Early treatment with Acyclovir will decrease the period of pain. In other patients postherpetic neuralgia may develop. (Note: The H. zoster/varicella virus is often dormant in the Gasserian ganglion and may be reactivated later in life.)

The following case is an example of trigeminal neuralgia.

CASE HISTORY 12.2

This 28-year-old, single, black, right-handed female reported approximately 21 days of sudden lancinating jabs of pain plus a duller more steady pain involving the right maxillary and mandibular distribution. She was very aware that she could trigger her pain by touching her nose or the skin over the maxillary or mandibular area. The pain was so severe that talking, chewing, or eating would all trigger episodes. As a result, she has not been eating a great deal. There was no clear-cut extension of pain into the eye, although some of the background pain did spread into the supraorbital area and back toward the interauricular line.

Two years prior to admission, she had a less severe episode in the same distribution that lasted 3 weeks. She denied any tearing of the eye or nasal stuffiness. She had no tingling of the face, change in hearing, facial paralysis, or diplopia.

Past history indicated (1) treatment for tuberculosis at age 7 or 8 years because of a positive skin test after exposure to a relative with the disease; (2) prior treated gonococcal infection; (3) an intake of 1 liter of whiskey on each weekend.

Neurological Examination
Mental status: Intact.
Cranial nerves were not remarkable except for findings relevant to the right fifth cranial nerve. Although touch and pain sensation over the face was normal, there were clear-cut exquisite trigger points producing sharp pains on light tactile stimulation of the nose or other maxillary areas as well as the mandibular skin areas and the mandibular supplied lower molars.
Motor system (including gait and cerebellar system): Intact.
Reflexes: All were normal except for an absence of the right patellar and both Achilles deep tendon stretch reflexes. Plantar responses were flexor.
Sensory system: Intact.
Clinical diagnosis: Trigeminal neuralgia: maxillary and mandibular divisions.
Laboratory Data

1. *Computerized tomography (CT) scan of the head, sinus X-rays, and a panoramic dental X-ray series* obtained in the emergency room 11 days prior to evaluation were not remarkable.
2. *White blood count* was normal.
3. *The erythrocyte sedimentation rate* was significantly elevated to 63 mm/hr.
4. *Antinuclear antibody* was positive at 1:1280 (anticentromere pattern), consistent with lupus erythematosus, an autoimmune disease.

Subsequent course: Evaluation by a dentist indicated no relevant dental disease. Treatment with phenytoin (Dilantin) produced partial improvement in symptoms so that she was now able to talk without pain. Subsequently the patient received carbamazepine and nerve blocks with greater relief of symptoms. In addition, she received treatment of her underlying autoimmune disease.

Comments

This patient had the classical symptoms of trigeminal neuralgia. Patients with onset at this age often have an underlying disorder such as multiple sclerosis or in this case an autoimmune disorder. As regards the loss of deep tendon reflexes, this may have reflected nutritional causes related to the excessive intake of alcohol or may have related to effects on peripheral nerve of the autoimmune disease.

The following case is an example of Herpes zoster involving the ophthalmic division of the trigeminal nerve.

CASE HISTORY 12.3

This ophthalmic Herpes zoster developed over 24 hours in a 44-year-old, right-handed physician, with increasing pain in the right supraorbital and orbital areas. Edema of the eyelid developed within 36 hours (Fig. 12.8B). Erythematous, edematous vesicular skin lesions developed over the right supraorbital area and the anterior half of the right side of the scalp. Edema of the lid was sufficient to produce closure of the lid. Significant cervical lymphadenopathy, neck pain, and low-grade fever developed. The acute pain gradually subsided over 2 weeks, but the skin lesions persisted.

The skin lesions crusted and gradually cleared over 4 weeks. Occasional episodes of right supraorbital pain continued to occur for 1 year. Faded, depressed scars were still present 24 years after the acute episode.

Clinical diagnosis: Ophthalmic Herpes zoster.
Comments
The development of pain followed by the characteristic skin lesions is consistent with the diagnosis of trigeminal neuralgia involving the

ophthalmic division of the trigeminal nerve. In some cases the cornea is involved with residual scarring. This complication is more likely to occur when the nasociliary branch of the ophthalmic nerve, supplying the midline nose, is involved. This patient did not have this pattern of involvement and did not have corneal involvement. Postherpetic neuralgia (persistence of pain greater than 1 year after the acute event) as discussed earlier is more likely to occur in older patients and did not occur in this middle-aged individual. As indicated previously, this disorder represents a reactivation of the varicella virus residual in sensory ganglia such as the trigeminal. In rare instances, H. zoster ophthalmicus may be complicated by involvement of the intracranial arteries, resulting in infarction of brain.

CRANIAL NERVE VI: ABDUCENS

The nucleus of cranial nerve VI (Fig. 12.7) and the fibers of nerve VII form a prominent structure in the floor of the IV ventricle of the pons, *the facial colliculus*. The abducens nucleus is a large purely motor nucleus surrounded by the looping fibers of nerve VII.

The fibers of nerve VI leave the nucleus medial to the rootlets of nerve VII. Associated with the nucleus of nerve VI is the parabducens nucleus, or nucleus of the parapontine reticular formation, that integrates impulses via the medial longitudinal fasciculus. This center coordinates movements of the lateral rectus muscle of one side with the medial rectus muscle (cranial nerve III) of the other eye, producing conjugate horizontal deviations of the eyes. The parapontine reticular nucleus is also referred to as the lateral gaze center.

The fibers of cranial nerve VI pass inferiorly and emerge from the pons near the midline at the pontomedullary junction. The roots pierce the dura and enter the cavernous sinus (see Fig. 12.7) below and medial to nerve III and lateral to the internal carotid artery. The fibers enter the orbit via the superior orbital fissure and innervate the lateral rectus muscle, which abducts or deviates the eye laterally.

Stimulation of the frontal eye fields in the posterior part of the middle frontal gyrus produces contralateral innervation to the parapontine reticular formation. Stimulation of the occipital lobe also produces conjugate movement to the contralateral side. Movement originating from the occipital lobe is different from that originating in the frontal lobes, as it is primarily an involuntary fixation and tracking of moving objects. The cortical control of eye movement is discussed in Chapter 18.

CLINICAL DISORDERS

This nerve has a long intracranial course; thus, it is commonly affected by any increase in intracranial pressure (the involvement may be unilateral or bilateral) and by nasopharyngeal tumors invading the base of the skull in adults. Pontine gliomas produce similar effects in children.

CASE HISTORY 12.4

This 75-year-old white male had the onset in March of diplopia (double vision). Examination in April revealed only a variable possible lag in movement of the left medial rectus muscle. A Tensilon (edrophonium) test (see Chapter 8) and brain stem auditory evoked potentials were normal. In retrospect, a CT scan in April revealed a very small enhancing lesion at the level of the facial colliculus. Chest X-ray did reveal pleural thickening and a somewhat reticular nodular change of a nonspecific type. The erythrocyte sedimentation rate was elevated to 82 mm/hr, a sign of systemic disease.

The diplopia initially improved, but the patient then developed weight loss, cough, and headache pains. On readmission in June, there was now a clearly defined left abducens nerve paralysis and nystagmus on right lateral gaze. A left peripheral facial paresis was now also noted. Cerebrospinal fluid examination was negative. He was readmitted in July because of progression of the left facial paralysis. On examination he was unable to close the left eye and he was drooling from the left side of the mouth. He was also complaining of diplopia on gaze to either left or right side.

Neurological examination of eye movements: Several severe problems were now demonstrated:

1. On attempted gaze to the left; a total paralysis of left CN VI plus a lesser paresis of conjugate lateral gaze as regards the right eye.
2. On gaze to the right (a) full abduction of the right eye, (b) some adduction of the left eye but this was incomplete, and (c) coarse nystagmus of the abducting right eye.
3. In primary gaze, the left eye was pulled to the right.
4. Convergence was intact for both eyes.
5. Upgaze was intact but minor vertical nystagmus was present.

Conclusions were as follows:

1. Left CN VI paralysis.
2. Left lateral gaze center involved.
3. Left medial longitudinal fasciculus involved.

Except for the left peripheral facial paralysis, the neurological examination was otherwise normal. The CT scan now indicated a more prominent enhancing lesion at the level of the facial colliculus. Despite extensive evaluation of the pulmonary disorder, including bronchoscopy and open lung biopsy (nonspecific fibrosis and chronic inflammation), a specific diagnosis could not be established. The patient was treated both for tuberculosis (chemotherapy) and for possible metastatic tumor to brain stem (radiation therapy). Pulmonary status continued to deteriorate and the patient expired on November.

Postmortem examination: A metastatic tumor nodule was found to have destroyed the left abducens nucleus and part of the adjacent paramedian pontine reticular formation (Fig. 12.7B). Severe degenerative changes were present in the left MLF at the level of rostral pons and midbrain. Sections through the pons at and just below the lesion demonstrated secondary degeneration of the left abducens and left facial nerve.

CRANIAL NERVE VII: FACIAL

The facial nerve (Fig. 12.9A) consists of a large motor nerve with a smaller nerve, the intermediate (intermedius) nerve, located between the motor division of the facial and the vestibuloacoustic nerve component. The intermediate nerve contains taste and somatic sensory fibers from the oropahrynx, and a parasympathetic component. Figure 12.9B demonstrates the peripheral distribution of the sensory (chorda tympani for taste) and motor division (parasympathetic *to submandibular and sublingual glands, and* somatic *motor to muscles of facial expression*) of the facial nerve. In the pons there is one large motor nucleus controlling the muscles of facial expression and a sensory nucleus that reaches the hiatus of the facial canal, while peripherally there is one sensory ganglion the geniculate. The motor fibers supply the muscles associated with the second branchial arch (hyoid arch).

The branchial motor fibers originate from the motor nucleus of nerve VII in the lateral part of the reticular formation at the caudal pontine levels. The fibers leave the nucleus and pass medially and dorsally toward the fourth ventricle. Under the floor of the fourth ventricle, they pass over the dorsal surface of the nucleus of nerve VI and then turn anteriorly, forming the internal genu of the facial nerve. The fibers then pass laterally and anteriorly through the lateral portion of the pontine reticular formation and exit from the pons at its caudal-most border between the rootlets of nerves VI and VIII in the cerebellopontine angle. The nerve enters the posterior cranial fossa and passes into the internal acoustic meatus, where the motor and sensory divisions and nerve VIII lie separated from one another by only the arachnoid sheaths on the nerves. In the meatus the motor and sensory roots of nerve VII combine and enter the facial canal of the temporal bone. The nerve then continues until it reaches the hiatus of the facial canal, then bends

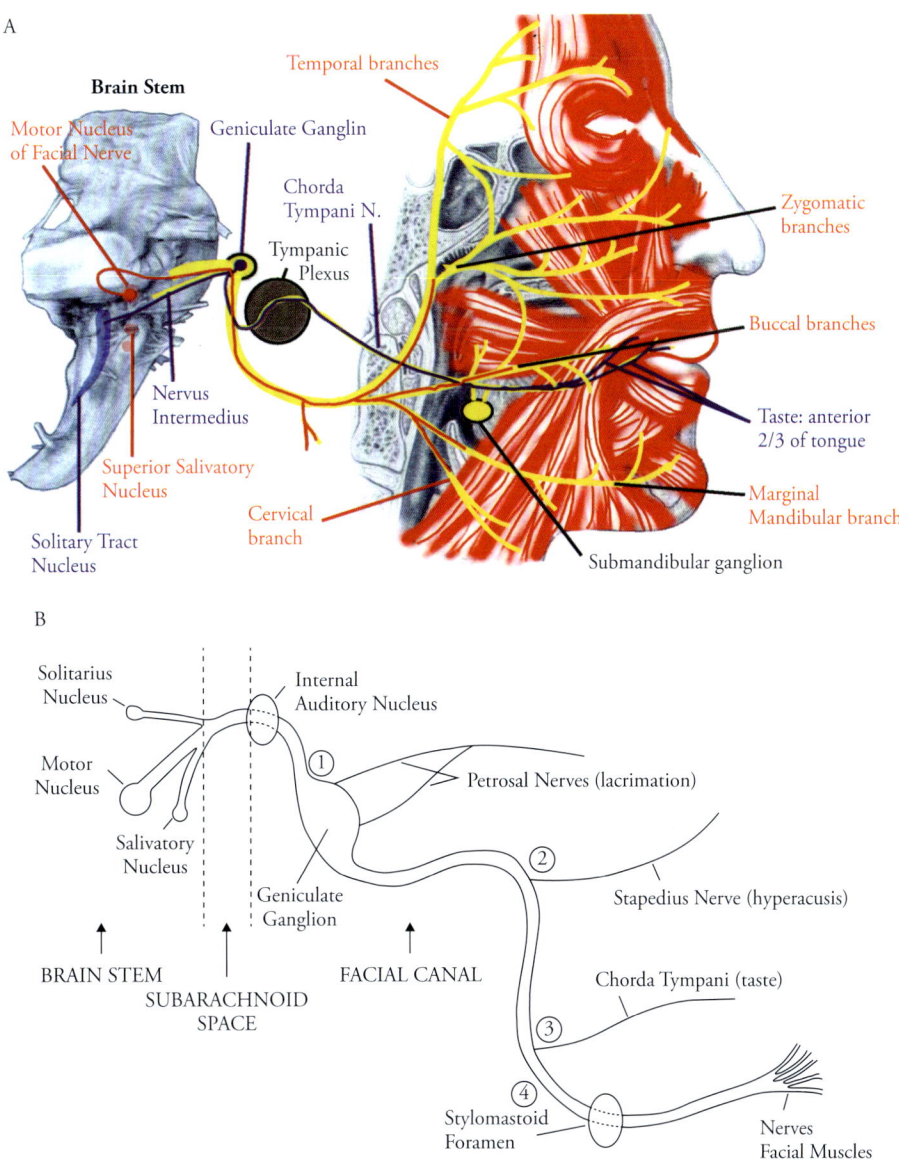

Figure 12.9 The facial nerve: cranial nerve VII. (*A*) Connections from pons onto muscles of facial expression. (*B*) Distribution of Facial Nerve into geniculate ganglion and onto lacrimal glands, chorda tympani for taste buds on anterior 2/3 of tongue, and finally to muscles of facial expression.

around the vestibule of the inner ear, forming the external genu of nerve VII. The geniculate ganglion, located at the external genu, contains the primary cell bodies of the intermediate or sensory root of nerve VII that innervates the external ear.

The *motor root* innervates:

1. The stapedius muscle
2. The posterior belly of the digastric muscle
3. The muscles of facial expression, which are innervated by the five branches of the facial nerve that arise in the parotid gland—temporal, zygomatic, buccal, marginal mandibular, and cervical.

The mimetic muscles are the following: the frontal, orbicularis oculi, anterior auricular, corrugators supercilium, zygomatic, orbicularis oris, depressor labi, levator labi, and levator anguli oris, nasalis, mentalis, platysma, buccinator, and risorius muscles.

Within the facial nucleus in the pons there is a separation into subnuclei representing each of these muscle groups.

Sensory Ganglion—Geniculate

The small sensory root originates from the geniculate sensory ganglia in the inner ear; fibers run through the facial canal into the internal acoustic meatus and then enter the pons. The fibers then pass through the lateral part of the reticular formation, and enter the tractus solitarius, which is found just lateral to the sulcus limitans. The tractus solitarius is separated from the ventricular cavity by the aqueductal gray on the floor of the fourth ventricle. The sensory root of nerve VII carries gustatory impulses from the taste buds in the anterior two-thirds of the tongue and cutaneous sensations from the anterior surface of the ear and the soft palate. The motor and sensory roots continue in the facial canal between the inner and middle ear and then turn and descend to the stylomastoid foramen, where they emerge from the temporal bone.

Chorda Tympani

Just before leaving the stylomastoid foramen, the chorda tympani, carrying taste fibers, separates from motor portion of nerve VII. It enters its own small canal in the petrotympanic fissure, then enters the tympanic cavity and runs on the medial surface of the tympanic membrane (from whence it gets its name), and onto the medial side of the manubrium. The nerve leaves the tympanic cavity and then emerges from the skull near the medial surface of the spine of the sphenoid and joins the lingual nerve at the medial surface of the lateral pterygoid muscle.

Taste Sensation

In the nucleus solitarius the taste sensitive cells are located as follows: (1) HCl (sour cells) are posterior, (2) sweet and salty are anterior, (3) cells responsive to bitter are diffusely located. The secondary axons ascend in the medial lemniscus to the parabrachial nucleus. The taste information then ascends near the central tegmental tract to the parvocellular ventral posterior medial nucleus of the thalamus. This information is then projected onto the parietal operculum. For regulation of feeding behavior, the information enters the lateral hypothalamus and central amygdaloid nuclei.

PARASYMPATHETIC GANGLIA OF CRANIAL NERVE VII: SUBMANDIBULAR AND PTERYGOPALATINE

1. *Submandibular ganglia* are suspended from the lingual nerve on the lateral surface of hypoglossal muscle. The chorda tympani contain parasympathetic preganglionic fibers from the submandibular ganglia, the submaxillary and sublingual glands to the anterior two-thirds of the tongue.

2. The *pterygopalatine ganglia* is suspended from maxillary nerve in pterygopalatine fossa and provides innervation to glands and blood vessels in the nasal cavity, palate, and paranasal air sinuses (maxillary, ethmoid, sphenoid), as well as the lacrimal glands.

   1. *Injury in the brain stem*. A central injury to the facial nucleus in the pons produces ipsilateral paralysis of the facial muscles. Injury to just the nucleus or tractus solitarius, although rare, produces a loss of taste on half of the tongue because the taste fibers from nerves VII and IX are found together in the tractus solitarius.

   2. *Peripheral injury*. Injury to the facial nerve near its origin or in the facial canal produces:

      a. paralysis of the motor, secretory, and facial muscles,

      b. a loss of taste in the anterior two-thirds of the tongue, and

      c. abnormal secretion in the lacrimal and salivary glands.

      As a result, the patient has sagging muscles in the lower half of the face and in the fold around the lips and nose and widening of the palpebral fissure.

      Voluntary control of facial and platysmal musculature is absent. The patient is unable to close the eyelid. When the patient smiles, the lower portion of the face is pulled to the unaffected side. Saliva and food tend to collect on the affected side. When the injury is distal to the ganglion, an excessive accumulation of tears occurs because the eyelids do not move but the lacrimal glands continue to secrete.

      Injury to the facial nerve may also interrupt the reflex arc for the corneal blink reflex, which includes the motor component to the orbicularis from nerve VII and the sensory corneal nerves of the ophthalmic division of the trigeminal nerve. The muscles eventually atrophy.

   d. *Injury to nerve VII at the stylomastoid foramen* produces ipsilateral paralysis of the facial muscles without affecting taste.

   e. *Injury to the chorda tympani* results in absence of taste in the anterior two-thirds of the tongue.

3. Other peripheral sites and other disorders with injury to VII:

   a. *Tumors of the parotid gland* often involve the facial nerve.

   b. *H. zoster (the Ramsey-Hunt syndrome)*: involvement of the sensory geniculate ganglion, associated with the facial nerve will result in a facial nerve paralysis. The cutaneous vesicular lesions involve the small sensory distribution of the facial nerve in the external auditory canal and tympanic membrane. The adjacent CN VIII nerve is often involved, producing vertigo, tinnitus, and deafness. In some patients the dorsal root ganglion of cervical nerves II or III may also be involved.

   c. *Bilateral facial nerve involvement (facial diplegia):*

      1. Guillain-Barré syndrome

      2. Sarcoidosis—uveoparotid fever

   d. *Hemifacial spasm:* spontaneous contractions of the facial muscles occur, often triggered by attempted movement. There is often synkinesis, an overflow of movement, so that attempts to smile result in closure of the eye, and so on. Hemi-facial spasm usually relates to a previous facial nerve paralysis that has partially recovered but in which anomalous reinnervation has occurred. In the majority of cases in which the etiology is unrelated to a previous Bell's palsy, the etiology relates to a compression of the facial nerve root close to the brain stem by a blood vessel such as the anterior inferior cerebellar artery or posterior inferior cerebellar artery. With compression, demyelination will occur with subsequent ephaptic transmission between adjacent fibers. The treatment, both medical (carbamazepine) and surgical (decompression of the nerve placing a soft implant between the vessel and the nerve), is similar to the treatment of trigeminal neuralgia.

   e. *Facial myokymia* is sometimes confused with hemifacial spasm. This is a fine rippling of muscles—arrhythmic involuntary fibrillations.

Etiology: pontine glioma, or multiple sclerosis -producing demyelination of the nerve within the brain stem. However a similar localized effect involving the eyelid or the orbicularis oculi muscle may occur without clinical significance.

Central/Cerebral Innervation of VII. The corticobulbar pathway to the lower half of the facial nucleus is a crossed unilateral innervation, whereas the upper half of the facial nucleus receives a bilateral innervation. A unilateral lesion in the appropriate part of the precentral gyrus will thus paralyze the lower half on the opposite side, sparing the forehead and eye closure, while a bilateral cortical involvement paralyzes both the upper and lower facial musculature. The cerebral cortical control of the muscles of facial expression through the motor strip is especially important in communication. If these upper motor neurons are destroyed or their fibers interrupted in a bilateral manner, other cortical areas, including the limbic system, will now cause inappropriate and excessive facial expressions. This is referred to as pseudobulbar palsy. Pseudobulbar palsy represents excessive uninhibited brain stem activity. External stimuli will then trigger excessive response, for example, excessive crying to a sad story or excessive laughter. The following case is an example of one of the more common disorders of the facial nerve, Bell's palsy.

CASE HISTORY 12.5

This 37-year-old, previously healthy, right handed, white housewife and registered nurse was referred for emergency consultation regarding left facial paralysis. Three days prior to evaluation the patient had developed a dull pain above and behind the left ear. She then noted occasional muscle twitching about the left lower lip and a vague stiffness of the left side of the face. On the morning of the evaluation, the patient noted that she had difficulty with left eye closure and was drooling from the left side of her mouth. She denied any alteration in taste or in hearing and she had no tinnitus. She had no crusting or any pain within the ear canal.

General physical examination: This was within normal limits, including skin. The external auditory canal and tympanic membrane were normal with no rash, etc.

Neurological examination: The complete examination was normal except for findings limited to the left seventh cranial nerve: The patient had an incomplete paralysis of the entire left side of the face. She had sufficient eye closures sitting or recumbent to cover the cornea. She was able to have minor elevation of the eyebrow in forehead wrinkling. She had minimal elevation of the lower lip in smiling. The patient was unable to wrinkle her forehead. Taste for sugar was slightly decreased but not absent on left side of the tongue (anterior two-thirds).

Clinical diagnosis: Bell's palsy: left peripheral seventh cranial nerve palsy.

Laboratory data: Routine blood counts, erythrocyte sedimentation rate, blood chemistries, and chest X-ray were all normal.

Subsequent course: The patient was treated with a 1-week course of prednisone and was seen in follow-up at weekly intervals. Over the next 2–3 weeks a complete recovery occurred, related or unrelated to the therapy.

Comments

This patient had an uncomplicated palsy of the seventh cranial nerve, of uncertain etiology. Specific causes such as sarcoid, H. zoster, and immunological disorders were ruled out by the examination and basic laboratory data. An underlying diabetes was not present. No specific tests for Lyme disease were performed, but there was no exposure to ticks, no history of tick bites, or of skin manifestations. Note that 75% of cases of Bell's palsy recover completely without any specific therapy, particularly where the paralysis is incomplete. Patients with insufficient eye closure to cover the cornea in a recumbent position should be provided with an eye patch to protect the cornea.

This usually transient impairment of a facial nerve is the result of swelling of the nerve within the relatively narrow bony facial canal. More precise localization depends on whether this motor function alone is involved, as opposed to additional involvement of taste or the anterior two-thirds of the tongue, or of parasympathetic supply to the facial and salivary glands. This has been discussed earlier.

The overall annual incidence of Bell's palsy has been estimated as 23 cases per 100,000 persons. As such, this syndrome is one of the more common acute disorders involving the cranial nerves. The etiology of this swelling is often uncertain, but infections with the herpes simplex virus or the spirochetal agent producing Lyme's disease have been implicated. Any treatment of the disorder must take into account the fact that in untreated cases 70% recover completely within 1–2 months and in 85% of cases relatively normal function is achieved. If electromyographic (EMG) studies are performed, evidence of denervation continuing after 10 days suggests a long delay in recovery of function. From a practical standpoint early recovery of motor function in the first 5–7 days usually indicates that an excellent recovery will occur. Most experts recommend treatment with a corticosteroid such as prednisone 40–60 mg per day for 7 days. The basis of this treatment is to reduce swelling within the narrow bony facial canal. The routine use of the H. simplex antiviral agent acyclovir has not been demonstrated to be of value. Routine use of anti Lyme disease antibiotics is not indicated unless Lyme disease titers are elevated.

CRANIAL NERVE VIII: VESTIBULOCOCHLEAR NERVE

The vestibulocochlear nerve has two divisions: the vestibular and cochlear nerves, which are attached to the medulla at its border with the pons lateral to the root of nerve VII. The cochlear nerve is smaller than the vestibular nerve and is lateral to it. (See also discussion on Auditory and Vestibular Pathways in Chapter 15.)

COCHLEAR NERVE

The cochlear nerve (Fig. 12.10A) is concerned with hearing and originates from the spiral ganglion of Corti in the petrous portion of the temporal bone. The peripheral process originates from the hair cells in the spiral ganglion. The cochlear division of cranial nerve VIII originates from the spiral ganglion and terminates in the dorsal and ventral cochlear nuclei located on the external surface of the inferior cerebellar peduncle. The primary auditory fibers enter the cochlear nuclei and bifurcate, ending in the dorsal and ventral cochlear nuclei. Throughout the auditory system a tonotopic arrangement occurs. The secondary auditory fibers arise from the dorsal and ventral cochlear nuclei and form the three acoustic striae. The *ventral acoustic stria* originates from the ventral cochlear nucleus and courses through the ventral boundary of the pontine tegmentum (the medullary-pontine junction), forming the *trapezoid body*.

These fibers pass through the medial lemniscus, reach the *superior olive,* and migrate laterally to form *the lateral lemniscus*. The *dorsal and intermediate striae* arise from the *dorsal cochlear nucleus* and the dorsal half of the ventral cochlear nucleus. The *dorsal stria* crosses the midline ventral to the medial longitudinal fasciculus and joins the contralateral *lateral lemniscus* (Fig. 12.10A). The *intermediate stria* runs through the center of the reticular formation, crosses the midline, and enters the contralateral lateral lemniscus.

Some secondary auditory fibers end in the superior olivary, trapezoid, and lateral lemniscus nuclei and the reticular formation. In these three nuclei tertiary axons originate which ascend, primarily crossed, to the *inferior colliculus*, where many of the axons terminate or send collaterals into the inferior collicular nuclei. Fibers from the inferior colliculus and lateral lemniscus form the *brachium of the inferior colliculus*

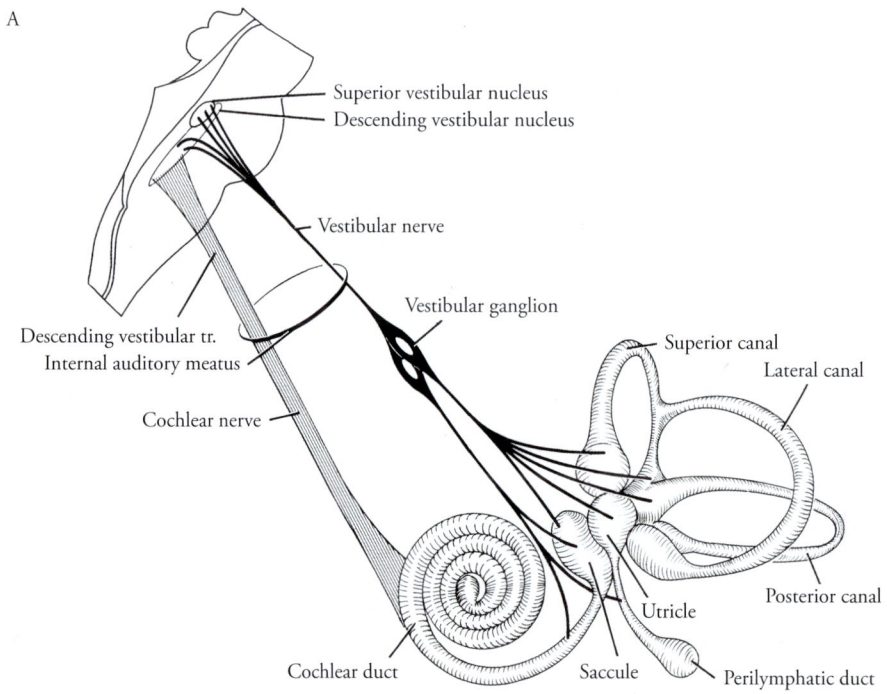

Figure 12.10A Central and peripheral location of the vestibular and cochlear portions of cranial nerve VIII.

that ends in the *medial geniculate nucleus of the thalamus*. Auditory information ascends bilaterally to the medial geniculate nucleus, with the contralateral information forming the largest component. All auditory fibers synapse in the medial geniculate nucleus and are then projected to the auditory cortex, *areas 41 and 42 (the transverse temporal gyri of Heschl)*.

One of the most fascinating pathways in the central nervous system is the *olivocochlear bundle of Rasmussen*, or the efferent cochlear bundle. Crossed fibers originate from the areas dorsal to the accessory olivary nucleus, while uncrossed fibers originate from the superior olivary nucleus, join with the crossed pathway, exit with the inferior division of the cochlear nerve, and anastomose upon the hair cells in the cochlea. This prime example of central nervous control of peripheral receptors is most noticeable when loud sounds are quickly reduced to more moderate levels (e.g., the intensity of loud rock and roll is reduced to that of mood music). Note that similar mechanisms exist in the visual, olfactory, and gustatory systems. Throughout the auditory system there are crossed and uncrossed fibers, so that representation is bilateral throughout.

CLINICAL DISORDERS

Auditory Symptoms and Signs

Deafness: Classification.

Conductive: External and middle ear disease (loss of low-frequency sounds)

Sensory neural (nerve deafness—loss of high-frequency sounds)

1. Disease of cochlea

   a. Often bilateral, hereditary, or related to loud sound exposure.

   b. Antibiotic use—aminoglycosides, dihdrostreptomycin, and vancomycin.

   c. If sudden and unilateral, consider vascular etiology: occlusion of the internal auditory artery.

2. Disease of eighth nerve: small tumors (vestibular schwannoma) of eighth nerve within the bony canal may produce limited CN VIII symptoms. Large tumors, such as vestibular schwannomas, meningiomas, etc., at the cerebellar pontine angle produce involvement of a cluster of cranial nerves (VIII, VII, ±V, ±IX, X). Note that the old term "acoustic neuromas" is no longer used since these tumors arise from the Schwann cells of the vestibular divisions of the nerve. The more correct term is "vestibular schwannoma."

Tinnitus—various forms of ringing in the ear:

Etiology—middle or inner ear or eighth nerve.* Usually associated with hearing loss.

Note: Paroxysmal tinnitus may occur in association with various other symptoms of seizures—arising in the temporal lobe (transverse gyrus of Heschl—is the auditory projection area). Such symptoms may occur as part of other symptoms of the temporal lobe seizure, which will be discussed in Chapter 22.

Central Lesions of Cochlear Pathway

Note that beyond the cochlear nuclei, central connections of the auditory system are both crossed and uncrossed. Therefore, a unilateral lesion is unlikely to produce a unilateral hearing defect. Massive intrinsic lesions are required to produce "brain stem deafness."

VESTIBULAR NERVE

The vestibular nerve is concerned with equilibrium. The vestibular nerve originates from the vestibular ganglia (Fig. 12.10B,C).

Its *primary neurons* are bipolar and located in the vestibular ganglia in the internal acoustic meatus. The vestibular nerve originates from the hair cells in maculae of the saccule and utricle and from the cristae of the ampullae of the three semicircular canals. The fibers terminate in the vestibular nuclei located in the fourth ventricular floor of the rostral medulla and caudal pons. It has five branches.

The primary fibers terminate mainly in the *four secondary vestibular nuclei in the floor of the fourth ventricle*.

The secondary vestibular nuclei are the inferior (descending), lateral, medial, and superior nuclei (Fig. 12.10D).

The primary vestibular fibers bifurcate into ascending and descending portions. The *ascending axons* end in the superior, lateral, and rostral portions of the medial nucleus, while the *descending axons* run in the inferior nuclei and provide collaterals to the medial nucleus. The *lateral nucleus forms the vestibulospinal tract, which extends to sacral levels*.

The *inferior vestibular nucleus* extends from the entrance of the vestibular nerve root, at the medullopontine junction, through the lower medullary levels.

The *medial vestibular nucleus* is found medial to the inferior nucleus at the same levels. The medial and inferior vestibular nuclei form the prominent vestibular area on the floor of the fourth ventricle, lateral to the sulcus limitans. The myelinated bundles of the primary descending vestibular axons can delimit the inferior nucleus.

The *lateral vestibular nucleus* is found lateral to the roots of nerve VIII in the tegmentum.

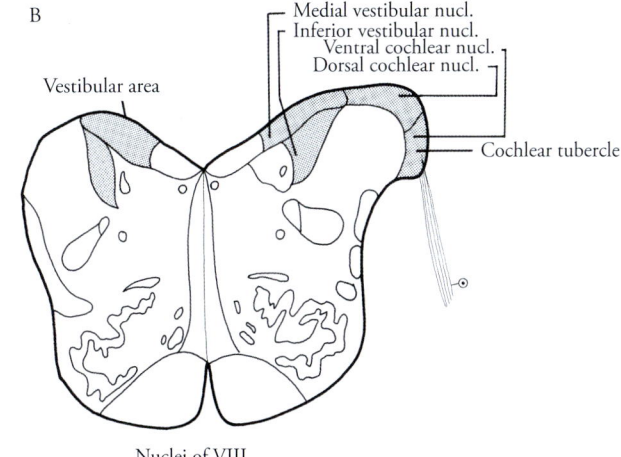

Figure 12.10B This figure identifies the location of the secondary vestibular and cochlear nuclei on the floor of the IV ventricle at medullary levels.

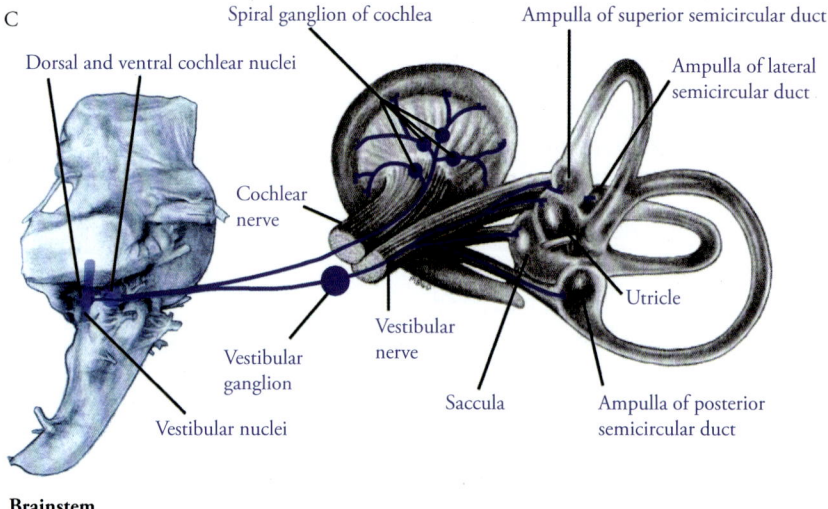

Figure 12.10C Vestibulocochlear nerve: cranial nerve VIII.

The *superior vestibular nucleus* lies in the angle formed by the floor and wall of the fourth ventricle and extends through the upper pontine levels in this position. The superior cerebellar peduncle forms its dorsal border.

Primary vestibular fibers also run directly into the ipsilateral cerebellum, forming the juxtarestiform body and projecting to the flocculus, nodulus, and uvula of the cerebellum (portions of the midline cerebellum, which are old from a phylogenetic standpoint).

The *secondary vestibular axons* originate from the secondary vestibular nuclei and project to the cerebellum, reticular formation, motor cranial nerve nuclei, and all levels of the spinal cord.

Fibers from all the vestibular nuclei join the medial longitudinal fasciculus and are crossed and uncrossed with ascending and descending branches.

Vestibular ascending pathway. The vestibulothalamic pathway fibers arise from the lateral vestibular nucleus and ascend with the cervical proprioceptive fibers in the medial lemniscus. They terminate in the ventral posterior nucleus and medial geniculate nucleus. The vestibular impulses and responses have been noted in the cervical area of the postcentral gyrus and temporal lobe of the cerebrum.

CLINICAL DISORDERS: VESTIBULAR

Symptoms

1. *Vertigo:* a sensation of movement (usually rotation) of the environment or of the body and head:

    a. When due to involvement of the horizontal (lateral) canals, the sense of movement is usually rotation in the horizontal plane.

    b. When due to involvement of the posterior or vertical canals, the sense of movement may be in the vertical or diagonal planes with a sense of the floor rising up or receding.

    c. Vertigo must be distinguished from the more general symptom of dizziness—or light-headedness, which has many causes. Simple light-headedness as a symptom of presyncope (the sensation one is about to faint) may accompany any process which produces a general reduction in cerebral blood flow (cardiac arrhythmia, decreased cardiac output, peripheral dilatation of vessels, decreased blood pressure, or hyperventilation). Hypoglycemia and various drugs also produce dizziness. *Some patients cannot make the distinction and a series of operational tests may be necessary to reproduce symptoms:* rotation, hyperventilation, orthostatic changes in blood pressure. Additionally, caloric testing, cardiac auscultation, EKG, and Holter monitor may be necessary in selected cases.

2. *Nausea and vomiting:* vertigo of vestibular origin is accompanied by these symptoms because of the connections of the vestibular system to the emetic center of the medulla.

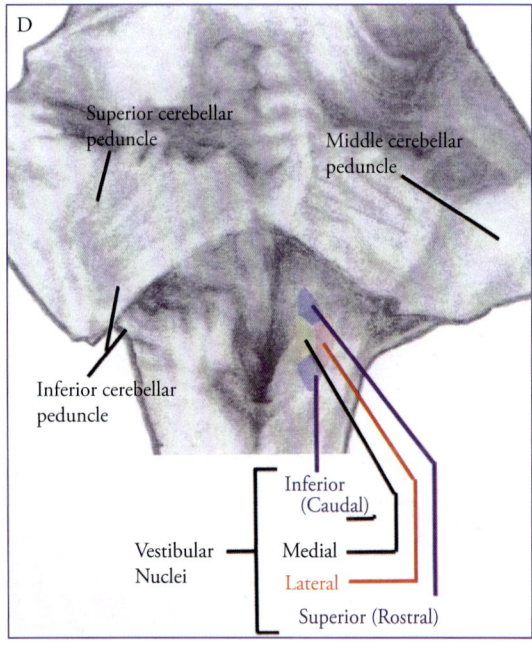

Figure 12.10D Location of secondary vestibular nuclei in the medulla, pons, and midbrain.

3. *Nystagmus*: a jerk of the eyes—slow component alternating with a fast component is associated with stimulation or disease of the vestibular system. Nystagmus is named from the fast component—and the direction of movement is specified: rotatory, horizontal, or vertical.

4. *Unsteadiness*: Severe or mild.

Etiology—Multiple.

Labyrinthine disease is the most common.

Benign positional vertigo (nonbenign forms of positional nystagmus may occur with brain stem disease, e.g., posterior fossa tumors). Sudden vertigo and associated symptoms of nystagmus, such as nausea, selectively occur on sudden tilting of head from the upright to recumbent position. This syndrome may occur as a late complication of head trauma. The proposed etiology relates to detachment of otolithic crystals from the macula of the utricle. When these calcium carbonate particles then enter and float free in the endolymph of the semicircular canals, the endolymph movement stimulates the ampulla of the semicircular canal. The ampullary nerve is thus stimulated and vertigo results. At times the particles may become stuck within the canal. In particular positions of the head, this debris intermittently blocks the flow of fluid into the cupula. This condition is the most frequent cause of recurrent vertigo. The posterior canal is involved in 85%–90% of cases; the horizontal canal in 10% of cases. It is also a condition that can be inexpensively diagnosed and treated with a series of head position maneuvers. As discussed by Neuhauser and Lempert, in a series of 100 unselected geriatric patients, 9% had a positive head maneuver test (the Dix-Hallpike maneuvers). In unselected primary care patients seen in consultation because of dizziness, 40% had both typical symptoms of benign positional vertigo and positive head tilt maneuver tests.

Meniere's disease: Paroxysmal attacks of vertigo, with or without vomiting and ataxia are associated with tinnitus and deafness. The etiology relates to endolymphatic hydrops—an increase in volume resulting in distention of the endolymphatic system of the semi circular canals.

Acute labyrinthitis: In this condition, cochlear as well as vestibular symptoms are present. As with vestibular neuritis discussed next, a viral etiology has been implicated.

Vestibular Nerve

Vestibular neuropathy is an acute, self-limited syndrome which follows a viral infection. Symptoms are vestibular without cochlear involvement. There is unilateral vestibular paresis. This is the most common cause of acute severe vertigo of the type seen in emergency departments. In addition to vertigo, severe nausea, vomiting, and imbalance will occur, the latter often of severe degree. Symptoms may persist for 1–6 weeks.

Antibiotic damage (streptomycin and aminoglycosides) may produce vestibular nerve damage.

Tumors—arising from or compressing vestibular nerve, so-called acoustic neuroma. Note that this tumor actually arises from the Schwann cells of the vestibular nerve, and the modern term is "vestibular schwannoma."

Brain stem and cerebellum: Infarcts or other lesions involving the vestibular nuclei or the cerebellar connections will produce vertigo and/or nystagmus. Almost always other brain stem signs are present. However, rarely, these symptoms alone will be present.

The following case represents a possible example.

CASE HISTORY 12.6

This 39-year-old, left-handed married white female medical clinic employee had experienced much of her life symptoms of car, air, or sea sickness. Three weeks prior to admission while at an amusement park, she had taken a ride on the "Tower of Terror," which involved a free fall of 200 feet. Following the vestibular stimulation, she developed significant but intermittent symptoms of several types of vertigo: rotational or horizontal and the particularly troublesome symptom that the floor was pitching up to meet her. When this latter symptom occurred, she would become diaphoretic and experience tingling in her hands and decreased vision. Loud noises were painful. On the day of admission she had a particularly severe episode and fell to the floor. Examination in the emergency room indicated that she tended to fall to the right when standing on a narrow base. Her symptoms had improved with meclizine, an antivertigo medication.

Neurological examination: No remarkable features were present except for (1) minimal weakness in the right lower extremity which had been present for 14 years related to a herniated disk at L5-S1. (2) On rotation with the head in the upright position, horizontal and rotational vertigo developed, reproducing that aspect of her symptoms. When rotated with the head down on the shoulder (a maneuver that places the vertical [posterior] canal in a horizontal position), the "floor pitching up" sensation was reproduced.

Clinical diagnosis: Labyrinthine vertigo.

Laboratory data: However, the magnetic resonance image (MRI) demonstrated a very minimal (5 mm) nonenhancing cyst within the inferior aspect of the right cerebellum located in the cerebellar tonsil.

Comments

This patient had a long history of vertigo and associated nausea and vomiting occurring in relationship to motion in cars, airplanes, and boats. In relationship to the significant vestibular stimulation, she developed intermittent episodes of severe vertigo. Her symptoms could be reproduced with rotational maneuvers, the type of vertigo and the accompanying nystagmus varying with the head position during the rotation. The MRI findings raised the possibility that a minor lesion in that sector of the cerebellum related to the vestibular system may have predisposed the patient to these symptoms. Although the patient had a sense that loud noises were painful, she had no clear-cut cochlear symptoms. The acute onset of vestibular symptoms often triggers the occurrence of autonomic symptoms such as diaphoresis, in addition to anxiety and hyperventilation syndrome with manifestations such as blurring of vision and tingling in the hands.

Other disorders of cranial nerve VIII such as vestibular schwannoma are considered below in relation to combined syndromes.

Cerebral cortex: Stimulation of temporal lobe in patients with seizures of temporal lobe origin produces dizziness.

CRANIAL NERVE IX: GLOSSOPHARYNGEAL

The glossopharyngeal nerve (Fig. 12.11A) is a mixed nerve with sensory and motor nuclei in the medulla. The functions of cranial nerve IX are often discussed with the vagus nerve (CN X), as is done here.

The *rootlets of nerve IX* are found in the medulla in a postolivary position. The nerve trunk exits from the skull via the jugular foramen, where it is located anterolateral to the vagus nerve.

In the jugular foramen are found two swellings on the nerve trunk of nerve IX, *the superior and inferior ganglia*.

Sensory Division (Fig. 12.11B). The primary sensory cell bodies are located in the superior and inferior ganglia and carry *gustatory sensations* from the taste buds in the posterior third of the tongue and *cutaneous sensations* from the pharynx, soft palate, auditory canal, middle ear, palatine tonsils, Eustachian tube, and carotid sinus. The *general and special visceral axons* enter the medulla and run in the tractus solitarius in the middle and posterior medullary level, and synapse in the *nucleus of the tractus solitarius*. Afferent fibers are derived from baroreceptors in the wall of the carotid sinus (BP regulation) and chemoreceptors in the carotid body (ventilatory response to hypoxia).

Motor Division. The *motor fibers of nerve IX* originate from the most superior part of the nucleus ambiguus in the medulla. They pass posteriorly and laterally into the jugular foramen and innervate the stylopharyngeus muscle.

The *preganglionic parasympathetic fibers originate from the inferior salvatory nucleus* in the medulla, join the rootlets of IX, and run via the lesser petrosal nerve *to the otic ganglion*.

The *postganglionic fibers* (Fig. 12.11B) pass via the auriculo-temporal nerve of the mandibular nerve to form the secretory pathway to the parotid gland.

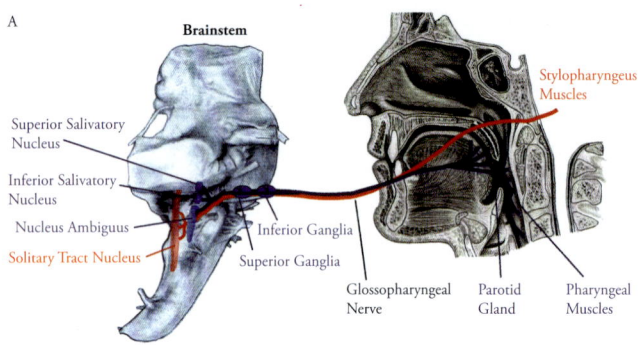

Figure 12.11A The glossopharyngeal nerve. The central and peripheral distribution of the glossopharyngeal nerve.

CLINICAL DISORDERS

Lesions restricted to the nuclei or nerve roots of nerve IX are rare, but if they occur, taste is lost on the posterior third of the tongue and the gag reflex is absent ipsilaterally. There is no response when the posterior pharyngeal wall and soft palate are stimulated. The function of the parotid glands may also be impaired but can be easily evaluated by placing a highly seasoned food on the tongue and seeing if a copious flow from the duct of the parotid gland occurs.

Isolated lesions are uncommon. A combined involvement with vagus and accessory nerves at the jugular foramen is more common and is discussed next.

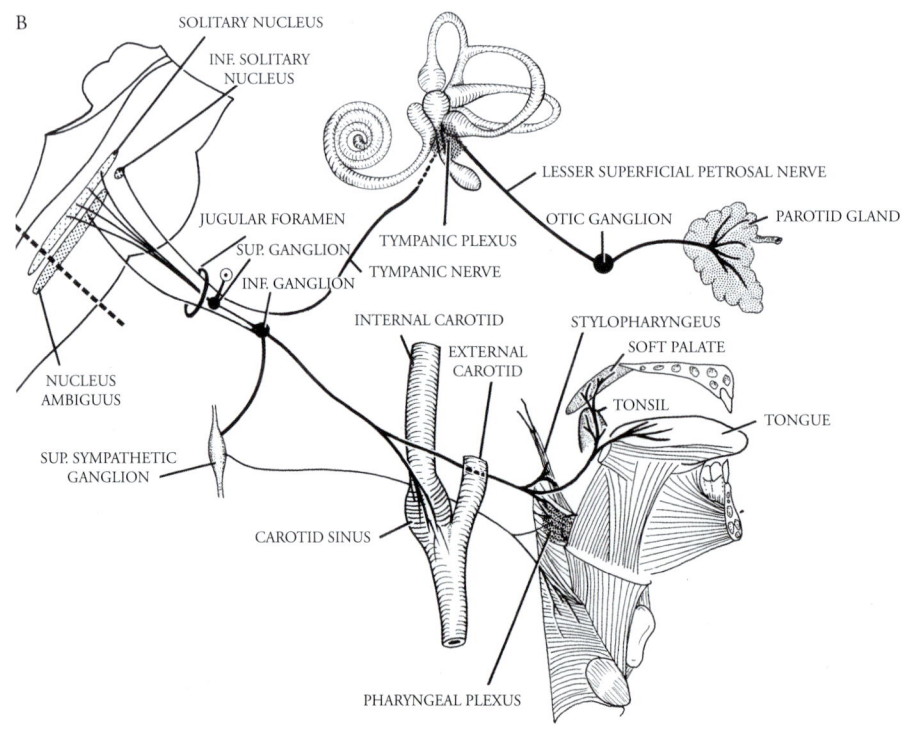

Figure 12.11B Glossopharyngeal nerve with the distribution of parasympathetic fibers to carotid sinus solitary nucleus (parasympathetic) and ambiguus (motor to pharynx and larynx) nucleus of the vagus in a cross section of the medulla.

Glossopharyngeal neuralgia is one of the few isolated syndromes. Symptoms are similar to those of trigeminal neuralgia but localized to the posterior tongue and pharynx with swallowing, coughing, or sneezing providing the trigger. However, syncope may also occur because of connections to the carotid sinus. Treatment is similar to trigeminal neuralgia.

CRANIAL NERVE X: VAGUS

The vagus nerve (Figs. 12.12A & 12.12B) has *one sensory and two motor nuclei in the medulla* and also has the most extensive peripheral distribution of any cranial nerve. Its roots are located in a postolivary position in the posterolateral sulcus of the medulla, in line with the fibers of nerve IX but inferior to them. The nerve formed from these roots exits from the posterior cranial fossa via the jugular foramen. *The superior ganglion, the jugular*, is found in the jugular foramen, while *the inferior ganglion, the nodose*, is found just as the nerve leaves the jugular foremen. In the neck the vagus nerve is found in the carotid sheath close to the common carotid artery and jugular vein.

Motor Nuclei (Fig. 12.12B): There are *two motor nuclei*: (a) *the dorsal motor nucleus/parasympathetic of the vagus* and (b) *the nucleus ambiguus or ventral motor nucleus of the vagus* to skeletal muscles of the soft palate, pharynx, and the intrinsic muscles of the larynx.

1. The *dorsal motor nucleus of the vagus nerve* forms the vagal trigone on the floor of the fourth ventricle at the medullary levels. This nucleus constitutes the cranial portion of the parasympathetic autonomic system. It provides *preganglionic parasympathetic innervation to the ganglion* in the walls of the pharynx, trachea, bronchi, esophagus, stomach, small intestine and ascending portions of the large intestine, and the heart. The *fibers of X end in the parasympathetic ganglia found in Auerbach's plexus (myenteric plexus) and Meissner's plexus (submucosal plexus)*. The actions of the parasympathetic nervous system are considered in greater detail in the chapter concerned with the autonomic nervous system (Chapter 16). The interactions of the dorsal motor nucleus of the vagus with the nucleus of the tractus solitaries and other brain stem, hypothalamic, and cortical centers is also discussed in Chapter 11 on the brain stem. The various actions may be briefly summarized here.

    a. Heart: The preganglionic fibers originate in the dorsal nucleus of nerve X, exit from the central nervous system, and run in the vagus nerve to the ganglia in the cardiac plexus and atria. The postganglionic axons reach coronary vessels and atrial musculature, causing cardiac deceleration. *In contrast*, the action of the sympathetic system is to produces cardiac acceleration.

    b. Lungs: The preganglionic fibers originate in the dorsal motor nucleus of nerve X and run in the vagus to the pulmonary ganglionic plexus in the bronchi and blood vessels. Stimulation causes constriction of the bronchi and decreased respiration. *In contrast*, the action of the sympathetic system is to produce dilation of the bronchi and increased respiration.

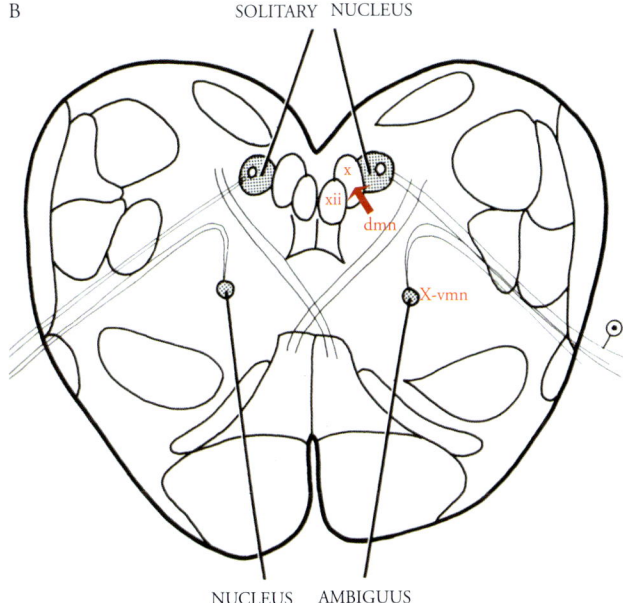

Figure 12.12 The vagus nerve. (*A*) The central and peripheral distribution of the vagus nerve. (*B*) Location of solitary nucleus (visceral) and dorsal motor nucleus of X (parasympathetic) and ambiguus (motor to pharynx and larynx) nucleus of the vagus in a cross section of the medulla. XII = hypoglossal nucleus.

c. Abdominal viscera: The preganglionic parasympathetic originate from the dorsal motor nucleus of nerve X and S2–S4, and end in the intrinsic ganglionic plexus of the organ (Meissner's submucosal plexus and Auerbach's myenteric plexus). From these plexuses postganglionic fibers originate. Stimulation produces general alimentary function by causing the secretion of gastric and pancreatic juices important in peristalsis. It also stimulates the liver and spleen and inhibits the suprarenal glands. The end result is increased peristalsis and increased gastrointestinal secretions. (S2–S4 supplies the pelvic organs.) In contrast, sympathetic action inhibits peristalsis and gastrointestinal secretion; stimulates secretion from the adrenal medulla and causes vasoconstriction of the visceral vessels.

CLINICAL AUTONOMIC EFFECTS

Peripheral Autonomic Neuropathies

Autonomic effects may occur in peripheral neuropathies related to diabetes mellitus and amyloidosis. The main manifestations are orthostatic hypotension, diarrhea, and urinary retention. Obviously not all of these manifestations relate to the vagal nerve per se.

However, normally when the blood pressure falls in relation to a change in posture from the recumbent to the up right position, the heart rate is increased in a compensatory action thus increasing overall (summated) cardiac output and thus maintaining cerebral perfusion. Failure to maintain cerebral perfusion results in syncope (faints). The failure of the heart rate to accelerate under these circumstances has been attributed to a dysfunction of the vagal system. Under normal circumstances, decreased blood pressure will result in decreased vagal efferent activity and increased heart rate (reflex cardio-acceleration), increased blood pressure will result in increased vagal efferent activity and decreased heart rate (reflex cardio de-acceleration).

Vagotomy: Before the development of effective agents to decrease the secretion gastric acid, this procedure was performed in patients with peptic ulcer disease.

Vagal nerve stimulation: This procedure has been employed in cases of poorly controlled epilepsy. There may also be some effects with regard to depression.

2. *The other motor division of the vagus nerve originates from the posterior two-thirds of the nucleus ambiguus in the reticular formation of the tegmentum of the medulla, the ventral motor nucleus,* and connects to the striate muscles of the soft palate and pharynx, and the intrinsic muscles of the larynx. It is thus important in swallowing and speech. The ambiguus portion of nerve X innervates the following muscles:

1. Esophagus: the upper third is skeletal muscle, middle third is skeletal and smooth; and the lower third is smooth.
2. Pharynx: the superior, middle, and inferior constrictors of the pharynx
3. Palate: the palatoglossus, palatopharyngeus, salpingopharyngeal, and levator palatine velum of the soft palate
4. Larynx: cricothyroid, the posterior cricoarytenoid, arytenoid, lateral cricoarytenoid, and thyroarytenoid

SENSORY FUNCTIONS

The primary cell bodies of the sensory fibers are located in the inferior ganglion and carry gustatory information from taste buds in the epiglottis and pharynx, cutaneous innervation from the base of the tongue and epiglottis, and general visceral sensation from all the structures receiving motor innervation (pharynx, larynx, heart, tracheal bronchi, esophagus, small and large intestines. external ear, and dura of the sigmoid venous sinus).

The fibers enter the medulla and *synapse in the nucleus solitarius.*

The secondary axons subserving pain and temperature ascend in close proximity to the medial lemniscus to the ventroposterior medial thalamic nuclei (VPM).

The taste fibers ascend ipsilaterally to the parabrachial nuclei in the central tegmental tract and terminate in the cranial (medullary) and spinal portions. The taste fibers synapse in the parvocellular region of VPM and are then projected to the cortical taste area in the parietal operculum.

Note that 80% of fibers in the peripheral segment of the vagus nerve are afferent. Stimulation of the vagus nerve has been employed in the treatment of cases of epilepsy that are refractory to pharmacological treatment.

REFLEXES

The vagus nerve is also important in many visceral reflexes: gag, vomiting, swallowing, coughing, sneezing, sucking, hiccupping, and yawning, and in the aortic sinus reflex.

Lesions producing abnormalities of these reflexes usually involve structures in addition to the vagus nerve.

CLINICAL DISORDERS

Bilateral lesions of the vagal portion of the nucleus ambiguus in the medulla are usually fatal because of its proximity to the pneumotaxic, apneustic, and medullary respiratory centers. In addition, bilateral paralysis of vocal cord abduction will result in CO_2 retention and decreased O_2 saturation. Both of these conditions will result in coma.

Unilateral lesions of the vagus nerve may or may not produce autonomic dysfunction. The heart rate, respiratory system, and gastrointestinal tracts appear to function normally, but there may be minor difficulty in swallowing. Injury to pharyngeal branches produces difficulty in swallowing.

LESIONS OF PERIPHERAL BRANCHES OF THE VAGUS NERVE

1. *Lesions of the superior laryngeal nerve* affect the motor innervation to the cricothyroid muscle and the inferior constrictor of the pharynx. However, such a lesion may also affect the internal laryngeal branch, the "watch dog

of the larynx." This innervation of the mucosa of the laryngeal region produces coughing when foreign particles lodge in this region, thus keeping the airway open. When this reflex is not present due to injury to the nerve or an overdose of drugs, foreign objects can then enter the trachea and block the airway. This may produce aspiration pneumonia or even lead to death.

2. *The recurrent laryngeal nerve* supplies all of the intrinsic muscles of the larynx (except for the cricothyroid muscle) and the mucosa of the larynx below the vocal cords. Interruptions of the recurrent laryngeal nerves produce paralysis of the vocal cords, hoarseness, and dysphonia.

Bilateral involvement of both recurrent laryngeal nerves produces aphonia and inspiratory stridor.

Isolated peripheral lesions are more frequent and occur especially with operations on the thyroid gland. When the recurrent laryngeal is injured, there is weakness in speech and anesthesia of the upper part of the larynx, resulting in a weak gag reflex, paralysis of the cricothyroid muscle, and easily fatigued laryngeal muscles. The recurrent laryngeal nerve may also be injured under the following circumstances:

a. Aneurysms of the arch of the thoracic aorta may involve the left recurrent laryngeal nerve.
b. Apical lung (superior sulcus) tumors, pharyngeal carcinoma, and metastatic involvement of cervical lymph nodes may all have effects on the vagus or recurrent laryngeal nerves.
c. Diphtheria toxin may involve the nerves, producing difficulty in swallowing.
d. Myasthenia or D. botulinum toxin may affect the relevant neuromuscular junctions.
e. Dissections of the neck for carotid endarterectomy or for thyroid surgery may damage the vagus or recurrent laryngeal nerves.

Central Lesions of the Vagus Nerve

Lesions in the upper medulla produce dysphagia, while lesions in the lower medulla cause dysarthria. The palate on the affected side is paralyzed and the uvula deviates to the unaffected side (see discussion of lateral medullary syndrome in Chapter 13).

Isolated central lesions are rare. The nucleus ambiguus may be affected in syringobulbia and vascular lesions of the lateral medulla in association with other findings, as noted later. The motor neurons of this nucleus are damaged in bulbar poliomyelitis or the bulbar variant of amyotrophic lateral sclerosis.

Supranuclear lesions involving the corticobulbar (corticonuclear) pathways to the ambiguus nuclei usually cause difficulty in swallowing but only become clinically significant when they are bilateral. Such bilateral lesions of these pathways produce a syndrome of pseudobulbar palsy. This syndrome to be discussed further may produce emotional lability and a hyperactive jaw jerk.

CRANIAL NERVE XI: SPINAL ACCESSORY

The spinal accessory nerve (Fig. 12.13) is a purely motor nerve that originates from both the medulla and spinal cord and is consequently divided into cranial (medullary) and spinal portions. It is appropriately named the accessory nerve as many of its functions are in cooperation with the vagus nerve.

The *cranial root* arises from the most posterior-part of the nucleus ambiguus, exits in a postolivary position, enters the jugular forarmen, and then combines with the spinal root. The cranial root innervates the uvula, levator veli palatini, and pharyngeal and laryngeal muscles in concert with cranial nerve X (*to which it is accessory*).

The *spinal rootlets* arise from the ventrolateral part of the ventral horn in the upper four cervical segments. *The innervation to the sternocleidomastoid muscle originates primarily from C2, while the innervation to the large trapezius muscle originates in C3 and C4.* The fibers from the spinal portion of XI pass up through the foremen magnum, combine with the cranial roots, and distribute to the sternomastoid and trapezius muscles. Branches of the trigeminal also carry general sensations from these muscles. Injury to the nucleus ambiguus in the medulla causes paralysis and atrophy of the trapezius and sternomastoid muscles (Figs. 12.16B and 12.16C), resulting in weakness affecting head movements to the opposite side and shrugging of the shoulder.

Supranuclear lesions of the corticobulbar system produce only paresis of the muscles.

CLINICAL DISORDERS

Isolated involvement of cranial nerve XI by intracranial lesions is rare. However, combined involvement with cranial nerves IX and X at the jugular foramen is more common (Fig. 12.16A). Injuries or malignant masses in the posterior triangle of the neck may also damage the nerve.

Figure 12.13 The spinal accessory nerve: cranial nerve XI.

CRANIAL NERVE XII: HYPOGLOSSAL

The hypoglossal nerve (Fig. 12.14) is a purely motor nerve that originates from the hypoglossal nucleus, which forms the hypoglossal trigone in the medullary floor of the fourth ventricle. The fibers pass anteriorly, passing inferiorly between the olive and pyramids of the medulla. The fibers exit from the cranium via the hypoglossal canal and supply all the extrinsic muscles (styloglossus, hypoglossus, and genioglossus) and the intrinsic muscles (superior and inferior longitudinal, transverse, and vertical) of the tongue with the exception of the palatoglossal, which is innervated by the vagus nerve.

Branches from V3 of the trigeminal nerve, the mandibular, carry general sensations from the tongue and taste sensation from the anterior two-thirds of the tongue.

CLINICAL DISORDERS

Unilateral injury to the nerve or nucleus produces atrophy and paralysis of the ipsilateral tongue with the tongue protruding toward the injured side. This is due to the unopposed action of the intact genioglossus muscle pushing the tongue up and out from below.

Bilateral paralysis of the nucleus or nerve causes difficulty in eating and a dysarthria.

Isolated lesions limited to this nerve are unlikely to occur with brain stem pathology. The hypoglossal nucleus may be involved as part of a more generalized somatomotor neuron process in poliomyelitis or amyotrophic lateral sclerosis (bulbar palsy). A limited lesion may occur along the extramedullary course of the nerve, in the jugular foramen (Fig. 12.16D), but rarely at the hypoglossal foramen, and more commonly with radical cervical dissections, or as a complication of carotid endarterectomy. Supranuclear lesions rarely produce paralysis of the tongue. The combination of an ipsilateral hypoglossal lower motor lesion of the tongue and a crossed hemiplegia has been named the syndrome of Hughlings Jackson and is due to a penetrating branch vertebral artery infarct. Compared to the other classical vascular syndromes such as the dorsolateral medullary syndrome of Wallenberg or the paramedian midbrain syndrome of Weber, it is rare.

The wide distribution of the cranial nerves in the head and neck is shown in Figure 12.15.

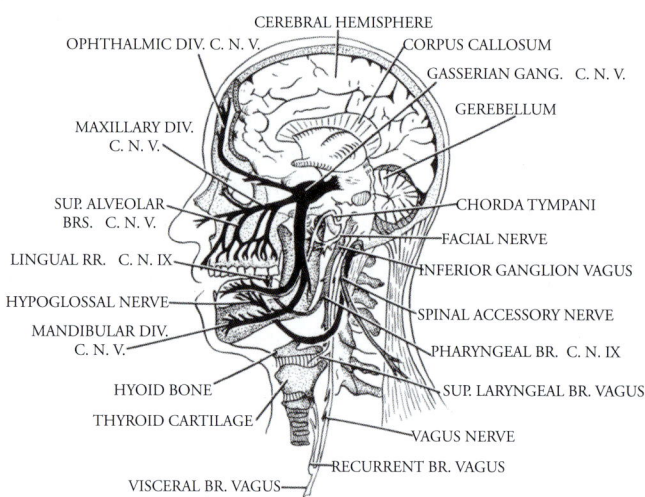

Figure 12.15 Peripheral distribution of the cranial nerves in the head and neck.

EFFECTS OF EXTRINSIC LESIONS ON CRANIAL NERVES

Cranial nerves are commonly affected by mass lesion and the syndromes produced by these extrinsic lesions are summarized in Table 12.5.

VOLUNTARY CONTROL OF THE CRANIAL NERVES: CORTICOBULBAR AND CORTICOMESENCEPHALIC PATHWAYS

This system distributes to the motor nuclei of the cranial nerves (cranial nerves V, VII, IX, X, XI, and XII) and provides voluntary and involuntary control of the muscles and glands.

Voluntary Control of Cranial Nerves V, VII, IX–XII (Fig. 18.22). The corticobulbar pathway controls the cranial nerves in the medulla and pons, the bulb. The cranial nerves controlled in the pons are V, VI, and VII, while in the medulla, IX, X, and XII. We have used the term *corticonuclear* because it reminds the student of the key role of the cranial nerve nuclei in movement.

These fibers are found anterior to the corticospinal fibers in the genu of the internal capsule and medial to the corticospinal tract in the cerebral peduncle, pons, and medullary pyramids.

The lower third of precentral gyrus, area 4 controls the neurons innervating the muscles of facial expression (motor nerve VII) and the muscles of mastication (motor nerve V) and deglutination (ambiguus nuclei of nerves IX and X). The inferior frontal

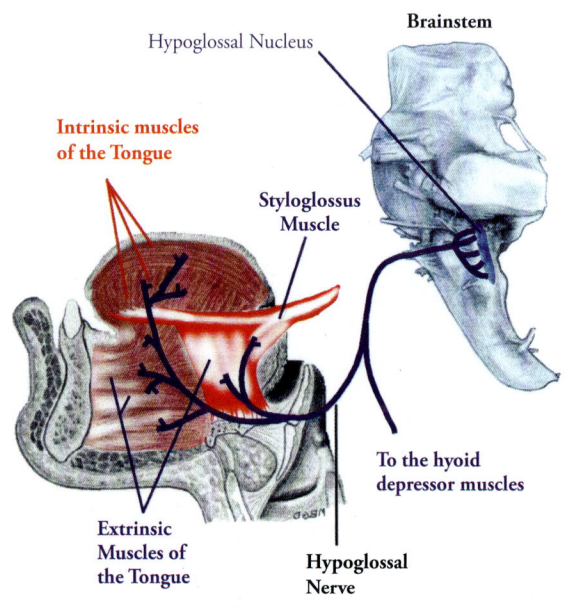

Figure 12.14 The hypoglossal nerve: cranial nerve XII.

Table 12.5 SYNDROMES OF THE ADJACENT CRANIAL NERVES DUE TO EXTRINSIC MASS LESIONS

SITE	CRANIAL NERVE INVOLVED	CAUSE
1. Superior orbital fissure	III, IV, VI, and V1	Meningioma Aneurysm
2. Optic foramen	II	Meningioma inner one-third of sphenoid wing
3. Cavernous sinus	III, IV, VI, and V1 (ophthalmic), V2 (maxillary nerve). Note: with pituitary, optic chasm also may be involved and CN findings may be bilateral.	Traumatic carotid cavernous fistula Intracavernous carotid aneurysm Thrombosis of cavernous sinus Invasive tumors of sinuses and pituitary
4. Apex of petrous bone	V, VI	Inflammation of bone (Gredenigo syndrome)
5. Internal auditory canal	VII, VIII	Tumors and chronic infection
6. Cerebellar pontine angle	VII, VII, + V, + IX	Tumors: vestibular schwannoma and meningiomas
7. Jugular foramen	IX, X, XI*	Tumors—e.g., neurofibroma

*Large lesions may also involve XII.
Source: Modified from Adams, Victor, and Ropper (1994).

gyrus and frontal operculum (the posterior part of the par triangularis—area 44) controls the neurons innervating the larynx.

It appears that most corticonuclear (bulbospinal) axons end on interneurons and not directly on the motor neuron of the cranial nerve. The cortical innervation of the majority of the cranial nerves is mostly bilateral with the exception of the contralateral control of the lower facial muscles; consequently, unilateral lesions in the cortical bulbar system produce usually only weakness and not paralysis.

CLINICAL DISORDERS

A bilateral supranuclear lesion of the corticonuclear system produces upper motor neuron signs, including hyperactive jaw jerk and gag reflex and pseudobulbar palsy characterized by a release of inappropriate behavioral signs, emotional lability, and often urinary incontinence.

Pseudobulbar Palsy

A bilateral corticobulbar lesion produces a pseudobulbar syndrome. This is characterized by a release of bulbar functions. This is an upper motor neuron lesion with hyperactive jaw jerk, spasticity- affecting speech, and gag reflexes. Cranial nerve components of emotions are released—emotional lability. This most likely represents the release from cortical control via the corticobulbar innervation of the muscles controlled by the cranial nerves, and now the limbic control to these same nuclei takes over via descending autonomic pathways with the emotional state being undampened by inhibition from the frontal lobes. Amyotrophic lateral sclerosis (ALS) produces upper and lower motor paralysis.

Voluntary control of eye movements: The corticomesencephalic pathway controls cranial nerves III, IV, and VI. Eye movements originate from the frontal eye fields (area eight) localized to the caudal part of the middle frontal gyrus and the adjacent inferior frontal gyrus.

In upper midbrain levels, fibers to cranial nerves III and IV leave the corticomesencephalic tract and then decussate. Bilateral stimulation of area 8, the frontal eye field, results in vertical eye movements. Conjugate vertical eye movements are mediated by *the pretectal area* of the rostral mesencephalon at the interface of mesencephalon and diencephalon. The structures in this area include the rostral interstitial nucleus of the medial longitudinal fasciculus and *the nucleus and fibers of the posterior commissure*. From the pretectal area neurons project to the *III and IV cranial nerve nuclei*.

Fibers to cranial nerve VI descend and terminate on the contralateral parabducens/*parapontine reticular nuclei of the horizontal (lateral) gaze center of the pons*. From this center neurons project *to the lateral rectus (abducens) nucleus*. This nucleus contains two groups of neurons. Group 1 are motor neurons, which supply the ipsilateral lateral rectus muscle. Group 2 neurons project via the contralateral medial longitudinal fasciculus to the neurons, supplying the contralateral medial rectus muscle neurons of the cranial nerve III. The end result is a coordinated (yoked) conjugate horizontal eye movement on lateral gaze.

(See also Chapter 18, where the occipito-parietal role in eye movements is also discussed.)

COMBINED CRANIAL NERVE SYNDROMES

These syndromes are summarized in Table 12.5. Examples are provided next.

CAVERNOUS SINUS SYNDROME

CASE HISTORY 12.7

This 61-year-old, right-handed, white female developed blurring of vision in the left eye 4 days prior to admission. Two days prior to admission, she noted a left eyelid droop, diplopia on forward gaze, and numbness of the left side of the face.

Past history: There was a past history of hypertension and congestive heart failure both treated and under good control. The patient had been a heavy smoker for over 30 years but had quit 14 years previously. There was a family history of lung cancer, hypertension, and congestive heart failure.

General Physical Examination
1. Minor proptosis of the left eye
2. Minor fullness of the left tonsillar area.

Neurological Examination
Findings were limited to the following left cranial nerves:

III: incomplete ptosis of the left eyelid; no significant medial or upward movement of the left eye was noted. Depression of the left eyeball was possible. Although the left pupil was slightly smaller than the right (2 mm vs. 3 mm), both responded to light.

VI: no lateral movement of the left eye was obtained.

V: pain sensation was decreased over all three divisions over the left side of the face. As regards the mandibular division, the left side of tongue, the oral mucosa and lip were also involved. However, touch sensation was intact and corneal reflex was normal.

Clinical diagnosis: Lesion of skull base involving left cavernous sinus plus possible involvement of foramen ovale region.

Laboratory Data
1. *CT scan of head* demonstrated a mass involving the left cavernous sinus extending into the left middle fossa, and as a soft tissue mass within the sphenoid sinus extending through the sphenoid bone into the nasopharynx. There was also destruction of the Vidian canal. Multiple lesions, probably metastatic, were also present in the calvarium of the skull with demonstrated extensive infiltration of the left skull base with extensive enhancing tumor within the dorsal sphenoid bone with extension into the sphenoid sinus and cavernous sinus. There was evidence of the skull lesions involving the parietal bone.
2. There also was apparent thrombosis of the left superior sphenoidal venous sinus.
3. *Chest X-rays and CT scan of the chest* revealed a 3 cm nodule in the right apical lung area, with enlarged paratracheal and paracarinal nodes.
4. *CT scan of the pelvis* indicated metastatic destruction of the right bony symphysis pubis and a left adnexal cystic mass.
5. *A biopsy of the paratracheal nodes* revealed poorly differentiated small cell carcinoma.

Subsequent course: The patient was begun on radiotherapy and chemotherapy as well as dexamethasone. At the time of hospital discharge, 8 days following admission, she had a minor ability to move the left eye medially but had no lateral, upward, or downward movement of the eye.

Comments
The simultaneous development of diplopia, and numbness of the left side of the face, suggested the possibility of involvement of the cavernous sinus or of multiple cranial nerves at the base of the skull or of the superior orbital fissure. All three of the cranial nerves supplying the motor action of the globe could be involved in these locations. The examination indicated pathology involving at least cranial nerves III and IV.

Whether cranial nerve IV was also involved is not certain. This nerve will act through the action of the superior oblique muscle to depress the eyeball (globe) when the action of the medial rectus has already resulted in adduction of the eye. With the eye in neutral position, the inferior rectus is the main depressor of the globe. In neutral position, the action of the superior oblique is to rotate the globe inward. This specific action was not noted in this patient.

In terms of the trigeminal nerve findings, both divisions V1 and V2 pass through the lateral wall of the cavernous sinus. Only V1 passes through the superior orbital fissure. All three divisions could be involved if the trigeminal ganglion were to be involved. A lesion at the base of the skull could involve V2 at the foramen rotundum and V3 at the foramen ovale (see Fig. 12 for relation of cranial nerves to skull base).

The fact that the extraocular findings developed simultaneously with the trigeminal findings makes the cavernous sinus location the more likely, although one would also have to postulate involvement also of the area of the foramen ovale or the trigeminal ganglion to explain the involvement of division 3. The underlying pathology was a small cell carcinoma arising in the lung. Such a pathology may also produce carcinomatosis of the meninges, with involvement of cranial nerves, and this could be complicating the analysis outlined earlier.

CEREBELLAR PONTINE ANGLE TUMOR (ACOUSTIC NEUROMA)

CASE HISTORY 12.8

This 64-year-old, white, right-handed housewife was admitted to the hospital for evaluation of progressive 10- to 15-year loss of hearing in the right ear with total deafness during the several months prior to admission plus progressive right facial numbness and weakness and increasing headaches. During the 2 years prior to admission the patient had noted the gradual development of an unsteadiness in walking (ataxia of gait). This had recently worsened, leading to several falls. During this same time a progressive numbness of the right side of the face had developed, and in recent months a weakness of the entire right side of the face had also occurred. During recent months, a bifrontal, or right-sided frontal and vertex headache developed, with occasional diplopia. A minor change in hearing in the left ear had also occurred.

Neurological examination: The following limited findings were present:

Mental status: Intact.

Cranial nerves:

II. Fundi—There was evidence of an increase in intracranial pressure with bilateral papilledema (elevation of the disks with old and new retinal hemorrhages).

V. There was a decrease in pain and light touch over the maxillary and mandibular divisions of the right trigeminal nerve. The right corneal reflex was absent and the patient did not feel touch over the cornea.

VII. A moderate right peripheral facial weakness was present with a droop to the right corner of the mouth, a widened right palpebral fissure, and an absence of blinking with the right eye.

VIII.

a. Hearing was markedly decreased in the right ear (both air and bone) compared to the left.
b. Ice water caloric labyrinthine stimulation indicated no response of the right ear; there was normal response of the left ear.
c. There was a fine nystagmus on gaze to the left and to the right.

Motor system: Gait was slightly broad-based with some weaving to the right or left. She was unable to walk a tandem gait (narrow-based heel to toe walking). However, no dysmetria was present in the upper extremities.

Clinical diagnosis: Cerebellar pontine angle tumor, most likely a vestibular schwannoma (acoustic neuroma).

Laboratory data: Neuroimaging studies revealed a mass lesion displacing the aqueduct and fourth ventricle posteriorly, slightly upward and to the left, consistent with a tumor at the right cerebellopontine angle, for example, a vestibular schwannoma.

Subsequent course: Dr. Samuel Brendler performed a right suboccipital craniotomy. When the right cerebellar hemisphere was retracted and the right lateral third of the cerebellum amputated, a large schwannoma was exposed, enveloping cranial nerves VII and VIII and extending into the internal auditory meatus. At its lower end, the capsule of the tumor was also loosely attached to nerves IX, X, and XI. At its superior end, the tumor was adherent to nerve V. A portion of the tumor extended superiorly through the hiatus of the tentorium. At several points, the tumor capsule was adherent to the brain stem. In the removal of the tumor, neither cranial nerve VII nor VIII could be spared. A small portion of nerve V was also removed with the tumor capsule. As the tumor was being freed from the tentorium and brain stem, there were several episodes of hypotension and cessation of spontaneous respiration. It was therefore necessary to terminate the procedure after 60% of the tumor had been removed.

Follow-up evaluation, 10 weeks and 9 months after surgery, revealed the following residual abnormalities:

Cranial nerves:

V: Pain and touch were decreased on the right side of the face and the right masseter was weak.

VII: A complete right peripheral facial palsy was present. (The right eyelids had been sutured closed to avoid injury to the right cornea—tarsorrhaphy.)

VIII: Hearing was completely absent in the right ear and decreased on the left.

IX and X: There was difficulty in swallowing; gag reflex was depressed and speech indistinct.

Motor system: The patient was able to walk with assistance. Her gait was unsteady. A slight appendicular ataxia was evident bilaterally on finger-to-nose and heel-to-shin tests.

Comments

The symptoms and findings presented by this patient were those to be expected with a large tumor in the right cerebellar pontine angle. There was a combination of cranial nerves VIII, VII, and V, in addition to cerebellar findings. The tumor, moreover, had displaced brain stem structures, distorting the aqueduct and fourth ventricle. A significant increase in intracranial pressure had been produced. The occasional diplopia reported by the patient may well have suggested some of the bilateral cranial nerve VI dysfunction to be expected when a significant increase in intracranial pressure occurs. As regards the origin of this large tumor, the earliest symptoms were related to cranial nerve VIII, but other cranial nerves had been involved as the tumor progressed and other cranial nerve symptoms therefore developed. Note that in occasional cases, neurofibromas (schwannomas) may arise from cranial nerves VII, V, and IX. The most common site, however, remains nerve VIII.

The patient had been seen relatively late in her disease course. The tumor at operation was certainly very large and presented a formidable problem for the neurosurgeon. The complications of the surgical procedure were not unusual, when one considers that nerve VII was completely surrounded by the tumor and that cranial nerve V was also attached to the tumor. In some of these cases, the best result involves a subtotal removal of the tumor, attempting to preserve the continuity of the involved cranial nerves. It should of course be noted that prime indications for neurosurgical intervention were present: increased intracranial pressure and distortion of brain stem structures.

At the present time the use of noninvasive techniques: CT scan, MRI, and brain stem auditory evoked potentials (BAEPs) allow early diagnosis in almost all patients who present with only mild changes in hearing. The least expensive of these techniques, the BAEP, is abnormal in 98% of patients with vestibular schwannomas (see Martuza et al., 1985, and Chiappa, 1989). If the study is abnormal demonstrating a delay between Wave I, which is generated in the cochlea, and the waves generated in the brain stem, then an MRI with contrast may be performed. Significant advances have also occurred in operative management related to the use of the operating microscope and intraoperative monitoring of the function of cranial nerves VII and VIII. In the series from the Mayo Clinic (Harner et al., 1987), facial nerve function was intact postoperatively in 81% of 162 cases and in all cases where the tumor was less than 2 cm in size. Since the tumor arises primarily from the Schwann cells of the vestibular portion of the nerve, it is theoretically possible in early cases to preserve cochlear function. In the Mayo Clinic Series, the cochlear nerve was preserved in 55 of the 162 cases, but only 14 patients had actual preservation of hearing. Thus, it is rare to see patients who present the far advanced natural history and complications observed in this patient.

The subject of the relatively rare entity of bilateral acoustic neuromas (neurofibromatosis 2) has been discussed in Chapter 9 (in relationship to the more common neurofibromatosis 1). This disease is usually manifested earlier in life than the more common unilateral acoustic neuroma. Inheritance is autosomal dominant, possibly related to a partial deletion in the long arm of chromosome 22 (see Martuza Eldridge, 1988; Wertelecki et al., 1988).

Other Tumors in the Cerebellopontine Angle: Although less frequent, other types of pathology are found in this location: meningiomas (Fig. 2.10) arising from arachnoidal cell nests and cholesteatomas (epidermoids). A series from the Mayo Clinic (Laird et al., 1985) indicated 20 meningiomas over a 6-year period compared to 160 vestibular schwannomas over a similar period (Harner et al., 1985), a ratio of 1:8. Specific neurological deficits were as frequent as in patients with acoustic neuromas. Diagnosis may be made with contrast enhanced MRI or if not available contrast enhanced CT scan.

JUGULAR FORAMEN SYNDROME

CASE HISTORY 12.9

This 28-year-old, right-handed, married, white, male, junior high school science teacher was referred for evaluation of weakness in movements at the left shoulder, which began approximately 5 years prior to evaluation with a sense of minor soreness in the left shoulder and scapula areas and an inability to abduct above 90 degrees with the left arm. The problem had progressed slowly since that time, with the subsequent development of atrophy in the shoulder area and winging of the scapula. He denied any actual tingling in the arm or any radicular pain, etc. (Fig. 12.16).

Figure 12.16A Case 12.8. There was a well-defined enhancing mass that extended from the jugular foramen superiorly to the height of the left petrous apex.

Figure 12.16B Case 12.8. Normal right sternocleidomastoid muscle. Atrophy of left sternocleidomastoid muscle.

Figure 12.16C Case 12.8. Winging of left scapula.

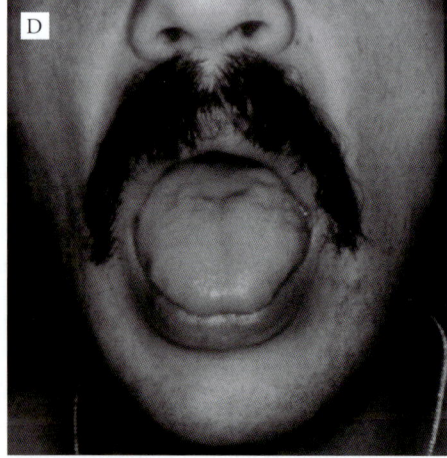

Figure 12.16D Case 12.8. Atrophy of left side of tongue.

Past history was negative except for problems related to vocal cords. Several months prior to the onset of the shoulder symptoms, he had an upper respiratory infection and developed severe hoarseness. Examination by an ENT specialist (Dr. Fine) at that time indicated a paralysis of the left vocal cord. The left vocal cord was fixed slightly off midline. The right vocal cord moved well but did not fully compensate.

Family history was not remarkable except that his mother died of rheumatic heart disease in her 40s.

General physical examination: There was a café au lait spot on the left forearm, 1 x 2 cm in size, and a large 8 x 5 cm café au lait spot on the right posterior leg just below the buttock.

Neurological Examination

Mental status: Intact.

Cranial nerves: The following abnormalities were present:

X: the uvula pulled very slightly to the right on gag. There was only a minimal suggestion of any hoarseness at this time. Gag was intact. Laryngoscopy by the ENT specialist indicated paralysis of the left vocal cord.

XI: There was significant weakness and marked atrophy of the left sternomastoid muscle (Fig. 12.16B). There was marked atrophy of the left trapezium seen in both elevation of the shoulder and in abduction of the scapula with involvement of both the middle and lower portions with winging of the medial edge of the scapula (Fig. 12.16C).

XII. Minor ridges of atrophy and fasciculations were seen on the left side of the tongue (Fig. 12.16D).

Motor system: There was questionable minimal weakness of muscles about the left shoulder: supraspinatus, infraspinatus, and serratus anterior.

Reflexes:

a. Deep tendon reflexes were hyperactive except for possible mild depression of finger jerks on the left compared to the right.
b. Plantar response on the right was equivocal; that on the left was flexor.

Sensory system: no definite abnormality was present.

Clinical diagnosis: Jugular foramen tumor, probably neurofibroma.

Laboratory Data

1. *Brain stem auditory evoked potential* was normal for the right ear but demonstrated a delay in the I-II interval for the left ear.
2. *Tomograms of the petrous bone* showed marked bone destruction in the region of the jugular foramen.

3. *CT scan of head:* The left skull base demonstrated marked erosion of the left jugular foramen, extending anteriorly to the carotid canal and laterally to the base of the petrous bone. There was a well-defined enhancing mass which extended from the jugular foramen superiorly to the height of the left petrous apex (Fig. 12.16A).

Sagittal and coronal reconstructions demonstrated the continuity of this mass with the jugular foramen. The fourth ventricle was compressed and shifted from left to right. There was a slight effacement of the left CP angle cistern.

Subsequent course: The neurosurgeon Dr. Bernard Stone performed a suboccipital craniotomy, revealing a large tumor mass in the lower inferior portion of the left cerebellar-pontine angle originating from the jugular foramen. All of the intracranial extent of the tumor was removed as was most of the tumor within the jugular foramen. However, the remainder of the tumor which extended through the foramen into the extracranial space could not be removed by this approach. Histological examination of the tumor confirmed the preoperative impression of a schwannoma (neurofibroma) of the ninth or tenth cranial nerves which had to be sacrificed during the procedures.

The patient did well and was readmitted 4 months later for removal of the extracranial portion of this dumbbell tumor at the base of the skull by the ENT surgeon, Dr. Fine. The tumor mass enmeshed the structures exiting from the jugular foramen.

CT scans 4 years later indicated recurrence of both of the intracranial and the extracranial portion of the tumor (extending again into the parapharyngeal space).

Comments

The schwannoma in this case presented initial symptoms relevant to cranial nerve 10, that is, paralysis of the left vocal cord. Occasionally patients will have a vocal cord paralysis following an upper respiratory infection, possibly due to involvement of the recurrent laryngeal nerve. In this case, however, within several months, the first signs of involvement of the eleventh cranial nerve appeared and progressed over the next 5 years. The CT scan demonstrated a large mass which extended from the jugular foramen into the cerebellar pontine angle. The surgical procedures also indicated the extension of this mass into the extracranial parapharyngeal space. Whether the involvement of cranial nerves 10 and 11 occurred in the extramedullary space proximal to the jugular foramen or within the foramen is unclear. Usually the syndrome of the jugular foramen includes signs relevant to cranial nerve 9 as well, but this patient had no involvement of sensation in the posterior pharynx and no clear-cut involvement of taste over the posterior third of the tongue. As regards the involvement of cranial nerve 12, this could have involvement by this large tumor mass in the intracranial area or the parapharyngeal area. This large tumor mass also produced minor subclinical compromise of cranial nerve VIII—evident on the brain stem auditory evoked potential with a delay between the cochlea and the cochlear nucleus. As regards the apparent minor weakness at the left shoulder, these findings may have reflected a failure of stabilization at the left shoulder due to the involvement of the trapezius muscle. The right-sided Babinski sign probably reflected the distortion of the left pyramidal tract due to the brain stem distortion produced by the tumor. As regards the question as to whether this patient had neurofibromatosis type I, the following may be noted: he had no peripheral neurofibromas, no family history, and had only two café au lait spots (six or more over 15 mm in diameter after puberty constitute a significant number). Moreover, the patient had none of the other cutaneous or bony abnormalities seen with this disorder.

Figure 12.17 The twelve cranial nerves.

PLAYBASIA, MALFORAMTION OF THE BASE OF THE SKULL

The following case history illustrates the effects of platybasia (malformation of the base of the skull), secondary to Paget's disease on the cranial nerves, spinal cord, and brain stem (Fig. 12.17).

CASE HISTORY 12.10

This 57-year-old, white salesman 5 years prior to admission first noticed difficulty in obtaining a standard-size hat. Two years prior to admission the patient first noted the gradual onset of a steadily progressive difficulty in walking, characterized by a loss of balance. He had experienced increasing difficulty in standing erect and had fallen on several occasions. The patient had noted increasing discomfort at the occipital area of the head. Two months prior to admission the patient had noted a hoarseness of his voice, a weakness or tremor of the tongue, a difficulty in articulating words, and a difficulty in swallowing, and more recently the patient had noted numbness of all fingers, the right more than the left, and a correlated clumsiness in the manipulation of small objects. In the several weeks prior to admission, the patient had noted difficulty in focusing his eyes. He had also noted diplopia, particularly when gazing to the right.

Neurological Examination

Mental status: Intact deep tendon reflexes and sensation over limbs and body were intact. Findings were limited to:

Cranial nerves:

a. A right lateral rectus weakness was present with diplopia on right lateral gaze.
b. Pain and to a lesser degree touch sensation was significantly decreased in the ophthalmic and maxillary divisions of the left fifth nerve, with a decreased left corneal reflex.
c. Hearing (both bone and air) was decreased bilaterally.
d. Horizontal nystagmus on lateral gaze to either side was present.
e. Gag reflex and pharyngeal tactile sensation were bilaterally decreased, particularly on the left. The uvula pulled to the right. The voice was hoarse and speech was dysarthric.
f. Lingual movements and lingual sounds were slowly performed, although no definite weakness or atrophy of the tongue was present.

Motor system:

a. Gait was grossly reeling and ataxic.
b. Ataxia was present on finger-to-nose and heel-to-shin tests of cerebellar function.

Reflexes: Intact and physiologic.
Sensory system: Intact.
Head and neck:

The head was large. The neck was short. There was limitation of movement on turning the head laterally.

Clinical diagnosis: Paget's disease. Platybasia with involvement of lower cranial nerves and cerebellum.

Laboratory data: The relevant findings included the following:

1. Skull X-rays showed marked thickening of the diploe with the changes characteristic of Paget's disease. Well advanced platybasia was present with the tip of the odontoid of the axis found to be 25 mm above McGregor's line. (This is a line drawn from the posterior margin of the hard palate to the inferior surface of the basal occipital bone; normally the odontoid should not extend above this line by more than 4 to 5 mm.)
2. Alkaline phosphatase was significantly elevated (2x the upper limit of normal).

Subsequent course: A suboccipital decompression was performed by Dr. Bertram Selverstone. The bone of the cranium was very thick. There was marked compression of the lower medulla and upper cervical cord by the anterior rim of occipital bone forming the posterior margin of the foramen magnum. The posterior arch of the first cervical vertebra was also compressing the underlying cervical spinal cord. Postoperatively, there was a significant improvement. Follow-up 1 month later indicated that the patient had regained fine movement skills in the hand. His gait was markedly improved, although still slightly wide based. Lower cranial nerve findings were no longer present. The sixth and eighth cranial nerve findings were unchanged.

Follow-up evaluation 1 year later indicated continued improvement in gait. Nystagmus was present but the weakness of nerve VI had resolved.

Several years after the surgery patient had increasing ataxia of gait, increasing diplopia, and decreasing vision in the left eye. Within 2 years bilateral medial rectus weakness was present. Re-evaluation over the next year indicated progression of ataxia. Skull X-rays indicated a progression of the degree of basilar invagination.

The patient refused any additional surgical procedures.

Comments

The findings in this case indicated involvement of the cerebellum and lower cranial nerves, particularly the vagus and glossopharyngeal nerves: hoarseness of voice, defect in elevation of the uvula, and defective sensation in the posterior pharynx. In addition, there was involvement of the sixth and trigeminal nerves. Whether the fifth nerve involvement related directly to platybasia or whether this reflected occlusion of the ostia of the skull by Paget's disease would not be certain. Involvement of nerve VIII usually reflects narrowing of the internal auditory foramen with compression of the nerve. Basilar impression occurs in conditions other than Paget's disease. In the majority of cases, the defect reflects a congenital malformation of the basal occipital bone. There are often associated malformations of bone: a fusion of the occipital bone with the atlas, a dislocation of the odontoid, a fusion of the vertebrae (Klippel-Feil abnormality), cervical spinal bifida, or a small foramen magnum.

Other abnormalities of the foramen magnum region: There may also be associated malformations of the central nervous system, for example, the Arnold-Chiari malformation that is elongation of the inferior portion of the cerebellum through the foramen magnum into the cervical canal or persistence of the embryonic cervical flexure with apparent downward displacement of the medulla and cervical cord. (Refer to the discussion of syringomyelia in the spinal cord chapter 9 for an illustration.) Malformations of the meninges (arachnoid cysts) or of the roof of the fourth ventricle, with absence of the foramina of Luschka and Magendie (Dandy-Walker syndrome; see Embryology chapter 4) may be present. In occasional cases, syringomyelia or hydrocephalus also will be found. Although many of these malformations will produce their effects in infancy or childhood, not infrequently the first neurological manifestation may be delayed until adult life.

BIBLIOGRAPHY

GENERAL

Akesson, E. J., and Stewart, P. A. 1988. Cranial Nerves. Anatomy and Clinical Comments. Philadelphia, PA: B. C. Decker.

Asbury, A. K., McKhann, G. M., and McDonald, W. I. (Eds.) 1992. Diseases of the Nervous System: Clinical Neurobiology. 2nd ed., Vol. 1.. Philadelphia, PA: W. B. Saunders (See particularly Chapter 21: Central Mechanisms of Initiation and Control of Movement, Chapter 26: Oculomotor Control: Normal and Abnormal, Chapter 31: Vertigo and Dizziness, Chapter 34: Pupillary Function and Dysfunction).

Brodal, A. 1965. The Cranial Nerves. Anatomy and Anatomical Clinical Correlation. London, UK: Oxford Blackwell.

Clemente, C. 1988. Gray's Anatomy. 30th ed. Philadelphia, PA: Lea and Febiger.

DeJong, R. N. 1978. The Neurologic Examination. New York, NY: Hoeber Medical Division, Harper & Row.

Haymaker, W. 1969. Bing's Local Diagnosis in Neurological Disease. 15th ed. St. Louis, MO: C. V. Mosby.

Herrick, C. J. 1948. The Brain of the Tiger Salamander. Chicago, IL: University of Chicago Press.

Specific Cranial Nerves: I: Olfactory (See also Chapter 22)

Doty, R. 2009. The olfactory system and its disorders. Semin. Neurol. 29: 74–81.

II: OPTIC NERVE (SEE ALSO CHAPTER 23)

Selhorst, J. B., and Chen, Y. 2009. The optic nerve. Semin. Neurol. 29:29–35.

I, IV, AND VI: EXTRAOCULAR MUSCLES

Brazis, P. W. 2009. Isolated palsies of cranial nerves III, IV and VI. Semin. Neurol. 29:14–28.

Bender, M. B. 1980. Brain control of conjugate horizontal and vertical eye movements: a study of the structural and functional correlates. Brain 103:23–69.

Breen, L. A. 1980. Pupil sparing oculomotor nerve palsy due to mid brain infarction. Arch. Neurol. 48:105–106.

Buttner-Ennever, J. A. (Ed.) 1988. Neuroanatomy of the oculomotor system. Rev. Oculomotor Res. 2:1–36.

Leigh, R. J., Averbuch-Heller, L., Thomsake, R. L., et al. 1994. Treatment of abnormal eye movements that impair vision. Strategies based on current concepts of physiology and pharmacology. [Review] Ann. Neurol. 36:129–141.

Leigh, R. J., and Zee, D. S. 2006. The Neurology of Eye Movements. 4th ed. Oxford, UK: Oxford University Press.

Rush, J. A., and Younge, B. R. 1981. Paralysis of cranial nerves III IV and VI: cause and prognosis in 1,000 cases. Arch. Ophthal. 99:76–79.

Schmidtke, K., and Buttner-Ennever, J. A. 1992. A nervous control of eyelid function: a review of clinical experimental and pathological data. Brain 115:227–247.

V: TRIGEMINAL SYSTEM

Gonella, M. C., Fischbein, N. J., and Yuen, Y. T. 2009. Disorders of the trigeminal system. Semin. Neurol. 29:36–44.

Rozen, T. D. 2004. Trigeminal neuralgia and glossopharyngeal neuralgia. Neurol. Clin. 22:185–206.

Sweet, W. H. 1986. Current concepts: the treatment of trigeminal neuralgia (tic douloureux). N. Engl. J. Med. 315:174–177.

VII: FACIAL NERVE

Adour, K. K. 1982. Current concepts in neurology: diagnosis and management of facial paralysis. N. Engl. J. Med. 15:346–351.

Gilchrist, J. M. 2009. Seventh cranial neuropathy. Semin. Neurol. 29: 5–13.

Sullivan, F. M., Swan, I. R., Donnan, P. T., et al. 2007. Early treatment with prednisolone or acyclovir in Bell's palsy. N. Engl. J. Med. 357: 1598–1607.

Kappos, L., and Mehling, M. 2010. Dissociation of voluntary and emotional innervation after stroke. N. Engl. J. Med. 363:e25.

VII: EIGHTH NERVE: ACOUSTIC AND VESTIBULAR

Fife, T. D. 2009. Benign paroxysmal positional vertigo. Semin. Neurol. 29:500–508.

Hain, T. C. 1995. Treatment of vertigo. The Neurologist 1:125–133.

Harner, S. G., Daube, J. R., and Ebersold, M. J. 1987. Improved preservation of facial nerve function with the use of electrical monitoring during removal of acoustic neuromas. Mayo Clinic Proc. 62:92–102.

Harner, S. G., and Ebersold, M. J. 1985. Management of acoustic neuromas 1978–1983. J. Neurosurg 63:175 179.

Kerber, K. A. 2009. Vertigo presentations in the emergency department. Semin. Neurol. 29:482–490.

Laird, F. J., Harner, S. G., Laws, E. R., Jr., et al. 1985. Meningiomas of the cerebellopontine angle. Otolaryngol. Head Neck Surg. 93:163–167.

Landau, M. E., and Barner, K. C. 2009. Vestibulocochlear nerve. Sem. Neurol. 29:66–73.

Lockwood, A. H., Salvi, R. J., and Burkard, R. F. 2002. Tinnitus. N. Engl. J. Med. 347:904–910.

Martuza, R. L., Parker, S. W., Nadol, J. B., et al. 1985. Diagnosis of cerebellopontine angle tumors. Clin. Neurosurg. 32:177–213.

Martuza, R. L., and Eldridge, R. 1988. Neurofibromatosis 2 (bilateral acoustic neurofibromatosis). N. Engl. J. Med. 318:684–688.

Neuhauser, H. K., and Lempert, T. 2009 Vertigo: epidemiologic aspects. Semin. Neurol. 29:473–481.

Rasmussen, G. L. 1960. Efferent fibers of the cochlear nerve and cochlear nucleus. In G. L. Rasmussen and W. F. Windle (Eds.). Neural Mechanisms of the Auditory and Vestibular Systems, pp. 105–125. Springfield, IL: Charles C Thomas.

Strupp, M., and Brandt, T. 2009. Vestibular neuritis. Semin. Neurol. 29: 509–519.

Wertelecki, W., Rouleau, G. A., Superneau, D. W., et al. 1988. Neurofibromatosis 2: clinical studies of a large kindred. N. Engl. J. Med. 319:278–283.

IX AND X: GLOSSOPHARYNGEAL AND VAGUS NERVES

Erman, A. B., Kejner, A. E., Hogikyan, N. D., and Feldman, E. L. 2009. Disorders of cranial nerves IX and X. Semin. Neurol. 29:85–95.

XI: SPINAL ACCESSORY NERVE

Massey, W. E. 2009. Spinal accessory nerve lesions Semin. Neurol. 29:82–84.

XII: HYPOGLOSSAL NERVE

Lin, H. C., and Barkhaus, P. E. 2009. Cranial nerve XII: the hypoglossal nerve. Semin. Neurol. 29:45–52.

MULTIPLE CRANIAL NEUROPATHIES

Carroll, C. G., and Campbell, W. W. 2009. Multiple cranial neuropathies. Semin. Neurol. 29:53–65.

Victor, M., and Ropper, A. H. 2001. Principles of Neurology. 7th ed. New York, NY: McGraw Hill.

Brodal, A. 1965. The Cranial Nerves. Anatomy and Anatomical Clinical Correlation. London, UK: Oxford Blackwell.

Clemente, C. 1988. Gray's Anatomy. 30th ed. Philadelphia, PA: Lea & Febiger.

DeJong, R. N. 1978. The Neurologic Examination. New York, NY: Hoeber Medical Division, Harper & Row.

Herrick, C. J. 1948. The Brain of the Tiger Salamander. Chicago, IL: University of Chicago Press.

Rasmussen, G. L. 1960. Efferent fibers of the cochlear nerve and cochlear nucleus. In G. L. Rasmussen and W. F. Windle (Eds.) Neural Mechanisms of the Auditory and Vestibular Systems, pp 105–125. Springfield, IL: Charles C. Thomas.

Wilson-Pauwels, L., Akesson, E. J., and Stewart, P. A. 1988. Cranial Nerves. Anatomy and Clinical Comments. Philadelphia, B. C. Decker.

13.

BRAIN STEM

CLINICAL CONSIDERATIONS

Of all sites in the central nervous system, the brain stem provides the best example of how the anatomical pattern of involvement may allow the prediction of the actual pathologic process. The student has, of course, already encountered several examples of this phenomenon at the level of the spinal cord. For example, the clinical finding of a selective dissociated loss of pain and temperature in a cape-like distribution over the shoulders and upper extremities implies an anatomical process in a pericentral location involving the anterior commissure. One could readily deduce that an intrinsic pathological process was present and, moreover, could assume that in most cases the pathological process was that of syringomyelia.

At the level of the brain stem, such examples of close correlation occur frequently. Thus, the progressive combined involvement of the ipsilateral cranial nerve VIII (auditory and vestibular), nerve VII (facial), and nerve V (trigeminal), with the manifestations of deafness, tinnitus (a buzzing or ringing sound in the ear), dizziness, peripheral facial paralysis, and unilateral facial numbness, not only indicates the location of the pathology (the cerebellar pontine angle) but also strongly suggests the actual nature of the pathology: vestibular schwannoma (*acoustic neuroma* was the old term). While other pathological lesions may occur at this site, they are much less common.

There are several possible approaches to the problem of localization of disease processes in the brain stem. We have already considered in Chapter 11 a number of guidelines for localization that should be reviewed at this time. We will now consider in greater detail the particular anatomical syndromes and the various types of pathology in terms of specific extrinsic and intrinsic syndromes. Many of the extrinsic syndromes related to cranial nerve syndromes have already been considered in Chapter 12 and are summarized in Table 12.5. When speaking of the anatomical syndromes of the brain stem in clinical neurology, we will limit our considerations to the medulla oblongata, pons, and midbrain. The thalamus, hypothalamus, and subthalamus represent a natural rostral continuation of the midbrain, and diseases involving the midbrain sometimes also involve the adjacent diencephalon. From the standpoint of vascular anatomy, the midbrain and the diencephalon do share a vascular supply from the penetrating branches of the posterior cerebral arteries

SPECIFIC SYNDROMES AND DISEASE ENTITIES

Specific syndromes and disease entities will now be considered. Our emphasis will be on various classic syndromes, each of which implies a single-level lesion. The reason for this emphasis in the teaching of clinical anatomical correlation is obvious. However, the student should realize that, in actuality, a number of the diseases involving the brain stem are not simply limited to a single level but rather affect multiple levels; that is, they are multifocal or they are system disorders. Thus, although we will consider in detail patients with limited focal infarcts, it is more frequent to have infarction at several levels of the brain stem in occlusive disease of the basilar-vertebral system (perhaps the most common disease involving the brain stem). Another rather common disease of the brain stem, multiple sclerosis, almost always follows a multifocal pattern.

DIFFERENTIATION OF EXTRINSIC VERSUS INSTRINSIC DISEASES

The same categories of disease already familiar to the student from his or her study of the spinal cord will be employed: extrinsic and intrinsic. At the level of the spinal cord, extrinsic diseases were much more common and were emphasized. At the level of the brain stem, the intrinsic diseases occur much more frequently. (This is also the case at the level of the cerebral hemisphere.) Nevertheless, extrinsic diseases have an importance outside of their actual frequency of occurrence. As we have already noted, at the level of the spinal cord, extrinsic diseases represent progressive compression-type problems such as tumors or degenerative disk disease. Early diagnosis and surgical relief of the compression will prevent the development of disability and will preserve life. All lesions compressing the brain stem are potentially life-threatening if they progress to the vital centers of the medulla involved in the control of respiration, blood pressure, swallowing, and changes in intracranial pressure (ICP), and so on. Moreover, involvement of those areas essential for motor control (reticular formation of pons and medulla) or those areas in the midbrain reticular formation essential for the maintenance of consciousness will result in a severe bedridden state.

In distinguishing extrinsic and intrinsic diseases, several differential points have already been mentioned (Table 13.1).

The development of techniques such as the computerized tomography (CT) and magnetic resonance imaging (MRI) scan has markedly increased our ability to confirm the anatomical localization of disease involving the brain stem. Magnetic resonance angiography has provided a noninvasive method of imaging the blood supply of the brain stem (see Chapter 2).

Table 13.1. PATTERNS OF EXTRINSIC VERSUS INTRINSIC DISEASE OF THE BRAIN STEM

PATTERNS OF EXTRINSIC LESIONS	PATTERNS OF INTRINSIC LESIONS
a. Successive unilateral involvement of multiple cranial nerves early in the course of the disease, with fiber systems involved only later in the disease.	a. Simultaneous segmental involvement of the cranial nerve nuclei and of long tracts, as in a lateral medullary infarction.
b. Early involvement of the eighth cranial nerve (as in acoustic neuroma).	b. Progressive bilateral involvement of cranial nerves and long tracts, as in infiltrating glioma.
c. A syndrome in which symptoms are limited to the midline cerebellum: loss of equilibrium and truncal ataxia.	c. Involvement of the fifth cranial nerve—descending spinal tract with selective involvement of pain sensation over the face. Involvement of the MLF, as in MS, glioma, or infarction with the occurrence of internuclear ophthalmoplegia and vertical nystagmus.
d. Symptoms of ICP of the disease—headache, nausea, and vomiting. Occasionally, as in midline cerebellar lesions, the symptoms of ICP (with or without truncal ataxia) may be the only symptom.	d. If an infiltrating tumor, occurring early in the course the symptoms of ICP tend to occur late in the disease.

ICP, intracranial pressure; MLF, medial longitudinal fasciculus; MS, multiple sclerosis.

EXTRINSIC DISEASES OF THE BRAIN STEM

EXTRINSIC TUMORS AND OTHER MASS LESIONS

As indicated, almost all of the problems within the extrinsic category are tumors. When we use the term "extrinsic" in the present context, we mean extrinsic to the actual substance of the brain stem. Some of the tumors to be considered are actually invasive tumors intrinsic to the cerebellum or arising from the ependymal cells lining the fourth ventricle that are secondarily compressing or infiltrating the brain stem. Some of these tumors are actually derived from cells of the glial series, for example, cystic astrocytomas of the cerebellum, medulloblastomas, and ependymomas. Some are locally invasive malignant tumors, for example, nasopharyngeal carcinoma infiltrating the bone of the skull or carcinoma of the lung or breast, metastatic to the cerebellum. (In general, carcinomas only rarely spread in a metastatic manner to the brain stem per se.)

1. The cerebellar pontine angle syndrome

   a. *Vestibular schwannoma (acoustic neuroma) (Figs. 13.1 and 13.2):* Tumors at the cerebellar pontine angle account for 10% of all central nervous system tumors. Most tumors encountered at the cerebellar pontine angle are vestibular neuromas arising from the Schwann cells about cranial nerve VIII. As already noted the tumor actually arises from Schwann cells within the vestibular component of cranial nerve VIII within the internal auditory canal. This is a disease of the middle-aged or older adult. (Onset of symptoms in the teens or early 20s should suggest the possibility of neurofibromatosis 2 in which bilateral acoustic neuromas occur (see Martuza and Eldridge, 1988, and Chapter 9.) The early symptoms and findings relate to a progressive involvement of nerve VIII (progressive loss of hearing of a neural type and a dead labyrinth on caloric stimulation). As the tumor enlarges, symptoms referable to nerves VII and V and to the cerebellum develop. An illustrative case has been presented in Chapter 12.

   b. *Other tumors in the cerebellar pontine angle:* Although less frequent, other types of pathology are found in this location: meningiomas (Fig. 2.10) arising from arachnoidal cell nests) and cholesteatomas (epidermoids). A large series from the Mayo Clinic (Laird et al., 1985) indicated 20 meningiomas over a 6-year period compared to 160 acoustic neuromas over a similar period (Harner et al., 1985). Specific neurological deficits were as frequent as in patients with acoustic neuromas. Diagnosis may be made with contrast enhanced MRI or, if not available, contrast-enhanced CT scan.

2. Syndromes of the cerebellum

   a. *Midline cerebellum (fourth ventricle) syndrome.* The midline cerebellar syndrome is frequently encountered

Figure 13.1 Vestibular schwannoma ("acoustic neuroma") at the cerebellar pontine angle. (Courtesy of Dr. Jose Segarra and Dr. Remedios Rosales, Boston Veterans Administration Hospital.)

Figure 13.2 Cerebellar pontine angle tumor: vestibular schwannoma. Magnetic resonance imaging. A large mass extends from an enlarged right internal auditory canal compressing and distorting the pons and medulla. (Courtesy of Dr. Milton Weiner and Dr. Alex Danylevich.)

Figure 13.3 Medulloblastoma. Magnetic resonance imaging (T1 weighted). This large tumor arising from the midline cerebellum in this 4-year-old child fills the fourth ventricle, producing hydrocephalus and compressing the medulla. (Courtesy Dr. Milton Weiner.)

in neurology. Clinical deficit: The patient is often a child and presents with a disturbance of balance and ataxia of the trunk and gait but no clearly lateralized symptoms. In general, the etiology is neoplastic. The type of tumor varies as a function of age. The most common cause in an infant or child is a medulloblastoma (Fig. 13.3). This tumor arises from nests of external granular cells in the nodulus, an older portion of the cerebellum relating to the vestibular system. Since this portion of the cerebellum projects as a roof into the fourth ventricle, early obstruction of the ventricle is to be expected. A typical case is presented in Chapter 19 (cerebellum). Occasionally this tumor may present in adolescents and young adults. The cells may seed via the cerebrospinal fluid (CSF), so that rarely the early symptoms may be those of a lumbar radiculopathy.

In children and young adults, the most common cause is the ependymoma that arises from ependymal cells in the floor or roof of the fourth ventricle (Fig.13.4). The tumor mass grows into the ventricle, obstructing this cavity but also exerting upward pressure on the midline nodulus (and other aspects of the cerebellar vermis). At times, however, the ependymoma may extensively invade the tegmentum of the medulla and pons. At times, the tumor is a mixture of ependymoma and astrocytic components. Taken together, the medulloblastoma and the ependymoma constitute the most common central nervous system tumors in the pediatric age group.

In the adolescent and young adult the low-grade cystic astrocytoma must also be considered, although a lateral hemisphere location is the much more common location.

In the middle-aged adult, the most common cause of the syndrome is a midline hemangioblastoma. These are tumors derived from embryonic vascular elements. In contrast to the medulloblastoma and the ependymoma, the hemangioblastoma and the cystic astrocytoma are surgically curable

Figure 13.4 Ependymoma of the fourth ventricle. Magnetic resonance imaging (T1 weighted). This 14-year-old male had a 4-month history of headache and neck pain, with gait ataxia and nystagmus. This large mass obstructs the fourth ventricle, producing hydrocephalus, displaces the cerebellar vermis, and extends out the fourth ventricular foramen then down through the foramen magnum to compress the spinal cord. (Courtesy of Dr. Gerald McGuillicuddy, Dr. Milton, Dr. Weiner, and Dr. Artinian.)

neoplasms. It is often found that a nodule of tumor exists within a nonneoplastic cystic cavity, allowing for removal of the tumor without sacrifice of a large amount of the cerebellum.

When the patient is 50 years old, hemangioblastomas and metastatic tumors constitute the major midline entities. Metastatic carcinomas in general, however, are more often found in a non–midline cerebellar hemisphere location.

b. *Lateral cerebellar hemisphere syndrome.* Clinical deficit: lateralized symptoms affecting the ipsilateral arm and leg have already been mentioned. The syndrome is discussed in greater detail with an illustrative case history in Chapter 20 on the cerebellum. As regards the specific mass lesions, this in large part depends on the patient's age:

- In the child and young adult, the most common lesion is probably the cystic astrocytoma.

- In the middle-aged and older age groups, the most common lesions are metastatic carcinoma and the hemangioblastoma. The metastatic carcinoma may represent a solitary metastasis from a primary lesion in lung, breast, ovary, or kidney or may be only one of multiple lesions. The cerebellar lesion in any case is often surgically removed since it does represent a relatively acute life-threatening lesion. The hemangioblastoma has already been discussed. Other mass lesions of the cerebellar hemisphere in the pre-antibiotic era included brain abscess (the source of infection was usually the adjacent middle ear and mastoid) and tuberculomas. Hypertensive cerebellar hemorrhages may also present as acute mass lesions as may acute edematous cerebellar infarcts.

3. Extrinsic midbrain syndromes

   a. *Syndrome of compression of the pretectal area and superior colliculus (Figs. 13.5 and 13.6).* These are essentially three causes of this syndrome: (1). tumors of the pineal (pinealomas) occurring primarily in men and boys; (2) hydrocephalus in infants; and (3) hypertensive hemorrhages of the posterior thalamus occurring most

Figure 13.6 Tumor of the pineal region. Magnetic resonance imaging. This 68-year-old female presented with apraxia of gait, urinary incontinence, and dementia. Symptoms resolved following a shunt procedure and radiotherapy.

commonly in middle-aged or older patients. Tumors of the pineal are of several types. (1) The most frequent (50%) are germ cell tumors: germinoma, or atypical teratomas: arising from congenital cell nests of a mixed type and occurring at any age but most commonly in males under 10 years. Histologically these tumors are identical to congenital tumors of the testes (seminoma) or dysgerminoma of the ovary. (2) In addition to the malignant germinoma, noninvasive congenital germ cell tumors may occur and may be resected: teratomas, dermoids, and epidermoids. (3) Other types are astrocytomas and ependymomas, pineal parenchymal tumors (pineocytomas), meningiomas, and arachnoid cysts. For additional discussion, see DeGirolami and Schmidek (1973), and Stein (1979).

An illustrative case history (11.2) has been presented in the brain stem Chapter 11 on functional localization.

b. Syndromes of the tentorium

The Tentorial Notch syndrome: Herniation of the medial aspects of the temporal lobe (uncus and parahippocampal gyrus) secondary to supratentorial mass lesions is the most common syndrome found in relation to the tentorium. More lateral supratentorial masses as in temporal lobe tumors produce a lateral herniation syndrome characterized initially by an ipsilateral fixed dilated pupil and then an ipsilateral cranial nerve (CN) 3 paralysis. Additional compression will shift the midbrain and compress the opposite cerebral peduncle against the rigid tentorial edge resulting in an ipsilateral hemiparesis in addition to the already present contralateral hemiparesis. As compression and displacement of the brain stem progresses, hemorrhages (Duret hemorrhages) into the substance

Figure 13.5 Tumor of the pineal. This is an enlarged nonmalignant cyst arising from the pineal gland (arrow). (Courtesy of Dr. John Hills and Dr. Jose Segarra.)

Figure 13.7 Herniation of the parahippocampal gyrus secondary to a subdural hematoma. Note residuals of Duret hemorrhages in pons. (Courtesy of Pathology Department at St. Vincent Hospital.)

of the midbrain and pons develop. A progressive sequence of midbrain, then pontine, and eventually medullary symptoms evolves. Supratentorial masses in a more parasagittal location produce central herniation with bilateral midbrain (CN III) and subsequently pontine-medullary involvement (Figs. 13.7, 13.8, and 13.9).

Tentorial meningiomas: These are rare. A variety of syndromes may occur: (1) midline obstructing mass with increased intracranial pressure but without definite localizing features, (2) mass lesion extending above the tentorium to involve the temporal and occipital lobes, (3) mass lesion

Figure 13.9 Duret hemorrhage. Multiple small hemorrhages are present in the pontine tegmentum and to a lesser extent in the basilar pons secondary to massive infarction of cerebral hemisphere, temporal lobe herniation, and brain stem compression. (Courtesy of Dr. John Hills.)

extending below the tentorium, displacing or invaginating the cerebellum and compressing the brain stem and cranial nerves.

4. Jugular foramen syndrome

   This is caused by neurofibromas or other tumors arising from the lower cranial nerves (CN IX, X, and XI) as these nerves pass together through the jugular foramen. An illustrative case history 12.7 is presented in Chapter 12.

5. Foramen magnum syndromes

   a. *Herniation syndrome (Fig. 13. 10).* This is the most common process at the foramen magnum and is sometimes referred to as cerebellar pressure cone. Any mass lesion in the posterior fossa may produce herniation of the cerebellar tonsils compressing the lower end of the medulla and the upper cervical spinal cord. When gradually acquired, head tilt, stiff neck, and pain in the neck may be early symptoms. When acutely acquired, a rapid and fatal arrest of respiratory and circulatory function is

Figure 13.8 Tentorial herniation with brain stem compression. A large intracerebral hematoma and hemorrhagic infarction (single arrow) in right cerebral hemisphere has produced herniation of the medial aspect of temporal lobe (double arrow). Shift of the brain stem has occurred with compression and infarction of the left cerebral peduncle against the tentorium (triple arrow). (Courtesy of Pathology Department, Tufts New England Medical Center.)

Figure 13.10 Herniation of the cerebellar tonsils. The cerebellar tonsils have been compressed downward through the foramen magnum (arrow), secondary to a teratoma of the pineal, compressing the caudal medulla and upper cervical spine. (Courtesy of Dr. John Hills and Dr. Jose Segarra.)

likely to occur. Such an acute event may be precipitated by the performance of a lumbar puncture in a patient with a posterior fossa mass lesion. At times in subacute cases, this final stage of arrest of respiration and fall in blood pressure is preceded by a period of irregular respiration, slow pulse, and rising blood pressure.

Once tentorial herniation has occurred in a supratentorial mass lesion, increased mass is present in the posterior fossa. In addition, hemorrhage into the brain stem and edema of the brain stem act to increase the mass in the posterior fossa. Tonsillar herniation with medullary compression would then in this situation also be the expected terminal event. (For a more complete discussion of the clinical pathophysiology of the tentorial and tonsillar herniation syndromes, the student is referred to Plum and Posner, 1980).

b. *Meningiomas.* These are rare in this location and produce a variable picture. Their growth may be primarily in the posterior fossa with compression of the lower cranial nerves, brain stem, and cerebellum. On the other hand, the tumor may extend down through the foramen magnum, compressing the upper and middle cervical roots and then the long tracts on one or both sides of the spinal cord. In some cases, a mixture of posterior fossa and cervical cord findings will be present.

SYNDROMES DUE TO DEVELOPMENTAL AND BONY ABNORMALITIES

These syndromes primarily occur at the foramen magnum.

1. The Arnold Chiari syndrome has been discussed and illustrated in Chapter 9.
2. Deformation of the bones at the base of the skull occurs in platybasia, a flattening of the sphenoid and occipital bones (sometimes referred to as basilar impression because the bones about the foramen magnum are pushed into the posterior fossa). There are essentially two causes for this deformation: Paget's disease and various developmental malformations.

Paget's disease is a chronic metabolic disease of bone occurring in the adult, in which there is both excessive and disorganized bone formation and excessive bone destruction. Bony overgrowth may result in pressure on nerve roots, on cranial nerve VIII and on the facial nerve. Involvement of the vertebrae may result in spinal cord compression. Involvement of the skull is common. When the disease process affects occipital and sphenoid bones at the base of the skull, a softening, flattening, and distortion occurs. As a result, the odontoid process projects up into the posterior fossa. The posterior fossa in its normal state is a relatively small cavity. The end result is a compression of the contents of the posterior fossa—medulla, cerebellum, and lower cranial nerves—in addition to the upper cervical spinal cord.

VASCULAR SYNDROMES AFFECTING THE BRAIN AS EXTRINSIC LESIONS

1. *Aneurysms:* At points of congenital weakness in the wall of an artery (usually points of bifurcation), a dilated thin-walled sac may form, termed an *aneurysm*. Intracranial aneurysms produce symptoms in several ways: (1) the dilated sac may act as a space-occupying lesion compressing adjacent structures such as cranial nerves; (2) rupture of the aneurysm may occur with leakage of blood into the subarachnoid space; (3) the sudden hemorrhage into this space may also dissect into the brain with the formation of a hematoma and/or rupture into the ventricular system may occur; (4) the circulation of blood in the artery beyond the point of the aneurysm may be impaired, producing ischemia and destruction of tissue supplied by the artery; (5) additionally blood in the subarachnoid space about arteries may produce vasospasm; and (6) blood in this subarachnoid space and ventricles may also block the circulation of CSF resulting in hydrocephalus.

The majority (85% to 90%) of aneurysms arise from what is termed the *anterior circulation* at essentially three locations: (1) the anterior cerebral-anterior communicating junction, (2) the middle cerebral artery bifurcation, and (3) the junction of the posterior communicating and internal carotid arteries. As already discussed in the cranial nerve Chapter 12, Case 12.1 at this last location, an enlarging saccular aneurysm, may compress cranial nerve III. The finding of a fixed, dilated pupil and ptosis of the lid in a patient with subarachnoid hemorrhage may provide a valuable clue for localization of the aneurysm at the junction of the posterior communicating internal carotid junction. Approximately 10% to 15% of saccular aneurysms are found in relation to the basilar vertebral system. Common sites include the bifurcation of the basilar artery. In addition to saccular aneurysms, fusiform dilatation of the basilar artery may occur in atherosclerosis, resulting in an enlarged tortuous vessel that may compress adjacent structures.

2. *Hypertensive cerebellar hemorrhage* (Chapter 20). The hematoma may secondarily compress the fourth ventricle and brain stem. The early symptoms of acute onset of headache, dizziness, vomiting, and ataxia are often followed by coma and evolving extraocular muscle findings. Similar symptoms and findings may also occur in acute large cerebellar infarcts due to the effects of edema.

INTRINSIC DISEASES OF THE BRAIN STEM

The disease entity affecting the brain stem that is most frequently encountered in clinical practice is vascular disease, predominantly of the ischemic-occlusive type. Ischemic-occlusive cerebrovascular disease usually produces its initial clinical manifestations in patients over the age of 50 years. The basic pathological process of atherosclerosis that underlies occlusive vascular disease (the deposition of lipids such as cholesterol in the walls of vessels) certainly may begin in an asymptomatic manner earlier in life. On the other hand, multiple sclerosis, which is the second most frequent brain stem disease entity encountered, usually produces its initial manifestations in the age group of 20–40 years. Of the other intrinsic diseases affecting the brain stem, the next most frequently encountered are brain stem gliomas (occurring predominantly in the pediatric age group under 20 years and the bulbar variety of amyotrophic lateral sclerosis (occurring predominantly in the age group over 40 years).

SCHEMIC-OCCLUSIVE DISEASE OF THE BASILAR VERTEBRAL ARTERIES

Stenosis (narrowing) or occlusion of the vertebral and basilar arteries may occur at a number of sites. In general, maximum areas of atherosclerosis disease occur at the points of origin, bifurcation, or angulation of the extracranial and intracranial portions of the large and medium-sized cerebral arteries. There is no one-to-one relationship of a particular site of stenosis or occlusion to a specific pattern of clinical symptoms. Thus, occlusion of a vertebral artery may occur with no resultant clinical symptoms in evidence. In other instances, such an occlusion may result in transient symptoms indicating ischemia that is a temporary decrease in blood flow (perfusion) below a critical level, within the distribution of a particular vessel or combination of vessels arising from the vertebral or basilar arteries. In still other instances, such an occlusion may result in actual tissue destruction or infarction (encephalomalacia) within the distribution of one or more vessels taking origin from the vertebral or basilar arteries, for example, the posterior inferior cerebellar artery arising from the vertebral artery or the posterior cerebral artery from the basilar artery.

In still other instances, one may find that infarction within the distribution of a particular vessel has occurred without actual occlusion of that particular vessel or even of the parent vessel. Instead, stenosis with a decrease in blood flow has occurred.

Factors accounting for this lack of correspondence between the state of a particular vessel and the vascular status of the region supplied by that vessel are as follows:

1. There are significant congenital variations with regard to the normal patency of the two vertebral arteries. One artery may be hypoplastic.

2. There are significant congenital variations in the circle of Willis often representing persistence of an earlier fetal pattern.

3. There are significant leptomeningeal anastomoses over the surface of the cerebellum between the posterior inferior, anterior inferior, and superior cerebellar arteries.

4. To a variable degree anastomoses between extracranial and intracranial arteries may occur.

5. Variations may also reflect the fact that often atherosclerosis affects more than one major artery.

6. Considerable variability may also occur because of certain general systemic and metabolic factors.

7. Certain mechanical factors may introduce a degree of variability. Thus, a patient may have stenosis of a vertebral artery without clinical symptoms when the head is in a neutral position. Hyperextension or rotation may produce symptoms. Postural effects may also occur related to a relative decrease in blood pressure in the upright position compared to the recumbent position.

Not all-occlusive disease is due to atherosclerosis. Emboli account for a significant proportion of disease involving the posterior circulation. Among the 407 well studied patients in a posterior circulation registry (Caplan, 2000), at least 40% had embolism as the single most likely diagnosis, as opposed to 32% with large vessel disease (atherosclerosis-thrombosis) and 14% with penetrating artery disease. The most common sources of embolism were cardiac (60%) and intra-arterial (35%), usually the vertebral arteries. Cardiogenic emboli were most likely to produce distal infarcts within the territory of the posterior cerebral and posterior inferior cerebellar arteries. Emboli originating from the external vertebral artery were more likely to produce proximal infarcts within the territory of the intracranial vertebral artery and the origin of the basilar artery plus or minus additional more distal infarcts. Overall, of the 156 patients with embolic infarcts, 53% had distal infarcts only (distal basilar artery-posterior cerebral and superior cerebellar), 17% had proximal infarcts only, and 6% had middle territory infarcts (basilar artery and branches). The remainder were mixed, including the distal field.

As regards large vessel disease, in terms of the location of sites of >50% stenosis due to atherosclerosis, among 260 patients, 44% involved the extracranial portion of the vertebral artery, 42% the intracranial portion of the vertebral artery, 42% the basilar artery, and 15% the posterior cerebral artery. Clearly some patients had stenosis or occlusion at multiple sites.

SPECIFIC VASCULAR SYNDROMES

Basic Anatomy

We will now consider syndromes involving the territories of particular arteries. In addition to the large vessels, the vertebrals and basilar, we will deal with the major branches of these vessels. There is a general plan of brain stem vascular architecture. The basilar artery and the two vertebral arteries are placed on the basal (ventral) surface of the brain stem. One can visualize a midline or paramedian wedge-shaped area extending into the brain stem with a base on this ventral area. Penetrating vessels, termed *paramedian*, supply this paramedian wedge. The lateral tegmental portions of the brain stem are supplied by branches, long circumferential arteries, named for their areas of supply over the surface of the cerebellum: posterior inferior, anterior inferior, and superior cerebellar arteries. In addition, at the upper midbrain level, quadrigeminal arteries arise from the posterior cerebral arteries which function as long circumferential arteries with regard to this area of the brain stem. Variable transverse arteries, termed *short circumferential*, supply ventral lateral portions of the pons and midbrain arising from the long circumferential arteries of the basilar artery (Fig. 13.11A). Short circumflex branches also arise from the vertebral arteries to supply ventral lateral medulla.

At each level of the brain stem, we will be dealing primarily with paramedian as opposed to lateral tegmental syndromes. The paramedian branches always supply the corticospinal tracts and the paramedian exiting motor cranial nerves III, VI, and XII. In the case of cranial nerve III, the paramedian artery arises from the posterior cerebral artery.

1. Vertebral arteries (Fig. 1.20). The vertebral arteries usually arise from the subclavian artery (the left vertebral artery may arise directly from the aorta in 6% of cases). The artery ascends to enter the foramen of the transverse process of the sixth cervical vertebra, and then passes upward through the foramina of the successive cervical vertebrae; then, after passing behind the superior articular process of the atlas, it enters the foramen magnum. After passing upward and medially, the artery unites with its opposite number at the lower border of the pons to form the basilar artery. During its course in the neck, the vertebral artery gives rise to radicular branches (which anastomose with the anterior and posterior spinal arteries) and to muscular branches whose anastomoses have already been considered. The intracranial branches are the posterior inferior cerebellar, the anterior spinal, the posterior spinal, and the paramedian arteries.

   a. Syndromes associated with occlusive disease of the vertebral artery are variable:

      1) Occlusion or absence of one vertebral artery, particularly at a proximal point in an otherwise intact individual, is usually well tolerated (as we have indicated, it is not unusual to find one vertebral artery hypoplastic).

      2) Stenosis or occlusion of the proximal portions of both vertebral arteries in the series of patients reported by Fisher (1970) was associated with transient symptoms: faintness, blurred vision, dizziness, loss of balance, diplopia, and numbness of an arm or of the face. The symptoms are essentially those of transient insufficiency of circulation in the more distal distribution of vertebral and basilar arteries.

      3) Stenosis or occlusion of the intracranial segment of the vertebral artery or arteries may result in infarction over a variable area: the distribution of the basilar artery, and/or the distribution of the paramedian branches of the vertebral, and/or the distribution of the posterior inferior cerebellar artery. Actually, occlusive disease of the intracranial segment of the vertebral artery is a much more frequent cause of the lateral medullary syndrome than is limited occlusion of the posterior inferior cerebellar artery.

      4) Medullary syndromes

Lateral (dorsolateral) medullary syndrome (syndrome of the posterior inferior cerebellar artery or Wallenberg's syndrome) (Fig. 13.11B). Of all the various classic vascular syndromes of the brain stem, this syndrome, either alone in a relatively pure form or in a modified form, is the one most frequently encountered. (It is important to emphasize that nonclassic vascular syndromes of the brain stem are more commonly encountered than the classic syndromes involving isolated vascular territories.)

The brain stem territory of the posterior inferior cerebellar artery (PICA) includes the following structures: (a) the restiform body (the inferior cerebellar peduncle) and the adjacent dorsal and ventral spinocerebellar pathway, (b) the descending spinal tract and nucleus of the trigeminal nerve, the lateral spinothalamic tract, (d) the descending sympathetic pathway, (e) the nucleus ambiguus and the fibers of cranial nerve X, and (f) the vestibular nuclei (primarily spinal and medial at this level). The clinical findings of a lateral medullary infarction are illustrated in the following case history. It is important to note that occlusion of the posterior inferior cerebellar artery may produce infarction of the lateral medullary territory or of the PICA

Figure 13.11 (*A*) Aneurysm of the basilar artery with the clinical syndromes of left lateral gaze, dizziness, decreased pain sensation over the face on the left and occasional episode of blindness. (*B*) Dorsal-lateral medullary infarct (arrows) due to occlusion of the posterior inferior cerebellar artery (arrow) in a 72-year-old diabetic with the correlated clinical syndrome of acute-onset nystagmus on left lateral gaze, decreased pain sensation on the left side of face and right side of body, with difficulty swallowing, slurring of speech, and deviation of the uvula to the right. (Courtesy of Dr. Jose Segarra.)

cerebellar territory or of both areas. Prior to CT scan and MRI, the cerebellar infarct in a patient who also had a lateral medullary syndrome would have been overlooked, since infarction of the cerebellar peduncle, as part of a lateral medullary syndrome, would produce effects similar to the cerebellar infarct.

CASE HISTORY 13.1

This 53-year-old male customer service representative on the morning of admission while seated had the sudden onset of vertigo accompanied by nausea and vomiting, incoordination of his left arm and leg, and numbness of the left side of his face. On standing, he leaned and staggered to the left. Several hours later, he noted increasing difficulty in swallowing and his family described a minor dysarthria. He had a two-pack-per-day cigarette smoking history for more than 10 years.

Physical examination: Elevated blood pressure of 166/90.

Neurologic Examination

Mental status: Intact.

Cranial nerves:

a. The right pupil was 3 mm in diameter; the left was 2 mm in diameter. Both were reactive to light. There was partial ptosis of the left eyelid. A horizontal nystagmus was present on left lateral gaze, but extraocular movements were full.
b. Pain and temperature sensation was decreased over the left side of the face but touch was intact.
c. Speech was mildly dysarthric for lingual and pharyngeal consonants. Secretions pooled in the pharynx. Although the palate and uvula elevated well, the gag reflex was absent.

Motor system:

a. Dysmetria was present on left finger-to-nose test and heel-to-shin tests.
b. He tended to drift to the left on sitting and was unsteady on attempting to stand, falling to the left.

Reflexes:

a. Ankle jerks which were absent.
b. Plantar responses were flexor.

Sensory system: Pain and temperature sensation were decreased on the right over the right arm and leg, but all other modalities were normal.

Clinical diagnosis: 1. Dorsolateral medullary infarct. 2. Decreased ankle jerks due to possible diabetic peripheral neuropathy.

Laboratory data: Blood sugar: random elevated to 225 mg; fasting elevated to 196 mg%. Total cholesterol: elevated to 340mg% compared to normal of <200mg%, with low-density lipoproteins (LDL) elevated to 261 mg%, and high-density lipoproteins (HDL) 42mg%.

MRI (Fig. 13.12): A significant acute or subacute infarct involved posterior inferior cerebellar artery territory of the left cerebellum and dorsolateral medulla. The MRA was normal; however, the vertebral arteries were not well visualized.

Subsequent course: a percutaneous endoscopic gastrostomy (PEG) tube was placed since he was unable to swallow for the first 6 days. By the time of transfer to a rehabilitation facility, 12 days after admission, finger-to-nose tests and gait had improved, and he could walk with a walker. Speech and sensory examination had returned to normal.

Figure 13.12 Total posterior inferior cerebellar artery syndrome. Magnetic resonance imaging. Both the lateral medullary territory and the posterior inferior cerebellum are infarcted. The magnetic resonance angiogram indicated decreased flow in the vertebral artery.

Comments

The initial symptoms in this case suggested involvement of the vestibular system (vertigo, nausea, and vomiting) and the cerebellum or cerebellar peduncle (incoordination of the left arm and leg). Subsequent symptoms suggested involvement of the trigeminal system on the left side and of the nucleus ambiguus or the tenth cranial nerve (dysarthria and dysphagia). The examination confirmed the involvement of these areas but also provided additional information. The involvement of the trigeminal system was more specific to the descending spinal tract and nucleus of the cranial nerve V, since pain but not touch sensation over the left side of the face was affected. In addition, the adjacent left spinal thalamic system was involved since pain and temperature sensation were selectively affected in the right arm and leg. In addition, a partial Horner's syndrome was present on the left side (the pupil was smaller and there was partial ptosis), suggesting involvement of the descending sympathetic pathway. Taken all together, this constellation of symptoms and signs suggests an upper medullary location involving the dorsolateral tegmentum.

Had cranial nerve 10 not been involved, the location of the lesion would have been less precise. A lesion in the lower half of the pons would have produced all of the other findings. However, such a lower pontine lesion would have been accompanied by involvement of the auditory nerve or cochlear nucleus and the facial nerve. Such an inferior dorsal lateral lesion of the pontine tegmentum would fall within the territory of the anterior inferior cerebellar artery (discussed later). In the era before CT and MRI scans, this patient would be classified as having only an infarct of the dorsolateral medulla; the involvement of the posterior inferior cerebellum would be concealed, since the effects of a lesion of the inferior cerebellar peduncle would be in general similar to a lesion of this area of cerebellum. With these new techniques, we are able to see the full extent of the lesion. Thus, occlusion of the posterior inferior cerebellar artery may produce an infarct of the lateral medulla, the appropriate cerebellar territory, or a combined infarct of both territories. Embolic occlusion is more likely to produce the limited cerebellar infarction.

Although this patient had been asymptomatic, multiple predisposing factors were discovered at the time of his hospitalization: heavy tobacco use hypertension, diabetes mellitus, and high cholesterol level. Prevention would have had to address all of these issues. It is more common to encounter variations of the syndrome rather than the pure syndrome.

Lateral medullary infarct: The following case history provides an additional example of this syndrome.

CASE HISTORY 13.2

This 66-year-old, retired white male 10 days prior to admission noted at his evening bath that he was unable to detect the temperature of the water with his left foot and ankle. Several hours later, he awoke from sleep to void and found that his balance was defective; he tended to fall to the right side. He also noted a strange altered sensation over his right ear and face. The following morning, a more marked numbness of the right side of the face was present, in addition to headache, dysarthria, and nausea and vomiting. The patient was admitted to his local hospital, where skull X-rays and lumbar puncture was essentially normal. His symptoms were beginning to clear at the time of his transfer to the neurological center.

Past history: 6 weeks prior to admission he had been treated for mild symptoms of congestive heart failure.

Neurological Examination

Mental status: Intact.

Cranial nerves:

a. There was a partial ptosis of the right eyelid as well as a smaller pupil on the right.
b. Nystagmus was present on lateral and forward gaze.
c. Pain but not touch sensation was decreased over the right half of the face. The right corneal reflex was absent.
d. The uvula deviated to the left, with right gag reflex depressed.
e. The voice was hoarse.

Motor system:

a. Strength: Intact.
b. The patient was ataxic standing on a narrow base, tending to fall to the right.
c. A side-to-side intention tremor was present in the right upper extremity on finger-to-nose testing. A similar dysmetria was apparent in the right lower extremity in heel-to-shin testing.

Reflexes:

a. Deep tendon reflexes were symmetrical and 2+.
b. Plantar responses were flexor.

Sensory system: Pain and temperature sensation was decreased over the left lower extremity, an improvement compared to the earlier finding of a decrease over the entire left side below the cervical 2 segment. All other modalities were intact.

Clinical diagnosis: Lateral (dorsolateral) medullary infarct.

Subsequent course: Almost all neurological symptoms and signs resolved over the next 15 days.

Comments

This patient presents essentially all the features found in an infarct involving the territory of the posterior inferior cerebellar artery: the dorsolateral medullary syndrome. The initial symptom suggested involvement of the right lateral spinothalamic pathway pain and temperature pathway, that is, the inability to detect the temperature of bath water with the left lower extremity. The subsequent examination confirmed such a deficit in sensation involving the entire left side below the level of cervical 2. Shortly thereafter, sensory symptoms developed on the right side of the face, suggesting possible involvement of the trigeminal system. The subsequent examination demonstrated the specific involvement of pain but not touch sensation on the right side of the face. Thus, the more specific involvement of the descending spinal tract/nucleus of the trigeminal system could be deducted. Both the lateral spinothalamic tract and the descending spinal tract are found closely located in the dorsolateral tegmentum of medulla and lower pons. The nausea and vomiting suggested possible involvement of the vestibular nuclei. The presence of nystagmus would be consistent with the involvement of the vestibular system. The vestibular nuclei are located in the lateral tegmentum of lower pons and medulla. The defect in balance could have suggested involvement of either the vestibular or cerebellar system. The findings on examination of lateralized intention tremor in right arm and leg would be consistent with the lateral tegmental location and would more specifically implicate the inferior cerebellar peduncle conveying the spinocerebellar and cuneocerebellar pathways). The partial Horner's syndrome—partial ptosis of right eyelid and smaller pupil on the right—would implicate the descending sympathetic pathway found in a lateral tegmental location in the medulla or lower pons. The symptom of dysarthria and the findings of depressed gag reflex on the right with the defect in uvula elevation on the right (so that the uvula pulled to the left), plus the hoarseness, all suggested involvement of the right nucleus ambiguus. This nucleus is the source of the vagal innervation of the larynx and pharynx and is located in the dorsolateral tegmental area of the upper medulla supplied by the posterior inferior cerebellar artery. In many cases the actual occlusion is located in the vertebral artery and not in the posterior inferior cerebellar artery. It is more common to encounter variations of the syndrome rather than the pure syndrome. (A more detailed discussion of course and prognosis will be found in Norrving, 1991.)

In some patients a combined lateral and paramedian medullary syndrome could be found.

Paramedian medullary syndrome (Fig. 13.13 and Fig. 13.14). Occlusion of the paramedian penetrating branches from the vertebral artery may result in a syndrome characterized by ipsilateral paralysis and atrophy of one-half of the tongue (hypoglossal fibers or nucleus) in addition to a contralateral hemiparesis (medullary pyramid). There may be involvement of the adjacent medial lemniscus as well, producing a contralateral deficit in position and vibratory sensation and a relative decrease in tactile sensation. This syndrome, which bears the name of Hughlings Jackson, is rarely encountered in its pure form.

Combined syndrome: lateral medullary plus paramedian + cerebellum (Fig. 13.15). An example of a patient with infarction of the paramedian vertebral territory in addition to partial involvement of the lateral medullary territory, cerebellum, and pons is presented in the MRI of Fig. 13.16.

Figure 13.13 Left vertebral and posterior inferior cerebellar artery occlusions: lateral plus paramedian medullary. This 65-year-old hypertensive male expired 5 years after an acute event characterized by difficulty swallowing, "dizziness," ataxia, numbness of the left side of the face and the right side of the body plus a left-sided Horner's syndrome, a decrease in pain sensation on the left side of the face, deviation of the tongue to the left but increased deep tendon reflexes on the right side.

Figure 13.14 Vertebral artery syndrome. Magnetic resonance imaging demonstrates extensive infarction in the paramedian vertebral artery territory with lesser involvement of the lateral medullary territory plus the cerebellum. Severe stenosis was present in vertebral artery.

THE BASILAR ARTERY

Anatomy

(Refer to Figs. 1.20 and 1.21.)

The union of the two vertebral arteries forms the basilar artery. As with the vertebral artery, it is customary to distinguish paramedian and circumferential branches. The initial long circumferential branch is the anterior inferior cerebellar artery, which supplies the dorsolateral tegmentum of the lower one-half of the pons (Fig. 13.18A), including the eight nerve and the cochlear nuclei, the vestibular nuclei, the facial nerve, the descending spinal tract and nucleus of the fifth nerve, the lateral spinothalamic tract, the sympathetic pathway, the middle and inferior cerebellar peduncles, and the anterior inferior portion of the cerebellum. The area of supply may also include the main sensory nucleus of the fifth nerve at a midpontine

Figure 13.15 Syndromes of the Basilar Artery circumferential branches. (*A*) Inferior Pons. The cross hatched portion of the lateral pons is the territory of the anterior inferior cerebellar artery, AICA. (*B*) Superior pons. The cross hatched portion of the lateral pons is the territory of the superior cerebellar artery, SCA. At times there is overlap with the paramedian tegmental artery.

Figure 13.16 Middle-lower pontine basilar infarct with locked-in-syndrome. Two weeks prior to death, this 74 y.o. female was found motionless and speechless in bed. She could however open and close her eyes on command. (Courtesy of Dr. John Hills.)

level. The internal auditory artery that supplies the inner ear may arise from this vessel or independently from the basilar artery. Whether there is some supply as well to the nucleus ambiguus is uncertain; this area may constitute a border zone.

The next long circumferential branch is the superior cerebellar artery, which supplies the tegmentum of the upper pons and caudal midbrain (Fig. 13.18B), including the brachium conjunctivum, the medial longitudinal fasciculus, the motor and main sensory nucleus of the trigeminal nerve, the medial lemniscus, the lateral spinothalamic tract, and the central tegmental tract, and then proceeds to supply the superior cerebellum.

POSTERIOR CEREBRAL ARTERY

The basilar artery then terminates at the pontine-midbrain border into two posterior cerebral arteries.[1] From the top of the basilar and from each posterior cerebral artery in its proximal segment arises a series of vessels to supply the midbrain: penetrating paramedian branches from this vessel supply the medial one-half of the cerebral peduncle, the third nerve fibers, the third nerve nucleus, and the medial one-half of the red nucleus. Other penetrating branches (thalamoperforating and thalamogeniculate) of the posterior cerebral artery and top of the basilar artery in this location supply the subthalamus hypothalamus and much of the thalamus: pulvinar, ventral lateral, ventral posterior, medial geniculate, lateral geniculate, centromedian, and the dorsal median nuclei. Short circumferential vessels from the posterior cerebral artery supply the remainder (lateral one-half) of the cerebral peduncle and red nucleus. Somewhat longer circumferential branches also called quadrigeminal arteries supply the lateral tegmentum and tectum of the midbrain.

The main posterior cerebral artery then passes around the cerebral peduncle and midbrain close to the tentorial opening, supplying branches to the medial aspect of the temporal lobe and then dividing into the parieto-occipital and calcarine branches to supply the occipital lobe.

The syndromes of the posterior cerebral arteries relevant to the thalamus, subthalamus, and the temporal and occipital lobes are discussed in the Chapters 17, 18 and 19 on the cerebral hemispheres and motor system.[2]

SYNDROMES OF THE BASILAR ARTERY AND ITS BRANCHES

As atherosclerosis involves the basilar and vertebral arteries, there may be transient symptoms suggesting ischemia in the distribution of the various vessels originating from these major arteries. In some cases, infarction may occur within the distribution of these branches. Thus, the patient may experience episodes of vertigo or dizziness and diplopia, a bilateral blurring of vision, or a weakness or numbness of one side of the body or face, and then in a later attack, of the contralateral side of the face or body. In some cases, the transient symptoms are precipitated by extension or rotation of the head that reduces blood flow in the vertebral arteries. Sudden drop attacks without loss of consciousness are not unusual, due to ischemia of paramedian branches supplying the motor pathways: corticospinal tracts and the pontine-medullary reticular formation. Episodes of bilateral blindness may occur due to ischemia of the territory supplied by the posterior cerebral arteries.

---

[1] Some authors refer to the short segment of posterior cerebral artery between the top of the basilar artery and the posterior communicating artery as the basilar communicating artery (see Caplan, 1986).
[2] The student should realize that this is an artificial separation; thus, 75% of patients with paramedian midbrain infarcts also have paramedian thalamic infarcts (see Jelliger, 1986).

With total occlusion of the basilar artery, various combinations of cranial nerve findings, coma, decerebrate rigidity, and quadriplegia will be found. Before we examine the situation of total basilar artery occlusion, we will consider the various syndromes of the branch territories. In general, the partial segmental syndromes of the circumferential branches are rare. In contrast, the branch syndromes of the paramedian arteries are relatively common, particularity in diabetic and hypertensive patients (see Caplan, 1986; Fisher and Caplan, 1971). The student, moreover, will recognize that the histories presented do not really provide pure examples. There will be some signs or symptoms in each case suggesting involvement at several segmental levels of the brain stem. As with the vertebral artery, we will distinguish between paramedian (penetrating branch) and lateral tegmental (circumferential branch) syndromes.

INFERIOR PONTINE SYNDROMES

Lateral Tegmentum (Syndrome of the Anterior Inferior Cerebellar Artery)

Infarction of the lateral tegmentum at a caudal pontine level results in a sudden unilateral deafness in association with an ipsilateral peripheral facial weakness, ipsilateral Horner's syndrome, vertigo (due to involvement of the vestibular nucleus), and ipsilateral cerebellar symptoms. There may be involvement of the descending spinal tract and nucleus of the trigeminal nerve, resulting in an ipsilateral loss of pain and temperature over the face; or the main sensory nucleus may be involved, resulting in involvement of facial tactile sensation as well. If the lateral spinothalamic tract is involved, a contralateral loss of pain and temperature will be evident over the arm, leg, and trunk (Figs. 13.15 and 13.16).

In the following case history the major area of infarction was the territory of the anterior inferior cerebellar artery involving both the brain stem and the cerebellum. However, the initial area of ischemia suggested a much wider area of the territory of the basilar artery.

CASE HISTORY 13.3

This 55-year-old, white, married salesman, while driving, had the sudden onset of pain on the left side of the head, accompanied by dizziness (counterclockwise vertigo). The headache soon became generalized and within a short time nausea, projectile vomiting, and anorexia developed. At the same time, the patient noticed that he could not hear sounds in the left ear. Diplopia was present on left lateral gaze. The patient was able to continue driving slowly to his home. When he reached home and walked from the car or sat on the edge of his bed, he noted that he tended to fall to the left. The symptoms were unrelieved by a night of rest; the patient was brought to the hospital emergency room and subsequently admitted to the hospital.

Past history: Two years previously, the patient had experienced a "dizzy spell" and headache requiring bed rest for 10 days. Elevated blood pressure had required treatment from that time with antihypertensive medication. Obesity of a marked degree had been present for 20 years.

General Physical Examination

1. The patient was an obese male who was alert and cooperative.
2. Blood pressure was elevated to 220/110.
3. Skin color was florid.

Neurological Examination

Mental status:

a. Orientation and recent and distant memory were all intact.
b. Although speech was dysarthric, there was no impairment of higher language functions.

Cranial nerves:

a. Fundi and visual fields were intact.
b. Pupillary responses were intact.
c. A marked coarse horizontal nystagmus was present at rest on forward gaze and in all directions of gaze but was most marked on left lateral gaze. On upward and downward gaze, vertical nystagmus was also noted. Eye movements were described as "unstable and rolling over" with lack of sustained fixation. One examiner felt that a bilateral weakness of the lateral rectus muscle was present. Convergence and upward gaze were noted to be intact.
d. Pain sensation was selectively decreased over the left trigeminal distribution, most significantly over the mandibular division. The left corneal reflex was absent and left corneal sensation was reduced. There was a marked weakness of the left masseter muscle.
e. An incomplete left peripheral facial palsy was present with greater involvement of the lower half of the face.
f. Taste sensation was absent on the anterior two-thirds of the left side of the tongue.
g. The left ear was totally deaf.
h. The gag reflex was absent on the left. The left half of the uvula and soft palate failed to move on elevation.
i. On protrusion, the tongue deviated to the left.

3. *Motor system:*

a. Strength was intact except for very minimal weakness extending the left wrist and elbow.
b. Tone was normal.
c. Alternating movements of the left hand and foot were impaired. There was an ataxia and side-to-side intention tremor apparent in the left upper extremity on finger-to-nose test and in the left lower extremity on heel-to-shin test.
d. On attempting to sit or stand, the patient fell to the left.

Reflexes:

a. Deep tendon reflexes were questionably more active on the left at the biceps, triceps, and quadriceps. The asymmetry was of minimal degree.
b. Plantar response on the right was extensor, on the left equivocal.

Sensory system: All modalities were intact.

Arteries: The carotid pulses in the neck were strong. The blood pressure in the two arms was equal.

Clinical diagnosis: Basilar artery ischemia and infarction with predominant involvement of the territory of the anterior inferior cerebellar artery.

Laboratory Data

a. Skull X-rays were negative.
b. Electroencephalogram was normal.
c. Electrocardiogram was abnormal and suggested left ventricular hypertrophy (presumed secondary to the patient's hypertension).
d. Lumbar puncture demonstrated an elevated CSF pressure of 275 mm of water. No cells were present and the protein was normal at 35 mg/100 ml.
e. Brachial arteriograms demonstrated an area of relative avascularity in the inferior one-half of the cerebellum. There was a marked tortuosity of the basilar artery secondary to atherosclerosis with an aneurysmal dilatation present at the apex of the basilar artery.

Hospital course: Because of the severe headache and elevated CSF pressure, arteriograms were performed to rule out an atypical but treatable space-occupying lesion in the posterior fossa (such as an intracerebellar hematoma) with the results as indicated. In actuality, both symptoms were most consistent with the edema that accompanies an acute cerebellar infarction (the area of relative avascularity in the inferior cerebellum) which must have been present in addition to the brain stem infarction. Within 6 days, eye movements were described as more stable and a left lateral rectus weakness could now be more clearly defined. The slight reflex asymmetry was no longer present, plantar responses were flexor, and strength was intact. The persistent findings at this time related to nystagmus; left cranial nerves V, VI, VII, and VIII; and to cerebellar findings involving the left arm and leg. Within an additional 10 days, the patient was able to walk with assistance, although he still tended to fall to the left. The patient had continued improvement and was transferred to the rehabilitation division. By the time of his eventual rehabilitation discharge, 9 weeks after the acute admission, the patient was able to walk with a cane. He was described as independent in dressing and shaving. A variable but improving diplopia was still present on lateral gaze to the left or right and at times on superior gaze. On upward gaze, the separation of images was vertical, suggesting an involvement of the superior rectus muscle.

Comments

The combination of vertigo, left-sided deafness, vomiting, left peripheral facial palsy, and left-sided ataxia suggests a disease process involving the lateral tegmentum of the caudal pons or the cerebellar-pontine angle. Thus, this particular combination of symptoms, accompanied by headache, might also be found in a tumor (a vestibular schwannoma) at the cerebellar-pontine angle. The suddenness of onset of symptoms, however, is more in favor of a vascular accident, in this case ischemia and infarction within the territory of the anterior inferior cerebellar artery. The vertigo and vomiting may be related to the acute involvement of the vestibular nuclei or nerve. The deafness was due to involvement of the entering auditory division of nerve VIII or of the cochlear nuclei. The left-sided ataxia suggests a lesion involving the inferior or middle cerebellar peduncle or the left half of the cerebellum. The facial palsy suggested damage to the left facial nerve or to the motor nucleus of this nerve. The partial nature of the palsy with greater involvement of the lower face but with some involvement of the upper face is usually more in favor of nuclear rather than peripheral nerve involvement.

The decrease in taste on the anterior two-thirds of the tongue in all likelihood indicates involvement of fibers which have entered the brain stem from the geniculate ganglion in company with the facial nerve to join the tractus solitarius (or involvement of the tractus solitarius per se). These fibers whose bipolar neurons are located in the geniculate ganglion have traversed in turn the lingual nerve, the chorda tympani, and then the facial nerve to the geniculate ganglion. The taste fibers as they pass from the geniculate ganglion to the brain stem often appear to be grouped in a separate bundle of fibers, the nervus intermedius. Taste sensation from the posterior one-third of the tongue is conveyed by the glossopharyngeal (superior petrosal ganglion); from the epiglottis, by the vagus nerve (nodosa ganglion). These fibers then enter the brain stem to join the tractus solitarius at the medullary level.

It was of course evident at once, from the time of onset, that additional structures outside the distribution of the anterior inferior cerebellar artery were involved by the disease process. It is this more widespread involvement of brain stem structures which makes a vascular process even more likely. Thus, the basic process of stenosis is not in the anterior inferior cerebellar artery per se (although its point of origin may be narrowed or occluded by the process of atherosclerosis) but in the parent basilar artery.

Thus, the patient had diplopia as a prominent symptom. At times early in his hospital course, a bilateral palsy of nerve VI was evident. At times, a palsy of left nerve VI was evident with failure of movement of the left lateral rectus muscle. Such findings suggested some involvement of the paramedian areas in the lower pons (abducens nucleus or more likely abducens nerve fibers), areas usually within the territory of the paramedian branches of the basilar artery in this region. The extraocular findings later in the hospital course suggested a definite vertical separation of images due to dysfunction of the left superior rectus and left inferior oblique muscles. Such findings then would implicate the paramedian branches of the posterior cerebral artery to the midbrain.

The involvement of pain sensation over the left side of the face, most prominent in the mandibular division, is certainly consistent with involvement of a portion of the descending spinal tract and nucleus of the trigeminal nerve in the lateral tegmentum of the caudal pons. The involvement of the masseter muscle, and the motor nucleus of nerve V, suggests involvement of the lateral tegmentum at a upper pontine level. This area is on the border between supplies of the anterior-inferior and the superior cerebellar arteries.

The deviation of the tongue to the left was of uncertain explanation and might have suggested that the hypoglossal nucleus (perhaps its rostral portion) was involved by the lesion. The deviation, however, was not accompanied by any actual atrophy. Thus, a significant lesion of the hypoglossal nucleus was unlikely. Some apparent deviation of the tongue is almost always seen where a significant degree of facial paralysis is present, whether central or peripheral. The patient may also have had involvement of the corticobulbar fibers to the hypoglossal nucleus before or after the decussation of these fibers.

The slight and transient reflex asymmetry with greater activity on the left, accompanied by an equivocal plantar response, suggested a transient involvement of the corticospinal tracts at a pontine location, implicating paramedian branches of the basilar artery.

The decreased gag reflex on the left with defect in movement of the uvula and soft palate on the left, indicating involvement of the nucleus ambiguus, suggests some extension of the area of ischemia and infarction into the adjacent lateral tegmentum of the rostral medulla, an area usually supplied by the posterior inferior cerebellar artery. This raises additional questions. Was the actual site of disease the vertebral artery? If so, this was not demonstrated by the arteriogram. Did the posterior inferior cerebellar artery originate as a branch of the basilar or anterior inferior cerebellar artery? If so, this was not demonstrated by the arteriogram. More likely is the possibility that the nucleus ambiguus may constitute a border zone with supply from both the anterior and posterior inferior cerebellar arteries.

As regards treatment of the cerebrovascular disease in this particular case, there was little specific or definitive therapy that could be undertaken. This case dates from the era prior to the introduction of CT scan imaging. A CT scan would certainly have confirmed the area of infarction within the inferior cerebellum and likely would have confirmed the infarction within the brain stem. An MRI would have clearly indicated the area of brain stem and cerebellum involved. Any progression of symptoms, such as drowsiness or the evolution of the extraocular findings, would have prompted a repeat imaging study with the possibility of surgical therapy, that is, shunting to relieve the hydrocephalus which often accompanies the compression of the fourth ventricle in these cases or removal of the infarcted cerebellar tissue.

We may indicate at the onset that the basic disease process was atherosclerosis with ischemia and infarction. The aneurysmal dilatation at the apex of the basilar artery was secondary to the atherosclerosis. This aneurysmal dilatation in any case was essentially above the level of the infarction and could not be implicated in the disease process from the standpoint of subarachnoid bleeding or brain stem compression. Surgical treatment of this aneurysm, even if feasible from a technical standpoint, would have little effect on the basic disease process. In cases where recurrent episodes of transient basilar vertebral ischemia occur, anticoagulation therapy may be instituted with a reduction in frequency of the attacks. Occasionally patients with an occlusion or infarction in evolution may benefit from this therapy. Such therapy has little or no value in a completed infarction. Although the patient had "dizzy spells" 2 years previously, this probably related in a nonspecific manner to hypertension and does not necessarily indicate an earlier ischemic episode. Hypertension (present in this case) and a past history of gastrointestinal bleeding are contraindications for anticoagulation therapy. The combination of hypertension and anticoagulation may result in a secondary hemorrhagic infarction. Therapy in the present case was nonspecific: gait training, reasonable reduction of blood pressure, weight reduction, and dietary control.

Paramedian Lower Pontine Syndromes: Infarction within the territory supplied by the paramedian vessels of the basilar artery supplying the lower half of the pons, if unilateral, results in the combination of an ipsilateral lateral rectus weakness and a contralateral hemiplegia due to involvement of the emergent fibers of nerve VI and the corticospinal tract in the basilar portion of the pons. If the area of infarction extends into the tegmentum, there would be evidence of involvement of the nucleus of nerve VI (with an ipsilateral paralysis of lateral gaze) and of the genu of nerve VII about the nucleus of nerve VI (with an

Figure 13.17 Paramedian syndrome of the upper pons. Case 13-8. This 64 y.o. patient had Transient ischemic attacks, TIA, characterized by left or right sided hemiplegia and then a thrombosis of the basilar artery. (Courtesy of Drs. John Hills and Jose Segarra.)

ipsilateral peripheral palsy of cranial nerve VII) (syndrome of Foville). The medial longitudinal fasciculus would often be involved, with a unilateral (or bilateral) internuclear ophthalmoplegia. Involvement of the medial lemniscus would produce a contralateral hemianesthesia with deficits in position and vibratory sensation. Damage to the central tegmental tract in the pontine tegmentum may result in rhythmical contractions of the palate (palatal myoclonus). Bilateral infarcts of the pons are more frequent. A bilateral paramedian midpontine infarct producing a locked-in syndrome is demonstrated in Figure 13.15.

SUPERIOR PONTINE SYNDROMES

Lateral Tegmental Superior Pontine Syndrome: Territory of the Superior Cerebellar Artery

Ischemia or infarction of the tegmentum of the rostral pons involves the medial lemniscus and the lateral spinothalamic pathways, producing a contralateral hemianesthesia and hemianalgesia (Figs. 13.17). Since the secondary trigeminothalamic (quintothalamic) fibers have already crossed the midline below this level and have essentially merged with the medial lemniscus, the sensory deficit involves the contralateral side of the face as well as the contralateral arm, leg, and trunk. There is, in addition, damage to the superior cerebellar peduncle (the brachium conjunctivum). The cerebellar symptoms are ipsilateral to the lesion when the damage to the brachium conjunctivum occurs below the level of decussation. However, since the superior cerebellar artery also supplies the lateral tegmentum of the midbrain at a caudal level, the brachium conjunctivum may be involved above its decussation. If so, the cerebellar symptoms will be contralateral to the lesion. Moreover, the disturbance of movement is likely to be more variable. Thus, a coarse tremor at rest or instability of sustained posture may be seen in addition to the expected intention tremor. As at lower levels of the pons, the central tegmental tract may also be involved. The lesion (and the territory of the superior cerebellar artery) may extend into the paramedian tegmentum. If so, damage to the medial longitudinal fasciculus may occur.

Paramedian Upper Pons

When unilateral infarction of the corticospinal and corticobulbar tracts of the basilar pons occurs, the clinical effect is a contralateral, upper motor neuron paralysis of the face, arm, and leg. This produces a relatively pure motor syndrome as demonstrated in the following case. Note that the more common location for a lacunar infarct producing a pure motor syndrome is the internal capsule. It is, moreover, important to realize, as demonstrated in Figures 13.18 and 13.20, that disease of the basilar artery often produces a bilateral paramedian syndrome with a bilateral infarction of the basilar pons. Basilar artery thrombosis thus occludes the paramedian branches in a bilateral manner.

CASE HISTORY 13.4

This 70-year-old, right-handed, white male retired salesman, on the day prior to admission while working in his garden, had the acute onset of weakness of the right arm and leg, a right central facial

Figure 13.18 (A) Paramedian infarct of the upper pons demonstrated on computerized tomography scan. (B) Magnetic resonance imaging, Case 13.5: Paramedian infarct of the upper pons.

weakness, and slurring of speech. A similar episode had occurred 2 months previously but had resolved over 2 weeks. There was a past history of non-insulin-dependent diabetes mellitus for which the patient had been receiving an oral hypoglycemic agent. He had been taking three aspirin tablets per day (325mgx3).

Neurological Examination

Mental status: Intact.

Cranial nerves: There was flattening of the right nasolabial fold and slurring of speech,

Motor system: There was pronator drift in the outstretched right arm with 4+/5 weakness in the right iliopsoas.

Reflexes: Deep tendon stretch reflexes were increased in the right arm. A Babinski sign was present on the right.

Sensory system: Intact.

Clinical diagnosis: Lacunar infarct: pure motor syndrome probable location left internal capsule with paramedian pons less likely.

Laboratory data: The MRI demonstrated a well-defined paramedian upper pontine infarct (Fig.13.22). The MRA study was within normal limits.

Hospital course: The following morning the right arm was now plegic, and the patient needed assistance with walking. By the fourth hospital day, dysarthria and strength in right leg were improving. He was discharged to a rehabilitation facility on the fifth hospital day.

Comments

This patient presented a relatively pure motor syndrome, one of several types of lacunar infarction. If all cases of a pure motor vascular syndrome involving the face, arm, and leg are considered (Fisher and Curry, 1965), it is found that the most frequent site of infarction is the posterior limb of the internal capsule. The paramedian upper pons is the second most common site. The most common predisposing conditions for these small vessel occlusions are hypertension and diabetes. Often there is a considerable improvement from the effects of the lacunar infarction. In this case the most definitive study was the MRI. Note that the MRA essentially ruled out any large vessel disease. It is, moreover, important to realize, as demonstrated in Figures 13.19 and 13.20, that disease of the basilar artery often produces a bilateral

Figure 13.19 Weber's syndrome. An area of infarction is noted in the right cerebral peduncle (arrow), so located as to involve the fibers of the right third cranial nerve. This 61-year-old patient with rheumatic heart disease, endocarditis, and auricular fibrillation had the sudden onset of paralysis of the left face, arm, and leg, plus a partial right third nerve palsy. (Courtesy of Dr. John Hills and Dr. Jose Segarra.)

Figure 13.20 Posterior cerebral artery ischemia and infarction paramedian midbrain and medial temporal. This 86-year-old male had a transient episode of bilateral blindness, then transient bilateral weakness and dysarthria followed by a left facial weakness, left hemiplegia, bilateral medial rectus weakness, and a nonresponsive right pupil. (Courtesy of Dr. Joel Kaufman.)

paramedian syndrome with a bilateral infarction of the basilar pons. Basilar artery thrombosis thus occludes the paramedian branches in a bilateral manner.

MIDBRAIN SYNDROMES

Paramedian Syndromes (Weber's Syndrome)

A unilateral infarction in the territory supplied by paramedian-penetrating branches from the proximal posterior cerebral artery (or basilar communicating artery) involves the cerebral peduncle, the ipsilateral third nerve fibers, and, to a variable degree, the substantia nigra. The resultant clinical syndrome is that associated with the name Weber (Figs. 13.21 and 13.22): contralateral upper motor neuron paralysis of the face, arm, and leg, in association with an ipsilateral paralysis of third nerve function. The clinical effects of the damage to the substantia nigra may not be apparent. (Refer to Chapter 19.) At times, the symptoms related to the cerebral peduncles may be bilateral since the basic process of ischemia may have involved the upper basilar artery. In other cases both the penetrating (paramedian) branches and the cortical branches of the posterior cerebral artery may be involved, resulting in a Weber's syndrome plus a homonymous hemianopsia (due to involvement of the calcarine artery branch supplying the occipital/visual cortex). In addition, confusion may be present due to involvement of the cortical branches supplying the mesial temporal structures. As noted earlier, thalamic infarcts may also be found in patients with paramedian midbrain infarcts because the same process may occlude the penetrating branches to both areas.

Figure 13.21 Pontine hemorrhage. This 58-year-old hypertensive patient had had a presumed brain-stem infarct 4 weeks previously and then this massive pontine hemorrhage, possibly related to anticoagulant therapy. (Courtesy of Dr. John Hills.)

The following case presents an example of the more limited midbrain syndrome.

CASE HISTORY 13.5

This 66-year-old white male awoke 2 days prior to admission with weakness of both his legs. He attempted to stand but fell to the floor.

Neurological Examination

Mental status: Intact.

Cranial nerves: The right pupil was slightly larger than left; both were reactive to light. Ptosis of the right lid was present.

Motor system: Weakness of the left upper extremity and minor weakness of both lower extremities was present, more marked on the left. The patient was unable to walk without support. When supported, the patient walked with a left hemiplegic gait.

Reflexes: A left Babinski sign was present.

Sensory system: Intact.

Clinical diagnosis: Possible paramedian midbrain infarct: Weber's syndrome.

Laboratory data: A lumbar puncture demonstrated normal CSF.

Hospital course: Two days following admission, the patient demonstrated neurological progression with more complete third nerve palsy, progression with a significant dilation of the right pupil and weakness of the right superior rectus, right medial rectus, right inferior oblique, and levator palpebrae muscles. During the subsequent 1 month improvement occurred. By the following 1 month, the patient had equal pupils, no ptosis, and no extraocular palsies with the only residual a minimal weakness of the left leg and a left Babinski sign.

Comments

The initial symptoms in this case of bilateral weakness of the lower extremities, taken in isolation, did not allow for localization, in terms of spinal cord, medulla, pons midbrain, or even bilateral parasagittal motor cortex. However, the findings of a ptosis and a slightly larger pupil on the right in association with a left hemiplegia (although minor weakness was also present in the right lower extremity) all suggested a possible Weber's syndrome of the paramedian penetrating branch territory of the posterior cerebral artery. The subsequent progression 2 days later to a more complete cranial nerve III syndrome confirmed the diagnosis. In retrospect, the initial bilateral lower extremity weakness suggested that the initial ischemic process involved the penetrating branches in a bilateral manner. The lumbar puncture was performed to rule out a possible subarachnoid hemorrhage secondary to an aneurysm of the posterior communicating artery and was negative.

The following case history provides an example of a patient in whom symptoms and signs involved the larger territory of the posterior cerebral artery: both paramedian branches to midbrain and cortical branches were involved.

CASE HISTORY 13.6

This 73-year-old white housewife, without a previous history of neurological disease, awoke on the morning of admission complaining of diplopia. She was noted by her husband to be drowsy and mumbling. She was brought to the emergency room at 9:20 a.m., where she was found to have a dilated and fixed right pupil with associated paralysis of right levator palpebrae, superior rectus, medial rectus, and inferior rectus. The left pupil was pinpoint. A left facial weakness and a minor weakness of left hand were also present. Although drowsy, the patient was able to respond to commands.

Past history: Rheumatoid arthritis had been present for many years. Iron deficiency anemia noted 1 year previously.

Neurological Examination (approximately 11:50 a.m.)

Figure 13.22 Pontine hemorrhage. This 67-year-old obese and hypertensive female collapsed with sudden onset of deep coma, with no purposive responses to painful stimuli. The right pupil was fixed and dilated; the left pupil was pinpoint (1 mm) and minimally responsive to light. No oculocephalic or corneal responses were present. Bilateral Babinski signs were present. Respirations, which initially were spontaneous and rapid (central neurogenic hyperventilation), subsequently became irregular and shallow. She expired within 24 hours.

Mental status:

a. The patient was drowsy—responding poorly to commands.
b. She was disoriented to time and place.
c. She reported the president incorrectly.
d. There was no evidence of an aphasia.

Cranial nerves:

a. II: A questionable left homonymous hemianopsia was present.
b. III, IV, VI: The right globe was in a lateral position; no medial, upward, or downward movement of the right eye was possible. The right pupil measured 6 mm. The left pupil was pinpoint. Horizontal movements of the left eye were intact. Vertical movements of the left eye were difficult to test.
c. Pain sensation was decreased on the left side of the face.
d. A left central facial weakness was present.

Motor system:

a. A complete paralysis of left upper extremity, except for slight movement at left shoulder was now apparent.
b. Tone was slightly decreased in left upper extremity.
c. Cerebellar tests were negative.

Reflexes:

a. Deep tendon reflexes were hyperactive bilaterally at biceps(4+) and triceps(4+). Patellar reflexes were 2+ bilaterally.
b. The left plantar response was markedly extensor; the right was also extensor but less markedly so.
c. No release of grasp or such was apparent.

Sensory system:

a. Position and vibratory sense were decreased in the left hand.

Clinical diagnosis: Posterior cerebral artery syndrome most likely embolic (top of the basilar syndrome) with predominant involvement of the right paramedian midbrain and right occipital and mesial temporal areas.

Laboratory Data

1. Hematocrit was 35–40.
2. CSF exam demonstrated pressure of 90 mm; no significant cells were present. Protein was normal at 31 mg%.
3. Right common carotid arteriogram demonstrated that reflux occurred into the right basilar and right vertebral artery. No aneurysm was present.

Hospital course: Examination approximately 10 days after admission indicated essentially a persistence of the following findings:

1. There was an inability to detect stimuli in the left visual field.
2. The right pupil was now 3-4 mm in diameter and responsive to light. However, a marked ptosis of the right lid was present with a partial paralysis of medial, upward, and downward movements of the right eye.
3. A left central facial weakness was present.
4. A left hemiparesis was present with arm more involved than leg.
5. The plantar responses were extensor bilaterally, the left more markedly than the right.

Comments

The sudden onset of the total third cranial nerve paralysis associated with drowsiness, and confusion, and with a left homonymous hemianopsia, left central facial, and left arm and left leg weakness could raise the possibility of several diagnoses:

1. A right hemisphere tumor or hemorrhage, which was producing via temporal lobe herniation pressure effects on the right third cranial nerve and brain stem.
2. An aneurysm of the junction of the posterior communicating and internal carotid artery with secondary subarachnoid hemorrhage.
3. A hemorrhage within the substance of the midbrain involving the right cerebral peduncle and the adjacent third nerve. This was actually the pathology responsible for the initial patient described by Weber (see Wolf, 1971).
4. Basilar-vertebral ischemic occlusive disease with predominant involvement of the penetrating paramedian vessels of the proximal posterior cerebral artery on the right, and of the distal posterior cerebral artery supplying the calcarine (visual cortex). The right common carotid arteriogram served to essentially rule out the right hemisphere mass lesion, temporal lobe herniation, and an aneurysm of the posterior communicating–internal carotid artery junction. The normal CSF examination also served to rule out a subarachnoid hemorrhage (today the diagnostic procedure to confirm the localization and diagnosis would be MRI and MR angiography—both noninvasive).

The persistent findings in this case consisted of a right third nerve paresis, which was partial plus a paralysis of left face, arm, and leg. These findings alone would be consistent with a Weber's syndrome of the right midbrain, peduncle, and third nerve due to proximal posterior cerebral paramedian artery involvement. The persistent left field defect reflected involvement of the cortical territory of the right posterior cerebral artery due to ischemia or an embolus.

What then is the explanation for the other transient findings?

1. The drowsiness and confusion may have reflected involvement of any of the following structures:

    a. Paramedian tegmentum of the midbrain. The integrity of the reticular formation at this level is essential for maintaining an alert state.
    b. The upward extension of these same structures into the diencephalon: hypothalamus, the medial thalamus, and intralaminar nuclei. These also are supplied by the paramedian branches of the proximal posterior cerebral artery.
    c. The hippocampal structures: The blood supply is derived from the longer medial temporal branches of the posterior cerebral arteries. When damage occurs, the patient is often confused.

2. The left pinpoint pupil undoubtedly reflected involvement of the descending sympathetic fibers from the hypothalamus at some point on the left side of the brain stem, for example, midbrain or pons.
3. The sensory findings: decreased pinprick on the left side of the face and decreased position and vibration probably reflected ischemia of the medial lemniscus at midbrain level or possibly of thalamic nuclei. Weber's original description included mention of but not emphasis on such sensory findings.
4. That the right Babinski sign was less evident than the left Babinski sign probably indicated involvement of the opposite cerebral peduncle. Thus, the basic process may have been at the level of the

upper basilar artery with multiple branches at the "top of the basilar" involved (see Caplan, 1980, and Mehler, 1989, for additional discussion of rostral brain stem syndromes).

The following case illustrates a patient with thrombosis of the basilar artery in which several midbrain and pontine syndromes were present.

CASE HISTORY 13.7

This 64-year-old, white, right-handed, male beginning 6 months prior to admission, had experienced a series of 15 to 20 attacks of unsteadiness of gait, attributed to transient weakness of the right or left side of the body (predominantly the left side) and associated with vertigo and occasional tinnitus ("motor sounds") of the left ear. Initially, head turning precipitated the vertigo. Six months prior to admission, because of a sensation of dizziness when climbing his ladder, the patient had been forced to stop his work. Seven days prior to admission, the patient was admitted to his local community hospital with acute onset of paralysis and numbness of the left arm and leg of several hours duration. The patient was noted to be slightly confused and unable to speak clearly (dysarthric). These symptoms apparently improved; but approximately 7 days later, the patient had an onset of weakness of the right arm and leg accompanied by increased difficulty in speech, necessitating his transfer to a neurological center.

Past history: Hypertension had been present for at least 6 months. Weakness and cramps in the legs on walking, relieved by rest, had been present for 1 year (suggesting the intermittent claudication of the peripheral vascular disease).

General Physical Examination
a. Blood pressure was elevated to 200/90.
b. Pulses in the lower extremities were decreased or absent.

Neurological Examination

Mental status: Although speech was severely dysarthric (speech was hardly intelligible to observers), the patient was alert and cooperative. He was able to follow commands and to identify objects. There was no evidence of left-right confusion.

Cranial nerves:

a. The left pupil was slightly larger than the right.
b. A right lateral rectus weakness was present.
c. Horizontal nystagmus was present on gaze to the left or right.
d. Pain sensation was decreased about the right corner of the mouth. The right corneal response was decreased.
e. The jaw jerk was hyperactive.
f. There was a paralysis of the lower half of the right side of the face.
g. The gag reflex was decreased; the patient was unable to swallow on command. The uvula did elevate on phonation.
h. The tongue was midline, but lateral tongue movements were weak.

Motor system:

a. Strength was uniformly decreased in the right arm and leg, but intact on the left.

b. Truncal ataxia was apparent in the sitting position.
c. Ataxia was evident on the right in finger-to-nose and heel-to-shin tests. Interpretation of these findings was clouded by the presence of right-sided weakness.

Reflexes:

a. Deep tendon reflexes were hyperactive throughout with clonus apparent at the patellar. As noted earlier, the jaw jerk was 3–4+.
b. Plantar responses were extensor bilaterally (bilateral Babinski signs).

Sensory system:

a. Pain sensation was decreased in the left leg.
b. Vibratory sensation was decreased in both lower extremities.
c. Position sense was defective in the toes of the left foot.

Clinical diagnosis: Transient ischemic attacks followed by infarction basilar-vertebral system. Possible thrombosis of basilar artery.

Laboratory Data

a. Blood and spinal fluid serology were normal.
b. CSF was normal, with no cells. The protein content, however, was increased to 120 mg/100 ml (explanation never certain).

Skull X-rays were negative except for calcifications in the internal carotids adjacent to the sella turcica.

Hospital course: The patient's inability to swallow progressed so that by the third day in the hospital, it was necessary to make use of a nasogastric feeding tube. On the fifth day, a temperature elevation occurred, related to aspiration pneumonitis. Death occurred 14 days after admission.

Postmortem examination of the brain: The major supply of the basilar artery was derived from the left vertebral artery. The right vertebral artery was rudimentary (hypoplastic). In the lower portion of the basilar artery, significant atherosclerosis and calcification was present with narrowing of the lumen. The lower-middle segment of the vessel was occluded by thrombus. The proximal (caudal) portion of the thrombus was older, fibrous, and well organized; the distal portion was more recent. This suggested distal propagation from the more proximal thrombus.

The pons was soft to palpation. Serial sections revealed a recent area of infarction (with swelling and some hemorrhagic component) involving the entire left cerebral peduncle at the level of the midbrain, extending in a massive manner into the basilar pontis on the left (Fig. 13.21). The areas of softening extended into the left and right paramedian areas of the pontine tegmentum. A similar but possibly older lesion was present involving the right cerebral peduncle and right basilar pons. On the right the infarct extended up to the capsule of the red nucleus, to the subthalamus nucleus, and into the posterior and lateral portions of the thalamus. Old small infarcts (lacunae) were also noted in the right lenticular nucleus and the head of the left caudate nucleus. In addition, the right occipital cortex demonstrated old infarction.

Comments

The symptoms and signs in this case would appear to be well correlated with the findings at postmortem examination. Thus, the appearance of the basilar artery and of the brain stem suggests several events from a chronological standpoint. The recent massive lesion in the left cerebral peduncle and basilar pons corresponded to the right hemiparesis and right central facial weakness. The previous episodes of primarily left-sided involvement of the arm and leg would correlate with the older infarcts on the right side of the brain stem. The bilateral involvement of the basilar pons and cerebral peduncles must have resulted in a pseudobulbar syndrome, as regards the hyperactive jaw jerk and the movements of the tongue and the pharynx (reflecting bilateral corticobulbar involvement). The bilateral hyperactivity of deep tendon reflexes and the bilateral extensor plantar responses reflected bilateral corticospinal tract damage. The infarction of the right paramedian area of the pontine tegmentum must presumably correlate with the right lateral rectus muscle weakness and with deficit in position sense in the left toes. At some point, the infarction must have extended sufficiently lateral in the right pontine tegmentum to have involved the descending portion of the spinal tract and nucleus of the right fifth cranial nerve in addition to the lateral spinothalamic tract (decreased pain sensation in the left foot). In addition, the vertigo and tinnitus would suggest that the territory of the anterior inferior cerebellar artery had been involved to produce these symptoms in the lower pontine tegmentum.

The examination of the basilar artery indicated an old well-organized thrombus in the caudal portion of the artery that may have correlated with the earlier transient ischemic attacks. Presumably sufficient collateral circulation was present to prevent infarction until additional more recent thrombus extended to the middle portion of the artery. The specific syndromes associated with stenosis of the middle and distal segments of the basilar artery are discussed by Pessin et al. (1987). Patients with basilar artery thrombosis may infarct the pons but leave the midbrain intact producing—"un-locked-in syndrome." The patient remains awake but is able to communicate only with eyelid and vertical eye movements (refer to Fig.13.15). This condition must be differentiated from coma and is discussed in Chapter 29.

The major vascular syndromes of the brain stem are reviewed in Table 13.1.

Paramedian syndrome with associated tegmental involvement (Benedikt's syndrome): Involvement of the adjacent midbrain tegmentum (red nucleus, dentatorubrothalamic fibers) will produce a contralateral tremor and movement disorder in association with an ipsilateral third nerve lesion. The involvement of the cerebral peduncle produces a contralateral hemiparesis.

Paramedian periventricular mesencephalic-diencephalic junction: This involves the periaqueductal, pretectal, posterior-medial thalamic, and subthalamic areas. Bilateral infarction of this territory supplied by the penetrating branches of the proximal posterior cerebral arteries results in a drowsy, relatively immobile state (apathetic akinetic mutism) from which the patient can be roused with strong stimulation. The lesion interrupts the ascending reticular system within the upper mesencephalon and its intralaminar diencephalic extension. Third cranial nerve findings are often present as associated findings, due to involvement of the third nerve nuclei. This syndrome has been considered in greater detail by Segarra (1970), Plum and Posner (2007), and Castaigne et al. (1981). (Refer to Chapter 28 for additional discussion and illustrations.)

TREATMENT

Prevention is of major importance. Control of hypertension and of elevations of the low-density lipid component of cholesterol (LDL) and of the triglycerides should be beneficial. If dietary alterations are insufficient, then the use of lipid-lowering drugs (the statins) should be considered. Increase in the high-density lipoprotein (HDL) produced by common-sense exercise may also be beneficial. In patients with cardiac disease (valvular disease, mural thrombi, and particularly atrial fibrillation) long-term anticoagulation may prevent cerebral emboli. In addition, for cardiac arrhythmias, other measures will be considered by the cardiologist. The use of aspirin or related compounds to alter platelet aggregation may be of value to prevent additional ischemic attacks events. In patients with symptomatic disease of the subclavian or proximal vertebral artery, surgical procedures to bypass sites of occlusion may be considered. The treatment of a basilar artery thrombosis presents a major problem. Previously intravenous heparin, an anticoagulant, was utilized in patients with evolving basilar artery thrombosis, but the results were often disappointing. Because of the poor prognosis of these patients, intra-arterial thrombolysis with urokinase has been utilized. In a series from the Mayo Clinic (Wijdicks et al., 1997), recanalization of the thrombosed basilar artery was achieved in 7 out of 9 patients treated within 2–13 hours with 5 of the 7 recanalized patients recovering fully, including 2 patients who had a locked-in syndrome. Failure to recanalize resulted in coma and death. A complication is the occurrence of hemorrhage in a small number of patients. An additional study of 22 patients (Cross et al., 1997) confirmed the beneficial effects of recanalization achieved by this method, in terms of survival and improvement in neurologic status. Patients with distal clots did significantly better than those with proximal or mid basilar clots.

The major vascular syndromes of the brain stem are reviewed in Table 13.2.

HEMORRHAGE

INTRAPONTINE HEMORRHAGE

The most common location of hypertensive hemorrhages is intracerebral (putamen predominantly, thalamus and cerebral white matter somewhat less commonly). In a small percentage of cases, the pons is the primary location of the hemorrhage. A large hemorrhage in the relatively small space of the pons produces rapid effects: coma and bilateral involvement of the long tracts within seconds or minutes, and death within minutes or hours. Rupture into the ventricular system is common. Although the illustrations present the typical course of such large hemorrhages, small pontine hemorrhages have been recognized in the era of CT and MRI scan.

Arteriovenous malformations of the brain stem may produce repeated small hemorrhages and infarct with a course characterized by a variable progressive series of stroke-like episodes. At times such cases have been mistaken for multiple sclerosis (Stahl et al., 1980).

Primary Intracerebellar Hemorrhages. See earlier and Chapter 20.

SUBARACHNOID HEMORRHAGE

Intrinsic Tumors

The substance of the brain stem is a relatively uncommon site for metastatic tumors (however, see example earlier in this chapter). Almost all tumors found within the substance of the brain stem are intrinsic, arising from glial elements, generally the astrocyte. Various histological grades of malignancy may be encountered. In contrast to gliomas of the cerebral hemisphere, the majority of which are of a very malignant variety (the glioblastomas), the majority of those involving the brain stem are astrocytomas with a lower grade of malignancy and with a longer course. The tumor slowly infiltrates the pons and medulla, producing a gross external enlargement of these structures (Fig. 13.24). On section, the distinctions between gray and white matter are obliterated. Areas of necrosis may be found within the tumor. The essential clinical syndrome is characterized by the progressive development of bilateral long tract and bilateral cranial nerve findings. The cranial nerve findings suggest involvement over adjacent segments of the brain stem, rather than a single segmental level. This tumor occurs primarily in children, adolescents, and young adults. At the present time the diagnosis is easily confirmed by MRI scan, which has replaced the earlier techniques of CT scan, pneumoencephalograms, ventriculograms, and posterior fossa-myelograms.

Figure 13.23 Brain stem glioma. Marked enlargement of the pons has occurred with obscuration of the usual anatomical landmarks and obstruction of the fourth ventricle. (Courtesy of Dr. John Hills.)

CASE HISTORY 13.8

This 20-year-old single female had the onset of occasional horizontal diplopia and headache. Five months later clumsiness and weakness of the left arm and leg developed accompanied by increased intracranial pressure. CT and subsequently MRI demonstrated a mass within the pons with compression of the fourth ventricle and cerebellum. After treatment with dexamethasone (a powerful corticosteroid) ventriculoperitoneal shunt at the Massachusetts General Hospital to reduce hydrocephalus and radiotherapy (5400 rads) at the St Vincent Hospital, all neurological signs resolved and the tumor shrank on imaging studies. Symptoms recurred 30 months later, with diplopia, progressive ataxia, left hemiparesis occipital headache, and projectile vomiting.

Neurological examination: The following abnormal features were now present:

Mental status: Intact except for marked emotional lability.
Cranial nerves:

a. Bilateral lateral rectus palsy.
b. Horizontal nystagmus on gaze to left or right, vertical nystagmus on upward gaze.

Motor system:

a. Left hemiparesis.
b. Ataxia on attempting to sit or stand.

Reflexes: Bilateral Babinski signs were now present.
Clinical diagnosis: Progression of pontine glioma.
Laboratory data: MRI (Fig. 13.23) demonstrated additional enlargement of the pons with compression of the fourth ventricle and with extension of tumor and edema on the right side into the cerebellar peduncle, medulla, midbrain, and thalamus.
Subsequent course: Treatment with dexamethasone and chemotherapy produced temporary clinical and MRI improvement.
Comments

The occurrence of headache and diplopia in a 20-year-old certainly raises the question of an intracranial tumor. The localization is not certain based only on these symptoms. Thus, sixth nerve palsy may occur with an increase in intracranial pressure without clear-cut localization to the brain stem or even the posterior fossa. The subsequent development of clumsiness of the left arm and leg could have raised the question of cerebellar mass except that these symptoms occurred in the context of a left-sided weakness. Thus, the clumsiness could have been a nonspecific tumor in relationship to the fourth ventricle such as medulloblastoma, or ependymoma, or cerebellar hemisphere lesion such as a cystic astrocytoma, but these tumors would not produce a left hemiparesis. The combination of a left hemiparesis and cranial sixth nerve palsy, if progressive in nature, would then suggest a pontine glioma. The findings at the time of her recurrence left little doubt as to the diagnosis but did not entirely indicate the much more extensive nature of the tumor now present.

The following case history indicates the total course to be seen with a brain stem (medullary and pontine) glioma.

CASE HISTORY 13.9

This 24-year-old white housewife and secretary was referred for evaluation of progressive headache, diplopia, and left-sided weakness. Approximately 2 weeks after the delivery of her second child, the patient had an onset of diplopia with an apparent horizontal separation of images. Her family noted that the right eye was "turned in." The symptom was intermittent for a week, then persistent and static for approximately 1 year. Fifteen months later, 1 year prior to admission, the double vision worsened. Moreover, a weakness of the left leg, an unsteadiness of gait, and clumsiness of the left hand were now noted. These symptoms steadily progressed so that the patient 8 months later fell, sustaining a fracture of the left ankle. Skull X-rays and lumbar puncture at that time were normal and the diagnosis of multiple sclerosis was entertained (this was before the era of CT and MRI). As the previous symptoms worsened, the patient in the 3 months prior to admission noted a progressive numbness of both sides of her face and of the oral cavity. She had lost all of her ability to taste food or even to tell

Figure 13.24 Pontine glioma. Magnetic resonance scan. Case 13.9: (*A*) normal for comparison; (*B*) pontine glioma.

where food was located in the mouth. She had experienced increasing difficulty in attempting to swallow food. Liquids such as coffee were frequently regurgitated into the nasopharynx on swallowing. Her speech had developed a nasal quality, and hoarseness had been noted. A bilateral occipital headache had developed, at times precipitated by flexion of the neck. In recent days, the headache had been accompanied by vomiting (Fig. 13.24).

General physical examination: No remarkable features were present.

Neurological Examination

Mental status: The patient was alert with intact memory and orientation. Although speech was slurred and the voice was low and hoarse, language function per se was intact with no evidence of aphasia.

Cranial nerves:

a. Bilateral papilledema was evident on examination of the fundus with marked blurring of disk margins, elevation of the disks, and retinal hemorrhages. Visual acuity was intact.
b. Bilateral lateral rectus weakness was present, more marked on the right than on the left.
c. Vertical nystagmus was present on upward gaze.
d. Pain and touch sensation were decreased over all three divisions of the trigeminal nerve, more marked on the right than the left. Corneal reflexes were absent bilaterally.
e. A mild right central (supranuclear) facial weakness was present.
f. The uvula deviated to the left on attempted elevation. The gag reflex was decreased bilaterally. Speech was of low tone and slurred.
g. A bilateral weakness of the sternocleidomastoid muscles was present. The upper half of the left trapezius was weak.
h. The tongue deviated to the right on protrusion.

Motor system:

a. Marked weakness accompanied by spasticity was noted in the left arm and leg.
b. Gait was unsteady with a spastic quality evident in the movements of the left leg.
c. Coordination was poor on the left side. Whether this reflected cerebellar deficits in addition to weakness was not certain.

Reflexes:

a. Deep tendon reflexes were symmetrical and physiologic.
b. Plantar response extensor on the left, flexor on the right.

Sensory system: Except for the findings over the face, no deficits were present.

Clinical diagnosis: Brain stem glioma.

Laboratory Data

a. Skull and chest X-rays were negative.
b. Electroencephalogram was normal.
c. Left brachial arteriogram indicated a probably low position of the posterior inferior cerebellar artery, suggesting the possibility of cerebellar tonsillar herniation. Basilar and vertebral arteries were in a normal position.
d. A Pantopaque ventriculogram revealed an intrinsic pontine and medullary tumor. The fourth ventricle and aqueduct were midline but were displaced posteriorly. This study was performed by instilling a radioopaque dye (Pantopaque) into the ventricular system by means of a needle placed in the frontal horn.

Hospital and subsequent course: A suboccipital craniotomy and removal of the lamina of C1 and C2 was performed by Dr. Samuel Brendler with the aim of decompressing the cerebellum, brain stem, and cervical cord. The cerebellar hemispheres were found to be under marked tension. The medulla oblongata was markedly enlarged to twice the normal size, displacing the cerebellar hemispheres laterally. The upper cervical cord was also markedly enlarged. Although a firm yellow discolored mass could be visualized within the medulla, no definite delineation from the surrounding normal tissue could be made. No cyst was present within the tumor mass. The upward extent of the tumor could not be visualized because the suboccipital approach allowed only limited inspection of the upper pons.

Surgical decompression was followed by X-ray therapy (total of 4846 roentgens). An improvement in neurological status was subsequently noted. At the time of hospital discharge, 10 weeks after surgery, papilledema had disappeared. Corneal reflexes had returned. Gag reflex was now present and swallowing was intact. Sternocleidomastoid muscles and tongue were intact. Bilateral lateral rectus weakness and bilateral facial weakness were still present. There was still a slight bilateral decrease in pain sensation over the face. The patient was able to ambulate using a walker. Strength in the left upper extremity had improved. Improvement continued to such an extent that the patient returned to her job as a secretary and walked to work each day. Her only residual symptoms were a minor degree of diplopia and a minor ataxia of gait. Progression occurred 3.5 years after surgery and radiotherapy with increased symptoms of diplopia and vertigo plus findings of nystagmus of a rotary type in all directions of gaze, moderate weakness of the sternocleidomastoid muscles, and fasciculations bilaterally in the tongue. Shortly thereafter the patient was readmitted to the hospital because of increasing ataxia, slurred speech, numbness of the right side of the face (pain and touch were now decreased over all three divisions of the trigeminal nerve), loss of taste, and decreased hearing in the right ear. In addition, the gag reflex was decreased on the right. A greater degree of hoarseness was now evident, and laryngoscopy demonstrated no movement of the right vocal cord. The sternocleidomastoid muscles were weak. Atrophy and fasciculation involving the right half of tongue was now evident. Intention tremor was now present. A pneumoencephalogram demonstrated an enlargement of the substance of the brain stem with posterior displacement of the fourth ventricle and narrowing of the pontine cistern. High-voltage radiotherapy was started but had to be discontinued when symptoms progressed. Follow-up evaluation over the next 5 months demonstrated continued progression with additional neurological findings. Adduction and convergence of the right eye was now defective. A right peripheral facial weakness was now present. A marked intention tremor was present in the right upper extremity with a marked heel-to-shin ataxia in the right lower extremity. Re-evaluation 1 month later now indicated additional progression. A bilateral peripheral facial weakness was now present. Bilateral Babinski signs were present. In addition to the marked right-sided cerebellar findings previously noted, a significant involvement of the trunk and, to a lesser degree, of the left arm and leg was now apparent. Despite treatment with steroid therapy (Decadron) and with an intraventricular infusion of an experimental chemotherapeutic drug, 8-azaguanine, progression of the basic disease process continued at the time of hospital discharge with atrophy of the muscles of the left upper extremity. The patient was unable to stand and unable to arise from bed. The patient was transferred to a chronic disease hospital, where death occurred 6.5 years after onset of symptoms.

Comments

The course of events in this case over a 6.5-year period clearly indicates the progressive involvement of cranial nerves and long fiber systems over a wide extent of the brain stem. In the later stages, the cervical spinal cord was involved as well. The initial diplopia was related to involvement of the right sixth nerve. The long duration of this finding, its unilateral nature, the fact that headache and other symptoms and signs of increased intracranial pressure were absent (despite examinations by ophthalmologists and neurologists) all suggested that this was not the nonspecific effect of increased intracranial pressure. Such an increase in internal pressure may produce bilateral sixth nerve palsy.

With the subsequent development 1 year later of left-sided cerebellar findings, involvement of both sides of the brain stem was suggested, which would have been a somewhat unusual combination for a focal extrinsic compressive lesion. The subsequent development 3 months prior to admission of bilateral fifth nerve symptoms more clearly suggested a bilateral intrinsic lesion involving the pons. The difficulties in swallowing and the hoarseness in speech suggested involvement of the nucleus ambiguus or the vagus nerve at a medullary level. The loss of all sense of taste may have indicated bilateral involvement of the tractus solitarius or, less likely, of the various entering fibers passing via the facial and glossopharyngeal nerves. At later stages, the motor neurons or associated fibers at a medullary level supplying the tongue and sternocleidomastoid muscles were involved, as indicated by the significant atrophy and fasciculations present in these muscles. In very late stages, defects in adduction and convergence of the right eye suggested spread to a midbrain level with involvement of the third nerve nucleus supply to the right medial rectus muscle. The atrophy of muscles in the left upper extremity suggested spread to a spinal cord level.

Eventually increased intracranial pressure (with headache, vomiting, papilledema) was certainly present at the time of hospital admission. Thus, diplopia was present for 2 years without evidence of an increase in pressure. This is the usual situation in intrinsic tumors of the brain stem—increased intracranial pressure is absent in early stages. In contrast, extrinsic tumors involving the brain stem usually manifest increased intracranial pressure early in their course.

Having concluded that an intrinsic lesion is present, the identification of the type of pathology as glioma should be evident when one considers the differential diagnoses. Vascular disease, multiple sclerosis, amyotrophic lateral sclerosis, and syringobulbia represent other intrinsic diseases of the brain stem. Vascular disease would be unlikely in view of the gradual but progressive nature of the problem and the age of the patient. Multiple sclerosis would be unlikely since both neurons and long tracts were involved. Moreover, the symptoms were limited to the brain stem (although certainly involving several rostral-caudal segments of the brain stem and upper cervical spinal cord). The progressive nature of the problem without definite remissions would also be against the diagnosis of multiple sclerosis. A bulbar form of amyotrophic lateral sclerosis would be unlikely in view of the early age of onset of symptoms, the presence of sensory signs and symptoms, and the presence of cerebellar symptomatology. The relatively rare disorder syringobulbia is also unlikely. It is often associated with a relatively typical syndrome of syringomyelia. The brain stem involvement, which tends to be localized to several wedge or slit-type areas extending in from the fourth ventricle at a medullary level, is often associated with a relatively typical syndrome of syringomyelia. As regards treatment of brain stem gliomas, the general principles are similar to those considered for intrinsic tumors of the spinal cord. For most patients there is no surgical cure. Surgery often confirms the diagnosis and eliminates the possibility of extrinsic tumor. In occasional patients surgery may produce subtotal resection of or drainage of a focal cystic component. In addition, surgical decompression provides greater room for expansion of the brain stem. At times, when the tumor has produced obstruction of the fourth ventricle or aqueduct, the use of a bypass shunt will produce a considerable reduction in those symptoms related to a reduction in intracranial pressure. The tumor often has a significant response to radiation with the production of a temporary remission, as in the present case.

DEMYELINATING DISEASES

A general discussion of demyelinating diseases, particularly multiple sclerosis, will be found in Chapters 9 and 27. In one of the illustrative cases, there were several episodes suggesting discrete lesions at various levels of the brain stem in addition to lesions involving the spinal cord.

Multiple sclerosis, the most common type of demyelinating disease, frequently involves the white matter of the brain

Figure 13.25 Multiple sclerosis affecting the brain stem. Multiple irregular areas of myelin loss and gliosis are evident in a 58-year-old male with a long history of progressive multiple sclerosis. (*A*) Myelin stains; (*B*) glial stain (darkly staining areas). See also spinal cord section in Figure 9.21A. (Courtesy of Dr. Jose Segarra.)

stem and cerebellum (Fig. 13.26). The classic triad of Charcot includes nystagmus, intention tremor, and scanning speech—symptoms which are often present in the later stages of progressive cases but which may be absent early in the disease course or in nonprogressive cases.

The following example (Figs. 13.25A and 13.25B) illustrates a case of multiple sclerosis with predominant involvement of brain stem and cerebellar pathways early in the course of the disease.

CASE HISTORY 13.10

This 38-year-old, divorced, right-handed, white female employed as a tape library supervisor had been in excellent health until 1 year prior to admission when she developed vomiting, vertigo, numbness of her right leg, and difficulty walking. All symptoms cleared over 1 month. One year later, she awoke to find that she had diplopia, divergence of both eyes, limited upgaze, blurring of vision in the left eye, and ataxia.

Figure 13.26 Multiple sclerosis. Multiple areas of demyelination in the white matter of brain stem and cerebral hemispheres are demonstrated in this myelin stain. (Courtesy of Dr. Harry Zimmerman, Montefiore Hospital.)

Neurological Examination
Mental status: A mild degree of indifference to her difficulties was present.
Cranial nerves: On primary gaze, the left eye was divergent (exotropia). Neither eye could adduct past the midline. Dissociated nystagmus was present in the abducting eye on attempted lateral gaze to right or left. Vertical gaze up and down was now intact.
Motor system:
a. Rapid alternating hand movements were somewhat slow.
b. The gait was slightly broad based and mildly ataxic. She would fall to either side on attempted tandem gait.
Reflexes:
a. Deep tendon reflexes were bilaterally hyperactive.
b. The left plantar response was extensor.

Clinical diagnosis: Acute exacerbation of multiple sclerosis with predominant involvement of brain stem and cerebellar system.

Laboratory Data
MRI (Fig. 13.27) revealed that there were well-defined foci of increased signal, particularly in the T2-weighted images in the periventricular white matter, the corpus callosum, the subcortical white matter of the right parietal lobe, the left midbrain, and the cerebellar peduncles. CSF: protein was high (60 mg%), 1 oligoclonal band was present; 3 lymphocytes were present (normal).

Subsequent course: The patient was treated with a 5-day course of high-dosage intravenous methylprednisolone (1000 mg/day for 5 days) followed by a tapering course of oral prednisone. Within 10 days of the intravenous therapy, the patient had significant improvement: diplopia disappeared and walking improved. She was subsequently treated with beta interferon and had no significant exacerbations for the next 5 years. When last evaluated she did have residual symptoms of 2x/month fecal incontinence, more persistent cerebellar dysarthria and a hypophonia, increased reflexes on the left, and a slightly broad-based gait. She had persistent symptoms over the years related to the common symptom in patients with multiple sclerosis of fatigue that improved when treated with methylphenidate (Ritalin) and amantadine (Symmetrel). She had a persistent but stable complaint that her memory and cognitive processes were not as good as before her illness. Urinary frequency responded to the use of oxybutynin (Ditropan), an anticholinergic.

Comments
This patient clearly met the criteria for a diagnosis of definite multiple sclerosis. Her symptoms and signs clearly indicated a disease

Figure 13.27 Multiple sclerosis affecting brain stem and cerebellum on clinical evaluation. Magnetic resonance imaging demonstrates brain stem, cerebellar peduncle, and cerebral involvement.

process disseminated in time and space. Her major symptoms had clear-cut correlations on the MRI scan. The divergent position of the left eye and the inability to converge must have correlated with the left-sided rostral midbrain lesion at the floor of the cerebral aqueduct involving the area of the left third nerve complex. This lesion extended across the midline and certainly was in a position to involve the convergence center and the medial longitudinal fasciculus. The cerebellar symptoms correlated with involvement of the cerebellar peduncles. The complaints relevant to cognitive function most likely correlated with the changes in the lesions in cerebral white matter.

As regards treatment, acute exacerbations often respond to the intravenous administration of high-dosage corticosteroids (5 days of 1000mg/day of methylprednisolone is the usual therapy). This therapy reduces the inflammatory response and the edema of acute lesions. Oral therapy is not effective. The use of beta interferons has been demonstrated to significantly reduce exacerbations and to decrease progression of the disease. Serial MRI studies also confirm that beta interferon therapy also reduces the incidence of new lesions.

The following case demonstrates a problem of progressive multiple sclerosis that initially presented with brain stem symptoms but then pursued a course resulting in a terminal bedridden state.

CASE HISTORY 13.11

This 43-year-old, right-handed housewife was referred for evaluation of acute symptoms of ataxia, dizziness, diplopia, and tinnitus. In retrospect, the patient had experienced urinary frequency and possible symptoms of a spastic bladder for several years. Two months prior to admission, the patient experienced pain and a vague numbness-tingling on contact in both lower extremities followed by decreased strength in both legs. Examination by a neurosurgeon was reported to be negative.

Two to three weeks prior to admission, transient unsteadiness/ataxia was noted. Three days prior to admission, the patient reported a poorly defined "dizziness"—not clearly vertigo—present all the time but clearly accelerated by any attempt to roll over or to sit up. She could not walk without feeling "drunk."

Two days prior to admission tinnitus was noted in the right ear and diplopia was first reported.

General physical examination: Normal.
Neurological Examination

Mental status. Normal as regards orientation, memory function, and language function. However, a considerable blunting of mood was present.

Cranial nerves

a. The patient had diplopia on gaze to either left or right with a horizontal separation of images. Red glass testing suggested bilateral involvement of medial rectus.
b. In addition, nystagmus was present on lateral gaze, particularly to the left. Although usually conjugate, at times, there was greater nystagmus in the abducting left or right eye. The total pattern suggested a possible bilateral internuclear ophthalmoplegia.
c. The jaw jerk was hyperactive.

Motor system

a. Strength was intact.
b. Cerebellar function: The patient was ataxic when sitting; when standing or when attempting to walk, even on a broad or normal base.

Finger-to-nose testing was intact but heel-to-shin test demonstrated a dysmetria with a problem in placement of heel to knee.

Reflexes

a. Deep tendon reflexes were everywhere hyperactive, including the finger jerks (Hoffman signs).
b. Bilateral Babinski signs were present and more marked on the left than on the right.

Sensory *system:*

a. Vibration was decreased distally at toes and fingers.
b. Pain and position sensation were intact.

Clinical diagnosis: Multiple sclerosis: predominantly brain stem.
Laboratory Data

a. The sedimentation rate, vitamin B12 level, and serological tests for neurosyphilis and lupus erythematous were all negative.
b. CT scan of the brain and pneumoencephalography were normal.
c. Lumbar puncture demonstrated normal pressure and no significant cells. Although the total protein was normal at 27mg%, gamma globulin at 15mg% constituted 55% of the total protein (normal less than 14%). The serum gamma globulin was not significantly increased; thus, the increased gamma globulin in the CSF must have been produced in relation to the central nervous system.

Subsequent course: Several days after admission the patient developed tingling paresthesias on the right side of the face involving the upper and lower lip in a pattern that suggested involvement of the descending spinal tract of the fifth cranial nerve. Despite treatment for several weeks with prednisone, a corticosteroid, some progression occurred with the development of numbness of left side of face, a left central facial weakness, and slurring of speech. Eventually over 2–3 weeks a minor improvement in gait occurred. Within months she was able to walk without assistance, although she remained ataxic. On follow-up 2 months later, in addition to an internuclear ophthalmoplegia, a gaze paralysis for conjugate lateral gaze to the right was present, as well as the prior cerebellar and pyramidal tract findings.

When seen 1 year after the acute episode, diplopia was no longer present, and gait although ataxic and slightly broad based, was stable. However, complaints of emotional liability and changes in memory began to appear followed by periods of depression. Evaluation 2 years later indicated persistence of a spastic ataxic gait and a marked heel-to-shin ataxia. Over the years minor exacerbations occurred with incomplete remissions. With a severe exacerbation in 4 years after initial admission, the patient was readmitted to the hospital with urinary incontinence and worsening gait. Mental status indicated marked emotional lability and poor recall of recent events. A homonymous left upper quadrant field defect was present. Nystagmus was present on gaze to the left and right. A left peripheral facial weakness was present. Speech was scanning and dysarthric. Weakness of left arm and leg was present with marked spasticity and clonus of left knee and ankle. The gait was broad based and unstable. The patient was confined to a wheelchair. Bilateral Babinski signs and frontal release signs were present.

CT scan with enhancement demonstrated multiple white matter lesions in both hemispheres as well as left pons. During the hospitalization a bilateral internuclear ophthalmoplegia, vertical nystagmus, and worsening of gait occurred only to subsequently improve. The urinary incontinence related to an atonic bladder with overflow incontinence. The patient returned home but subsequently had increasing motor disability affecting all four limbs, resulting in a bedridden state. Progressive changes in mental status occurred with severe impairment of memory, hallucinations, and agitation. She expired in a chronic case facility, 7 years after the initial admission.

Comments

The diagnosis of definite multiple sclerosis is based on evidence in the history and on the examination of lesions disseminated in time and space. Eventually there was then little question of the diagnosis in this case. However, at the time of initial hospital admission, the patient had evidence of cerebellar, pyramidal tract, and lower pontine findings. The dissociated nystagmus, greater in the abducting eye, on right or left lateral gaze, suggested a bilateral lesion of the medial longitudinal fasciculus. Multiple sclerosis is the most common cause of such a bilateral lesion. (Vascular disease with infarction may produce either a unilateral or bilateral type of internuclear ophthalmoplegia.) A pontine glioma may also produce this syndrome. Initially there was little evidence of disease except at the possible pontine location. The pneumoencephalograms was performed to rule out a pontine glioma. This was prior to the clinical availability of the MRI scan. Today the MRI would be performed. In only a minority of cases (usually in far advanced cases) will the CT scan reveal lesions.

At the time of the patient's second hospital admission, evidence of multiple sites of involvement was evident both from the clinical and CT standpoint.

Initially this patient presented with an evolving brain stem syndrome. The symptoms never completely resolved. The diagnosis would be secondarily progressive multiple sclerosis. In view of remission and exacerbations in the initial course, this would be a more likely diagnosis than primary progressive multiple sclerosis. Today she would have been treated with a 5-day course of high-dosage (1000 mg per day) methyl prednisolone and then would have started on a beta interferon. This might have reduced subsequent exacerbations and reduced progression of the disease. See discussions in cases of this chapter and Chapter 9. Oral corticosteroids are no longer employed in therapy.

DEGENERATIVE DISEASES

1. Focal disease: syringobulbia: Discussed in Chapter 9 in relation to syringobulbia

2. System diseases

   a. Amyotrophic lateral sclerosis: This disorder has been discussed in detail in Chapter 9 on the spinal cord. Case 9.8 provides ample evidence of bulbar and corticobulbar involvement.

2. Spinocerebellar degenerations: Discussed in detail in Chapter 20 on the cerebellum, and Chapter 9.

TOXIC METABOLIC DISORDERS

1. Wernicke's encephalopathy: Discussed in detail in Chapter 30 in relation to memory.

2. Central pontine myelinolysis (refer to Case History 13.12).

CASE HISTORY 13.12

This 49-year-old male with a long history of alcoholism and poor nutrition was confused and lethargic with a low serum sodium of 99 mEq/liter, which was corrected to 123 mEq/liter over 24 hours. He developed a mute, akinetic state with bilateral spasticity, bilateral Babinski signs, and difficulty in swallowing and respiration. MRI demonstrates an extensive area of demyelination involving the central areas of the pons and midbrain (courtesy of Dr. Carl Rosenberg).

INFECTIONS OF THE BRAIN STEM

1. Poliomyelitis: discussed in detail in Chapter 9 on the spinal cord.

2. H. simplex and other infections.

BIBLIOGRAPHY

SUGGESTED READINGS

Asbury, A. K., McKhann, G. M., and McDonald, W. I. (Eds.). 1992. Diseases of the Nervous System: Clinical Neurobiology. 2nd ed., Vol. 1. Philadelphia, PA: W. B. Saunders.

Atlas, S. W. (Ed.). 1995. Magnetic Resonance Imaging of the Brain and Spine. New York, NY: Raven Press.

Black, P. M. C. L. 1991. Medical progress: brain tumors. N. Engl. J. Med. 324:1471–1476, 1555–1564.

Buttner-Ennever, J. A. (Ed.). 1988. Neuroanatomy of the oculomotor system. Rev. Oculomotor Res. 2:1–25.

Hain, T. C. 1995. Treatment of vertigo. The Neurologist 1:125–133.

Haymaker, W. 1969. *Bing's Local Diagnosis in Neurological Disease*. 15th ed. St. Louis, MO: C. V. Mosby.

Kunze, K., Zangemeister, W. H., and Artt, A. (Eds.). 1986. *Clinical Problems of Brain Stem Disorders*. New York, NY: Thieme Verlag.

Leigh, R. J., Averbuch-Heller, L., Thomsake, R. L., et al. 1994. Treatment of abnormal eye movements that impair vision. Strategies based on current concepts of physiology and pharmacology. [Review] Ann. Neurol. 36:129–141.

Leigh, R. J., and Zee, D. S. 1991. The Neurology of Eye Movements. 2nd ed. Philadelphia, PA: F. A. Davis.

Plum, F., and Posner, T. B. 1980. The Diagnosis of Stupor and Coma. 3rd ed. Philadelphia, PA: F. A. Davis.

Rowland, L. (Ed.). 1989. Merritt's Textbook of Neurology. Philadelphia, PA: Lea & Febiger.

Ropper, A. H., and Samuels, M. A. (Eds.). 2009. Adams and Victor's Principles of Neurology. 9th ed. New York, NY: McGraw Hill.

Wolf, J. 1971. The Classical Brain Stem Syndromes. Springfield, IL: Charles C. Thomas.

SPECIFIC CITATIONS

Adour, K. K. 1982. Current concepts in neurology: diagnosis and management of facial paralysis. N. Engl. J. Med. 15:346–351.

Averbuch-Heller, L., Zivotofsky, A. Z., Das, V. E., et al. 1995. Investigations of acquired pendular nystagmus. Brain 118:369–378.

Bender, M. B. 1980. Brain control of conjugate horizontal and vertical eye movements: a study of the structural and functional correlates. Brain 103:23–69.

Breen, L. A. 1980. Pupil sparing oculomotor nerve palsy due to midbrain infarction. Arch. Neurol. 48:105–106.

PART II: VASCULAR DISEASE

Abe M., and Kuellberg, R. N. 1989. Clinical presentations of vascular malformations of the brain stem. J. Neuro. Neurosurg. Psychiatry 52:167–175.

Barnett, H. J. M., Mohr, J. R., Stein, B. M., and Yatsu, F. M. (Ed.). 1998. Stroke: Pathophysiology: Diagnosis and Management. 3rd ed. New York, NY: Churchill Livingstone.

Barrett, K. M., and Meschia, J. F. 2010. Acute ischemic stroke management: medical management. Semin. Neurol. 30:461–468.

Berguer, R., and Bauer, R. B. 1984. Vertebrobasilar Arterial Occlusive Disease: Medical and Surgical Management. New York, NY: Raven Press.

Black, P. M. L. 1991. Medical progress: brain tumors. N. Engl. J. Med. 324:1471–1476, 1555–1564.

Caplan, L. R. 1986. Vertebrobasilar Occlusion Disease. In H. J. M. Barnett, J. P. Mohr, B. M. Stein, and F. M. Yatsu (Eds.) Stroke: Pathophysiology: Diagnosis and Management, pp.549–619. New York, NY: Churchill Livingstone.

Caplan, L. R. 1979. Occlusion of the vertebral or basilar artery: follow-up analysis of some patients with benign outcome. Stroke 10:277–282.

Caplan, L. R. 1980a. "Top of the basilar" syndrome. Neurology 30:72–79.

Caplan, L. R. 1980b. Vertebrobasilar occlusive disease: time for a new strategy. Stroke 12:111–114.

Caplan, L. 2000. Posterior circulation ischemia: then now and tomorrow. The Thomas Willis Lecture-2000. Stroke 31:2011–2023.

Caplan, L. R., and Sergay, S. 1976. Positional cerebral ischemia. J. Neurol. Neurosurg. Psychiatry 39:385.

Castaigne, P., Lhermitte, F., Buge, A., Escourolle, R., Haia, J. J., and Lyon-Caen, O. 1981. Paramedian thalamic and midbrain infarcts-clinical and neuropathological study. Ann. Neurol. 10: 127–148.

Castaigne, P., Lhermitte, F., Gautier, J. C., et al. 1973. Arterial occlusions the vertebrobasilar system: a study of forty-four patients with post-mortem data. Brain 96:133–159.

Cross, D. T., Akins, P. T., Angtuaco, E. E., and Diringer, M. N. 1997. Relationship between clot location and outcome after basilar artery thrombolysis. Am. J. Neuroradiol. 18:1221–1228.

Dunne, J. W., Chakere, J., and Karmode, S. 1987. Cerebellar hemorrhage. Quart. J. Med. 64:739–754.

Ellison, P. H., and Hanson, P. A. 1977. Herpes simplex: a possible cause of brain stem encephalitis. Pediatrics 9:240–243.

Epstein, F. J., and Farmer, J. P. 1993. Brain stem glioma growth patterns. J. Neurosurg. 78:408–412.

Fisher, C. M. 1970. Occlusion of the vertebral arteries. Arch. Neurol. 22:13–19.

Fisher, C. M., and Caplan, L. R. 1971. Basilar artery branch occlusion: a cause of pontine infarction. Neurology 21:900–905.

Fisher, C. M., and Curry, H. B. 1965. Pure motor hemiplegia of vascular origin. Arch. Neurol. 13:30–44.

Fisher, C. M., Karnes, W. E., and Kubik, C. S. 1961. Lateral medullary infarction- the pattern of vascular occlusion. J. Neuropath. Exp. Neurol. 20:323.

Kaplan, A. M., and Koveleski, J. T.1978. St. Louis encephalitis with particular involvement of the brain stem. Arch. Neurol. 35:45–46.

Kase, C. S., and Caplan, L. R.1986. Hemorrhage affecting the brain stem and cerebellum. In H. J. M. Barnett, J. Mohr, B. M. Stein, and F. M. Yatsu (Eds.) Stroke: Pathophysiology: Diagnosis and Management. Vol. 1, pp. 621–641. New York, NY: Churchill Livingstone.

Kase, C. S., and Caplan, L. R. 1994. Intracerebral hemorrhage. Boston, MA: Butterworth Heinemann.

Kim, J. S., and Lee, H. 2009. Inner ear dysfunction due to vertebrobasilar ischemic stroke. Semin. Neurol. 29:534–540.

Kubik, C. S., and Adams, R. D. 1946. Occlusion of the basilar artery: a clinical and pathological study. Brain 69:73.

McKee, A. C., Levin, D. N., Kowall, N. W., and Richardson, E. P., Jr. 1990. Peduncular hallucinosis associated with isolated infarction of the substantia nigra pars reticulata. Ann. Neurol. 27:500–504.

Lehrich, J., Winkler, G., and Ojemann, R. 1970. Cerebellar infarction with brain stem compression: diagnosis and surgical treatment. Arch. Neurol. 22:490.

Mehler, M. F. 1989. The Rostral brain stem syndrome. Neurology 39:9–16.

Mokri, B., Houser, W., Sandok, B. A., and Piepgras, D. G. 1988. Spontaneous dissections of the vertebral arteries. Neurology 38:880.

Nakajima, K. 1983. Clinicopathological study of pontine hemorrhage. Stroke 4:485.

Norrving, B. 1991. Lateral medullary infraction: prognosis in an unselected series. Neurology 41:244–248.

Ojemann, R. G., Ogilvy, C. S., Crowell, R. M., and Heros, R. C. 1995. Surgical Management of Neurovascular Disease. 3rd ed. Baltimore, MD: Williams and Wilkins.

Ott, K. H., Kase, C. S., Ojemann, R. G., and Mohr, J. P. 1974. Cerebellar hemorrhage: diagnosis and treatment: a review of 56 cases. Arch. Neurol. 31:160–167.

Pessin, M. S., and Caplan, L. R. 1986. Heterogenicity of vertebrobasilar occlusive disease. In K. Kunze, W. H. Zangemeister, and A. Artt (Eds.) Clinical Problemsof Brain Stem Disorders, pp. 30–42. New York, NY: Thieme Verlag.

Pessin, M. S., Chimowitz, M. I., Levine, S. R., et al. 1989. Stroke in patients with fusiform vertebrobasilar aneurysms. Neurology 39:13:16–21.

Pessin, M. S., Gorelick, P. B., Kwan, E. S., and Caplan, L. R. 1987. Basilar artery stenosis middle and distal segments. Neurology 37:1742–1746.

Prasad, S., and Galetta, S. L. 2010. Eye movement abnormalities in multiple sclerosis. Neurol. Clin. 28:641–655.

Prasad, S., and Volpe, N. J. 2010. Paralytic strabismus. Neurol. Clin. 28:803–833.

Ropper, A. H., Fisher, C. M., and Kleinmann, G. M. 1979. Pyramidal infarction in the medulla. A cause of pure motor hemiplegia sparing the face. Neurology 21:91.

Rucker, J. C. 2007. Oculomotor disorders. Semin. Neurol. 27:244–256.

Rundek, T., and Sacco, R. L. 2008. Risk management to prevent first stoke. Neurol. Clin. 26:1007–1045.

Segarra, J. M. 1970. Cerebral vascular disease and behavior: I. The syndrome of the mesencephalic artery (basilar artery bifurcation). Arch. Neurol. 22:408–419.

Stahl, S. M., Johnson, K. P., and Malamod, N. 1980. The clinical and pathologial spectrum of brain stem vascular malformations: long course simulates multiple sclerosis. Arch. Neurol. 37:25–29.

Strank, A. R., Hoffman, H. J., Henrick, E. B., and Humphreys, R. P. 1986. Diagnosis and management of pediatric brain stem gliomas. J. Neurosurg. 65:754–760.

Waxman, S. G., Sabin, T. D., and Embree, L. J. 1974. Subacute brain stem encephalitis. J. Neurol. Neurosurg. Psychiatry 37:811–816.

Wijdicks, E. F. M., Nickols, D. A., Thielen, J. R., et al. 1997. Intra-arterial thrombolysis in acute basilar artery thromboembolism: the initial Mayo Clinic experience. Mayo Clin. Proc. 72:1005–1013.

Wijdicks, E. F., and St. Louis, E. 1997. Clinical profiles predictive of outcome in pontine hemorrhage. Neurology 49:1342.

Wilkins, R. H., and Brody, I. A. 1970. Neurological classics XXX. Wallenberg's syndrome. Arch. Neurol. 22:379–382, 408–419.

EYE MOVEMENTS

Carpenter, M. B., McMasters, R. E., and Hanna, G. R. 1963. Disturbances of conjugate horizontal eye movement in the monkey: I. Physiological effects and anatomical degeneration resulting from lesion of the abducens nucleus and nerve. Arch. Neurol. 8:232–247.

Chiappa, K. H. 1989. Evoked Potentials in Clinical Medicine. 2nd ed. New York, NY: Raven Press.

Christoff, N. 1974. A clinicopathologic study of vertical eye movements. Arch. Neurol. 31:1–8.

DeGirolami, V., and Schidek, H. 1973. Clinicopathological study of 53 tumors of the pineal region. J. Neurosurg. 39:455–462.

Fuchs, A. F., and Kaneko, C. R. S., and Suddar, C. A. 1985. Brain stem control of saccadic eye movements. Ann. Rev. Neurosci. 8:307–337.

Gamlin, P. D. R., Gnadt, J. W., and Mays, L. E. 1989. Lidocaine-induced unilateral internuclear ophthalmoplegia: effects on convergence and conjugate eye movements. J. Neurophysiol. 62:82–95.

Goebel, H. H., Komatsuzaki, A., Bender, M. B., et al. 1971. Lesions of the pontine tegmentum and conjugate gaze paralysis. Arch. Neurol. 24:431–440.

Gonyea, E. F. 1966. Bilateral internuclear ophthalmoplegia: association with occlusive cerebrovascular disease. Arch. Neurol. 31:29–34.

Harner, S. G., and Ebersold, M. J. 1985. Management of acoustic neuromas 1978–1983. J. Neurosurg. 63:175–179.

Harner, S. G., Daube, J. R., and Ebersold, M. J. 1987. Improved preservation of facial nerve function with the use of electrical monitoring during removal of acoustic neuromas. Mayo Clinic Proc. 62:92–102.

Hatcher, M. A., and Lintworth, G. K. 1966. The sylvian aqueduct syndrome. Arch. Neurol. 15:215–224.

Jackel, R. A., Gittinger, W., Jr., Smith, T. W., et al. 1986. Metastatic adenocarcinoma presenting as one-and-one-half syndrome. J. Clin. Neuro-ophthal. 6:116–119.

Jacobs, L., Anderson, D. J., and Bender, M. B. 1973. The lesions producing paralysis of downward but not upward gaze. Arch. Neurol. 28:319–323.

Laird, F. J., Harner, S. G., Laws, E. R., Jr., et al. 1985. Meningiomas of the cerebellopontine angle. Otolaryngol. Head Neck Surg. 93:163–167.

Martuza, R. L., Parker, S. W., Nadol, J. B., et al. 1985. Diagnosis of cerebellopontine angle tumors. Clin. Neurosurg. 32:177–213.

Martuza, R. L., and Eldridge, R. 1988. Neurofibromatosis 2 (bilateral acoustic neurofibromatosis). N. Engl. J. Med. 318:684–688.

Nakada T., and Kwee, I. L. 1986. Oculopalatal myoclonus. Brain 109:431–441.

Pasik, P., Pasik, T., and Bender, M. B. 1969. The pretectal syndrome in monkeys: II. Spontaneous and induced nystagmus and lightening eye movements. Brain 115:227–247.

Perrot-Deseillgny, C., Chain, F., Serdau, M., et al. 1981. The one and a-half syndrome. Brain 104:665–669.

Schmidtke, K., and Buttner-Ennever, J. A. 1992. A nervous control of eyelid function: a review of clinical experimental and pathological data. Brain 115:227–247.

Stein, B. M., and Fetell, M. R. 1985. Therapeutic modalities for pineal lesion tumors. Clini. Neurosurg. 32:445–455.

Sweet, W. H. 1986. Current concepts: the treatment of trigeminal neuralgia (tic douloureux). N. Engl. J. Med. 315:174–177.

Wertelecki, W., Rouleau, G. A., Superneau, D. W., et al. 1988. Neurofibromatosis 2: clinical studies of a large kindred. N. Engl. J. Med. 319:278–283.

Zee, D. S., Friendlich, A. R., and Robinson, D. A. 1974. The mechanism of downbeat nystagmus. Arch. Neurol. 30:227–237.

Zee, D. S., Yamazaki, A., Butler, P. H., et al. 1981. Effects of ablation of flocculus and paraflocculus on eye movements in primate. J. Neurophysiol. 46:878–899.

VASCULAR DISESE OF THE BRAIN STEM
GENERAL REFERENCES

Adams, R. D., Victor, M., and Ropper, A. 1997. Principles of Neurology. 6th ed. New York, NY: McGraw Hill.

Berguer, R., & Bauer, R. B. 1984. Vertebrobasilar Arterial Occlusive Disease: Medical & Surgical Management. New York, NY Raven Press.

Caplan, L. R. 1986. Vertebrobasilar occlusion disease. In H. J. M. Barnett, J. P. Mohr, B. M. Stein, and F. M. Yatsu (Eds.) Stroke: Pathophysiology: Diagnosis and Management, pp. 549–619. New York, NY: Churchill Livingstone.

Jellinger, K. 1986. Neuropathology and clinical signs of brain stem disorders. In K. Kunze, W. H. Zangemeister, and A. Arrt (Eds.) Clinical Problems of Brain Stem Disorders, pp. 17–29. New York, NY: Stuttgart Thieme Verlag.

Kase, C. S., and Caplan, L. R. 1986. Hemorrhage affecting the brain stem and cerebellum. In In H. J. M. Barnett, J. P. Mohr, B. M. Stein, and F. M. Yatsu (Eds.) Stroke: Pathophysiology: Diagnosis and Management. Vol. 1, pp. 621–641. New York, NY: Churchill Livingstone.

Plum, F., and Posner, J.1980. The Diagnosis of Stupor and Coma. 3rd ed. Philadelphia, PA: F. A. Davis.

Wolf, J. 1971. The Classical Brain Stem Syndromes. Springfield, IL: Charles C. Thomas.

SPECIFIC CITATIONS
A. Ischemic Occlusive

Abe, M., and Kuellberg, R. N. 1989. Clinical presentations of vascular malformations of the brain stem. J. Neuro. Neurosurg. Psychiatry 52:167–175.

Caplan, L. R. 1979. Occlusion of the vertebral or basilar artery: follow-up analysis of some patients with benign outcome. Stroke 10:277–282.

Caplan, L. R. 1980. "Top of the basilar" syndrome. Neurology 30:72–79.

Caplan, L. R. 1980. Vertebrobasilar occlusive disease: time for a new strategy. Stroke 12:111–114.

Caplan, L. 2000. Posterior circulation ischemia: then now and tomorrow. The Thomas Willis Lecture-2000. Stroke 31: 2011–2023.

Castaigne, P., Lhermitte, F., Buge, A., Escourolle, R., Haia, J. J., and Lyon-Caen, O. 1981. Paramedian thalamic and midbrain infarcts-clinical and neuropathological study. Ann. Neurol. 10: 127–148.

Castaigne, P., Lhermitte, F., Gautier, J. C., et al. 1973. Arterial occlusions the vertebrobasilar system: a study of forty-four patients with post-mortem data. Brain 96:133–159.

Cross, D. T., Akins, P. T., Angtuaco, E. E., and Diringer, M. N. 1997. Relationship between clot location and outcome after basilar artery thrombolysis. Am. J. Neuroradiol. 18:1221–1228.

Fisher, C. M. 1970. Occlusion of the vertebral arteries. Arch. Neurol. 22:13–19.

Fisher, C. M., and Caplan, L. R. 1971. Basilar artery branch occlusion: a cause of pontine infarction. Neurology 21:900–905.

Fisher, C. M., and Curry, H. B. 1965. Pure motor hemiplegia of vascular origin. Arch. Neurol. 13:30–44.

McKee, A. C., Levin, D. N., Kowall, N. W., and Richardson, E. P., Jr. 1990. Peduncular hallucinosis associated with isolated infarction of the substantia nigra pars reticulata. Ann. Neurol. 27:500–504.

Mehler, M. F. 1989. The rostral brain stem syndrome. Neurology 39:9–16.

Norrving, B. 1991. Lateral medullary infraction: prognosis in an unselected series. Neurology 41:244–248.

Pessin, M. S., and Caplan, L. R. 1986. Heterogenicity of vertebrobasilar occlusive disease. In K. Kunze, W. H. Zangemeister, and A. Artt (Eds.) Clinical Problems of Brain Stem Disorders, pp. 30–42. New York, NY: Thieme Verlag.

Pessin, M. S., Chimowitz, M. I., Levine, S. R., et al. 1989. Stroke in patients with fusiform vertebrobasilar aneurysms. Neurology 39(13):16–21.

Pessin, M. S., Gorelick, P. B., Kwan, E. S., and Caplan, L. R. 1987. Basilar artery stenosis middle and distal segments. Neurology 37:1742–1746.

Segarra, J. M. 1970. Cerebral vascular disease and behavior: I. The syndrome of the mesencephalic artery (basilar artery bifurcation). Arch. Neurol. 22:408–419.

Wijdicks, E. F. M., Nickols, D. A., Thielen, J. R., et al. 1997. Intra-arterial thrombolysis in acute basilar artery thromboembolism: the initial Mayo Clinic experience. Mayo Clin. Proc. 72:1005–1013.

Wilkins, R. H., and Brody, I. A. 1970. Neurological classics XXX: Wallenberg's syndrome. Arch. Neurol. 22:379–382.

Wijdicks, E. F. M., Nickols, D. A., Thielen, K. R., et al. 1997. Intra-arterial thrombolysis in acute basilar artery thromboembolism: the initial Mayo Clinic experience. Mayo Clin. Proc. 72:1005–1013.

B. Pontine and Cerebellar Hemorrhages (see also Chapter 26)

Abe, M., and Kjellberg, R. N. 1989. Clinical presentations of vascular malformations of the brain stem. J. Neuro. Neurosurg. Psychiatry 52:167–175.

Dunne, J. W., Chakere, J., and Karmode, S. 1987. Cerebellar hemorrhage. Quart. J. Med. 64:739–754.

Ott, K. H., Kase, C. S., Ojemann, R. G., and Mohr, J. P. 1974. Cerebellar hemorrhage: diagnosis and treatment: a review of 56 cases. Arch. Neurol. 31:160–167.

Stahl, S. M., Johnson, K. P., and Malamod, N. 1980. The clinical and pathologial spectrum of brain stem vascular malformations: long course simulates multiple sclerosis. Arch. Neurol. 37:25–29.

C. Other Intrinsic Diseases of the Brain Stem: Tumors (see Earlier and Chapter 27)

Black, P. M. L. 1991. Medical progress: brain tumors. N. Engl. J. Med. 324:1471–1476, 1555–1564.

Epstein, F. J., and Farmer, J. P. 1993. Brain stem glioma growth patterns. J. Neurosurg. 78:408–412.

Strank, A. R., Hoffman, H. J., Henrick, E. B., and Humphreys, R. P. 1986. Diagnosis and management of pediatric brain stem gliomas. J. Neurosurg. 65:754–760.

Demyelinating Disorders: Multiple Sclerosis (See Chapter 9); Focal Degenerations: Syringobulbiar System Disease and Degenerations (See Chapter 9 and Chapter 27); Infections of the Brain Stem (see also Chapter 27)

Ellison, P. H., and Hanson, P. A. 1977. Herpes simplex: a possible cause of brain stem encephalitis. Pediatrics 9:240–243.

Kaplan, A. M., and Koveleski, J. T. 1978. St. Louis encephalitis with particular involvement of the brain stem. Arch. Neurol. 35:45–46.

Waxman, S. G., Sabin, T. D., and Embree, L. J. 1974. Subacute brain stem encephalitis. J. Neurol. Neurosurg. Psychiatry 37:811–816.

14.

CASE HISTORY PROBLEM SOLVING

PART II: BRAIN STEM AND CRANIAL NERVES

Lesion Diagrams: For each of the following diagrams, indicate the structures involved by the crosshatched lesion(s). For each structure involved, indicate the expected clinical signs or symptoms with appropriate lateralization, that is, left or right (ipsilateral or contralateral). Where appropriate, indicate the vascular territory involved, the designation of the type of pathology, and/or the various names of the syndrome (Figs. 14.1–14.10).

CASE HISTORY PROBLEM SOLVING PART II. BRAIN STEM

Each of the following case histories deals with disease at the level of the brain stem or of the cranial nerves. In some cases, it will be evident that the disease process involves the spinal cord as well as the brain stem. Some of the cases deal with intrinsic disease, and some deal with extrinsic disease. For each case indicate and diagram the location of the lesion and indicate the nature of the pathological process. Where appropriate, indicate the name(s) of the syndrome and/or the vascular territory.

Figure 14.1

Figure 14.3

Figure 14.2

Figure 14.4

281

Figure 14.5

Figure 14.6

Figure 14.7

Figure 14.8

Figure 14.9

CASE HISTORY 14.1 (PATIENT OF DOCTOR JOHN SULLIVAN)

A 31-year-old white policeman entered the hospital with symptoms of progressive difficulty in speech, in swallowing, and with weakness of his grip in both hands. Fifteen months before admission, he first noted hoarseness, fatigability of his voice, and faulty articulation. This has been slowly, steadily progressive, such that now speech was barely intelligible. Three months after onset of symptoms, he noted difficulty in swallowing both solids and liquids. He had a tendency to regurgitate liquids through his nose. Finally, 3 months before entry, the patient began to note

R L

Figure 14.10

increasing weakness of handgrip. He had no complaints referable to his legs. He denied any sensory symptoms. Six months before admission, he noted the presence of muscle twitching with a diffuse distribution, but particularly in the arms and shoulders. He had lost 10 pounds in weight and was easily fatigued. System review was otherwise entirely negative and general physical examination was well within normal limits.

Neurologic Examination

Mental status: Normal.

Cranial nerves: Positive findings in cranial nerve function were as follows:

a. Stiffness and weakness of jaw muscles, with jaw clonus.
b. Weakness of facial musculature, including eye closure and incomplete retraction of the corners of the mouth.
c. Fasciculations were seen in the facial muscles.
d. Gag reflex was very brisk, but palate moved weakly.
e. Tongue would not be protruded; it was atrophic with fibrillations seen beneath the mucous membrane.
f. Speech, as noted, was slurred, slow, and strained.

Motor system:

a. Weakness of handgrips was present.
b. Atrophy was present in the thenar eminence and dorsal interosseus spaces. The proximal muscles were strong, without atrophy; leg muscles were strong and revealed no atrophy.
c. Widespread muscle fasciculations were seen in both upper and lower extremities.

Reflexes:

a. Deep tendon reflexes were increased symmetrically in the lower extremities.
b. Plantar responses were extensor bilaterally (positive Babinski sign).

Sensory system: Normal.

Questions

1. Does this patient have a level lesion or a system disease? If it is a system, which system or systems are involved?
2. Indicate the significance of the hyperactive jaw jerk and of the hyperactive gag reflex.
3. Indicate the significance of the fasciculations in the facial muscles, the atrophy of the tongue, and fibrillations seen in the tongue.
4. Indicate the significance of the atrophy in the hands and the widespread fasciculations.
5. Indicate the significance of the hyperactive deep tendon reflexes in the lower extremities and the bilateral Babinski signs.
6. Where is the pathology?
7. What is the pathology? Indicate the postulated pathophysiology.
8. Name the disease. Whose name is attached to the disease in the United States?
9. Which diagnostic laboratory studies would assist in the diagnosis?
10. What would a muscle biopsy reveal?
11. Which neuroimaging studies, if any, are indicated in this case? What results are expected?
12. What is the prognosis? Discuss in terms of this patient in particular and then in terms of patients in general with this disease.

CASE HISTORY 14.2 (PATIENT OF DR. JOHN SULLIVAN)

This is a 63-year-old, right-handed woman, who on the day before admission was suddenly seized by a sensation as though a weight had descended upon her head. She felt dizzy, staggered to a chair, and called for help. It was noted that her speech was slurred and indistinct. As she looked at an object, it seemed to her to be out of focus. Since then she has had great difficulty in swallowing liquids because of a tendency to regurgitate through her nose. Solid foods did not seem to pass down. She also noted clumsiness of her right hand and of the right leg with staggering to the right side.

General examination: Blood pressure was 210/100 and she was obese with cardiomegaly.

Neurological Examination

Mental status: Brief mental status examination revealed her to be alert and cooperative, exactly oriented, and rather apprehensive. There was no evidence of any intellectual deficit.

Cranial nerves:

a. Examination of the fundi showed marked tortuousity of the retinal vessels; disks were normal; there were no hemorrhages or exudates.
b. Visual fields were full.
c. Left pupil was 7 mm in size; the right 4 mm; both reacted briskly to light and accommodation; there was a partial ptosis of the eyelid on the right and slight enophthalmos on the right.
d. There were no ocular palsies, but there were fairly well-sustained quick nystagmoid jerks on gaze to either side.
e. Right corneal reflex was absent. Pain and temperature sensation on the right side of the face were lost, but touch sensation was intact.
f. Hearing was acute bilaterally.
g. Voice was somewhat hoarse; speech was slightly slurred and scanning. The right vocal cord was paralyzed. The gag reflex was not elicited on the right, but it was present on the left. The uvula pulled to the left.
h. The eleventh and twelfth cranial nerve functions were normal.

Motor examination:

a. There was instability of posture of the right arm with dyssynergia and intention tremor, which was also present in the right leg.
b. Strength of arms and legs was approximately normal.

Reflexes:

a. Deep tendon reflexes in upper and lower extremities were equal.
b. Right and left plantar responses were flexor.

Sensory system:

a. There was a loss of pain and temperature sensibility throughout the left half of the body.
b. Position and vibration sensation were intact.

Questions

1. Diagram the lesion using anatomical diagrams—be specific. Mark this Case 14.2. Be certain to indicate laterality. Prepare a list of symptoms and signs in one column and anatomical structures involved in the opposite column.
2. Select the diagram in the selection which best corresponds to this case.
3. What is the nature of the pathological process?
4. If vascular, indicate the vascular territory in terms of specific vessel.
5. Which labels or names are attached to this overall syndrome? Is there another named syndrome also present?

CASE HISTORY 14.3

This 54-year-old, right-handed, obese white female was referred for evaluation of diplopia and ataxia. The patient had a 19-year history of diabetes mellitus initially treated with insulin and more recently with diet alone. The patient also had experienced significant pain in both lower extremities related to intermittent claudication, initially occurring on exercise but more recently occurring also at rest. Evaluation by the vascular surgery service had also indicated bilateral carotid bruits.

On the night prior to admission, the patient had the acute onset of a diplopia. At the same time, she noted that she was no longer able to move her eyes upward and that in order to look up she had to turn her head back. At the same time, she developed a sense of unsteadiness. This morning she had a persistence of symptoms.

Neurological Examination

Mental status: All areas were intact but a marked degree of anxiety was present.

Cranial nerves:

a. She had significant bilateral impairment of upward gaze.
b. As she attempted to gaze upward, she had significant lid retraction.
c. In addition, there was an indication of a weakness of right medial rectus.
d. The pupils were equal and responded to light.
e. There was now no evidence of ptosis. There was no definite fatigue of the lids by repetitive movement.

Motor system:

a. Strength was intact.
b. On examination of gait, the patient walked on a broad base. She tended to fall to the left. She was unable to walk a tandem gait.
c. She had a minor tremor of outstretched hands but no definite appendicular cerebellar findings.

Reflexes:

a. Deep tendon reflexes were 2+ except Achilles, which were absent (probably related to diabetes mellitus).
b. Plantar responses were flexor.

Sensory system:

All modalities were intact except for a decrease in vibration of toes (consistent with diabetes mellitus).

Hospital course: The patient had no additional progression. By day 5, she had shown improvement in right medial rectus function and had improvement in her ability to look up.

Questions

1. The bilateral lid retraction and the bilateral impairment of conjugate upward gaze in this case probably reflect involvement of which area or nucleus?
2. Indicate the blood supply of this area.
3. In this case, impairment of upward gaze was due to an ischemic event; however, impairment of conjugate upward gaze is also commonly noted in relation to other pathological processes. Consider the following:
   a. An infant of several weeks of age is found to have not only an impairment of upgaze but also one of the "setting sun" signs of neurology. The eyes are downcast. What is the most likely diagnosis? (*Be specific.*) What do you measure?
   b. A boy of 8 or 9 years has a 2-month disease course characterized by progressive impairment of upgaze, progressive ataxia, increasing headache, nausea, and vomiting. In addition to these findings, he has papilledema and impairment of hearing. What is the nature of the pathology? (*Be specific.*)

CASE HISTORY 14.4 (PATIENT OF DR. JOHN SULLIVAN)

This 65-year-old man entered another hospital complaining of headaches, severe vertigo, and nausea and vomiting. The diagnosis of labyrinthitis was made and the patient seemed to recover after a few days. He remained well, however, only a few days when he again had severe vertigo and vomiting. The latter was so persistent and severe that he became dehydrated.

On the morning of transfer to this hospital, at about 3:00 a.m., the patient noted the sudden onset of weakness and numbness of his right thigh.

Physical examination: The patient had a blood pressure of 110/80. There was a cold, clammy perspiration over his entire body. No other gross physical abnormalities were discovered.

Neurologcial Examination

Mental status: The patient was extremely restless and confused.

Cranial nerves:

a. He had a paralysis of left external (lateral) rectus muscle.
b. There was a coarse, irregular nystagmus on gaze to either side.
c. His fundi were quite normal.
d. The pupils and pupillary reflexes were normal.
e. There was a selective diminution of pain sensation on the left side of the face. The left corneal reflex was diminished.
f. He had a left facial paralysis of peripheral type.
g. Hearing was markedly diminished on the left.
h. Gag reflex on the left was diminished. The uvula pulled to the right. The patient's speech was hoarse, and he had a left vocal cord paralysis. He was unable to swallow without choking.
i. His tongue protruded slightly to the right.

Motor system:

a. On examination of his limbs, there was an intention tremor on the left involving both arm and leg.
b. His arms and legs were strong, and there seemed to be no increased resistance to passive movement.

Reflexes:

a. Deep tendon reflexes were increased on the right side throughout.
b. Both plantar responses were extensor (positive Babinski signs).

Sensory system:

a. There was a loss of pain and temperature sensibility throughout the entire right side of the body, arm, and leg.
b. Other forms of sensation could not be adequately tested because of the patient's inability to cooperate.

QUESTIONS

1. Consider, in isolation, the left peripheral facial weakness, the decrease in hearing in the left ear, the severe vertigo, and the decrease in pain sensation on the left side of the face and right side of body. Diagram this specific lesion at the proper level. Label this Case 14.4.
2. Select the appropriate diagram from the group above which best corresponds to this type of lesion. *You may have to disregard laterality to answer this question only!*
3. What specific artery supplies the area you have outlined above?
4. Now take into account those additional findings in this case that were not included in the consideration of Question 1. List those additional findings and indicate the artery responsible for the entire episode (there are two possibilities).

CASE HISTORY 14.5

This right-handed, 43-year-old white female had the onset of deafness in the right ear. Rapid progression of deafness was noted; some tinnitus (sensation of ringing) was also noted. Caloric testing of labyrinthine function at that time indicated no response to cold or hot water on the right side.

During the following month, the onset of a minor unsteadiness of gait was noted. Approximately 5 months later the patient noted defects in coordination of the right hand, particularly in typing, with a progression of unsteadiness of gait. At the same time "numbness" sensation of "pins-and-needles like Novocain given by a dentist" was noted over the entire right side of the face. Relatively continuous pain was noted, extending from the right side of the neck to the suboccipital area and right postauricular area. One month later difficulty in swallowing solids and liquids was noted.

Past history: Episodes of vertigo had occurred 5 to 6 years prior to admission. Right frontal headache had been present since age 33.

Neurological Examination
Mental status: Intact.

Cranial nerves:

a. Pain and touch sensation were decreased over all divisions of the trigeminal nerve on the right side, including the face, cornea, and the right side of the tongue.
b. There was minimal flattening of the right nasolabial fold and a poorer degree of eye closure on the right side than the left (orbicularis oculi).
c. There was no perception of voice in the right ear.
d. No vestibular response was present to ice water caloric testing in the right ear.
e. Minimal rotatory nystagmus was present on horizontal gaze with a minor degree of vertical nystagmus on upward gaze.
f. A minimal degree of dysarthria was apparent as regards guttural sounds.

Motor system:

a. Strength and tone were intact.
b. Cerebellar tests revealed a slight clumsiness in fine finger movements of the right hand.
c. Gait was slightly ataxic when performed on a narrow base with eyes open.

Reflexes:

a. Deep tendon reflexes were symmetrical and physiologic.
b. Plantar responses were flexor.

Sensory system: All modalities were intact.

Laboratory Data

Cerebrospinal fluid protein was slightly elevated to 50 mg/100 ml. Skull X-rays were reported as negative.

QUESTIONS

1. This patient presents a typical example of a classic neurological syndrome. Locate the lesion.
2. What is the most likely pathology to be found by the neurosurgeon in this location? Which pathological processes are also possible but less likely?
3. The initial involvement of the functions of cranial nerve VIII prior to involvement of other cranial nerves should provide a clue as to the structure from which this lesion arises.
4. Does the pattern of sensory disturbance over the right side of the face indicate primary involvement of the trigeminal nerve extrinsic to the brain stem or of the descending spinal tract and associated nucleus of the trigeminal nerve within the brain stem?
5. Were long sensory and motor tracts within the brain stem involved by this lesion?
6. Predict the clinical picture that would have occurred if the lesion had progressed.
7. During the course of surgery, aimed at total resection in these cases, the facial nerve must often be sacrificed or damaged. Based on your understanding of the anatomical considerations in these cases, indicate why this occurs. Which studies may be performed during surgery in early cases to preserve residual hearing or facial nerve function?
8. Which critical diagnostic studies would you perform?
9. When should these studies be performed?

CASE HISTORY 14.6

This 57-year-old housewife 1 day prior to admission suddenly developed double vision and a drooping of the right eyelid. In addition, she had difficulty walking. Examination of the patient in the emergency room revealed weakness of adduction of the right eye, ptosis of the right eye, and a left extensor plantar response. She was admitted to the neurology service.

Past History
1. Moderate hypertension had been present for many years.
2. Four years previously, the patient had begun to have sudden 30-minute episodes of right-handed weakness and dysarthria. Twenty-six months prior to admission, she had a 15–20 minute episode of bilateral blurred vision, unsteadiness of gait, and tingling paresthesias of the right hand and face. Twenty-two months prior to admission, she had an episode of paresthesias involving either the left leg and arm or the right arm and leg. Examination at that point demonstrated increased deep tendon reflexes on the right side.

   Eighteen months prior to admission, she experienced 10-minute episodes of numbness of the left hand and face accompanied by renewed numbness of the right hand. Three days prior to admission she had a brief episode of right hand weakness.
3. The patient had been receiving anticoagulant therapy (Coumadin) for phlebitis for several months prior to admission.

General examination: The patient was obese and anxious with blood pressure elevated to 160/100.

Neurological Examination
Mental status: The patient was alert and oriented. Recent memory was poor and delayed recall was limited to 2/4 objects. (All similar to 18 months previously)

Cranial nerves:
a. Ptosis of the right eyelid was present, but pupillary responses were intact.
b. At rest, the right eye was deviated out to the right and down. No medial or upward movement of the right eye was possible. (Note change.)
c. A mild left central (supranuclear) facial weakness was now present.

Motor system: Strength was intact.

Reflexes: There were changes compared to examinations 22 and 18 months previously.

a. Deep tendon reflexes were now increased in the left lower extremity.
b. A left Babinski sign was now present with an absent left abdominal reflex.

Sensory system: All modalities were intact.
Carotid pulses: Strong bilaterally.

Laboratory Data
1. Skull X-rays demonstrated calcifications in the cavernous carotid arteries.
2. Electrocardiogram was normal.
3. Electroencephalogram demonstrated scattered multifocal slow waves.
4. Blood studies: Complete blood counts, serology, blood sugar, and total cholesterol were normal.
5. Prothrombin time was close to normal.
6. The patient refused lumbar puncture and angiography.

QUESTIONS
1. This is clearly a more complex case. However, the new symptoms of diplopia, ptosis of the right eyelid, plus the new findings of a paralysis of medial and upward movement of the right eye, increased deep tendon reflexes in the left lower extremity, a left Babinski sign, and a left central facial weakness should allow for the diagnosis and localization of at least one syndrome. What name do you assign to this syndrome? Does this syndrome involve a specific vascular territory? If so, name the artery involved.
2. Which diagram best indicates the lesion? For this purpose only, you may disregard laterality.
3. How do you explain the earlier episodes?
    a. Episodes of right hand weakness and dysarthria.
    b. Bilateral blurring of vision, plus unsteadiness plus tingling of the right hand and face.
    c. Paresthesias left leg and arm followed by paresthesias of the right arm and leg.
4. Are there any additional questions that you might pose for this patient?
5. If this patient had a severe headache at the time of admission, why might a lumbar puncture have been considered?
6. Why was angiography considered?
7. The patient refused both lumbar puncture and angiography. Would you have requested these studies or would you have requested other noninvasive studies? If so, present your plan of workup justifying each study.
8. Present your working diagnosis and final diagnosis. (There are several possible ways to tie together all of the episodes.)
9. **ADVANCED QUESTION**: If this patient had a series of miscarriages earlier in life plus the cerebral arterial episodes and thrombo-phlebitis, indicate a possible diagnosis. Which diagnostic studies would you perform?

CASE HISTORY 14.7

This 69-year-old white male was seen for outpatient neurological re-evaluation. His neurological problems began 4 years previously. The patient had a history of intermittent ptosis of the left lid. In addition, at times significant ptosis of both lids had been noted. Over the years, he had intermittent episodes of diplopia. He had also noted weakness of his jaw in chewing and weakness in shoulders or in his neck on exercise of these muscle groups.

Neurological Examination
Mental status: Intact.
Cranial nerves:

a. The patient demonstrated a significant bilateral ptosis that was variable; it was significantly increased by exercise, and it was more marked in the left eye.
b. The patient showed a significant bilateral defect in upward movement and of lateral movement of the right eye. These deficits were all more marked on exercise.
c. The patient was able to smile for 8 seconds and then his smile began to evaporate bilaterally.
d. The patient had weakness in jaw muscles on repetitive opening and closure of jaw.

Motor system: The patient had weakness in shoulder abduction, which developed after 10 repetitive movements. He had weakness in forward head movement, which developed after 4 repetitive movements.

No definite atrophy was present.

No definite persistent weakness was otherwise present in the extremities.

Reflexes: Deep tendon reflexes were intact; plantar responses were flexor.

Sensory system: Intact.

QUESTIONS

1. Indicate the diagnosis. Be specific.
2. Where is the defect located in this disease? Be specific.
3. Discuss the underlying pathophysiology.
4. Which tests would confirm the diagnosis and might produce temporary improvement?
5. Outline therapeutic approaches. Consider both symptomatic relief and more specific management of the underlying pathology.
6. **ADVANCED QUESTION:** In this case, the intermittent weakness was made worse by repetitive exercise. There is, however, another syndrome in which weakness is improved by exercise. Name and discuss that syndrome in terms of etiology and pathophysiology. Be specific.

CASE HISTORY 14.8

This 56-year-old white housewife was admitted for evaluation of episodes of stupor and cyanosis associated with severe laryngeal stridor (high-pitched and harsh respiratory sounds) and stertorous breathing.

Laryngeal stridor had been present for 20 years and had grown worse during the last 5 to 6 years. An episode of anoxia during a Cesarean section 18 years prior to admission may have been a complication of this problem.

Sixteen years prior to admission numbness and weakness of the right leg had been noted. Progression had occurred in the last 2 years and episodic unsteadiness of gait had been noted. During this same period, weakness of the right hand had developed.

During the 1 year prior to admission the patient had three hospital admissions related to episodes of coma and cyanosis. Each had followed a several-week period in which there was increased temperature, stridor, and increased accumulation of tracheal and bronchial secretions with frequent periods of daytime sleepiness.

Neurological Examination

Mental status: Intact.

Cranial nerves:

a. Pain sensation was selectively decreased over all three divisions of the right side of the face with a decreased right corneal reflex.
b. Laryngoscopy revealed paralysis with atrophy of the left vocal cord. The right cord moved but was inhibited on abduction, indicating partial paresis.
c. Horizontal nystagmus was present on lateral gaze with minimal vertical nystagmus on upward gaze.

Motor system:

a. Atrophy of the right upper extremity was present, including the shoulder, arm, and hand.
b. Weakness was present in the right upper extremity—approximately 50% of normal strength at shoulder, elbow, wrist, and fingers. Weakness without atrophy was present in the right lower extremity and to a lesser degree in the left lower extremity.
c. Spasticity was present on passive movement at the right knee and ankle and to a lesser degree at the left knee.
d. Gait: There was circumduction of the right leg with unsteadiness on rapid turns.
e. Cerebellar tests were negative.

Reflexes:

a. Deep tendon:
  Biceps: right, 0; left, 0
  Triceps: right, 0; left, 0
  Radial: right, 0; left, 0
  Patellar: right, 4+; left, 3+
  Achilles: right, 4+; left, 3+
b. Superficial reflexes:

  Plantar: extensor on the right and possibly extensor on the left
  Abdominal: right, 0; left, 0

Sensory system:

a. Position, vibration, and touch were intact.
b. Pain decreased in a cape-like distribution over the shoulders.

Laboratory Data

1. Cerebrospinal fluid: normal (pressure 150, cell count 0, protein 45 mg/100 ml)
2. Skull X-rays were negative.
3. Cervical spine X-rays revealed minor nonsignificant degenerative changes at C5–C7.

Subsequent course: The patient was readmitted to the hospital 10 weeks later in a semicomatose and cyanotic condition. She required an emergency tracheostomy and 48 hours of respiratory assistance. Subsequent neurological examination was unchanged from that recorded earlier.

QUESTIONS

1. Where is the lesion? Does this lesion involve a single localized segment or are several segments involved?
2. Is the pathology limited to the brain stem or to the spinal cord?
3. Indicate what structures are involved to produce:
   a. laryngeal paralysis,
   b. cape-like deficit in pain and temperature but sparing touch and vibration,
   c. atrophy of all muscle groups in right upper extremity,
   d. absence of deep tendon reflexes in both upper extremities, and
   e. defective pain sensation on the right side of the face.
4. Indicate the most likely pathology and the probable prognosis.
5. What diagnostic tests should be undertaken to establish the diagnosis?
6. Why did the patient have episodes of coma and excessive daytime sleepiness? (There are several explanations. The most likely, however, has a purely mechanical explanation.)

15.

DIENCEPHALIC NUCLEI, FUNCTIONAL LOCALIZATION, AND ATLAS OF THE DIENCEPHALON

The diencephalon appears as a large region at the upper end of the brain stem. All the ascending fiber pathways from the spinal cord and brain stem terminate upon nuclei in the diencephalon. From these nuclei the information is relayed onto the cerebral cortex. Due to the convergence of all major ascending sensory, motor, autonomic, and reticular systems, consciousness for general sensations is first realized at this level. In addition, the ascending motor information from the cerebellum mixes with the striatal and cortical motor fibers in the dorsal thalamus, producing a motor thalamic region. Finally, the hypothalamus and limbic cortical regions have major input onto the anterior and dorsomedial nuclei of the thalamus.

DIENCEPHALIC BOUNDARIES

The border between the diencephalon and the midbrain is indistinct and may be arbitrarily defined by passing a line from the inferior surface of the mammillary bodies to the posterior border of the habenula. Portions of the substantia nigra and red nucleus are also seen in the posterior portion of the diencephalon. In order to identify the region containing the nuclei in the diencephalon and basal nuclei, the cerebral cortex and corpus callosum are carefully separated and removed, revealing the diencephalon (Figs. 15.1 and 15.2). Then one finds the slit-like third ventricle in the midline. At the rostral end of the diencephalon we can identify the anterior tubercle (containing the anterior thalamic nuclei) and at the posterior margin the pulvinar. The major new white matter bundles at this level are the internal capsule, fornix, and stria terminalis. The basal nuclei of the cerebrum can now also be visualized (Fig. 15.2), and they consist of caudate, putamen, and globus pallidus. The globus pallidus is found lateral to the internal capsule, and the putamen is adjacent to it. The caudate nucleus is found medial to the internal capsule. In the posterior levels of the diencephalon, the caudate is relatively small, but as one proceeds anteriorly, the diencephalon becomes smaller and the caudate enlarges.

The body of the lateral ventricle along with the corpus callosum and fornix form the superior border of the diencephalon (Fig. 15.3). The posterior limb of the internal capsule and the optic tract mark its lateral boundary, and the slit-like third ventricle denotes its medial border. Inferiorly, the hypothalamus of the diencephalon is continuous with the tegmentum of the midbrain, while rostrally it ends at the lamina terminalis. (This is the rostral end of the embryological neural tube/central nervous system.) The organum vasculosum of the lamina terminalis, which regulates the osmolality of the blood, is also present at this level (Fig. 15.4).

The diencephalon consists of five distinct nuclear subdivisions: thalamus, epithalamus, hypothalamus, metathalamus, and subthalamus (Fig. 15.3). As can be seen from the terminology associated with the regions in the diencephalon, all structures are described by their spatial relationship to the thalamus, being above (epithalamus), below (hypothalamus and subthalamus), or behind this region (metathalamus). The epithalamus and hypothalamus are discussed in Chapter 16. The hypothalamic sulcus is about a third of the way up from the floor of the third ventricle. All nuclear structures superior to the sulcus are included in the dorsal thalamus, and all nuclei below it are included in the hypothalamus (Fig. 15.3).

NUCLEI OF THE THALAMUS

The thalamus and metathalamus are the major relay center between the brain stem and the cerebral cortex. The thalamus is the largest portion of the diencephalon. It is ovoid in shape. Its boundaries are as follows: laterally by the posterior limb of the internal capsule, medially by the third ventricle, inferiorly by the subthalamus and hypothalamus, and superiorly by the body of the lateral ventricle and corpus callosum.

Figure 15.1 Brain in sagittal plain demonstrating the relationship between brain stem, diencephalon, and cerebrum. (Magnetic resonance imaging [MRI], T1 weighted.) Location of thalamus. MRI.

Figure 15.2 Dorsal view of gross specimen of brain stem, diencephalon, and basal ganglia. Medulla, pons, midbrain, thalamic regions, and internal capsule labeled.

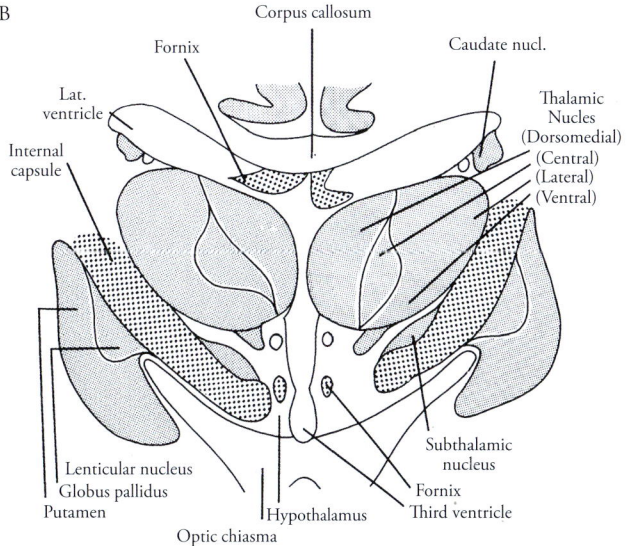

Figure 15.3 Mid thalamic level. (*A*) Magnetic resonance imaging (MRI), (*B*) Schematic coronal section showing nuclei of thalamus, hypothalamus, subthalamus, basal ganglia, and the white matter internal capsule.

THALAMIC BORDERS

The external medullary lamina forms the lateral boundary of the thalamus and separates it from the reticular nucleus of the thalamus. There is also an intrinsic bundle of white matter, the internal medullary lamina, which divides the thalamus into three major nuclear masses: the anterior, medial, and lateral. The boundary between the thalamus and hypothalamus (Fig. 15.3) is the hypothalamic sulcus on the medial wall of the third ventricle.

The anterior mass includes the anterior nuclei, the medial mass includes the dorsomedial nuclei and the midline nuclei, and the lateral mass includes all of the other nuclei. Cell and fiber stains are used to further subdivide the thalamus. With these stains the following nuclei are identifiable: anterior, medial, midline, intralaminar, lateral, posterior, reticular, and metathalamus.

Each of these nuclear groupings can be further subdivided as follows (Table 15.1).

FUNCTIONAL ORGANIZATION OF THALAMIC SENSORY AND MOTOR RELAY NUCLEI—THE VENTROBASAL COMPLEX, LATERAL POSTERIOR

These nuclei (Fig. 15.4) are part of the somatic brain as they receive direct input from the ascending sensory and motor systems, from the cerebellum, and from the optic tract. The special sensory medial and lateral geniculate nuclei are discussed later.

The *lateral nuclear mass* is divided into three parts: lateral dorsal, lateral posterior, and pulvinar. It occupies the upper half of the lateral nuclear grouping throughout the thalamus. It is bounded medially by the internal medullary lamina of the thalamus and laterally by the external medullary lamina of the thalamus. In a stained preparation its ventral border with the ventral nuclear mass is distinct. The lateral nuclear mass starts near the anterior end of the thalamus and runs the length of the thalamus with its posterior portion, the pulvinar, overhanging the geniculate bodies and the midbrain.

The lateral posterior part of the lateral nuclear mass projects to the superior parietal lobule and receives input from specific thalamic nuclei. The lateral dorsal part is included above with the limbic nuclei.

The *ventral basal nuclear mass* consists of three distinct regions: ventral anterior, ventral lateral, and ventral posterior.

The *ventral anterior (VA) nucleus* is the smallest and most rostral nucleus of this group. It can be identified by the

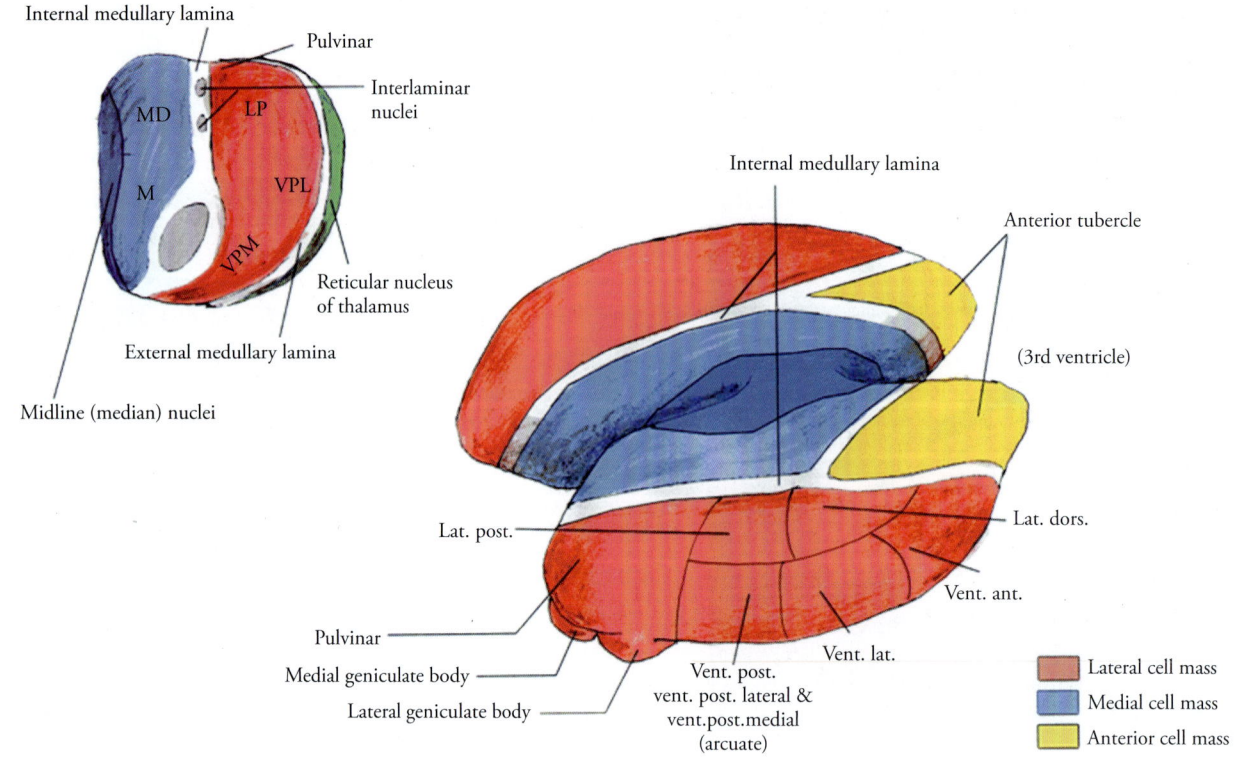

Figure 15.4 Three-dimensional reconstruction of the thalamic nuclei with the upper portion showing the three major nuclear subdivisions and the lower portion showing individual nuclei. (Modified after Carpenter Core Text, Williams and Wilkins, 1992.)

Table 15.1 NUCLEI IN THE THALAMUS

A. **ANTERIOR NUCLEI (Limbic)**
   1. Anterior dorsal
   2. Anterior medial
   3. Anterior ventral (Anterior principalis)

B. **MEDIAL NUCLEI (Limbic and Specific Associational)**
   1. Nucleus medialis dorsalis
      a. Pars parvocellulares
      b. Pars magnocellularis

C. **MIDLINE NUCLEI (Nonspecific Associational)**
   1. Nucleus parataenialis
   2. Nucleus paraventricularis
   3. Nucleus reuniens
   4. Nucleus rhomboideus

D. **INTRALAMINAR NUCLEI**—in the internal medullary lamina (Nonspecific Associational)
   1. Nucleus centrum medianum
   2. Nucleus parafascicular
   3. Nucleus paracentralis
   4. Nucleus centralis lateralis
   5. Nucleus centralis medialis

E. **LATERAL NUCLEI**
   1. Pars dorsalis (Specific Associational)
      a. Nucleus lateralis posterioris
      b. Nucleus lateralis dorsalis
   c. Pulvinar
      (1) Pars inferioris
      (2) Pars lateralis
      (3) Pars medialis
   2. Pars ventralis/Ventrobasal complex (Motor and Sensory Relay)
      a. Ventralis anterior
      b. Ventralis lateralis
      c. Ventralis ventralis
      d. Ventralis posterior
         (1) Posterolateral
         (2) Posteromedial

F. **RETICULAR NUCLEI (Nonspecific Associational)**

G. **METATHALAMIC NUCLEI (Sensory Relay)**
   1. Lateral geniculate (Vision-opticothalamic)
   2. Medial geniculate (Audition-auditothalamic)

H. **POSTERIOR NUCLEI (Nonspecific Associational)**
   1. Limitans
   2. Suprageniculate
   3. Posterior (Nociceptive System)

presence of numerous myelinated bundles. The magnocellular portion of this nucleus receives fibers from the globus pallidus, via the lenticular and thalamic fasciculi, and from the intralaminar nuclei and has some projections to areas 4 and 6.

Stimulation of this nucleus produces the same effects as stimulation of the intralaminar nuclei.

The *ventral lateral* and *ventral posterior nuclei* contain cell bodies that project onto the motor and sensory cortex. In the thalamus the head region is found medial and posterior and the leg anterior and lateral.

The *ventral lateral (VL, somatic motor thalamus) nucleus* occupies the middle portion of the ventral nuclear mass. It is a specific relay nucleus in that it receives fibers from the contralateral deep cerebellar nuclei (via the superior cerebellar peduncle/ dentatorubrothalamic tract) and the ipsilateral red nucleus. This nucleus also receives fibers from the globus pallidus and from the intralaminar nuclei. This nucleus projects to area 4 and to area 6 and has a topographic projection to the motor cortex. This nucleus is important in integrative somatic motor functions because of the interplay between the cerebellum, basal ganglia, and cerebrum in this nucleus.

The *ventral posterior nucleus* occupies the posterior half of the ventral nuclear mass and consists of two parts: the ventral posterior medial nucleus and the ventral posterior lateral nucleus. Both of these nuclei receive input from the specific ascending sensory systems.

The *ventral posterior medial (VPM) nucleus*, arcuate or semilunar, is located lateral to the centromedian nucleus and medial to the ventral posterior lateral nucleus. The secondary fibers of the trigeminal and gustatory pathways terminate in this nucleus; thus, this nucleus is concerned primarily with taste and with general sensation from the head and face. The basal region of the ventromedial nucleus receives the taste fibers and probably some of the vagal input. General sensation from the face, including pain, temperature, touch, pressure, and proprioception, terminate in the other portions of this nucleus. This nucleus projects information from the face, ears, and head, and tongue regions onto the inferior part of the postcentral gyrus, areas 3, 1, 2.

The *ventral posterior lateral (VPL) nucleus* receives fibers from the posterior columns and the direct spinothalamic tracts with the bulk of the input originating in the upper extremity. The VPL nucleus projects to the body and neck regions on the postcentral gyrus (areas 3, 1, 2).

The *lateral dorsal nucleus* and the anterior nucleus are surrounded by the rostral portion of the internal medullary lamina of the thalamus and should be considered a caudal continuation of the anterior nuclear group. This nucleus projects to the rostral cingulate cortex and onto the parahippocampal gyrus.

LIMBIC NUCLEI—THE ANTERIOR, MEDIAL, LATERAL DORSAL, MIDLINE, AND INTRALAMINAR NUCLEI

The limbic nuclei may also be called the nuclei of the emotional brain due to the strong input from the hypothalamus, cingulate, and orbital regions of the frontal lobe.

Anterior nuclei (Fig. 15.4) are at the most rostral part of the thalamus and form the prominent anterior tubercle in the floor of the lateral ventricle. The tubercle includes a large main nucleus (anteroventral) and small accessory nuclei (anterodorsal and anteromedial). The internal medullary lamina of the thalamus surrounds the anterior nuclei. The mammillothalamic fibers form the bulk of the fibers in the internal medullary lamina. This zone is an important relay station in the limbic brain and receives input from the subiculum, presubiculum, and mammillary body via the mammillothalamic tract.

The anterior nuclear complex is part of the Papez circuit: hippocampal formation → fornix → mammillary body → mammillothalamic tract → anterior thalamic nucleus → anterior thalamic 11, 12 (see Chapter 22).

Medial nuclear complex or the dorsomedial nucleus consists of both a large-celled and a small-celled division. This medial thalamic region is found between the internal medullary laminae and the midline nuclei lining the third ventricle (Fig. 15.4).

The *magnocellular* portion of the dorsomedial nucleus is interconnected with the hypothalamus, amygdala, and midline nuclei and connects to the orbital cortex. The large *parvicellular* division is interconnected with the temporal, orbitofrontal, and prefrontal cortices (areas 9, 10, 11, and 12; see also Chapter 22).

The medial nuclear complex is an important relay station between ascending input from the brain stem on to the hypothalamus, amygdala, and the prefrontal cortex and is concerned with the multimodal associations between the limbic, visceral, and somatic impulses that contribute to the emotional makeup of the individual. Destruction of this nucleus in cats results in a lower threshold for rage so that the animal is easily aroused. In human beings, infarction of the medial nucleus or a prefrontal lobotomy has been used as a therapeutic procedure to relieve emotional distress. (See Chapter 22.)

Lateral dorsal nucleus. This nucleus and the anterior nucleus are surrounded by the rostral portion of the internal medullary lamina of the thalamus and should be considered a caudal continuation of the anterior nuclear group. This nucleus projects to the rostral cingulate cortex and onto the parahippocampal gyrus. This nucleus projects to the anterior cingulate gyrus (areas 23, 24, 32) and receives input from the hypothalamus, habenula, and cingulate cortex. Stimulation or ablation of this nuclear complex alters blood pressure and may have an effect on memory.

SPECIFIC ASSOCIATIONAL—MULTI MODAL/ SOMATIC NUCLEI: THE PULVINAR NUCLEI

Pulvinar Nuclei

1. The pulvinar (Fig. 15.4) is the largest nucleus in the thalamus and is continuous with the posterior part of the lateral division. All the major ascending sensory pathways have some terminations in the medial and lateral nuclei; the pulvinar, therefore, is the major multimodal associational.

    a. The pulvinar is divided into three major nuclei: the medial pulvinar nucleus, the lateral pulvinar nucleus, and the inferior pulvinar nucleus:

1) The medial pulvinar nucleus projects onto the prefrontal and anterior temporal limbic cortex.

2) The lateral pulvinar nucleus projects onto supramarginal, angular, and posterior temporal lobe. Because of the strong projections of the lateral pulvinar nucleus onto the cortex surrounding the posterior end of the lateral sulcus, lesions in the pulvinar in the dominant hemisphere produce disturbances in language.

3) The inferior pulvinar nucleus projects onto the visual association cortex, areas 18 and 19, V2 and V3.

b. Pulvinar and the dorsal visual stream. Humans possess two distinct visual systems (Milner and Goodale, 2008) that exit the occipital lobe: the ventral stream and dorsal stream: (1) the ventral stream, ("what pathway") travels to the temporal lobe and is involved with object identification and recognition, while the (2) dorsal stream ("how pathway") terminates in the parietal lobe and is involved with processing the object's spatial location (Ungerleider and Mishkin, 1982).

c. Blindsight: *Awareness without sight*. The dorsal stream that bypasses V1, and goes from the retina—superior colliculus—pulvinar—parietal cortex and areas 18 and 19 may be the basis of awareness without sight. The primate retina, including that of humans, sends its major neural output (after a relay in the LGN of the thalamus) to the visual cortex ("V1," "striate cortex"). When the striate cortex is removed or blocked in monkeys, the animals can still carry out visual discriminations, although their capacity changes in certain ways. That they can still do so is perhaps not surprising because the output from the eye also reaches a number of other brain targets lying in the midbrain and thalamus that remain intact even when V1 is entirely removed. In recent years it has become evident that monkeys without primary visual cortex, area V1, can discriminate shapes, demonstrate contrast sensitivity, and have measurable acuity, although reduced from normal. Human subjects with lesions in V1 are phenomenally blind, and they do have some residual function (Weiskrantz, Cowey, and LeMare, 1998).

Patient GY has a lesion in left V1 (De Gelder, Pourtois, and Weiskrantz, 2002). He reports being blind to objects in the right visual field, yet he can correctly point to and grasp them. Functional magnetic resonance imaging (fMRI) scans of patient GY shows activity in extrastriate visual areas (areas 18 and 19) when stimuli were presented in the "blind" region. Without V1, these signals probably go through the dorsal pathway. So damage to V1 can lead to sight without awareness (blindsight). But damage to the (usually right) parietal lobe can lead to the opposite problem, called *anosognosia*. These patients can be blind, but they insist that they can see. They will often confabulate stories or excuses to prevent them from demonstrating their disability.

d. Diffusion MRI, also referred to as diffusion tensor imaging or DTI, has been applied clinically in the study of neurological disorders, especially for the management of patients with acute stroke (Oppenheimer et al., 2007; Vargas et al., 2009). It can reveal abnormalities in white matter fiber structure and provide models of brain connectivity; therefore, it is rapidly becoming a standard for white matter disorders. The ability to visualize anatomical connections between different parts of the brain, noninvasively and on an individual basis, has emerged as a major new focus on neural pathways leading to the *Human Brain Connectome* project (NIH, NINCDS). DTI tractography study in humans reveals connections between the pulvinar and cortical and subcortical areas, including the superior colliculus and caudate, as also noted in previous primate studies. The connections to the superior colliculus and caudate were observed in DTI tractography, suggesting that the pulvinar plays an important role in human visual information processing and visual spatial attention as it does in nonhuman primates and cats.

e. Pulvinar sign: diagnosing variant of Creutzfeldt-Jakob disease.

Creutzfeldt-Jakob disease (vCJD) causes a rapidly progressive dementia that may be associated with other neurologic and psychiatric features such as cerebellar or visual disturbance (see also Chapter 3 discussion on prions) and is similar to bovine spongiform encephalopathy. Presently, the diagnosis of variant CJD can be confirmed only at postmortem examination. However, there is a characteristic abnormality seen in the posterior thalamic region (the "pulvinar sign"), which is highly sensitive and specific for variant CJD. In cases of CJD, symmetrical hyperintensity in the pulvinar nuclei of the thalamus (pulvinar sign) on brain magnetic resonance images was described as a specific, noninvasive, diagnostic sign of vCJD. Electroencephalography and cerebrospinal fluid analysis for 14-3-3 protein are also useful as diagnostic aids. The pulvinar sign has been found in more than 90% of pathologically proven CJD cases. The differential diagnosis for abnormal findings in this region of the thalamus includes bilateral thalamic infarcts, vasculitis, perinatal ischemic insult, deposition of iron or copper, and neoplastic infiltration—particularly of lymphoma or glioma.

SPECIAL SENSORY NUCLEI—METATHALAMUS: VISION AND AUDITION, THE LATERAL GENCULATE, AND MEDIAL GENCULATE NUCLEI

1. *Audition* (also see Chapter 11). The medial geniculate nucleus (MGN) is located on the most caudal portion of the thalamus receives the ascending auditory fibers originating from the following nuclei: cochlear, trapezoid,

superior olivary, lateral lemniscal, and inferior colliculus. Auditory fibers end on the medial geniculate pars parvocellular.

Vestibular fibers end in the magnocellular portion of the medial geniculate and are projected onto postcentral gyrus. This nucleus projects to area 41 in the temporal lobe, the transverse temporal gyrus of Heschl. The ventral nucleus of the medial geniculate receives input from the inferior colliculus.

2. *Vision* (also see Chapter 23)

   a. Cortical projections. The lateral geniculate nucleus (LGN) is a horseshoe-shaped six-layered nucleus with its hilus on its ventromedial surface. The LGN receives the optic tract and projects to areas 17 and 18. Figure 15.5 demonstrates the visual radiation onto the calcarine cortex of the occipital lobe. This nucleus contains the six neuronal layers separated by bands of myelinated axons. The four outer layers contain small- to medium-sized cells that project onto layer IV of the striate cortex; the two innermost layers contain large cells (magnocellular) projecting onto layer I and the deep portion of layer IV of area 17. Crossed fibers of the optic tract terminate in laminae 1, 4, and 6, while uncrossed fibers end in laminae 2, 3, and 5. This nucleus also connects with the inferior pulvinar, ventral, and lateral thalamic nuclei.

   b. Connections to midbrain. Some optic fibers proceed directly to the pretectal area and the superior colliculus with or without synapsing in the lateral geniculate nucleus. There they partake in the light reflex and accommodation reflex (see Chapter 23).

   c. Retino-hypothalamic fibers from the optic nerve go directly to the suprachiasmatic nucleus of the hypothalamus. This nucleus regulates circadian rhythms, and couples the rhythms to the light/dark cycles.

NONSPECIFIC ASSOCIATIONAL

The thalamic reticular nucleus forms a cap around the thalamus, medial to the internal capsule. All fibers systems leaving the thalamus and projecting onto the cerebral cortex and the fibers coming back from these same cortical areas pass through this nuclear complex with many specific systems terminating in this nucleus. This nucleus contains GABA-ergic neurons and has a modulating effect on thalamic neurons.

The midline thalamic nuclei (Fig. 15.4) are located in the periventricular gray above the hypothalamic sulcus. They are small and difficult to delimit in human beings, but these nuclei are intimately connected to the hypothalamus and the intralaminar nuclei, and their function must be interrelated. The intralaminar nuclei (Figs. 15.3 and 15.4) are found in the internal medullary laminae of the thalamus. The most prominent intralaminar nucleus is the posteriorly placed centromedian, which is located in the metathalamic region between the medial and ventral posterior nuclei and receives many nociceptive fibers. The centromedian nucleus has a strong projection to VA and VL and has a direct projection to the caudate and putamen, which permits interrelationship with the extrapyramidal motor system (see Chapter 17).

The parafascicular nucleus is also easily delimited because it is at the dorsomedial edge of the habenulopeduncular tract. The intralaminar nuclei receive input from many regions throughout the central nervous system, including ascending axons from the reticular nuclei, indirect spinothalamic pathways, midbrain limbic nuclei, subthalamus, and hypothalamus, as well as other thalamic nuclei. The intralaminar nuclei have some direct projections onto the frontal lobe; however, their major influence is on the cerebral cortex by their connections to the specific thalamic nuclei.

Recruiting Response

Electrical stimulation of the intralaminar nuclei activates neurons throughout the ipsilateral cerebral hemisphere. As the stimulation continues, more and more cortical neurons fire, which is called the recruiting response, and there is a waxing and waning, with the response finally peaking then decreasing, but it may increase again.

In Table 15.2, the principal thalamic nuclei are grouped as to the type of modality that reaches the individual nuclei. This table demonstrates that the thalamus receives input from gray matter in the spinal cord, brain stem, cerebellum, and cerebrum. The type of input is identified functionally as sensory, motor, limbic, or associational.

WHITE MATTER OF THE DIENCEPHALON

At the lateral margin of the diencephalon is the major white matter bundle that connects the diencephalon and the cerebrum: the internal capsule (Fig. 15.6).

The internal capsule is a large myelinated region that marks the border between the diencephalon and telencephalon. The internal capsule, consisting of the anterior limb, genu, and posterior limb, is best visualized in a horizontal

Figure 15.5 Horizontal section, demonstrating the ant. limb, genu, and post limb of the internal capsule. Note the putamen and globus pallidus are external to the internal capsule. Magnetic resonance imaging (MRI), T2 weighted.

Table 15.2 FUNCTIONAL GROUPS OF THALAMIC NUCLEI

MODALITY	NUCLEI
Sensory relay	Nuclei: ventral posterior medial (touch and taste), ventral posterior lateral (touch and vestibular), medial geniculate (hearing), and lateral geniculate (vision). Input from ascending specific sensory modalities and project to cortical area subserving that modality.
Motor relay	Nuclei: ventral lateral and ventral anterior. Input from the contralateral cerebellar hemispheres, superior cerebellar peduncle, medial globus pallidus, and the nigrostriatal fibers from the area compacta of the substantia nigra.
Limbic	Nuclei: dorsal medial, anterior, and lateral dorsal. Input well-defined from the mammillothalamic tract of the Papez circuit and project onto the prefrontal and cingulate gyrus.
Specific associational	Nuclei: dorsal medial, lateral, and pulvinar. Forms the bulk of the thalamus. Input multimodal and projects onto cortical areas that also receive a multimodal intracortical associational input.
Nociceptive	Nuclei: dorsomedial, VPL, and posterior. Input from ascending anterolateral system, spinothalamic, spinoreticular and spinomesencephalic.
Nonspecific associational	Nuclei: intralaminar, midline, and reticular. Input from diverse subcortical regions, including the reticular formation, visceral brain, and corpus striatum, project to specific thalamic nuclei or associational areas in the cortex.

section, where it forms an obtuse angle. All fibers projecting from the thalamus onto the cerebral hemispheres must pass through this region, while all fibers leaving the cerebral cortex and going either to the diencephalon, basal nuclei, brain stem, or spinal cord must also pass through its parts. In the following diagrammatic horizontal section, the three major parts of the internal capsule are identified and their constituent fiber systems discussed: the anterior limb, genu, and posterior limb (Fig. 15.6).

1. *Anterior limb of internal capsule* lies between the caudate nucleus and putamen, and this portion of the capsule contains the anterior thalamic radiation and the frontopontine fibers.

2. *Genu of internal capsule* is found at the rostral end of the diencephalon on the lateral wall of the lateral ventricle and is the point at which the fibers are displaced laterally by the increasing bulk of the diencephalon. The corticobulbar fibers are found in the genu.

3. *Posterior limb of the internal capsule* consists of three subdivisions: thalamolentiform, sublenticular, and retrolenticular:

   a. The thalamolenticular portion (between the thalamus and lenticular nuclei) contains the corticospinal, corticorubral, corticothalamic, thalamoparietal, and superior thalamic radiations.

   b. The sublentiform portion (passing inferiorly and posteriorly) includes the posterior thalamic radiations that include optic radiation (Fig. 15.6), acoustic radiation, corticotectal, and temporal pontine fibers.

   c. The retrolenticular portion (passing posteriorly into the temporal and occipital lobes) contains the posterior thalamic radiation to the occipital and temporal lobes and the parieto-occipital fasciculus. Within the diencephalon many other myelinated fiber bundles can be identified (Table 15.3).

Table 15.3 MAJOR FIBER BUNDLES ASSOCIATED WITH THE DIENCEPHALON

PATHWAY	CONNECTIONS
External medullary lamina	Includes fibers of medial lemniscus, superior cerebellar peduncle, spinothalamics, and pathways Between cerebral cortex and thalamus
Fornix	Subiculum and hippocampus to septum and hypothalamus (part of Papez Circuit)
Habenulopeduncular	Habenula to interpeduncular nucleus and tegmentum of midbrain
Internal capsule i	Includes, anterior, genu, and posterior limbs. Connects thalamus and cerebral cortex, and cerebral cortex to brain stem and spinal cord
Internal medullary lamina	Contains mammillothalamic, ascending reticular and spinothalamic fibers
Mammillothalamic	Mammillary bodies with anterior thalamic nuclei (part of Papez Circuit)
Mammillary peduncle	Mammillary nuclei with tegmentum of midbrain

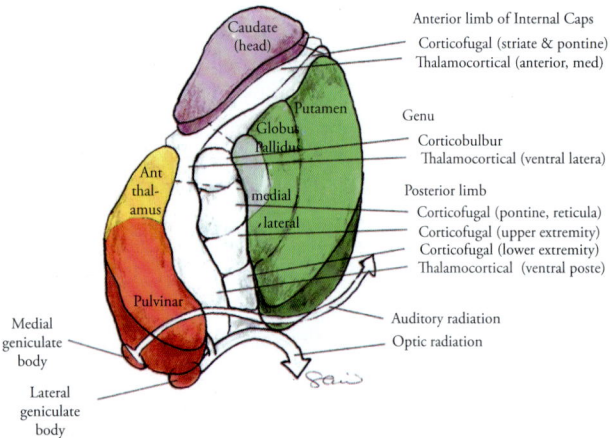

Figure 15.6 Horizontal section through diencephalon. The major fiber tracts in the right internal capsule are labeled. (Modified after Carpenter Core Text, Williams and Wilkins, 1992.)

RELATIONSHIP BETWEEN THE THALAMUS AND THE CEREBRAL CORTEX

The thalamus has several major roles (Table 15.4):

1. To receive input from the brain stem, cerebellum, and corpus striatum
2. To project this information, after some processing, onto the cerebrum
3. To receive reciprocal projections from the same cerebral areas. The relationship between many thalamic nuclei and specific cortical areas is so intimate that when a cortical region is destroyed the neurons in a particular thalamic nucleus atrophy (Walker, 1938). This degeneration is a consequence of the thalamic projection and its reciprocal from the cortex, being restricted to only a single specific cortical region, and is seen in portions of the following nuclei: anterior, ventral lateral, ventral posterior, lateral geniculate, medial geniculate, and magnocellular portion of the medial, dorsal, and pulvinar. The intralaminar, midline, posterior portions of the pulvinar, and medial nuclei are unaffected by cortical lesions (Fig. 15.7).

THALAMIC INPUT ONTO THE SIX-LAYERED CEREBRAL CORTEX

The most important input the cerebral cortex receives is from the thalamus onto layer iv of the six-layered neocortex; the densest input from the specific relay projectional nuclei (e.g., VPL, VPM) is to granular cells in layer iv, but pyramidal cells in layers iii and v many also receive direct or indirect inputs.

Layer i receives from the nonspecific nuclei (midline and intralaminar).

Layers ii and iii receives input from the opposite hemisphere via the corpus callosum and from adjacent ipsilateral areas.

Layer v projects subcortically to spinal cord and brain stem, while layer vi projects back to the thalamus.

There is a modality-specific columnar arrangement. With many nuclei having an extensive input onto the cortex, there is always a reciprocal cortical input.

THALAMIC RADIATIONS AND THE INTERNAL CAPSULE

The fibers that reciprocally interconnect the cortex and the thalamus form the thalamic radiations (Fig. 15.6). The thalamic radiations are grouped in the internal capsule into four peduncles: anterior, superior, posterior, and inferior.

1. Anterior radiation: connects frontal lobe and cingulate cortex with median and anterior thalamic nuclei. This is an extensive projection.
2. Superior radiation: connects motor sensory strip and adjacent frontal and parietal lobes with fibers from the ventrobasal nuclei. This is also a large projection.
3. Posterior radiation: connects occipital and posterior parietal areas with pulvinar, and lateral geniculate nucleus (geniculocalcarine radiations—optic radiations). This is an extensive radiation due to the optic radiations.
4. Inferior radiation: connections from medial geniculate (auditory radiations) and pulvinar with temporal lobe. This is the smallest group of fibers between the thalamus and cortex.

In Figure 15.7 the afferents and efferents of the individual thalamic nuclei are presented.

In Figure 15.8 we have shown the cortical projections of the same thalamic nuclei.

In Figures 15.9, 15.10, 15.11, and 15.12 we discuss the major afferent pathways to the thalamus and metathalamus.

Table 15.4 CORTICAL PROJECTIONS OF MAJOR THALAMIC NUCLEI

NUCLEUS	CORTICAL PROJECTION	FUNCTION
Anterior and lateral dorsal	Cingulate and parahippocampal gyrus	Limbic
Medial dorsal	Prefrontal and limbic rostral temporal	Limbic
Lateral geniculate	Calcarine cortex of occipital lobe area 17	Vision
Medial geniculate	Transverse temporal gyri of superior temporal gyri, areas 41 and 42	Audition
Lateral posterior	Superior parietal lobule	Sensory associational (body image)
Pulvinar	Medial pulvinar N.>prefrontal and anterior temporal. Lateral pulvinar N.>language areas- supramarginal, angular, and post temp. Inferior pulvinar N.>visual associational areas 18 and 19	
Ventral anterior	Premotor area 6 and 8	Motor organizational
Ventral lateral	Precentral area 4	Primary motor cortex
Ventral posterior	Postcentral area 3-1-2	Primary somatic sensory area

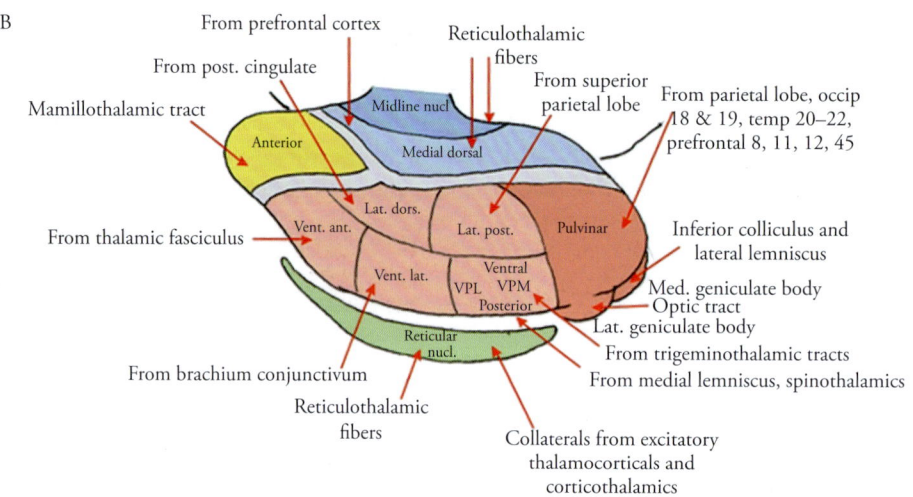

Figure 15.7 Representation of the thalamic nuclei: (*A*) showing connections of ventrobasal, midline, anterior, lateral nuclei, and geniculate nuclei; (*B*) demonstrating connections of lateral dorsal, lateral posterior, and pulvinar nuclei. (After Truex, R.C., and Carpenter, M.B.: Human Neuroanatomy. Baltimore, Williams and Wilkins, 1970.)

In Table 15.4, we have summarized the cortical projections of the major thalamic nuclei and also included the functions of these regions.

OTHER POSSIBLE INPUTS TO THE THALAMUS

In addition to the major pathways discussed earlier, there are other subcortical sources of input onto the cerebral cortex that pass through the diencephalon, and they may well have modulating effects on the thalamus (see discussion in Chapter 17). These include the following:

1. Noradrenergic (norepinephrine) pathway from the locus ceruleus of the midbrain projecting in primates predominantly to layer vi of the motor and somatosensory cortex and related frontal and parietal association cortex.
2. Serotoninergic pathway from the raphe nuclei in the pons and medulla and the pontine reticular formation.
3. Dopaminergic pathways from ventral tegmental—rostral mesencephalic nuclear groups. The strongest projection is to the prefrontal cortex and limbic system.
4. Cholinergic pathways from the basal forebrain nucleus of Meynert project widely to cerebral cortex.
5. GABA-ergic pathways from basal forebrain, ventral tegmental area, and zona incerta to sensory and motor cortex.

THALAMIC CLINICAL CONSIDERATIONS

The thalamus is the final processing station for systems that project to the cerebral cortex; thus, it serves an important integrative function. Many sensations are first crudely appreciated at thalamic levels, including pain, touch, taste, and vibration. The discriminative processes associated with these sensations, as well as tactile discrimination, vision, audition, and taste, are elevated to consciousness in the cerebral hemisphere. Glutamate is the principal transmitter in the thalamus.

Thalamic Syndrome (of Dejerine)

In the human a large lesion in the thalamus results in the thalamic syndrome, causing diminished sensation on the contralateral half of the head and body. (Complete anesthesia results from injury to the ventral posterior lateral nucleus.)

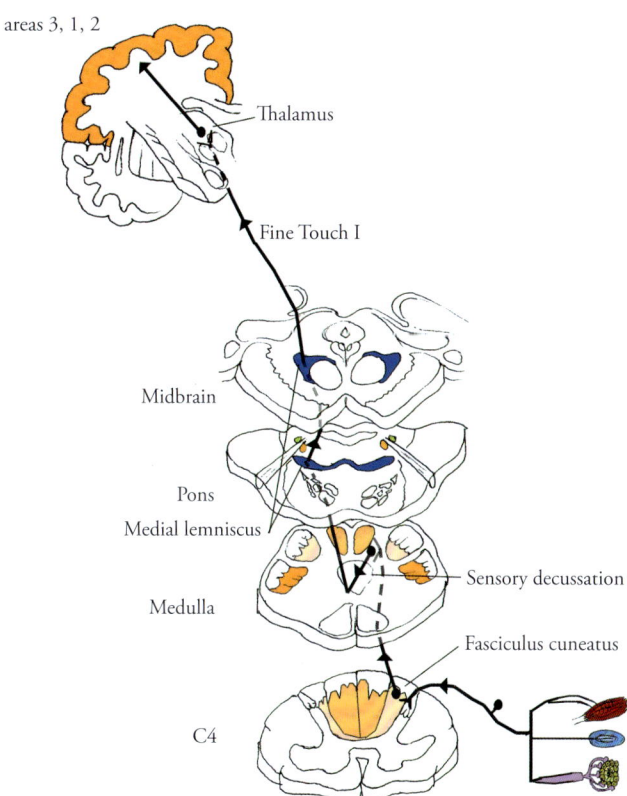

Figure 15.10 Medial lemniscus—general somatic tactile sensation.

Some pain and temperature sensation from the contralateral side of the body may be retained. The internal capsule is usually involved, producing an upper-motor-neuron lesion of the contralateral limb. The thresholds for pain, temperature, touch, and pressure are usually elevated contralaterally. A mild sensory stimulus now produces exaggerated sensory responses on the affected side and may even cause intractable pain.

A change in emotional response may also be noted. Lesions restricted to the medial thalamic nucleus produce memory (Chapter 30) and personality disturbances (Chapter 22); lesions in the lateral nuclei produce sensory deficits (see Chapter 21).

The following case (Fig. 15.9) is an example of the thalamic syndrome of Dejerine from a patient of Dr. Thomas Sabin.

Figure 15.8 Thalamic projections onto cerebral cortex. (*A*) Projections onto lateral surface of a cerebral hemisphere; (*B*) projections onto medial surface of cerebral hemisphere.

Figure 15.9 Computerized tomography (CT) of a 63-year-old patient with the thalamic syndrome of Dejerine. (Courtesy of Dr. Thomas Sabin, Tufts University School of Medicine.)

CASE HISTORY 15.1

A 63-year-old man reported that while taking his morning shower, he noted a sensation of numbness over the right side of his body. This persisted while he shaved and combed his hair. He had no visual symptom or paralysis. He could not feel the shower striking the right side of the body and face nor could he perceive its temperature. He had a history of type 2 diabetes mellitus and hypertension. He was taken by ambulance to Tufts Medical Center and emergency head computerized tomography (CT) scan revealed a thalamic hemorrhage on the left side. He admitted to not being fully compliant with his medications. These included valsartan 160 mg daily, metformin, rosuvastatin, and glyburide. He noted hourly improvement of his numbness, but he was "nowhere near normal." He had a 15-pack-per-year history of smoking. He had no fever, chest pain, palpitations, cough, rashes, or bladder-bowel dysfunction.

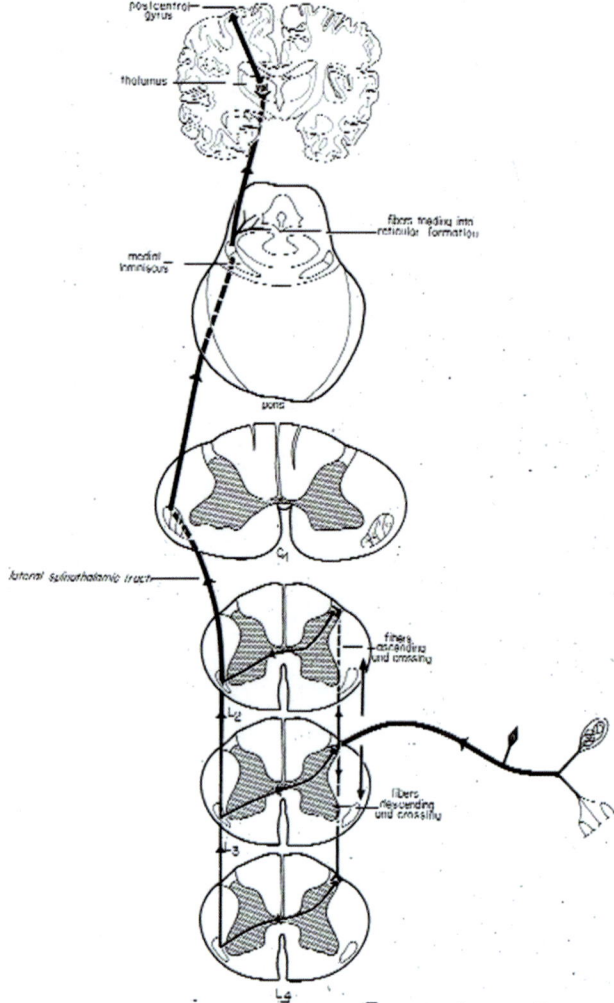

Figure 15.11 Trigeminal lemniscus—general somatic tactile sensation and pain from the head and neck.

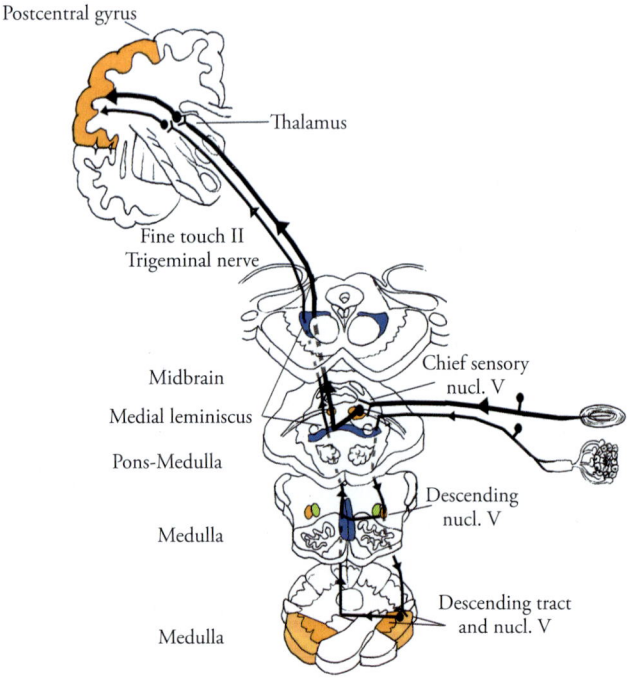

Figure 15.12 Trigeminal lemnsicus, showing the trigeminothalamic pathway.

Physical Examination

Vital signs: P 78; BP 148/92; RR 18 T afebrile. Alert, pleasant, and cooperative.

HEENT: Conjunctiva clear; sclera nonicteric.

Neck: No stiffness. No carotid bruit.

CVS: Normal rhythm and no murmurs.

Pulmonary: Clear to auscultation.

Abdomen: Soft without masses or tenderness.

Neurological Examination

Fully oriented without aphasia, apraxia, or agnosia. No right-left confusion or extinction.

Cranial nerves: Fundi showed AV nicking but no hemorrhages or papilledema.

Pupils round, equal, and responsive to light and accommodation. Extraocular movements full and conjugate. There was decreased sensation to temperature pinprick and touch over the right face.

Motor exam showed normal strength tone and bulk bilaterally. The deep tendon reflexes were 2+ throughout. There was diminished temperature, position, and touch sensation on the right side.

Gait testing showed a tendency to drift to the right when standing with feet together and eyes closed.

Laboratory Data

His routine labs were all normal, and no coagulation abnormality was found. A transthoracic echocardiogram was normal. His CT scan showed a 2.3 cm intraparenchymal hemorrhage in the region of the left thalamus with surrounding edema and minor mass effect without extension into the ventricles or subarachnoid space.

Hospital course: He was admitted to the neurointensive care unit to observe for extension of bleeding or edema. He became mildly confused for 36 hours, but then he was transferred to rehabilitation for help with his gait. The sensory loss improved, but he became very bothered by a sensation of numbness which he could not further describe. This feeling was most intense in the right face and hand.

A month after discharge he was seen in the outpatient department and was still obsessing about the abnormal sensations. He did get some relief from large doses of gabapentin. After a year and trials of other anticonvulsant medications and amitriptyline he was still complaining about the disturbing sensations and transferred his care to another institution to seek further relief.

SUBTHALAMUS

The subthalamus region is included in the diencephalon, but functionally it is part of the basal ganglia. The subthalamic nucleus, zona incerta, and prerubral field together form the subthalamus. This region is medial to the posterior limb of the internal capsule, lateral to the hypothalamus, and below the thalamus. The ansa lenticularis, subthalamic fasciculus, lenticular fasciculus, and thalamic fasciculus provide input from the globus pallidus to the subthalamus. The zona incerta lies between the thalamus and lenticular fasciculus. The adjacent substantia nigra also projects onto the subthalamus. The medial portion of the globus pallidus provides the principal input to the subthalamus via the subthalamic fasciculus, which runs through the internal capsule. The motor and premotor cortex also project to this region. The subthalamus projects back to both segments of

Table 15.5 **MAJOR SUBCORTICAL PATHWAYS WITHIN THE BRAIN STEM AND DIENCEPHALON**

	FUNCTIONS
I. SENSORY PATHWAYS:	
Anterolateral system: spinothalamic, spinoreticular tract (Fig. 15.12)	Pain (fine and crude) and Temperature from body
Cerebellar peduncles: Figure 11.1; Chapter 20 – superior cerebellar>thalamus and basal ganglia, – middle cerebellar<input from cerebrum via pons, – inferior cerebellar peduncles<>spinal cord and brain stem.	Proprioception and modulation of movements
Cranial nerve VIII: Auditory pathway—cochlear nuclei via lateral lemniscus > inferior colliculus, brachium of inferior colliculus > medial geniculate > auditory cortex (Chapter 11), Figure 15.13	Audition and auditory reflexes
Cranial nerve VIII: Vestibular pathway (part of proprioceptive pathway); lateral vestibular nucleus to ventral posterior and MGN then to postcentral gyrus (Chapter 11); Figure 15.14	Proprioception
Medial lemniscus (Fig. 15.10)	Tactile discrimination and proprioception from body
Solitary tract	Taste (via CN VII, IX, X) and general sensation from the viscera
Spinocerebellar and cuneocerebellar (Fig. 6.34A)	Unconscious proprioception to cerebellum
Trigeminothalamic (Fig. 15.11)	Pain and temperature and tactile discrimination from head and neck (CN V, VII, IX, X)
II. MOTOR PATHWAYS	
Corticospinal (Fig. 18.22)	Voluntary control of muscles in limbs, thorax and abdomen
Corticonuclear/corticobulbar (Fig. 18.21)	Voluntary control of muscles of: – Facial expression by innervation of cranial nerves V, VII, and IX-XII – Larynx and pharynx by CN IX and X – Tongue by CN X and XII
Corticomesencephalic (Fig. 18.21)	Voluntary control of eye movements by innervation of CN III, IV, and VI.
Descending sympathetic and parasympathetics	Autonomic modulation of CN VII, IX, X: T12-L2; and S2-S4
Medial longitudinal fasciculus (MLF)	Coordinate eye movements in brain stem via CN III, IV, VI
Monamine containing norepinephrine, dopaminergic, serotonergic	Set tone in motor system, affect limbic system
Reticular	Limbic (emotional)
Rubrospinal, rubronuclear, tectospinal, and tectonuclear	Backup to voluntary motor system

the globus pallidus, and substantia nigra via the subthalamic fasciculus, and projects to the thalamus and contralateral subthalamus. The glutaminergic cells in the subthalamus form the main excitatory projection from the basal ganglia. In the human, a lesion in the subthalamus, usually vascular in origin, produces hemiballismus: purposeless, involuntary, violent, flinging movements of the contralateral extremity. These movements persist during wakefulness but disappear during sleep. This lesion represents underactivity in the indirect pathway in contrast to overactivity that produces Parkinsonism (see Chapter 18).

THE MAJOR SENSORY PATHWAYS ENDING IN THE THALAMUS

This discussion will focus on the sensory systems that form the bulk of the afferents to the thalamus. The voluntary motor pathways (corticospinal and corticobulbar) are discussed in Chapter 18, and the sensory and motor system related to the cerebellum are discussed in Chapter 20.

1. Basic principle of sensory system: All sensory systems have three neurons:

   a. *First-order neuron* in periphery in the dorsal root ganglion or ganglion of cranial nerves V, VII, IX, X, with their axons ipsilateral.

   b. *Second-order neuron* within central nervous system, spinal cord, or brain stem; its axon crosses to the contralateral side.

   c. *Third-order neuron* within thalamus is the final neuron in the sensory systems and its axons reach the cerebral cortex.

The ascending sensory fibers from the body for touch (posterior columns), from the face for touch and pain (trigeminothalamic), and from the viscera for general and special sensation ascend in the medial lemniscus to the dorsal thalamus.

2. The major sensory pathways ending in the thalamus.

POSTERIOR COLUMNS (FASCICULUS GRACILIS AND CUNEATUS)

This fiber bundle originates from tactile and proprioceptive receptors. *The primary and secondary cell bodies are on the ipsilateral side of the spinal cord. The secondary neurons are found in the medulla.* The posterior columns—the fasciculus gracilis and the fasciculus cuneatus (Fig. 15.10)—conduct proprioception (position sense), vibration sensation, tactile discrimination, object recognition, deep touch (pressure) awareness, and two-point discrimination from the neck, thorax, abdomen, pelvis, and extremities. The sensory receptors for the system are the Golgi tendon organs, muscle spindles, proprioceptors, tactile discs, and Pacinian corpuscles (deep touch or pressure). The *primary cell body* is located in the dorsal root ganglion.

The well-myelinated fibers of this system enter the spinal cord as the medial division of the dorsal root and bifurcate into ascending and descending portions, which enter the dorsal column. The fasciculus gracilis contains fibers from the sacral, lumbar, and lower thoracic levels, while the fasciculus cuneatus contains fibers from the upper thoracic and cervical levels. Fibers from the sacral levels are the first to enter and lie most medial, followed by lumbar, thoracic, and finally, cervical fibers. The primary axons ascend in the dorsal columns of the spinal cord to the secondary cell body of this system located in the nucleus gracilis and the nucleus cuneatus in the lower medullary levels.

From the *secondary cell bodies* the fibers cross the midline, join the medial lemniscus, and ascend to the ventral posterior lateral nucleus in the thalamus. From this thalamic nucleus these fibers are projected to the postcentral gyrus (areas 1, 2, 3). Fibers also descend in the dorsal columns, but their functional significance is unknown. The fibers responsible for proprioception cross in the medial lemniscus. The fibers for vibration sensation and tactile discrimination ascend bilaterally in the medial lemniscus to the ventral posterior lateral nucleus. Consequently, a unilateral lesion can abolish proprioception, but tactile discrimination and vibration sensation will not be entirely lost.

Clinical Lesions

The secondary axons cross the midline and ascend in the contralateral medial lemniscus to the ventral posterior lateral nucleus (VPL) in the thalamus. In the spinal cord the posterior columns are uncrossed and divided into the medial gracile fasciculus (lower extremity) and the lateral cuneate fasciculus (upper extremity). Fibers from the upper extremity form 50% of the posterior columns with the lower extremity 25% and the remainder from the thorax and abdomen. These fibers cross in the sensory decussation and form the bulk of the medial lemniscus along with trigeminal and other fibers.

Injury to the posterior column appears not to affect pressure sense, but vibration sense, two-point discrimination, and tactile discrimination are diminished or abolished, depending on the extent of the lesion. Interruption of the medial fibers (cervical-hand region) affects the ability to recognize differences in the shape and weight of objects placed in the hand. Since the extremities are more sensitive to these modalities than any other body regions, position sense is impaired more severely in the extremities than elsewhere, and the person has trouble identifying small passive movements of the limbs. Consequently, performance of voluntary acts is impaired and movements are clumsy (sensory ataxia). Lesions in lateral fibers of the posterior column, gracilis, may be devastating due to the interruption of one of the most important sensory mechanisms: the ability to detect the sole of the foot. This is a major handicap in walking in a dimly lit or dark room, in driving a car, and so on. The discussion of the analysis of tactile information in the cerebral cortex is found in Chapter 21 with several cases also illustrating lesions in this region of the brain.

ANTEROLATERAL/SPINOTHALMIC PATHWAYS-PAIN PATHWAY

Anterolateral pathways: pain pathways (Fig. 15.12). Anterolateral pathway = spinothalamic, spinotectal, spinoreticular. This tract conducts pain and temperature sensation from the neck, thorax, abdomen, pelvis, and extremities. The receptors for pain are the naked free nerve endings, and the corpuscles of Ruffini and of Krause detect warmth and cold. The primary cell bodies are located in the dorsal root ganglion; the axons enter the spinal cord and ascend or descend one segment ipsilaterally before ending on neurons in the dorsal horn lamina 1 to 3. The axons of the secondary cells cross in the anterior commissure of the spinal cord and ascend in the ventrolateral part of the lateral funiculus in the spinal cord and medulla. In the pons they are found at the lateral margin of the medial lemniscus and continue up to the ventral posterior lateral nucleus and the intralaminar nuclei of the dorsal thalamus. The axons in this tract convey information from the contralateral side.

The pain fibers in this tract are arranged segmentally with the most lateroposterior fibers representing the lowest part of the sacral levels of the body, and the more medioanterior fibers representing the upper extremities and neck. The temperature fibers have this same arrangement but are internal to the pain fibers. For surgical relief of pain this tract is located by identifying the denticulate ligament and then sectioning about 1 mm below the ligament (Fig. 6.29). The sharp pain noted with most injuries is associated with the heavily myelinated direct, or spinothalamic, pathway to the ventral posterior lateral nucleus. In addition to the stabbing pain, dull throbbing pain is usually noted; it is carried up more slowly by a multisynaptic pathway, probably via the reticular system, and is called the spinoreticulothalamic pathway. A unilateral lesion of the spinothalamic tract in the spinal cord produces an almost complete absence of pain (analgesia) and temperature sensation (thermoanesthesia) on the contralateral side. At the upper pontine levels, the lateral spinothalamic tract is usually closely associated with the medial lemniscus. Consequently, a unilateral lesion at these levels diminishes pain and temperature sensation from the opposite side of the body—as well as touch, vibration sensation, and proprioception.

a. Anterior spinothalamic tract—light touch. Light touch awareness from the neck, thorax, pelvis, and extremities is carried up the anterior spinothalamic tract (Fig. 15.11). The primary neuron is located in the dorsal root ganglion; the secondary neuron is located in the dorsal horn of the same side. The secondary fibers ascend contralaterally in the lateral funiculus, joining the medial lemniscus at the upper pontine levels. Stroking a hairless area of the skin with cotton evokes light touch. Lesions involving this tract produce no definite clinical deficiencies, probably because somewhat similar sensations are also carried in the uncrossed dorsal columns (fine touch, pressure).

b. Anterolateral pathway—lateral spinothalamic fibers. The pain pathway. Originate from pain and temperature receptors in the skin. Primary cell bodies are dorsal root ganglia of the spinal cord; the entering fibers ascend and descend for several levels in Lissauer's tract on the surface of the dorsal horn. The axons synapse in the secondary nuclei, in nucleus proprius in lamina II and III of the ipsilateral dorsal horn nuclei, cross within three spinal cord segments, and form the spinothalamic fibers in the anterolateral region of the spinal cord. These fibers pass into the thalamus.

The direct pathway, for localizing the pain on the body, ends in VPL, which projects onto postcentral gyrus. How one responds to pain comes from the indirect pain pathway that ascends to the dorsomedial thalamic nucleus and is then projected onto the prefrontal gyrus.

TRACTS ORIGINATING FROM SECONDARY TRIGEMINAL NUCLEI IN THE BRAIN STEM

Above all, remember that the primary cells of the trigeminal nerve are located in the trigeminal ganglion in Meckel's cave in the middle cranial fossa. This is the largest cranial nerve in the brain stem and has three divisions: ophthalmic (V1), maxillary (V2), and mandibular (V3). Each of these divisions brings in sensation from pain, temperature, touch, and pressure receptors in the skin, muscles, and sinuses they innervate.

1. *Proprioception from the head: mesencephalic nucleus of V.* These unique primary cell bodies are located not only in the trigeminal ganglion but also within the pons and midbrain along the ascending trigeminal rootlets, where they form the mesencephalic nucleus of nerve V. The primary axons project to the motor nucleus of nerve V and the reticular formation. Axons are also projected to the cerebellum and inferior olive.

The origin of the secondary neuron is unclear (but probably the descending nucleus of nerve V). The secondary axons ascend near the medial lemniscus to the ventral posterior medial nucleus of the thalamus.

2. *Pain and temperature from the head: descending nucleus of nerve V.* This information is carried by the descending nucleus and root of nerve V. The cell bodies of primary neurons are located in the trigeminal ganglion, and the primary axons are numerous. The primary cell bodies are found in the trigeminal ganglion located in Meckel's cave in the middle cranial fossa, and the secondary cell bodies originate in the descending nucleus of nerve V. These fibers enter the pons, lie on the external surface of the descending tract of nerve V, and then terminate in the descending nucleus of nerve V. The ophthalmic fibers descend to C3, the maxillary to C1, and the mandibular to The descending or spinal nucleus is very large and extends from pons into medulla and upper cervical spinal cord. This nucleus is divided into three regions—pars-oralis (in pons), pars-interpolar (in medulla), and pars-caudalis (in cervical cord)—and are somatotopically organized with V3 dorsal, V1 ventral, and V2 intermediate. These fibers enter the spinal trigeminal nucleus external to the descending nucleus on the lateral surface of the pons (in pons and upper medulla). Fibers of cranial nerves VII, IX, and X are dorsal to V3. These fibers descend and end in the spinal trigeminal nucleus with V1 ending in pars caudalis in cervical levels, V2 to interpolar nucleus in medulla, and V3 to pars oralis in upper medulla and pons. The secondary axons ascend contralaterally in the dorsal region of the medial lemniscus to the ventral posterior medial nucleus of the thalamus or to the intralaminar nuclei.

3. *Touch and pain from the head.* The tactile fibers synapse with the chief sensory nucleus in the pons. The proprioceptive fibers (not shown) enter and ascend through pontine and midbrain levels and synapse on the mesencephalic nucleus of nerve V, which then synapses on the motor nucleus of V in the pons for the "jaw jerk." The secondary axons ascend in the medial lemniscus to the ventral posterior medial nucleus (VPM) in the thalamus. The pain fibers cross while the touch fibers run bilateral up to the thalamus and end in VPM, and are then projected onto the lower third of the postcentral gyrus.

The secondary axons leave the descending nucleus of nerve V and ascend bilaterally in the medial lemniscus to the ventral posterior medial nucleus of the thalamus. The predominant component is crossed.

4. *Tactile discrimination, vibration sensation, and pressure sense from the head: chief nucleus of V.* The cell bodies of the primary neurons are located in the trigeminal ganglion. The primary axons enter the pons and end on the main sensory nucleus of nerve V, from which the secondary axons ascend contralaterally in the medial lemniscus or ipsilaterally in the dorsal trigeminothalamic tract to the ventral posterior medial nucleus, primarily on the contralateral side of the brain stem.

Lesions in the sensory nuclei cause an absence of sensation on the same side of the head, while lesions of the tracts produce diminished sensation.

SPECIAL SENSORY: CRANIAL NERVE II AND VIII

Cranial nerve II and the visual pathway are discussed in Chapter 23, Figures 23.6 and 23.7.

a. *Cranial nerve VIII, auditory division* (Fig. 15.13). The auditory fibers terminate in the dorsal and ventral cochlear nuclei in the medulla. Each sound has a specific location on the cochlea. The termination is in a tonotopic pattern in each nucleus with the low-frequency fibers terminating ventrally and the high-frequency fibers dorsally creating a series of frequency-sensitive layers. The frequency of sounds is from 100 to 15,000 Hz. The dorsal cochlear nucleus projects contralaterally through the lateral lemniscus to the inferior colliculus, while the ventral cochlear nucleus projects bilaterally to the medial superior olivary nucleus and ipsilateral lateral superior olivary nucleus. Frequencies above 2000 Hz are recorded in the lateral superior olivary nucleus. The lateral superior olive projects to the contralateral inferior colliculus, while the medial superior olivary nucleus projects ipsilaterally to inferior colliculus, medial geniculate, and auditory cortex.

Cortical projection. The laminated ventral medial geniculate projects onto the primary auditory cortex area 41, while the dorsal medial geniculate projects onto auditory association areas 42.

b. Cranial nerve VIII–vestibular pathway. These fibers should be considered part of the proprioceptive system. The vestibular fibers originated from two ganglia: the superior and inferior ganglia of Scarpa. There are four major vestibular nuclei: superior (SVN), lateral (LVN), medial (MVN), and inferior (IVN). Trunk and limb somatosensory pathways send information to LVN, MVN, and IVN. Visual information also indirectly reaches these same nuclei. The semicircular input reaches SVN, MVN, and LVN. The utricle projects mainly to LVN, the saccule to IVN. The fastigial nucleus of the cerebellum is excitatory to the vestibular nuclei, while the cerebellar cortex is inhibitory. The vestibular nuclei project to deep layers of the superior colliculus adjacent to projections from cervical proprioceptive endings.

Cortical projection. From the LVN there is a small contralateral input to ventroposterior and medial magnocellular of MGN. Ventroposterior projects to SI arm region of 3a, while the MGN projects to area 5 and the neck region of area 2. Stimulation of either of these cortical regions produces vestibular sensations. The cortical neurons respond to both vestibular and proprioceptive stimuli from neck trunk and proximal joints and the response are excitatory for one rotation in one direction and inhibitory in the other.

TASTE AND GENERAL SENSATION FROM THE VISCERA

General sensation from the gastrointestinal system (cranial nerve X) and from the taste buds on the tongue (cranial nerves, VII, IX, and X) enters the brain stem to terminate on the nucleus solitarius in the medulla. Fibers ascend primarily uncrossed either in the central tegmental pathway or in the medial lemniscus to reach basomedial portion of ventral posterior medial (VPM) nucleus in the dorsal thalamus. Many of

Figure 15.13 Projections of the auditory portion of cranial nerve VIII onto pons, midbrain, thalamus (MGN), and finally onto the auditory cortex of the temporal lobe.

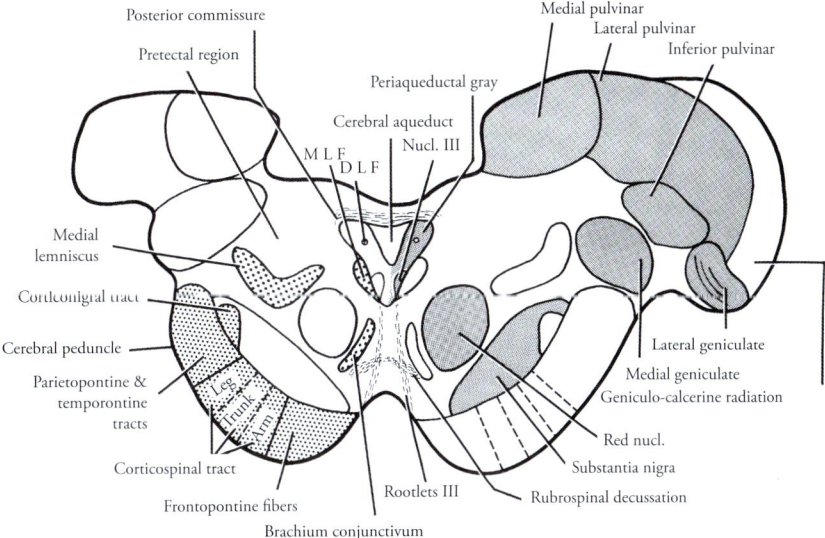

Figure 15.14 Level midbrain and posterior thalamus illustration of the junction between midbrain and thalamus showing cerebral peduncle on basis of the midbrain and the subdivisions of the pulvinar nucleus, medial geniculate (receives from cranial nerve VIII), and lateral geniculate nuclei (receives from cranial nerve II) in the posterior thalamus.

the gustatory fibers terminate in the ipsilateral parabrachial nucleus before reaching the ventrobasal portion of the VPM nucleus. The cortical region for taste is in the parietal lobe in the upper banks of the lateral sulcus.

Figure 15.13. Cranial Nerve VIII, Central connections of Auditory Division.

ATLAS OF THALAMIC LEVELS VII. THALAMIC ATLAS

The sections that follow include three levels of the thalamus and one level of the definitive caudate and putamen. In these levels note their location within the thalamus and discusses their functions (Figs. 15.14 to 15.18). At each level there will a myelin-stained section (B) with a labeled diagrammatic section (A).

Gross features. This level is near the caudal end of the thalamus with elements from the midbrain and diencephalon present.

Diencephalon occupies the bulk of this section, with the corpus callosum, fornix, and lateral ventricles forming its superior surface, and the third ventricle its medial surface. The lateral wall of the diencephalon is formed by the posterior limb of the internal capsule. The cerebral peduncles are prominent on the inferior surface; adjacent to them are the substantia nigra and more medially the red nucleus. The laminate lateral geniculate nucleus is prominent on the left side lateral to the cerebral peduncle.

Epithalamus. This nuclear grouping with its associated tracts is functionally part of the visceral brain. The habenular nuclei and stria medullaris are present on the medial surface protruding in the third ventricle. The habenulopeduncular tract is seen on the left side connecting the medial habenular nucleus to the interpeduncular nucleus. At more posterior levels, the pineal gland is seen above the habenular nuclei and commissure.

Thalamus. The bulk of the thalamus at this level consists of the pulvinar nuclei.

Which connect to the sensory associative cortex in the superior and inferior parietal lobule? A large ovoid nucleus is present about one-third of the way in from the third ventricle. This is the central median nucleus of the intralaminar group. The ascending tract of the reticular system ends here and makes this nucleus important in determining our level of consciousness. Lateral to this nucleus is the ventral posterior medial nucleus. It receives the second-order gustatory and trigeminal fibers carried up to the thalamus in the medial lemniscus. This nucleus projects to the inferior one-third of the postcentral gyrus, areas 3, 1, 2 (see Chapter 20). Thus, we have reached the final subcortical center for gustatory and trigeminal impulses.

Optic thalamus. On the left side, the laminate lateral geniculate nucleus is present. It receives the third-order fibers which stem from the ganglionic cell layer of the retina via the optic nerve, chiasm, and tract. This thalamic nucleus projects to the striate cortex on the medial surface of the occipital lobe.

Red nucleus. This nucleus is conspicuous near the wall of the third ventricle, and receives input from the cerebellum via the superior cerebellar peduncles. It connects to the ventral lateral nucleus of the thalamus and also to the alpha and gamma motor neurons in the spinal cord via the rubrospinal tract.

Substantia nigra. This large pigmented nucleus is an important part of the extrapyramidal system. It connects with the globus pallidus, hypothalamus, and midbrain tegmentum, and probably also the caudate-putamen.

Deep telencephalic gray. Although the caudate nucleus is a part of the telencephalon, its tail is found in diencephalic levels on the most lateral wall of the lateral ventricles separated from the thalamus by the external laminae of the thalamus. The stria terminalis is found on its medial surface; it is unrelated to the caudate nucleus and interconnects the amygdaloid

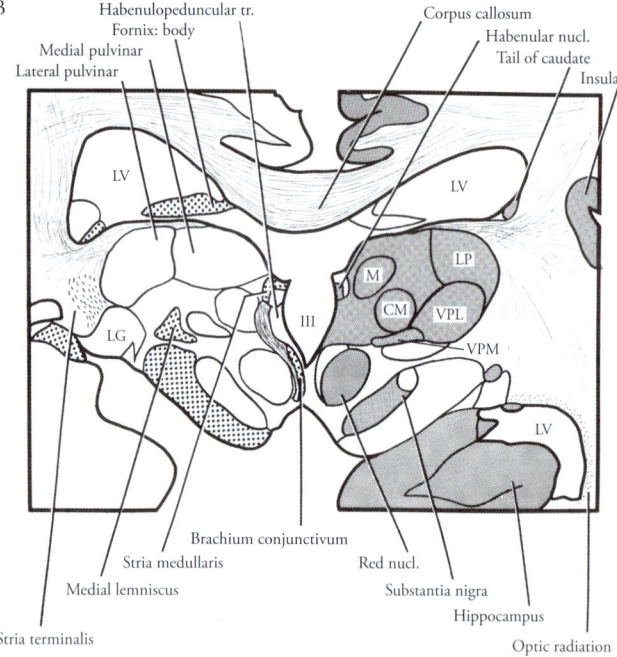

Figure 15.15A and B Level: Midbrain—diencephalic junction.

nuclei. The caudate nucleus is an important part of the extrapyramidal system having to do with supporting volitional motor functions.

Cranial nerve nuclei. Cranial nerves are found only in the medulla, pons, and midbrain. They are absent from diencephalic levels.

Fornix. This tract is an important part of the limbic or visceral brain. The fornix originates from the hippocampus located in the medial surface of the temporal lobe. It takes a circuitous pathway, following the inferior horn and body of the lateral ventricle, through or around the internal capsule to reach the aforementioned nuclei.

Fornix. The fornix connects the hippocampus with the septum, habenula, lateral hypothalamic nucleus, and mammillary bodies. The fornix originates from the hippocampus in the medial portion of the temporal lobe. It is suspended from the undersurface of the corpus callosum up to the most anterior portion of the thalamus, where it enters the hypothalamus

and passes to the mammillary body. In this cross section, it is seen under the corpus callosum and in the substance of the hypothalamus. The hippocampus is an important part of the visceral brain and participates in recent memory.

Gross features. The diencephalon occupies the bulk of this section with the corpus callosum, fornix, and lateral ventricles forming its superior surface, the third ventricle, its medial surface, and the posterior limb of the internal capsule, its lateral surface. The optic tract is prominent inferiorly and it is below the lateral geniculate, nucleus where it will terminate. Lateral to the internal capsule are found the deep telencephalic nuclei, the globus pallidus, and the putamen.

Epithalamus. The stria medullaris is seen on the superior margin of the third ventricle. This tract connects habenula with septum, amygdala, and hippocampus.

Thalamus. The thalamus at this level consists of two prominent divisions: the medial and lateral nuclei separated by the internal medullary laminar of the thalamus.

The medial portion, the medial nucleus, connects to the prefrontal and orbital cortices and receives reciprocal innervation from these same regions as well as the hypothalamus. It is an important subcortical nucleus in the visceral brain.

The lateral, more heavily myelinated portion consists of dorsal and ventral regions. Posteriorly the pulvinar is the continuation of this dorsal group. The ventral half consists of the nuclei, which receive the specific ascending tracts from lower levels of the central nervous system. The ventral posterior medial nucleus receives the ascending gustatory and cutaneous and proprioceptive fibers from the head. Present also is the ventral posterior lateral nucleus, which receives the cutaneous (spinothalamic and dorsal columns), proprioceptive (dorsal columns), and visceral information via the medial lemniscus, which projects to the upper two-thirds of the postcentral gyrus. The ventral lateral nucleus receives the superior cerebellar peduncle and projects to the motor and premotor cortices, areas 4 and 6 (see Chapter 9). Consequently in this section we have reached the final subcortical center for the dorsal columns, the spinothalamic and dentatorubrothalamic tracts.

Awareness of pain and temperature and crude touch are located in the ventral posterior lateral nucleus. More specialized sensory awareness is found in the postcentral gyrus, that is, the position of digits in space and tactile discrimination.

Hypothalamus. The hypothalamic sulcus, at the midpoint of the third ventricle, marks the separation between the thalamus above and the hypothalamus below. At this level a cell stain would show several hypothalamic nuclei at or near the ventricular surface. On the right side, even in this fiber stain, the mammillary body is conspicuous with the mamillothalamic and mammillotegmental fibers forming a capsule on its medial surface. On the left side the fornix is seen anterior to the mammillary body. Near the ventricular surface a prominent pathway, the mammillothalamic tract, is present. This connects the mammillary body with the anterior thalamic nuclei.

Subthalamus. This zone lies medial to the cerebral peduncle, below the medullary laminae of the thalamus and lateral to the hypothalamus. It has three principal nuclei: (1) subthalamic, touching the cerebral peduncle; (2) zone incerta,

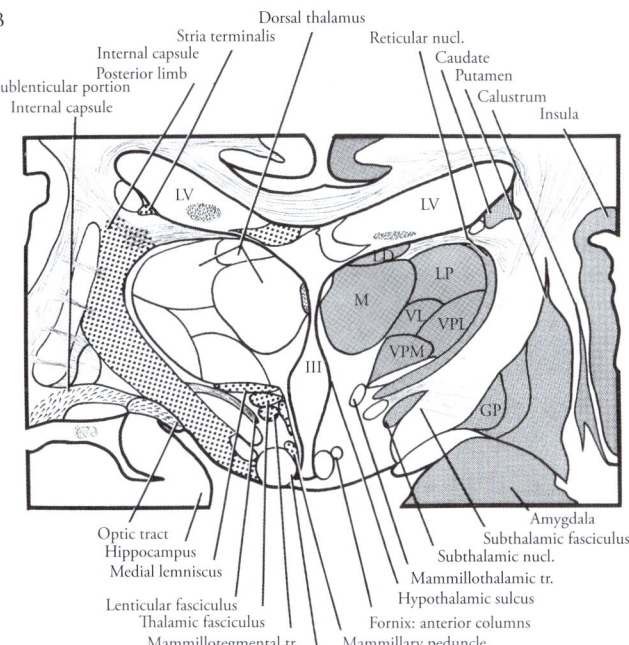

Figure 15.16A and B Level: Midthalamus.

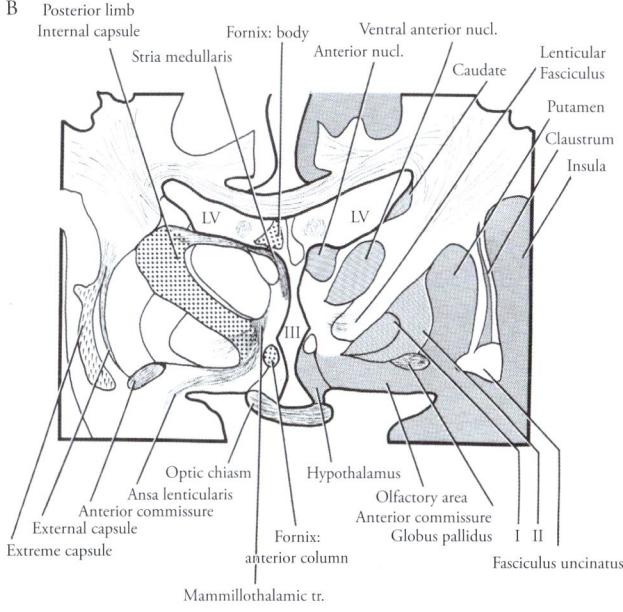

Figure 15.17A and B Level: Anterior tubercle of thalamus.

below the external medullary lamina; and (3) the tegmental nucleus of Forel (or prerubral nucleus), lateral to the mammillothalamic tract. The lenticular fasciculus separates the zona incerta above from the subthalamic nucleus below. This region is an important region for relay in the extrapyramidal system because of its connections with the globus pallidus, thalamus, and hypothalamus. Fibers reach the subthalamic zone from the globus pallidus by going through the internal capsule.

Temporal lobe. This lobe of the cerebrum forms the inferior region of the cerebrum and contains the hippocampus.

Fornix. This tract connects the hippocampus with the septum, habenula, lateral hypothalamic nucleus, and mammillary bodies. The fornix originates from the hippocampus in the medial portion of the temporal lobe. It is suspended from the undersurface of the corpus callosum up to the most anterior portion of the thalamus, where it enters the hypothalamus and passes to the mammillary body. In this cross section, it is seen on the dorsla surface of the hippocampus, the fimbria of the fornix. We next find it under the corpus callosum and the column of the fornix, where it enters the substance of the hypothalamus. The hippocampus is an important part of the visceral brain and participates in recent memory.

Deep telencephalic gray. The caudate (tail) nucleus, the putamen, and the globus pallidus are present in this section. The caudate nucleus is seen near the superior surface of the thalamus. The globus pallidus and putamen are found lateral to the posterior limb of the internal capsule. The globus pallidus is the heavily myelinated nucleus just lateral to the internal capsule. It receives input from the caudate nucleus and putamen while it provides the only efferents from the basal ganglia to the subthalamus, the ventral anterior and the ventral lateral nuclei in the thalamus, hypothalamus, the substantia nigra, and the midbrain tegmentum. The fibers leave the globus pallidus and cut through or around the internal capsule to reach the aforementioned nuclei.

Ventricular system. In this section we find the following parts of the ventricular system: inferior horn of the ventricle medial to the hippocampus, the body of the ventricle above the thalamus, and the third ventricle between the diencephalic halves.

Gross features. This section is near the rostral end of the thalamus. The optic chiasm is prominent on the base of the third ventricle.

The diencephalon is much smaller than in the previous levels, while the deep telencephalic nuclei, the globus pallidus, and the putamen are much larger than in the previous section. The boundaries of the diencephalon are laterally the posterior limb of the internal capsule; medially, the third ventricle; and superiorly, the lateral ventricle and corpus callosum.

Epithalamus. The stria medullaris is conspicuous on the medial surface of the thalamus.

Thalamus. The thalamic nuclei at this level consist of two prominent divisions: the anterior nuclei and the ventral anterior separated by the internal medullary. The anterior nuclei are important subcortical nuclei in the visceral brain because of their connections to the cingulate cortex and the mammillary bodies. The internal medullary laminae which separate the anterior nucleus from the ventral anterior nucleus consist primarily of mammillothalamic fibers, while the external medullary lamina, which touches the superior surface of the anterior nucleus, contains fibers interconnecting the anterior nuclei and the cingulate cortex. The ventral anterior nucleus receives fibers from the intralaminar nuclei, the ventral anterior nucleus, and globus pallidus and projects to areas 4 and 6 (see Chapter 10), the motor and premotor cortices.

Hypothalamus. In this cross section the fornix has just entered the hypothalamus. The optic chiasm forms the floor of the third ventricle. Note that a portion of the fornix is also seen under the corpus callosum.

Subthalamus. This is absent from this cross section. The subthalamus is seen in mid- and posterior thalamic sections (see preceding levels).

Deep telencephalic gray. The globus pallidus and putamen are conspicuous lateral to the posterior limb of the internal capsule. Fibers can be seen leaving the globus pallidus and sweeping around the internal capsule, as the ansa lenticularis, or cutting through the internal capsule, the pallidothalamic fibers.

Anterior commissure. The anterior commissure is seen on the inferior border of the globus pallidus and putamen. This level is just caudal to the actual decussation of the anterior commissure. The anterior commissure interconnects portions of the rostral temporal lobe, olfactory bulb, and olfactory cortex, as well as the amygdaloid nuclei (see Fig. 15.4).

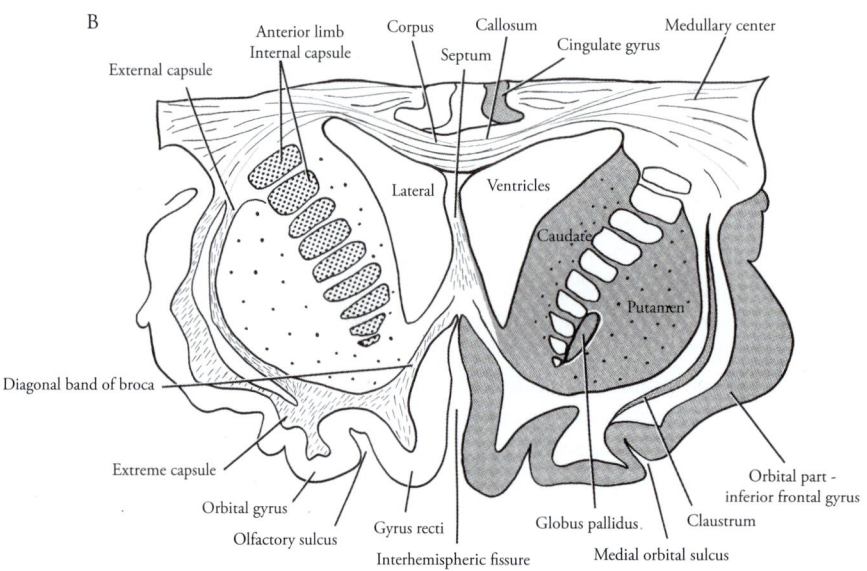

Figure 15.18A and B Level: Anterior limb of internal capsule.

Telencephalic cortex. In this section the uncus containing the amygdala with olfactory cortex forms the medial surface of the temporal lobe.

This section only contains telencephalon, the embryonic regions from which the cerebrum develops. In mammals, the dorsal telencephalon, or pallium, develops into the cerebral cortex, and the ventral telencephalon, or subpallium, becomes the basal ganglia. The cerebrum is divided into a left and right hemisphere with different functions.

The anterior limb of the internal capsule separates the caudate nucleus from the globus pallidus. In this white matter region one finds the anterior thalamic projection from the dorsal medial nuclei, anterior and ventral lateral thalamic nuclei upon the frontal lobe. Note the cellular bridges between the caudate and the putamen. The septum which receives fibers from the hypothalamus and limbic cortex separates the anterior poles of the body of the lateral ventricles.

Cerebrum. The cingulate gyri are seen above the corpus callosum.

The orbital region and the gyrus rectus are present on the base of the frontal lobes.

BIBLIOGRAPHY

Suggested Readings

Goldman-Rakic, P. S., and Porrino, L. J. 1989. The primate mediodorsal (MD) and its projection to the frontal lobe. J. Comp. Neurol. 242:535–560.

Guillery, R. W. 1995. Anatomical evidence concerning the role of the thalamus in corticocortical communications: a brief review. J. Anat. 187:583–592.

Jones, E. G. 1989. A new parcellation of the human thalamus on the basis of histochemical staining. Brain Res. Rev. 14:1–34.

Jones, E. G. 2007. The thalamus. Vols. 1-2. Cambridge, UK: Cambridge University Press.

Purpura, D. P., and Yahr, M. D. 1966. The thalamus. New York, NY: Columbia University Press.

Trojanowski, J. Q., and Jacobson, S. 1976. Areal and laminar distribution of some pulvinar cortical efferents in rhesus monkey. J. Comp. Neurol. 76:371–391.

Van Buren, J. M., and Borke, R. C. 1972. Variation and Connections of the Human Thalamus. Springer-Verlag.

Walker, A. E. 1938. The primate thalamus. Chicago, IL: University of Chicago Press.

Citations

Collie, D. A., Summers, D. M., Sellar, R. J., et al. 2003. Diagnosing variant Creutzfeldt-Jakob disease with the pulvinar sign: MR imaging findings in 86 neuropathologically confirmed cases. Am J Neuroradiol. 24:1560–1569.

De Gelder, B., Pourtois, G., and Weiskrantz, L. 2002. Fear recognition in the voice. Proceedings Nat. Academ. of Sciences. USA. 99:4121–4126.

De Wulf, A. 1971. Anatomy of the Normal Human Thalamus, Topometry and Standardized Nomenclature. Amsterdam, The Netherlands: Elsevier.

Goldman-Rakic, P. S., and Porrino, L. J. 1989. The primate mediodorsal (MD) and its projection to the frontal lobe. J. Comp. Neurol. 242:535–560.

Guillery, R. W. 1995. Anatomical evidence concerning the role of the thalamus in corticocortical communications: a brief review. J. Anat. 187:583–592.

Jones, E. G. 1989. A new parcellation of the human thalamus on the basis of histochemical staining. Brain Res. Rev. 14:1–34.

Jones, E. G. 2007. The Thalamus. Vols. 1-2. Cambridge, UK: Cambridge University Press.

Milner, A. D., and Goodale, M. A. 2008. Two Visual Systems, reviewed. Neurosych. 46:774–785.

Molloy, S., O'Laoide, R., Brett, F., and Farrell, M. 2000. The "pulvinar" sign in variant Creutzfeldt-Jakob disease. AJR 175:555–556.

Oppenheim, C., Ducreux, D., Rodrigo, S., et al. 2007. Université Paris Descartes. Radiol. 88:510–520.

Purpura, D. P., and Yahr, M. D. 1966. The Thalamus. New York, NY: Columbia University Press.

Trojanowski, J. Q., and Jacobson, S. 1976. Areal and laminar distribution of some pulvinar cortical efferents in rhesus monkey. J. Comp. Neurol. 76:371–391.

Ungerleider, L. G., and Mishkin, M. 1982. Two cortical visual systems. In D. Ingle, M. A. Goodale, and R. J. W. Mansfield (Eds.) Analysis of Visual Behavior, pp. 549–586. Cambridge, MA: MIT Press.

Van Buren, J. M., and Borke, R. C. 1972. Variation and Connections of the Human Thalamus. Springer-Verlag.

Vargas, M. I., Delavelle, J., Jlassi, H., et al. 2008. Review. Diffusion-weighted imaging, diffusion-tensor imaging, and fiber tractography of the spinal cord. [Magn Reson Imaging Clin N Am. 2009]. Neuroradiology 50(1):25–29.

Walker, A. E. 1938. The Primate Thalamus. Chicago, IL: University of Chicago Press.

Weiskrantz, L., Cowey, A., and Hodinott-Hill, I. 2002. Prime-sight in a blindsight subject. Nature Neurosci. 5:101–102.

Weiskrantz, L. 1986. Blindsight: A Case Study and Implications. Oxford: Oxford University Press.

Weiskrantz, L. 1997. Consciousness Lost and Found. Oxford: Oxford University Press.

SECTION III

MAJOR SYSTEMS

16.

HYPOTHALAMUS, NEUROENDOCRINE SYSTEM, AND AUTONOMIC NERVOUS SYSTEM

HYPOTHALAMUS

The hypothalamus is a very small nuclear mass found at the base of the third ventricle in the diencephalon. Its functional potency is related to its control of the hypophysis and its descending autonomic fibers, which affect preganglionic parasympathetic and sympathetic nuclei in the brain stem and the thoracic, lumbar, and sacral spinal cord. In addition, this diencephalic region with its important tracts form part of the Papez circuit and must be included in any discussion of the limbic (or emotional) brain in Chapter 22.

The hypothalamus bilaterally forms the medial inferior part of the floor of the diencephalon and is located on the wall of the third ventricle, extending from the anterior margin of the optic chiasm to the posterior margin of the mammillary bodies. It is bounded dorsally by the dorsal thalamus and laterally by the subthalamus and internal capsule. It is connected to the hypophysis by the hypothalamic-hypophyseal tract and the hypothalamic-hypophyseal portal system. The hypothalamus consists of more than a dozen nuclei with their associated fiber systems. Although the hypothalamus weighs only 4 g, this small area controls our internal homeostasis and influences emotional and behavior patterns.

HYPOTHALAMIC NUCLEI

Anatomically, the hypothalamus is divided into a medial and a lateral zone (Fig. 16.1).

The medial zone consists of three regions:

1. The anterior zone, including the preoptic, supraoptic, pariventricular, anterior, and suprachiasmatic nuclei (Fig. 16.2).

2. The middle zone, including the dorsomedial, ventromedial, and suprachiasmatic nucleus.

3. The posterior zone (Fig. 16.3), including the posterior hypothalamic nuclei and mammillary nuclei (both large and small celled).

The lateral zone includes the lateral nucleus, the lateral tuberal nucleus, and the medial forebrain bundle. In addition, periventricular nuclei are adjacent to the third ventricle at all levels of the medial region (Table 16.1).

Anterior Group

The preoptic, suprachiasmatic, supraoptic, and pariventricular nuclei are found in this region (Fig. 16.2). The supraoptic and periventricular nuclei contain secretory granules (containing oxytocin and vasopressin) that leave these nuclei and pass down the hypophyseal pathway, which terminates at the capillaries in the posterior lobe of the pituitary, or neurohypophysis.

The supraoptic nucleus functions as an osmoreceptor; it releases vasopressin in response to an increase in osmotic pressure in the capillaries. Vasopressin or ADH (antidiuretic hormone) increases water resorption in the kidneys.

The suprachiasmatic nucleus, which receives direct input from optic fibers in the chiasm, is important in the endocrine response to light levels and may well be the location of the biological clock.

Middle Group

This region includes the dorsomedial, ventromedial arcuate (Infundibular), lateral, and lateral tuberal nuclei (Fig. 16.3). The ventromedial nucleus has extensive projections onto the diencephalon, brain stem, and spinal cord. Lesions here affect feeding behavior (e.g., obesity or anorexia). Arising from the tuberal nuclei, the tuberoinfundibular pathway terminates on the hypophyseal portal veins, permitting releasing factors produced in the hypothalamus to reach the anterior lobe of the pituitary.

Posterior Group

This region consists of the mammillary (medial and lateral nuclei) and the posterior hypothalamic nuclei (Fig. 16.4). A major part of the fornix projects onto this region with the mammillary nuclei then projecting via the mammillothalamic tract on the anterior

Figure 16.1 The zones and nuclei of the hypothalamus. The hypophysis and the nuclei of the hypothalamus.

311

Table 16.1 REVIEW OF FUNCTIONAL LOCALIZATION IN THE HYPOTHALAMIC NUCLEI

HYPOTHALAMIC NUCLEI	FUNCTION
Supraoptic and pariventricular	Osmoregulation—release of vasopressin or oxytocin. Lesion here produces diabetes insipidus.
Ventromedial nucleus and lateral hypothalamus	Feeding centers. Lesion in ventromedial nucleus produces overeating; lesion in lateral hypothalamus produces anorexia.
Anterolateral region and posterior hypothalamus	Lesions in anterolateral produce sympathetic response, while lesion in posterior produces parasympathetic response. Stimulation of anterolateral region excites parasympathetic nervous system and inhibits sympathetic nervous system, hypothalamus (posterior region), and produces slow-wave sleep. Stimulation of posterior hypothalamus excites sympathetic and inhibits parasympathetic and is important in arousal and waking from sleep.

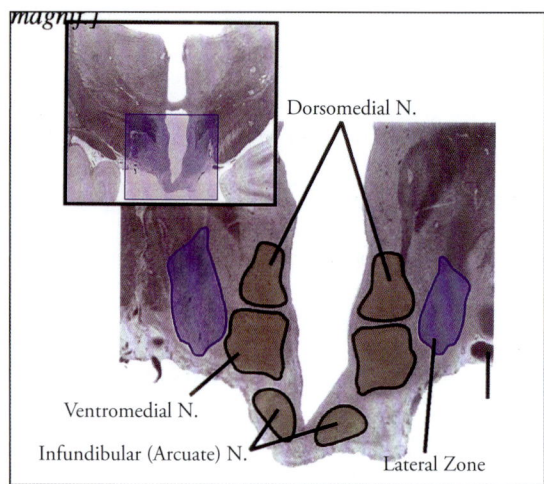

Figure 16.3 Myelin and cell stain (Kluver-Berrera) of diencephalon at mid-hypothalamus, demonstrating tuberal nuclei and mammillary bodies. (110×)

nuclei of the thalamus. The mammillary nuclei also project onto the brain stem tegmentum through the mammillary peduncle. Lesions in these nuclei are seen in Korsakoff's psychosis with accompanying retrograde amnesia (see Chapter 30).

AFFERENT PATHWAYS

The hypothalamus is so situated that it functions as an important integrating center between the brain stem, reticular system, and the limbic forebrain structures.

The major subcortical (afferent) inputs into the hypothalamus include the following (Fig. 16.5):

1. Reticular input from the ascending multisynaptic pathways in the mesencephalic reticular nuclei via the medial forebrain bundle, dorsal longitudinal fasciculus, and mammillary peduncle.

2. The globus pallidus through lenticular fasciculus and ansa lenticularis (see Chapter 18).

3. Thalamic input from the dorsal medial nucleus and intralaminar nuclei via direct connections onto the hypothalamus.

4. Fibers from the optic nerve, retinohypothalamic fibers, which end in the suprachiasmatic nucleus (see Chapter 23).

5. The major cortical input into the hypothalamus comes from the temporal lobe-hippocampal formation (fornix), amygdala (stria terminalis), cingulate gyrus (cingulohypothalamic), and frontal associational cortex (corticohypothalamic fibers). Thus, we see that the hypothalamus is so situated that it serves as an important integrating center between the brain stem reticular system and the limbic forebrain structures.

Figure 16.2 Myelin stain of diencephalon at the level of the anterior hypothalamus and optic chiasm, showing corpus callosum, precommissural anterior commissure, and corpus striatum. Medial, ventromedial, lateral, and tuberal nuclei.

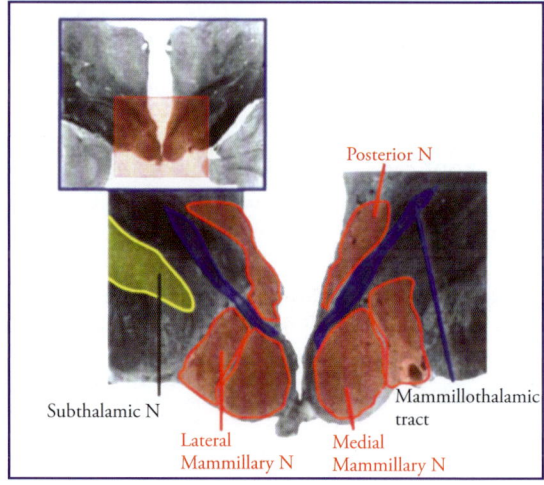

Figure 16.4 Myelin and cell stain (Kluver-Berrera) of diencephalon at posterior hypothalamus. (Corpus callosum removed.)

Figure 16.5 Map of location of hypothalamic sections 16.2, 16.3, and 16.4.

EFFERENT PATHWAYS

Fiber tracts and the neurosecretory system mediate the output of the hypothalamus (Figs. 16.6 and 16.7). The efferent pathways from the hypothalamus are as follows:

1. *Mammillothalamic tract*, which interconnects the medial mammillary nucleus with the anterior thalamic nucleus and, ultimately, with the cingulate cortex.
2. *Periventricular system*, which arises in the supraoptic, tuberal, and posterior nuclei in the hypothalamus to supply the medial thalamic nucleus and joins the medial forebrain bundle and dorsal longitudinal fasciculus.
3. *Mammillotegmental tract*, which connects the medial mammillary nuclei with the midbrain reticular nuclei and autonomic nuclei in the brain stem.
4. *Medial forebrain bundle and dorsal longitudinal fasciculus*, which receive fibers from the lateral hypothalamic nucleus and periventricular nuclei and connect to the midbrain tegmentum and autonomic neurons in the brain stem associated with cranial nerves VII, IX, and X and the spinal cord.
5. *Hypothalamic-hypophyseal tracts, or neurosecretory system* (Fig. 16.8), which connects the supraoptic, periventricular,

Figure 16.7 Hypothalamic efferent pathways.

and magnocellular nuclei via the hypophyseal stalk with the neural hypophysis.

6. *Hypothalamic-hypophyseal portal system*, which permits releasing factors made in the hypothalamus to reach the adenohypophysis (see later discussion).

FUNCTIONAL STABILITY

The hypothalamus through its relation with the autonomic nervous system and hypophysis, maintains a more-or-less

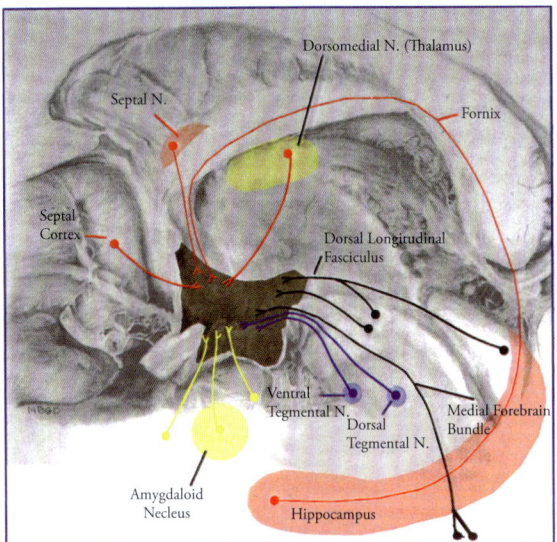

Figure 16.6 Hypothalamic afferent pathways.

Figure 16.8 The hypothalamic-hypophyseal tract (neurosecretory system). This tract provides a direct connection between the hypothalamus and the neurohypophysis. The neurosecretory granules pass down the axons of this tract and are stored in the neural lobe until they are released into the blood stream.

stable, controlled, internal environment regardless of the external environment. It affects body temperature, water balance, neurosecretion, food intake, sleep, and the parasympathetic and sympathetic nervous systems.

NUEROENDOCRINE SYSTEM, THE HYPOTHALAMUS, AND ITS RELATION TO THE HYPOPHYSIS

In addition to the direct control of the autonomic nervous system by central pathways, the hypothalamus has a powerful influence on other homeostatic mechanisms of the human by its direct control of the hypophysis. The discussion that follows is an overview of this information flow that is the basis of the neuroendocrine system (Fig. 16.9).

HYPOPHYSIS CEREBRI

The hypophyseal gland or pituitary gland consists of two major divisions: the anterior lobe or adenohypophysis and the posterior lobe, the neurohypophysis. There is also a smaller pars intermedia associated with the anterior lobe. The adenohypophysis is the larger component and contains cords of different cell types closely associated with capillaries of the hypothalamic-hypophyseal portal system. The neurohypophysis consists of the infundibular stalk and the bulbous neurohypophysis and includes neuroglia like pituicytes, blood vessels, and some finely myelinated axons. The hypophysis is directly connected to the hypothalamus by the hypophyseal stalk (Figs. 16.4 and 16.6) and indirectly connects to the hypothalamus by the hypothalamic hypophyseal venous portal system. The hypophysiotrophic area of the hypothalamus is necessary for hormone production in the adenohypophysis. The hypophysiotrophic area includes parts of the ventromedial and other hypothalamic nuclei. These peptidergic neurons are termed parvicellular (composed of small cells). The cells forming the neurohypophyseal tract are magnocellular neurons.

HYPOTHALAMIC-HYPOPHYSEAL PORTAL SYSTEM

The *hypothalamus and adenohypophysis* are connected by the hypothalamic- hypophyseal venous portal system (Fig. 16.9). Releasing factors travel from the hypothalamus to the adenohypophysis by this means.

The *hypophysis* receives its blood supply from two pairs of arteries: the superior hypophyseal arteries and the inferior hypophyseal arteries. The superior hypophyseal arteries leave the internal carotid and posterior communicating arteries and supply the median eminence, Infundibular stalk, and adenohypophysis.

In the infundibular stalk and median eminence the arteries terminate in a capillary network, which empties into veins that run down the infundibular stalk. In the anterior lobe these veins form another capillary network, or sinusoid.

The *inferior hypophyseal arteries* leave the internal carotid and distribute to the posterior lobe, where they form a capillary network that flows into the sinus in the adenohypophysis. The hypophyseal veins finally drain into the cavernous sinus. The releasing factors enter the venous drainage of the hypothalamus, which drains into the median eminence and hypophyseal stalk. These factors are then carried via the hypophyseal portal system to the adenohypophysis. The *capillary loop*s in the infundibular stalk and neural hypophysis drain in close proximity to the cortiotrophin neurosecretory axons of the hypothalamic-hypophyseal tract.

HYPOPHYSIOTROPHIC AREA

The hypophysiotrophic area is a paramedian zone that extends rostrally at the level of the optic chiasm dorsally from the ventral surface to the paraventricular nuclei. Caudally this area narrows down to include only the ventral surface of the hypothalamus at the level of the mammillary recess of the third ventricle. The hypophysiotrophic center includes neurons in the following hypothalamic nuclei: paraventricular, anterior, arcuate, ventromedial, and tuberal. Releasing and inhibitory factors, listed in Table 16.2, are produced in the parvicellular hypophysiotrophic area and stimulate the adenohypophysis to produce and release hormones into the circulation.

HORMONES PRODUCED BY HYPOTHALAMUS

Two hormones, vasopressin and oxytocin, are manufactured in the hypothalamus, carried down the hypothalamic-hypophyseal tract, and stored in the neurohypophysis before being released into the bloodstream.

Vasopressin is an antidiuretic hormone (ADH) formed primarily in the supraoptic nucleus and to a lesser degree in the paraventricular nucleus and carried down the hypothalamic-hypophyseal tract. This substance acts on the distal convoluted tubules and collecting ducts in the kidney, causing resorption of water.

Oxytocin is formed primarily in the paraventricular nucleus and to a lesser degree in the supraoptic nucleus and is carried down the hypothalamic-hypophyseal tract. This substance stimulates the mammary gland, causing it to contract and

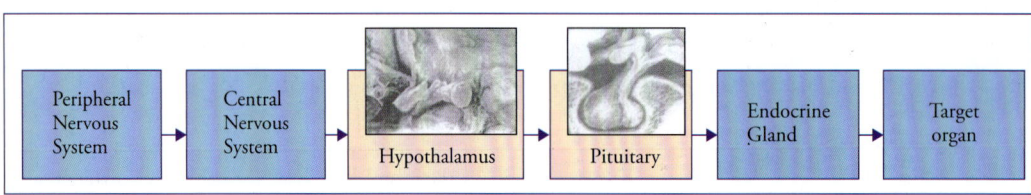

Figure 16.9 Information flow between the brain and endocrine system.

Table 16.2 **RELEASING FACTORS AND HORMONES PRODUCED IN THE HYPOTHALAMUS**

Releasing factors produced in parvicellular region of hypothalamus:
Corticotrophin
Growth hormone (somatotropin hormone)
Growth hormone–inhibiting factor
Luteinizing hormone
Melanocyte-stimulating hormone
Melanocyte-stimulating hormone–inhibiting factor
Prolactin-inhibitory factor
Thyrotropin

Hormones produced or stored in neurohypophysis:
Vasopressin from paraventricular nucleus
Oxytocin from supraoptic nucleus

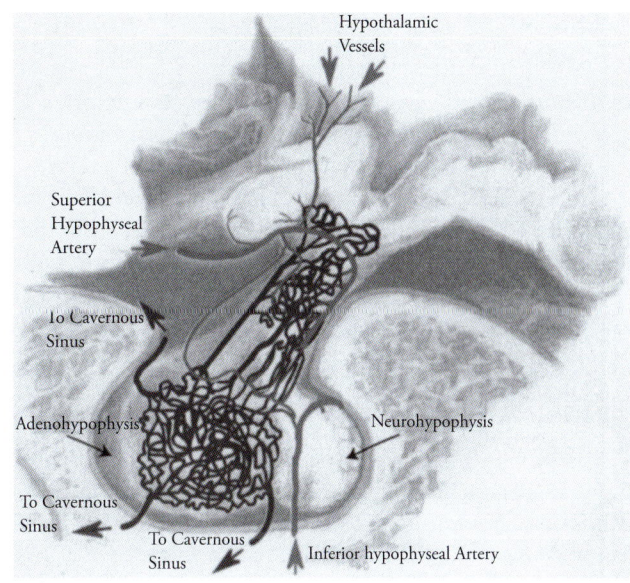

Figure 16.10 The hypothalamic-hypophyseal venous portal system. These venous channels provide vascular continuity between the hypothalamus and the adenohypophysis. The releasing factors from the hypophysiotrophic area of the hypothalamus drain into the veins of the hypothalamus, which connect to the capillary bed in the infundibular stalk and median eminence. The factors are then carried to the adenohypophysis.

expel milk concomitant with suction on the nipple. During delivery, oxytocin also contracts the smooth muscle in the uterus and dilates the uterus, cervix, and vagina.

HORMONES PRODUCED IN ADENOHYPOPHYSIS

Releasing factors from the hypothalamus traverse the hypothalamic-hypophyseal portal system and trigger the formation and eventual release of the glandotropic or tropic hormone (see Table 16.3). All of the tropic (switch on) hormones produced in the anterior lobe are at the same time trophic (growth promoting or maintaining) hormones, in whose absence their target organs atrophy (Fig. 16.10).

Hormones produced in the adenohypophysis:

1. *Adrenocorticotrophic hormone (ACTH).* This hormone is produced by basophilic cells and stimulates the formation of adrenal glucocorticoids (hydrocortisone) and, to a lesser degree, mineral corticoids (aldosterone). In conditions of stress (cold, heat, pain, fright, flight, inflammation, or infection), ACTH is produced. Cushing's disease is caused by excessive secretion of ACTH, while Addison's disease results from ACTH insufficiency.

2. *Lactogenic hormone (prolactin).* This substance in combination with the growth hormone promotes development of the mammary glands and lactation.

3. *Gonadotropin* (luteinizing hormone [LH] in females; or interstitial cell-stimulating hormone [ICSH] in males). In females, gonadotropin is necessary for ovulation. It causes luteinization of follicles after they are ripened by follicle-stimulating hormone (FSH). In males, gonadotropin activates the interstitial cells of the testis to produce testosterone, which is essential for the development and maturation of the sperm.

4. *Follicle-stimulating hormone* (FSH). This substance stimulates growth of the ovarian follicle in the female and stimulates spermatogenesis in males.

5. *Growth hormone* (somatotropin, or STH). This hormone is important for growth after birth. It specifically affects the growth of the epiphyseal cartilage but is also important in the metabolism of fat, protein, and carbohydrates. Cessation of growth follows hypophysectomy. The inhibitory form of this hormone controls the release of the hormone. Gigantism results from an excessive somatotropin before the epiphyseal plate's close (Case 16.1). Case 16.2 is different from Case 16.1 as the pituitary tumor in this instance produces defects in vision and an increase in the growth hormone after the epiphyseal plates have

Table 16.3 **HORMONES PRODUCED IN ADENOHYPOHYSIS**

Releasing Hormones
Adrenocorticotropic (ACTH)
Lactogenic (prolactin)
Gonadotrophic
Luteinizing (LH) in females
Interstitial cell stimulating in males (ICSH)
Follicle-stimulating (FSH) in females
Melanocyte-stimulating (MSH)
Somatotropin hormone (STH)
Thyrotrophic hormone (TSH)

Inhibitory Hormones
Lactogenic (dopamine)
Melanocyte
Somatotopic

closed, with resultant acromegaly (enlarged extremities) gigantism and effects on the libido (review also Fig. 23.9).

6. *Thyrotrophic hormone (TSH). TSH stimulates the thyroid gland to prod*uce triiodothyronine (T3) and thyroxine (T4), which regulate the rate of breakdown of fats and carbohydrates. When circulating levels of T3 and T4 rise, thyrotrophic-releasing hormone (TRH) release from the adenohypophysis is inhibited by a drop in TRH production in the hypothalamic neurons until the preferred levels returns to normal.

CASE HISTORY 16.1

A 25-year-old male autobody mechanic, in July, developed numbness in the median nerve distribution of the left hand with pain at the left wrist, shooting into the index, middle, and ring fingers. He also had aching pain in his finger joints. To a lesser degree, similar symptoms had developed in the right hand. The clinical impression of bilateral carpal tunnel syndrome was confirmed by nerve conduction studies. In addition, the patient presented many of the facial features of acromegaly: coarse lips, large jaw, and nose. None of his family had similar facial features, and according to his mother, these features had emerged about age 12 years.

Growth hormone levels were consistently elevated to 17–20 ng/ml (normal is less that 5 ng/ml fasting and recumbent). A glucose load produced no suppression. Prolactin level was moderately increased to 37 ng/ml (normal in men if less than 1–20 ng/ml). Magnetic resonance imaging (MRI) demonstrated an enlarged pituitary gland with a hypodense lesion, consistent with an adenoma (Fig. 16.11). A partial agenesis of the corpus callosum (splenium and posterior one-third of the body) was also present and may have related to long-standing learning disabilities. A trans-sphenoid excision of the pituitary adenoma was performed. Except for transient diabetes insipidus, he did well and all symptoms disappeared.

Comments

The patient presented with a chief complaint relevant to compression of the median nerve at the carpal tunnel. Usually the carpal tunnel syndrome occurs in one hand or the other and may reflect local swelling in the tendons and soft tissues. This is at times a result of occupation-related repetitive motion at the wrist. In occasional cases, an underlying systematic condition is present; these include rheumatoid arthritis, pregnancy, myxedema of the hypothyroid state, and acromegaly associated with excessive secretion of growth hormone by pituitary adenomas.

In this case, the neurologist noted the facial feature characteristic of acromegaly. In retrospect, the patient's mother was able to date these changes to his teen years. Excessive production of growth hormone, prior to closure of the epiphyseal plates in long bones, results in excessive growth or gigantism, including enlargement of facial bones, jaw, hands, and feet. The pain in the finger joints may have reflected an early stage of enlargement of the fingers. In the present case, the adenoma had enlarged the pituitary gland, but the tumor had not expanded out of the sella turcica. The pituitary gland sits in the sella turcica, which is part of the sphenoid bone. Suprasellar, or upward extension of the tumor, may result in compression of the optic chiasm. A characteristic visual field defect occurs: a bitemporal hemianopsia (loss of the outer halves of both visual fields). Lateral extension of the tumor into the cavernous sinus may compress cranial nerves III, IV, and VI, resulting in diplopia (double vision). Headaches may reflect unusual pressure on the diaphragm sella. Acute headache may reflect sudden increase in mass within the tumor due to infarctions of hemorrhage (so-called pituitary apoplexy). Eye pain may reflect compression of the maxillary or ophthalmic division of the trigeminal nerve with the cavernous sinus.

Careful removal of the tumor, in this case utilizing the trans-sphenoidal approach and the operating microscope, allowed preservation of residual pituitary function. Transient diabetes insipidus often is present, reflecting temporary damage to the posterior pituitary or pituitary stalk.

CASE HISTORY 16.2 (PATIENT OF DR. ELLIOTT MARCUS)

This 51-year-old married salesman was admitted for evaluation of a progressive disturbance of vision. Approximately 8 years previously, the patient noted blurring of print on the labels of paint cans. Glasses

Figure 16.11 Adenomas. (*A*) Magnetic resonance imaging (MRI), T1-weighted midline sagittal sections; (*B*) control MRI, T1 weighted: Case 16.1.

were obtained and produced improvement, but within a short time, symptoms recurred. During the succeeding years, the glasses had to be changed eight times. For 6 to 7 months, the patient had noted diplopia, especially on right lateral gaze when driving at night. For 3 to 4 months, a left frontoparietal and left orbital headache had been present. One month prior to admission, progression of visual symptoms occurred. The patient had a marked decrease in visual acuity and was unable to find objects on shelves. He reported also that he was unable to drive his automobile because he was unable to see the sides of the road. The patient consulted an ophthalmologist who noted visual field defects and referred the patient for neurological evaluation.

History

The patient denied any significant change in physical appearance, appetite, or fluid intake. The patient's sexual interests had declined. He had no sexual intercourse for the last 10 years.

General Physical Examination

1. The patient was obese with large puffy hands and feet, a prominent jaw, and prominent frontal skull area.
2. Pallor of skin and mucous membranes was noted.
3. Axillary hair was absent; pubic hair was normal.
4. Testes were of normal size but were described as soft.

Neurological Examination

1. *Cranial nerves:*
   a. *Visual acuity wa*s reduced bilaterally; however, the patient could read 1 cm print at 14 inches.
   b. On visual field examination a complete bitemporal defect was present, cutting the central vision (Fig. 23.10).
   c. Examination of the fundi revealed pallor of the left optic disk, suggesting optic atrophy.
   d. On testing extraocular movements, a diplopia was present in a pattern that suggested bilateral medial rectus involvement (that is, bilateral third-nerve damage).

Clinical diagnosis: Pituitary adenoma/acromegaly.

Laboratory Data

The following studies were abnormal:

1. Thyroid studies indicated borderline low function with a protein-bound iodine of 4.0 μg/dl (normal = 4–8 μg/dl) and radioactive iodine of 23.3% in 24 hours (normal = 20% to 50%).
2. Adrenal-function studies indicated subnormal values. Urinary 17-hydroxysteroids were 2.1 to 2.3 mg/24 hr (normal = 3–10 mg/24 hr).
3. Urinary 17-ketosteroids were 4.0 mg/24 hr (normal = 10–25 mg/24 hr).
4. Despite these low urinary steroid levels, no FSH was detectable in the urine.
5. Skull X-ray revealed marked enlargement of the sella turcica (length 3 cm, depth 2 cm) without calcification.
6. Electroencephalogram was abnormal with bilateral frontal, slow (5 cps) waves, suggesting a bilateral frontal dysfunction.
7. Bilateral carotid arteriograms demonstrated a marked elevation of the distal segment of the internal carotid arteries, with elevation of the origins of both the anterior and middle cerebral arteries; this was consistent with a large tumor extending superiorly out of the pituitary fossa.
8. Pneumoencephalograms: large lesion extending out of the pituitary fossa was again demonstrated.
9. Cerebrospinal-fluid protein was elevated to 85 mg/dl.

Hospital course: Replacement therapy with cortisone acetate and thyroid was begun. Dr. Bertram Selverstone performed a right frontal craniotomy and removed a cystic necrotic chromaphobe adenoma compressing optic nerves and chiasm. Vision improved in the right eye.

Comments

Although the patient did not emphasize an acute history of a bitemporal hemianopsia, he did mention that his ability to drive had been limited not only by the decrease in visual acuity but also by his inability to see the road at the sides of the car, that is, the peripheral temporal fields.

The patient presented with many of the stigmata of acromegaly but claimed that he had large hands, feet, jaw, and so on, for all of his adult life.

Changes in libido had apparently been present for at least 16 years. Axillary hair had never been present. One may only speculate that perhaps a mixed tumor of the pituitary had been present almost all of the patient's life, only becoming symptomatic once extrasellar (that is, suprasellar) extension had compressed the optic nerves and chiasm. Today, blood levels of growth hormone and prolactin would be obtained and, in all likelihood, would have been found to be elevated long before the visual symptoms appeared. Today such symptoms would have prompted neuroimaging studies such as MRI or computerized tomography (CT) with the diagnosis probably being established much earlier.

Tables 16.2 and 16.3 review the functions of the anterior and posterior lobes of the pituitary.

HYPOTHALAMUS AND THE AUTONOMIC NERVOUS SYSTEM

An individual performing daily functions usually has a balance between the parasympathetic and sympathetic nervous system. Stimulation of the anterior hypothalamus (anterolateral region) excites the parasympathetic nervous system and inhibits the sympathetic nervous system. The heartbeat and blood pressure decrease (the vagal response), the visceral vessels dilate, peristalsis and secretion of digestive juices increase, the pupils constrict, and salivation increases.

Stimulation of the posterior hypothalamus (posteromedial region) excites the sympathetic nervous system and inhibits the parasympathetic nervous system. The heartbeat and blood pressure increase, the visceral vessels constrict, peristalsis and secretion of gastric juices decrease, pupils dilate, and sweating and piloerection occur.

A lesion in the anterior or parasympathetic zone produces a sympathetic response; destruction of the posterior or sympathetic zone may produce a parasympathetic response. The effects on blood vessels are produced by stimulation of the smooth muscles in the tunica media, and the effects on the sweat glands result from the stimulation of the glands through the cranial or peripheral nerves.

FUNCTIONAL LOCALIZATION

The hypothalamus, through its relation with the autonomic nervous system and hypophysis, maintains a more-or-less stable, controlled, internal environment regardless of the external environment. It affects body temperature, water balance, neurosecretion, food intake, sleep, and the parasympathetic and sympathetic nervous system.

Food Intake

Bilateral lesions restricted to the ventromedial hypothalamic nuclei produce hyperplasia, resulting in obesity. Stimulation of this center inhibits eating. Experiments have shown that animals with ventromedial lesions are not motivated to eat more; they just do not know when to stop eating. For this reason it is thought that the satiety center is located here.

Bilateral lesions in the lateral hypothalamic region produce anorexia; the animal refuses to eat and eventually dies. However, if this region is stimulated but not destroyed, the animal overeats. Appetite, the stimulus for eating, is dependent on many factors, including glucose concentration in the blood, stomach distension, smell, sight, taste, and mood. Lesions in other portions of the limbic system may also affect appetite. Although obesity in humans usually does not have a neurological cause, in rare cases some overweight individuals have had a ventromedial nuclei lesion.

Sleep Cycle

The hypothalamus helps set our level of alertness with the assistance of input from the reticular system and cerebral cortex (see Chapters 11 and 30). The medial preoptic region can initiate slow-wave sleep. The lateral hypothalamus receives input from the ascending reticular system that produces arousal. The posterior portion, including the mammillary body, is important in controlling the normal sleep cycle. Lesions in this region may produce an inversion in the sleep cycle, or hypersomnia. Lesions in the anterior hypothalamus may produce insomnia.

The amount of light is monitored in the hypothalamus by input from the optic nerve directly to the suprachiasmatic nucleus. The sympathetic innervation to the pineal monitors the dark levels, and melatonin release from the pineal is part of the sleep mechanism.

Body Temperature

Maintenance of a constant body temperature is vital to a warm-blooded animal. The hypothalamus acts as a thermostat, establishing a balance between vasodilation, vasoconstriction, sweating, and shivering. It does this by means of two opposing thermoregulatory centers: one regulates heat loss, and the other regulates heat production. Lesions in either of these centers interfere with the regulation of body temperature.

Control Center for Heat Loss

A destructive lesion in the anterior hypothalamus at the level of the optic chiasm or in the tuberal region renders an animal incapable of controlling its body temperature in a warm environment; a tumor in the third ventricle may produce a similar result. The human can no longer control the heat-loss mechanism, which consists of cutaneous vasodilation and sweating. Without this mechanism the body temperature rises (hyperthermia), and the patient becomes comatose and may even die.

Control Center for Heat Production and Conservation

Lesions in the posterior hypothalamus above and lateral to the mammillary bodies disrupt an animal's ability to maintain normal body temperature in either a warm or cold environment. Normally, exposure to cold produces vasoconstriction, shivering, piloerection, and secretion of epinephrine in mammals, all of which tend to increase body temperature. Following a lesion in the posterior hypothalamus, the body temperature tends to match that of the environment, whether warmer or colder, relative to 37°C. (poikilothermic). Poikilothermy probably reflects damage to the fibers descending from the heat-loss center as well as direct injury to the heat production and conservation center.

The thermoreceptors are located in the skin (end bulbs of Krause and end bulbs of Golgi-Mazzoni; see Fig. 3.22) or in the hypothalamus itself, which monitors the temperature of the cranial blood. Some receptors respond to cold and others to warmth. Cold receptors excite the caudal heat production and conservation center and inhibit the rostral heat-loss center. Warm receptors reverse this pattern.

WATER BALANCE AND NEUROSECRETION

Water balance is regulated by the hypothalamic-hypophyseal tract, which originates in the supraoptic and paraventricular nuclei and runs through the median eminence and hypophyseal stalk to terminate in close proximity to blood vessels in the neural hypophysis. A lesion in the region of the supraoptic nucleus or in the hypothalamic-hypophyseal system causes diabetes insipidus with polyuria (excessive formation of urine). The patient drinks copious amounts of water (polydipsia) and may excrete 20 liters of urine a day. The symptoms of diabetes insipidus may be relieved by the administration of vasopressin (Pitressin), an antidiuretic hormone (ADH), or extract from the hypophysis.

The hypothalamic-hypophyseal tract controls the formation and release of ADH, which causes water to be reabsorbed from the distal convoluted tubules and collecting duct of the kidneys into the bloodstream, thereby limiting the amount of water lost in the urine. Ingestion of large amounts of water causes a drop in the ADH level and reduces tubular reabsorption with resultant diuresis. Water deprivation increases the ADH level and causes increased reabsorption and concentrated urine. The cells in the supraoptic nuclei form much of the ADH or its precursors. ADH is formed in the cell body, travels down the axons of the hypothalamic-hypophyseal tract, and is stored in the posterior lobe of the hypophysis as neurosecretory granules. The osmoreceptor in the aortic and carotid body and in the hypothalamus itself detect the concentration of water in the blood. This information is passed on to the hypothalamic nuclei, which then control the release of ADH into the circulation.

Water intake is also controlled by hypothalamic neurons, with the area dorsal to the paraventricular nuclei being one of the water intake centers.

Hypothalamus and Emotions

As noted earlier in Case 16.2 and in Chapter 21, the hypothalamus sets the foundation for emotional responses and controls visceral functions. It exerts these powerful influences through the multisynaptic descending autonomic pathways in the lateral margins of the reticular formation and by controlling the release of the catecholamine—epinephrine (adrenaline) and norepinephrine (noradrenalin)—from the adrenal medulla.

Most postganglionic sympathetic fibers release a substance that is 80% epinephrine and 20% norepinephrine, which acts on alpha- and beta-adrenergic receptors in the organs; these are called adrenergic fibers. Small doses of acetylcholine injected into the bloodstream produce the same effect as stimulation of the cholinergic endings of craniosacral column.

Norepinephrine causes constriction of the peripheral vessels, with resultant increased blood flow in the large vessels. The blood pressure and pulse rate rise and blood flow to the coronary muscles increases. Epinephrine increases the heart rate and the force, amplitude, and frequency of heart contractions. It also dilates the pupils and the urinary and rectal sphincters, causing voiding and defecation. It inhibits the motility of the gut and causes the bronchial musculature to relax, thereby dilating the bronchial passages.

Epinephrine increases oxygen metabolism and the basic metabolic rate, causes hyperglycemia by increasing phosphorylase activity, which accelerates glycogenesis in the muscles and liver. And it increases the rate of synthesis of lactic acid to glycogen, thereby prolonging the contraction of the skeletal muscle.

HYPOTHALAMUS AND LIGHT LEVELS

Light produces dramatic effects that are mediated by the hypothalamus via the retinohypothalamic tract to the suprachiasmatic nucleus. In many animals abnormal variations in light levels alter the sexual cycle and prevent estrus. Light levels also affect the formation of melanin.

Epithalamus

The epithalamus is part of the limbic system and is located on the dorsal surface of the diencephalon above the thalamus. It consists of the pineal gland, habenular nuclei, stria medullaris thalami, and the habenular peduncular tract (fasciculus retroflexus of Meynert). Through these tracts the habenular nuclei have extensive connections to the septum and hypothalamus via the stria medullaris thalami and to the interpeduncular nuclei and onto somatic and autonomic nuclei in the brain stem and spinal cord, via the habenulopeduncular tract. Through these same pathways neuromodulators (especially the melatonin) produced in the pineal have considerable influence on the development of the gonads, the release of pituitary hormones, and the functions of the autonomic nervous system.

Pineal Body

The pineal, or epiphysis cerebri, is a small pinecone-shaped gland found in the roof of the third ventricle. This richly vascularized gland contains glial cells and pinealocytes and is innervated by the sympathetic nervous system from the superior cervical sympathetic ganglion with synapses on the pinealocytes.

Pinealocytes contain serotonin, melatonin, and norepinephrine. The pineal makes melatonin from serotonin; the enzyme levels necessary for this transformation are controlled by the suprachiasmatic nucleus. This nucleus sends fibers via the descending sympathetic pathway into the medial forebrain bundle, and via the descending spinal fibers to the intermediolateral cell column of the upper thoracic cord and then on to the superior cervical ganglion. The pinealocytes are related to the photoreceptor cells seen in this region in fish and amphibians. Pinocyte secretion of serotonin and melatonin is a cyclic response to stimulation from the optic system. These 24-hour circadian rhythms may well be the biological clock.

AUTONOMIC NERVOUS SYSTEM

Langley's description of the autonomic nervous system includes three parts: the sympathetic, parasympathetic, and enteric nervous systems.

The enteric nervous system, the second brain (Gershon, 1981, 1998), is recognized as a separate portion of the autonomic nervous system. It is considered a second brain because peristalsis and other spontaneous movements persist after it is isolated from all nervous input.

Much of the effectiveness of the hypothalamus is due to its innervation of the nuclei in the central nervous system that form the autonomic nervous system. In this section we identify these neurons in the central and peripheral nervous systems and list the responses produced by the autonomic nervous system in each organ. Note that normally an antagonistic balance exists between the functions of the parasympathetic and sympathetic systems. However, this equilibrium may be modified by environmental stresses or disease processes.

The somatic nervous system has its own receptors and effectors, which provide cutaneous and motor innervation to the skin and muscles in the head, neck, and body. The visceral, or autonomic, nervous system also has its own receptors and effectors, which provide dual motor and sensory innervation to the glands, smooth muscles, cardiac muscles, viscera, and blood vessels. These axons run part of the way with somatic fibers, but they also have separate pathways.

In the somatic nervous system the efferent neuron is the ventral horn cell or motor cranial-nerve nucleus. Its axon leaves the central nervous system to innervate a skeletal muscle.

In the visceral nervous system, two efferent neurons are found: the preganglionic neuron and the postganglionic neuron.

The preganglionic neuron is found in the intermediate horn at the thoracic and lumbar levels of the spinal cord. The axon of this cell leaves the central nervous system via the ventral root and ends in an autonomic ganglion, which parallels the spinal cord or is found near the target organ.

The preganglionic cell bodies are found in the central nervous system at the following sites:

Parasympathetic (Craniosacral)

1. Cranial parasympathetic (cranial nerves III, VII, IX, and X).
2. Sacral parasympathetic (sacral segments 2 to 4).

Sympathetic (Thoracolumbar)

1. All thoracic segments and lumbar segments 1 and 2. The postganglionic neuron, or the motor ganglion cell, is located outside the central nervous system and ends in the appropriate gland, smooth muscle, or cardiac muscle.

The nerve fibers are further classified as being adrenergic or cholinergic, depending on which nerve transmitter is involved—epinephrine or acetylcholine. The lumbar sympathetic preganglionic axons to the adrenal gland activate chromaffin cells (modified nerve cells) in the adrenal medulla, which release epinephrine (80%) and norepinephrine (20%) into the circulation and act on alpha- and beta-adrenergic receptors in the hollow organs, glands, and skin. Injections of epinephrine into the bloodstream produce an effect similar to the stimulation of the thoracolumbar or sympathetic nervous system. Small doses of acetylcholine injected into the bloodstream produce the same effect as stimulation of the craniosacral column. Most postganglionic parasympathetic fibers release acetylcholine at their terminals, receive innervation from the thoracolumbar system, and are cholinergic. Pilomotor axons, which also receive thoracolumbar innervation, are adrenergic.

The two systems provide dual innervation to glands and viscera and act to produce optimal balances of internal conditions under any environmental condition.

ENTERIC NERVOUS SYSTEM

In the alimentary canal (esophagus, stomach, intestines, and rectum) there are about 100 million neurons (Gershon, 1981, 1998). One network of neurons, Meissner's (submucosal) plexus, lies in the connective tissue between the longitudinal muscle coat and the circular musculature coat in the alimentary canal. Another, Auerbach's (myenteric) plexus, lies in the connective tissue between the circular muscle coat and the muscularis mucosa. Each plexus consists of multipolar, bipolar, and unipolar neurons. The enteric nervous system includes glia that appears similar to the astrocytes in the central nervous system. The astrocytes enwrap the neurons and their processes and also form a barrier between the blood and the enteric nervous system. There are extensive connections within the enteric nervous system and projections onto the pancreas, gallbladder, and elsewhere. The unipolar and bipolar neurons appear to function as sensory neurons with the multipolar cells forming many of the connections. The noradrenergic sympathetic postganglionic fibers project onto the submucosal and myenteric plexus, where they are inhibitory to the cholinergic neurons. (The cholinergic vagal input from the dorsal motor nucleus of the vagus to the submucosa and mucous membrane is excitatory.)

PARASYMPATHETIC SYSTEM: CRANIAL NERVES III, VII, IX, AND X

Cranial nerve III. The fibers originate in the Edinger-Westphal nucleus in the midbrain and innervate the constrictors of the pupil via the ciliary ganglion.

Cranial nerve VII. The axons originate in the superior salvatory nuclei of the pons and innervate glands in the nasal

Table 16.4 **COMPARISON BETWEEN SYMPATHETIC AND PARASYMPATHETIC SYSTEMS**

	SYMPATHETIC	PARASYMPATHETIC
Function	Energy expenditure, emergency	Protective, restorative
Effect	Generalized, long lasting	Local, short lasting
Preganglionic neuron	Thoracolumbar cord, T1 to L3	Cranial nerves III, VI, IX, X Sacral cord, S2 to S4
Ganglion	Paravertebral Prevertebral	Near end organ
Preganglionic myelinated fiber	Short	Long
Preganglionic neurotransmitter	Acetylcholine	Acetylcholine
Postganglionic unmyelinated fiber	Long	Short
Distribution	Throughout body	Specific organs
Innervation of limbs	Yes	No
Postganglionic neurotransmitter	Norepinephrine (except sweat) glands	Acetylcholine
Receptors	Alpha- and beta-adrenergic	Muscarinic
Neurotransmitter inactivation	Slow	Fast
Transmitter	Neuropeptide Y ATP	Vasoactive intestinal Polypeptide ATP

cavity and palate, and in the lacrimal glands (pterygopalatine, submandibular, and sublingual glands).

Cranial nerve IX. The fibers originate in the inferior salivatory nucleus in the medulla. The axons exit with nerve IX and end in the otic ganglion, which innervates the parotid gland.

Cranial nerve X. The dorsal motor nucleus of the vagus nerve provides preganglionic parasympathetic innervation to the pharynx, larynx, esophagus, lungs, heart, stomach, and intestines up to the transverse colon. The postganglionic fibers originate from ganglia in the respective organs and in the nodes of the submucosal plexus of Meissner and the myenteric plexus of Auerbach in the enteric nervous system associated with the alimentary tract.

SACRAL SEGMENTS S2–S4

The parasympathetic sacral plexus originates from sacral segments S2 and S4 and supplies the genitalia, sigmoid colon, rectum, bladder, and ureter. The ganglia are located in the organ and are named for the organ.

SYMPATHETIC SYSTEM

The preganglionic fibers originate in the intermediolateral column of gray matter in the spinal cord from T1 to L2; they exit in the white rami and enter the paravertebral sympathetic ganglionic chain (Fig. 16.12). The student is reminded that cranial nerves are not part of the sympathetic nervous system. The ganglia form a continuous paravertebral trunk in the cervical, thoracic, lumbar, and sacral segments.

The postganglionic fibers originate in the ganglia and exit via the gray communicating rami. The postganglionic fibers reach their destinations via plexuses enwrapping the arteries or via cranial and spinal nerves.

CERVICAL SYMPATHETIC GANGLIA

The cervical ganglia extend posterior to the great vessels from the level of the subclavian artery to the base of the skull. There are usually three ganglia in the cervical region: superior, middle, and inferior.

The superior cervical ganglion is flat and the largest (25 to 35 mm). The internal carotid nerves leave the superior border of the superior cervical ganglion and pass into the cranial cavity with the carotid artery in the carotid canal. These fibers form the plexus around the carotid artery and in the cavernous sinus. This ganglion provides postganglionic innervation to the eye, lacrimal gland, parotid gland (otic ganglia), submaxillary and sublingual glands (sublingual ganglia), and some branches to the heart.

The middle cervical ganglion is small and variable and is found at the level of the cricoid cartilage. It provides postganglionic fibers to the heart.

The inferior cervical ganglion is usually fused with the first thoracic ganglion to form the stellate ganglion. It is also small and irregular in shape and lies posterior to the vertebral artery. The postganglionic fibers innervate the heart.

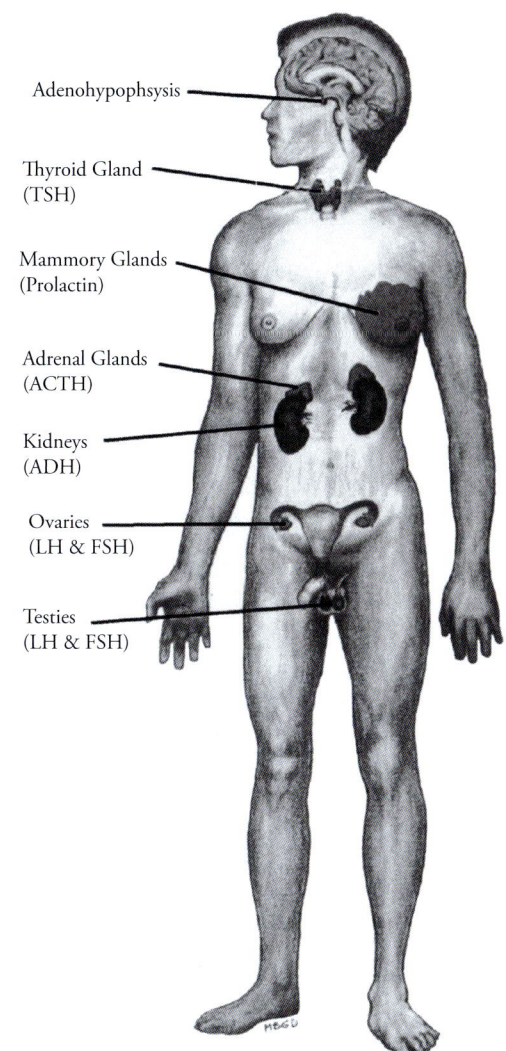

Figure 16.12 Target glands for adenohypophysis hormones.

THORACIC SYMPATHETIC GANGLIA

The thoracic portion of the sympathetic trunk extends anterior to the heads of the first ten ribs and then passes along the sides of the lower two thoracic vertebrae. The number of thoracic ganglia varies from 10 to 12.

The ganglia of T1 to T4 provide postganglionic fibers to the heart and lungs. The postganglionic fibers from T5 to T12 form the splanchnic nerves. The greater splanchnic nerve is formed by preganglionic rootlets from T5 to T10; the axons pass through the thoracic ganglia and end in the celiac ganglion. From there postganglionic axons run above the aorta, esophagus, thoracic duct, and azygos vein to reach the stomach, small intestine, and adrenal glands. The lesser and least splanchnic nerves arise from spinal cord segments T11 and T12 and run through the paravertebral ganglion to the celiac and superior mesenteric ganglia. From there the postganglionic axons run to the small intestine, the ascending portion of the colon, and the kidneys.

LUMBAR SYMPATHETIC GANGLIA

The lumbar sympathetic trunk consists of small ganglia that lie along the anterior border of the psoas muscle. The preganglionic fibers originate from the intermediate column of spinal cord, segments L1 and L2, pass through the lumbar ganglia, and end in the inferior mesenteric ganglion, where they innervate the descending colon, rectum, urinary bladder, ureter, and external genitalia.

AUTONOMIC DUAL INNERVATION OF SPECIFIC STRUCTURES

Eye

The major structures receiving dual sympathetic and parasympathetic innervations are listed in Table 16.4.

Parasympathetic

The preganglionic cell bodies are found in the Edinger-Westphal nuclei associated with cranial nerve III (Fig. 16.13). These fibers run on the outside of the third nerve and end in the ciliary ganglion. The postganglionic fibers run in the short ciliary nerve, providing innervation to the ciliary muscle and the constrictor of the iris, which permit accommodation for near vision.

Sympathetic

Preganglionic axons originate from the intermediolateral nucleus at cord levels C8 to T2 (Fig. 16.13). The fibers ascend in the sympathetic chain to the postganglionic neurons in the superior cervical ganglion. The postganglionic axons join the carotid plexus and then the ophthalmic branch of nerve V to innervate the dilator muscle of the iris and the levator palpebrae and radial ciliary muscles, producing eye opening (lifting of the lid) and dilation of the pupil for distant vision.

Lacrimal Glands

Parasympathetic

Preganglionic fibers originate in the superior salivatory nucleus of nerve VII and run to the pterygopalatine ganglion. The postganglionic fibers join the maxillary division of nerve V, resulting in vasodilation and secretion.

Salivary Glands

Parasympathetic

The preganglionic axons to the submaxillary and sublingual glands originate in the superior salivatory nucleus of nerve VII (pons) and enter the submandibular gland from which the postganglionic axons enter the salivary glands.

The preganglionic axons to the parotid originate in the inferior salivatory nucleus of nerve IX and leave the central nervous system and enter the otic ganglion. The resulting action is vasodilation and secretion.

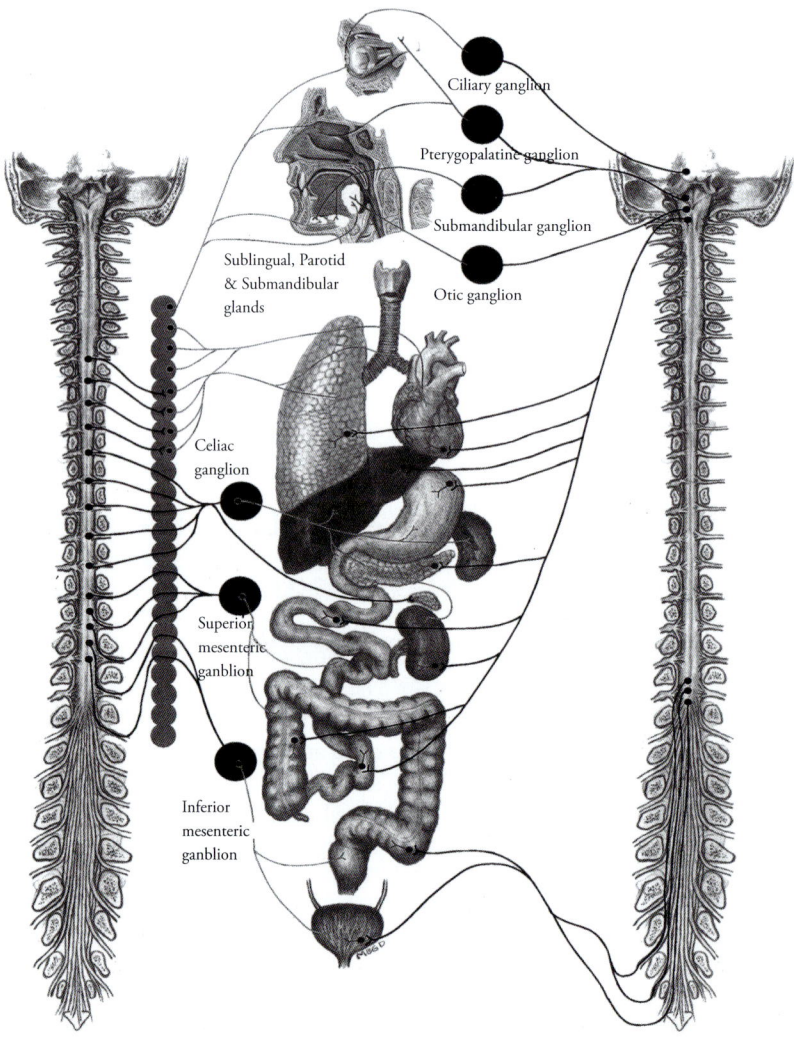

Figure 16.13 Autonomic nervous system. (Left) Sympathetic (thoracolumbar). (Right) Parasympathetic (craniosacral).

Sympathetic

These fibers originate from the intermediolateral column at the upper thoracic level, exit from the central nervous system, run up to the superior cervical ganglion, and then proceed to the glands. Vasoconstriction and reduced secretion result.

Heart

Parasympathetic

The preganglionic fibers originate in the dorsal nucleus of nerve X, exit from the central nervous system, and run in the vagus nerve to the postganglionic ganglia in the cardiac plexus and atria. These axons reach coronary vessels and atrial musculature, causing cardiac deceleration.

Sympathetic

The preganglionic fibers originate in the T1 to T4 segments, exit from the central nervous system, and reach the postganglionic neurons in the upper thoracic ganglion and all three cervical ganglia. The fibers form the cardiac nerves and enter the cardiac plexus. The resulting effect is cardiac acceleration.

Lungs

Parasympathetic

The preganglionic fibers originate in the dorsal motor nucleus of nerve X and run in the vagus to the pulmonary plexus in the bronchi and blood vessels. They cause constriction of the bronchi and decreased respiration.

Sympathetic

The preganglionic fibers originate in T1 to T4. The postganglionic fibers originate in the upper thoracic and lowest cervical ganglia. The result in this case is dilation of the bronchi and increased respiration.

Abdominal Viscera

Parasympathetic

These fibers originate from the dorsal motor nucleus of nerve X and S2 to S4, and end in the intrinsic plexus in the organ. They stimulate peristalsis and gastrointestinal secretions.

Sympathetic

The sympathetic fibers originate from the lower thoracic and lumbar segments, pass through the paravertebral ganglia, and form the splanchnic nerves, which end in the celiac and superior and inferior mesenteric ganglia. Postganglionic fibers from these ganglia end on smooth muscle or glands. They inhibit peristalsis and gastrointestinal secretion, stimulate secretion from the adrenal medulla, and cause vasoconstriction of the visceral vessels (see earlier discussion of enteric nervous system).

Pelvis

Parasympathetic

These fibers originate from segments S2 to S4 and end in ganglia in the organs. Postganglionic fibers supply the uterus, vagina, testes, erectile tissue (penis and clitoris), sigmoid colon, rectum, and bladder. They cause contraction and emptying of the bladder and erection of the clitoris or penis.

Sympathetic

These fibers originate from the lowest thoracic segments and segments L1 to L3 and run in the hypogastric nerves to the target viscera, where the ganglia are found. They cause vasoconstriction and ejaculation of semen, and inhibit peristalsis in the sigmoid colon and rectum.

Cutaneous and Deep Vessels, Glands, and Hair

Blood vessels receive only sympathetic postganglionic innervation from the appropriate paravertebral ganglion. Activation of this system produces vasoconstriction (cooling of the skin), sweating, and piloerection.

The innervation of the peripheral blood vessels and glands is summarized in Table 16.5.

DISORDERS OF THE AUTONOMIC NERVOUS SYSTEM

Disorders of the autonomic nervous system can affect any of the organs innervated by the autonomic nervous system. Only a few will be discussed here. The student is referred to any standard neurology text for further details.

EYE

A lesion in the nucleus or nerve root of cranial nerve III injuring the fibers from the Edinger-Westphal nucleus produces pupillary dilation (due to only sympathetic input).

Injury to the descending sympathetic fibers produces an ipsilateral Horner's syndrome (pupillary constriction and drooping of the

Table 16.5 INNERVATION OF THE PERIPHERAL BLOOD VESSELS AND GLANDS

REGION	LOCATION OF PREGANGLIONIC NEURONAL CELL BODY	LOCATION OF POSTGANGLIONIC NEURONAL CELL BODY
Head and neck	T1–T2	Superior cervical ganglion
Forelimb	T5–T9	Middle and inferior ganglion T1 and T2 of paravertebral chain
Hind limb	T10–L2	Lumbar and sacral ganglion
Thorax	T1–T5	Thoracic ganglion, T1–T5
Abdomen	T6–L2	Abdominal ganglion, T6–T12

eyelid). The Argyll-Robertson pupil does not react to light but will accommodate and is commonly seen in neurosyphilis in the central nervous system. (See discussion of tabes dorsalis in Chapter 9.)

BLOOD VESSELS

Reynard's disease (vasomotor disease), most common in young women, causes the patient to be abnormally sensitive to cold. On exposure to cold the extremities become cyanotic and then red and very painful. Sympathetic innervation does not seem to dilate the vessels. Vasodilators help, but resection of the preganglionic sympathetic innervation to the limb usually brings permanent relief.

HEART AND GASTROINTESTINAL TRACT

These organs respond to any change in our emotional state. Consequently, psychosomatic diseases, for example, hypertension and ulcers, affect them.

Bladder

The bladder is a reflex organ and contracts in response to stretch. The afferents are carried into the sacral spinal cord; efferent are supplied by the parasympathetic (S2–S4) and sympathetic (L1+L2) ganglia. The parasympathetic axons initiate the reflex contraction of the bladder during urination (micturition)—a voluntary action initiated through the nerve to the external sphincter (striated in males, essentially the whole urethra in females). Sympathetic axons do not participate in micturition but control blood vessels and closure of the internal sphincter during sexual intercourse.

Normally, the bladder fills and expands, stretching the receptors in the bladder walls. The pressure buildup is carried into the central nervous system by the sensory nerves. Following the voluntary contraction of the external sphincter, the bladder contracts reflexively; the internal and external sphincters open and the muscles in the pelvic floor relax (control from cerebral cortex). The urine passing through the urethra continues the stimulation until the bladder is empty. The external sphincter then closes. We can also initiate closing voluntarily with the assistance of the abdominal muscles.

The urine passing through the urethra continues the stimulation until the bladder is empty (can be interrupted by enlarged prostate). The external sphincter then closes, the bladder fills and becomes distended, and it voids suddenly without cortical control.

Autonomic Bladder
Destruction of the parasympathetic supply by injury to the motor roots produces the autonomic bladder, in which there is no sensation and no longer any reflex or voluntary control. The need to void arises from abdominal discomfort produced by increasing intra-abdominal pressure.

Sensory Bladder
Injury to the sensory roots or ganglia or to the dorsal column produces the sensory paralytic bladder, in which there is no sensation and no reflex ability to void. The bladder visibly enlarges and then (overflows) dribbles. Voiding is also difficult without sensory feedback.

Uninhibited Bladder
Interruption of the cortical pathways (bilateral involvement of the cerebral hemispheres) produces the uninhibited bladder, in which sensation is normal, but the patient no longer has control over voiding. Thus, as the bladder fills and becomes distended, it voids suddenly without cortical control.

Reflex Bladder
Isolation of the bladder from the upper motor neurons either by transection of the spinal cord above the sacral level or by extensive brain disease produces the reflex bladder. In this condition the descending autonomic fibers are interrupted as well as the corticospinal fibers, but the spinal reflex circuit remains intact. Micturition is involuntary and results from just the stretch reflex alone. When the volume reaches above 250 ml or so, voiding is sudden and uncontrollable, closing voluntarily with the assistance of the abdominal muscles voiding can be stopped.

BIBLIOGRAPHY

Bodian, D. 1963. Cytological aspects of neurosecretion in opossum neurohypophysis. Bull. Johns Hopk. Hosp. 113:57.

Bodian, D. 1966. Herring bodies and neuroapocrine secretion in the monkey: an electron microscopic study of the fate of the neurosecretory product. Bull. Johns Hopk. Hosp. 118:282.

Becker, K. L. Principles and Practice of Endocrinology and Metabolism 2001. 3rd ed. Philadelphia, PA: Lippincott, Williams and Wilkins.

Brownstein, M. J. 1989. Neuropeptides. In G. J. Siegel, B. W. Agranoff, R. W. Albers, and P. B. Molinoff (Eds.) Basic Neurochemistry. Molecular, Cellular and Medical Aspects, pp. 287–309. New York, NY: Raven Press.

Gershon, M. D. 1981. The enteric nervous system. Ann. Rev. Neurosci. 4: 227–272.

Gershon M. 1998. The Second Brain: The scientific Basis of Gut instinct and a ground breaking Understanding of Nervous Disorders of the Stomach and Intestines. Harper p. 338.

Green, J. D. 1966. The comparative anatomy of the portal vascular system and of the innervation of the hypophysis. In G. W. Harris and B. T. Donovan (Eds.) The Pituitary Gland, Vol. 1, p. 127. Berkely: University of California Press.

Haymaker, W., Anderson, E., and Nauta, W. J. H. 1969. The Hypothalamus. Springfield, IL: Charles C. Thomas.

Karczmar, A. G., Koketsu, K., and Nishi, S. (Eds.) 1986. Autonomic and Enteric Ganglia. New York, NY: Plenum Press.

Martin, J. B., Reichlin, S., and Brown, G. M. 1987. Clinical Neuroendocrinology. 2nd ed. Philadelphia, PA: F. A. Davis.

McGeer, P. L., and McGeer, E. G. 1989. Amino acid neurotransmitters. In G. J. Siegal, B. W. Agranoff, R. W. Albers, and P. B. Molinoff (Eds.) Basic Neurochemistry. Molecular, Cellular and Medical Aspects, pp. 123–131. New York, NY: Raven Press.

Muller, E. E., and Nistico, G. 1989. Brain Messengers and the Pituitary. New York, NY: Academic Press.

Palay, S. L. 1957. The fine structure of the neurohypophysis. In H. Waelsch (Ed.) Progress in Neurobiology: II. Ultrastructure and Cellular Chemistry of Neural Tissue, p. 31. New York, NY: Paul B. Hoeber.

Siegal, G. J., Agranoff, B. W., Albers, R. W., and Molinoff, P. B. 1989. Basic Neurochemistry. Molecular, Cellular and Medical Aspects. New York, NY: Raven Press.

Scharrer, E. 1966. Endocrines and the Central Nervous System. Baltimore, MD: Williams and Wilkins.

Szentagothai, J., Flerko, B., Mess, B., and Halasy, B. 1968. Hypothalamic Control of the Anterior Pituitary. Budapest, Hungary: Akademiai Kiado.

Wislocki, G. B.1938. The vascular supply of the hypophysis cerebri of the rhesus monkey and man. Proc. Assoc. Res. Nerv. Dis. 17:48.

17.

CEREBRAL CORTEX

CYTOARCHITECTURE, PHYSIOLOGY, AND OVERVIEW OF FUNCTIONAL LOCALIZATION

For correlations with the regions in the brain, refer to the gross brain sections in Chapter 33. Figures 33.1 to 33.7 are coronal sections of the gross brain, and Figure 33.8 is a horizontal section showing the relationship between the cerebral cortex, caudate, and putamen. Once the student has reviewed the chapters on the functions of the cerebral cortical regions (Chapters 17–22), it is then appropriate to examine these sections for further correlation of structure with functions. The gyri and sulci of the brain are labeled in these sections. The position of the ventricular system should be noted in each section with the lateral ventricles found in sections of the cerebrum, the third ventricle found between the diencephalic halves, and the fourth ventricle found at levels of the medulla and pons. The cerebral aqueduct can be seen in the center of the midbrain levels. The position of the cerebellum should also be noted in the more posterior sections (see Figs. 33.6, 33.7, and 33.9). In Figure 33.9 these relationship can also be seen in the gross brain sections of levels through the cerebrum and diencephalon, midbrain, pons, and medulla.

ANATOMICAL CONSIDERATIONS

A firm knowledge of the structure and function of the cerebral cortex and the relationship of the cerebral cortex to the subcortical centers is of crucial importance for all who wish to understand the behavior and accomplishments of humans as opposed to other animal forms. The use of the thumb and fingers for fine manipulations with tools, the use of linguistic and mathematical symbols for communication in the auditory and visual spheres, and the capacity for postponement of gratification all reflect the evolution of the cerebral cortex. This development of the cerebral cortex has led to a laminar arrangement of 16 billion nerve cells with an almost infinite number of synapses. Beaulieu and Colonnier have estimated that in a cubic millimeter of neocortex there are 2.78×10^8 synapses, 84% of which are type I (excitatory) and 16% type II (inhibitory).

The almost infinite number and variety of circuits present not only has provided the anatomical substrate for the recording of an infinite number of past experiences but has also allowed for a plasticity of future function projected both in time and in space.

The attempt to relate functional differences to the differences in structure of the various areas of the cerebral cortex was a scientific outgrowth of the earlier philosophical arguments concerning the relationship of mind and body. We may indicate at the onset that to a certain degree cytoarchitectural differences do reflect functional differences. This is never, however, a one-to-one relationship. Moreover, at times, architectural differences are not sharp; strict borders may not be present.

The various areas of cerebral cortex differ on several parameters:

1. Thickness, evident on simple visual inspection (average thickness is 2.5 mm; motor cortex: 4.5 mm; visual cortex: 1.45 to 2.0 mm). In addition to differences in overall thickness, some areas differ in the thickness of the various layers that constitute the laminar pattern.

2. Relative density of the various cell types (evident in Nissl stains for cells or Golgi silver stains) to be discussed later, for example, pyramidal versus stellate. It must also be noted that within a given area of cortex, the various layers of cortex differ as regards the relative distribution of these various types of cells (Fig. 17.1).

3. Density of horizontal fiber plexuses (stripes) (evident on myelin and silver stains) and density of axodendritic and other synapses (evident on Golgi stain and Fink-Heimer stains).

4. Degree of myelination of intracortical fiber systems (evident on myelin stain). To some extent, the various myelinated bands may be seen with the naked eye in freshly cut sections of the cerebral cortex. For example, Gennari in 1782 and Vicq d'Azyr in 1786 independently had noted a white line in the cortex near the calcarine fissure. The various features to be noted in the several types of stains are demonstrated in Figure 17.1.

CYTOLOGY

From the standpoint of cytology the neurons within the cerebral cortex may be classified into two major categories: pyramidal and stellate (Fig. 17.2). The axons of pyramidal cells

Figure 17.1 Diagram of the structure of the cerebral cortex. The results obtained with a Golgi stain, a Nissl stain or other cellular stain, and a myelin stain are contrasted. I = molecular layer; II = external granular layer; III = external pyramidal layer; IV = internal granular layer; V = large or giant pyramidal layer (ganglionic layer); VI = fusiform layer. The following features should be noted in the myelin stain: 1a = molecular layer 3a1 = band of Kaes-Bechterew; 4 = outer band of Baillarger; 5b = inner band of Baillarger. (After Brodmann, from Ranson, S. W., and Clark, S. L.: The Anatomy of the Nervous System, Philadelphia, W. B. Saunders, 1959, p. 350.)

(type I cells/neurons with long axons) form the majority of association, callosal, and subcortical projections, while the stellate cells (type II cells/neurons with short axons) form the local circuits (refer to Chapter 3 for additional discussion).

Neurons may also be classified on the basis of whether the dendrites have spines or an absence of spines.

From the standpoint of electrophysiology the neurons may be classified as fast spiking, regular spiking, or bursting (repetitive discharge).

1. Neurons whose dendrites have spines (spiny neurons) account for the majority of the neurons in the cerebral cortex. These are excitatory and are of two types:

    a. Pyramidal cells: these constitute two-thirds of all neurons in the neocortex. These cells are defined by a prominent apical dendrite extending through all layers of the cortex to layer 1. Pyramidal neurons have cell bodies of variable height—small, 1 to 12 μm; medium, 20 to 25 μm; large, 45 to 50 μm; and giant, 70 to 100 μm. The giant pyramidal cells are characteristic of the motor cortex. The upper end of the pyramidal cell continues on toward the surface as the apical dendrite. Numerous spines are found on the dendrite, providing

Figure 17.2 Pyramidal and stellate cells as demonstrated in Golgi stain of cat cerebral cortex. Arrow indicates stellate cell; AD, apical dendrite of pyramidal cell; AX, axons of pyramidal cell; BD, basal dendrite of pyramidal cells; PC, pyramidal cells.

sites for synaptic contact. The pyramidal neurons have the largest dendritic trees and also contain axons that form associational, callosal, and projectional connections. In general, the larger the cell body, the larger the apical dendrite and the wider the spread in terms of ramifications of the terminal horizontal branches. The wider the spread of the apical dendrite, the greater the number of possible axodendritic synapses. The larger the cell body, the greater the number of possible axosomatic synapses. In addition to the apical dendrite, shorter basal dendrites arise from the base of the cell body and arborize in the vicinity of the cell body. The axon emerges from the base of the cell body and descends toward the deeper white matter. In general, the axons of small- and medium-sized pyramidal cells terminate as association fascicles within the cortex. The axons of large and giant pyramidal cells enter the deeper white matter as (a) association fibers to other cortical areas, (b) commissural fibers to the contralateral hemisphere, or (c) projection (efferent) fibers to subcortical, brain stem, and spinal cord areas. In addition, recurrent collateral association fibers may branch off from these axons within the cortex. They also function as the main efferent outflow of the cerebral cortex to subcortical areas (thalamus, basal ganglia, brain stem, and spinal cord) and to other cerebral cortical areas (ipsilateral and body [soma]). These neurons are found primarily in layer 4 of the sensory cortex. Their axons project locally within the area and not to distant sites.

Physiology: Most spiny neurons/pyramidal cells utilize glutamate as a synaptic transmitter and demonstrate "regular" spiking that is an adapting pattern of discharge in response to a constant current injection. These cells generally demonstrate a significant after hyperpolarization (AHP). Some of the pyramidal cells located in deeper layers, primarily layer 5, may demonstrate a bursting pattern at low threshold. These neurons respond to depolarization by generating repetitive spikes, usually three in sequence. The regular firing pyramidal cells are contralateral hemispheres; the pyramidal cells also provide a massive collateral network to other neurons within the local area. Each pyramidal cell also receives multiple inputs on to its dendritic spines. The Betz cells, the giant pyramidal neuron of the motor cortex, have at least 10,000 spines, each with a type I excitatory synapse.

  b. Spiny stellate neurons: the prominent apical dendrite is not present. Instead dendrites of almost equal length radiate out from the cell, characterized by thin apical dendrites that do not branch extensively in layer 1. In contrast, the burst firing pyramidal cells have thick apical dendrites and extensive branching in layer 1. As we will discuss next, this may have considerable significance for the difference in excitability of the various cortical areas, for example, motor cortex compared to visual cortex.

2. Smooth neurons without spines, formerly referred to as smooth stellate cells. Multiple types have been described. The most common is the basket cell that has axons that form baskets around the soma of the pyramidal cells. The Retzius-Cajal neurons are horizontally oriented cells found in layer 1. The Martinotti cell, the double bouquet cell of Cajal, and the chandelier cell have a vertical orientation.

Physiology: The smooth cells are generally fast spiking and make type II inhibitory connections utilizing gamma amino butyric acid (GABA) as the transmitter. In contrast to pyramidal neurons, the action potentials of these fast-spiking cells are brief; the repolarization phase is rapid and followed by a significant under shoot. This has been correlated with very large, fast repolarizing potassium current.

The interrelationship of neurons within the neocortex is demonstrated in Figure 17.3.

BASIC DESIGN AND FUNCTIONAL ORGANIZATION OF CEREBRAL CORTEX

The cerebral cortex is characterized by two essential design principles: (1) the neurons have a horizontal laminar arrangement, and (2) connections occur in a vertical columnar manner. These vertical columns extend from pial surface to white matter. A specific region, a specific stimulus, or a specific stimulus orientation activates each cylindrical column. Activation of a specific column also activates inhibition in adjacent columns, the concept of inhibitory surround (see Angevine and Smith, 1982). In the primary sensory, each column is concerned with a particular modality of sensation for a particular representation of the body or specific sector of a field of

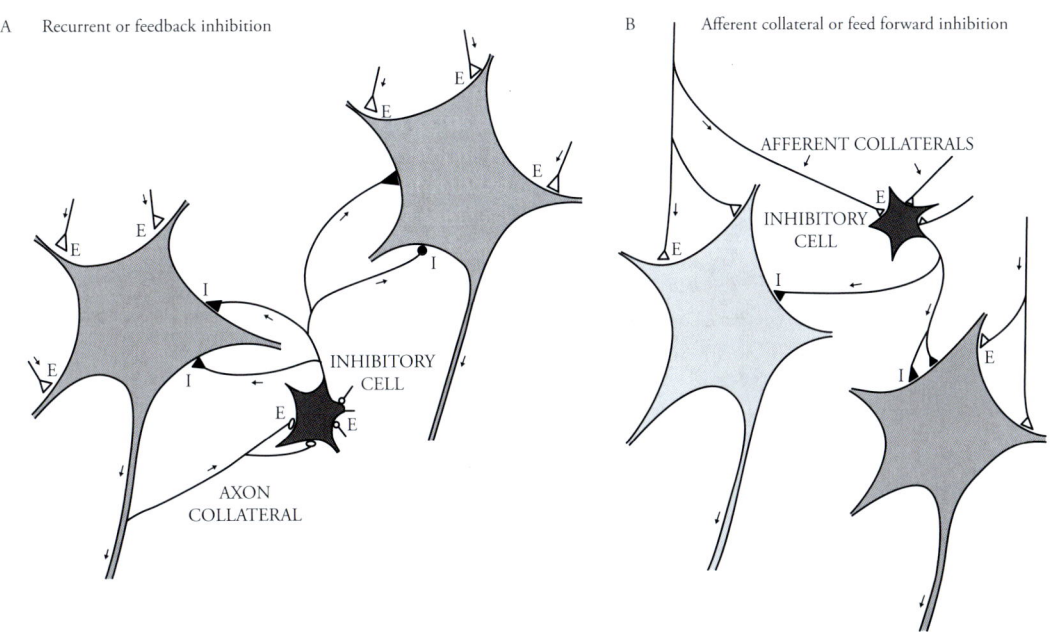

Figure 17.3 Diagram indicating possible function of stellate cells as inhibitory interneurons. Two mechanisms are demonstrated. (*A*) Recurrent or feedback inhibition and (*B*) afferent collateral or feedforward inhibition. (Modified from Eccles, J.C. in Jasper, H. et al. Basic Mechanisms of the Epilepsies. Boston, Little, Brown & Company, p. 249, 1969.)

stimulation. This columnar organization first was described by Mountcastle for somatosensory cortex and has been subsequently found in other sensory and associational cortex. As discussed by Rakic (1988), this columnar or radial organization may be a reflection of the ontogenetic ingrowth of neurons from the ependymal surface via glial guide to the cortical surface, which was discussed in Chapter 4. A similar columnar organization of the callosal system has also been demonstrated (see Jones, 1985).

FUNDAMENTAL TYPES OF CEREBRAL CORTEX

Brodmann in 1903 distinguished two fundamental types of cerebral cortex: homogenetic or heterogenetic.

1. *Homogenetic.* This type, as already illustrated in Figure 17.1, has a six-layer pattern at some time during development recognizable by the end of the third fetal month. This type of cortex is also called neocortex or isocortex; neopallium; or supralimbic.
2. *Heterogenetic.* This type of cortex does not have six layers at any time during development or during adult life. This type of cortex is also called allocortex and has three layers. There is a transitional zone between allocortex and the neocortex: the mesocortex that corresponds to the cingulate gyrus, the parahippocampal gyrus, the piriform area, and the anterior perforated substance (Fig. 17.4).

Figure 17.4 Frontal section through the diencephalic part of the prosencephalon of an 87 mm (crown to rump), 3-1/2-month-old embryo. a and a1 = anlage of the hippocampus (heterogenetic or rhinal allocortex); b = anlage of the parahippocampal cortex (limbic mesocortex); c = supra limbic isocortex (or homogenetic). Mg, marginal layer; Mt, mantle layer; Mx, matrix layer. (From Yakovlev, P.I.: Res. Publ. Assn. Nerv. Ment. Dis., 39:3-46, 1962, Williams and Wilkins.)

SUMMARY OF THE FUNDAMENTAL SIX-LAYERED SCHEME OF NEOCORTEX

Layer I: the molecular or plexiform layer. This layer primarily consists of dendrites and axons from other cortical area, deeper layers, and nonspecific thalamic input. A tangential plexus of fibers composed of the apical dendrites, ascending axons, and axon collaterals provides a dense collection of axodendritic synapses.

Layer II: the external granular layer. This layer is a relatively densely packed layer of small stellate granule cells and small pyramidal cells whose apical dendrites terminate in the molecular layer and whose axons are sent to lower cortical layers.

Layer III: the external pyramidal layer. This layer is composed of medium and large pyramidal cells whose apical dendrites extend to layer I. The axons of these cells may function as association, commissural, or intracortical association fibers.

Layer IV: the internal granular layer. This layer is densely packed with granular/stellate cells. A dense horizontal plexus of myelinated fibers, the external band of Baillarger is also present and is composed of the branches of the specific thalamo-cortical projection system. These fibers synapse with the stellate cells of this layer, with the basilar dendrites of the pyramidal cells of layer III, or with the apical dendrites of the pyramidal cells of layers V and VI.

Layer V: internal or large and giant pyramidal cell layer; also called the ganglionic layer. This layer serves as the major source of outflow fibers, particularly to motor areas of the basal ganglia, brain stem, and spinal cord and possibly to the projection nuclei of the thalamus. Although corticocortical output arises primarily from the more superficial pyramidal cells of layer 3, layers 5 and 6 also provide such an output. Note that there is some overlap of the functions of pyramidal cell of layers 5 and 6. Collaterals of the axons also function as intracortical association fibers. In the deeper portion of this layer a dense horizontal plexus of fibers is present: the internal band of Baillarger.

Layer VI: the fusiform or spindle cell multiform layer. This layer is composed of a mixture of spindle-shaped cells, pyramidal cells, and stellate cells. Dendrites ascend to various cortical levels. The axons enter the white matter as short association fibers or ascend to other cortical layers. However, the corticothalamic outflow usually occurs from pyramidal cells in this layer.

CLASSIFICATION OF THE VARIOUS TYPES OF NEOCORTEX

It is evident that in the adult not all areas of neocortex have the same appearance. Brodmann termed those areas of homogenetic neocortex that demonstrated the typical six-layered pattern seen in Figure 17.1 as homotypical.

At one extreme is the agranular motor cortex. This has many giant pyramidal cells present in layer 5 but with a virtual absence of an internal granular layer 4. At the opposite extreme is the granular primary sensory projection cortex. Layers 2, 3, and 4 appear as an almost continuous granular layer. Layers of 5 and 6 are thin and few large pyramidal cells are present.

Von Economo divided the cerebral cortex into five basic categories (Fig. 17.5):

Type 1 is the agranular motor cortex.

Type 2 is referred to as homotypical or frontal granular cortex and is found in the superior frontal gyrus of the prefrontal area.

Type 3 is the midpoint and is best seen in the inferior parietal lobule.

Type 4 is referred to as polar and is represented by the nonstriate visual association cortex of area 18 close to the occipital pole.

Type 5 is the granular striate occipital visual projection cortex. Because the large number of granule cells in this type of cortex resembles a cloud of dust, the Greek word *konios* is employed—thus the term *koniocortex*.

Figure 17.6 demonstrates the distribution of these various cortical types. Von Economo and Koskinis then developed a classification that dealt in a logical manner with the variations of cytoarchitecture in terms of definable histologic gradations using a letter terminology. Thus, motor cortex received the designation FA; premotor cortex, FB; and the frontal eye field, FC; and so on. In this textbook we will follow the classification of Brodmann that has been most commonly

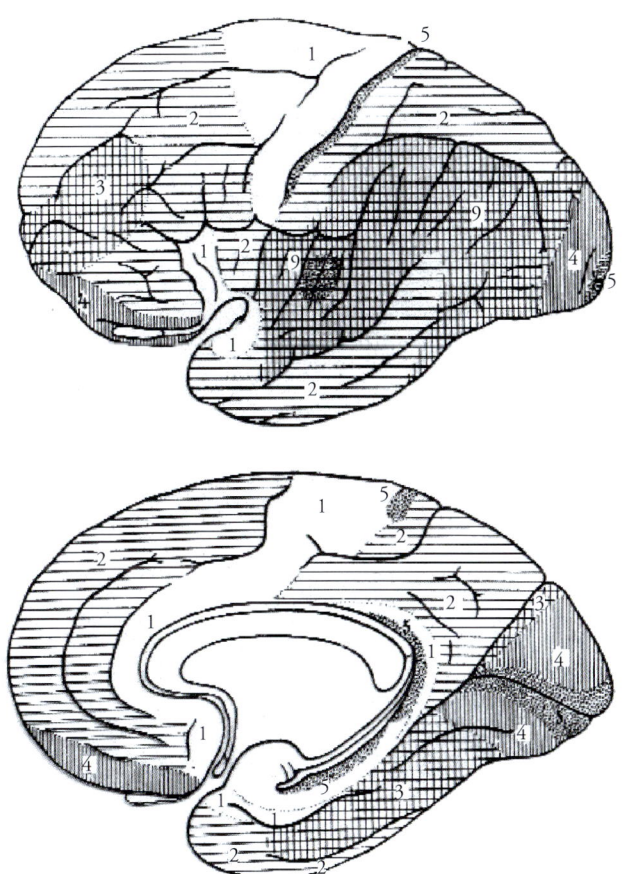

Figure 17.6 Distribution of the five cortical types of Figure 17.5 over the lateral and medial surfaces of the cerebral surface. The Sylvian fissure has been laid open. (From Von Economo, C.: The Cytoarchitectonics of the Human Cerebral Cortex. London, Oxford University Press, 1929, p. 18.)

employed (Fig. 17.7).[1] Numbers were initially assigned as histologically distinct areas were identified in successive horizontal slices moving in anterior and posterior directions from the central sulcus. The crest of the postcentral gyrus would then appear in the first horizontal section and would be assigned the number 1. The primary motor cortex is assigned 4; the premotor cortex, 6; and the frontal eye field, 8. Thus, there is no logical reason why the numbers 6 and 8 are assigned to areas of the frontal lobe and 5 and 7 to areas in the parietal lobes. Nevertheless, some of the numbers are used with sufficient frequency in everyday neurological language that the student should commit these to memory. Before we review these areas with their correlated function, it is necessary to consider the methods employed in the study of functional localization.

METHODS FOR THE STUDY OF FUNCTIONAL LOCALIZATION IN CEREBRAL CORTEX

HOW DO WE STUDY FUNCTION?

In considering functional localization, and the correlation with cytoarchitecture, it has been customary to consider the effects of two general categories: stimulation and ablation.

Figure 17.5 The five fundamental types of cortical structure: Type 1 = agranular motor cortex. Type 2 = frontal homotypical (frontal granular). Type 3 = parietal homotypical. Type 4 = polar, for example, area 18. Type 5 = granular koniocortex. (From Von Economo, C.: The Cytoarchitectonics of the Human Cerebral Cortex. London, Oxford University Press, 1929, p. 16.)

[1] For a comparison of the two systems in the monkey, see Figure 17.8.

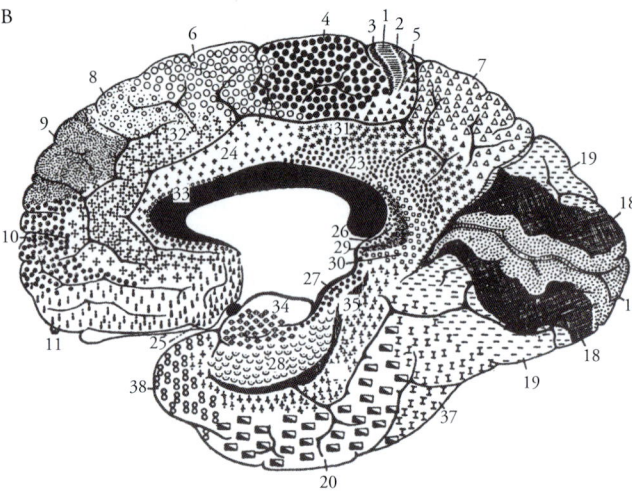

Figure 17.7 Cytoarchitectural areas of cerebral cortex as designated by Brodmann. (*A*) Lateral Surface and (*B*) Medial Surface. (From Curtis, Jacobson and Marcus. 1972: An Introduction to the Neurosciences: Filmstrip. Philadelphia, W.B. Saunders.)

Stimulation

Various disease processes in humans involving the cerebral cortex may produce a local area of excessive discharge, in a sense, a local area of stimulation resulting in focal seizures.

Actually, our first understanding of cortical function was derived from the systematic study of such cases of focal discharge (termed *focal seizures, focal convulsions, focal epilepsy,* or *epileptiform seizures*) by Hughlings Jackson in 1863 and 1870. Jackson was able to predict that an area existed in the cerebral cortex that governed isolated movements of the contralateral extremities. Such focal seizures are also referred to as *partial seizures* in the International Classification. These partial seizures are subdivided into *simple partial* (simple motor or sensory or psychic symptoms), as contrasted with *complex partial* (complex motor sequences of automatic behavior and/or alterations in mental function as regard perception, memory, and affect) accompanied by impairment of consciousness, confusion, and amnesia.

Partial seizures or partial epilepsy must be distinguished from those seizures which are nonfocal, that is, bilateral or generalized in their onset (*generalized or idiopathic epilepsy* in the International Classification).

Other Methods of Stimulation

Electrical stimulation of the cerebral cortex may be carried out in the human patient undergoing operative procedures on the cerebral cortex to identify specific cortical areas or may be employed on animal preparations in the experimental laboratory. Transcranial electrical and magnetic stimulation of the cerebral cortex has been developed as a clinical technique.

Evoked potentials: stimulation of afferent pathways may be utilized to identify short latency responses evoked from specific cortical areas. When stimulating the lower extremity (or sciatic nerve), response is limited to that specific area of the contralateral postcentral gyrus devoted to the representation of the lower extremity. Stimulation of the upper extremity will elicit a similar response from a different portion of the contralateral postcentral gyrus: that devoted to representation of the upper extremity. Eventually it is possible to prepare a map of the somatosensory projection cortex of the postcentral gyrus. It is possible to refine this technique at the response end by using microelectrode recordings from within or just outside neurons at particular depths of the cortex. It is also possible to define more carefully the parameters of stimulation, as Hubel and Wiesel have done in their analysis of responses in the visual cortex to specific types of visual stimuli (see Chapter 23). The evoked potential method has been subsequently developed as a practical noninvasive method to study conduction in the visual, auditory, and somatosensory systems.

By stimulating particular thalamic nuclei, one may map out specific thalamocortical relationships.

A modification of the technique is that of antidromic stimulation of an efferent pathway, such as the pyramidal tract, to map out the cortical nerve cells of origin of fibers in this tract.

Chemical agents locally applied to the pial responses of the patient with seizure discharges surface of cerebral cortex may be employed in the laboratory preparation to produce an acute or chronic focus of discharge. The most common agent employed for the acute focus is penicillin. Chronic foci are produced by cobalt or alumina cream.

Interpretation of results: The results obtained by the method of stimulation are subject to several possible interpretations from the standpoint of functional localization:

1. The effect observed may be clearly related to the actual function of the area stimulated; for example, stimulation of the motor cortex results in discrete movements.

2. The effect observed may be in part related to the spread of discharge to other cortical areas via corpus callosum to the opposite hemisphere or association pathways, within the same hemisphere.

   The effects observed may in part reflect the spread of discharge to various subcortical and brain stem centers. The generalized convulsive seizure that may develop secondary to the focal seizure represents such a spread.

   At times, the secondary spread to other cortical and subcortical areas may be so rapid that the focal origin of the seizure discharge may be difficult to ascertain and it may be difficult on clinical grounds to separate such seizures from nonfocal (primary, generalized) epilepsy.

3. The effects observed may indicate that the remainder of the central nervous system is functioning without the participation of the area stimulated. Thus, if all the neurons of a given cortical area are involved in a seizure discharge, they may be unable to participate in their usual activities, be they of an afferent, integrative, or efferent nature. Thus, the effects of seizure discharges involving prefrontal or hippocampal areas may be in some aspects quite similar to the effect of ablation of these areas as regards intellectual functions, personality, and memory or learning. This concept also implies, in a sense, to release of function in other areas (cortical and subcortical). Therefore, certain emotions involving the prefrontal or temporal lobe areas are also similar to the effects obtained on ablation of these areas and suggest release of other centers.

4. In the interpretation of the relationship of location of the pathology to the seizure manifestation, the threshold for discharge of the underlying cortex must be considered. Thus, in the large series of parasagittal meningiomas reported by Cushing and Eisenhardt (1938), seizure invariably accompanied those overlying the Rolandic cortex ("middle third parasagittal") at a relatively early point in the clinical history, whereas anterior or posterior one-third of parasagittal lesions had seizure manifestation at a much later point corresponding to a larger size of tumor. Motor cortex has a much lower threshold for seizure discharge than other areas of cerebral cortex.

Ablation

This method involves destruction of a specific area by operative resection, coagulation, or freezing to the point of tissue death. In man, the method of clinical pathological correlation has produced considerable information. The destructive lesions have been the result of a local area of tissue destruction due to blood vessel occlusion, hemorrhage, solitary metastatic tumor, or intrinsic tumor. In the laboratory transient focal depression may be produced by focal cooling or by application of KCl.

Interpretation of results:

1. The observed effects may indicate deficits directly related to a failure of a positive function normally subserved by the area destroyed. For example, after destruction of parietal somatosensory projection areas, deficits in stereognosis and position sense occur.

2. The effects may reflect the release of centers in other cortical areas or at other levels of the neural axis. This presumes that the area ablated usually inhibits certain functions of these other centers. The end result then is an enhancement of certain functions. Spasticity several days, weeks, or months after ablation of the motor cortex is an example.

3. A temporary loss of function of a lower center may follow acute ablation of higher centers. For example, following acute unilateral ablation of all motor cortex in human, there will be observed a temporary loss or depression of deep tendon reflexes and of other stretch reflexes in the contralateral extremities. There will be initially a flaccid paralysis. This state (referred to as the "diaschisis of Von Monakow") is analogous to spinal shock or pyramidal shock. As recovery from this state occurs, deep tendon reflexes return and become progressively more active. The flaccid paralysis is replaced by a spastic paresis. Transhemispheric effects also occur.

HOW DO WE CONFIRM THE LOCATION OF THE PATHOLOGY?

Initially, data as to the actual location of the disease process and its nature (old scar from traumatic injury; old area of tissue damage due to ischemia, infection, local compression, or invasive brain tumor) were dependent on final examination of the brain at autopsy. One may then speak of the method of clinical pathological correlation. With the development of neurosurgery it became possible to define and to confirm during life the anatomical boundaries of the disease process, often allowing for treatment or cure of the basic disease process.

The specialized techniques of electroencephalography, arteriography, pneumoencephalography, and radioactive brain scan were developed during the 1930s, 1940s, and 1950s, to provide some information about localization prior to surgery.

The subsequent development of the more precise noninvasive imaging techniques of computerized axial tomography (CT scan), magnetic resonance imaging (MRI scan), and positron emission tomography (PET scan) during the 1970s and 1980s now provides the closest correlation of clinical findings and anatomical location of the lesion in the living patient, supplanting the earlier radiological techniques of arteriography, pneumoencephalography, and radioactive brain scans.

The techniques of CT scan, MRI, PET, and SPECT have been discussed previously (see Chapter 2).

Concept of representation and re-representation of function: In considering functional localization, one must keep in mind that a given function may be represented and re-represented at the various levels of the neural axis.

Ontogenetic factor. In considering the effects of ablation, one must also consider the ontogenetic factor. Bilateral ablation of the prefrontal cortex in the adult monkey produces impairment in the capacity to delay responses. Bilateral prefrontal ablation at 1 week of age in the infant monkey does not have this effect. Such a monkey when tested at 4 months, the usual age when the capacity to delay response appears, is able to manifest this capacity. Similar observations may be made with regard to somatosensory and visual pattern discrimination in the infant cat as compared to adult cats following the appropriate resection of the somatosensory or visual projection cortex. Similar observations may be made in humans. Thus, extensive destruction in most adults of the speech areas in the left hemisphere will result in a marked and lasting deficit in linguistic expression (so-called Broca's expressive aphasia). Destruction of this same area in the infant or young child does not produce an enduring defect.

CORRELATION OF THE NEOCORTICAL CYTOARCHITECTURE AND FUNCTION

General observation: Those neocortical areas with specialized cytoarchitecture deviating from the classical six-layered cortex have very specialized function, for example, primary motor or sensory cortex. In contrast, the classical six-layered pattern tends to occur in association areas such as prefrontal, which have more complex and not such limited highly specialized functions.

The more commonly used Brodmann numbers are listed in the following outline with a brief note as to function. The corresponding terminology of Von Economo and Koskinis is indicated in parentheses. The list is not all inclusive and does not include the areas of mesial temporal lobe. Since many studies have been performed in the monkey, a comparison guide for cytoarchitecture is provided in Figure 17.8.

Figure 17.9 demonstrates the lobes, gyri, and major sulci visible on the lateral surface of the cerebral hemisphere. Figure 17.10 demonstrates the lobes, gyri, and major sulci visible on the medial surface of the cerebral hemisphere. The orbital surface is illustrated in Figure 22.1.

FRONTAL LOBE

The following cortical areas, according to Brodmann (Fig. 17.7), are noted in the frontal lobe: primary motor area, 4; premotor, 6 and 8; inferior frontal (Broca's), 44, 45, and 47; frontal eye fields area, 8; prefrontal/orbital, 46, 9, 10, 11, 12, 13, and 14 (Table 17.1). It is customary to divide the frontal lobe into those more posterior areas devoted to motor functions and those more anterior areas devoted to nonmotor functions.

MOTOR AREAS

Area 4 (FA) corresponds in general to the precentral gyrus and functions as the primary motor cortex. It is continued onto the medial surface as the paracentral lobule (Figs. 17.10 and 17.11).

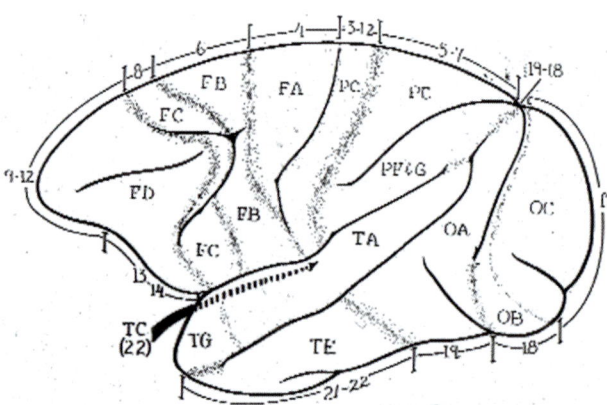

Figure 17.8 Reference diagrammatic cytoarchitectural map of monkey brain relating number system terminology of Brodmann to the letter system terminology of Von Bonin and Bailey (after Von Economo and Koskinis). The borders are only approximate. (From Ruch, T.C., and Patton, H.D.: Physiology and Biophysics. 19th Edition, Philadelphia, W.B. Saunders, 1965, p. 156.)

Stimulation: discrete repetitive focal movements are produced based on the area stimulated, for example, repetitive jerks of the thumb or of the foot. A march of focal movements may occur, for example, starting in the thumb, then spreading to hand, then to arm, then to face and leg, and so on.

Ablation: an upper motor neuron type weakness occurs with a contralateral monoplegia or hemiparesis.

Area 6 (FB) located anterior to area 4 and thus referred to as premotor cortex, functions as motor association or elaboration area (Figs. 17.8 and 18.6). This area also functions to inhibit certain functions of the primary motor cortex. The supplementary motor cortex represents the continuation of this area onto the medial aspect of the hemisphere (Figs. 17.11 and 18.12).

Stimulation: patterns of movement occur, for example, tonic rotation of head, eyes, and trunk to the opposite side associated with tonic abduction of the arm at the shoulder and flexion of the arm at elbow. Stimulation of the supplementary motor cortex produces similar complex patterns of tonic movement. In addition, there are bilateral movements of the trunk and lower extremities.

Ablation: Transient release of "primitive" automatic reflexes mediated by the primary motor cortex such as instinctive grasp and suck occurs. A more persistent release of these instinctive reflexes follows the combined ablation of areas 6, 8, and supplementary motor cortex. Such lesions also produce a significant gait apraxia, an impairment of the ability to walk without actual weakness or sensory deficit. Other deficits in the initiation of patterns of movement in relationship to somatosensory or visual stimuli may also occur.

Area 8 (FC) (Fig. 18.18) located anterior to area 6 in the middle frontal gyrus in the human is often grouped with area 6 as premotor cortex. This area functions in relation to conscious eye turning and is often referred to as the frontal eye field or frontal center for adversive or contraversive eye movement. This area is involved when the subject responds to the command "turn your eyes to the left (or right)." The effects are mediated by descending crossed connections to the pontine center for lateral gaze.

Stimulation (Fig. 18.18): a conscious repetitive conjugate eye movement to the opposite field occurs. More specific effects can also be achieved by discrete stimulation within this area, for example, eyelid opening and repetitive eyelid movements' pupillary dilatation (Fig. 18.19). Bilateral stimulation will result in conjugate upward eye movements.

Ablation: transient paralysis of voluntary conjugate gaze to the contralateral visual field occurs. In general, in humans, this paralysis of voluntary gaze does not occur in isolation but is associated with those processes such as infarction which have also produced a severe hemiparesis. The patient then lies in bed with the contralateral limbs in a hemiplegic posture and with the head and eyes deviated toward the intact arm and leg. This deviation most likely reflects the unbalanced effect of the adversive eye center of the opposite intact hemisphere. The effect is usually transient, clearing in a matter of days or weeks. A transient neglect syndrome primarily involving the contralateral visual field occurs, although contralateral tactile and auditory stimuli may also be neglected. Bilateral ablations within this area in the monkey resulted in animals that had a

Figure 17.9 Lobes, gyri, and major sulci. Lateral surface.

Figure 17.10 Lobes, gyri, and major sulci. Medial surface.

Table 17.1 MAJOR GYRI IN THE FRONTAL LOBE

GYRUS	MAJOR FUNCTION
Precentral	Origin of volitional motor pathways, the corticospinal and corticonuclear pathways (upper motor neurons)
Superior frontal	Premotor and prefrontal regions
Middle frontal	Prefrontal and frontal eye fields
Inferior frontal	Broca's motor and speech area in the dominant hemisphere
Orbital	Limbic
Gyrus rectus	Limbic

bilateral neglect of the environment, remained apathetic, and continued to have a "wooden expression." Similar findings may occur in the human patient with degenerative disorders involving these frontal areas.

Areas 44 and 45 (FCB). These areas correspond in general to the inferior frontal gyrus triangular and opercular portions. In the dominant (usually left) hemisphere this constitutes Broca's motor speech center or the anterior speech center (Fig. 24.1).

Stimulation (Fig. 24.2): arrest of speech occurs. Occasionally, simple vocalization occurs. A similar arrest of speech may also occur on stimulation of the other speech centers: posterior and superior.

Ablation: a nonfluent aphasia occurs. The patient is mute. With limited lesions, considerable language may return. While isolated lesions (for example, embolic infarcts) involving this area may occur, more often this type of language defect is associated with a contralateral hemiparesis.

PREFRONTAL-NONMOTOR AREAS

Areas 9, 10, 11, and 12 (FD), the prefrontal areas, are concerned with emotional control and other aspects of cognitive function (Fig. 18.21). Areas 13 and 14 (FE, FF, FG, FH) are also often included in this group.

Stimulation: Complex partial seizures with alteration of personality, emotion, and behavior occur, often accompanied by tonic motor components. Note that 25% of complex partial seizures originate in frontal lobe structures, but 75% originate in temporal lobe.

Ablation: An alteration in personality, affect, and control of emotion may occur and/or there may be an alteration in cognitive/executive function.

PARIETAL LOBE

Areas 3, 1, and 2 (PA, PB, and PC). These areas correspond to the *postcentral gyrus* and function as the somatosensory projection areas (continue into paracentral lobule). *Stimulation:* Episodes of localized tingling paresthesias occur which may spread as with focal motor seizures.

Ablation: Deficits in cortical sensory (discriminative sensory) modalities will occur, for example, stereognosis, position sense, graphesthesia, and tactile localization.

Areas 5 and 7 plus in human 39 and 40 (PD, PE, PF, and PG): the parietal lobules. About halfway up the postcentral sulcus, the *intraparietal sulcus* extends posteriorly, dividing the parietal lobe into superior and inferior parietal lobules. The *inferior parietal lobule* consists of the supramarginal and angular gyri. The *supramarginal gyrus* surrounds the posterior ascending limb of the lateral sulcus. The *angular gyrus* is behind the supramarginal gyrus and surrounds the posterior end of the superior temporal sulcus (Table 17.2).

Areas 39 and 40 (PG and PF) correspond to the inferior parietal lobule (the angular and supramarginal gyri). These areas in the dominant hemisphere function in relation to reading and

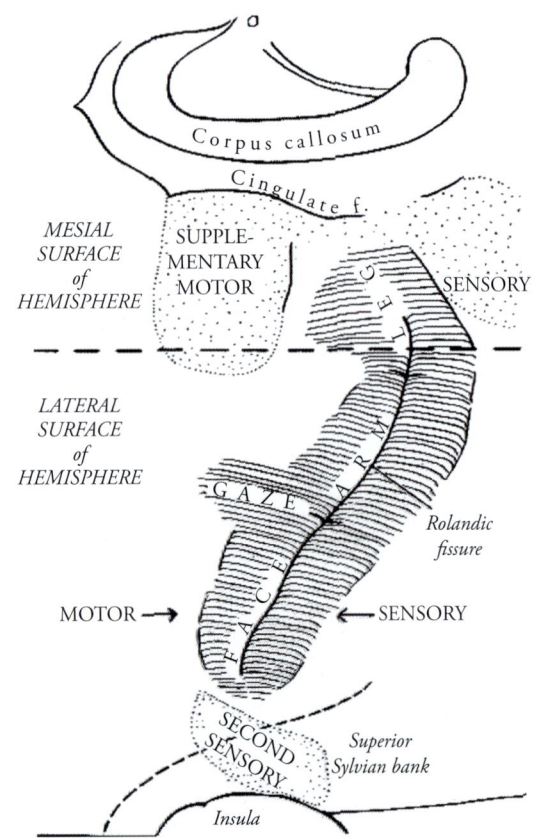

FIGURE 17.11 Map of somatic motor and sensory areas. Note that the primary motor and sensory areas extend into the depth of the rolandic fissure and extend onto the medial surface of the hemisphere. Note that the premotor cortex, area 6, also extends onto the medial surface of the hemisphere as the supplementary motor cortex. Note the location of the adversive gaze field in relation to motor cortex. (From Penfield, W., and Jasper, H.: Epilepsy and the Functional Anatomy of the Human Brain. Boston, Little, Brown & Company, 1954, p. 103.)

Table 17.2 MAJOR GYRI IN THE PARIETAL LOBE

GYRUS	MAJOR FUNCTIONS
Postcentral	Sensory cortex
Superior parietal lobule	Sensory associational
Inferior parietal lobule: – Pars supramarginal – Pars angular	Sensory language areas in the dominant hemisphere
Precuneus	Sensory associational

writing as higher integrative areas for language. This area is part of the posterior speech area. In the nondominant hemisphere these areas relate to our concepts of visual space.

Stimulation: In the dominant hemisphere, arrest of speech occurs.

Ablation: In the dominant hemisphere, defects in reading, writing, and calculations occur. These deficits along with difficulty in finger identification and left/right confusion constitute aspects of the Gerstmann's syndrome. A variety of fluent aphasia occurs. In the nondominant hemisphere, a denial or neglect syndrome occurs.

TEMPORAL LOBE

The temporal lobe is a complex structure that includes neocortex, allocortex, mesocortex, and a subcortical nucleus (the amygdala). At its posterior borders, it merges into the parietal and occipital lobes.

Major areas in the temporal lobe (see Fig. 17.7) include the following: auditory (transverse temporal), 41; auditory associational, 42 and 22; middle temporal, 21; inferior temporal, 20; posterior temporal, 37; and entorhinal, 27, 28, and 35.

The temporal lobe lies below the lateral sulcus and on its lateral surface has a sequence of three anterior to posterior arranged gyri: the superior, middle, and inferior temporal gyri.

The inferior temporal gyrus extends onto the ventral surface of the cerebrum. The superior temporal gyrus forms the temporal operculum. Near its posterior end two gyri are seen running into the lateral fissure (Table 17.3). These are the transverse temporal gyri, consisting of the primary receptive auditory cortex, area 41.

One of the first conclusive bits of evidence on the significance of anatomic asymmetry in the cerebrum was noted by Geschwind and Levitsky (1968) in the temporal lobe. They made a horizontal section through the lateral sulcus and removed the overlying parietal and occipital cortex. They called this exposed region of the superior temporal gyrus the *planum temporale*. They noted a larger planum temporale in the left temporal area than on the right side in right-handed humans. In left-handed individuals the area was the same on both sides. Their observations on the anatomical basis of cerebral dominance have since been supported by radiological and other anatomical studies.

Areas 41 and 42 (TC and TB): the transverse gyri of Heschl's function as primary auditory projection areas.

Stimulation: Episodic tinnitus (a ringing sensation) occurs. Usually such seizures are not limited to this symptom in isolation, since other aspects of the temporal lobe are involved to produce the more complex phenomena of the temporal lobe seizure.

Ablation: Limited unilateral lesions may produce a disturbance in the ability to localize sounds. Bilateral lesions of a limited nature would be rare but could produce "cortical deafness."

Area 22 (TA) corresponds to the superior temporal gyrus and surrounds areas 41 and 42. This is an auditory higher association center. In the dominant hemisphere, the posterior half of this area represents an auditory association area concerned with the reception and interpretation of spoken language. This is one component of the posterior speech area. The area is often referred to as Wernicke's receptive aphasia center. In the nondominant hemisphere this area is more concerned with visual aspects of space.

Stimulation: Stimulation of the posterior speech (Wernicke's) area (Fig. 24.2) produces an arrest of speech. Seizures originating in the superior temporal gyrus are also characterized by "experiential "phenomena: distortions of auditory and visual perception alterations in the sense of time and in well-formed visual and auditory hallucinations (psychical seizures). As will be discussed in Chapter 22, complex partial seizures may begin with these phenomena but subsequently proceed to impairment of awareness; amnesia and automatisms (unconscious stereotyped patterns of movement) reflect involvement of or spread to the mesial temporal areas of hippocampus and amygdala. Fear that may also accompany these seizures reflects involvement of the amygdala. Olfactory hallucinations that may also accompany these seizures reflect involvement of the mesial temporal structure, the uncus.

Ablation: Damage to Wernicke's area, a part of the posterior speech area, produces a deficit in the comprehension of speech, a type of fluent aphasia.

Additional information about more extensive unilateral or bilateral damage to the temporal lobe will be considered in Chapters 22 and 30. Suffice it to say that bilateral damage to the hippocampus will produce severe deficits in the ability to record new memories. Damage to the amygdala will alter emotional control.

OCCIPITAL LOBE

The lateral occipital gyri consist of visual associative cortex. The visual receptive cortex (calcarine-cortex) is found on the medial surface of the hemisphere (Table 17.4).

Table 17.3 **GYRI IN THE TEMPORAL LOBE**

GYRUS	MAJOR FUNCTIONS
Hippocampal formation	Limbic and memory
Amygdala	Limbic
Parahippocampal	Limbic
Occipitotemporal	Limbic
Inferior temporal	Limbic
Middle temporal	Limbic and facial recognition
Superior temporal Transverse temporal gyri	Sensory language area in the dominant hemisphere Auditory area

Table 17.4 **MAJOR GYRI IN OCCIPITAL LOBE**

GYRUS	FUNCTIONS
Lateral occipital	Visual associational
Lingula	Superior visual field
Cuneus	Inferior visual field

Areas in the occipital lobe include visual (calcarine), 17, and visual association, 18 and 19.

Area 17 (OC) corresponds to the striate cortex bordering the calcarine fissure and functions as the primary visual projection area. In modern physiological terms the designation V1 is utilized.

Stimulation: Seizures originating in this area produce simple unformed visual hallucinations such as flashing lights, stars, or jagged lines. The phenomena may be localized to the contralateral visual field or at times to the contralateral eye.

Ablation: Homonymous visual deficits are produced, for example, a homonymous hemianopsia or quadrantanopsia.

Areas 18 and 19 (OB and OA) form surrounding stripes around area 17. These areas function as visual association areas of varying complexity. The terms V2–V4 are utilized. These areas are also involved in the fixation and following of objects in the contralateral visual field. Note that visual areas V4 and V5 extend into the adjacent temporal-parietal cortex.

Stimulation: Some of the effects are similar to stimulation of area 17. In addition, conjugate deviation of the eyes to the contralateral field will occur.

Ablation: Selective lesions may produce deficits in some of the more complex visual activities. In addition, defects in visual fixation and following may occur. (See Chapter 23.)

DEVELOPMENTAL ASPECTS OF NEOCORTEX

The topics of prenatal development, postnatal development, and abnormalities of cortical neuronal migration are discussed in Chapter 4.

SUBCORTICAL WHITE MATTER AFFERENTS AND EFFERENTS

Essentially three types of fiber systems occupy the subcortical white matter: (1) projection fibers, (2) commissural fibers, and (3) association fibers.

Projection fibers consist of the corticopetal afferent fibers, such as the thalamocortical radiations, and the corticofugal efferent fibers such as the corticospinal, corticoreticular, and corticorubral tracts (Fig. 17.12).

The major commissural systems are the corpus callosum, anterior commissure, and hippocampal commissure. The corpus callosum is the major commissure for the neocortical areas (except the middle and inferior temporal gyri) (Fig. 17.13) and the rostral portions of the superior and inferior temporal gyrus (see Pandya and Rosene, 1985, for a more detailed discussion). In general, homologous areas of the two hemispheres are interconnected. However, there are significant regional variations between homologous areas as regards fiber density (Fig. 17.14). Thus, there is a high density of callosal fibers connecting the premotor areas of the two cerebral hemispheres. On the other hand, the primary visual projection area—area 17—has almost no direct callosal connection to the contralateral hemisphere.

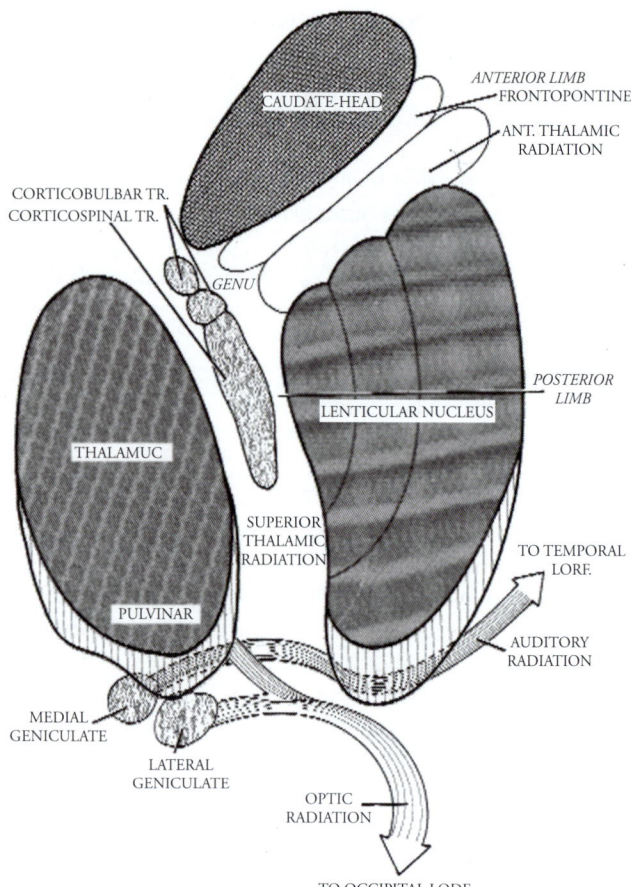

Figure 17.12 Projection fiber systems passing through the internal capsule. The superior thalamic radiation includes fibers projecting from ventral thalamus to sensory and motor cortex.

Area 17 transmits to the adjacent area 18 that has connection to contralateral area 18.[2]

Cortical areas also differ as regards the spread of fibers to asymmetrical as well as to symmetrical points in the contralateral hemisphere. Thus, area 6 has widespread connections in the contralateral hemisphere not only to area 6 but also to areas, 4, 5, 7, and 39, whereas area 4 has discrete contralateral connection only to the homotypic points.

The anterior commissure interconnects the rostral portions of the superior, middle, and inferior temporal gyri; and inferior-posterior orbital gyri and paleocortex (parahippocampal gyrus). The hippocampal commissure[3] interconnects the hippocampal formation and dentate gyri (archicortex) and the

---

[2] The organization of callosal projections is more complex than the picture provided by the early degeneration maps. Thus, within somatosensory cortex callosal connections are most dense in area 2, less dense in area 1, and least dense in area 3B. Within each of those areas, differences also occur. In area 3B, relatively dense connections are present for trunk and head but relatively sparse connections for hand and foot. In contrast, within area 2 relatively dense connections are present for all parts of the body. Significant changes occur during development, in part related to the overlap with thalamocortical afferent input. For a more complete discussion, see Killackey (1985), Killackey and Chalupa (1986), and Dehay et al. (1988). The end result is in part a complementary relationship to the distribution of thalamocortical fibers.

[3] In the monkey two hippocampal commissures have been identified based on relationship to the fornix. (For a more complete discussion of the topography of commissural fibers, see Pandya and Rosene, 1985.)

Figure 17.13 Radiation of fibers from corpus callosum as dissected in human brain.

Figure 17.15 Dissection of long fiber systems; the uncinate fasciculus (*C*) passing from orbital frontal (*A*) to anterior temporal areas (*B*).

surrounding presubiculum, entorhinal, and adjacent inferior temporal gyrus. These fibers are conveyed via the fimbria of the fornix and cross at the point beneath the splenium of the corpus callosum, where the posterior pillars of the fornix converge.

Two types of subcortical association fibers may be distinguished (excluding from this discussion the intracortical association fibers): (a) short subcortical U or arcuate fibers, which interconnect adjacent gyri, and (b) long fiber bundles, which reciprocally interconnect distant cortical areas. The following long fiber bundles may be distinguished on blunt dissection of the cerebral hemisphere:

1. The *uncinate fasciculus* interconnects the orbital and medial prefrontal areas and the anterior temporal area (Fig. 17.15).

2. The *superior longitudinal fasciculus* interconnects the superior and lateral frontal, parietal and temporal, and occipital areas (Fig. 24.5). The extension of this fiber system into the temporal area, passing through the subcortical white matter of supramarginal and angular gyri, is often distinguished as the arcuate fasciculus. This fasciculus has considerable importance because of its role in connecting the receptive language centers of the temporal lobe with the expressive motor speech centers of the inferior frontal gyrus. Such a connection must be made if a sentence that has been heard is to be repeated.

3. The *cingulum* passes within the subcortical white matter of the cingulate gyrus; it interconnects the subcallosal, medial-frontal, and orbital-frontal with the temporal lobe, occipital areas, and cingulate cortex.

4. The *inferior longitudinal fasciculus* interconnects the occipital and inferior temporal areas.

5. The *inferior frontal occipital fasciculus* interconnects the frontal and occipital areas. It is often difficult to clearly differentiate this fiber system from the uncinate fasciculus.

MAJOR AFFERENT INPUTS AND EFFERENT PROJECTIONS OF NEOCORTEX

AFFERENT INPUTS: THALAMUS

The thalamus is the major source. The transmitter is glutamate. With the exception of the olfactory system, all sensory information passes through the thalamus.

In many classifications, the thalamus has been divided into three major divisions: (1) the dorsal thalamus, (2) the ventral thalamus, and (3) the epithalamus.

The **dorsal thalamus** is by far the largest component and at times the term *thalamus* has been applied only to the dorsal thalamus. This structure is composed of a series of relay nuclei that connect in a reciprocal manner with the cerebral cortex and the striatum (refer to Chapter 15); these nuclei can be subdivided into specific projection (or relay) nuclei and nonspecific or diffuse projection (or relay) nuclei.

The *specific nuclei* have specific afferent inputs and project in a relatively precise topographic manner to specific areas of cerebral cortex. Experience, or functional disuse, may modify

Figure 17.14 Pattern of distribution of commissural fibers over the cortical surface of the left hemisphere of the monkey (*Macaca mulatta*) as studied following section of major commissures. (From Myers, R. E.: In Ettlinger, E. G. (ed.): Functions of the Corpus Callosum. Boston, Little, Brown & Company, 1965, p. 142.)

the precise cortical areas devoted to the topographic representation of a given sensory area. Examples of specific nuclei and their cortical projections have been provided in Chapter 15.

The densest input from the specific relay projection nuclei is to layer 4, but as indicated earlier, pyramidal cells in layers 3 and 5 many also receive direct or indirect inputs. There is a modality-specific columnar arrangement.

The *nonspecific nuclei* have a more diffuse input and a more diffuse but not necessarily a generalized cortical interaction. Examples include the following: midline nuclei (massa intermedia), central-medial, intralaminar nuclei, and the medial dorsal (which is diffuse to frontal areas).

The nonspecific nuclei project mainly to layer 1.

The **ventral thalamus** is a thin shell nucleus that is external to the external medullary lamina. It does not project directly to cerebral cortex, but it receives innervation from cerebral cortex. The subnuclei grouped as the thalamic reticular nucleus have specific reciprocal relationships with projection (relay) nuclei in the dorsal thalamus. As we will see next in discussing the basis of the electroencephalogram, these nuclei have a significant effect on thalamocortical interactions. These nuclei in the rodent (but not in the primate) have a high concentration of GABA-ergic neurons. The drive on the relay nuclei is therefore inhibitory.

The **epithalamus** includes the pineal body, the stria medullaris, and the habenular trigone. These structures relate primarily to the hypothalamus and are not relevant to a discussion of thalamocortical interactions.

NONTHALAMIC SOURCES OF INPUT

There are multiple other subcortical sources of input including the following:

1. *Noradrenergic (norepinephrine)* pathway from the locus ceruleus of the midbrain projecting in primates predominantly to layer 6 of the motor and somatosensory cortex and related frontal and parietal association cortex. This pathway functions in relationship to arousal responses induced by sensory stimuli, and activity in this system is altered during the rapid eye movement stage of sleep.

2. *Serotoninergic pathway* from the raphe nuclei in the pons and medulla and the pontine reticular formation. Although these neurons project to all cortical areas, the predominant projection in the primate is to layer 4 of area 17, the primary visual cortex. This system may be involved in the onset of the slow-wave stage of sleep. During rapid eye movement sleep, there is decreased activity in this system. Damage to the system produces insomnia.

3. *Dopaminergic pathways* from ventral tegmental rostral mesencephalic nuclear groups. The strongest projection is to the prefrontal cortex and limbic system. The fibers extend to all cortical layers except for IV. The projection is primarily inhibitory. This system is probably involved when psychotic behavior occurs in schizophrenia.

4. *Cholinergic pathways* from the basal forebrain nucleus of Meynert project widely to cerebral cortex. In addition, cholinergic neurons in the septum project to the hippocampus. In addition, cholinergic neurons in the brain stem tegmentum project to the thalamus and will be discussed in the chapter on sleep (Chapter 29). Electrical stimulation of brain stem reticular formation (resulting in desynchronization/arousal of the EEG) results in an increase in rate of liberation of acetylcholine from the surface of cerebral cortex. This effect may be mediated through the reticular formation projection to the basal forebrain.

5. *GABAergic inhibitory pathways* from basal forebrain, ventral tegmental area, and zona incerta to sensory and motor cortex.

6. *Claustrum* projects to all sensory, limbic, and motor areas with an excitatory input.

EFFERENT PROJECTIONS

Projections occur in a reciprocal manner with many subcortical areas (thalamus, basal ganglia, brain stem, and spinal cord). However, these projections are estimated to account for only 0.1% to 1% of all fibers in the white matter. Instead, most fibers are involved in intrahemispheric and interhemispheric connections, pyramidal neurons to pyramidal neurons and to interneurons.

NEUROPHYSIOLOGY OF THE CEREBERAL CORTEX: CORRELATES OF CORTICAL CYTOARCHITECTURE AND THE BASIS OF THE ELECTROENCEPHALOGRAM

The cerebral cortex of humans and of other mammals is characterized by continuous rhythmic sinusoidal electrical activity of variable frequency. This electrical activity may be recorded through the scalp of humans in the form of the electroencephalogram (EEG) or directly from the cerebral cortex during surgery in the form of the electrocorticogram (ECG). The term *EEG* will be used during the subsequent discussion to refer to the activity found in either the EEG or the ECG. The electroencephalogram provides a physiologic correlate of the various states of consciousness.

The normal electroencephalogram (EEG) in the awake adult who is recorded while resting with eyes lightly closed is characterized by a dominant activity in the posterior (parietaloccipital) recording areas of continuous 8–13 Hz sinusoidal waves of 25–75 μv (Fig. 2.18). Amplitudes recorded directly from the cortex are higher. This pattern is referred to as the alpha rhythm since this was the first pattern discovered. The second described pattern, the beta rhythm, is found predominantly in the frontal recording areas and consists of low-amplitude, 14–30 Hz activities. Many sedative medications will produce increased amounts of generalized beta activity and eventually generalized slow-wave activity. The frequency of the basic background activity is also influenced by the age and level of consciousness of the patient. Any pattern slower than alpha is referred to as composed of slow waves (theta = 4–7 Hz; delta = 0.5–3 Hz), as illustrated in Figures 2.24 and 2.25. Many sedative medications will produce increased amounts of generalized beta activity and eventually generalized slow-wave activity (Fig. 2.21). The frequency of the basic background activity is also influenced by the age and level of consciousness of the patient (Figs. 2.19 and 2.20). In general, the activity of the two cerebral hemispheres is relatively symmetrical and synchronous.

The electrical activity recorded is not a result of axon potentials and does not represent the activity of individual neurons and synapses. Instead, EEG rhythms represent the summated electrical activity of a large number of synapses located in the more superficial layers of the cerebral cortex. Seizure discharges do not originate in single neurons but instead are generated in a group of neurons that manifest increased excitability and synchronization (the epileptic focus). Nevertheless, certain mutations involving the neuronal membrane and the synaptic receptor provide the basis for several types of genetically determined seizure disorders (see Chapter 29). The difference between axonal and synaptic activity has been discussed in Chapter 5.

THE ACTIVITY OF ISOLATED CEREBRAL CORTEX

In considering the basis of the electroencephalogram, it is of value to first consider the activity of large blocks of cerebral cortex isolated from all subcortical interactions but retaining pial blood supply. The basic activity of such preparations in the cat, the monkey, and in the human is characterized by bursts of electrical activity composed of mixed-frequency sharp waves, spikes, slow waves, and fast activity alternating with periods of relative electrical silence. In the chronic studies of Kellaway et al. (1966), the bursts of activity were correlated in large part with unit discharges in the depths of cortex at the level of the large pyramidal cell bodies. In a related preparation, large homologous blocks of cerebral cortex were isolated in each hemisphere along with the interconnecting corpus callosum (Fig. 17.16A) (Marcus and Watson, 1966). The basic pattern is composed of bilateral relatively synchronous and symmetrical bursts of activity with intervening periods of relative electrical silence (Fig. 17.16B). Similar burst suppression type activity is obtained in preparations in which all thalamic, hypothalamic, and rostral mesencephalic structures have been ablated. The burst suppression pattern may be seen in several clinical circumstances: (1) very deep anesthesia, (2) diffuse encephalopathies as in anoxic encephalopathy or encephalitis, (3) following intractable status epilepticus, or (4) in the premature brain.

THE ACTIVITY OF ISOLATED THALAMUS

In contrast in the studies of Kellaway et al. (1966), the electrical activity of isolated thalamus was characterized by continuous sinusoidal waves of 8 Hz. The more recent studies of Steriade and Llinas (1988) have demonstrated that all thalamic reticular neurons can spontaneously generate rhythmic discharges at a rate of approximately 10 Hz. Groups of such cells even when

Figure 17.16 Isolated cerebral cortex. (A) The anatomical bilateral cortical callosal preparation. (B) The electrical activity of the preparation. The upper six channels are bipolar recordings from the isolated areas. The lower two channels are recorded from the nonisolated cortex. (From Marcus, E. M. In Reeves, A. Epilepsy and the Corpus Callosum. New York, Plenum Press, p. 158, 1985.)

deafferented can generate synchronized oscillations. These neurons have a strong inhibitory input to the thalamic relay (projection) neurons and thus could entrain these neurons in a similar oscillation. This could then be reflected in a similar entrainment of cortical neurons and synapses in a 10 Hz oscillation. (See later discussion.)

In brief, the continuous rhythmic activity seen in the electroencephalogram must indicate the effects of thalamic neurons on the activity of cortical neurons and synapses. As we will see next, brain stem structures are also of importance in modifying cortical activity.

MODIFICATION OF CORTICAL ACTIVITY BY STIMULATION OF VARIOUS STRUCTURES: EVOKED POTENTIALS

The background cortical electrical activity may be modified by stimulation at various levels. These evoked responses include the superficial cortical response, the direct response, the transcallosal response, the primary evoked response, the recruiting response, and the generalized arousal response.

Primary evoked response: Stimulation of the sciatic nerve or of other specific sensory pathways produces after a 10–15 msec latency surface positive wave followed by a surface negative wave (Fig. 17.17). A similar response of much shorter latency (1–5 msec) is produced by stimulation of the specific thalamic nucleus involved in the primary evoked response.

Augmenting response: With repetitive stimulation of the same nucleus at 6–12 Hz, the amplitude and latency of each successive response increase (Fig. 17.17).

Recruiting response: In contrast, repetitive 6–12 Hz stimulation of the nonspecific thalamic nuclei, such as the intralaminar, the medial or midline groups, or the thalamic reticular nucleus, produces a predominantly surface negative response of greater latency (15–60 msec) termed *the recruiting response* (Figs. 17.17 and 17.18). The response waxes and wanes and is

Figure 17.17 Laminar analysis of the various cortical evoked responses in terms of the type and magnitude of response recorded with an external microelectrode at various depths. Specific afferent fibers terminate in layer IV and are shown making synaptic contact with both granule cell interneurons and adjacent pyramidal cells. Nonspecific afferent fibers are shown terminating in many layers, including layer I. The SCR (superficial cortical response) is limited to the superficial layers of cerebral cortex. The initial surface positive component of the primary evoked response (specific stimulus, recording from specific cortical projection) originates in the deeper cortical layers (the vertical lines represent cell discharges). The subsequent surface-negative wave originates in superficial cortical layers. The transcallosal response would have a similar form and analysis. Specific thalamic nucleus stimulation results in the augmenting response. The origin of the recruiting response to stimulation of nonspecific thalamic nuclei is complex (see text). (Reproduced with modifications from an unpublished diagram by Purpura.)

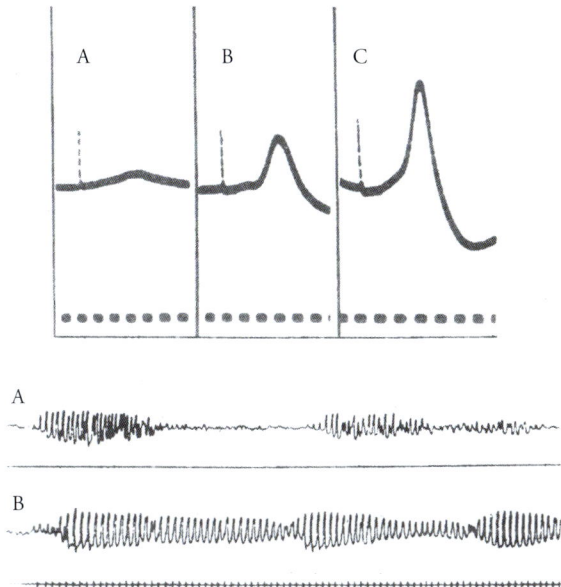

Figure 17.18 The recruiting response. (Top) Cortical responses in anterior sigmoid gyrus of cat to successive stimulation of intralaminar nuclei of thalamus (A, B, C) at 8 Hz characterized by long latency and a progressive increase in amplitude of the surface negative response. The time marks indicate 10 msec. (From Morison, R.S., and Dempsey, E.W.: Amer. J. Physiol., 135:288, 1942.) (Bottom) The similarity of the waxing and waning amplitude of the recruiting response to the spontaneous 8–12 cps spindles, which characterize sedation or anesthesia with Nembutal or other barbiturates, is also demonstrated. Recordings from middle suprasylvian gyrus of cat. (A) Spontaneous spindle bursts. (B) Recruiting response to stimulation (stimulus marker) or intralaminar areas of thalamus. (From Dempsey, E. W., and Morison, R. S.: Amer. J. Physiol., 135:297, 1942, Amer. Physiol. Soc.)

similar to the 8–12 Hz spindle response that characterizes light anesthesia in the cat. In the human, a similar spindle occurs at 14–15 Hz during stage 2 sleep. Although this system is referred to as the diffuse thalamocortical system, in the monkey, the response is obtained predominantly from the frontal and parietal association cortex. The recruiting response represents summated excitatory postsynaptic potentials (EPSPs) generated in the more superficial layers of cerebral cortex and the waves are therefore surface negative. At times a small initial surface positivity may be present. Under particular conditions of anesthesia with stimulation of these same thalamic nuclei, a longer duration (100–200 msec) surface negative wave may follow the initial wave of the recruiting response. This is, however, correlated with a prolonged hyperpolarization in the deeper cortical layers. In the cat preparation, this combination of the initial recruiting wave (the spike) and the subsequent slow wave provides a model of the thalamic induced spike wave complex and has been correlated with behavioral changes (arrest of activity, myoclonus) similar to the absence seizures of idiopathic epilepsy (see Chapter 29).

Arousal or activation or desynchronization response: Stimulation of the sciatic nerve or other sensory pathways or eye opening or intense mental activity will also have a significant generalized effect on the background activity of the EEG. The alpha rhythm is replaced by a low-voltage fast activity (Fig. 2.18C). This response can be reproduced by high-frequency (50–300 Hz) stimulation of the brain stem ascending reticular activating system. The response occurs with a latency of approximately 40 msec and outlasts the period of stimulation. The long latency suggests a pathway involving several synapses as opposed to the classic short latency lemniscal sensory pathway. This system has diffuse effects on the cerebral cortex via two systems: the nonspecific thalamic nuclei and the pathway from basal diencephalon to the basal forebrain. The intralaminar nuclei of the thalamus represent an upward continuation of the ascending reticular formation. Stimulation of these thalamic nuclei, for example, centrum medianum, at high frequency (300 Hz) produces the same effects on cortical electrical activity as stimulation of ascending reticular formation at a brain stem level Thus, sciatic stimulation produces not only the short latency, localized, primary evoked response but also the long latency, generalized, arousal response. This reflects the fact that sensory data enter the reticular formation via collaterals from the specific sensory pathways, particularly the spinothalamic system. Moreover, multiple sensory modalities may synapse on the same neuron in the reticular formation. The system then is in a sense nonspecific as to the modality identity of the incoming stimulus.

The role of the reticular formation and other brain stem areas in sleep, consciousness, and attention will be considered in greater detail in Chapter 29.

THE INTERACTION OF CORTICAL NEURONS AND THALAMIC RELAY NUCLEI

The interaction is complex. Thalamic relay nuclei function in two possible states: (1) a transmission mode when the neuron is near firing threshold in which the discharge reflects the sensory input. (2) A burst mode when the neuron is hyperpolarized by inhibitory input. The thalamic relay neurons have a special voltage-gated calcium channel (transient or T type) that is inactive when the membrane potential is near threshold. However, when the cell is hyperpolarized, incoming excitatory synaptic potentials trigger transient opening of this calcium channel. The resulting calcium current then brings the neuron potential above threshold. The neuron then fires a burst of action potential until the calcium that has entered the cell activates potassium current that again produces a hyperpolarized state. During burst firing the thalamic relay neurons cannot transmit sensory information to the cerebral cortex. The source of the hyperpolarization of the thalamic relay neurons is the reticular thalamic nucleus that is composed of GABA-ergic inhibitory neurons. In turn, the neurons of the reticular nucleus receiving collateral input from cortical thalamic and thalamocortical relay neurons (Fig. 17.19). The thalamic reticular nucleus also has the property of the burst mode of discharge when hyperpolarized. The burst firing of the thalamic relay cells is reflected in rhythmic waves of excitatory postsynaptic potentials in the dendrites of cortical neurons and is expressed in the surface EEG as rhythmic slow waves. This pattern of slow-wave activity may be seen in sleep or in diffuse encephalopathies.

During states of wakefulness, the thalamus remains in the transmission mode because of cholinergic input from rostral

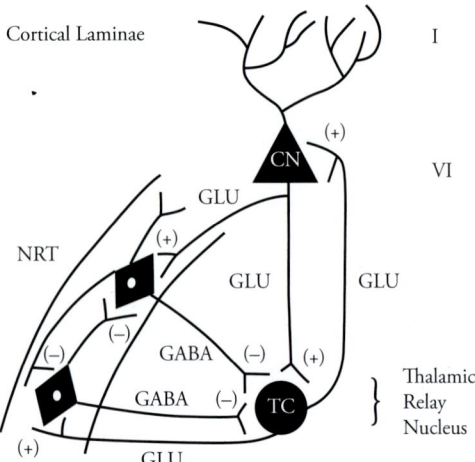

Figure 17.19 The interaction of cortical pyramidal cell (CN), thalamic relay nucleus (TC), and thalamic reticular nucleus (NRT). GABA, gamma amino butyric acid; GLU, glutamate. (Modified from Snead, O.C. III, In Malafossa, A. Idiopathic Generalized Epilepsies: Clinical, Experimental and Genetic Aspects. London, John Libbey.)

pons to the thalamic relay and thalamic reticular neurons. There are also cholinergic inputs to the thalamic reticular nucleus from the basal forebrain.

CLINICAL AND PHYSIOLOGICAL CORRELATES OF CYTOARCHITECTURAL VARIATION

THE CAPACITY FOR FOCAL SEIZURE DISCHARGE

Anatomical observation: In the monkey as in the human, the motor cortex (area 4) of the precentral gyrus is characterized by the presence of giant and large pyramidal cells. These giant and large pyramidal cells are characterized by a long apical dendrite. Associated with these pyramidal cells, there is noted in the Golgi stain the presence of a massive tangential plexus in the molecular layer with the presence of many axodendritic synapses. In contrast, the striate occipital cortex (area 17) has a dense external line of Baillarger in layer IV but only a thin tangential plexus in the molecular layer. In general, similar differences were found in studies of McCulloch and his associates (1944) employing a local area of seizure discharge (strychnine neuronography) rather than direct electrical stimulation. Both series of studies also indicated that significant regional differences existed as regards the diffuseness of callosal projection. Thus, certain cortical areas (e.g., motor cortex) had projection only to the symmetrical area of the contralateral hemisphere. Other areas, such as the premotor area (area 6), had widespread projection to many points in the contralateral hemisphere (areas 6, 4, 1, 5, and 39 as regards area 6) (Fig. 17.20).

Clinical correlation: Experimental or clinical seizures originating from the premotor cortex will have widespread bilateral effects, whereas seizures originating from the striate occipital cortex will have limited focal effects (Fig. 17.21). The

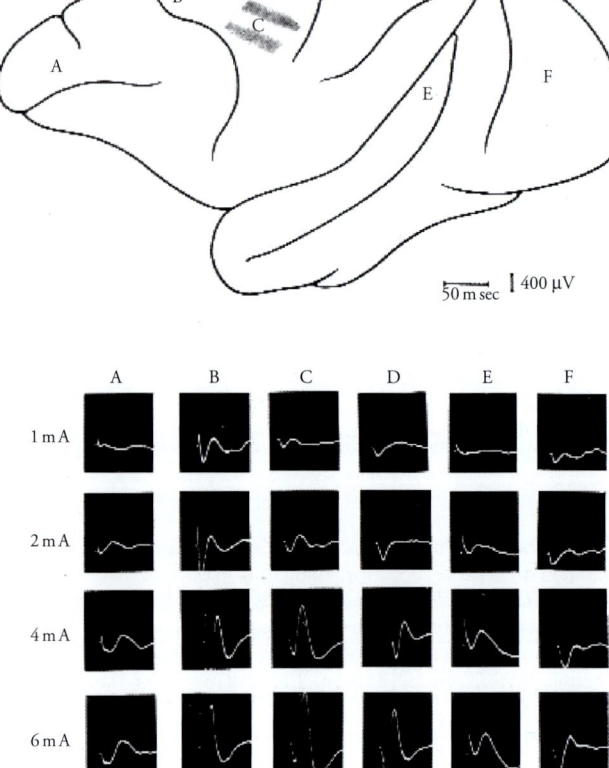

Figure 17.20 Variations in thresholds and amplitude of superficial cortical response (local cortical response) as a function of locus of stimulation in the monkey. Note the low threshold and relatively higher amplitude of the premotor and motor cortex responses (B, C, D) compared to those obtained in area 17 (F) posterior temporal (E) and prefrontal areas (A). The stimulation intensities were the same in all areas (0.10 msec single shocks). (From Eidelberg, E., Konigsmark, B., and French, J.D.: Electroenceph. Clin. Neurophysiol. 11:123, 1959. Elsevier.)

widespread intra- and interhemispheric spread of discharge from a unilateral experimental focus in area 6 is demonstrated in Figure 17.22A. Compare this to the limited spread of discharge from a similar focus in areas 17 of occipital cortex (Figs. 17.22B and 17.22C).

Figure 17.21 Regional differences in seizure susceptibility in the monkey cortex. Note the low threshold of the motor cortex of sectors in premotor cortex and of anterior medial temporal lobe, in contrast to occipital striate, prefrontal, posterior temporal, and parietal areas. Compare with Figure 17.30. (From French JD, Gernandt BE, and Livingston RB, Arch. Neurol. Psychiatr. 75:270, 1956.)

Figure 17.22 Capacity for spread of an experimental focal discharge. (*A*) Unilateral focus in the left premotor area 6 of the monkey results in a wide intrahemispheric and interhemispheric spread. (*B*) Production of the same unilateral focus in area 17 of the right occipital area results in a restricted unilateral discharge which even when prolonged as in (*C*) fails to spread. IP, intraparietal; OC, occipital; PC, precentral; PF, prefrontal; PM, premotor.

THE CAPACITY FOR BILATERAL SYNCHRONOUS DISCHARGES: ANATOMICAL AND PHYSIOLOGICAL OBSERVATIONS

Experimental Epilepsy Correlation

1. *Bilateral foci of epileptic discharge in symmetrical cortical areas of the two hemispheres*: an interaction soon occurs, resulting in the synchronization of the seizure discharges in the two hemispheres. However, in the monkey there are significant regional variations in the capacity for this interaction. In the premotor and precentral areas, a close and well-developed interhemispheric synchrony is evident (Fig. 17.23); in striate occipital and superior temporal areas, bilateral synchrony is poorly sustained (Fig. 17.24). Section of major commissures markedly disrupts the synchrony of discharge. Refer to Marcus (1985).

2. *Intravenous injection of a threshold amount of pentylenetetrazol (Metrazol)* provides an example of a diffuse toxic disease (Marcus, 1985): following injection in the monkey, bilateral synchronous discharges developed first in the premotor and precentral areas. Discharges in the temporal and striate occipital areas develop later and are independent and multifocal (Fig. 17.25). Synchrony is lost following section of the corpus callosum (Fig. 17.26) but is maintained in the cortical callosal preparation (Fig. 17.27).

The role of the corpus callosum in other generalized models of epilepsy is discussed in Chapter 28.

Figure 17.23 Capacity for bilateral synchrony in premotor area of monkey cerebral cortex. Experimental design of bilateral symmetrical discharging premotor foci (1% conjugated estrogen). Recordings from superior frontal (S.F.) and precentral gyri (Pre C). Note the repetitive bilaterally synchronous discharges of spikes and spike slow-wave complexes. Compare to Figure 17.24. (From Marcus, E. M., and Watson, C. W.: Arch. Neurol. 19:102, 1968, AMA.) See also Chapter 29.

Figure 17.24 Lack of capacity for bilateral synchrony in area 17 of monkey cerebral cortex. Experimental design of bilateral symmetrical discharging foci as in Figure 17.23. Recordings from left and right occipital area. Note independence of discharge, particularly when prolonged (*A* and *C*). Occasional bilateral discharges relatively synchronous at onset could occur (*B*), particularly discharges when triggered as in (*D*) by an extrinsic source, for example, photic stimulation (PS). (From Marcus, E. M., and Watson, C. W.: Arch. Neurol. 19:107, 1968, AMA.)

Figure 17.25 Regional variations in capacity for discharge and bilateral synchrony following administration of a threshold dosage of an intravenous convulsant agent (15 mg/kg) in a monkey. Discharges begin in a bilateral synchronous manner in the precentral areas (Pre C U). Only later do discharges begin in the occipital area (Oc), and these are not synchronous or symmetrical. (From Marcus, E. M. in Reeves, A. G. Epilepsy and the Corpus Callosum. New York: Plenum Press, 1985, p. 169.)

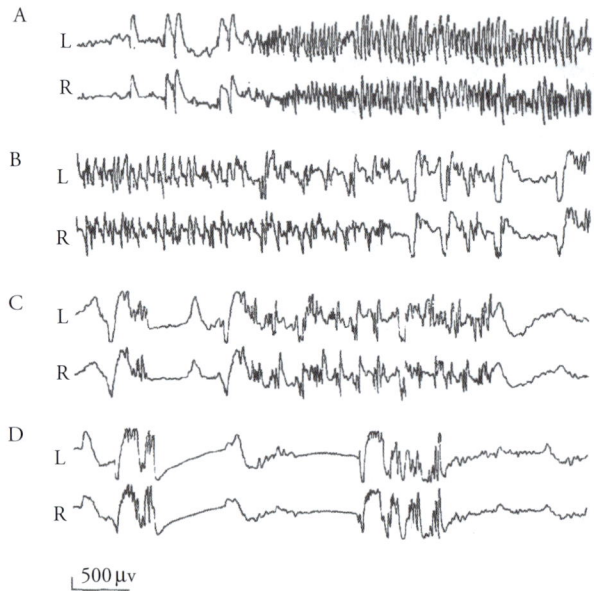

Figure 17.26 Intravenous pentylenetetrazol at threshold dosage 6 days after complete section of major commissures in the monkey. Bipolar recordings from upper-middle precentral gyrus. All bilateral synchrony is lost. (A) Anatomy. (B) Electroencephalogram (EEG) recording. (From Marcus, E. M. in Reeves, A. G. Epilepsy and the Corpus Callosum. New York, Plenum Press, p. 183.)

Figure 17.27 Intravenous pentylenetetrazol at threshold dosage (20 mg/kg). (i) Intact cat; (ii) bilateral cortical callosal isolation. The apparent amplitude differences between the intact and the isolate reflect differences in the degree of amplification.

Clinical correlation: Seizure discharges, as recorded in the human electroencephalogram, may be focal, multifocal, or generalized with bilateral symmetry and synchrony of discharge. When the latter category of bilateral discharges is examined, it is evident that the bilateral synchrony is usually best developed in the frontal and central and parietal parasagittal recording areas. On the other hand, bilateral discharges in the temporal and occipital areas often appear to be independent, that is, multifocal. Section of the corpus callosum has been employed to limit spread of seizure discharge or to prevent the interaction of multiple foci of epileptic seizure discharge when seizures could not otherwise be controlled (see Reeves, 1985).

BIBLIOGRAPHY

CYTOARCHITECTURE, NEUROPHYSIOLOGY, AND CORRELATIONS, GENERAL (SEE ALSO CHAPTER 29)

Bailey, P., and von Bonin, G. 1951. The Isocortex of Man. Urbana: University of Illinois Press.
Brazier, M. A. B. 1977. The Electrical Activity of the Nervous System. 4th ed. Baltimore, MD: Williams and Wilkins.
Brodal, A. 1981. Neurological Anatomy in Relation to Clinical Medicine. 3rd ed. New York, NY: Oxford University Press. (Chapter 6: The Reticular Formation and Some Related Nuclei, pp. 394–441, Chapter 12: Cerebral Cortex, pp. 778–848)
Brodmann, K. 1994. Localization in the Cerebral Cortex (L. J. Garey, Trans.). London, UK: Smith-Gordon.
Colonnier, M. L. 1966. The structural design of the neocortex. In J. C. Eccles (Ed.) Brain and Conscious Experience, pp. 1–23. New York, NY: Springer-Verlag.
Conel, J. 1939–1968. The Postnatal Development of the Human Cerebral Cortex. Vols. 1–6. Cambridge, MA: Harvard University Press.
Eccles, J. C. (Ed.). 1966. Brain and Conscious Experience. New York, NY: Springer Verlag.
Engel, J., Jr. 1989. Seizures and Epilepsy. Philadelphia, PA: F.A. Davis.
Lorente de No, R. 1949. Cerebral cortex: architecture, intracortical connections, motor projections, In J. F. Fulton (Ed.) Physiology of the Nervous System. 3rd ed, pp. 288–330. New York, NY: Oxford University Press.
Peters, A., and Jones, E. G. (Eds.). 1984. Cerebral Cortex I: Cellular Components of the Cerebral Cortex. New York, NY: Plenum.
Rakic, P., and Singer, W. (Eds.). 1988. Neurobiology of Neocortex. New York, NY: Wiley.

SPECIFIC REFERENCES AND CITATIONS

Angevine, J., and Smith, M. S. 1982. Recent advances in forebrain anatomy and their clinical correlates. In R. A. Thompson and J. R. Green (Eds.) New Perspectives in Cerebral Localization, pp. 105–135. New York, NY: Raven Press.
Clemente, C. D., and Sterman, M. B. 1967. Basal forebrain mechanisms for internal inhibition and sleep. Res. Publ. Assn. Nerv. Mental Dis. 45:127–147.
Curtis, H. H. 1940. Inter cortical connections of corpus callosum as indicated by evoked potentials. J. Neurophysiol. 3:407–413.
Dehay, C., Kennedy, H., Bullier, J., et al. 1988. Absence of interhemi-spheric connections of area 17 during development in the monkey. Nature 331:348–350.
Duchowny, M., Jayakar, P., and Levin, B. 2000. Aberrant neural circuits in malformation of cortical development and focal epilepsy. Neurology 55:423–428.
Eidelberg, E., Konigsmark, B., and French, J. D. 1959. Electrocortical manifestations of epilepsy in monkey. Electroenceph. Clin. Neurophysiol. 11:121–128.
Enna, S. J. 1993. Gamma aminobutyric acid A receptor subunits in the mediation of selective drug action. Curr. Opin. Neurol. Neurosurg. 6:597–601.
French, J. D., Gernandt, B. E., and Livingston, R. B. 1956. Regional differences in seizure susceptibility in monkey cortex. Arch.Neurol. Psychiat. 72:260–274.
Jacobson, S., and Marcus, E. M. 1970. The laminar distribution of fibers of the corpus callosum: a comparative study in rat, cat, monkey and chimpanzee. Brain Res. 24:517–528.
Jacobson, S., and Trojanowski, J. Q. 1974. The cells of origin of the corpus callosum in rat, cat and rhesus monkey. Brain Res. 74:149–155.
Jasper, H. 1949. Diffuse projection system: the integrative action of the thalamic reticular system. Electroenceph. Clin. Neurophysiol. 11:121–128.
Jones, E. G. 1985. Anatomy, development and physiology of the corpus callosum. In A. G. Reeves (Ed.) Epilepsy and the Corpus Callosum, pp. 102–155. New York, NY: Plenum.
Kellaway, P., Goi, A., Proler, M. 1966. Electrical Activity of the isolated cerebral hemisphere and isolated thalamus. Exp. Neurol. 14: pp. 281–304.
Killackey, H. P. 1985. The organization of somato-sensory callosal projections: a new interpretation. In A. G. Reeves (Ed.) Epilepsy and the Corpus Callosum, pp. 41–53. New York, NY: Plenum.
Killackey, H. P., and Chalupa, L. M. 1986. Ontogenetic changes in the distribution of callosal projection neurons in the post central gyrus of the fetal rhesus monkey. J. Comp. Neurology 244:331–348.
Marcus, E. M. 1985. Generalized seizure models and the corpus callosum. In A. G. Reeves (Ed.) Epilepsy and the Corpus Callosum, pp. 131–206. New York, NY: Plenum.
Marcus, E. M., and Watson, C. W. 1968. Symmetrical epileptogenic foci in monkey cerebral cortex: mechanisms of interaction and regional variations in capacity for synchronous discharges. Arch. Neurol. 19:99–116.
Marcus, E. M., Watson, C. W., and Jacobson, S. 1969. Role of the corpus callosum in bilateral synchronous discharges induced by intravenous pentylenetetrazol. Neurology 19:309.
Martin, J. H. 1985. Cortical neurons, the EEG and the mechanisms of epilepsy. In E. R. Kandel and J.H. Schwartz (Eds.) *Principles of Neural Science*. 2nd ed, pp. 636–647. New York, NY: Elsevier.
McCulloch, W. S. 1944. Cortico-cortical connections. In P. C. Bucy (Ed.) The Precentral Motor Cortex, pp.211–242. Urbana: University of Illinois Press.
McNamara, J. C. 1993. Excitatory amino acid receptors and epilepsy. Curr. Opin. Neurol. Neurosurg. 6:583–587.
Meyer, B. U., Roricht, S., Grafin von Einsiedel, H., et al. 1995. Inhibitory and excitatory interhemispheric transfers between motor cortical areas in normal humans and patients with abnormalities of the corpus callosum. Brain 118:429–440.
Morrison, R. S., and Dempsey, E. W. 1942. A study of thalamocortical relations. Amer. J. Physiol. 135:281–292.
Myers, R. E. 1965. General discussion: phylogenetic studies of commissural connections. In E. G. Ettlinger (Ed.) Functions of the Corpus Callosum, pp. 138–142. Boston, MA: Little Brown & Company.
Pandya, D. N., and Rosene, D. L. 1985. Some observations on trajectories and topography of commissural fibers. In A. G. Reeves (Ed.) Epilepsy and the Corpus Callosum, pp.21–39. New York, NY: Plenum Press.
Prince, D. A. 1978. Neurophysiology of epilepsy. Ann. Rev. Neurosci. 1:395–415.
Purpura, D.P. 1959. Nature of electrocortical potentials and synaptic organizations in cerebral and cerebellar cortex. Int. Rev. Neurobiol. 1:47–163.
Purpura, D. P. 1964. Relationship of seizure susceptibility to morphologic and physiologic properties of normal and abnormal immature cortex.In F. Kellaway and I. Petersen (Eds.) Neurological and Electroencephalographic Correlative Studies in Infancy, pp. 117–157. New York, NY: Grune and Stratton.
Reeves, A. G. (Ed.). 1985. Epilepsy and the Corpus Callosum. New York, NY: Plenum.
Scheibel, M. E., and Scheibel, A. B. 1967. Structural organization of non-specific thalamic nuclei and their projection toward the cortex. Brain Res. 6:60–94.
Skinner, J. E., and Lindsley, D. B. 1967. Electrophysiological and behavioral effects of blockade of the non-specific thalamocortical system. Brain Res. 6:95–118.
Spencer, W. A., and Kandel, E. R. 1961. Electrophysiology of hippocampal neurons: IV fast prepotentials. J. Neurophysiol. 24:272–85.
Spencer, W. A., and Kandel, E. R. 1968. Cellular and integrative properties of hippocampal pyramidal cells and the comparative electrophysiology of cortical neurons. Int. J. Neurol. 6:266–296.

Starzl, T. E., and Whitlock, D. G. 1952. Diffuse thalamic projection system in the monkey. J. Neurophysiol. 15:449–468.

Steriade, M., and Llinas, R. 1988. The functional states of the thalamus and the associated neuronal interplay. Physiol. Rev. 68: 649–742.

Velasco, M., and Lindsley, D. B. 1965. Role of orbital cortex in regulation of the thalamocortical electrical activity. Science 149: 1375–1377.

Von Economo, C. 1929. The Cytoarchitectonics of the Human Cerebral Cortex. London, UK: Oxford University Press.

Walker, A. E. 1964. The patterns of propagation of epileptic discharge. In G. Schaltenbrand and C. W. Woolsey (Eds.) Cerebral Localization and Organization, pp. 95–111. Madison: University of Wisconsin Press.

18.

MOTOR SYSTEM AND MOVEMENT

PART I: REFLEX ACTIVITY, CENTRAL PATTERN GENERATORS, AND CEREBRAL CORTICAL MOTOR FUNCTIONS

In studying the motor system, we will consider reflex activity, central generators of patterns of movement, voluntary movement, and learned movements. We will also consider two interrelated aspects: posture and movement. Under posture we will be studying static or tonic reactions. Under movement we will be studying short-duration phasic reactions. We should keep in mind, as Sherrington has indicated, that the reflexes involved in posture and movement are the same. There are no reflexes exclusively for the maintenance of a correct posture, as opposed to those reflexes involved in a movement. We should note that with more detailed microelectrode studies we may find that some neurons in the cerebral cortex or spinal cord are predominantly involved in phasic activities and other predominantly in tonic activities. In the following discussion, we will examine motor function at the level of the spinal cord, the brain stem, and cerebral cortex. It is important to realize that motor functions are represented at successively higher physiological and anatomical levels of the neural axis. As we go higher in the neural axis, we are utilizing and modifying mechanisms that have been integrated at a lower level of the neural axis, a concept first expressed in the modern era by Jackson. Thus, pattern generators make use of the motor mechanisms involved in reflexes without the necessity of afferent input. In turn, voluntary and learned movements incorporate or impose a higher level of a more complex cortical control of these reflex and central pattern mechanisms.

In subsequent chapters the role of the basal ganglia and the cerebellum in modulating movement will be considered.

REFLEX ACTIVITY—CONCEPT OF CENTRAL PATTERN GENERATORS

The terms utilized in defining a reflex are presented in Table 18.1.

Specific neural circuits or neuronal clusters or centers may be responsible for the generation of simple and complex patterns of movement in the absence of afferent input. In actuality, such central patterns are modified or modulated by afferent input, utilize many of the reflex components to be discussed later, and are controlled and/or modified by descending control motor systems from higher centers. Such pattern generators have been described at the level of the spinal cord and the brain stem (mesencephalic locomotor system) for more complex behavior related to locomotion. The latter system is also involved in the motor components of emotional expression, as well as chewing, licking, and sucking behavior. For the accurate performance of complex patterned movements involving the limbs, afferent input and reflex activity are essential. In the absence of such afferent input, the movements while repetitive are not as well coordinated (see DeLong, 1971; Harris-Warrick and Johnson, 1989).

1. *The spinal pattern generator.* This is probably composed of bilateral clusters of interneurons in the intermediate gray matter at the base of the posterior horn. These interneurons are the same interneurons involved in the flexion reflex to be described later. In the spinal cord preparation to be discussed later, the effects of dopaminergic and adrenergic agents in triggering behavior can be demonstrated.

2. *The mesencephalic locomotion pattern generator.* This center is located in the periventricular tegmentum at the junction of midbrain and pons. Axons from this region descend to the medullary medial reticular formation. From this region axons descend as the medial reticulospinal tract in the ventrolateral funiculus to the spinal locomotor system of the lumbar spinal cord. In the decerebrate preparation to be discussed later, glutaminergic effects can be demonstrated. Glutamate receptor antagonists will prevent the locomotion effects that occur on stimulation of the mesencephalic center.

Table 18.1 DEFINITION OF A REFLEX

TERM	EXAMPLES
Adequate stimulus	Nociceptive, proprioceptive, tactile, visual
Synapses involved	Monosynaptic in the stretch reflex; polysynaptic in the flexion reflex
Segments involved	Segmental-stretch reflex, intersegmental-interlimb reflexes. Suprasegmental-brain stem-tonic neck/labyrinthine. Cerebral cortex, placing and long loop reflexes
Movement or response	Flexion, extension, righting, standing, walking, grasp, avoidance, placing
Aim or purpose	Avoidance of pain, escape from predator, acquisition of food

Figure 18.1 High spinal cat: flexion and crossed extension reflexes. (1) The initial posture of the animal. (2) Nociceptive stimulation of the left hind foot produces flexion of the left hind limb and crossed extension of the right hind limb. (3) Nociceptive stimulation of both right and left hind limbs leads to flexion of both hind limbs. Flexion reflex then remains prepotent. (From Sherrington, C.: The Integrative Action of the Nervous System. New Haven: Yale University Press, 1947, p. 226).

3. *Other motor pattern centers.* The premotor cortex for visually guided movements, the subthalamic nucleus, the pontine reticular formation, and the cerebellum will be discussed later (Fig. 18.1).

EFFECTS OF SPINAL AND BRAIN STEM LESIONS ON THE MOTOR SYSTEM

TRANSECTION OF THE SPINAL CORD IN THE HUMAN

In humans, transection of the spinal cord reflects (1) the effects of spinal shock and (2) the prepotency of flexion reflexes as reflex recovery occurs.

Transection of the spinal cord in the human is reviewed in Table 18.2 and in Chapter 9.

TRANSECTION OF THE BRAIN STEM— THE DECEREBRATE PREPARATION

(See Chapter 11 for discussion of anatomical basis.)

The decerebrate preparation involves a transection of the brain stem between the vestibular nuclei and the red nucleus, usually at the intercollicular midbrain level.

In the human the decerebrate state may reflect several pathological processes such as basilar artery thrombosis with brain stem infarction, temporal lobe herniation with midbrain compression, or massive destruction of both cerebral hemispheres.

Decerebrate Rigidity

A state described as decerebrate rigidity develops almost immediately. Decerebrate rigidity may be defined as the exaggerated posture of extension of the antigravity muscles due to the enhancement of proprioceptive stretch reflexes. In four-legged animals, such as the cat and dog, the enhancement of these stretch reflexes results in extensor posture in all four limbs with extension of the tail and arching of the back and neck. This posture is also referred to as opisthotonos (Fig. 18.2). Sherrington has described the posture of decerebrate rigidity as "an exaggerated caricature of standing." This is most intense in those muscles that normally counteract the effect of gravity. In an animal such as the sloth that normally hangs upside down, it is the flexor posture that is exaggerated.

It is important to realize that with transection of the brain stem, the decerebrate rigidity develops almost immediately. Spinal shock does not result. It is important to note that

Table 18.2 COMPLETE TRANSECTION OF THE SPINAL CORD IN THE HUMAN

ONSET	EVENT	MANIFESTATIONS
Immediate	Spinal shock	Below lesion: flaccid paralysis of limbs, no DTRs, atonic bladder and bowel (overflow incontinence)
		Loss of autonomic control: hypotensive if erect[*]
	Sensory loss	Absence of all sensation below lesion
	If section C1–C4	No spontaneous respiration (phrenic outflow—C4)
1–6 weeks	Recovery of flexion reflexes. Note that flexion reflexes usually remain prepotent.	Sign of Babinski, initially dorsiflexion of great toe and fanning of small toes, later flexor withdrawal of foot, leg and thigh
3–4 weeks	Onset of detrusor and bowel function. Minimal return of DTRs	Reflex voiding and defecation begins to occur Achilles and patellar DTRs now present
2–3 months	Mass reflex	Flexion reflexes now exaggerated without local sign with flexor spasms, bladder emptying and profuse sweating, erection and ejaculation
	Autonomic reflexes	Sweating below level of lesion returns
6+ months	Local sign develops	Mass reflex less prominent, flexion reflexes more specific for point of stimulus (may recur with fever)
	Hyperactive extensor reflexes	Deep tendon reflexes become hyperactive; spasticity develops. Crossed extension (Fig. 18.1) and alternate stepping may occur. Occasionally positive support reaction is sufficient for spinal standing

[*] Other aspects of autonomic control are also affected, including sympathetic control of blood pressure, noted particularly with
DTR, deep tendon reflex.

Figure 18.2 The posture of the decerebrate cat when suspended. The hyperextended, rigid posture of neck, back, limbs, and tail is to be noted (opisthotonos). (From Pollack, L.J., and Davis, L.: J. Comp. Neurol., 50:384, 1930, Wiley.)

Figure 18.3 Tonic neck reflexes modify decerebrate rigidity (monkey preparation). Upper figures: flexion of head results in flexion of upper extremities; extension of head produces extension of upper extremities. Lower figures: rotation of head produces extension of upper limb on side to which face is turned and flexion of contralateral upper limb. Correlated adjustments occur in the lower extremities. (From Twitchell, T.E.: J. Amer. Phys. Ther. Ass. 45:413, 1965.)

though the extensor tone is sufficient to allow the animal to stand, the animal is pillar-like. The pillar-like limb seen in this extensor posture is indicative of the positive supporting reaction already seen in the "spinal" cat and dog. This is the tonic form of the extensor thrust reaction previously noted. The animal lacks righting reflexes and has no reactions to sudden displacement.

Modification of Decerebrate Rigidity

The posture of decerebrate rigidity may be modified by several influences: tonic neck reflexes, tonic labyrinthine reflexes, noxious stimuli, and time.

Tonic Neck Reflexes (Fig. 18.3). Tonic neck reflexes are studied best after destruction of the hypotension occurring in the upright position (orthostatic) and parasympathetic control of intestinal peristalsis (ileus occurs). labyrinth or after bilateral section of nerve VIII. These procedures eliminate various labyrinthine influences. The afferents for the tonic neck reflexes are conveyed via the upper cervical dorsal roots from joint receptors—for example, those located in the atlanto-occipital joint. The tonic neck reflexes produce several types of modification of the decerebrate posture. Rotation of the head produces a fencer's posture with extension of the forelimb on the side to which chin, nose, and eyes have rotated with flexion of the forelimb on the contralateral side. Correlated interlimb adjustments may occur in the lower extremities. Extension of the head at the neck produces extension of the forelimbs and flexion of the hind limbs. One may imagine the posture of a cat that is attempting to look at objects upon a table. Flexion of the head onto the chest produces flexion of the forelimbs and extension of the hind limbs. One may imagine the posture of a cat that is attempting to look under a shelf or door.

Tonic Labyrinthine Reflexes (Fig. 18.4). These tonic labyrinthine reflexes are studied best after the head has been immobilized in a plaster cast or after section of the upper cervical dorsal roots. The afferents are conveyed from the otoliths via the vestibular nerves to the vestibular nuclei.

Noxious stimulus to a limb produces the classic interlimb reflex figure (Fig. 18.4).

Time. With time (7–14 days), rigidity decreases and righting reflexes begin to emerge.

The anatomical basis of decerebrate rigidity: Refer to Chapter 11.

THE MIDBRAIN PREPARATION

This involves transection above the superior colliculus with red nucleus and portions of subthalamic nucleus and posterior hypothalamus intact (Fig. 18.5). In this preparation, proprioceptive reflexes are modified by contactual stimuli.

In the dog or cat midbrain preparation, a sequence of righting reflexes occurs. Righting responses in the animal with intact central nervous system are demonstrated in Figures 18.6 and 18.7. Kinetic reactions such as standing and walking may also occur. In contrast, the primate midbrain preparation is unable to stand. There are some fragments of a traction grasp.

Role of hypothalamus: The motor responses for rage are represented at a brain stem level. Stimulation of the midbrain of the decerebrate preparation will produce all of the motor

Figure 18.4 Tonic labyrinthine reflexes modify decerebrate rigidity. (Upper figure) With the animal held in the supine position and the head facing upward, the limbs extend. (Lower figure) With the animal held in the prone position (face downward), the limbs flex. The tonic neck influences must be eliminated by immobilization of the neck or by section of the upper cervical dorsal roots. Note that in a human with neurological disease, the opposite pattern may occur so that a flexion posture predominates when the patient is supine and an extensor posture when prone. (From Twitchell, T.E.: J. Amer. Phys. Ther. Ass. 45:414, 1965.)

components of anger. The hypothalamus, however, is essential for the sham rage reaction of the decorticate animal (Bard).

THE DECORTICATE PREPARATION

The cat and dog preparations are similar to the midbrain animal. In the primate, the tonic grasp reflex may be present. The decorticate human or primate manifests a considerable degree of spasticity often referred to as *decorticate rigidity*. The posture of the decorticate primate or human involves extension of the lower extremities and flexion of the upper extremities (Fig. 18.8). In a sense, this is a double hemiplegic posture.

Figure 18.5 Reflex figures in the decerebrate cat preparation. Effects of nociceptive stimulation. (*A*) Prior to stimulation. (*B*) Change produced by stimulation of left fore foot. (*C*) Change produced by stimulation of left hind foot. (From Sherrington, C.S.: The Integrative Action of the Nervous System. New Haven, Yale University Press, 1947, p. 167.)

Figure 18.6 Righting reflexes in intact cat. Diagram showing series of maneuvers that a cat executes in order to turn itself in the air: (1) free fall; (2) head turns, forelimbs drawn in, hind limbs extended; (3), (4), (5), continued turning with gradual extension of forelimbs while hind limbs are drawn closer to axis of rotation; and (6) turning completed. (Redrawn from Marey, C.R.: Acad. Sci. Paris, 1894, 119:714-717: From Fulton, J.F.: A Textbook of Physiology, 17th Edition. Philadelphia, W.B. Saunders, 1955, p. 221.)

Reactions Dependent on Cerebral Cortex

The cerebral cortex may be considered as providing for a complex reaction to the external environment. The cerebral cortex analyzes afferent information from many sources and utilizes reactions which have been integrated at lower levels of the neural axis. Thus, the presence of the cerebral cortex allows for the accurate projection of the limb in space and for the interaction of various reflex activities with visual and tactile stimuli. The following reflexes are associated with the cerebral cortex:

1. The *optical righting reflex* (Fig. 18.7). This results in the righting of the head in relation to a visual stimulus. This response continues to occur after elimination of the labyrinths and dorsal roots from the upper cervical neck proprioceptors. The response can still be demonstrated after bilateral ablation of the motor and premotor areas in the primate. We should, of course, note that righting of the head when the head and body have been turned on to the side is dependent not only on visual cues but also on labyrinthine cues and asymmetrical body contact stimuli.

2. *Placing reactions.* A number of placing reactions are also noted in the intact animal. When the animal approaches a visible edge, the forelimb is advanced to be precisely placed on the surface. This is termed *the visual placing reaction.* On the other hand, if the animal is blindfolded and the dorsum of the foot or hand touches the edge of a surface, appropriate adjustments are then made to place the plantar or palmar

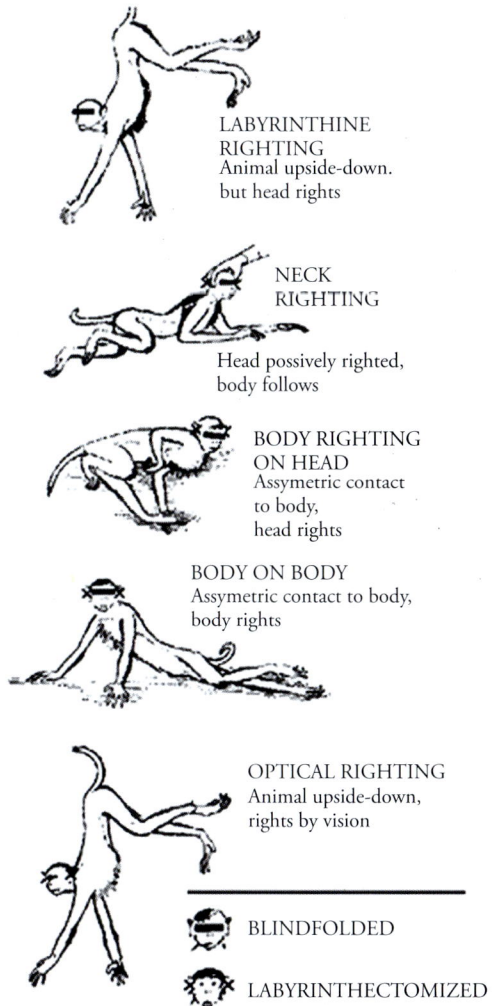

Figure 18.7 Righting reflexes in the monkey. With the exception of the optical righting reflex (which depends on cerebral cortex), all of the righting reflexes demonstrated above are within the capacity of the midbrain preparation. (From Twitchell, T.E.: J. Amer. Phys. Ther. Ass. 45:415, 1965.)

Figure 18.8 Decorticate rigidity in the human. The differences in humans between (*A*) decorticate rigidity in neutral position (both arms are flexed) and (*D*) true decerebrate rigidity (legs are extended arms are rigidly extended and pronated). (*B* and *C*) Alterations produced in the decorticate human by head turning due to tonic neck reflexes. (From Fulton, J.F., A Textbook of Physiology. Philadelphia, W.B. Saunders, 1955, p. 217.)

surface of the extremity on the surface. This is termed *the tactile placing reaction*. Also noted in the intact preparation is a hopping response. If the animal's body is displaced to one side, the animal abducts the leg to that side to regain stability.

3. The *grasp reflex*, as defined by Seyffarth and Denny-Brown, consists of a stereotyped progressive forced closure of the subject's hand on the slowly moving stimulus of the examiner's fingers across the palm. These authors considered the tactile pressure to be the appropriate stimulus. This reflex had emerged following frontal lobe ablation in the monkey (Rushworth and Denny-Brown, 1959). Local anesthesia infiltration of the palm abolished the reflex.

4. *Instinctive grasp*. A more complex and variable response was also described by Seyffarth and Denny-Brown: the instinctive tactile grasp reaction (Fig. 18.9).[1] This response is also triggered by a tactile (or contactual) stimulus to the hand. The hand orients so as to grasp the object. Often the hand follows a moving object making moment-to-moment adjustments so as to grasp onto the object. This instinctive tactile grasping reaction allows for the exploration of space with the hand. The grasp reflex and instinctive tactile grasping reaction are, of course, seen normally when the intact individual attempts to grasp onto an object or to reach for an object. It is not surprising that intact motor and parietal cortex is required. The movements involve distal finger and thumb movement and require precise feedback information.

At times, however, the reaction is seen to be released in abnormal form and degree and to occur in a context where voluntary grasping is inappropriate. Patients with release of the tactile grasp reaction usually have damage to the premotor cortex (areas 6 and 8) and the adjacent supplementary motor cortex and cingulate area on the medial surface of the hemisphere. The instinctive tactile grasp reaction, then, although requiring an intact motor and parietal cortex is released in an abnormal form by lesions of the premotor, supplementary motor, and cingulate areas. This is a form of transcortical release. The same lesion, of course, also acts to release various subcortical areas.[2]

---

[1] Seyffarth and Denny-Brown (1948) also described a group of behavioral responses to the same stimulus, which are more variable and appear to be more subject to factors of attention, distraction, and so on. These were grouped together as the *instinctive grasp reaction*: (a) the closing reaction, (b) the final grip, (c) the trap reaction, (d) the magnet reaction (the hand moves to follow the object), and (e) instinctive groping (if the stimulus moves without capture, the hand pursues).

[2] A recent clinical review of the grasp reflex, in which computerized tomography (CT) scans were used to locate lesions (DeRenzi and Barbieri, 1992), indicates the strongest association with damage to medial frontal areas: predominantly, anterior cingulate gyrus, and supplementary motor cortex and a lesser correlation with damage to the lateral premotor areas. Usually, the release was bilateral, unless the damage to adjacent motor cortex had produced a severe paresis of the contralateral hand. In such cases, only the ipsilateral hand could be tested. Considerable research data reviewed by DeRenzi and Barbieri suggest that the anterior cingulate area not only interconnects with the supplementary motor cortex but also has a similar pattern of connection to basal ganglia, cortical areas, and spinal cord.

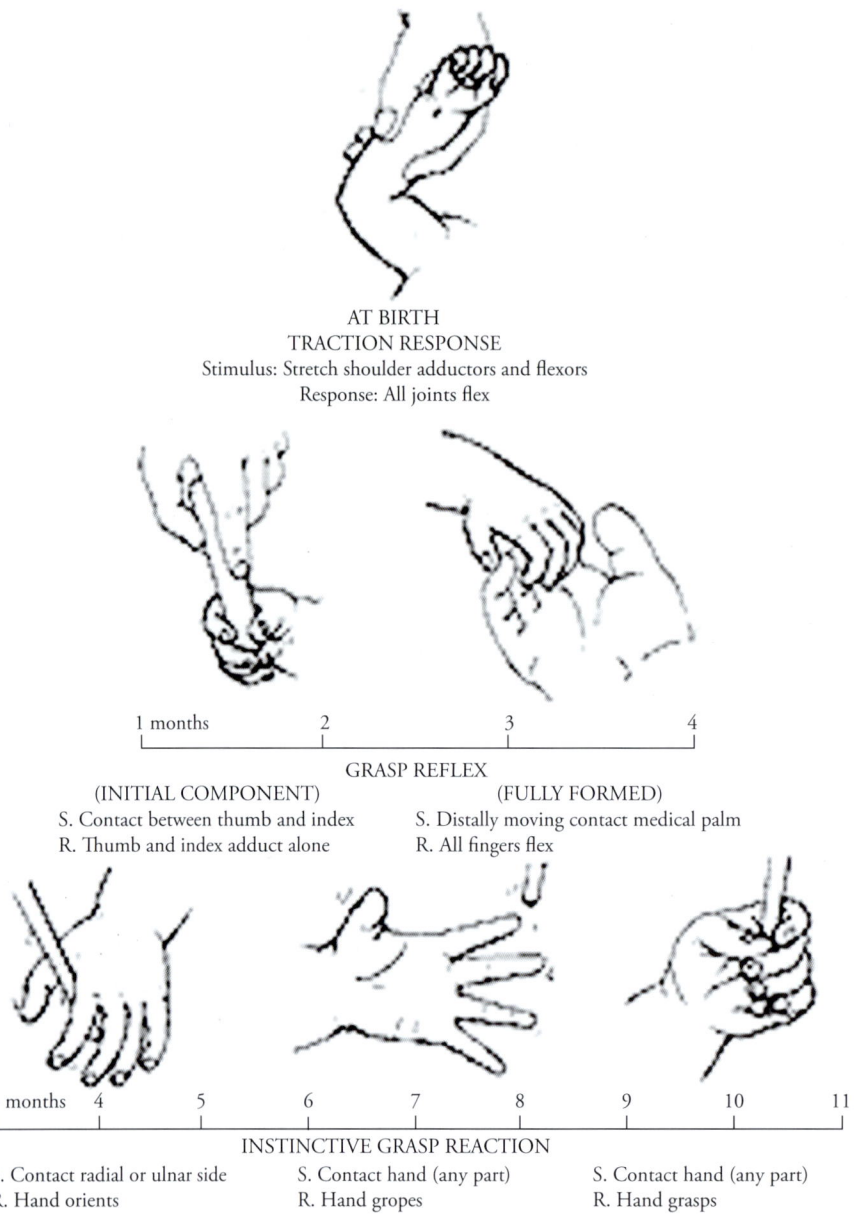

Figure 18.9 Evolution of the automatic grasping responses of infants. (From Twitchell, T.E., Neuropsychologia 3:251, 1965, Elsevier.)

Figure 18.10 Avoiding responses. (*A*) Elicitation of the avoiding response by contact stimulus to the ulnar border of hand as a normal response in infant of 4 to 6 weeks. (From Twitchell, T.E., Neuropsychologia, 3:250, 1965, Elsevier.) (*B*) Avoiding response as a pathological phenomenon. Overextension and abduction of fingers as hand approaches object (child with infantile spastic hemiparesis). (*C*) Avoiding response as a pathological phenomenon in another patient with infantile spastic hemiparesis. Reaction of hand to contact stimulation of the palm. (From Twitchell, T.E.: Neurology, 8:17, 1958, Lippincott/Williams and Wilkins.)

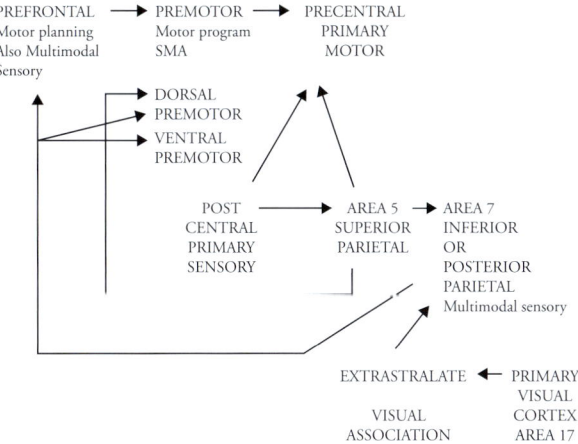

Figure 18.11 Interrelation of motor, premotor, prefrontal, and posterior parietal multimodal sensory areas. The input of the somatosensory and visual systems to the multimodal posterior parietal area is presented. The input of the auditory system and the relationship of the multimodal sensory system to the limbic system are not demonstrated. In a general sense the basis for reaching and grasp is demonstrated.

The instinctive tactile grasp reaction is to be compared to the instinctive tactile avoiding reaction (Fig. 18.10). The stimulus for this reaction is a distally moving tactile stimulus to the outer (ulnar) border of the hand or to the palmar surface of the hand or to the dorsum of the hand. This stimulus leads to a nontonic orientation of the hand away from the stimulus. This is a more precise form of the tonic avoiding response noted in a decorticate preparation. The instinctive tactile avoiding response does not require the pyramidal system. The integrity of the cingulate area, area 8, and the supplementary motor cortex are required. The reaction is released in abnormal degree by damage to the parietal lobe (and adjacent motor cortex). The instinctive grasp and avoidance responses normally are in equilibrium from an anatomical and physiological standpoint.

Other Reflexes Associated with the Cerebral Cortex

In addition to these tactile instinctive grasp and instinctive avoiding responses, various visual triggered responses of a similar nature may be seen. One may speak of a visual instinctive grasp reaction. This requires the integrity of the posterior parietal areas, the visual mechanisms, and the motor cortex. As discussed later, the integrity of the lateral premotor cortex is undoubtedly required for visually triggered reaching and grasping. Damage to the temporal lobe releases this reaction in an abnormal form. The response does occur, of course, in a normal form as one normally reaches for an object, using visual stimuli. This type of phenomenon occurs in the Kluver-Bucy syndrome, which follows the production of bilateral lesions of the temporal lobe in the monkey. The release of various visual automatisms occurs. The animals tend to pick up all objects that appear in their field of vision and to bring these objects to their mouth. (See limbic system chapter 22 for additional discussion). Magnani et al. (1987) studied the anatomical correlation of release of the visually triggered grasping and groping response in humans. In contrast to the experimental studies, the computerized tomography (CT) scan evidence suggested a medial frontal location of lesion responsible for such release.

Another variety of visually cued reaction is the visual instinctive avoiding reaction. This requires the integrity of the temporal lobe and visual mechanisms. The response apparently is independent of the pyramidal system. Again, in the intact individual, equilibrium of grasp and avoidance is to be noted.

While our discussion has focused on the upper extremity, similar grasp and avoiding reactions may also be noted in the lower extremities. Lesions of premotor cortex also affect gait, producing an apraxia in walking termed a *frontal lobe gait apraxia*. This will be discussed later in this chapter.

POSTNATAL DEVELOPMENT OF MOTOR REFLEXES

Some reflexes are present at birth and disappear with time: the startle reflex, sucking, rooting, and the extensor plantar response. A sequence of reflex activities is noted in the developing human infant as regards the use of hands and fingers. In addition, a sequence of changes occurs with respect to sitting, standing, and walking, as summarized in Table 18.2.

OVERVIEW OF THE RELATIONSHIP OF PRIMARY MOTOR, PREMOTOR, AND PREFRONTAL CORTEX

In order to understand voluntary and learned behavior, it is necessary to explore the relationship of primary motor, premotor (including supplementary motor), and the prefrontal areas (Fig. 18.11). Voluntary and learned behaviors also reflect the motivational role of limbic structures to be considered in subsequent chapters.

The large and giant pyramidal cells in the *primary motor cortex* discharge, producing movements in specific directions (flexion, extension, abduction, adduction) resulting from the contraction of muscles at a specific joint. Among other sources of input, the primary motor cortex receives information from somatosensory cortex of the postcentral gyrus and the ventral lateral nucleus of the thalamus. This input may allow the response of motor cortex to peripheral stimuli in what are termed *long loop reflexes*.

In contrast, *the premotor cortex* is concerned with patterns of movements, that is, motor programs neurons in the premotor cortex discharge during the preparation phase prior to movement. The premotor cortex projects in parallel pathways to motor cortex, to basal ganglia, and to spinal cord. The premotor cortex receives projections among other sources from the unimodal sensory association cortex (somatosensory, auditory, and visual) as well as the primary somatosensory cortex and the ventral lateral nucleus of the thalamus.

The *prefrontal areas* have functions that relate to the limbic system and the motor system. While the orbital and mesial regions of the prefrontal cortex are related to the limbic system and will be considered in a later chapter, the dorsal region of the prefrontal cortex is concerned with the executive functions involved in the planning, regulation, and sequencing of behavior and movement over time. In this regard, movement is simply the expression of behavior. This same area of prefrontal cortex functions as the anterior multimodal association cortex and receives projection from the posterior multimodal association cortex located at the intersection of the major sensory association areas. In turn, this dorsal prefrontal area projects to the premotor cortex.

PRIMARY MOTOR CORTEX (AREA 4)

Area 4 is distinguished by the presence of giant pyramidal cells in layer V. Occasionally giant pyramidal cells may also be found more anteriorly in area 6. In humans, much of area 4, particularly its lower half, is found on the anterior wall of the central sulcus. More superiorly, area 4 appears on the lateral precentral gyrus and continues onto the medial aspect of the hemisphere in the anterior half of the paracentral lobule.

It is important to note that the pyramidal tract is not named because of its cells of origin but rather on the basis of its passage through the medullary pyramid. Of the approximately 1 million fibers in the pyramidal tract, 31% arise from area 4; 29% arise from the premotor cortex of area 6; and 40% arise from areas 3, 1, 2, 5, and 7 of the parietal lobe. Fibers with a large diameter (9 to 22 µm) number about 30,000 and correspond roughly to the number of giant pyramidal cells. Most of these large fibers originate from area 4. It is also important to note that the same cortical areas that give rise to the pyramidal tract also give rise to other descending motor pathways: corticoreticular and corticorubral (as well as corticostriate and corticothalamic). From a phylogenetic standpoint this is a logical arrangement, since this relatively new control center, the motor cortex, has available a relatively new fast conducting pathway to the anterior horn cells. At the same time, the motor cortex also has available pathways to certain older brain stem centers, which formerly exercised primary control, for example, the reticular formation and the red nucleus. Note that 70%–90% of the fibers passing through the medullary pyramid will decussate and continue as the lateral corticospinal tract. These fibers originate primarily from those portions of area 4 representing the distal extremities and synapse directly on alpha motor neurons in the lateral sector of the ventral horn.

In contrast, the remaining uncrossed fibers arise from area 6 and the portions of area 4 representing the trunk and neck areas. These uncrossed fibers, as they descend through the brain stem, give off collaterals to the bilateral medial brain stem areas of the reticular formation. These uncrossed fibers continue as the anterior corticospinal tract and terminate bilaterally on interneurons, which in turn will synapse on neurons in the ventral medial cell column of motor neurons.

The fibers originating in the parietal cortex synapse in relationship to interneurons that in turn synapse in relationship to neurons of the dorsal horn.

The premotor sector of area 6 projects primarily to the medial pontomedullary areas. The spinal projections of this area consist of the ventromedial descending reticulospinal system and the vestibulospinal tracts.

The red nucleus receives inputs from the rostral (proximal) arm and leg sectors of area 4 and the adjacent premotor cortex and projects as the rubral-spinal system.

Area 4: Stimulation. Electrical stimulation of the motor cortex at threshold level produces isolated movements of the contralateral portions of the body. The movements may be described as a twitch or small jerk. With increased strength or increased frequency of stimulation, repetitive jerks occur; the movements involve a larger part of the contralateral side of the body and an orderly sequence of spread may occur. The repetitive jerks are similar to the movements of a focal motor seizure. The orderly sequence of spread is duplicated in the "Jacksonian March" of a focal motor seizure.

In the conscious patient, these movements, which can be evoked by stimulation of the motor cortex during surgery, are not clearly the same as consciously willed voluntary movements. According to Penfield, the patient recognizes that these are not voluntary movements of his or her own and will often attribute them to the actions of the neurosurgeon.

There was considerable controversy as to whether muscles or movements were represented in the motor cortex. Single-unit recording studies have suggested a close topographic grouping of all the neurons for a given muscle. Occasionally stimulation will evoke the movement of a single muscle, usually a distal finger muscle, such as an interosseous. In general, however, stimulation produces contraction of a group of muscles concerned with a specific movement. Voluntary actions also involve the integrated contraction of several muscles rather than the isolated contraction of a single muscle. It should then be apparent that the motor cortex "thinks" in terms of movements. This is, in a sense, inherent in the intracortical connections between the neurons representing the various muscles related to a given movement.

Although there is considerable overlap and plasticity in the representation of movements on the surface of the motor cortex, a certain sequence is apparent (Fig. 18.12). In the classical homunculus, the representation of the pharyngeal and tongue movements is located close to the sylvian fissure. Unilateral stimulation of these areas results in bilateral movements. Next in upward sequence are movements of the lips, face, brow, and neck. In the middle third of the precentral gyrus, a large area is devoted to the representation of the contralateral thumb, fingers, and hand. In the upper third, the sequence of the contralateral wrist, elbow, shoulder, trunk, and hip is found. The remainder of the lower extremity in the sequence (knee, ankle, and toes) is represented on the medial surface of the hemisphere in the paracentral lobule. The representation of the anal and vesicle sphincters has been located lowest on the paracentral lobule. It is important to note how large the areas devoted to the thumb, fingers, and face (particularly the lips and tongue) are in the human, reflecting the evolution in use of these structures as regards speech, writing, tool making, and manipulation.

It is also important to note that not all areas of the motor cortex have the same threshold for discharge. As studied in the baboon (Phillips, 1966), the thumb and index finger are the areas of lowest threshold. Slightly stronger shocks are required

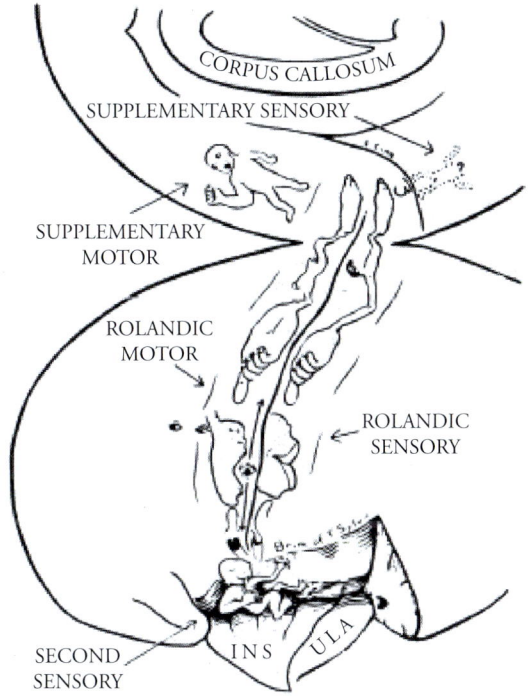

Figure 18.12 Somatic figurines. The primary motor and sensory representation and the effects produced by supplementary motor and second sensory stimulation are demonstrated. (From Penfield, W. and Jasper, H. Epilepsy and the Functional Anatomy of the Human Brain. Boston, Little, Brown & Company, 1954, p. 105.)

to produce a movement on stimulation of the great toe area; at slightly greater intensities of shock, movements of the face begin to occur on stimulation of the appropriate area. These findings may relate in part to the fact that those pyramidal fibers making direct connection to anterior horn cells are primarily those mediating cortical control of the distal finger and thumb muscles.

It must also be noted that at times on stimulation of the postcentral gyrus discrete movements will be produced similar to those elicited from the motor cortex. There is some evidence that such discrete movements are produced at a higher threshold than in the precentral cortex and that the ability to obtain such discrete movements is lost after ablation of the primary motor cortex. However, not all of these neurosurgical data on stimulation of postcentral gyrus in the human are consistent.

Modern concepts of the plasticity of the primary motor cortex: More recent studies reviewed by Sanes and Donoghue (2000) indicate a considerable dynamic plasticity in the primate primary motor cortex. Thus, although modules for the head region, upper extremity, and lower extremity can be distinguished, there is within each module a considerable overlap and plasticity with less of the specific localization for each movement suggested by the earlier maps. Instead, a mosaic is present. The area devoted to specific movement representations may be modified by trauma to peripheral nerves, central nervous system damage, and most important by motor skill learning and cognitive motor actions.

Area 4: Ablation. The effects of ablation of the motor cortex must be distinguished from the more selective effects of limited section of the pyramidal tract in the cerebral peduncle or medullary pyramid. Damage to or ablation of the motor cortex affects not only the pyramidal tracts but also the corticorubral, corticostriate, corticothalamic and corticoreticular pathways.

Studies of the recovery of function following motor cortex lesions in the monkey are most useful in illustrating many aspects of the integration of reflex activity at successive levels of the neural axis and are reviewed and in Table 18.3.

The sequence of events in the human following partial vascular lesions (infarcts) of the precentral cortex or of the motor pathways in the internal capsule has been studied by Twitchell (1951).

Table 18.3 DEVELOPMENTAL CHANGES IN MOTOR RESPONSES

RESPONSE	POSTNATAL TIME
Sucking and rooting reflexes	Present at birth
The Moro (startle) reflex	Present at birth and persisting until 2 months
Tonic neck reflexes	May be present at birth, fragments at 1–2 months
Traction response grasp elicited by traction at shoulder	May be present at birth
Grasp reflex: all fingers flex briefly as unit	Birth–8 weeks
Instinctive grasp reaction	Begins at 4–5 months
Projected grasp (pincer). Then thumb-finger opposition. Subsequently this is voluntary.	Begins at 6–8 months
Plantar grasp response	Present at birth disappears at 9–12 months
Extensor plantar response on lateral plantar stimulation	Present at birth, disappears at 9–12 months (due to immature corticospinal pathway)
Plantar flexion on lateral plantar stimulus (dorsiflexion) and normal through life	Present at 9–12 months
Sitting	Infants usually sit unsupported at 6–7 months
Standing with support	– At 8–9 months
Pulls self to standing position holding onto object	– At 10–12 months
Walking	Begins to walk with support at 10–12 months. Begins to walk independently at 9–16 months

Note. We have not considered here the prenatal motor development of the human fetus. Wolff and Ferber (1979) review many of the earlier studies (which demonstrated considerable capacity for swimming movements) and discuss the use of high-resolution ultrasound to study movements intrautero in a noninvasive manner. Such studies allow more precise establishment of actual fetal maturation. The suck reflex is actually present in the prenatal state.

1. *Flaccid paralysis.* Particularly with a large lesion there is a transient period of flaccid paralysis of the contralateral arm and leg and the lower half of the face, with a transient depression of stretch reflexes. The duration of this flaccid state (reflecting "cortical shock") is variable; it may be quite fleeting depending on the extent of the lesion (which is usually less than total). The sign of Babinski is present with an extensor plantar response on tactile or painful stimulation of the lateral border of the foot.

2. *Return of deep tendon reflexes/stretch reflexes.* After a variable period of time, the deep tendon reflexes in the affected limbs return and become hyperactive. There is increased resistance on passive motion at the joints (when there are severe lesions even this stage may not be reached). This does not affect all movements equally but tends to have its greatest effect on the flexors of the upper extremity. *A hemiplegic posture and gait is noted:* the upper extremity is flexed at the elbow, wrist, and fingers and the leg is extended at the hip, knee, and ankle and externally rotated at the hip with circumduction in walking. Walking is possible with the hemiplegic limb as movement of the proximal limb begins to return. In general, recovery of function in the lower extremity is usually greater than in the upper extremity. Following the return of stretch reflexes, variation in the relative degree of spasticity in the flexor and extensor muscles in relation to tonic neck reflexes may be noted. With the return of tonic neck reflexes one will begin to note proximal limb movements.

3. *Return of traction response.* Abduction of the arm and shoulder will result in stretch of the abductors. There will then be an adduction of the arm at the shoulder. In addition, synergistic flexion of the arm at the elbow, wrist, and fingers will occur, and objects may be grasped in this manner. This flexion synergy, however, results in a whole hand grasp; all of the fingers flex together.

4. *Return of selective ability to grasp.* This stage of recovery involves a more selective grasp of the entire hand albeit a tonic grasp. There is some dissociated synergy so that the hand alone tends to grasp. Finger and thumb opposition begin to return.

5. *Return of the instinctive tactile grasp reaction with the capacity for projected movement.* This occurs with incomplete lesions. If a massive lesion is present, the instinctive grasp reflex does not return.

6. *Return of distal hand movement.* Eventually, depending on the extent of the lesion, some return of distal hand movement may occur but such recovery is usually less than that which occurs for movements at more proximal joints, for example, at the shoulder and hip.

From a physiological and anatomical standpoint, the logic of this pattern of recovery should be evident. One sees in this sequence a recovery of spinal reflex activities, then of brain stem reflex activities, as noted in the decerebrate preparation, then those noted in the decorticate preparation, and finally those reflexes integrated at a cortical level. (This analysis of recovery of function is to some extent an oversimplification: A small hemispheric lesion of the internal capsule in the adult may produce as great a deficit as a hemi-spherectomy performed on a hemisphere damaged extensively early in life; [Freund, 1991].)

More recent studies by Freund of lesions limited to the precentral gyrus in the human indicate that the essential deficit consists of deficits in force generation and execution of independent finger movements. After partial recovery, force is regained and finger movements, although clumsy and slow, are purposive and appropriate to the object. It should be noted that in the human, following massive lesions of the motor cortex, a long delay may occur before spasticity develops and deep tendon reflexes return. Such a long delay in the reappearance of stretch reflexes usually signifies a poor prognosis for complete recovery.[3]

The recent study of Warabi et al. (1990) utilized the CT scan to predict recovery of voluntary movement based on the degree of shrinkage of the cerebral peduncle. When the peduncle had shrunk to less than 60% of normal, recovery of distal limb function was incomplete. When cerebral peduncle was greater than 60% of normal, recovery of distal movement occurred.

Additional discussion regarding the possible reorganization of sensory and motor function at a cortical level that follows damage to these systems is provided in the review of Kaas (1991) and the study of Jacobs and Donoghue (1991). Damage may unmask a considerable degree of latent cortical plasticity, as discussed earlier. The intrinsic horizontal fibers within the primary motor cortex interconnect large areas and could provide the substrate for this reorganization. Some of the changes occur within hours, suggesting some degree of prewiring. In the studies of Nudo et al. (1996), experimental destruction of part of the hand area in the monkey resulted in loss of discrete finger movements. The monkey relied on proximal arm movements and the area of representation of the shoulder and elbow expanded into the otherwise undamaged hand and forearm areas. However, if the lesioned animals were trained to use the hand, the remaining undamaged area of cortex representing the hand and digits expanded into the area of representation of elbow and shoulder. The trained animals regained the ability to use discrete finger movements in retrieving small objects in 3–4 weeks. The untrained animals did not achieve this level of recovery. These studies certainly indicate the potential role of rehabilitation (occupational and physical therapy) in helping patients recover from the effects of cerebrovascular accidents, trauma, and other pathology involving the motor cortex. Positron emission tomography (PET) scan studies indicate increased functional activity in other areas of the same and contralateral hemisphere in patients who have recovered from a hemiparesis due to an infarct involving the internal capsule. This was noted in the posterior cingulate

---

[3] The studies of Patano et al. (1995) utilizing CT/MRI and SPECT scan have demonstrated that patients with a prolonged flaccid hemiparesis as opposed to a spastic hemiparesis had a greater structural involvement of the lentiform nucleus and lower perfusion in the lentiform nucleus, thalamus, and cerebellum as well as cortical motor areas.

area on the side of the lesion and the premotor and caudate nucleus of the opposite intact hemisphere. During movement there was increased bilateral activation of anterior insular cortex, ventral premotor, anterior cingulate, and inferior parietal areas (39 and 40), as well as premotor cortex of the intact hemisphere (Weiller et al., 1992).

The following case history illustrates the effects of focal disease involving the motor cortex.

CASE HISTORY 18.1

Three months prior to admission, this 29-year-old, right-handed, white female developed an intermittent "pulling sensation" over the anterior aspect of the left thigh, lasting a few minutes, which recurred about twice a week. On the evening of admission she again had the onset of this same sensation, then had numbness followed by "jerky movements" in her left foot which progressed to involve the whole left lower extremity. She was then observed to have tonic extension and then clonus of all four limbs with loss of consciousness for a minute or less. She still appeared dazed and slightly confused for the next 5 minutes and was subsequently amnestic for the secondarily generalized seizure

Physical examination: Normal except for bite marks on the left lateral aspect of the tongue.

Neurologic examination: Significant only for a slight asymmetry of deep tendon reflexes, left > right.

Clinical diagnosis: Focal seizures originating right parasagittal motor cortex (foot area), with question of parasagittal meningioma.

Laboratory Data

Electroencephalogram (Fig. 29.1B) demonstrated rare focal spikes, right Rolandic parasagittal consistent with the focal source of the secondarily generalized seizure.

CT scan (Fig. 18.13) demonstrated an enhancing lesion in the right parasagittal region just anterior to the central sulcus.

Arteriograms (Fig. 18.14) were consistent with a right parasagittal meningioma.

Figure 18.13 Parasagittal meningioma. Case 18.1. Computerized tomography (CT) scan demonstrates an enhancing lesion in the most rostral sections of the CT scan, just anterior to the right rolandic sulcus. See text for details.

Subsequent course: The patient did well after removal of a well-circumscribed right parasagittal meningioma by Dr. Bernard Stone. The patient received diphenylhydantoin (Phenytoin) to prevent additional seizures.

SELECTIVE LESIONS OF THE PYRAMIDAL TRACT

We have previously indicated that the student should consider as the primary manifestations of an upper motor neuron lesion a spastic paralysis with increased deep tendon reflexes and the sign of Babinski. A more detailed analysis indicates that the effects of selective pyramidal tract damage are not quite the same or equivalent to those which follow, in a general sense, upper motor neuron lesions. We should note that the ablation of the motor cortex destroys not only the origin of the pyramidal tract (the corticospinal tract) but also the origin of the corticoreticular, the corticorubral, the corticothalamic, and the corticostriatal fibers. The effects of such a cortical ablation are to release these various subcortical and brain stem centers from cortical control and also to produce the effects of damage to the corticospinal tract. We should note that section of the pyramidal tract in the medullary pyramid or in the cerebral peduncle does not have the same anatomical and physiological effects as ablation of the motor cortex, which has been previously summarized.

Furthermore, selective section of the pyramidal tract or cerebral peduncle may yield different effects than section of the lateral column in the spinal cord. The descending rubrospinal and the lateral reticulospinal tract (from the bulbar inhibitory center of the medulla) are closely related to the corticospinal tract in the lateral column. In addition, the medial reticulospinal tract from the pontine extensor facilitatory center descends in the anterior column and thus would be left undamaged by a lesion of the lateral column.

The studies of Bucy suggest that both the human and the monkey were capable of useful movements after section of the pyramidal tract in the cerebral peduncle. Thus, locomotor abilities returned. The monkey could use his hand in feeding and in manipulating small objects. With bilateral section, however, the hand was used as a claw with some deficiency in independent finger movements. It should be stressed that spasticity and increased deep tendon reflexes were not noted. The sign of Babinski was found in the human patient. In the human patient, the retention of discrete finger movements was remarkable. Somewhat different results were obtained by Denny-Brown (1966) following section of the pyramidal tract in the medullary pyramid. There was a moderate increase of deep tendon reflexes and a mild spasticity. Schwartzman (1978) found no spasticity 3 years after section of the medullary pyramid in the monkey. (A recent study by Jagiella and Sung [1989] does suggest the eventual development of spasticity in a patient with the bilateral ischemic infarction of the medullary pyramids.)

What was clearly defective after section in all of these studies was the discrete fractionated distal finger movements required for the instinctive tactile grasp reaction that normally would allow for the precise orientation of fingers to a moving

Figure 18.14 Parasagittal meningioma. Case 18.1. Arteriograms demonstrate the characteristic features of a circumscribed vascular tumor in the parasagittal rolandic area, supplied by the right anterior cerebral artery and meningeal branches of the external carotid artery. (*A*) Arterial phase lateral common carotid injection. (*B*) Arterial phase anteroposterior view of common carotid injection. (*C*) Selective injection of the external carotid artery. (*D*) Common carotid injection: venous phase—tumor blush with large draining vein. See text for details.

three-dimensional stimulus. The pyramidal tract fibers mediating cortical control of these distal muscles make direct connection to the anterior horn cell. These direct fibers of the corticospinal system elicit predominantly flexor facilitation and extensor inhibition. In contrast, the indirect corticospinal fibers (those which do not synapse directly on anterior horns cells) synapse predominantly in relation to interneurons, which make synaptic contact with anterior horn cells innervating more proximal muscles. Additional discussion will be found in Kuypers (1987).

We have not considered in our discussion the possible role of the pyramidal tract in modifying transmission of sensory information at the spinal cord (posterior horn) and brain stem levels (nucleus gracilis and nucleus cuneatus). The various studies, which have suggested such a role, are considered in the review of Bizzi and Evarts (1971).

CORTICORUBRAL SPINAL SYSTEM

In the monkey and cat, if the pyramidal tracts are intact, destruction of the rubral spinal system produces no definite motor deficit. However, in monkeys and cats that have already had bilateral section of the pyramidal tract (a section which has produced very little qualitative change in limb movement) a complete loss of distal limb movement may occur after additional bilateral destruction of the rubrospinal tract. In the intact monkey, complex coordinated movements may be evoked by stimulation of the red nucleus. Flexor excitation predominates with extensor inhibition. The studies of Lawrence and Kuypers (1968) suggested that the rubrospinal tract is mainly concerned with steering movements of the extremities, particularly distal segments. On the other hand, the ventromedial brain stem reticulospinal tract is mainly concerned with steering movements and posture of head or body and synergistic movements of the extremities (Kuypers, 1987).

PREMOTOR CORTEX (AREAS 6 AND 8)

Overview of the functions of the premotor and supplementary motor cortex (Fig. 18.15).

Penfield grouped area 6, area 8, and the supplementary motor cortex (the continuation of areas 6 and 8 onto the medial surface of the hemisphere) on clinical grounds as intermediate frontal areas. These areas may also be grouped from the functional standpoint as concerned with the preparation

Figure 18.15 The motor cortical fields of the human as determined by Foerster employing cortical stimulation. Stimulation of the area indicated in black produced discrete movements at low threshold and was designated pyramidal. Lines or cross-hatching indicate other areas producing movements and were designated in a broad sense as extrapyramidal. These movements were usually more complex synergistic and adversive movements and included the adversive responses obtained by stimulation of area 19. Each of the areas extending to the midline is continued on to the medial surface. (Modified from Foerster, O.: Brain, 59:137, 1936, Oxford University Press.)

for movement and the temporal sequencing of movements (Passingham, 1987).

These areas receive a polysensory input from sensory association areas. These are widespread connections of these areas both within and between the hemispheres (see Pandya and Kuypers, 1969; Pandya and Vignolo, 1971; Ward et al., 1946).

There is considerable rationale for grouping these areas from the standpoint of the results of stimulation studies. Moreover, there is also considerable justification for such an approach from the cytoarchitectural standpoint. Histologically, area 6 is similar to area 4 but lacks, in general, giant pyramidal cells. Area 8 has some similarity to area 6 but is also transitional to the granular prefrontal areas. There are considerable variations when the several cytoarchitectural maps are compared as to the exact boundaries of area 8 in both human and monkey. Areas 44 and 45 in the inferior frontal convolution (Broca's motor speech or expressive aphasia centers) should also be included within this motor association or intermediate frontal grouping, from both the functional and cytoarchitectural standpoints. For simplicity of presentation, these areas will be considered later in relation to language function.

Note that clinical lesions, such as vascular infarcts and tumors, usually do not respect cytoarchitectural borders. Thus, vascular lesions that involve the lateral premotor aspect of area 6 usually also involve the primary motor cortex. Tumors such as parasagittal meningiomas may involve both the lateral premotor and the supplementary motor cortex or may involve the prefrontal and the several premotor areas.

With increasing research, there has come recognition that there are differential functions for the various sectors of these premotor areas (Wise et al., 1997).

An initial distinction may be made between the supplementary motor cortex (SMA) and the lateral premotor areas (PMA).

1. *The Supplementary Motor Area.* SMA is concerned with the sequencing of movements that are initiated internally without triggering from external sensory stimuli. SMA is concerned with the performance of learned sequences of movement. The area just anterior to the SMA, the pre-SMA, is involved along with other prefrontal areas such as area 46 in the actual process of learning the sequences (training of a motor skill). This same pre-SMA area is also involved when the same complex movement sequence is imagined. Once a sequence has been fully and usually over learned, control may be centered in primary motor cortex.

   The Readiness Potential (Bereitschafts Potential): In humans, surface electrodes placed on the scalp are able to record 1–2 seconds prior to voluntary movements, a significant surface negative potential with maximum amplitude over the midline of the frontal area corresponding primarily to the supplementary cortex. The process of initiation of more complex actions enhances this potential. In contrast, when the same movements were triggered by external stimuli, there was no such readiness potential. These noninvasive studies in humans (as well as blood flow studies) confirm much earlier experimental data derived in studies of the monkey (Papa et al., 1991).

2. *The Lateral Premotor Area.* In contrast to the SMA, the lateral PMA is concerned with the sequencing of movements that are triggered by external stimuli. In this regard, there is a close relationship of the lateral PMA to the sensory association cortex of the superior parietal cortex (area 5) and the posterior parietal multimodal sensory areas, which are directly connected, with the extrastriate visual cortex. This relationship is complex, as demonstrated in reaching for and grasping precisely an object presented at a particular point in visual space.

   The lateral PMA has been divided into two major functional areas: the dorsal and the ventral:

   a. *The dorsal lateral PMA* neurons are involved in reaching for that object. This area is also involved in learning to associate specific stimuli particularly visual with the motor response of reaching for that stimulus. As opposed to the learning of a repetitive motor act (pressing a key) involving the supplementary motor cortex, this is a different type of learning referred to as associative learning. Multiple bits of information must be integrated for this reaching activity, visual position of object, position of gaze, position of arm, and so on, and this involves information received from various posterior parietal areas adjacent to the extrastriate cortex discussed in greater detail by Wise et al. (1997).

   b. *The ventral lateral PMA* is concerned with grasping. This area also must receive information from the extrastriate cortex regarding size and shape of the object as well as other multimodal and sensory association data so that an effective grasp of the object may occur.

Area 6 stimulation: Essentially stimulation of PMA and SMA results in a pattern of movement characterized by tonic abduction of the contralateral arm at shoulder with flexion at elbow plus deviation of head and eyes to the contralateral field. In addition with SMA stimulation bilateral lower extremity movements may occur (Fig. 21.12). *Ablation* of these areas will result in a release of grasp reflex and an apraxia in limb movements. Bilateral lesions of the SMA may result in an akinetic mute state.

The following case provides an example of a low-grade glioma involving the premotor and supplementary motor cortex from the standpoint of focal seizure activity. The motor effects of frontal lesions are presented in case histories 22.2 and 22.3, which follow the discussion of the prefrontal areas.

CASE HISTORY 18.2

This 57-year-old, right-handed, at age 47, had the onset of observed generalized convulsive seizures, which occurred without warning with sudden loss of consciousness. Shortly after the onset of the grand mal seizures, the patient began to have focal seizures, which increased in frequency to one per week. She described these as beginning with the abduction and raising of the right arm at the side, over her head, then a jerking of the right arm, and then she would fall to the ground. She would remain fully conscious but she would be unable to talk. She would have an awareness that something strange was occurring. She had a sinking sensation. She denied any impairment of memory after the episode. However, she would be aware that her right arm and leg were tingling and weak for perhaps 5 minutes afterward, and she would be unable to speak for 10–30 minutes afterward. These focal seizures occurred once a month, but for the last 2 years, they had been occurring once a week. The patient indicated that over the last 10 years she has had problems with her memory.

She was reported to have had three "negative" CT scans over the years, and yearly EEGs, which did not reveal focal features or electrical seizure discharges.

Neurological Examination

Mental status: Delayed recall without assistance was 0 out of 5 and with assistance 2 out of 5.

Motor system: Intact except for a decreased swing of the right arm in walking.

Reflexes: Deep tendon reflexes were increased on the right at biceps and patellar. Plantar response was extensor on the right and equivocally extensor on the left.

Clinical diagnosis: Seizures of focal origin left premotor/supplementary motor cortex, possibly secondary to low-grade glioma. A meningioma was less likely due to the reports of "normal CT scans."

Laboratory data: CT scan (Fig. 18.16) demonstrated an area of calcification with surrounding edema in the left premotor area. Magnetic resonance imaging (MRI) scan (Fig. 18.17) demonstrated extensive involvement of the premotor and supplementary areas by tumor and edema.

Subsequent course: Dr. Bernard Stone performed subtotal resection of this tumor. Histological examination of the tissue confirmed the preoperative impression of an infiltrating glioma—predominantly oligodendroglioma in type. The patient received postoperative radiotherapy, 5000 rads to the left hemisphere and an additional 1000 rads to area of tumor. When last seen in follow-up 4 years after surgery, the

Figure 18.16 Case 18.2. Oligodendroglioma of premotor and supplementary motor cortex. Computerized tomography (CT) scan. The noncontrast CT scan demonstrated an area of calcification with surrounding edema, involving the premotor cortex. See text for details.

patient was still experiencing infrequent (1–2 per month) short focal seizures of the same type involving focal movements of right arm, plus speech arrest. The neurological examination demonstrated some decrease in spontaneous speech and some blunting of affect. Bilateral extensor plantar responses were present. She had a moderate frontal type apraxia of gait and required a cane to avoid falls.

CORTICAL CONTROL OF EYE MOVEMENT: FRONTAL (AREA 8) AND PARIETO-OCCIPITAL EYE FIELDS

Overview of Eye Movements

In Chapters 11 and 12 the basic cranial nerve and brain stem mechanisms for eye movement were considered. In this section, the mechanisms for control from other centers will be considered. This is a complex subject and has been presented in great detail in the studies of Goldberg (2000).

Vision is sharpest at the fovea, the center of the macular area of the retina. There are various mechanisms for moving the eyes so that points of interest are centered on the fovea of the two eyes. These may be listed as follows: saccadic eye movements, smooth eye movements, vergence eye movements, fixation system, vestibulo-ocular responses, and optickinetic responses.

Definitions and Anatomical Localization

1. *Saccadic eye movements: Rapid movements of gaze that shift the fovea rapidly to a point of interest are termed saccades.* These movements may be triggered by attending to

Figure 18.17 Case history 18.2. Oligodendroglioma of premotor and supplementary motor cortex, magnetic resonance imaging (MRI) nonenhanced (*A*) horizontal T2-weighted study demonstrates the wide extent of tumor and edema involving the premotor and frontal cortex. (*B*) Coronal section T2-weighted MRI demonstrates the involvement of the supplementary motor cortex. (*C*) Reference diagram for coronal section (slice 13). See text for details.

a visual point of interest, by memories, or by commands. The brain stem substrate for all horizontal saccades is the lateral gaze center of the paramedian pontine reticular formation. Several types of neurons are present in this center. Neurons referred to as medium lead burst cells provide direct excitation to motor neurons in the ipsilateral abducens nucleus and to the interneurons in that nucleus which give rise to the medial longitudinal fasciculus. Long lead burst cells drive the medium lead burst cells and receive excitatory input from the higher centers to be discussed later. The medium lead burst neurons also excite inhibitory burst neurons, which in turn suppress the discharge of contralateral abducens neurons. In addition, there are neurons located in the dorsal raphe nucleus of the pontomedullary area, which cease firing during saccades (omnipause neurons). These neurons, if stimulated during a saccade, will stop the saccadic movement. Additional neurons provide tonic discharges relevant to eye position and maintain the eyes in a position set by the saccade: the flocculus of the old vestibular portion of the cerebellum, the vestibular nucleus, and the nucleus prepositus hypoglossi.

For vertical saccades, burst and tonic neurons are found in the rostral interstitial nucleus of the medial longitudinal fasciculus in the mesencephalic reticular formation.

Central control of saccades: A complex system with redundant features is present. Essentially, two major cortical areas are involved: the contralateral frontal eye field (area 8) and the contralateral lateral intraparietal area of the posterior parietal area at the border of the extrastriate cortex. Area 8 provides the motor input for the response to the command (e.g., "look to the left or right field"). The frontal eye field has major interconnections in a topographic manner with areas that participate in the streams of information that flow out of the extrastriate visual cortex. These two streams, the dorsal and ventral, will be discussed in the visual system, Chapter 23. The posterior parietal area, in contrast, is involved with visual attention, with representations of the location of objects of interest. Beyond a simple representation, there is a transformation of this information by parietal neurons into motor coordinates (Colby and Goldberg, 1999). There is a significant interconnection with area 8 with an exchange of information. Both areas project to the intermediate and deep cell layers of the superior colliculus. The superior colliculus in turn projects to the mesencephalic and pontine reticular formation. The same areas of the superior colliculus also receive inputs from the prestriate areas of the posterior temporal gyri. The superficial layers of the superior colliculi receive input from both the striate cortex and the retina. The frontal eye field (area 8) projects not only to the superior colliculus but also directly to the pontine and mesencephalic reticular formation. Lesions of either area 8 or of the superior colliculus would produce a defect in saccades to the contralateral field and a transient visual neglect. The defect, however, would be temporary, since the alternative system would be intact. Lesions of the parietal cortex tend to produce longer lasting visual neglect syndromes. The interaction of area 8 and the superior colliculus is even more complex. Area 8 projects to the caudate nucleus. The caudate nucleus inhibits the S. nigra pars reticularis, which in turn acts to inhibit the superior colliculus.

Other cortical areas are also involved in saccades include the SMA eye field and the dorsolateral frontal cortex. The former area has neurons that direct movement to part of a target. The latter contains neurons that discharge when the saccade is made to a remembered target.

2. *Smooth pursuit in contrast to saccades keeps the image of a moving target on the fovea.* Eye movement velocity must match the velocity of the target. The medial vestibular nucleus, the nucleus prepositus hypoglossi, and the paramedian pontine reticular formation receive information from the vermis and flocculus of the cerebellum and project to the abducens nucleus and the oculomotor nucleus. Morrow and Sharpe (1993) discuss the deficits in smooth pursuit after unilateral frontal lesions.

The cortical inputs for smooth pursuit arise from area 8: the frontal eye field. In the monkey, stimulation of area 8 produces ipsilateral pursuit. Area 8 receives input from the posterior sectors of the superior and middle temporal gyri. This area in turn receives input from the visual cortex. In humans the posterior parietal area may serve this same function. Both the frontal and temporal (or posterior parietal) areas project to the dorsolateral pontine areas.

3. *The fixation system holds the eyes still during intentional gaze on an object.* During fixation, saccades must be suppressed. The most rostral segment of the superior colliculus has a representation of the fovea and neurons here are active during fixation. These neurons act to inhibit neurons in the more caudal superior colliculus. In addition, these neurons excite the omnipause neurons in the lateral gaze center, which, as discussed earlier, inhibit saccades.

4. *Vergence movements (convergence and divergence) and accommodation* are controlled by neurons within the third nerve complex of the midbrain.

5. *Vestibulo-ocular movements* hold images stable on the retina during brief head movements. Input occurs from the vestibular system.

6. *Opticokinetic movements hold images stable during sustained head rotation.* Visual input is required. In rabbits, retinal neurons project to the nucleus of the optic tract in the pretectum, which then projects to the medial vestibular nucleus. These neurons can distinguish between visual and vestibular stimuli. In primates, there is, in addition, a "cortical system" that includes the magnocellular layers of the lateral geniculate, striate cortex, and the posterior portions of the middle and superior temporal gyri. Compared to the noncortical system, which responds to stimuli moving slowly in a temporal to nasal direction, this "cortical system" can respond to stimuli moving with higher velocities in a nasal to temporal direction. This evolution in the system may reflect the changes, which have occurred in the placement of the orbits in the skull when the primates are compared to the rabbit.

Opticokinetic nystagmus occurs when a pattern of vertical black-and-white lines is moved slowly in front of the eyes. A similar nystagmus occurs as one sits in a moving train looking out the window at the series of telephone poles flashing by. A lesion in the cortical system produces defective opticokinetic nystagmus to visual stimuli moving toward the side of the lesion.

Area 8: Stimulation: there is disagreement regarding the exact boundaries of area 8 in the human. Some investigators (Vogts, Foerster, and Penfield) (Figs. 17.10, 18.10, and 21.15) have limited area 8 to those portions of middle frontal and inferior frontal gyri just anterior to the precentral gyrus. These authors have then designated all of the superior frontal gyrus between the prefrontal areas and the motor cortex as area 6. It is clear that conscious, adversive eye and head movements to the contralateral field occur most frequently in relation to

Figure 18.18 (*A*) Simple (conscious) adversive seizures at onset. The epileptogenic lesion localizes to the middle frontal gyrus anterior to motor cortex. (From Penfield, W., and Kristiansen, K.: Epileptic Seizure Patterns, Springfield, Ill., Charles C. Thomas, 1951, p. 30.) (*B*) Unconscious adversive seizures at onset. The epileptogenic focus in 16 patients whose seizures began with unconscious aversion of head and eyes localizes predominantly to the anterior portion of the frontal lobe. (From Penfield, W., and Kristiansen, K.: Epileptic Seizure Patterns. Springfield, Ill., Charles C. Thomas, 1951, p. 22.)

stimulation of that portion of the middle frontal gyrus just anterior to the precentral gyrus. In actuality, in the studies of Penfield and Jasper (1954) and confirmed more recently by Luders et al. (1988), the eye field for gaze actually extended onto the motor strip between the face and hand areas, as demonstrated most particularly in Figure 17.11. Adversive head and eye movements may also occur, of course, as part of a more complex movement on stimulation of area 6 or of the supplementary motor cortex. Moreover, adversive head and eye movements, as a seizure phenomenon following loss of consciousness, may occur with foci of seizure discharge more anteriorly placed in the prefrontal areas (compare Figs. 18.18a and 18.18b), but these have less localizing significance. Quesney concluded that seizures arising in parasagittal frontal area are more likely to involve conscious head turning; seizures originating in anterolateral dorsal-frontal convexity—unconscious head turning. In addition, stimulation in areas 18 and 19 will also produce eye turning. Thus, the clinical neurologist must in each case weigh the localizing significance of seizures characterized by head and eye turning. Such seizure components do not always have the more specific localizing significance of the focal motor seizure or of the olfactory hallucination (refer also to the paper of Ochs, which discusses the variability of localization in terms of ipsilateral versus contralateral deviation of the eyes).

In addition to head and eye turning, opening and closing of the eyelids may occur on area 8 stimulation. At times, pupillary dilatation and eye movements, other than conjugate aversion, may occur, for example, upward deviation of the eyes (Fig. 18.19).

Area 8: Ablation. Ablation of area 8, or (in humans) infarction of this area following occlusion of the blood supply, results in a transient paralysis of voluntary conjugate gaze to the contralateral visual field. In general, in humans, this paralysis of voluntary gaze usually does not occur in isolation but is associated with a sufficient degree of infarction to have produced a severe hemiparesis. The patient then lies in bed with the contralateral limbs in a hemiplegic posture and with the head and eyes deviated toward the intact arm and leg. This deviation may perhaps reflect the unbalanced effect of the adversive eye center of the intact hemisphere. The effect is usually transient, clearing in a matter of days or weeks. Neglect these patients at times also appear to neglect objects introduced into the visual field contralateral to the lesion. The patients also neglect contralateral tactile and auditory stimuli. In the past, such a unilateral neglect has been attributed to associated involvement of the inferior parietal lobule. However, suggest that these unilateral neglect syndromes may also occur as transient phenomena following ablation of area 8 in monkeys (area within the superior limb of the arcuate sulcus). These animals also had conjugate deviation of head and eyes to the side of the lesion and forced circling. Bilateral ablations within this area resulted in animals that, in a sense, had a bilateral neglect of the environment, remained apathetic, and neglected visual, auditory, and tactile stimuli, although they could follow moving objects. Although some recovery occurred over a period of weeks to months, the animals continued to have a "wooden expression" and a fixed gaze. Some of these findings are seen in the human following bilateral frontal lobe damage. In addition, however, a similar state may occur in Parkinson's disease or in brain stem lesions, producing akinetic mutism, which will be discussed later. Note also that bilateral discharge of this area may produce a similar state of "neglect of the environment" and arrest of movement.

SUPPRESSOR AREAS FOR MOTOR ACTIVITY (NEGATIVE MOTOR RESPONSE)

Dusser de Barenne and McCulloch found in the monkey that stimulation of that portion of area 4, adjacent to area 6 (designated area 4S), resulted in a suppression of the motor response elicited by stimulation of area 4. In addition, thresholds for obtaining responses from area 4 were raised and, after discharge, were aborted. Stretch reflexes and muscle tone were decreased. It was soon discovered that these effects could be obtained by stimulation of a number of other cortical areas: areas 8 (8S), 2S, and 19S. On the medial aspect of the hemisphere, similar effects could be obtained from the anterior sector of the cingulate gyrus: areas 24S and 32. These "suppressor" areas cannot be distinguished on cytoarchitectural grounds from adjacent cortical areas. Similar effects have been elicited from stimulation of the caudate nucleus and of the bulbar medullary inhibitory center. There has been some evidence that the cortical motor suppressor effects are mediated via cortical reticular and corticostriate connections. In subsequent studies, indicated that arrest of movement could occur from stimulation of a number of distinct neocortical and rhinencephalic points. Note must of course be made that a nonspecific interference with voluntary movement may occur in relation to stimulation of the motor cortex. Thus, the patient who is experiencing a focal motor seizure involving the hand cannot use that hand in the performance of voluntary skilled movements. Similarly, arrest of speech is frequently produced by stimulation of the various speech areas of the

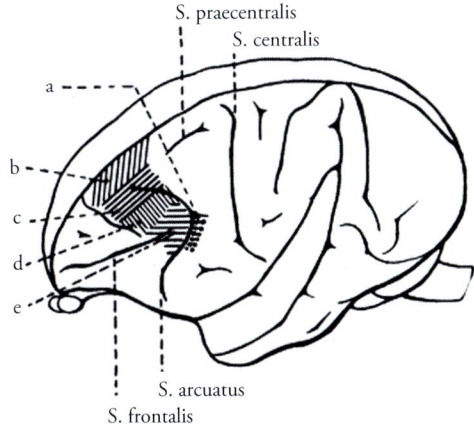

Figure 18.19 Functional subdivision of the frontal eye fields in the monkey under relatively light anesthesia: (*a*) closure of eyes; (*b*) pupillary dilatation; (*c*) eyelid opening (awakening reaction"); (*d*) conjugate deviation to the opposite side; and (*e*) nystagmus to opposite side. (From Smith, W.K., in Bucy, P.: The Precentral Motor Cortex. Urbana, University of Illinois Press, 1944.) In the studies of Crosby, E.C., et al. (J. Neurol. 97:357-383, 1952) oblique and vertical movements were also observed.

dominant hemisphere, whereas vocalization is only rarely produced.

Recent studies by Luders et al. (1988) with precise stimulation of the cerebral cortex of human in preparation for epilepsy surgery have revisited the concept of suppressor areas renaming the phenomena as "negative motor response"—an inability to perform or sustain a voluntary movement at a stimulation intensity that did not produce any symptoms or signs. The areas of cortex included (a) the inferior frontal gyrus, immediately anterior to primary motor area for face; (b) less often, the premotor cortex just anterior to the frontal eye field or the hand area; and (c) the supplementary motor cortex. The authors speculate that these effects are produced because the stimulation interferes with the preparation for movement.

PREFRONTAL CORTEX (AREAS 9, 10, 11, 12, 46, 13, AND 14)

Additional discussion will be found in Chapter 22.

The term *prefrontal* refers to those portions of the frontal lobe anterior to the agranular motor and premotor areas (areas 9, 10, 11, and 12). Three surfaces or divisions are usually delineated: (1) lateral-dorsal convexity, (2) medial, and (3) orbital or ventral. All three are concerned with executive function and relate to the mediodorsal thalamic nuclei. In general, the lateral-dorsal relates to motor association executive function, and the orbital-ventral and the medial to the limbic-emotional control executive system. Recent studies have questioned this simplistic approach. Thus, certain functions previously considered to be associated with dorsolateral location have been now localized to a medial location. In addition, there is evidence that dorsal-lateral lesions also alter affect and motivation. Moreover, as the clinical examples of Chapter 22 will demonstrate, most pathological processes involve the functions associated with more than one division either directly or through pressure effects.

Most studies of stimulation or of ablation lesions involving the prefrontal areas have included, within the general meaning of the term *prefrontal*, areas beyond areas 9, 10, 11, and 12. Posterior orbital cortex (area 13) and the posteromedial orbital cortex (area 14) have been added to the orbital frontal group (Fig. 18.20). These areas all share a common relationship to the medial dorsal nucleus of the thalamus. Areas 46 and 47, located in humans on the lateral surface of the hemisphere, are also included. The anterior cingulate gyrus (area 24) is also included in the prefrontal area, although it may be considered part of the limbic system and relates to the anterior thalamic nuclei.

Overview of the Role of the Prefrontal Area in Motor and Cognitive Function

Our concern here is primarily with the dorsal prefrontal subdivision. The ventral/orbital and medial subdivisions also will be considered here but also in the limbic system, Chapter 22. We are concerned with the sequencing of behavior, the planning of motor function, and with a very short type of memory referred to as working memory. *Working memory* provides for the temporary storage of information that is needed for

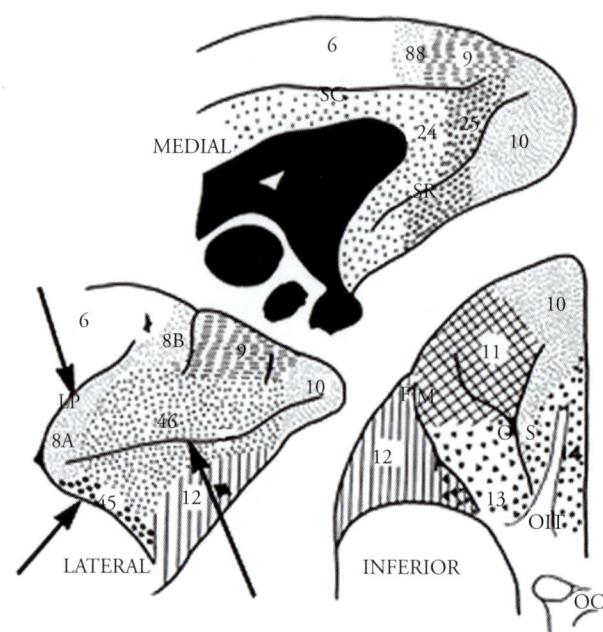

Figure 18.20 Prefrontal areas of the monkey (*Macaca mulatta*). Note location of orbital areas 13 and 14, anterior cingulate area 28, in addition to motor prefrontal areas 9, 10, 11, and 12. (Modified from Walker, E.A.: J. Comp. Neurol. 73:81, 1940, Wiley.)

ongoing behavior. This may be verbal, visual, or central executive. The concept of working memory is best demonstrated in the delayed response test in the monkey. Bilateral removal of prefrontal areas in monkeys and chimpanzees produced significant effects on two separate aspects of behavior: (1) delayed response and delayed alternation response; and (2) emotional responses, particularly aggression (Jacobsen, 1935). In the delayed response test, the hungry test subject observes food placed under one of two containers. A solid opaque screen is then interposed and after a delay of at least 5 seconds, the screen is raised—allowing the animal to select the appropriate container. Normal primates rapidly learn this task and a more complex task of delayed spatial alternation in which the choices must be alternated between the left and right containers. Both tasks, however, are difficult for the lesioned animal to perform if delays are imposed. Subsequent studies have demonstrated that a relatively small lesion around the middle one-third of the principal sulcus is sufficient to produce the deficit. Although Jacobsen initially attributed the disorder to a general deficit in short-term memory, subsequent studies have indicated that this is not necessarily the case, since such animals can learn discriminations involving the selection of a specific object from among several presented. When appropriate tests are selected, similar deficits can be demonstrated in humans. In the human, the digit span test utilizes working memory.

Additional studies have defined three sectors of the dorsal subdivision, which are concerned with different aspects of working memory and motor planning. These areas may be specified based on their relationship to the principal sulcus in the monkey dorsolateral prefrontal cortex (Fig. 18.20).

The *area surrounding the principal sulcus* contains neurons that begin to fire as the initial visual cue of food is presented in a particular position in the contralateral visual field, and continue to fire during the delay period. Lesions in the area of the principal sulcus will interfere with delayed response.

Neurons in the *cortex ventral to the principal sulcus* code information about what the object is in terms of shape and color. This area receives information via a ventral pathway from the visual cortex involving the inferior temporal lobe.

The *cortex dorsal to the principal sulcus* codes information regarding the location of the object. This area receives visual information via the posterior parietal area adjacent to the extrastriate cortex, as discussed earlier.

There are other neurons that respond to both types of stimulus information.

In the human, aspects of prefrontal function are tested with a variety of tests. These include more complex forms of the delayed response and delayed alternation tests. The Luria motor sequences can be easily utilized in the office: the patient must reproduce a demonstrated sequence of hand movements (strike the thigh with the open hand, then with the ulnar aspect of the open hand, and then with the ulnar aspect of the closed fist). In the Wisconsin Card Sorting test, the patient must sort 60 cards based on color, symbol, or number of symbols. By changing the rules once the patient has developed a pattern set, it is possible to also determine how readily set can be changed. Failure to change set is termed *rigidity*.

Fletcher and Henson have summarized PET scan and functional MRI studies, which suggest a role for lateral prefrontal areas both in working memory and long-term memory. Activation of the ventrolateral region (inferior to the inferior frontal sulcus) has been correlated with the updating and maintenance of information. Activation of the dorsolateral region (dorsal to the inferior frontal sulcus) has been correlated with the selection/manipulation/monitoring of that information. Activation of the anterior prefrontal cortex (anterior to a line drawn vertically from the anterior edge of the inferior frontal sulcus) has been correlated with the selection of processes/subgoals.

DISORDERS OF MOTOR DEVELOPMENT

Nonprogressive disorders of motor function or control recognized at birth or shortly after birth are referred to as cerebral palsy. Little, in 1862, first described "spastic rigidity." He was describing the most common form of cerebral palsy: spastic diplegia: severe bilateral spastic involvement of the lower extremities or a double hemiplegia. Other types of spastic cerebral palsy include quadriplegia and infantile hemiplegia.

In addition to the spastic varieties of cerebral palsy, other types have been identified: (a) double athetosis, (b) ataxic, and (c) dystonic.

As reviewed by Paneth (1986), cerebral palsy affects at least 1 of 500 school-aged children. More severely affected patients may die in infancy. Severely affected children may have subnormal intelligence (50%) and seizure disorders (25%).

Little related the motor deficits to the circumstances of birth: premature delivery, breech presentations, or prolonged labor. Often respiration was impaired at birth. Convulsions often occurred in the neonatal period. Little's hypothesis regarding causation has had serious medical and legal implications for the practice of obstetrics.

Sigmund Freud (1897) prior to his investigations into hysteria and the psychoneuroses undertook detailed clinical and neuropathological studies of these developmental motor syndromes. Freud unified the various disorders into a single syndrome and proposed the classification, which is presented earlier. He also proposed that the abnormalities of the birth process, noted by Little, were in actuality the consequence and not the cause of the perinatal pathology.

The National Collaborative Perinatal Project followed 54,000 pregnancies and the subsequent offspring to age 7. The conclusions of that study (Nelson and Ellenberg, 1986) tend to support Freud's hypothesis. Major prenatal malformations such as microcephaly and prenatal rubella infection were more common in the 189 children with cerebral palsy. Maternal mental retardation and low birth weight below 2000 grams were also significant predictors of cerebral palsy as was breech presentation but not breech delivery. In contrast, birth asphyxia did not add predictive power in the analysis.

GAIT DISORDERS OF THE ELDERLY

The older patient is frequently at risk for progressive disability in two areas of neurological function: (a) motor function, primarily manifested by disturbance of stance and gait, and (b) higher cortical functions of cognition and memory manifested by dementia. (The latter problem will be considered in Chapter 30.) These major problems of geriatrics—both alone or in combination directly and indirectly—account for many of the prolonged admissions to acute care hospitals and constitute the major reason for eventual placement of the elderly patient in chronic care facilities such as nursing homes. The cost impact on the health care system is massive because of the increasing age of the population and because of the frequency of the disorders.

Sudarsky (1990) discusses the several studies that indicate (a) 15% of patients over the age of 60 years have some abnormality of gait; (b) 200,000 hip fractures occur annually in the United States—most due to falls by older individuals; (c) accidental death is the sixth leading cause of death among the elderly—with the majority of these deaths the results of falls; (d) 40%–50% of patients in nursing homes have difficulty with walking; and (e) surveys of older patients (of average age 78 years) indicate a considerable fear of falling and insecurity of gait resulting in a self-imposed limitation of activities in 50%. (Tinettei and Speechley [1989] estimate the annual incidence of falls in the community: 25% at age 70 and 35% after age 75 years. For institutionalized patients fall incidence is 50%.)

Not all falls and not all gait disorders are related solely to neurological disorders. Joint and skeletal disorders may impair gait and result in falls. Age-related changes in vision, hearing, and vestibular function may all impair gait and postural stability. In terms of the nervous system, changes in the peripheral nervous system—those related to aging and to such disorders as diabetes mellitus, and nutrition may all result in impaired proprioception with resultant changes in balance and gait. The deficits are compounded by concurrent changes in vision, hearing, and vestibular dysfunction (see also Tinetti et al., 1988). It is the frequent central nervous system changes resulting in falls which concern us here. Sixteen percent of these patients have a cervical myelopathy, 10% Parkinson's disease, and 20% a frontal gait disorder due to normal pressure hydrocephalus, multiple strokes, or involvement of white matter (leukoaraiosis or Binswanger's disease; Thompson and Marsden, 1987). Cerebellar degeneration occurs in 8%, sensory imbalance in 18%, and toxic metabolic in 6%.

An example of a treatable cause, normal pressure hydrocephalus (NPH), will be found in case history 18.3 and Figures 18.21 and 18.22 presented on CD-ROM. These patients present with a triad of gait impairment (apraxia or ataxia), urinary incontinence, and dementia. The gait impairment usually predates and is more severe than the disorder of memory. In normal pressure hydrocephalus, a block is present in the subarachnoid space high over the convexity so that absorption of cerebrospinal fluid (CSF) fails to occur. In such cases, there is no obstruction to CSF flow within the ventricular system or within the CSF cisterns at the base of the brain. Such cases may be secondary (previous head traumatic or subarachnoid hemorrhage with the late effects of blood within the subarachnoid space) or primary, no prior history. The designation of "normal pressure" refers to the measurement of CSF pressure at lumbar puncture in those cases. Classically, removal of 20–30 cc of CSF produces a remarkable improvement. Not all cases of hydrocephalus in the elderly are of the "normal pressure" communicating variety. In some cases, also presenting with a similar gait disorder, there is a long-standing obstructive hydrocephalus, secondary to stenosis of the aqueduct of Sylvius, which was well compensated earlier in life but has become symptomatic late in life. Rarely, a pineal region tumor or midline cerebellar tumor may produce obstructive hydrocephalus in the elderly. For additional discussion of NPH, refer to Adams et al. (1965) and Fisher (1982).

MAJOR VOLUNTARY MOTOR PATHWAYS

In the older literature the motor pathways were divided into pyramidal (corticospinal and corticonuclear) and extrapyramidal (rubrospinal, tectospinal, and so on). These terms are no longer used, and each pathway is now usually described in terms of its function.

BASIC PRINCIPALS OF MOTOR SYSTEM

1. The descending volitional motor system consists of two portions: an upper and lower motor neuron. The portion originating in the gray matter of the motor sensory strip of the cerebral cortex is called upper motor neurons. The pathway from the upper motor neurons, corticospinal or corticonuclear, descends and crosses over to innervate the lower motor neurons in the brain stem or spinal cord.

   The axons of the upper motor neurons either synapse on interneurons or end directly on the lower motor neurons. The axons of the lower motor neurons leave the central nervous system and form the motor division of the peripheral nervous system.

2. Lower motor neuron lesions of motor cranial nerves and ventral horn cells. A lesion of the motor nucleus or rootlet produces a lower motor neuron syndrome with paralysis, muscle atrophy, and decreased reflexes. Supranuclear lesions produce upper motor neuron symptoms. Associated with bilateral lesions of the corticonuclear system is pseudobulbar palsy with bilateral upper motor neuron signs and inappropriate behavioral. This probably represents the release of cortical control via the corticonuclear innervation of the muscles controlled by the cranial nerves. Limbic control to these nuclei takes over, via descending autonomic pathways, and the emotional state is undamped by the frontal lobes.

CEREBRAL CORTICAL PATHWAYS TO LOWER MOTOR NEURONS IN THE SPINAL CORD

Corticospinal Tract: Voluntary Control of the Limbs, Thorax, and Abdomen

This tract innervates the motor neurons that control the skeletal muscles in the neck, thorax, abdomen, pelvis, and the extremities (see Fig. 18.21). It is essential for accurate voluntary movements and is the only direct tract from the cortex to the spinal motor neurons.

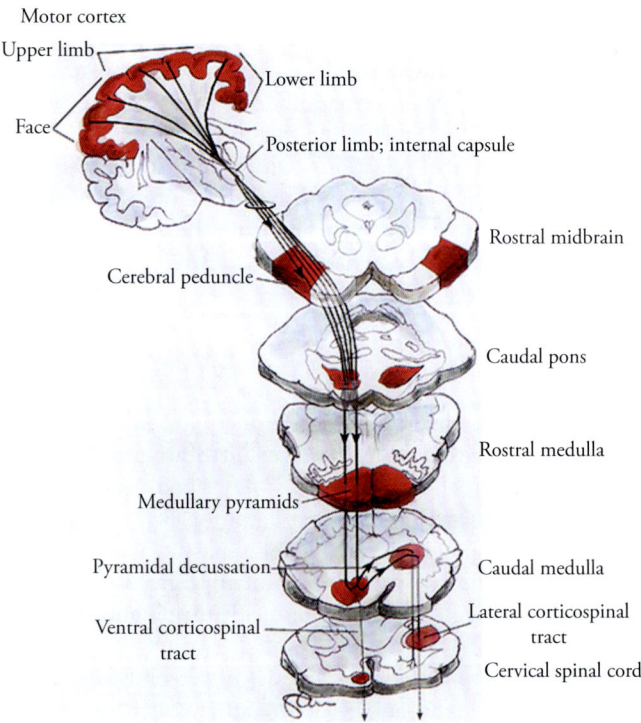

Figure 18.21 Corticospinal pathway: voluntary movement of the muscles in the upper and lower extremities, thorax, and abdomen. This system originates from the pyramidal cells and giant cells of Betz in the upper two-thirds of the precentral gyrus, area 4, and to a lesser degree from area 6 and parts of the frontal, parietal, temporal, and cingulate cortices. The fibers pass through the genu of the internal capsule into the middle third of the cerebral peduncles and enter the pons, where they are broken into many fascicles and are covered by pontine gray and white matter. In the medulla, the fibers are again united and are found on the anterior medial surface of the brain stem in the medullary pyramids.

About 75% to 90% of the corticospinal tract fibers cross at the medullospinal junction and are thereafter found in the lateral funiculus of the spinal cord. (The majority of fibers from the dominant hemisphere cross at the medullospinal junction.) Some corticospinal fibers remain uncrossed in the anterior funiculus but will slowly cross at cervical levels. About 50% of the corticospinal fibers end at the cervical levels, about 30% go to the lumbosacral levels, and the remainder goes to the thoracic levels. Most of the corticospinal fibers end on internuncial neurons in laminae 7 and 8 of the spinal cord, but in regions in the spinal cord where the digits are represented (in the cervical and lumbosacral enlargements) the corticospinal fibers sometimes end directly on the motor horn cells. The internuncial neurons are located in lamina 7 of the spinal cord. Lesions in the corticospinal tract produce contralateral upper motor neuron symptoms, while lesions in the spinal motor neurons or rootlets cause lower motor neuron symptoms.

CEREBRAL CORTICAL PATHWAYS TO LOWER MOTOR NEURONS IN THE BRAIN STEM

Corticonuclear System—Voluntary Control of the Muscles Controlled by Cranial Nerves V, VII, and IX to XII

This system distributes to the motor nuclei of the cranial nerves V, VII, IX, X, XI, and XII and provides voluntary and involuntary control of the muscles and glands innervated by these nerves (Fig. 18.22). In the older literature this pathway was called corticobulbar because the medulla and pons containing these nuclei are collectively called the bulb. We prefer the term *corticonuclear* because it makes the student realize the key role of the cranial nerve nuclei in movement. These fibers are found anterior to the corticospinal fibers in the genu of the internal capsule and medial to the corticospinal tract in the cerebral peduncle, pons, and medullary pyramids. With the exception of the lower facial muscles, which are innervated by the contralateral cortex and the innervation to the tongue which is primarily ipsilateral, this is a bilateral system. Consequently, unilateral lesions in the corticonuclear system produce only weakness and not paralysis. Paralysis results only from bilateral lesions in the corticonuclear system.

The fibers supplying the cranial nerves have the following cortical origin:

a. Muscles of facial expression (motor nerve VII), mastication (motor nerve V), and deglutition (ambiguous nuclei of nerves IX and X) originate from pyramidal cells in the inferior part of the precentral gyrus, area 4.

b. Muscles in the larynx are controlled from the inferior frontal gyrus and from the frontal operculum (the posterior part of the pars triangularis, area 44). It appears that many corticonuclear axons end on interneurons and not directly on the motor neuron of the cranial nerve.

Corticomesencephalic System—Voluntary Control of Eye Movements: Cranial Nerves III, IV, and VI

(See also Chapter 12.) The fibers controlling eye movements originate from the frontal eye fields in the caudal part of the middle frontal gyrus and the adjacent inferior frontal gyrus (area 8). At upper midbrain levels, fibers to cranial nerves III and IV leave the cerebral peduncles and take a descending path through the tegmentum, usually in the medial lemniscus (corticomesencephalic tract). Fibers to cranial nerve VI also descend in this way to the parabducens and parapontine reticular nuclei of the pons, which coordinate movements under the control of cranial nerves III and VI ascending through the medial longitudinal fasciculus.

Corticomesencephalic pathway controls the cranial nerves (III, IV, and VI that move the muscles) of the eyes. Table 15.5 lists the major sensory and motor pathways in the human central nervous system.

BIBLIOGRAPHY

PART I: REFLEX ORGANIZATION, THE PYRAMIDAL TRACT DEVELOPMENT, AND GAIT DISORDERS OF THE ELDERLY

(PART II: CORTICAL LOCALIZATION FOR THE MOTOR AREAS WILL BE FOUND IN THE MASTER CORTICAL LOCALIZATION BIBLIOGRAPHY)

GENERAL

Alexander, G. E., and Delong, M. R. 1992. Central mechanisms of initiation and control of movements. In A. K. Asbury et al. (Eds.) Diseases of the Nervous System, pp. 285–308. Philadelphia, PA: W. B. Saunders.

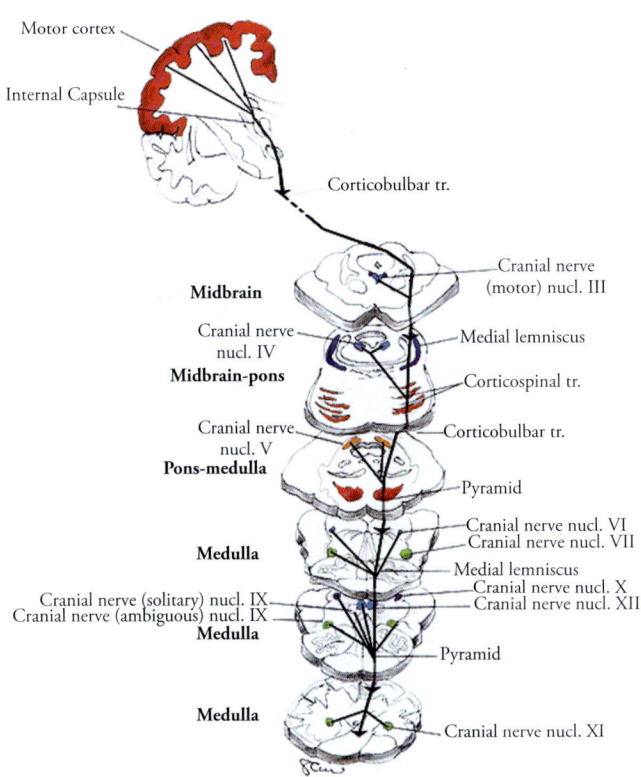

Figure 18.22 Corticobulbar/corticonuclear pathway: voluntary movements of the muscles associated with cranial nerves V, VII, IX, X, XI, and XII.

Carew, T. J., and Kelley, D. B. 1989. Perspectives in Neural Systems and Behavior. MBL Lectures in Biology 10. New York, NY: Alan Liss.

Denny-Brown, D. 1960. Motor mechanisms: introduction, the general principles of motor integration. In Handbook of Physiology, Section 1. Neurophysiology, pp. 781–796. Washington, DC: American Physiologic Society.

Denny-Brown, D. 1966. The Cerebral Control of Movement. Springfield, IL: Charles C. Thomas.

Desmedt, J. E. (Ed.). 1983. Motor Control Mechanisms in Health and Disease. New York, NY: Raven Press.

Fulton, J. F. 1951. Physiology of the Nervous System. 3rd ed. New York, NY: Oxford University Press.

Ghez, C. 1991. The Control of Movement. In E. R. Kandel, J. H. Schwartz, and T. M. Jessell (Eds.) Principles of Neural Science. 3rd ed., pp.553–547. New York, NY: Elsevier.

Humphrey, D. R., and Freund, H. J. 1991. Motor Control Concepts and Issues. New York, NY: John Wiley and Sons.

Klemm, W. R., and Vertes, R. P. (Eds.). 1990. Brain Stem Mechanisms of Behavior. New York, NY: Wiley Interscience.

Lance, J. W., and McLeod, J. G. 1981. A Physiological Approach to Clinical Neurology. 3rd ed., London, UK: Butterworths. (Chapter 4: Spinal Reflexes, pp.73–100, Chapter 5: Muscle Tone and Movement, pp.101–127, Chapter 6–Disordered Muscle Tone, pp.28–152)

Ruch, T. C., and Patton, H. D. (Eds.). 1965. Physiology and Biophysics. Philadelphia, PA: W. B. Saunders. (Chapters 6 and 7: Spinal Reflexes and Synaptic Transmission, pp.153–180, 181–206, Chapter 8: Transection of the Spinal Cord, pp. 207–214, Chapter 9: Pontobulbar Control of Posture and Orientation in Space, pp. 215–225)

Sherrington, C. 1947. The Integrative Action of the Nervous System. New Have, CT: Yale University Press.

Willis, W. D., and Grossman, R. G. 1981. Medical Neurobiology: Neuroanatomical and Neurophysiological Principles of Basic Clinical Neuroscience. 3rd ed. St. Louis, MO: C. V. Mosby. (Chapter 8: Motor Systems, pp. 347–402.)

CITATIONS

Bizzi, E., and Evarts, E. V. 1971. Translational mechanisms between input and output. Neurosci. Res. Prog. Bull. 9:31–59.

Burke, R. E. 1971. Control systems operating on spinal reflex mechanisms. Neurosci. Res. Prog. Bull. 9:60–85.

Delong, M. 1971. Central patterning of movement. Neurosci. Res. Prog. Bull. 9:10–30.

Grillner, S., and Wallen, P. 1985. Control pattern generators for locomotion with special reference to vertebrates. Ann. Rev. Neurosci. 8:233–261.

Harris-Warrick, P. M., and Johnson, B. R. 1989. Motor pattern networks: flexible foundations for rhythmic pattern production. In T. J. Carew and D. B. Kelley (Eds.) *Perspectives in* Neural Systems and Behavior. MBL Lectures in Biology, Vol. 10., pp. 51–71. New York, NY: Alan R. Liss.

Nudo, R. J., Wise, B. M., SiFuentes, F., Milliken, G. W. 1996. Neural substrates for the effects of rehabilitative training on motor recovery after ischemic infarct. Science 272:1791–1794.

Stein, P. S. G. 1978. Motor systems with specific reference to the control of locomotion. Ann. Rev. Neurosci. 1:61–81.

SPINAL CORD (INCLUDES SPASTICITY) (SEE ALSO CHAPTER 9)

Dimitrijevic, M. R., Faganel, J., Lehmkuhl, D., and Sherwood, A. 1983. Motor Control in Man After Partial or Complete Spinal Cord Injury. In E. Desmedt (Ed.) Motor Control Mechanisms in Health and Disease, pp.915–926. New York, NY: Raven Press.

Granit, R., and Kaada, B. R. 1952. Influence of stimulation of central nervous structures on muscle spindle in cat. Acta Physiol. Scan. 27:130–160.

Hutlborn, H., and Illert, M. 1991. How is motor behavior reflected in the organization of spinal systems?. In D. R. Humphrey & H. J. Freund (Eds.) Motor Control: Concepts and Issues, pp.49–73. New York, NY: John Wiley and Sons.

Young, R. R. 1989. Treatment of spastic paresis (Editorial). N. Engl. J. Med. 320:1517–1525.

BRAIN STEM (SEE ALSO CHAPTERS 15 AND 16)

Denny-Brown, D. 1962. The midbrain and motor Integration (Sherrington Memorial Lecture) Proc. Roy. Soc. Med. 55:527–538.

Klemm, W. R. 1990. Historical and introductory perspectives on brain stem mediated behavior. In W. R. Klemm and R. P. Vertes (Eds.) Brain Stem Mechanisms of Behavior, pp. 3–32. New York, NY: Wiley.

Magoun, H. W., and Rhines, R. 1946. An inhibitory mechanism in the bulbar reticular formation. J. Neurophysiol. 9:161–171.

McCulloch, W. S., Graf, C., and Magoun, H. W. 1946. A cortical bulbar reticular pathway from area 4S. J. Neurophysiol. 9:127–132.

Morgenson, G. J. 1990. Brainstem systems for the control of behavioral acts. In W. R. Klemm and R. P. Vertes (Eds.) Brain Stem Mechanisms of Behavior, pp. 171–195. New York, NY: Wiley.

Peterson, B. W. 1979. Reticulospinal projections to spinal motor nuclei. Ann. Rev. Physiol. 41:127–140.

Twitchell, T. E. 1965. Attitudinal reflexes. J. Amer. Phys. Ther. Assn. 45:411–418.

CEREBRAL CORTEX (SEE ALSO CORTICAL LOCALIZATION REFERENCES)

Alexander, G. E., DeLong, M. R., and Strick, D. L. 1986. Parallel organization of functionally segregated circuits linking basal ganglia and cortex. Ann. Rev. Neurosci. 9:357–381.

Andersen, R. A., Snyder, L. H., Bradley, D. C., and Xing, J. 1997. Multimodal representation of space in the posterior parietal cortex and its use in planning movements. Ann. Rev. Neurosci. 20: 393–330.

Colby, C. L., and Goldberg, M. E. 1999. Space and attention in parietal cortex. Ann. Rev. Neurosci. 22:319–351.

Decke, L. Bereitschaft potential as an indicator of movement preparation in Supplementary motor area and motor cortex. In Ciba Foundation Symposium 132. Motor Areas of the Cerebral Cortex, pp. 231–250. Chichester, UK: Wiley.

DeRenzi, E., and Barbieri, C. 1992. The incidence of the grasp reflex following hemispheric lesions and its relation to frontal damage. Brain 115:293–313.

Dum, R. P., and Strick, P. L. 1991. Premotor areas: nodal points for parallel efferent systems involved in the central control of movement. In D. R. Humphrey and H. J. Freund (Eds.) Motor Control: Concepts and Issues, pp. 383–397. New York, NY: John Wiley & Sons.

Georgopoulos, A. P. 1991. Higher motor control. Ann. Rev. Neurosci. 14: 361–377

Gilman, S., Lieberman, J. S., and Marco, L. A. 1974. Spinal mechanisms underlying the effects of unilateral ablation of areas 4 & 6 in the monkey. Brain 97:49–64.

Graziano, M. S. A., Yap, G. S., and Gross, C. G. 1994. Coding of visual space by premotor neurons. Science 266:1054–1056.

Humphrey, D. R., and Tanji, J. 1991. What features of voluntary motor control are encoded in the neuronal discharge of different cortical motor areas? In D. R. Humphrey and H. J. Freund (Eds.) Motor Control Concepts and Issues, pp. 413–443. New York, NY: John Wiley and Sons.

Kalaska, J. F., and Crammond, D. J. 1992. Cerebral cortical mechanisms of reaching. Science 255:1517–1523.

Magnani, G., Mazzucchi, A., Dolett, A., et al. 1987. Involuntary grasping and groping responses to space related visual stimuli. Mov. Disord. 1:9–24.

Papa, S. M., Artieda, J., and Obeso, J. A. 1991. Cortical activity preceding self initiated and externally triggered voluntary movement. Mov. Disord. 6:217–224.

Passingham, R. E. 1987. Two cortical systems for directing movements. In CIBA Foundation Symposium 132. Motor Areas of the Cerebral Cortex, pp. 151–164. New York, NY: John Wiley & Sons.

Phillips, C. G., and Porter, R. 1977. Corticospinal Neurons: Their Role in Movement. London, UK: Academic Press.

Rushworth, G., and Denny-Brown, D. 1959. The two components of the grasp reflex after ablation of frontal cortex in monkeys. J. Neurol. Neurosurg. Psychiatry 22:91–98.

Sanes, J. N., Donoghue, J. P., Thangaraj, V., et al. 1995. Shared neural substrates controlling hand movements in human motor cortex. Science 268:1775–1777.

Seyffarth, H., and Denny-Brown, D. 1948. The grasp reflex and the instinctive grasp reaction. Brain 71:109–183.

Twitchell, T. E. 1951. The restoration of motor function following hemiplegia in man. Brain 74:443–480.

Twitchell, T. E. 1958. The grasping deficit in infantile spastic hemiparesis. Neurology 8:13–21.

Twitchell, T. E. 1965. The automatic grasping responses of infants. Neuropsychologia 3:247–259.

Weisendanger, M., Hummelshein, H., Bianchetti, M., et al. 1987. Input and output organization of Supplementary motor area. In CIBA Foundation Symposium 132. Motor Areas of the Cerebral Cortex, pp. 40–62. New York, NY: John Wiley & Sons.

Wise, S. P. 1985. The primate premotor cortex: past, present and preparatory. Ann. Rev. Neurosci. 8:1–19.

Wise, S. P., Boussaoud, D., Johnson, P. B., and Caminiti, R. 1997. Premotor and parietal cortex: corticocortical connectivity and combinational computations. Ann. Rev. Neurosci. 20:25–42.

RECOVERY FROM CEREBRAL LESIONS AND PLASTICITY OF CORTEX

Buonomano, D. V., and Merzenich, M. M. 1998. Cortical plasticity: from synapses to maps. Ann. Rev. Neurosci. 21:149–186.

Freund, H. J. 1991. What is the evidence for multiple motor areas in the human brain. In D. R. Humphrey and H. J. Freund (Eds.) *Motor Control: Concepts and Issues*, pp. 399–411. New York, NY: John Wiley & Sons.

Jacobs, K. M., and Donoghue, J. P. 1991. Reshaping the cortical motor map by unmasking latent intracortical functions. Science 251:944–947.

Kaas, J. H. 1991. Plasticity of sensory and motor maps in adult mammals. Ann. Rev. Neurosci. 14:137–67.

Pantano, P., Formisano, R., Ricci, M., et al. 1995. Prolonged muscular flaccidity after stroke. Morphological and functional brain alterations. Brain 118:1329–1338.

Sanes, J. N., and Donoghue, J. P. 2000. Plasyicity and primary motor cortex. Ann. Rev. Neurosci. 23:393–416.

Twitchell, T. E. 1951. The restoration of motor function following hemiplegia in man. Brain 74:443–480.

Warabi, T., Inove, K., Noda, H., and Murakam, S. 1990. Recovery of voluntary movement in hemiplegic patients: correlation with degenerative shrinkage of the cerebral peduncle in CT images. Brain 113:177–189.

Weiller, C., Chollet, F., Friston, K. J., et al. 1992. Functional reorganization of the brain in recovery from striatocapsular infarction in man. Annal. Neurol. 31:463–472.

THE PYRAMIDAL TRACT AND OTHER DESCENDING MOTOR SYSTEMS

Bucy, P. C., Ladpli, R., and Ehrlich, A. 1966. Destruction of the pyramidal tract in the monkey. J. Neurophysiol. 25:1–20.

Jagiella, W. M., and Sung, J. H. 1989. Bilateral infarction of the medullary pyramids in humans. Neurology 39:21–24.

Kuypers, H. G. J. M. 1987. Some aspects of the organization of the output of the motor cortex. In G. Bock, M. O'Connor, and J. Marsh (Eds.) CIBA Foundation Symposium 132. Motor Areas of the Cerebral Cortex, pp.63–82. New York, NY: John Wiley & Sons.

Lawrence, D. G., and Kuypers, H. G. J. M. 1968. The functional organization of the motor system in the monkey. I. The effects of bilateral pyramidal lesions. Brain 91:1–14.

Nathan, P. W., Smith, M., and Deacon, P. 1996. Vestibulospinal, reticulospinal and descending propriospinal nerve fibres in man. 119:1809–1833.

Nathan, P. W., and Smith, M. C. 1982. The rubrospinal and central tegmental tracts in man. Brain 105:223–269.

Schwartzman, R. J. 1978. A behavioral analysis of complete unilateral section of the pyramidal tract at the medullary level in Macaca mulatta. Ann. Neurol. 4:234–244.

Wall, P. D. 1970. The sensory and motor role of impulses traveling in the dorsal columns towards cerebral cortex. Brain 95:503–524.

THE CENTRAL CONTROL OF EYE MOVEMENT BY CEREBRAL CORTEX (See also cerebral cortex and cortical localization)

Goldberg, M. 2000. The control of gaze. In E. R. Kandel, J. H. Schwartz, and T. M. Jessell (Ed.) Principles of Neural Science. 4th ed, pp.782–800. New York, NY: McGraw Hill.

Morrow, M. J. and Sharpe, J. A. 1993. Retinotopic and directional deficits of smooth pursuit initiation after posterior cerebral hemispheric lesions. J. Neurol. 43:595–603.

POSTNATAL DEVELOPMENT AND DISORDERS OF DEVELOPMENT

Adams, R. D., and Victor, M. 1993. Principles of Neurology. Seventh Editon Mc Graw Hill. (Chapter 28: Normal development and deviations in development of the nervous system, pp. 493–525)

Bodensteiner, J. G. 1992. Plantar responses in infants. J. Child. Neurol. 7:311–313.

Freud, S. 1968. Infantile Cerebral Paralysis (L. A. Russin, Trans.). Coral Gables, FL: University Miami Press. (1897 Original Date of Publication)

Gesell, A., and Amatruda, C. S. 1954. Developmental Diagnosis: Normal and Abnormal Child Development. 2nd ed. New York, NY: Hoeber Harper.

Little, W. J. 1862. On the influence of abnormal parturition, difficult labours, premature birth and asphyxia neonatorum with mental and physical conditions of the child especially in relation to deformities. Trans. Obstetrical. Soc. London 3:293–344.

Myers, G. J., and NcBride, M. C. 1993. Clinical neurological examination of the preterm and term neonate. Semin. Neurol. 13:1–9.

Nelson, K. B., and Ellenberg, J. H. 1986. Antecedents of cerebral palsy: multivariate analysis of risk. N. Engl. J. Med. 315:81–86.

Paneth, N. 1986. Birth and the origins of cerebral palsy (Editorial). N. Engl. J. Med. 315:124–126.

Wolff, P. H., and Ferber, R. 1979. The development of behavior in human infants, premature and newborn. Ann. Rev. Neurosci. 2: 291–307.

Yakolev, P. I., and LeCours, A. R. 1967. The myelogenetic cycles of normal development of the brain. In A. R. Minkowski (Ed.) Regional Development of the Brain in Early Life, pp. 3–70. Oxford, UK: Blackwell.

GAIT DISORDERS OF THE ELDERLY

Adams, R. D., Fisher, C. M., Hakim, S., et al. 1965. Symptomatic occult hydrocephalus with "normal" cerebrospinal fluid pressure: a treatable syndrome. N. Engl. J. Med. 273:117–126.

Fisher, C. M. 1982. Hydrocephalus as a cause of disturbances of gait in the elderly. Neurology 32:1358–1363.

Fishman, R. A. 1985. Normal pressure hydrocephalus and arthritis (Editorial). N. Engl. J. Med. 312:1255–1256.

Hachinski, V. C., Potter, P., and Merskey, H. 1987. Leuko-araiosis. Arch. Neurol. 44:21–23.

Inzitar, D., Diaz, F., Fox, A., et al. 1987. Vascular risk factors and leuko-araiosis Arch. Neurol. 44:42–47.

Jacobs, L., Conti, D., Kinkel, W. R., and Manning, E. J. 1976. "Normal pressure" hydrocephalus: relationship of clinical and radiographic findings to improvement following shunt surgery. JAMA. 235:510–512.

Masdeu, J. C., Wolfson, L., and Lantos, G., et al. 1989. Brain white matter changes in the elderly prone to falling. Arch. Neurol. 46:1292–1296.

Rasker, J. J., Jansen, E. N. H., Haan, J., and Oostrom, J. 1985. Normal pressure hydrocephalus in rheumatic patients: a diagnostic pitfall. N. Engl. J. Med. 312:1239–1241.

Steingart, A., Hackinski, V. C., Lau, C., et al. 1987. Cognitive and neurological findings in subjects with diffuse white matter changes on computed topographic scan (leukoariosis). Arch. Neurol. 44:32–34.

Sudarsky, L. 1990. Current concepts—geriatrics: gait disorders in the elderly. N. Engl. J. Med. 322:1441–1446.

Sudarsky, L., and Ronthal, M. 1983. Gait disorders among elderly patients: a survey study of 50 patients. Arch. Neurol. 40:740–743.

Thompson, P. D., and Marsden, C. D. 1987. Gait disorder of subcortical arteriosclerotic encephalopathy: Binswanger's disease. Mov. Disord. 2:1–8.

Tinetti, M. D., and Speechly, M. 1989. Current concepts: geriatrics: prevention of falls among the elderly. N. Engl. J. Med. 320:1055–1059.

Tinetti, M. D., Speechly, M., and Ginter, S. F. 1988. Risk factors for falls among elderly persons living in the community. N. Engl. J. Med. 319:1701–1707.

19.

MOTOR SYSTEMS

PART II: BASAL GANGLIA AND MOVEMENT DISORDERS

ANATOMICAL BACKGROUND

The term "basal ganglia" originally included the deep telencephalic nuclei, caudate, putamen, globus pallidus, claustrum, and nucleus accumbens. The globus pallidus and putamen are lens shaped and are called *lenticular nuclei*. Collectively, the putamen and caudate are called the *corpus striatum*. Additional structures now included within this group are the substantia nigra, the subthalamic nuclei, the ventral tegmental area, and the ventral pallidum. The caudate and putamen have the same structure and are continuous anteriorly. The globus pallidus has two sectors: a medial or inner, and a lateral or outer. The substantia nigra has two components: a ventral pars reticularis, which is identical in structure and function to the medial sector of the globus pallidus, and a dorsal darkly staining component, the pars compacta, which contains large dopamine- and melanin-containing neurons.

The nuclei of the basal ganglia may be categorized as (1) *input nuclei* (caudate, putamen, and accumbens); (2) *intrinsic nuclei* (lateral segment of the globus pallidus, subthalamic nucleus, pars compacta of the substantia nigra, and the ventral tegmental area); and (3) *output nuclei* (medial segment of the globus pallidus, pars reticularis of the substantia nigra, and the ventral pallium). The consideration of the chemical and pharmacological anatomy of transmitters and circuits within the system will provide an understanding of function and dysfunction within this system.

It should be noted that the nuclei of the basal ganglia, the circuits involving the basal ganglia, the cortical areas projecting to the basal ganglia, the cerebellar nuclei relating to the basal ganglia, and the reticular formation (which has connections with both the cortex and the basal ganglia) were once grouped together as an extrapyramidal system. The term "extrapyramidal disorders"—was used to refer to the effects of lesions within the basal ganglia system. However, the term "extrapyramidal" was also utilized to refer to the descending pathways: corticorubral spinal and cortical-reticulospinal that were alternative descending systems to the pyramidal system. The term *extrapyramidal* then becomes very nonspecific and confusing and had best not be utilized. It is important to note, moreover, that the cortical areas giving rise to this extrapyramidal system are also, in part, the same areas giving rise to the pyramidal system.

Additional discussions of the gross anatomy will be found in Chapters 1, 15, and 17 and in Noback et al. (1991), Alexander et al. (1986), and Young and Penney (1988).

The connections and transmitters within this system are presented in Figure 19.1 and are summarized as follows.

The essential pathways are the following: cerebral cortex (+) to striatum (caudate/putamen) (−) to globus pallidus (−) to ventrolateral thalamus (+) to cerebral cortex. Additional circuits involve subthalamus and substantia nigra.

Adding greater detail to the outline indicates the following sequence:

1. *The major input into the basal ganglia is from the cerebral cortex to the striatum (caudate nucleus/putamen/accumbens).* This input is excitatory—utilizing the transmitter glutamate and arises primarily from the supplementary motor premotor and motor cortices (areas 8, 6, and 4). However, the projection from the neocortex occurs from many other areas. In general, frontal and parietal, lateral temporal, and occipital areas project to the caudate nucleus; supplementary motor, premotor and motor primary cortex, and primary somatosensory cortex project to the putamen. The hippocampal areas, medial and lateral temporal, project to the nucleus accumbens. Alexander, Delong, and Strick (1986) have distinguished the following segregated basal ganglia-thalamocortical circuits based on the origin of the initial cortical input: (1) motor, (2) oculomotor, (3) prefrontal, (4) orbital frontal, and (5) cingulate-limbic. These are outlined in Table 19.2.

2. There are local circuits within the striatum, which involve the excitatory transmitter acetylcholine.

3. *The striatum also receives a major dopaminergic input from the substantia nigra compacta.* Based on the type of receptor, this input may be either excitatory (D1) or inhibitory (D2). Dopamine receptors have been classified based on the dopamine-mediated effects on the enzyme adenylate cyclase (which is involved in the ATP to cyclic AMP transformation). D2 receptors are involved in the inhibition of the enzyme; D1 receptors in stimulation of the enzyme. Note that five dopamine receptors have now been identified. This complex and still evolving topic has been reviewed by Cooper (1991), Guttman (1992), and Gerfen and Engber (1992).

4. Because of this differential input two pathways have been identified: the direct and the indirect.

5. *The major direct outflow pathway arises from those striatal neurons receiving excitatory dopaminergic input (D1)*

Table 19.1 ANATOMICAL DIVISIONS OF CORPUS STRIATUM

BASAL GANGLIA–TELENCEPHALIC NUCLEI	FUNCTION
NEOSTRIATUM	Input nuclei—neocortical and substantia nigra
Dorsal-caudate/putamen	
Ventral-nucleus accumbens	Nigra compacta
PALEOSTRIATUM (globus pallidus)	Input nucleus limbic system
	Intrinsic nucleus
Dorsal portion:	Output nucleus
Lateral segment	Output nucleus
Medial segment	
Ventral portion	
Ventral pallidum	
Basal Ganglia–Associated Nuclei	
Subthalamic nucleus of diencephalon	Intrinsic nucleus
	Intrinsic nucleus
Substantia nigra of midbrain	Output nucleus
– dorsal- pars compacta (dopaminergic)	
– ventral- pars reticularis	

and passes to the medial globus pallidus—mediated by the inhibitory transmitter gamma aminobutyric acid (GABA). Substance P is also involved as a transmitter or modulator in this pathway. The major outflow is to the inner (medial) segment of the globus pallidus. There is a lesser outflow of fibers from the striatum to the substantia nigra reticularis, which has the same microscopic structure

Figure 19.1 Diagram of the connections of the basal ganglia with transmitters and major transmitter action, (+) excitatory or (−) inhibitory. GABA, gamma aminobutyric acid (−); GLU, glutamate (+); Dopamine, Dopa (+). The action of acetylcholine within the striatum has been omitted. The sites of surgical lesions or of stimulator placement to relieve symptoms of Parkinson's disease are also shown. X1 =medial globus pallidus, X2= ventral lateral nucleus of thalamus, and X3= subthalamic nucleus. See text for details.

as the globus pallidus. *The outflow of the neurons of these structures is to the ventral lateral and ventral anterior thalamic nuclei,* mediated again by the inhibitory transmitter GABA. This outflow passes via two fiber systems: the fasciculus lenticularis and the ansa lenticularis. The fasciculus lenticularis penetrates through the posterior limb of the internal capsule; the ansa lenticularis loops around the undersurface of the most inferior part of the internal capsule and then passes upward to join the fasciculus lenticularis. These two fiber systems join at a point known as the Field H2 of Forel, then curve back toward the thalamus in the Field H1 of Forel, where they are known as the thalamic fasciculus. This fasciculus then enters the ventrolateral and ventral anterior nuclei of the thalamus. *The outflow of these thalamic nuclei is excitatory to the motor areas of the cerebral cortex predominantly to the premotor and supplementary motor areas.*

6. *The indirect outflow pathway arises from those striatal neurons receiving inhibitory dopaminergic input (D2) and passes to the lateral (or external) sector of the globus pallidus* mediated by the inhibitory transmitter GABA. Enkephalin is also involved as a transmitter or modulator in this pathway. *The neurons of the lateral globus pallidus give rise to inhibitory fibers, again utilizing GABA, which connect to the subthalamic nucleus.* This nucleus gives rise to excitatory fibers utilizing glutamate, which provide additional input to the medial (inner) sector of the globus pallidus and the substantia nigra reticularis. *As in the direct pathway, the subsequent connection of these structures is inhibitory to the ventral lateral and ventral anterior nuclei of the thalamus. The subsequent step in the sequence, as in the direct pathway, is excitatory to the motor areas of the cerebral cortex utilizing the transmitter glutamate.* In the case of both the direct and the indirect pathways, a loop has been completed: cerebral cortex to striatum to globus pallidus to ventrolateral and ventral anterior thalamus back to cortical motor areas.

7. In terms of final effect of this system on the thalamus, if one starts the analysis at the striatum, the end result of the direct system on the thalamus is excitatory. Inhibition of inhibitory drive is referred to as disinhibition. In contrast, following through the sequences of the indirect system, one finds that the end result is inhibitory.

If one begins at the substantia nigra compacta and follows through the direct and indirect circuits, it is evident that both have the same end result as regards the final effect at the thalamic and the cortical level.

8. It is then possible to analyze the eventual thalamic and cortical effects of *a decrease in dopaminergic* input at the level of the striatum: the thalamus and cortex will receive less excitation. The results are the same whether the direct or indirect pathway is considered. Movement then will be decreased or slowed down. The terms *akinesia* or *bradykinesia* are employed.

On the other hand, if there is *increased dopaminergic activity,* the end results at the thalamic or cortical level will be an increase in motor activity irrespective of whether the direct

Table 19.2 CEREBRAL CORTEX TO BASAL GANGLIA TO THALAMUS TO CEREBRAL CORTEX CIRCUITS

LOOP SEQUENCE	MOTOR	OCULOMOTOR	PREFRONTAL	ORBITAL	LIMBIC
1A. Major cortical inputs	Area 6/ SMA	Frontal eye field/ area 8	Dorsolateral Prefrontal	Lateral orbital frontal	Anterior cingulate (area 24)
1B. Additional cortical inputs	Areas 4, 6/PMA, 1,2,3, (post central)	Dorsolateral Prefrontal Posterior parietal	Posterior parietal, arcuate/ frontal, PMA	Limbic / anterior cingulate *See* Limbic	Hippocampus, parahippocampal amygdala entorhinal, temporal neocortical
2. Striatum	Putamen	Caudate (body)	Caudate (head)	Caudate (head)	N. accumbens
3. Pallidum/ substantia nigra reticularis	Globus pallidus/ substantia nigra/ reticularis	Globus pallidus (caudal) Dorsomedial Substantia nigra reticularis	Globus pallidus (lat. dorso medial)/substantia nigra reticularis	Globus pallidus (dorsomed)/ substantia nigra reticularis	Ventral pallidum, globus pallidus, (rostral lat.) substantia nigra reticularis
4. Thalamic nuclei	Ventro-lateral (pars oralis/ medialis)	Ventral anterior (magnocellularis) Medial dorsal (parvocellularis)	Medial dorsal (parvocellularis), ventral anterior (parvo cellularis)	Medial dorsal (magnocellularis) Ventral Anterior (parvo cellularis)	Medial dorsal (postmedial)
5. Projection to cortical area	6/SMA	Frontal eye field/ area 8	Dorsolateral prefrontal	Lateral orbital	Anterior cingulate

Source: Modified from Alexander et al., 1986.

or indirect pathway is considered. The terms *hyperkinesia* or *dyskinesia* are employed.

The ultimate effect of dopamine then is to facilitate movement (Bergman et al., 1990; Cote and Crutcher, 1991).

The striatum also has GABA-mediated inhibitory outflow to substantia nigra compacta. Specific sites in the striatum project to the substantia nigra compacta (and receive afferent input from the substantia nigra compacta).[1]

Now let us consider the more complex nature of the microanatomy of the striatum. From a histochemical and histological standpoint, distinct areas may be noted, referred to as patches within the larger background matrix. The patch areas have a high density of neurons; matrix areas are less dense. Patch zones contain little acetylcholine esterase, and matrix areas are rich in acetylcholine esterase. Patch areas are associated with bundles of dopamine fibers early in development. Later in development there are less dense dopaminergic inputs to the matrix (Graybiel and Ragsdale, 1978). Neurons within the striatum may be additionally categorized on the basis of size and morphology of the dendrite and size as (a) medium-sized, spiny neurons or (b) large or small aspiny neurons. The different properties of these regions and neuron types are presented in Table 19.3.

There is considerable evidence that the dopamine-containing terminals and their related synapses and the cholinergic synapses in the striatum have essentially antagonistic actions. Normally, however, they remain in a particular balance. We will discuss the problem of an imbalance when we come to discuss Parkinson's disease (Duvoisin, 1967; Hornykiewicz, 1970). As discussed earlier, both tend to be found in specific sites in striatum (striasomes). These sites exist in a larger matrix of the striatum.

Several additional loops and circuits must now be considered:

1. In addition to its major input from the cerebral cortex, the caudate-putamen also receives a lesser afferent input from the nucleus centrum medianum (CM) (excitatory transmitter presumed to be glutamate or aspartate). It should be noted that the CM represents a major interlaminar nucleus of the thalamus and is the main thalamic extension of the reticular formation. The centrum medianum, however, also receives fibers from the globus pallidus (inhibitory transmitter: GABA). This again completes an additional loop, relating the basal ganglia to the reticular formation.

2. It should also be noted that some fibers leave the ansa lenticularis and, rather than passing into the thalamus, descend to the pedunculopontine nucleus within the tegmentum of the mesencephalon. This nucleus then projects back to the globus pallidus.

3. There is also evidence for a direct excitatory input from motor and premotor areas to the subthalamic nucleus providing an additional circuit for modulating motor activity.

---
[1] A more detailed examination of the striatum in terms of microscopic neuroanatomy and neuropharmacology suggests a much more complex story (Albin et al., 1989; Martingusella, 1986; Wexler et al., 1991).

Table 19.3 **THE COMPLEX NATURE OF THE MICROANATOMY OF THE STRIATUM**

MATRIX REGIONS	PATCH REGIONS

1. Matrix areas form large background regions with a low density of neurons.
2. Receive afferent input from superficial cortical layers and multiple sites (motor, sensory, motor, premotor, frontal, parietal, and occipital) and intralaminar thalamic sites (Young and Penney, 1988).
3. Matrix areas are rich in acetylcholine esterase.
 	
SPINY NEURONS
 	
Spiny neurons in general project outside. The striatum and account for 90% of striatal neurons.
 	
Spiny neurons contain a transmitter and a neuropeptide modulator.
Types of Spiny Neurons:
  a. Spiny matrix neurons containing GABA and the neuropeptide substance P and projecting to medial globus pallidus and substantia nigra pars reticularis.
  b. Spiny, matrix neurons, containing GABA and other neuropeptide: dynorphin projecting to the medial globus pallidus and substantia nigra pars reticularis.
  c. Spiny matrix neurons containing GABA and the neuropeptide enkephalin and projecting to the lateral globus pallidus.
  d. Patch neurons containing GABA and substance P and projecting to the substantia nigra compacta.
	1. The patch areas are smaller and have a high density of neurons.
	2. Patch neurons receive input from deeper cortical layers in prefrontal and limbic cortex.
	3. Patch zones contain little acetylcholine esterase.
	4. Patch neurons contain GABA and substance P and project to the substantia nigra compacta.
	5. Patch neurons receive a dense dopaminergic input from the substantia nigra compacta.
	
	ASPINY NEURONS
	
	Aspiny neurons in general are interneurons, form 10% of the neurons, and are intrinsic to the striatum.
	
	Large aspiny interneurons within the matrix contain the transmitter acetylcholine.
	Small aspiny interneurons within the matrix contain the neuropeptides somatostatin and Y.

OVERVIEW OF THE DOPAMINERGIC SYSTEMS

In addition to the dopaminergic nigral-striatal pathways, which are of major concern in our discussion of motor function, there are other major dopaminergic pathways. These other pathways, however, are of importance when one begins to utilize L-Dopa (the precursor of dopamine) in therapy of Parkinson's disease. In addition, these pathways are of importance when agents (such as neuroleptics employed in the treatment of psychoses or other psychiatric syndromes) are used to block the dopamine receptor or to prevent the storage of dopamine. In addition, the overall disease state in Parkinson's disease may also involve these pathways.

a. *The mesolimbic system*—originating in the ventral tegmental area—medial and superior to the substantia nigra and projecting to the nucleus accumbens (ventral striatum); the stria terminalis septal nuclei; the amygdala; hippocampus; mesal frontal, anterior cingulate; and entorhinal cortex. A major role in emotion, memory, and perception is postulated for this system. Hallucinations are a side effect of a high dose of L-Dopa in the Parkinsonian patient.

b. *The mesocortical system*—originating in the ventral tegmental area and projecting to neocortex, particularly dorsal prefrontal cortex, with a role in motivation, attention, and organization of behavior.

c. *Hypothalamic* (arcuate nucleus) to infundibular stalk of pituitary involved in hypothalamic inhibition of prolactin release.

OVERLAP WITH THE CEREBELLAR SYSTEM

It is also important to remember that the major outflow from the cerebellum (via the superior cerebellar peduncle) terminates in relation to the same ventrolateral and ventral anterior nuclei of the thalamus.[2] This thalamic nucleus receives a projection from both the cerebellum (predominantly the dentate nucleus) and the globus pallidus. However, the information from the cerebellum is projected in a more limited manner primarily via ventrolateral to the motor areas of cerebral cortex, predominantly the premotor and motor cortices. The basal ganglia differ from the cerebellum in several important respects. In contrast to the more limited relationship of cerebellum to ventral lateral nucleus of thalamus (projection to motor areas of cortex—and projections from motor areas of cortex via pontine nuclei to the cerebellum), the basal ganglia have widespread inputs from the cerebral cortex and via several thalamic nuclei back to multiple cortical areas. These cortical basal ganglia relationships are not diffuse or overlapping but instead are organized in parallel systems.

It should be very clear then that patients with disease of the basal ganglia may have significant manifestations not only of motor function but also of cognitive and emotional function (see Cooper [1991] and Starkstein et al. [1989] in relationship

---

[2] It should be noted that the dentate nucleus of the cerebellum also has some outflow (via the superior cerebellar peduncle) to the red nucleus. After synapsing at the red nucleus, fibers are also conveyed to the ventrolateral nucleus of the thalamus. The major outflow, however, apparently is directly to these thalamic nuclei from the dentate and, to a lesser degree, from the emboliform nucleus of the cerebellum.

to Parkinson's disease and Laplane et al. [1989] with regard to obsessive-compulsive behavior change).

There is considerable overlap with frontal lobe, premotor, and supplementary motor dysfunction, as one might predict, based on the anatomical connections discussed earlier. An understanding of the basic anatomical interrelationships will aid in an understanding of the effects of the various medical and surgical modalities of treatment in Parkinson's disease. Thus, when dysfunction develops in the circuit, lesions at specific critical points, such as ventrolateral thalamic entry area or the subthalamic nucleus may allow restoration of considerable function. The usual location of surgical lesions for the relief of the tremor and rigidity of Parkinson's disease is shown in Figure 19.2. It should be evident that this lesion in the ventral lateral nucleus of the thalamus would also be extremely effective in eliminating tremor originating in the cerebellum, since such a lesion would prevent a disordered cerebellum from acting on the circuits passing through this nucleus and this disordered cerebellum would no longer influence motor activities originating at a cortical level.

We must consider the circuits through the basal ganglia as modulators of cortical function, particularly as regard movement. For voluntary movement, these circuits clearly provide a complex modulation acting on the premotor/ supplementary motor cortex. This modulation represents a focused equilibrium of opposing influences. When one of these influences acts to a disproportionate degree, dysfunction in the main circuit from the cortical motor cortex to the anterior horn cells and to the reticular formation will result.

SPECIFIC SYNDROMES

CLINICAL SYMPTOMS AND SIGNS OF DYSFUNCTION

Based on the anatomical circuits considered earlier, a variety of symptoms and signs may occur.

1. A lack of movement, an inability to initiate movement, or a slowness of movement because of excessive inhibition (a lack of excitation) so that the excitatory effect of ventral lateral nucleus of the thalamus on supplementary motor neurons fails to occur due to a decrease in dopamine. This lack of movement and slowness of movement is defined as *akinesia and bradykinesia*, as discussed earlier.

2. Elimination of inhibition at a critical point in the system may result in a release of disordered movement. The disordered movements are defined as *dyskinesia and tremor*.

3. The relationship of muscle tone in antagonists and agonists may be altered so that excessive tone is present, defined as *rigidity*. Tremor superimposed on this rigidity produces cogwheel rigidity.

4. A specific extreme of posture may be defined as *dystonia*.

5. Problems in the sequencing of movements as in walking or of posture as in standing may occur.

6. Disorganization of those higher level *righting reflexes* discussed in Chapter 18 may occur.

Not all of these symptoms and signs occur in a given disease or case. Some of these symptoms and signs occur with disease at other sites. As already discussed, akinesia or bradykinesia is frequently seen in patients with disease of frontal premotor and supplementary motor areas. (Refer to Delwaide and Gance [1988] for additional discussion of correlation of symptoms and signs with anatomy/physiology.)

There is considerable overlap with frontal lobe, premotor, and supplementary motor dysfunction, as one might predict, based on the anatomical connections discussed earlier. An understanding of the basic anatomical interrelationships will aid in an understanding of the effects of the various medical and surgical modalities of treatment in Parkinson's disease. Thus, when dysfunction develops in the circuit, lesions at specific critical points, such as ventrolateral thalamic entry area or the subthalamic nucleus, may allow restoration of considerable function. The usual location of surgical lesions for the relief of the tremor and rigidity of Parkinson's disease is shown in Figure 19.2.

We must consider the circuits through the basal ganglia modulators of cortical function, particularly as regard movement. For voluntary movement, these circuits clearly provide complex modulation acting on the supplementary motor cortex. This modulation represents a focused equilibrium of opposing influences. When one of these influences acts to a disproportionate degree, dysfunction in the main circuit from the cortical motor cortex to the anterior horn cells and to the reticular formation will result. Based on the anatomical consideration of multiple sequential circuits involving inhibitory synapses, certain clinical symptoms could be predicted.

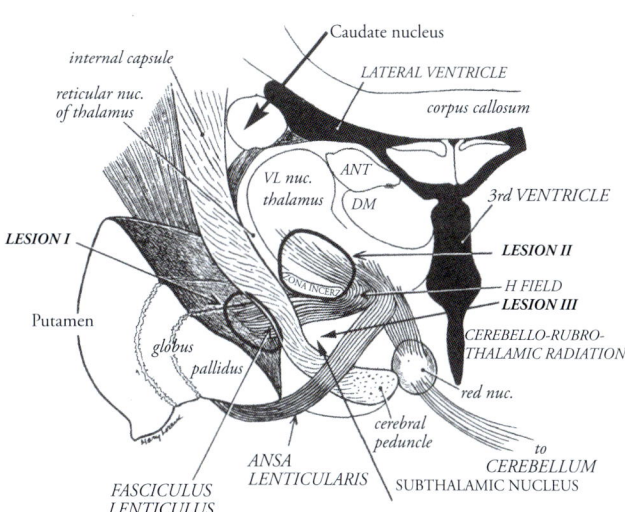

Figure 19.2 Major connections of the basal ganglia with the sites of surgical lesions or of sites of implantation of stimulators in Parkinson's disease and in other disorders. Lesion I globus pallidus: Lesion II ventral lateral nucleus of the thalamus (the sector of VL involvement is termed VIM = nuclear ventral inferior medial). Lesion III subthalamic nucleus. (Modified from Lin, LH, Okumura, S and Cooper IS: Electroenceph. Clin Neurophysiol. 13: 633, 1961.)

Table 19.4 **CLINICAL SIGNS IN PARKINSON'S DISEASE**

CLINICAL SIGNS	CLINICAL APPEARANCE
Rhythmic tremor at rest: Alternating type, initially fine, 4–5 Hz, and then, as the disease progresses, often coarse. The tremor disappears on movement but may re-emerge when a posture is maintained.	The tremor affects not only the extremities but also the eyelids, the tongue, and voice. The alternate movements of thumb against opposing index finger are often referred to as "pill rolling."
Clinical rigidity, which must be differentiated from decerebrate rigidity, which is primarily spasticity with the jack-knife quality of spasticity (a sudden resistance is encountered, which, as additional force is applied, suddenly gives way).	Comparable to the resistance of a lead pipe bending under force in which the resistance is relatively constant throughout the range of motion. As with spasticity, rigidity may reflect increased activity of the gamma system.
Akinesia, lack of spontaneous movement and the difficulty in initiating movement. A corollary term is *bradykinesia*, which refers to a slowness of spontaneous movement.	Seen in the fixed facies of the Parkinsonian patient, lack of spontaneous blinking and movement, loss of associated movements (the swing of the arms in walking). Correlated as discussed earlier with the reduction in dopaminergic input.
Defects in posture righting reflexes are best noted as the patient stands, walks, and attempts to turn.	Normally, as an individual turns, the eyes move initially in the direction of the turn, his head moves, then shoulders and arms, and the body then follows. The patient with Parkinson's disease, however, turns "en bloc." In walking at times, develops forward propulsion, seems to tilt forward and develop increasing speed—producing loss of balance with falls and injuries, and instability when turning.

PARKINSON'S DISEASE AND THE PARKINSONIAN SYNDROME

(Recent reviews are provided by Dunnett and Bjorklund [1999], Lang and Lozano [1998], Olanow and Tatton [1999], Quinn [1995], Riley and Lang [2000], Schapira [2009], and Stacy [2009].)

The most common disease involving the basal ganglia is Parkinson's disease, first described by James Parkinson in 1817.[3] Parkinson's disease, after Alzheimer's disease, is the most common degenerative disorder of the central nervous system, affecting approximately 1.5 million individuals in the United States with an incidence of new cases diagnosed of 70,000 per year. As regards epidemiology, the following statistics may be cited, taking into account the usual long duration of the disease. The age-adjusted prevalence is approximately 115 per 100,000. Under age 45 years the prevalence is 1.3 per 100,000. However, in the age group 75–85 years of age, the prevalence is 1193 per 100,000 (Mayeau et al., 1995).

The basic pathology is the progressive loss of the dopamine-producing neurons in the pars compacta of the substantia nigra. A certain mixture of symptoms then develops, each of which may vary in severity. *The essential (cardinal) signs and symptoms consist of tremor, rigidity, akinesia, and defects in postural and righting reflexes.* This total picture was essentially described by Charcot, and he named the disease after Parkinson (Goetz, 1986). The cardinal signs and symptoms are summarized in Table 19.4.

Some cases, throughout their course, may continue to manifest primarily tremor as the major symptom, and such cases tend to have a more favorable prognosis. Several types of Parkinson's disease and syndromes may be specified. The most common as regards variety is the idiopathic or primary Parkinson's disease, a degenerative disease arising insidiously in the patient of age 40, 50, or 60 years. In a series of 1644 patients with Parkinsonism, evaluated by Jankovic (1989) at a movement disorder clinic, 82% were found to have idiopathic Parkinson's disease. At times, there is a family history of the same disease; the relative risk for Parkinson's disease among first-degree relatives is 2–3 fold.

The relative risk among young-onset cases is much higher and is discussed later.

1. *Pathology of Parkinsonian lesions*. The basic pathology involves a progressive loss of the pigmented neuromelanin-containing neurons of the pars compacta of the substantia nigra (Fig. 19.2). (The pigmented neurons of the locus ceruleus are also affected.)[4] (The student will recall that both melanin and dopamine are steps in the metabolic pathway involving phenylalanine.) A long preclinical period estimated at 5 years occurs in this progressive disease. *Various estimates suggest that when symptoms first occur, 70%–80% of striatal dopamine*

---

[3] As we will discuss later, other disease entities may overlap with many of the same symptoms and signs, and it is appropriate to refer to the larger group as the Parkinsonian syndrome. The term "Parkinsonism" has also been employed for this larger group.

[4] Whether the dopamine-nigral-striatal-(mesostriatal) system involvement is the entire story in Parkinson's disease is unclear. The mesolimbic cortical dopaminergic system is also affected (50%-60% decrease). Noradrenergic, serotoninergic, and cholinergic systems are also affected; for example, there is a 50%–60% decrease in noradrenalin concentrations in cerebral cortex, locus ceruleus, limbic system, hypothalamus, and cerebellum; and a 58% loss of serotonin in dorsal raphe nucleus. There is also cholinergic nerve cell loss of 32%–87% in nucleus basalis of Meynert. In general, none of these systems show the degree of degeneration found in the nigral-striatal-dopaminergic system. (Estimated as 80%–90% depletion of striatal dopamine and 60%–70% degeneration of substantia nigral neurons when symptoms first emerge). For extensive reviews and discussions, see Agid et al. (1987, 1989).

Figure 19.3 Parkinson's disease. The substantia nigra in Parkinson's disease. (*A*) Normal substantia nigra. (*B*) Similar region in case of idiopathic Parkinson's disease. A marked loss of pigmentation is evident. (Courtesy Dr. Thomas Smith, Neuropathology, University of Massachusetts.)

is depleted. In terms of neurons in the pars compacta of the substantia nigra, 50% (compared to age-matched controls) to 70% (compared to young individuals) is already lost. Normally the rate of cell loss in the nigra during normal aging is 5% per decade. In patients with Parkinson's disease the rate of cell death is subsequently 45% per decade (Fig. 19.3).

On histologic examination (Fig. 19.4), there is a characteristic, specific finding of Lewy bodies: round, eosinophilic bodies surrounded by a clear halo within the cytoplasm of surviving neurons of the substantia nigra. In many cases, these Lewy bodies are found in other neurons, for example, cerebral cortex. Immunocytochemistry has demonstrated that a small protein, *a-synuclein*, is a major component of the Lewy body (Fig. 19.5). Under normal circumstances this protein is located in presynaptic nerve terminals. It is therefore likely that the Lewy body represents degenerated and aggregated neurofilaments. The Lewy body may also be found diffusely in cerebral cortex in Lewy body dementia.

Figure 19.4 Lewy body in a pigmented neuron of the substantia nigra. H&E stain, original at 125×. (Courtesy of Dr. Thomas Smith.)

Figure 19.5 Lewy body. Slide stained for alpha synuclein, 100×. (Courtesy of Dr. Thomas Smith.)

2. *Etiology of Parkinson's disease.* Why do the neurons degenerate? The long time answer suggested both genetic and environmental causes. The etiology now emphasizes the underlying genetic factors. Recent research has begun to uncover the underlying genetic factors not only in the early-onset cases but also links to those factors in sporadic cases. Nevertheless, the majority of cases with L-Dopa-responsive Parkinson's disease do not have a clear-cut genetic basis. However, mutations in the alpha synuclein gene have been found in several families of Italian or Greek origin with early-onset autosomal dominant Parkinson's disease mapping to locus 4Q21-25 (Duvoisin, 1998). Other families with autosomal recessive juvenile-onset disease have implicated the parkin gene at locus 6q25.2-27. Other gene loci are discussed by Dunnett and Bjorklund (1999) and by Schapira (2009).

Park 1: Alpha-synuclein. This was the first described familial cause and was attributed to a mutation. Multiplications of the wild-type gene have been described. The clinical variation includes not only early-onset but late-onset cases in an autosomal dominant pattern of inheritance. Overexpression of the wild type alpha-synnuclein protein is toxic to dopaminergic neurons. The mutation results in increased fibrillar protein formation, the end stage of many degenerative disorders.

Parkin (Park 2). This mutation is commonly see in the autosomal recessive early aged onset Japanese population. The Parkin mutation of deletions in this gene carries over into apparently sporadic cases.

PINK 1 (Park 6). These patients have a recessive mutation with onset of the typical Parkinsonian disorder before age 40 years. The gene encodes a mitochondrial kinase. Altered phosphorylation of target proteins leads to an abnormal stress response and degeneration.

LRRK2 (Park 8). Mutations in this kinase are of considerable interest in view of the frequency of this mutation. This accounts for 1% of sporadic cases and 4% of familial cases. Inheritance of the LRKK Gly 2019 Ser mutation is 28% at age 59 years, 51% at 69 years, and 74% at age 79 years. The occurrence of the mutant gene is frequent among those of North African origin (Healey et al., 2008).

Glucocerebrosidase mutations. Gaucher's disease is an autosomal recessive lysosomal storage disease which results from a deficiency of the enzyme glucocerebrosidase A (GBA). Mutations in the gene produce several medical and neurological syndromes. However, there is a significant risk factor for Parkinson's disease. Mutations in this gene were found in 2.9% of sporadic Parkinson's disease cases versus 0.4% of controls. A higher density of the mutations was found among Ashkenazi Jewish patients from Israel with Parkinson's disease in whom 31% had the mutation. A mutation in GBA was also identified in 4.3% of Chinese patients with Parkinson's disease.

Other mutations are discussed by Schapira (2009).

Environmental factors. These are less clear. Cigarette smoking (not good for overall health) and coffee drinking apparently lower the risk of Parkinson's disease. The use of nonsteroidal inflammatory drugs more than two times per week also can lower the risk of Parkinson's disease.

Neuroleptic agents. The use of neuroleptic agents may unmask an underlying genetic predisposition to Parkinson's disease. A significant percentage (15%–60% depending on age) of patients who receive neuroleptic tranquilizers also will develop symptoms of Parkinsonism. These agents include phenothiazides such as chlorpromazine, haloperidol, and reserpine. Reserpine interferes with the storage of dopamine within the nerve cells and, thus, depletes the brain of this neurotransmitter. Phenothiazides and related compounds, on the other hand, block the postsynaptic receptors at dopaminergic synapses. In general, of the symptoms produced by these agents, the akinesia, rigidity, and tremor will disappear when the agent has been cleared from the body. However, in some cases, the Parkinsonian features appear to remain as a permanent deficit. In such patients, one may find evidence in the family history of other cases of Parkinson's disease (Schmidt and Jarcho, 1966). As discussed by Koller (1992), there is then a clear indication that neuroleptic-induced Parkinsonism represents early or latent Parkinson's disease made evident by antidopaminergic medications.

Toxic agents. The major impetus for the study of possible toxic exposure has come from the study of cases of Parkinson's disease developing in miners exposed to manganese and more recently in cases exposed to the agent MPTP.

Manganese Poisoning. A relatively rare cause of a Parkinsonian syndrome is manganese poisoning. Manganese apparently accumulates in the melanin-containing neurons of the substantia nigra and interferes with the enzyme systems involved in the production of dopamine (Mena et al., 1970).

MPTP Toxicity. Another form of Parkinson's disease induced by the drug MPTP has provided major insights in the possible etiology of the degeneration of the dopamine-containing neurons in the substantia nigra. (MPTP is the abbreviated term for 1-Methyl- 4 phenyl-1,2,3,6, tetrahydropyridine). This agent is a by-product of the chemical process for the production of a reverse ester of meperidine (demerol): 1-methyl-4 propionoxypiperidine (MPPP). Meperidine is a controlled narcotic; MPPP is not controlled, has narcotic action, and can be produced in clandestine laboratories. MPTP had been recognized shortly after its legitimate synthesis in 1947 to produce a severe—rigid—akinetic state in monkeys. However, it was not until the summer of 1982, when MPPP was produced on a large scale in Northern California, for illicit mass distribution, that significant numbers of young drug abusers began appearing at emergency rooms with an acute Parkinsonian syndrome. The investigation of these cases has been presented in a series of papers by (Ballard et al., 1985). Essentially, the compound MPTP has selective toxicity on the dopaminergic neurons of the pars compacta of the substantia nigra, not only in human but also in subhuman primates, such as the Rhesus monkey, *Macaca mulatta*, and the squirrel monkey. Both in the human and the monkey, MPTP reproduces the clinical disease, the pathological findings, and the effects of pharmacological therapy of Parkinson's disease to a relatively complete degree, including in older animals, the presence of Lewy bodies. With such an animal model, experimental medical and surgical therapy can be studied with a clear-cut correlation with the human disease (for example, see Aziz et al., 1991; Kopin, 1988; Langston and Ballard, 1984). Moreover, since there were many patients exposed to the agent but not all exposed patients and not all acute cases developed the chronic Parkinsonian state, prospective studies can be performed as to the natural history and factors influencing the onset of the disease. In part because of MPTP, increased attention has been focused on other environmental exposures that may be involved in producing neurotoxic effects culminating in Parkinson's disease (Olanow and Tatton, 1999; Tanner and Langston, 1990).

Other pathological processes also will produce some of the symptoms of Parkinson's disease without the presence of Lewy bodies (Gibbs, 1988):

1. *Bilateral necrosis of the globus pallidus* may produce akinesia. Such a necrosis could occur in carbon monoxide poisoning, or anoxia, or in relation to infarction. Rigidity in flexion may also follow bilateral necrosis of the putamen or the globus pallidus.

2. A tremor at rest may occur with destructive lesions involving the ventromedial tegmentum of the midbrain. Such lesions, apparently, interrupt the pathway from the substantia nigra to the striatum. A degeneration of neurons in the substantia nigra and a decrease in dopamine in the corpus striatum occur.

3. *"Arteriosclerotic or vascular (multi-infarct)"* variety in which bilateral infarcts occur in the putamen. Usually this is the accompaniment of a lacunar state in which multiple small infarcts occur in the basal ganglia and internal capsule. The resultant syndrome affects the lower half of the body and thus can be clearly distinguished from the classical idiopathic L-Dopa-responsive Parkinson's disease.

4. *Von Economo's encephalitis in the years 1916–1926.* A certain proportion of cases may be termed postencephalitic. These cases had a clear onset in relation to the epidemic of Von Economo's encephalitis in those years. Approximately 50% of the survivors of this devastating disease developed a Parkinson's syndrome due to severe loss of neurons in the substantia nigra. In such cases, Lewy bodies are not found but neurofibrillary tangles are present in surviving cells (see Alzheimer's disease in Chapter 30 for a discussion

of neurofibrillary tangles). In addition to the aforementioned Parkinsonian symptoms and signs, these patients presented other evidence of involvement of the central nervous system, including oculogyric crises (tonic vertical gaze), chorea, dystonia, and sleep disorders. The symptoms and signs indicated the involvement not only of the substantia nigra but also of multiple other sites, including the midbrain, hypothalamus, and hippocampus (see Gibb, 1988). The essential distribution of the pathology was in the periventricular areas about the aqueduct and third ventricle. A dramatic example of postencephalitic Parkinsonism and its treatment is presented in the movie *Awakenings*, based on the book by Oliver Sacks.

Management. (Refer to Lang and Lozano [1998], Riley and Lang [2000], and Stacy [2009].) When one considers that the basic pathology in Parkinson's disease represents a marked loss of dopamine-containing neurons in the substantia nigra and a marked decrease in dopamine concentration in the striatum, whereas other transmitters and neurons are affected to a much lesser degree (e.g., cholinergic system within corpus striatum now has a relatively unopposed action), then the possible types of treatment are very evident.

1. *Early medical treatment*: For many years, the standard treatment involved the use of anticholinergic compounds such as belladonna and atropine or of synthetic analogs. Trihexyphenidyl (Artane) and benztropine (Cogentin) are examples of such agents. The anticholinergic compounds affect primarily the tremor and to some extent the rigidity of Parkinson's disease and in many cases may produce limited improvement.

2. *Early approaches to surgical intervention*: Various surgical procedures were attempted in the 1940s and 1950s, involving limited ablations of area 4 or area 6 or section of the cerebral peduncle. In 1952, while attempting to section the cerebral peduncle, Cooper accidentally occluded the anterior choroidal artery, and the Parkinsonian patient showed a significant improvement in contralateral symptoms, presumably as a result of infarction of the inner section of the globus pallidus. Cooper soon came to employ stereotaxic techniques for the direct production of lesions in the globus pallidus (Fig. 19.2, lesion 1). The procedure produced a significant reduction in contralateral tremor and, to a lesser extent, a decrease in the contralateral rigidity. Cooper was able to demonstrate later that lesions in the ventrolateral thalamus were much more effective (Fig. 19.2, lesion 2). Initially, the stereotaxic lesions were produced by the injection of alcohol or coagulation. In later procedures, a freezing cannula was employed.

3. *Transmitter replacement*: With the increasing knowledge of the neurotransmitters involved in the substantia nigra and corpus striatum and with reports of deficits of dopamine in these structures in patients with Parkinson's disease, the use of replacement therapy with L-Dopa (dihydroxyphenylalanine) subsequently developed (Cotzias et al., 1967, 1969). As we have indicated, the anticholinergic drugs had a limited effect primarily on the tremor rigidity; surgery affected primarily the tremor; the use of L-Dopa, which was more a physiological technique, improved the severe akinesia in addition to decreasing the tremor and rigidity. The use of L-Dopa required large amounts of medication since much of the administered dosage was decarboxylated to dopamine at peripheral systemic sites and never crossed the blood–brain barrier to be converted to dopamine (*note that L-Dopa crosses the blood–brain barrier; dopamine does not*). There were significant side effects due to the peripheral actions of the drug. By combining L-Dopa with a peripheral Dopa decarboxylase inhibitor, Carbidopa (in the form of Sinemet), a much lower dosage of L-Dopa was required with fewer gastrointestinal and blood pressure side effects. Central side effects continued to occur, for example, peak dose-related dyskinesias such as chorea and myoclonus. The short duration of action also continued to provide problems in terms of wearing off of dose. Other sudden on-off effects with sudden arrests of movement that were not entirely related to time of dose also occurred as the disease progressed. Individual titration of dosage, specific to the particular patient, is often required. The basic problem is that Parkinson's disease is progressive. Once the neurons in the substantia nigra have all died off or have become dysfunctional, there is no capability to convert L-Dopa to dopamine.

4. *Other therapeutic maneuvers* have been developed for such patients. Various dopamine agonists have been developed to bypass the problem of conversion of L-Dopa to dopamine. Additional surgical procedures involving the implantation of stimulators in deep brain structures such as the globus pallidus, thalamus, and subthalamic nucleus have also been developed. Transplantation of fetal mesencephalic cells into the striatum has benefit in younger patients but eventually increases dyskinesias. Therefore, this procedure has been abandoned. These are reviewed in the following patient who was followed for 19 years.

CASE HISTORY 19.1

This 48-year-old, married, left-handed white male school teacher and administrator, 3 months prior to evaluation in 1982, developed a sense of fatigue, stiffness, and lack of control in the left arm. After a period of prolonged writing, he would have to make a conscious effort to continue writing. Approximately 1 month prior to the evaluation, he first noted a slowing down in movements of the left leg. "I have to remember to lift it."

Neurological Examination

Cranial nerves: He had a tremor of the closed eyelids and a positive glabellar sign (he was unable to suppress eyelid blinking on tap of forehead).

Motor system: In walking there was a tendency to turn en bloc and a decreased swing of the left arm. There was a slight increase in resistance to passive motion at the left elbow, wrist, and knee (rigidity without definite cogwheel component). Although the patient was

Figure 19.6 Parkinson's disease. Case 19.1. See text. Handwriting sample: on 05/03/83 before therapy with L-dopa/Carbidopa and 05/10/83—1 week after starting therapy.

left-handed, there was a slowness of alternating finger movements of the left hand. No tremor was present. Handwriting was intact with no evidence of micrographia.

Clinical diagnosis: Early Parkinson's disease, predominantly unilateral.

Laboratory data: All studies were normal, including computerized tomography (CT) scan of the brain and thyroid studies.

Subsequent course: (This patient was followed for a total of 19 years after disease onset, initially for the first 13 years by the author, subsequently by Dr. Paula Ravin at the University of Massachusetts Medical Center, Dr. David Standeart at the Massachusetts General Hospital, and Dr. Warren Olanow at the Mount Sinai Hospital in New York.)

Initially the patient did not wish to begin any treatment; re-evaluation at 3 months indicated progression. One year after onset of symptoms there was significant micrographia (Fig. 19.6A) and cogwheel rigidity at left shoulder, elbow, and wrist. Therapy with Sinemet (10–100 mg, 3 times per day)[5] was begun. Re-evaluation 1 week later demonstrated a marked improvement in handwriting (Fig. 19.6B) and decreased cogwheel rigidity.

As the dose of Sinemet was increased to (10/100) mg 5x/day over the next week, occasional choreiform movements of the fingers of the left hand and occasional backward flinging (hemiballistic) movements of the left arm occurred at 60–90 minutes after later doses of Sinemet. As the dose reached 10–100 mg 6x/day, the patient reported that his handwriting now was back to normal. Examination confirmed the significant improvement in all findings. The patient did experience, 90 minutes after a Sinemet dose, a tremor of the left shoulder and an exaggerated grasp of the left foot toes on lifting the leg (possible form of dyskinetic or dystonic reaction). He was aware that some symptoms of his underlying disease would emerge 3–4 hours after a dose of Sinemet. *Five years after onset of symptoms*, despite a higher dosage of Sinemet of 25/100 mg tablets, 7 or 8 x/day, more resting pill rolling tremor of the left hand had emerged. (In actuality 75–100 mg of carbidopa is probably sufficient to saturate the peripheral dopa decarboxylase system.) Moreover, choreiform movements of the left arm occurred 60 to 90 minutes after each dose of Sinemet. The choreiform movements disappeared when the dosage of Sinemet was reduced to 25/100 mg 6/day. The increased rigidity and tremor responded to the addition of a Dopa agonist bromocriptine (Parlodel). Over the subsequent years other agents were employed, but the disease continued to progress with all of the problems in management discussed earlier. Eventually, in 1997 he underwent mesencephalic fetal cell transplantation. Evaluation 3 years after the transplant demonstrated a little improvement but a marked increase in the dyskinesias. Some improvement in dyskinesias occurred after dopaminergic medications again were reduced.

Comments

Parkinson's disease is a progressive disorder of motor function, with variable manifestations of tremor, rigidity, akinesia, bradykinesia, and impairment of postural reflexes. Patients vary in the type of major involvement and in the rate of progression. Pharmacological management has rapidly evolved and in the process has provided considerable insights into the nature of basal ganglia function. For the specific patient, therapy must still be individualized. As this case history illustrates, the pharmacological effects are time limited.

Evaluation of therapy must always record the time of drug intake and the time of examination. It is important to note that the disease remains progressive, despite the impressive pharmacological achievements. To prevent progression would require arresting or reversing the loss of the nigral cells producing dopamine or of introducing another source of dopamine-producing neurons into the basal ganglia, as discussed earlier. Surgical procedures, particularly deep brain stimulation involving the subthalamic nucleus or the globus pallidus, may offer benefit to specific patients.

DIFFERENTIAL DIAGNOSIS OF PARKINSON'S DISEASE

1. *In considering the akinesia and bradykinesia of Parkinson's disease, the major differential diagnosis in the older population are the syndromes of gait apraxia related to frontal lobe,* as discussed in Chapter 18. These may be outlined as follows:

   a. Normal pressure hydrocephalus

   b. Other types of hydrocephalus: late decompensation of aqueductal stenosis

   c. Multiple lacunar infarcts (the lacunar state)

   d. Leukoariosis or Binswanger's disease involving the periventricular white matter and seen in elderly hypertensive patients

   e. Alzheimer's disease. Note, however, that Mayeux et al. (1985) found that 34% of patients with Alzheimer's disease had some extrapyramidal signs. To confound the picture, 44% of patients with Parkinson's disease have dementia, with 29% found to have Alzheimer's disease and 10% Lewy body dementia. Studies were performed before the entity of Lewy body dementia was clearly established.

---

[5] This is a combination of 10 mg of carbidopa (Dopa decarboxylase inhibitor) and 100 mg of L-Dopa. Higher dosage combinations are (a) 25 mg of carbidopa with 100 mg L-Dopa, and (b) 25 mg carbidopa with 250 mg L-Dopa. A sustained-release form is also available (50 mg of carbidopa with 200 mg of L-Dopa) and is marketed as Sinemet CR.

Table 19.5 PARKINSONISM PLUS SYNDROMES

NAME	ABBREVIATION	PATHOLOGY-TYPE	LOCATION	CLINICAL SYNDROME
1. Progressive supranuclear palsy (the most common)	PSP	Neuron loss and abnormal tau protein in neurofibrillary tangles in neurons and glia cortex and subcortex	Midbrain tegmentum and tectum, substantia nigra, globus pallidus, subthalamic nuc. basal nuc. cortex	Parkinsonism plus supranuclear impairment of gaze, particularly in vertical plane Imaging = atrophy of midbrain
2. Corticobasal degeneration	CBD	Ballooned and achromat-ic neurons plus abnormal neurofibrillary tangles tangles with tau protein. Linked to chromosome 17 in familial cases	Asymmetrical involvement of frontal-parietal cortex (superior frontal), substantia nigra, caudate, thalamus	Akinetic-rigid Parkinsonism plus, dementia plus lateralized apraxia, useless hand, and lateralized myoclonus Overlap with Pick's, Frontal dementia and PSP. Imaging = focal atrophy of frontal-parietal cortex
3. Multiple-system atrophy Incorporates three previously separate disorders a. striatal nigral degeneration b. olivopontocerebellar atrophy c. Shy-Drager syndrome	MSA	Neuronal loss—gliosis, and oligodendroglial inclusions in neuronal cytoplasm, nuclei and glia containing filaments derived from cytoskeletal proteins: tau, ubiquitin, and alpha synnuclein	Substatia nigra, striatum, olivopontocerebellar pathways plus intermediolateral cell column of spinal cord	Akinetic–rigid Parkinsonism (predominant in 80%) plus cerebellar ataxia (predominates in 20%) plus dysautonomia (with neurogenic orthostatic hypotension) + *p* Imaging = atrophy of striatum or pons/cerebellum depending on predominant symptoms

    f. Frontal lobe tumors, for example, subfrontal or parasagittal meningiomas

    g. Myxedema with hypothyroid state

    h. General paresis and tabes dorsalis of neurosyphilis, now uncommon.

In general, frontal lobe syndromes do not have a prominent tremor (unless a coincident essential or senile tremor is present). Rigidity may be present, but this variable rigidity is of the frontal lobe type referred to as gegenhalten. A cogwheel component (to this frontal lobe rigidity) is usually not present unless there is a superimposed tremor of other cause. The rigidity and akinesia predominantly affect the lower extremities.

2. *In considering the tremor of Parkinson's disease, the major differential diagnosis is essential or senile or familial tremor.* In general, this is a tremor of the outstretched hand with some increase as termination of movement or when a sustained posture is maintained. The tremor is not present at rest and there is *no* pill rolling quality. Rigidity is not present, and gait is normal with a good swing of the arm. The tremor is usually long-standing without major disability. Note that there is a small group of Parkinson's disease patients with favorable outcome who have a resting tremor as a predominant symptom over many years. They will, however, have to a minor degree, on careful examination, many of the other cardinal symptoms of Parkinson's disease.

3. *Secondary Parkinsonism: Neuroleptic, toxic, or vascular induced.* In the series of Jankovic (1989) and Siemer and Reddy (1991), these cases accounted for 10% of all cases of Parkinsonism.

4. *Parkinsonism plus syndromes.* In the same series these cases accounted for 10% of all cases of Parkinsonism. These latter patients all share the following characteristics:

    a. A progressive disorder is present.

    b. From a clinical and pathological standpoint, the pathology of primary neuronal degeneration is much more widespread than in idiopathic Parkinson's disease. The term *multisystem atrophy* is often applied to some of these cases.[6]

    c. Lewy bodies are not found.

    d. In general, the patients are all poorly responsive to Levodopa (since the pathology extends far beyond the dopaminergic producing neurons of the substantia nigra).

    e. Some of the patients have a familial disorder.
    The more frequent types may be briefly noted (excellent, more detailed discussions are found in Jankovic [1989] and Riley and Lang [2000]) (Table 19.5).

---

[6] Many patients with Parkinson's disease have some symptoms, usually minor, that suggest some degree of involvement beyond the substantia nigra and beyond the dopaminergic nigral-striatal system, for example, orthostatic hypotension, which is present in the untreated patient. Idiopathic Parkinson's patients also may have some minor degree of upward gaze impairment.

5. Other neurological syndromes with rigidity and akinesia:

   a. Early-onset Huntington's disease and Wilson's disease (see below).

   b. Hallavorden Spatz disease: A rare familial (autosomal recessive disorder with linkage to chromosome 20P) in which prominent iron deposits and neuronal degeneration in globus pallidus and substantia nigra are associated with childhood onset of Parkinsonian syndrome, dementia, spasticity, dystonia, and chorea.

   c. Parkinsonism-dementia-ALS complex found in the Chamorros of Guam (and several other Pacific groups)—a probable toxic disease involving an excitatory amino acid (beta N methyl-amino L-alanine) derived from the cycad seed once used in the production of flooring.

   d. Creutzfeldt-Jakob disease: See discussion of dementia (Chapter 30).

CHOREA, HEMICHOREA, AND HEMIBALLISMUS

Chorea[7] may be defined as "excessive spontaneous movements irregularly repeated randomly distributed and abrupt in character." These movements, although involuntary, consist of fragments or sequences of normal, coordinated movements. Face, mouth, head, and proximal or distal limbs may be involved.

Two types of processes must be distinguished: (1) lateralized hemichorea and (2) generalized chorea. The lateralized hemichorea merges into a remarkable disorder called hemiballismus, which is characterized by sudden flinging or ballistic movements at the proximal joints such as throwing or sudden swinging movements at the shoulder joint. Patients may start with hemichorea and evolve into hemiballismus. In discussing this topic, we will deal first with the focal problem and then with the generalized type. We will see in both varieties abnormalities of the anatomic sequences discussed earlier in this chapter.

HEMICHOREA AND HEMIBALLISM

Initial clinical and experimental studies correlated these disorders with lesions of the contralateral subthalamic nucleus (see Carpenter et al., 1950; Whittier and Meller, 1947; Whittier et al., 1949). It was recognized that the underlying lesion could be a small infarct due to posterior cerebral penetrating branch involvement, often on a lacunar basis, in a patient with hypertension or diabetes mellitus. At times, the adjacent thalamic areas were involved, as well, for example, the ventral posterior lateral or ventral lateral nucleus. At times, the responsible lesion was a small hemorrhage in the subthalamic nucleus (Fig. 19.7) and, rarely, a small metastatic tumor.

Figure 19.7 Hemichorea. Case 19.2. See text. Magnetic resonance imaging (MRI) demonstrates a hyperdense area of the head of the right caudate, adjacent putamen, and external capsule, consistent with a hemorrhage. (*A, B*, and *C*) Sequential horizontal sections at 5 mm intervals—T1-weighted. (*D*) Sagittal section 12.5 mm to right of midline.

As regards the explanation for such contralateral excessive movement, hemichorea or hemiballismus, one needs only to consult Figure 19.1. Decreasing the excitatory drive from the subthalamic nucleus acting on the medial globus pallidus and the substantia nigra reticularis would decrease the inhibitory drive from those structures acting in the thalamus. Therefore, the thalamic/premotor-SMA circuit would be more active and more movement would result.

There were other clinical studies that did suggest other possible localization in the striatum (Cooper, 1969; Goldblatt et al., 1974; Martin, 1957; Meyers, 1947; Schwarz and Barrows, 1960). In experimental studies Crossman et al. (1988) demonstrated that local injection of a GABA antagonist into the border of the lateral segment of the globus pallidus and the adjacent medial segment of the putamen would produce hemichorea in the monkey. Such lesions interrupt the inhibitory afferent input to the lateral globus pallidus from the putamen. The lateral globus pallidus would then have greater inhibitory drive on the subthalamic nucleus. The overall effect then would be equivalent to producing a lesion of the subthalamic nucleus; hemichorea or hemiballismus would result (see Mitchell et al., 1989).

Another factor to be considered in chorea and other induced dyskinesias is the possible unopposed action of the nigral striatal dopaminergic circuits, as discussed earlier in this chapter. L-Dopa will exacerbate choreiform disorders.[8] Agents

---

[7] At times the adjective *choreiform* is used to describe the movement rather than employing the noun *chorea*.

[8] L-Dopa-induced dyskinesias are not observed in intact monkeys and humans who have normal dopaminergic and normal basal ganglia function. Parkinsonian patients, monkeys with MPTP lesions, and patients with a predisposition to Huntington's disease will develop dyskinesias after receiving L-Dopa (see later discussion and Suguin et al., 1992).

that block dopamine receptors, for example, the butyrophenones (such as haloperidol), are often very effective in alleviating hemichorea, hemiballismus, and chorea (see Crossman, 1990; Klawans et al., 1970).

HEMICHOREA

The following case history provides an example of hemichorea with magnetic resonance imaging (MRI) correlation of lesion location in the striatum (caudate/putamen) following a hemorrhage into those structures.

CASE HISTORY 19.2

This 88-year-old, right-handed, widowed white female with a past medical history of profound hearing impairment, adult-onset diabetes, euthyroid goiter, coronary artery disease, and hypertension, 5 days prior to admission, developed the insidious onset of involuntary rotary movement in the left foot, which increased in intensity and progressed to involve the left shoulder. The movements were constantly present; even during sleep and with progression, her ability to ambulate with a walker was impaired. She also had a dull headache greater on the left side than on the right during the previous few days.

Neurological Examination

Cranial nerves: Intact except for left eye blindness (cataracts) and gross impairment of hearing such that shouting was necessary to communicate.

Motor system:

a. There was minimal weakness in the left upper extremity (5-/5).
b. There was a persistent hemichorea: involuntary twisting movements of her left foot and upward and rotary movements of her left shoulder. The movement was exacerbated by motor tasks but did dissipate with sleep.
c. Gait was slightly unsteady due to hesitant placement of the left foot. She did quite well with minimal assistance.

Reflexes:

a. Deep tendon reflexes were symmetrical and physiologic, except for decreased Achilles secondary to diabetes.
b. The left plantar response was extensor.

Sensation: Symmetrically diminished vibration sense in toes.
Clinical diagnosis: Hemichorea.
Laboratory data: MRI scan 3 days after admission revealed mild cortical atrophy and a hyperdense area in the right basal ganglia (particularly the head of caudate and putamen) and external capsule consistent with subacute hemorrhage (Fig. 19.8).
Hospital course: The patient was begun on haloperidol 0.5 mg by mouth every morning and advanced to 1 mg by mouth three times per day with improvement in the hemichorea, particularly in the upper extremity over the next 2 weeks.

HEMIBALLISM

As we have previously indicated, the movements of hemichorea may evolve or merge into more violent, uncoordinated, rotatory, flinging movements at the shoulder joint and other

Figure 19.8 Hemiballismus. Myelin stain of basal ganglia demonstrating a discrete hemorrhage into the right subthalamic nucleus. The arrow points to the subthalamic nucleus of the normal left hemisphere. (From Luhan, J.A.: Neurology, Baltimore, Williams & Wilkins, 1968, p. 334.)

proximal joints, termed *hemiballistic*. The responsible lesion was located in the subthalamic nucleus or in the putamen or at the border of lateral pallidum-putamen, as discussed earlier.

The following case history illustrates this movement disorder in a patient seen prior to the era of CT and MRI scans in which the localization is relatively clear.

CASE HISTORY 19.3

This 79-year-old, right-handed, white housewife had the abrupt onset in the early morning hours, 2 days prior to admission, of almost constant flinging movements of the right arm over which she had no control. At the same time, she noted that her right arm felt numb and heavy. Over the next 2 days, the movements decreased markedly and she regained more control of the arm.

Past history: The patient had been a known diabetic for 21 years, receiving insulin—most recently, lente insulin, 25 units each morning.

Neurological Examination
Mental status: Intact.
Cranial nerves: Intact.
Motor system:

a. Minimal weakness was present in the right upper extremity at the elbow, wrist, and fingers. Alternating movements and finger-to-nose testing in the right hand were markedly impaired.
b. Occasional involuntary flinging movements occurred at the right shoulder.

Sensory system: Pain, touch, vibration, and position sense were all absent in the right upper extremity to the elbow and decreased in this extremity above the elbow.
Clinical diagnosis: Hemiballismus due to a lesion of penetrating branches of the posterior cerebral artery which involved the subthalamic nucleus and ventral posterior lateral nucleus of thalamus.
Laboratory data: Chest and skull X-rays, electroencephalogram (EEG), and cerebrospinal fluid studies were all normal.
Subsequent course: The flinging movements of the right arm subsided spontaneously, shortly after admission. Position sense returned and pain sensation showed a mild improvement. The ataxia on finger-to-nose testing disappeared.

Comments

The loss of pain, touch, vibration, and position sense in the right upper extremity, at the onset of symptoms in this case, would suggest a lesion involving the ventral posterior lateral nucleus of the thalamus, presumably as a result of occlusion of the penetrating branches of the posterior cerebral artery. Such a lesion could have damaged the subthalamic nucleus as well. The severe dysmetria in the right upper extremity could well have reflected the severe sensory deficit in the right upper extremity. This would appear to be more likely than postulating a lacunar ataxic hemiplegia, due to involvement of the corona radiata in which the origin of the hemiballistic movements could have been in the adjacent caudate putamen. This, however, would not explain the severe sensory deficit. Note that the use of antidopaminergic agents will decrease or eliminate hemiballismus or hemichorea; however, many patients as in this case resolve spontaneously.

GENERALIZED CHOREA

Bilateral generalized chorea may occur under the following circumstances:

1. Acute onset with an immunological basis: (a) one aspect of rheumatic fever (plus or minus carditis and arthritis) in any entity still labeled Sydenham chorea. This is the most common cause of chorea in childhood. (b) In relationship to various autoimmune disease such as lupus erythematosus.

2. As an acute complication of L-dopa therapy in patients with compromise of the dopaminergic system or with disease of the basal ganglia—as discussed earlier. Overall, this is probably the most common situation in which chorea is seen by physicians such as neurologists.

3. As an acute or chronic complication of various metabolic disorders: hepatic, renal, hypocalcemia, and so on rarely occurring in pregnancy. In acute hepatic encephalopathy, a number of toxic substances that would normally be removed from the portal venous system on passage through the liver are not removed. Instead, in patients with liver disease, portal hypertension may develop, portal-systemic shunting develops, and toxic substances such as ammonia may accumulate in blood and brain. In addition to depression of consciousness (hepatic coma), a hepatic "flap" or "asterixis" may develop. With the arms extended at elbows, and the hands extended at wrist, an irregular flexion extension movement will develop at the wrists and at the metacarpal-phalangeal joints. A similar "asterixis" may also be noted in other metabolic diseases such as uremia and pulmonary disease with CO_2 retention. In all of these disorders, ataxia, dysarthria, and action tremor of hands may also occur. With uremia and hypocalcemia, myoclonus (sudden jerks of the extremities) or generalized convulsions may occur.

With repeated episodes or prolonged periods of hepatic encephalopathy, more profound and lasting changes in neurological function occur—producing a syndrome characterized by chorea and athetosis, ataxia, dysarthria, tremor, and dementia. Neuropathological examination of the brain demonstrates cavities within the basal ganglia, cerebellum, and cerebral cortex. Swollen astrocytes are found, particularly within basal ganglia. This chronic irreversible syndrome was initially described as the acquired non-Wilsonian type of hepatocerebral degeneration (Victor et al., 1965).

4. As a chronic progressive disorder—indicating a degenerative disease—affecting the striatum and other sectors of basal ganglia and cerebral cortex.

HUNTINGTON'S DISEASE

The most frequent disease in this category is Huntington's disease. Huntington's disease is of importance beyond its prevalence in the population of 3–7/100,000. The disease was originally described in 1872 by George Huntington, based on clinical observations made by his grandfather, his father, and himself on an apparent autosomal dominant syndrome of high penetrance that occurred in families living on Long Island in New York State. The syndrome was characterized by the development in midlife of a progressive psychological change (depression, paranoia, psychoses), dementia, and involuntary choreiform movements. The disease often affects multiple members of a family over a number of generations. Genetic studies have confirmed that the pattern of inheritance follows an autosomal dominant pattern with extremely high penetrance. In large series, 50% of offspring will manifest the disease; that is, all who carry the affected gene will manifest the trait. The expression of the gene may vary. Mean age of onset in a large sample as defined by choreiform movements was 42 years. However, behavioral changes, including depression and suicide attempts, may precede the movement disorder by 10 years or more.

Earlier onset of disease is associated with a more rapid course and with the earlier development of features of rigidity. The juvenile-onset type with rapid progression to a rigid state has received the designation as the Westphal variant. Such patients, for unknown reasons, are more likely to have inherited the gene from the father.

Late-onset cases (onset between 50 and 70 years of life) have a much more prolonged course and choreiform movements are often the predominant feature (see Sax and Vonsattel, 1992). At times the term *senile chorea* has been utilized for these late-onset cases, which are more likely to have involved cases in the maternal line.

Modern genetic analysis using recombinant DNA techniques and studying families with large numbers of affected individuals or large numbers at risk have allowed the localization of the marker site for the gene on the short arm of chromosome 4. (See Gusella et al. [1983]; Martin and Gusella [1986]; Penny and Young [1988]; Roberts [1990]; Wexler et al. [1992].) The specific mutation has now been identified as an unstable trinucleotide repeat in the CAG series coding for polyglutamine tracts at the 4p16.3 locus on this chromosome. Normal individuals have 6–35 repeats; patients with

Huntington's disease have 40 or more expansions). Individuals with 36–39 repeats may also develop the disease but penetrance is incomplete. *The gene product is huntingtin.* Patients with onset at an early age or with a more severe form of the disease have a greater number of repeats. As we have already discussed in Chapter 9 on the spinal cord, similar mutations involving an excessive number of CAG repeats have also been found in a number of other neurological disorders, including several of the spinocerebellar degenerations and spinobulbar muscular atrophy. Other disorders such as myotonic dystrophy and Friedreich's ataxia have an excessive number of repeats in other trinucleotide sequences. Presymptomatic detection is possible, but this should be done under circumstances where a full gamut of genetic counseling is available. The underlying gross pathology has been well established (Fig. 19.9). Marked atrophy of caudate nucleus and putamen are the pathologic and neuroimaging hallmarks. This gross pathological feature allows for diagnosis and subsequent monitoring of progression by means of CT scan and MRI scan (Fig. 19.10) (Myers et al., 1985; Vonsattel et al., 1985). In addition, significant cortical atrophy also occurs as the disease progresses. The gene product huntingtin is expressed widely throughout the brain. There are high levels in both large striatal interneurons and medium spiny neurons, as well as cortical pyramidal cells and cerebellar Purkinje cells.

Additional analysis has indicated that not all cells and transmitters in the caudate and putamen are involved in the process of degeneration. The extensive studies have been reviewed by Albin et al. (1990); Martin and Gusella (1986); Penney and Young (1988); Young et al. (1988). The cells affected are classified as medium-sized, spiny neurons that project to sites outside the striatum and which constitute approximately 90% of all striatal neurons. All contain the transmitter GABA.[9] However, different subtypes are distinguished based on the specific associated neuropeptide that they contain, for example, enkephalin, substance P, and/or dynorphin and based on the projection destinations. On the other hand, other cells

Figure 19.10 Huntington's disease. Case 19.4. Magnetic resonance imaging (MRI). Refer to text. Marked atrophy of cerebral cortex and of caudate nucleus is evident in this patient with a familial history of the disorder and a significant increase in the CAG trinucleotide repeats.

with interneuron functions are not affected: (a) the large, spiny acetylcholine-containing interneurons and (b) the small aspiny interneurons containing the neuropeptides somatostatin and substance Y. Refer to Table 19.2.

Early in the course of the disease there is a loss of those spiny neurons which contain the GABA and enkephalin transmitters and which project to the lateral globus pallidus. At this point in the disease, the loss of these striatal inhibitory inputs to the lateral globus pallidus results in increased activity (inhibitory) of the lateral globus pallidus neurons. Since the lateral globus pallidus is the main input to the subthalamic nucleus and this input is inhibitory, an increased inhibition of the subthalamic nucleus results. As a result, the excitatory output from the subthalamic nucleus to the medial globus pallidus (MGP) and substantia nigra reticularis (SNR) is reduced. The output of neurons in MGP and SNR is reduced. This output is inhibitory and destined for ventrolateral thalamus. The output of ventrolateral thalamus is no longer inhibited—and increased activity occurs in the ventrolateral to supplementary motor cortex circuit. Abnormal excessive movements due to increased activity of supplementary motor area (SMA) then results as discussed earlier under the section on hemichorea.

The following case history provides an example of Huntington's disease.

Figure 19.9 Huntington's disease. Marked atrophy of the caudate and putamen with secondary dilatation of the lateral ventricles is evident. Cortical atrophy was less prominent in this case. (Courtesy of Doctor Emanuel Ross, Chicago.)

CASE HISTORY 19.4

This 54-year-old, right-handed white female was referred for evaluation of a movement disorder. The patient lived alone and it was difficult to obtain much of any history from the patient. She denied any neurological or psychiatric disorders except for a problem with memory during the last year. She did indicate that she had worked for 10 years as a secretary/computer operator but had been fired 10 years ago because "she did not work fast enough." She had a past history of hypertension but had not been reliable in taking her prescribed medication. The patient's son was aware that changes in emotion,

---

[9] These neurons are located in the matrix. Matrix neurons that appear late in development are the earliest affected; it is not until very late in the disease that patch neurons are affected.

personality, speech, and gait and a movement disorder had been present for at least 3 years.

Family history: The patient denied any neurological family history except for a maternal uncle who had the "shakes" (actually a maternal aunt with essential tremor); additional investigation revealed that her father clearly had Huntington's disease with onset of choreiform movements at age 30, and of irritability, paranoia, and gait disturbance in his early 50s. The patient's eldest daughter, age 34, had been depressed for 5 years and had problems with speech and walking for a number of years.

Neurological Examination

Mental status: The patient often avoided eye contact. Affect was usually inappropriate, with laughter as the response to many questions. The overall mini-mental status score was 27/30. The only deficit related to delayed recall portion of the test (0/3 objects).

Cranial nerves: The patient had a hyperactive jaw jerk. She had frequent facial grimacing.

Motor system:

a. The patient had decreased tone at wrists and elbows.
b. As she sat, she had frequent restless and at times choreiform movements of hands and feet.
c. Gait was often "bizarre" in terms of occasional sudden movements of a leg as she moved down the hall and came to a stop. These same movements occurred as she remained standing.
d. In addition, in standing or walking, there were intermittent dystonic postures of either left or right arm.

Reflexes: Deep tendon stretch reflexes were everywhere hyperactive but plantar responses were flexor.

Sensory system: Intact.

Clinical diagnosis: Huntington's disease.

Laboratory data: *MRI scans of head* (Fig. 19.10): The heads of the caudate nuclei were very atrophic. Cortical sulci were wide, consistent with cortical atrophy. The lateral and third ventricles were secondarily dilated.

PCR testing for the CAG trinucleotide repeats of the huntingtin gene indicated one allele normal at 17; and the second excessive at 42 repeats.

Subsequent course: The patient refused any treatment for the movement disorder. According to the son, the patient's neurological status worsened to a moderate degree over the subsequent 3 years as regards speech, unsteadiness of gait, and mood swings.

Comments

Occasionally patients are encountered who, due to changes in psychological function, are limited in the information that they can provide. In other cases denial of illness has a neurological as well as a psychological basis. In this case it was evident that this patient had not only symptoms relevant to the basal ganglia but also changes in cognitive function relevant to the cerebral cortex, particularly the frontal areas. In such cases, information must be sought from other sources. In this case, the patient was willing to provide permission to contact those possible sources.

The clinical presentation in this case was clear-cut. In retrospect, many of the neurological features were similar to her father's findings on his admission 30 years previously. When did the patient's disease begin? This was uncertain, but we may presume that serious problems had been present at least 10 years earlier when she had been fired from her long-time employment. Did this relate to motor problems, to changes in personality and interpersonal relations, or to cognitive changes? Most likely, there were problems in all of these areas. According to her family, symptoms had been present for 2–3 years, suggesting onset at age 51 or 52 years.

The following case history provides an example of a patient with Huntington's disease followed over a longer period of time.

CASE HISTORY 19.5

This 32-year-old, right-handed, married white male spray painter at a computer factory was referred for evaluation of a possible hereditary movement disorder. The patient was unclear about the reasons for his evaluation and much of the history was provided by his wife. She reported that the patient had undergone a personality change in the last several months. He had noticeable mood swings and on one occasion he reported people outside the window when no one actually had been there. He had some problems with remembering incidental matters, but no major problems, and his job performance had remained intact. He was described as always having been "fidgety."

Past medical history: Mild hypertension for 3 years.

Family history: The patient's initial history indicated that the family supposedly had Parkinson's disease and his father had died in his 40's at the state hospital after a 10- to 15-year illness. The patient indicated that he was a child at the time and his mother never really told him much about the father or let him visit the father in the hospital, but he did recall that perhaps his father had some excessive movements of the hands and face. The records were subsequently obtained, and these indicated the father had been admitted to Worcester State Hospital in 1968 at age 37. At that time, he had already had three previous hospitalizations for "nervous breakdowns." At the time of his final admission, he had developed hallucinations, seeing people in his room. He had threatened his wife and other relatives. He had difficulty sleeping and he had also developed a problem with his legs, that is, "they are jumping." The father's examination had demonstrated a mumbled speech with repetition of the same phrases. His responses would often be tangential and then incoherent with impairment of memory and judgment. His mood was depressed. He was noted to have involuntary movements of the fingers and occasional facial grimacing. The deep tendon reflexes were hyperactive and the plantar responses were extensor. His gait was ataxic. The subsequent course indicated increasing ataxia, choreiform movements, and rigidity with increasing weakness, difficulty swallowing, and the final development of bronchial pneumonia with death at age 42. *The diagnosis of Huntington's disease was confirmed at autopsy.*

The paternal grandfather had expired at age 67 with a diagnosis of Huntington's disease, manifested by "nervous breakdowns, inability to sleep, and movement disorder." The father's three siblings apparently did not manifest the disease. The patient had two siblings—a brother, age 28, and a sister, age 35—all without known disease. He had two children, ages 9 and 5.

Neurological Examination

Mental status: The patient was anxious and often appeared blunted in emotional expression or in answering questions. He avoided eye contact. He was oriented for time, place, and person. He was able to name objects and colors. His delayed recall was 2/5 without assistance and 4/5 with assistance.

Cranial nerves II–XII were intact, except for the occurrence of occasional, sudden darting movements of the eyes to either left or right. In addition, occasional facial grimacing was noted, occurring in a rather irregular manner.

Motor system:

a. Strength and gait were intact.
b. There were occasional, sudden, irregular, lateral, tremulous movements of the fingers of a choreiform type.

Reflexes:

a. Deep tendon reflexes, including the jaw jerk, were everywhere hyperactive.
b. Plantar responses were bilaterally extensor (bilateral Babinski signs).

Sensory system: Intact.

Clinical diagnosis: Huntington's disease.

Laboratory Data

All blood chemistries, including glucose, BUN, calcium, electrolytes, liver function studies, ceruloplasmin level, thyroid studies, and serological test for syphilis were within normal limits. Ceruloplasmin levels are low in Wilson's disease but normal in Huntington's disease.

Electroencephalogram was normal with a dominant awake background activity of 10 Hz alpha rhythm.

CT scan of the head demonstrated enlargement of the ventricles with particular atrophy of the caudate. In addition, the sulci were prominent for the age, suggesting some degree of cortical atrophy. The study was considered consistent with the clinical diagnosis of Huntington's disease.

The *MRI scan* demonstrated mild enlargement of the ventricles and deepening of the cortical sulci, as well as a very significant atrophy of the head of the caudate nucleus. The MRI from this patient is compared to a similar section from a patient without signs of neurological disease.

Subsequent course: The patient subsequently developed increased paranoid ideation, increasing dependency with regard to his wife. He was treated with haloperidol (a neuroleptic, tranquilizer) with considerable improvement with regard to personality. When evaluated, 3 years after onset of disease, it was evident that in the interim, the patient's personality problems had decreased. Attacks of anger and paranoid features had subsided. Mood swings were less. Memory problems, however, were worse and choreiform movements were worse. Dysarthria was now present. The patient had been divorced in the interim, and he was on Social Security disability and no longer working. The examination now showed an exacerbation of many of those features noted at the time of his initial evaluation. He had occasional, sporadic movements of head or eyes of a choreiform nature. He had frequent choreiform movements involving the fingers as he was sitting; also a similar type of movement appeared to involve the abdominal musculature. He had a moderate degree of dysarthria. He could walk a tandem gait but as he did so, the left arm came up in a somewhat flexed position.

When last seen 4 years after onset of disease, he had more dysarthria and his speech was more difficult to interpret. There had been some increase in degree of rigidity, but this had decreased when the dose of haloperidol had been decreased. The decrease in this medication, however, then resulted in a greater prominence of the choreiform movements. He could still handle a deck of cards, although he was dropping objects more often than previously. His neurological examination showed a significant degree of dysarthria, a greater degree of facial akinesia, and more frequent choreiform movements of hands and face. He had difficulty in mimicking facial expression. As before, all of his deep tendon reflexes were hyperactive and the plantar responses were extensor. The patient walked in a flexed position and tended to turn en bloc. He had a mild degree of cogwheel rigidity at wrist and elbows. His memory remained remarkably good for delayed recall.

Final telephone follow-up with his primary physician (approximately 7 years after apparent clinical onset of disease) indicated that the patient was no longer able to drive. He had continued weight loss. He had a marked dysarthria so that his speech was barely intelligible. Choreiform movements had increased. His gait was ataxic, but he could still walk without stumbling. He was relatively stable from a psychiatric standpoint. He was now living with his mother and brother.

Comments

This patient and his family demonstrate the relatively typical course of most patients with Huntington's disease. Patients and families do vary as to whether it is the psychiatric features or the movement disorder features that first bring the patient to medical attention. In this case, the psychiatric features, that is, the change in personality and the increasing paranoid ideation, were the first features noted. Subsequently, involvement of the motor system became the most prominent feature. As in the previous case, the patient was unclear as to why he had come for neurological evaluation. Was this a neurological or a psychological denial of illness? Most likely both factors were operational. It was of considerable interest that this patient when first seen, although he was aware of some neurological problem that had occurred in the family, was unclear as to the specific diagnosis. It was also evident that almost no genetic counseling had been done in a disorder that was very clearly an autosomal dominant disorder. The significant family impact of the disease, both socially and economically, is clearly evident in this patient. The implications of presymptomatic detection are discussed by Klawans (1972).

OTHER MOVEMENT DISORDERS ASSOCIATED WITH DISEASES OF THE BASAL GANGLIA

Double Athetosis

Athetosis may be described as instability of posture, a relatively continuous alternation or swing between two positions. For example, in the hand, this would involve a swing from hyperextension of the fingers and thumb with pronation at the wrist to full flexion of the fingers with flexion and supination of the wrist. In a sense, there is an alternation between grasp and avoidance. Occasionally, following cerebral infarction at various ages, athetosis may occur as a unilateral phenomenon admixed with hemichorea. In general, athetosis occurs as a bilateral congenital phenomenon with involvement not only of the upper extremities but also of the lips, tongue, and lower extremities. Double athetosis is one of the varieties of cerebral palsy discussed in Chapter 18. The pathology of double athetosis is found in the putamen that may have a marbled or mottled appearance as a result of the presence of excessive numbers of abnormally situated myelin sheaths. To a lesser degree, the thalamus may also be involved. The etiology is not certain: anoxia at birth or other perinatal or prenatal pathology is considered the likely cause. Some of the cases can be related to kernicterus—the rise in bilirubin that occurs in the perinatal period owing to hemolysis of red blood cells when an Rh factor or other incompatibility of blood type has been present.

Hepatolenticular Degeneration (Wilson's Disease)

This is a familial disorder (recessive inheritance) that affects, to a variable degree, the liver and the central nervous system and, in many cases, the kidney and bones. In the central nervous system, the most severe involvement occurs in the basal ganglia: the putamen and globus pallidus (cavitation, loss of neurons, and an increased number of swollen astrocytes). To a lesser extent, the cerebellum and cerebral cortex are involved.

The basic etiology has now been clearly established as a metabolic defect. There is a deficient plasma level of the circulating copper-binding globulin, ceruloplasmin.[10] As a result, there is an excessive serum level of unbound copper. Normally, the binding of copper to ceruloplasmin prevents the passage of copper out of the serum. In Wilson's disease, however, the increased amount of unbound copper results in passage of this metal into the brain,[11] liver, and kidney (The total combined level of both bound and unbound serum copper is less than normal.) In some cases, usually of early onset, the symptoms of liver involvement predominate. Wilson's disease should always be suspected when hepatocellular disease develops in a child or adolescent. In other cases, the central nervous symptoms predominate and hepatic disease may be only minor. Deposition of copper also occurs in the cornea at the scleral junction. The resultant greenish-brown pigmentation is referred to as the Kaiser-Fleischer ring. This ring is almost always present when central nervous system involvement is present. Overall, 54% of cases present with neurological onset, 31% with hepatic dysfunction, 14% with psychiatric symptoms, 2% with eye symptoms, 1% to 2% with hemolytic anemia, and 1% with heart disease (see Patten, 1988). In patients with hypersplenism as a complication of the hepatic disease, thrombocytopenia may develop.

The actual symptoms referable to the neurological involvement depend on the age of the patient. In early-onset cases (late childhood and early adolescence) rigidity predominates. When cases begin in early adult life, movement disorders predominate (tremor and choreoathetosis). The tremor is coarse and best described as sustained postural. The term "wing beating" is often used. The copper also produces damage to the renal tubules, resulting in glycosuria and aminoaciduria. Diagnosis can be based on the clinical findings, ceruloplasmin levels (normal levels are 200 to 400 mg/liter), serum copper (normal total levels are 11 to 24 μmol/liter versus 3 to 10 in Wilson's disease). The most definitive study involves analysis of copper content in a liver biopsy. The CT scan and MRI may demonstrate the lesions in the putamen and globus pallidus.

The treatment of Wilson's disease is dependent on a reduction of copper in the diet or the administration of an agent that will bind copper. Penicillamine (B.B-dimethyl-cysteine) is an effective chelator of copper. It is well absorbed on oral administration and promotes the urinary excretion of copper, resulting in a decreased level of copper in the serum, central nervous system, and liver.

The following case history illustrates the clinical problem of hepatolenticular degeneration in a 21-year-old female who developed progressive neurologic syndrome characterized by mood swings, a wing-beating tremor, choreoathetosis, dysarthria, ataxia, and a Kayser Fleischer ring. Her brother had died at age 16 with hepatic disease, a Kayser Fleischer ring, and choreoathetosis. The patient had serum elevation of free copper and a decrease in protein-bound copper and an abnormal liver biopsy. She was successfully treated with penicillamine.

CASE HISTORY 19.6 (PATIENT OF DR. HUNTINGTON PORTER)

This 21-year-old, single, white female shoe worker in January 1954 had the onset of a "shaking," or trembling of the fingers and hands, which progressed to involve both arms and legs. The degree of involvement increased sufficiently to force her to give up her work. Nine months after onset of symptoms, she began to note increasing difficulty with balance and coordination and a slurring of speech. She had also noted increasing weakness and difficulty in doing repetitive tasks. One year after onset, the patient noted blurring of vision, occasional diplopia, and periods of "staring." She also had experienced increasing urgency and occasional urinary incontinence.

Family history: A brother of the patient had died in 1952, at age 16, of a disease with manifestations similar to this patient's. Evaluation of the sibling 2 years before his death by Drs. John Sullivan, Raymond Adams, and D. Denny-Brown, had indicated the presence of choreoathetosis with lapses in posture of the hands. In addition, a brownish-green ring at the corneal scleral junction was noted. Liver disease was present in this sibling and possibly other members of the family.

Neurological Examination
Mental status:

a. The patient was anxious, at times crying and at other times euphoric.
b. Digit span was limited to 6 forward, 3 in reverse.
c. Serial 7 subtractions were poorly performed.

Cranial nerves:

a. A brown rim was present at the limbus of the cornea, more evidence inferiorly and superiorly.
b. Extraocular movements were impaired by involuntary jerk movements. The patient was unable to track a moving finger.
c. Facial expression was mask-like.
d. Speech was dysarthric and of a nasal quality with slurring and slowness of articulation.

---

[10] In a few cases, ceruloplasmin levels are just within normal limits, but biliary excretion of copper is low. Absorption of copper is normal in all cases.

[11] The distribution of copper in the normal brain corresponds in general to the distribution of catecholamine-containing neurons. Dopamine B hydroxylase is a copper-containing enzyme with considerable localization to the basal ganglia. However, copper is also found in cytochrome C-oxidase, which is found throughout the brain.

Motor system:

a. No actual weakness was present. However, this patient had difficulty maintaining the limbs in a fixed posture.
b. There was a rigidity to passive movement of the limbs.
c. A coarse arrythmic tremor was present which was most marked proximally and more marked on sustained posture and on movement than at rest.
d. Alternating movements were poorly performed.
e. Gait was ataxic. Romberg test was negative.

Reflexes: Deep tendon stretch reflexes were hyperactive, but plantar responses were flexor.

Sensation: Intact.

Clinical diagnosis: Wilson's disease: hepatolenticular degeneration.

Laboratory data:

a. *Liver function tests* were normal.
b. *Glucose tolerance test* was normal, but glycosuria occurred.

Total plasma copper: 52 µg/100 ml (normal range in a young adult is 65 to 150 µg/100 ml).

Direct reacting copper (unbound to ceruloplasmin): 31 µg/100ml (normal 10 µg/100 ml). *Indirect copper* (ceruloplasmin bound): 21 µg/100 ml (normal 105 µg/ml).

Subsequent course: The patient did relatively well following the use of the chelating agents, BAL, and calcium versenate and the institution of a copper-free diet. A liver biopsy performed at the time of a cesarean section 18 months after beginning treatment was compatible with perihepatitis with a question of postnecrotic cirrhosis.

Re-evaluation 6 years after onset revealed, in addition to the earlier findings, the presence of "continual spontaneous involuntary movements of the limbs; at the feet, characterized by alternating flexion and extension at the ankle and a waving of the toes." A broad-amplitude coarse tremor was noted when the patient was asked to abduct arms, flex elbows, and hold hands just before her nose (wing-beating position). A side-to-side tremor of the head was also present. The gait was slightly wide-based and associated with continual dystonic movements of the hands and arms. Treatment with d-penicillamine (which had just become available) was begun at that time. Urine copper excretion increased from 700 µg per 24 hours to 3240 µg per 24 hours. Normal 24-hour urinary copper in the adult is less than 40 µg. Neurological symptoms soon demonstrated improvement from the previously noted status. The patient was now able to do her housework and take care of her children.

Follow-up 2 years later indicated significant improvement as regards the findings noted in 1960; dystonic facies and dysarthria were less marked. No tremor was present in the left hand; that in the right hand was evident only when under tension. Dystonic posturing of the hands was present only to a minimal degree. At last report 4 years later, and 12 years after onset of the disease, the patient continued to do well. She had remarried and was expecting another child.

Comments

This patient presents a typical case of Wilson's disease with onset in the young adult years and with a definite familial background. The copper levels were consistent with the diagnosis (an increased unbound fraction and a decreased bound fraction). At the time that this patient was seen in the mid 1950s and early 1960s, ceruloplasmin levels were not available. Early establishment of a specific diagnosis in this case allowed for specific therapy with improvement of neurological symptoms and the prevention of progression of hepatic disease. With a specific diagnosis established in the patient, periodic blood tests were performed on her offspring to determine whether they also had inherited this genetic disease. (The child born 18 months after onset of the disease did not have the disorder.)

An acquired form of non-Wilsonian hepatic and cerebral degeneration occurs in patients who have had multiple episodes of hepatic coma. Degenerative changes occur in the astrocytes and neurons of the basal ganglia. This disorder, which was first described by Adams and Victor, is discussed in greater detail earlier in this chapter.

Dystonia

Dystonia is a hyperkinetic disorder dominated by sustained muscle contractions frequently causing twisting and repetitive movements or abnormal postures (Jankovic and Fahn, 1988). Dystonia may be focal (43%), segmental (30%), generalized (22%), or unilateral (5%). Focal dystonias are more common than the generalized form. Classifications may also include the terms early-onset versus late-onset and limb versus cranial location for that onset.

Focal and Segmental Idiopathic Dystonias

Focal dystonia affects predominantly a single body part, primarily cranial and cervical muscles. Involvement of limbs is less common. *Segmental* refers to dystonia involving multiple segments, usually cranial and cervical. Included within this category of cervical dystonia is the relatively common entity of spasmodic torticollis in which sudden movements of the head to one side occur. The movement may be intermittent or sustained. Focal or segmental dystonia involving the cranial nerves is termed *Meige's syndrome*.

The most frequent of the cranial dystonias is blepharospasm, in which there is forced eye closure. Other aspects of cranial dystonia may involve the tongue and jaw; lingual and oromandibular. Other overlapping variants may involve the larynx (spasmodic dysphonia) or the pharynx, with the latter producing difficulty in swallowing. Other focal dystonias known as occupational dystonias involve the more specific muscles of the hand and arm utilized in specific actions: writers, typists, violinists, and pianists. The underlying neuropathology has never been clearly established in idiopathic cases. However, blepharospasm, or dystonia of the foot, does occur in Parkinson's disease; retrocollis and oculogyric crises occur in postencephalitis Parkinson's disease. L-dopa and neuroleptic agents may both induce focal dystonias. The most effective treatment of focal/segmental dystonia is botulinum toxin injections that must be repeated every 3–4 months.

Generalized Dystonia

The terms "primary generalized idiopathic dystonia" and "idiopathic torsion dystonia" have replaced the older term "dystonia musculorum deformans." Most cases begin in childhood or adolescence and are familial. Autosomal dominant inheritance is now considered predominant in both Ashkenazi Jewish and non-Jewish families, with a mutation in a gene on chromosome 9. The most common cause of early limb onset primary dystonia is the autosomal dominant mutation in the DYT1 gene, which codes for Torsin A that codes for a protein *torsin A*. This mutation has been identified for the majority of cases of juvenile limb onset cases. Torsin A is a member of a family of ATPases concerned with cellular activities. There is a CAG deletion. This mutation is five times more frequent in Ashkenazi compared to non-Ashkenazi Jews. Overexpression of mutant Torsin A leads to the formation of membrane inclusions. Among gene carriers of this autosomal dominant mutation, 70% have no definite signs of dystonia. The remaining 30% have a dystonia that ranges from focal to generalized.

Anticholinergic drugs at high dosage levels may improve the symptoms of generalized dystonia in some patients. Approximately 10% of juvenile-onset cases beginning in the lower extremities described by the expression of dystonia range from mild focal to severe generalized.

Segawa Disease

This is a childhood-onset variant which begins in the lower extremities with a stiff gait. This is an autosomal dominant disorder coding to chromosome 14 and involving guanosine triphosphate cyclohydrolase 1 gene (GCH1) on chromosome 14 and is referred to as DYT 5. The disorder has a remarkable response to low dosage of L-Dopa (termed the L Dopa-responsive variant of progressive generalized dystonia). It has therefore been recommended that all juvenile-onset cases receive a trial of the L-Dopa/carbidopa combination.

The full spectrum of the genetics of dystonia has been recently reviewed by Schwarz and Bressman (2009), to whom the reader is referred. Their conclusion is that it is advisable to assume a genetic etiology for most early-onset primary torsion dystonia, especially those beginning in childhood or adolescence where there is onset in an arm or leg, which subsequently generalizes, or in those of Ashkenazi Jewish descent. It is important also to recognize overlap with other types of movement disorders.

Hemidystonia

Approximately 75% of patients in the hemidystonia group do have the history, findings, or CT or MRI evidence of a contralateral neuropathology involving the striatum, usually the putamen or striato-pallido-thalamic pathway. The corticospinal pathways are not usually involved. There is then presumably an excessive input into premotor/supplementary motor cortex, resulting in the excessive contralateral movement.

Movement Disorders Induced by Dopamine-Blocking Agents

Sethi (2001) has provided a comprehensive review of this topic.

These agents produce frequent acute and chronic complications in psychiatric patients:

1. *Acute dystonic reactions*: These occur in 2%–5% of patients within hours or days after onset of therapy with neuroleptic agents. Note that this complication occurs not only in psychiatric patients but also in patients receiving agents of this class as antiemetics.

2. *Acute akathesia*: Acute restlessness and an inability to sit still occur in 20% of patients receiving dopamine-blocking agents.

3. *Acute drug-induced Parkinsonian syndrome* discussed earlier. Although symptoms may appear in any patient given a sufficient amount of dopamine-blocking agents to block 80% of receptors, there does appear to be a predisposition to develop symptoms at a lower, more therapeutic range in patients with a family history of Parkinsonism.

4. *Tardive dyskinesia and other tardive reactions*. In this context, tardive has been defined as 3 months of exposure to the agent (1 month for patients over the age of 60 years). There may be a genetic predisposition.

Tardive dyskinesias are hyperkinetic choreiform movements. Usually these are seen in the older patient involving the mouth, tongue, lips, and face[12]: oral buccolingual facial masticatory syndrome. Symptoms usually develop after 6–24 months of drug therapy, and in many patients the symptoms decrease after drug withdrawal.

In another group of patients, symptoms develop only after neuroleptic drugs have been withdrawn or dosage has been reduced again after prolonged use. In one series, such withdrawal or dose reduction resulted in tardive dyskinesia in 40% of patients receiving chronic neuroleptic therapy. The presumed pathophysiology is not entirely clear.

5. *Tics:* Motor tics are sudden, brief involuntary movements resembling jerks or gestures. The patient may experience a poorly defined sensation of an irresistible urge to move prior to the movement. These movements may be simple: an eye blink, a head jerk, or a facial grimace. In some cases, the movement is more complex and patterned, resembling a compulsive act. In some cases (syndrome of Gilles de la Tourette which has autosomal dominant transmission), multiple tics occur accompanied by vocalizations. The vocalization may consist of a simple sound or may involve the use of obscene four-letter words referring to defecation, genitalia, or sexual acts (coprolalia). In contrast to other movement disorders, voluntary effort accompanied by anxiety may serve to inhibit the occurrence of the tic or tics. Then a flurry of tics may occur after the suppression. Tics may continue to occur in sleep. The usual idiopathic tics are common in children and may persist into adult life. Lees and Tolosa (1988) indicate 1 of 10 schoolboys will have idiopathic tics.

The data presented by Jimenez-Shahed (2009) indicate that chronic motor or vocal tics have a prevalence of 2%–5%. Transient tics have a prevalence of 3%–15%. The overall worldwide prevalence of Tourette's syndrome is estimated at 1%. Males are affected three times as often as females both in idiopathic tics and in Tourette's syndrome. No specific neuropathology has been established. Use of dopaminergic receptor-blocking agents such as haloperidol, Primozide, or fluphenazine may often produce a significant decrease in the

---

[12] In younger individuals, the limbs and trunk are more often involved.

clinical symptoms; in contrast, dopaminergic agents (L-dopa, bromocriptine) and amphetamines may produce an exacerbation of symptoms (Jankovic, 1987; Singer, 2000).

Note that a high proportion of patients with Tourette's syndrome also will manifest attention-deficit disorder and obsessive-compulsive disorder.

6. *Restless legs syndrome:* In this common syndrome, there is an urge to move the legs which improves with activity and worsens at night. The problem occurs frequently in the elderly, perhaps as many as 57% in the elderly age group. The prevalence in the general population may be as high as 29%. There is often a family history, but the specific gene mutation has not been identified. There is a relationship to central nervous system iron metabolism. Dopamine agonists treat restless legs syndrome. Cases may also be seen after spinal cord injuries. Incidence is also higher in pregnancy and uremia. Ondo (2009) has reviewed the topic.

7. *Familial paroxysmal dyskinesias*: These disorders, although not common, are of significance because they undoubtedly occur on the basis of channelopathies. The specific genetic mutation has not yet been identified. In this regard, they are similar to the episodic ataxias discussed in Chapter 20, periodic paralysis, and familial hemiplegic migraine, in which the specific ion channel mutation has been identified (see Bhatia, 2001, and Bhatia et al., 2000). In all of the syndromes, the neurological examination is normal between attacks. In the majority, autosomal dominance occurs and males predominate. Two major entities may be identified: (1) paroxysmal kinesigenic choreoathetosis/dyskinesias (PKC/PKD) and (2) paroxysmal dystonic choreoathetosis/nonkinesigenic dyskinesias (PDC/PNKD).

The first type (PKC/PKD) is the most common. Attacks lasting less than 5 minutes begin in childhood with multiple attacks per day induced by movement of chorea, dystonia, and ballism. The attacks are significantly reduced by the administration of low doses of the anticonvulsant carbamazepine, which has action on the sodium/potassium channel. Several families have mapped to the pericentromeric region of chromosome 16, where a group of ion channel genes are present.

The second type (PDC/PNKD) begins in infancy or childhood with infrequent attacks that last from 10 minutes to 6 hours and are predominantly dystonic. The attacks are induced by stress, fatigue, alcohol, and caffeine. In a number of families (Jarman et al., 1997) the genetic defect has been mapped to chromosome locus 2q33-q35, an area where a number of ion channel genes are located.

Paroxysmal exercise-induced dyskinesia (PED) is a third less common variety.

BIBLIOGRAPHY

Agid, Y., Cervera, D., Hirsh, E., et al. 1989. Biochemistry of parkinson's disease 28 years later: a critical review. Mov. Disord. 4(Suppl. 1): 126–144.

Agid, Y., Javoy-Agid, F., and Ruberg, M. 1987. Biochemistry of neurotransmitters in Parkinson's disease. In C. D. Marsden and S. Fahn (Eds.) Movement Disorders 2, pp. 166–230. London, UK: Butterworths.

Albin, D., Young, A. B., and Penney, J. B. 1989. The functional anatomy of basal ganglia disorders. Trends Neurosci. 12:366–375.

Albin, R. I., Young, A. B., Penney, J. B., et al. 1990. Abnormalities of striatal projection neurons and N-methyl D-aspartate receptors in presymptomatic Huntington's disease. N. Engl. J. Med. 322:1293–1298.

Alexander, G. E., De Long, M. R., and Strick, P. L. 1986. Parallel organization of functionally segregated circuits linking basal ganglia and cortex. Ann. Rev. Neurosci. 9:375–381.

Alyward, E. H., Codori, A. M., Rosenblatt, A., et al. 2000. Rate of caudate atrophy in pre-symptomatic and symptomatic stages of Huntington's disease. Mov. Disord. 15:552–560.

Aziz, T. Z., Peggs, D., Sambrook, M. A., and Crossman, A. R. 1991. Lesion of the subthalamic nucleus for the alleviation of l-methyl-4 phenyl 1,2,3,6, tetrahydropyridine (MPTP) induced Parkinsonism in the primate. Mov. Disord. 6:288–292.

Ballard, P. H., Tetrud, J. W., and Langston, J. W. 1985. Permanent human Parkinsonism due to l-methyl-4 phenyl, 1,2,3,6, tetra-hydropyrine (mptp): seven cases. Neurology 35:949–956.

Bandmann, O., Sweeney, M. G., Daniel, S. E., et al. 1997. Multiple system atrophy is genetically distinct from identified inherited causes of spinocerebellar degeneration. Brain 49:1598–1604.

Berciano, J. 1988. Olivopontocerebellar atrophy. In J. Jankovic and E. Tolosa (Eds.) Parkinson's sisease and Movement Disorders, pp. 131–151. Baltimore, MD and Munich, Germany: Urban & Schwartzenberg.

Bergman, H., Wichmann, T., DeLong, M. R. 1990. Reversal of experimental Parkinsonism by lesions of the subthalamic nucleus. Science 249:1436–1438.

Bhatia, K. P. 2001. Familial (idiopathic) paroxysmal dyskinesias. an update. Semin. Neurol. 21:69–74.

Bhatia, K. P., Griggs, R. C., and Ptacek, L. J. 2000. Episodic movement disorders as channelopathies. Mov. Disord. 15:429–423.

Bloom, F. E., and Roth, R. H. 1991. The Biochemical Basis of Neuropharmacology. New York, NY: Oxford University Press. (See in particular Chapter 10: Dopamine, pp.285–337)

Brashear, A. 2001. The botulinum toxins in the treatment of cervical dystonia. Semin. Neurol. 21:85–90.

Brooks, D. J. 1991. Detection of preclinical Parkinson's disease with PET. Neurology 41(Suppl. 2):24–27.

Cardoso, F. 2009. Huntington disease and other choreas. Neurol. Clin. 27:719–736.

Cooper, I. S. 1969. Involuntary Movement Disorders. New York, NY: Hoeber Medical Division.

Cooper, J. R. 1991. Movement Disorders. New York, NY: Paul B. Hoeber.

Cote, L., and Crutcher, M. D. 1991. The basal ganglia. In E. R. Kandel, J. H. Schwartz, and T. M. Jessell (Eds.) *Principles of Neural Science*. 3rd ed., pp. 647–659. New York, NY: Elsevier.

Cotzias, G. C., Papavasiliou, P. S., and Gellen, R. 1969. Modification of Parkinsonism—chronic treatment with L-dopa. N. Engl. J. Med. 280:337–345.

Cotzias, G. C., Van Woert, M. H., and Schiffer, L. M. 1967. Aromatic amino acids and modification of Parkinsonism. N. Engl. J. Med. 276:374–379.

Crossman, A. R. 1990. A hypothesis on the pathophysiological mechanisms that underlie levodopa or dopamine agonist induced dyskinesia in Parkinson's disease: implications for the future strategies in treatment. Mov. Disord. 5:100–108.

Crossman, A. R., Mitchell, I. J., Sambrook, M. A., and Jackson, A. 1988. Chorea and myoclonus in the monkey induced by gamma amino butyric acid antagonism in the lentiform complex. The site of drug action and a hypothesis for the neural mechanism of chorea. Brain 121:1–33.

Daniel, S. E., de Bruin, V. M., and Lees, A. J. 1995. The clinical and pathological spectrum of Steele-Richardson Olszewski syndrome (progressive supranuclear palsy): a reappraisal. Brain 118:759–770.

De Bie, R. M. A., Schuurman, P. R., de Haan, P. S., et al. 1999. Unilateral pallidotomy in advanced Parkinson's disease: a retrospective study of 26 patients. Mov. Diosord. 14:951–957.

Delwaide, P. J., and Gance, M. 1988. Pathophysiology of Parkinson's signs. In J. Jankovic and E. Tolosa.(Eds.) Parkinson's Disease and Movement Disorders, pp. 59–73. Baltimore, MD and Munich, Germany: Urban and Schwarzenberg.

Denny-Brown, D. 1962. The Basal Ganglia and Their Relation to Disorder of Movement. London, UK: Oxford University Press.

Deuschl, G. 2000. Treatment options for tremor. N. Engl. J. Med. 342:505–507.

Dunnett, S. B., and Bjorklund, A. 1999. Prospects for new restorative and neuroprotective treatments in Parkinson's disease. Nature. 399(Suppl.):A32–A39.

Duvoisin, R. C.1998. Familial Parkinson's disease. NeuroSci. News 1:43–46.

Ebersbach, G., Sojer, M., Valladeoriopla, F., et al. 1999. Comparative analysis of gait in Parkinson's disease. Cerebellar ataxia and subcortical arteriosclerotic encephalopathy. Brain 122:1349–1355.

Eidelberg, D., Sortel, A., Joachim, C., et al. 1987. Adult onset Lallervorden-Spatz disease with neurofibrillary pathology. A discrete clinicalpathological entity. Brain 110:993–1013.

Fearnley, J. M., and Lees, A. J. 1990. Striatatonigral degeneration. A clinicopathological study. Brain 113:1823–1824.

Forno, L. S., and Alford, E. C. 1987. Pathology of Parkinson's disease. In W. C. Roller (Ed.) Handbook of Parkinson's Disease, pp.209–236. New York, NY: Marcel-Dekker.

Freed, C. R., Greene, P. E., Breeze, R. E., et al. 2001. Transplantation of embryonic dopamine neurons for severe Parkinson's disease. N. Engl. J. Med. 344:710–719. (see also editorial by Fischbach, G. D. and G. M. McKhann. 2001. Cell therapy for Parkinson's disease. N. Engl. J. Med. 344:763–765)

Furukawa, Y., annd Kish, S. J. 1999. Dopa responsive dystonia: recent advances and remaining issues to be addressed. Mov. Disord. 14:709–715.

Galvez- Jimenez, N. (Ed.). 2001. Movement disorders. Semin. Neurol. 21:1–123.

Gerfan, C. R., and Engbar, T. M. 1992. Molecular neuroanatomic mechanisms of Parkinson's disease. Neurol. Clin. 10:435–449.

Gibb, W. R. G. 1988. The Neuropathology of Parkinsonian disorders. In J. Jankovic and E. Tolosa (Eds.) Parkinson's Disease and Movement Disorders, pp. 205–223. Baltimore, MD and Munich, Germany: Urban & Schwarzenberg.

Gibb, W. R., Luthert, P. J., and Marsden, C. D. 1989. Corticobasal degeneration. Brain 112:1171–1192.

Goerdert, M., Jakes, R., and Spillantini, M. G. 1998. Alpha-synuclein and the Lewy body. NeuroSci. News 1:47–51.

Goetz, C. G. 1986. Charcot on Parkinson's disease. Mov. Disord. 1:27–32.

Goldblatt, D., Markesbery, W., and Reeves, A. G. 1974. Recurrent hemichorea following striatal lesions. Arch. Neurol. 31:51–54.

Graybiel, A. M., and Ragsdale, C. W. 1978. Histochemically distinct compartments in stratum of human, monkey and cat demonstrated by acetylthiocholinesterase ataining. Proc. Natl. Acad. Sci. USA 75:5723–5726.

Growdon, J. H., Hirsh, M. J., Wurtman, R. J., and Wiener, W. 1977. Oral choline administration to patients with tardive dyskinesia. N. Engl. J. Med. 297:524–527.

Guridi, J., and Obesco, J. A. 2001. The subthalamic nucleus, hemiballismus and Parkinson's disease: reappraisal of a neurosurgical dogma. Brain 124:5–19.

Gusella, J. F., Wexler, N. S., Conneally, D. M., et al. 1983. A polymorphic DNA marker genetically linked to Huntington's disease. Nature 306:234–238.

Guttman, M. 1992. Dopamine receptors in Parkinson's disease. Neurol. Clin. 10:377–386.

Hallett, M. 1991. Classification and treatment of tremor. JAMA. 266:1115–1117.

Hallett,M., Litvan, I., et al. 2000. Scientific position paper of the Movement Disorder Society evaluation of surgery for Parkinson's disease. 15:436–438.

Haymaker, W., Mehler, W. F., and Schiller, F. 1969. Extrapyramidal motor disorders. In W. Haymaker (Ed.) Bing's Local Diagnosis in Neurological Disease, pp.404–440. St. Louis, MO: C.V. Mosby.

Healey, D. G., Falchi, M., O'Sullivan, S. S., et al. 2008. Phenotype, genotype and world wide genetic penetrance of LRRK2 associated Parkinson's disease: a case controlled study. Lancet Neurol. 7:583–590.

Hornykiewicz, O. D. 1970. Physiological, biochemical and pathological backgrounds of levo dopa and possibilities for the future. Neurology 20 (Part 2):1–13.

Hornykiewicz, O., Kish, S., Beckler, L. E., et al. 1986. Brain neurotransmitters in dystonia musculorum deformans. N. Engl. J. Med. 315:347–531.

Huntington, G. 1872. On chorea. Med. Surg. Report 26:317–321.

Hurtig, H. I., and Stern, M. B. (Eds.). 2001. Movement Disorders. Neurol. Clin. 19:523–788.

Huw, R. M., Lees, A. J., and Wood, N. W. 1999. Neurofibrillaryte Parkinsonian disorders-tau pathology and tau genetics. Mov. Disord. 14:731–736.

Huw, R. M., Wood, N. W., and Lees, A. J. 1999. Progressive supranuclear palsy (Steele- Richardson- Olszewski disease). Postgrad. Med. J. 75:579–584.

Jankovic, J. 1987. The neurology of tics. In C. D. Marsden and S. Fahn (Eds.) Movement Disorders 2, pp. 383–405. London, UK: Butterworths.

Jankovic, J. 1989. Parkinsonism plus syndromes. Mov. Disord. 4(Suppl. l):95–119.

Jancovic, J. 2001. Tourette's syndrome. N. Engl. J. Med. 345:1184–1192.

Jankovic, J., and Fahn, S. 1986. The phenomenology of tics. Mov. Disord. 1:17–26.

Jankovic, J., and Fahn, S. 1988. Dystonic syndromes. In J. Jankovic and E. Tolosa (Eds.) Parkinson's Disease and Movement Disorders, pp.283–314. Baltimore, MD and Munich, Germany: Urban & Schwarzenberg.

Jankovic, J., and Tolosa, E. (Eds.). 1988. Parkinson's Disease and Movement Disorders. Baltimore, MD and Munich, Germany: Urban & Schwarzenberg.

Jarman, P. R., Davis, M. B., Hodgson, S. V., et al. 1997. Paroxysmal dystonic choreoathetosis: genetic linkage studies in a British family. Brain 120:2125–2130.

Jarman, P. R., Bhatia, K. P., Davie, C., et al. 2000. Paroxysmal dystonic choreoathetosis: clinical features and investigation of pathophysiology ina large family. Mov. Disord. 15:648–657.

Jimeenez- Shahed, J. 2009. Tourette syndrome. Neurol. Clin. 27:737–755.

Kandel, E. 1991. Disorders of thought: schizophrenia. In E. R. Kandel, J. H. Schwartz, and T. M. Jessell (Eds.) Principles of Neural Science. 3rd ed., pp. 853–868. New York, NY: Elsevier.

Keenen, R. E. 1970. The Eaton Collaborative Study of Levo Dopa Therapy in Parkinsonism. Neurology 20(Part 2):46–59.

Kertesz, A. 2000. Corticobasal degeneration. J. Neurol. Neurosurg. Psyciatry. 68:275–276.

Kertesz, A., Martinez-Lage, P., Davidson, W., and Munoz, D. G. 2000. The corticobasal degeneration syndrome overlaps progressive aphasia and frontotrmporal dementia. Neurology 55:1368–1375.

Klawans, H. L. 1988. The pathophysiology of drug-induced movement disorders. In J. Jankovic and E. Tolosa (Ed.) Parkinson's Disease and Movement Disorders, pp. 315–326. Baltimore, MD and Munich, Germany: Urban and Schwarzenberg.

Klawans, H. L., Moses, H., Nausieda, D. A., et al. 1976. Treatment and prognosis of hemiballismus. N. Engl. J. Med. 295:1348–1350.

Klawans, H. C., Paulson, G. W., and Barbeau, A. 1970. Predictive test for Huntington's chorea. Lancet 2:1185–1186. doi:10.1016/S0140-6736(70)90367-3.

Klawans, H. L., Paulson, G. W., Ringel, S. P., and Barbeau, A. 1972. Use of L-dopa in the detection of presymptomatic Huntington's chorea. N. Engl. J. Med. 286:1332–1334.

Kluger, B. M., Klepitskaya, O., and Okun, M. S. 2009. Surgical treatment of movement disorders. Neurol. Clin. 27:633–677.

Koller, W. C. (Ed.). 1992. Role of the controlled release formulation of carbidopa-levodopa in the treatment of Parkinson's disease. Neurology 42(Suppl. L):Sl–60.

Koller, W. C. 1992. Initiating treatment of Parkinson's disease. Neurology 42:(Suppl. 1):29–32.

Kopin, I. J. 1988. MPTP toxicity: implications for research in Parkinson's disease. Ann. Rev. Neurosci. 11:81–96.

Lamousin, P., Krack, P., Pollak, P., et al. 1998. Electrical stimulation of the subthalamic nucleus in advanced Parkinson's disease. N. Engl. J. Med. 339:1105–1111.

Lang, A. E., and Lozano, A. M. 1998. Medical progress: Parkinson's disease. N. Engl. J. Med. 339:1044–1053, 1130–1143.

Lang, A. E., Lozano, A. M., Duff, M. E., et al. 1997. Posteroventral medial pallidotomy in advanced Parkinson's disease. N. Engl. J. Med. 337:1036–1042.

Langston, J. W., and Ballard, P. 1984. Parkinsonism induced by 1-methyl,4-phenyl-1,2,3,6, tetrahydropyridine (MPTP): implications for treatment and pathogenesis of Parkinson's disease. Can. J. Neurol. Sci.11:160–165.

Langston, J. W., Ballard, P., Tetrud, J. W., and Irwin, I. 1983. Chronic Parkinsonism in humans due to a product of meperidine—analog synthesis. Science 219:979–980.

Langston, J. W., Widner, H., Goetz, C. G., et al. 1992. Case assessment program for intracerebral transplantation (CAPIT). Mov. Disord. 7:2–13.

Laplane, D., Levasseur, M., Pillone, B., et al. 1989. Obsessive compulsive and other behavioral changes with bilateral basal ganglia lesions. Brain 112:699–725.

Lees, A. J., and Tolosa, E. 1988. Tics. In J. Jankovic and E. Tolosa (Eds.) Parkinson's disease and Movement Disorders, pp.275–281. Baltimore, MD and Munich, Germany: Urban and Schwarzenberg.

Lees, A. J. 1987. The Steele-Richardson, Olszewski syndrome (progressive supranuclear palsy). In C. D. Marsden and S. Fahn (Eds.) Movement Disorders 2, pp. 272–287. London, UK: Butterworths.

Lowe, J., Lennox, G., and Leigh, P. N. 1997. Disorders of movement and system degenerations. In D. I. Graham and P. L. Lantos (Eds.) Greenfield's Neuropathology. Vol 2, pp. 281–366. Taylor and Francis: London.

Lewin, R. 1983. Trail of ironies to Parkinson's disease. Science 224: 1083–1085.

Lewin, R. 1984. Brain enzyme is the target of drug toxin. Science 225: 1460–1462.

Le Witt, D. A. 1992. Clinical studies with and pharmacokinetic considerations of sustained release levodopa. Neurology 42:(Suppl 1):29–31.

Lieberman, A. 1992. Emerging perspectives in Parkinson's disease. Neurology 42(Suppl. 4):5–7.

Lindvall, O. 1999. Cerebral implantation in movement disorders: state of the art. Mov. Disord. 14:201–205.

Lindvall. O., Brundin, P., Widner, H., et al. 1990. Grafts of fetal dopamine neurons survive and improve motor function in Parkinson's disease. Science 247:514–577.

Litwin, I. 2001. Diagnosis and management of progressive supranuclear palsy. Semin. Neurol. 21:41–48.

Litwin, I., Campbell, G., Mangone, C. A., et al. 1997. Which clinical features differentiate progressive supranuclear palsy (Steele- Richardson-Olszewski syndrome) from related disorders? A clinicopathological study. Brain 120:65–74.

Luquin, M., Scipioni, R. O., Vaamonde, J., et al. 1992. Levodopa induced dyskinesias in Parkinson's disease: clinical and pharmacological classification. Mov. Disord. 7:117–124.

Marsden, C. D., and Fahn, S. (Eds.).1987. Movement Disorders 2. London, UK: Butterworths.

Martin, J. B., and Gusella, J. F. 1986. Huntington's disease: pathogenesis and management. N. Engl. J. Med. 315:1267–1276.

Mathuranath. P. S., Xuereb, J. H., Bak, T., and Hodges, J. R. 2000. Corticobasal degeneration and/or frontal temporal dementia? A report of two overlap cases and review of the literature. J. Neurol. Neurosurg. Psychiatry. 68:304–312.

Mayeau, R., Marder, K., Cote, L. J., et al. 1995. The frequency of idiopathic Parkinson's disease group and sex in northern Manhattan 1988–1993. Am. J. of Epidemiology 142:820–827.

Mayeux, R., Stern, Y., and Spanton, S. 1985. Heterogeneity in dementia of the Alzheimer type: evidence of subgroups. Neurology 35:453–461.

Mena, I., Court, J., Fuenzalida, S., et al. 1970. Chronic manganeses poisoning: treatment with L-dopa or 5-OH tryptophane. N. Engl. J. Med. 282:5–10.

Martin, J. R. 1957. Hemichorea (hemiballismus without lesions in the corpus Luysii. Brain 80:1–10.

Meyers, R., Sweeney, D. B., and Swidde, J. T. 1947. Hemiballismus: etiology and surgical treatment J. Neurol. Neurosurg. Psychiatry. 58:672–692.

Mitchell, I. J., Jackson, A., Sambrook, M. A., and Crossman, A. R. 1989. The role of the subthalamic nucleus in experimental chorea. Evidence from 2-desoxyglucose metabolic mapping and horse radish peroxidase tracing studies. Brain 112:1533–1548.

Montastruc, J. L., Rascol, O., and Senard, J. M. 1999. Treatment of Parkinson's disease should begin with a dopamine agonist. Mov. Disord. 14:725–730.

Myers, R. H., Sax, D. S., Koroshetz, W. J., et al. 1991. Factors associated with slow progression in Huntington's disease. Arch. Neurol. 48:800–804.

Myers, R. H., Vonsattel, J. P., Stevens, T. J., et al. 1988. Pathologic assessment of severity in Huntington's disease. Neurology 38:341–347.

Noback, C. R., Strominger, N. L., and Demarest, R. J. 1991. The Human Nervous System: Introduction and Review. 4th ed., pp. 375–395. Philadelphia, PA: Lea & Febiger.

Olanow, C. W., and Calne, D. 1992. Does selegiline monotherapy in Parkinson's disease act by symptomatic or protective mechanisms. Neurology 42(Suppl. 4):13–26.

Olanow, C. W., and Tatton, W. G. 1999. Etiology and pathogenesis of Parkinson's disease. Ann. Rev. Neurosci. 22:123–144.

Ondo, W. G. 2009. Restless legs syndrome. Neurol. Clin. 27:779–799.

Oppenheimer, D. R. 1984. Diseases of the basal ganglia, cerebellum and motor neurons. In J. H. Adams, J. A. N. Corsellis, and L. W. Dicker (Eds.) Greenfield's Neuropathology, pp. 700–747. London, UK: Edward Arnold.

Papp, M. I., and Lantos, P. L. 1994. The distribution of oligodendroglial inclusions in multiple system atrophy and its relevance to clinical symptomatology. Brain 117:235–243.

Parkinson, J. 1817. An Essay on the Shaking Palsy. London, UK: Sherwood, Neely & Jones. (Reprinted—The Classics of Neurology Neurosurgery Library, Birmingham, Gryphen Editions, 1986)

Patten, B. M. 1988. Wilson's disease. In J. Jankovic and E. Tolosa (Eds.) Parkinson's Disease and Movement Disorders, pp. 179–190. Baltimore, MD and Munich, Germany: Urban & Schwarzenberg.

Pauls, D. L., and Leckman, J. F. 1986. The inheritance of Gilles de La Tourette's syndrome and associated behaviors: evidence for autosomal dominant transmission. N. Engl. J. Med. 315:993–997.

Pearce, R. K. B. 1999. L-dopa and dyskinesias in normal monkeys. Mov. Disord. 14(Suppl. 1):9–12.

Penney, J. B., Jr., and Young, A. B. 1988. Huntington 's disease. In J. Jankovic and E. Tolosa (Eds.) *Parkinson's Disease and Movement Disorders*, pp. 167–178. Baltimore, MD: Urban and Schwarzenberg.

Quinn, N. 1995. Fortnightly review: Parkinson's disease: recognition and differential diagnosis. BMJ. 310:447–452.

Rascol, O., and Lees, A. J. (Eds.). 1999. Dyskinesias. Mov. Disord. 14(Suppl.1):1–80.

Riley, D. E., and Lang, A. E. 2000. Movement disorders. In W. G. Bradley, R. B. Daroff, G. M. Fenichel, and C. D. Marsden (Eds.) Neurology in Clinical Practice, pp. 1889–1930. Boston, MA: Butterworth Heinemann.

Rinne, J. O., Lee, M. S., Thompson, P. D., and Marsden, C. D. 1994. Corticobasal degeneration. A clinical study of 36 cases. Brain 117:1183–1196.

Roberts, L. 1990. Huntington's gene: so near and so far. Science 247: 624–617.

Sarma, K., Waltz, J. M., Riklan, M., Koslow, M., and Cooper, I. S. 1970. Relief of intention tremor by thalamic surgery. J. Neurol. Neurosurg. Psychiat. 33:7–15.

Sax, D. S., and Vonsattel, J. P. 1992. Chorea and progressive dementia in an 88-year-old woman. N. Engl. J. Med. 326:117–124.

Schapira, A. H. V. 2009 Etiology and pathogenesis of Parkinson's disease. Neurol. Clin. 27:583–603.

Schmidt, W. R., and Jarcho, L. W. 1966. Persistent dyskinesias following phenothiazide therapy. Arch. Neurol. 14:369–377.

Schwarz, C. S., and Bressman, S. B. 2009. Genetics and treatment of dystonia Neurol. Clin. 27:697–718.

Schneider, J. S., Pope, A., Simpson, K., et al. 1992. Recovery from experimental Parkinsonism in primates with GM1 ganglioside treatment. Science 256:843–845.

Scheinberg, I. H., and Steinlieb, I. 1984. Wilson's Disease. Philadelphia, PA: W. B. Saunders.

Schuurman, P. R., Bosch, D. A., Bossuyt, P. M. M., et al. 2000. A comparison of continuous Thalamic stimulation and thalamotomy for suppression of severe tremor. N. Engl. J. Med. 342:461–468.

Schwarz, G. A., and Barrows, L. J. 1960. Hemiballism without involvement of Luy's body. Arch. Neurol. 2:420–434.

Sethi, K. P. 2001. Movement disorders induced by dopamine blocking agents. Semin. Neurol. 21:59–68.

Siemers, E., and Reddy, V. 1991. Profile of patients enrolled in a new movement disorders clinic. 6:336–341.

Singer, H. S. 2000. Current issues in Tourette's syndrome. Mov. Disord. 15:1051–1063.

Sladek, J. R., Redmond. B. E., Jr., Collier, T. J., et al. 1989. Transplantation advances in Parkinson's disease. Mov. Disord. 4(Suppl. 1):S120, S125.

Stacy, M. 2009. Medical treatment of Parkinson'disease. Neurol. Clin 27:605–631.

Starkstein, S. E., Preziosi, T. J., Berthier, M. L., et al. 1989. Depression and cognitive impairment in Parkinson's disease. Brain 112:1141–1153.

Storey, E., and Beal, M. F. 1993. Neurochemical substrates of rigidity and chorea in Huntington's disease. Brain 116:1201–1222.

Stover, N. P., and Watts, R. L. 2001. Corticobasal degeneration. Semin. Neurol. 21:49–58.

The Parkinson Study Group. 1989. Effect of deprenyl on the progression of disability in early Parkinson's disease. N. EngI. J. Med. 321:1364. (For updated report see also—N. EngI. J. Med.328:176–83, 1993)

Tanner, C. M., and Lanston, J. W. 1990. Do environmental toxins cause Parkinson's disease? A critical review. Neurology 40:17–30.

Tolosa, E., and Alom, J. 1988. Drug-induced dyskinesias. In J. Jankovic and E. Tolosa (Eds.) Parkinson's Disease and Movement Disorders, pp. 327–347. Baltimore, MD and Munich, Germany: Urban and Schwarzenberg.

Victor, M., Adams, R. D., and Cole, M. 1965. The acquired (non-Wilsonian) type of chronic hepatocerebral degeneration. Medicine 44:345–396.

Vonsattel, J. P., Meyers, R. H., Stevens, T. J., et al.1985. Neuropathological classification of Huntington's disease. J. Neuropathol. Exp. Neurol. 44:559–577.

Walshe, J. M. 1999. Penicillamine: the treatment of first choice for patients with Wilson's disease. Mov. Disord. 14:545–550. (See also G. J. Brewer,14: 551–554 and P. A. LeWitt 14:555–556)

Weiner, W. J. 1999. The initial treatment of Parkinsom's disease should begin with levodopa. Mov. Disord. 14:716–724.

Wenning, G. K., Scherfler, C., Stefanova, N., and Puschban, Z. 2001. Multiple system atrophy. Semin. Neurol. 21:33–40.

Wenning, G. K., Ben Shlomo, Y., Magalhaes, M., et al. 1994. Clinical features and natural history of multiple system atrophy. An analysis of 100 cases. Brain 117: 835–845.

Wenning, G. K., Litwin, I., Jankovic, J., et al. 1998. Natural history and survival of 14 patients with corticobasal degeneration confirmed at postmortem examination. J. Neurol. Neurosurg. Psychiatry. 64:184–189.

Wexler, N. S., Rose, E. A., and Houseman, D. E. 1992. Molecular approaches to heredity diseases of the nervous system: Huntington's disease as a paradigm. Ann. Rev. Neurosci. 15:402–442.

Young, A. B., Grenamyre, T., Hollingsworth, Z., et al. 1988. NMDA receptor losses in putamen from patients with Huntington's disease. Science 241:1–983.

Young, A. B., and Penny, J. B., Jr. 1988. Biochemical and functional organization of the basal ganglia. In J. Jankovic and E. Tolosa (Eds.) Parkinson's disease and Movement Disorders, pp.1–12. Baltimore, MD and Munich, Germany: Urban & Schwarzenberg.

Zesiewicz, T. A., and Hauser, R. A. 2001. Surgery for the treatment of Parkinson's disease. Semin. Neurol. 21:91–102.

Zoghbi, H. Y., and Orr, H. T. 2000. Glutamine repeats and neurodegeneration. Ann. Rev. Neurosci. 23:217–248.

20.

MOTOR SYSTEMS

PART III: CEREBELLUM AND MOVEMENT AND MAJOR FIBER PATHWAYS OF THE CEREBELLUM

The cerebellum is a cortical structure containing number of layers and it is attached to the brain stem by three peduncles. There are dollars of nuclei deep to the white matter which provide many of the connections.

ANATOMIC CONSIDERATIONS

SUBDIVISIONS OF THE CEREBELLUM

A number of schemes for dividing the cerebellum into various lobes and lobules have been devised. From a functional standpoint, it is perhaps best for the student to visualize the cerebellum as composed of various longitudinal and transverse divisions. In order to visualize these subdivisions, it is necessary to unfold and to flatten the cerebellum as shown in Figure 20.1.

LONGITUDINAL DIVISIONS

The major longitudinal divisions are the median (vermal cortex), the paramedian (paravermal), and lateral (remainder of the cerebellar hemispheres).

The major projections and functional correlations are outlined in Table 20.1. In general, the median (vermal) region is concerned with the medial descending systems and with axial control. The lateral and paramedian regions are concerned with the lateral descending systems and with the appendages (the limbs) (midline to axis; lateral to appendages).

TRANSVERSE DIVISIONS

The transverse subdivisions are essentially phylogenetic divisions.

1. The archicerebellum is composed of a flocculus and nodulus and is related primarily to the vestibular nerve and vestibular nuclei. Reflecting this anatomical relation, the archicerebellum has a role in control of equilibrium (balance), axial posture, and eye movement.

2. The paleocerebellum, or anterior lobe, relates primarily to the spinocerebellar system and to its analog for the upper extremities, the cuneocerebellar pathway (the lateral cuneate nucleus is the analog of the dorsal nucleus of Clarke). Its major function, however, appears more related to the lower extremities than to the upper extremities. The primary fissure separates the anterior lobe from the middle posterior lobe.

3. The middle, or posterior, lobe, the neocerebellum, relates primarily to the neocortex. The function of the neocerebellum is primarily the coordination of discrete

Table 20.1 LONGITUDINAL SUBDIVISIONS OF THE CEREBELLUM

MEDIAN	PARAMEDIAN	LATERAL
(Vermal cortex)	(Paravermal)	(Remainder of cerebellar hemisphere)
Projects to:	Projects to:	Projects to:
Fastigial nucleus (globus and emboliform)	Interpositus nuclei	Dentate nucleus lateral
Role in:	Role in:	Role in:
Posture and movements of body (axial)	Discrete ipsilateral extremity movements (appendicular)	Discrete ipsilateral extremity patterns of movement. Coordinated with cerebral cortex, thalamus, and red nucleus. Initiating, planning, and timing of movements

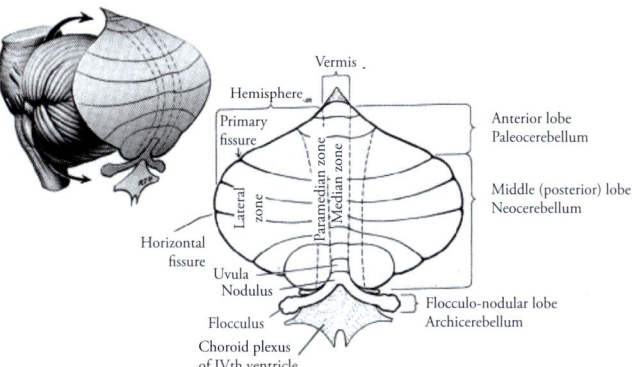

Figure 20.1 Major transverse and longitudinal subdivisions of the cerebellum. The surface has been unfolded and laid out flat. (From Noback, C.R. et al.: 1991. The Human Nervous System. 4th edition. Philadelphia, Lea & Febiger, p. 282.)

Table 20.2 **TRANSVERSE DIVISIONS OF THE CEREBELLUM**

ARCHICEREBELLUM (FLOCCULAR NODULAR LOBE)	PALEOCEREBELLUM ANTERIOR LOBE	NEOCEREBELLUM (MIDDLE, OR POSTERIOR, LOBE)
Connections:	Connections:	Connections:
Vestibular	Spinocerebellar and neocortex/cuneocerebellar and spino-olivary (inferior olive)	
Role:	Role:	Role:
Axial equilibrium (trunk primarily), posture, muscle tone, vestibular reflexes, eye movements	Equilibrium posture muscle tone in lower extremities; coordinated movements in lower extremities, e.g., heel to shin	Limb coordination in phasic posture movements (upper and lower extremities). Possible role in higher executive functions and emotion

movements of the upper and lower extremities (see Table 20.2). Transverse Divisions of the Cerebellum.

CYTOARCHITECTURE OF THE CEREBELLUM

In contrast to the cerebral cortex, all areas of the cerebellar cortex are relatively thin and have the same basic three-layered cytoarchitectural pattern, consisting of an outer molecular layer, a Purkinje cell layer, and an inner granule cell layer with an underlying medullary layer of white matter. The arrangement of cells and the basic synaptic connections are indicated in Figure 20.2. Afferent fibers enter the cerebellar cortex as *mossy fibers*. These fibers are so named because each terminates in a series of moss-like glomeruli, where axodendritic synaptic contacts are made with granule cells. The mossy fibers have already been encountered as spinocerebellar, cuneocerebellar, corticopontocerebellar, vestibulocerebellar, or reticulocerebellar pathways.

The granule-cell axon is sent into the molecular layer, where it divides into two long branches. These branches travel parallel to the long axis of the cerebellar folium and are designated as *parallel fibers*. These fibers make excitatory synaptic contact with the extensive dendritic arborizations of Purkinje cells, as well as with stellate cells, Golgi cells, and basket cells. The basket cells inhibit the Purkinje cells via axosomatic synapses as these projections are inhibitory in nature. The outflow of the Purkinje cells is inhibitory in nature. The target of the axons of the Purkinje cells is the neurons of the deep cerebellar nuclei. The axons of the neurons in these deep cerebellar nuclei are the major outflow from the cerebellum to the brain stem and thalamus.

Several additional systems must be considered. The *climbing fibers* are excitatory to the Purkinje-cell dendrites. These fibers originate in the contralateral inferior olivary nuclei and represent a long latency pathway from the spinal cord or cerebral cortex to the cerebellum (olivocerebellar). These fibers are so named because they climb and wrap around the

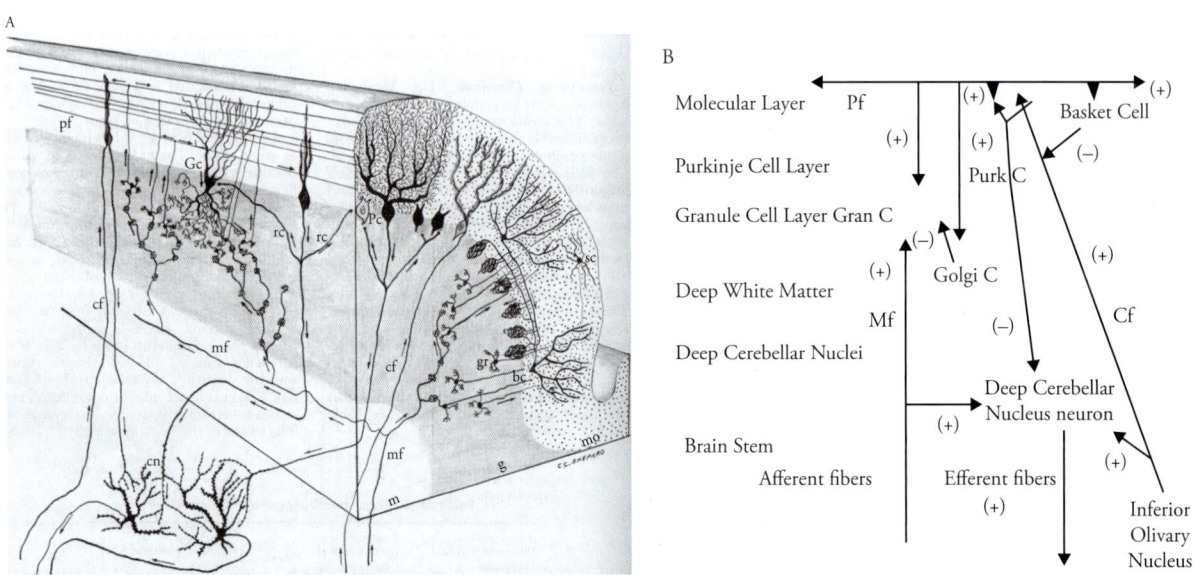

Figure 20.2 (*A*) Schematic view of a cerebellar folia. Demonstrating the relationships of moss fibers (mf) to granule cells (gr) and the synaptic relationships of the axons of granule cells as parallel fibers (pl) with Purkinje fibers (Pc), Golgi cells (gc), and basket cells (bs). The Purkinje cells also receive excitation from climbing fibers (cf). The major outflow from the cerebellum is to the deep cerebellar nuclei. g, granule cell layer; m, medullary layer; mo, molecular layer. (From Fox C.A. 1962. The structure of the cerebellar cortex. In Crosby FC, Humphrey T and E W. Lauer, Correlative Anatomy of the Nervous System. New York, Macmillan, p. 196.) (*B*) The most significant cells, connections, the afferents and efferent fibers in the cerebellar cortex. Arrows show direction of axonal conduction: (+) excitatory; (−) inhibitory; cf, climbing fibers; mf, mossy fibers; pf, parallel fibers.

dendrites and body of the Purkinje-cell neurons, making several hundred synaptic contacts. Stimulation of a single climbing fiber results in large postsynaptic potentials and in large high-frequency bursts of discharges.

The parallel fibers also have excitatory synapses in the molecular layer, but they synapse with the dendrites of the Golgi cells. The Golgi cell, in turn, is inhibitory to the granule cell with a synapse within areas of the molecular layer referred to as glomeruli. The parallel fibers also excite other interneurons (small stellate cells) in the molecular layer, which, in turn, are inhibitory to the dendrites of Purkinje cells.

GABA (gamma aminobutyric acid) is the inhibitory transmitter for the Purkinje, basket, stellate, and Golgi cells. Since the outflow from the cerebellar cortex occurs via the axons of Purkinje cells and since this outflow is inhibitory to the deep cerebellar nuclei, it is logical to ask what excitatory influences drive the neurons of these deep nuclei. The answer is that collaterals of the mossy fibers and climbing fibers serve this function.[1]

AFFERENTS

The inputs to the cerebellum may be summarized as follows:

A. Via the inferior cerebellar peduncle (restiform body):

1. Uncrossed dorsal spinocerebellar and cuneocerebellar
2. Crossed olivocerebellar
3. Uncrossed reticulocerebellar (from lateral reticular and paramedian nuclei)

B. Via the juxta-restiform body:

1. Uncrossed from vestibular nuclei are predominantly to the floccular nodular lobe, the archicerebellum, and the midline vermis.
2. Uncrossed from vestibular nerve (note that some fibers from the vestibular nerve bypass the vestibular nuclei and enter the cerebellum directly)

C. Via the middle cerebellar peduncle (brachium pontis): The corticopontocerebellar input (via the pontine nuclei) is primarily to the neocerebellum of the lateral hemisphere. This is crossed from the opposite cerebral hemisphere.

D. Via the superior cerebellar peduncle (brachium conjunctivum):

1. Crossed ventral spinocerebellar is primarily to the anterior lobe (paleocerebellum) and the intermediate area of the paraflocculus.
2. Tectal cerebellar
The superior cerebellar peduncle, then, serves only a minor role as afferent to the cerebellum. Its major role is as the efferent pathway.

EFFERENTS

A. Superior cerebellar peduncle (brachium conjunctivum)

1. Dentate nuclei and interpositus (globus and emboliform) nuclei; there is a major projection via the crossed brachium conjunctivum (superior cerebellar peduncle) to the ventral lateral (and ventral anterior) nucleus of the thalamus and to the red nucleus (dentatorubral-thalamic pathway).
2. Descending division of the brachium conjunctivum conveys impulses to the paramedian reticular nuclei.

B. Inferior cerebellar peduncle

1. The archicerebellum projects directly from the floccular nodular lobe and via the fastigial nuclei to the vestibular (lateral vestibular nucleus) and reticular areas of the brain stem.
2. The fastigioreticular and fastigiovestibular pathways hook around the superior cerebellar peduncle as the uncinate fasciculus. In addition, impulses are also conveyed via the juxtarestiform body.

C. Middle cerebellar peduncle. This contains only afferent connections from the cerebrum via the pons into the neocerebellum.

TOPOGRAPHIC PATTERNS OF REPRESENTATION IN THE CEREBELLAR CORTEX

Stimulation of tactile receptors or of proprioceptors results in an evoked response in the cerebellar cortex. There is a topographic pattern of representation. Visual and auditory stimuli evoke responses primarily in the midline vermis. Stimulation of the specific areas of the cerebral cortex also evokes responses from the cerebellar cortex in an appropriate topographic manner. Moreover, direct stimulation of the cerebellar cortex in the decerebrate animal will produce, in a topographic manner, movement or changes in tone of flexors or extensors. The general pattern of representation is consistent with the patterns of sensory and cortical representation previously noted.

A possible pattern of somatotrophic representation in the primate cerebellum is shown in Figure 20.3. It is important to recall that there is no conscious perception of stimuli arriving at the cerebellar level.

Vestibular stimulation evokes responses not only in the floccular nodular regions but also in the superior and inferior midline vermis.

FUNCTIONS OF THE CEREBELLUM AND CORRELATIONS

The cerebellum acts as a servomechanism, that is, as a feedback loop that dampens movements and motor power to prevent

---

[1] However, the mossy fibers from the pontine and brain stem reticular nuclei apparently do not serve this collateral excitatory function.

Figure 20.3 Topographic localization in cerebellum. (*A*) Summary of projections from the sensory area and the motor area in the monkey. (*B*) Summary of corticocerebellar projections in the monkey. Note that there is a unilateral representation on the dorsal surface and a representation within each paramedian lobule on the ventral surface. At the lateral margin the division between crus I and crus II is essentially the border between the dorsal and ventral surface. See Figure 20.1 for terminology in human cerebellum. (From Snider, R.S.: 1950. Arch. Neurol. Psych. 64:204, AMA.)

overshoot and oscillation (that is, tremor). In short, it acts to maintain stability of movement and posture. More recently, a role in higher motor function, such as the initiation of planning, the timing of movement, and motor learning, has been suggested for the cerebellum.

REGIONAL FUNCTIONAL CORRELATIONS

We have already discussed the functional relation of the longitudinal and transverse subdivisions of the cerebellum. It is evident that these two classifications overlap from a functional standpoint, and we may specify the following correlations:

Vestibular Reflexes and Eye Movement

a. Anatomic correlation: Floccular nodular lobe

b. Major input: Vestibular labyrinth (semicircular canals and otolith organs)

c. Major deep nucleus: Vestibular nuclei (lateral)

d. Major connections: Medial descending systems, vestibulospinal and medial longitudinal fasciculus, and extraocular motor nuclei

Posture and Equilibrium of the Trunk

A.
  a. Anatomic correlation: Flocular nodular lobe (vestibulocerebellum)
  b. Major input: Vestibular labyrinth as earlier
  c. Major deep nucleus: Vestibular nuclei (lateral)
  d. Major connection: Medial descending systems—vestibulospinal systems (medial and lateral)

B.
  a. Anatomic correlation: Midline vermis (spinocerebellum
  b. Major inputs:
    1. Vestibular labyrinth
    2. Dorsal spinocerebellar and cuneocerebellar from body and proximal limbs
    3. Trigeminal
    4. Visual and auditory
  c. Major deep nucleus: Fastigial
  d. Major connections: Medial descending motor systems:
    1. Via juxtarestiform body and central tegmental system to pontine and medullary reticular nuclei (origin of medial and lateral reticulospinal tracts) and to vestibular nuclei (origin of vestibulospinal tracts).
    2. Via superior cerebellar peduncle (decussated) to ventral nucleus of thalamus to motor cortex to anterior corticospinal tract

Distal Motor Control and Speech/ Voice Control

a. Anatomic correlation: Intermediate lobe (paravermal or paramedian zone-spinocerebellum)
b. Major input: Dorsal spinocerebellar and cuneocerebellar
c. Major deep nuclei: Interpositus (globose and emboliform)
d. Major connections: Lateral descending motor system, superior cerebellar peduncle via decussation to magnocellular sector of the red nucleus (origin of rubrospinal system) and to ventral lateral nucleus of thalamus and from the (lateral) thalamus to primary motor area and area 6 of supplementary motor cortex (origins of the crossed lateral corticospinal system)

Speech

Anatomic correlation: Superior paravermal area (more often left than right). Damage produces cerebellar dysarthria which affects prosody, harmony, and rhythm of speech rather than sequential or semantic aspects (see Amarenco et al., 1991; Lechtenberg and Gilman, 1978 for additional discussion).

Initiation, Planning, and Timing of Movement

a. Anatomic correlation: Lateral cerebellar hemisphere (cerebrocerebellum)
b. Major input: Motor and premotor cerebral cortex (areas 4 and 6) and parietal cortex (areas 1, 2, 3, 5) to pontine nuclei to lateral neocerebellum (after decussation) via the middle cerebellar peduncle
c. Deep nucleus: dentate
d. Major connection: Via decussation of superior cerebellar peduncle to
  1. Red nucleus (parvocellular) with subsequent rubro-olivary fibers
  2. Ventral lateral nucleus of thalamus, then projecting to motor and premotor cerebral cortex. From these areas, as already discussed, originate the lateral descending systems lateral corticospinal and corticorubrospinal and lateral reticulospinal and the anterior corticospinal systems.

EFFECTS OF DISEASE ON THE CEREBELLUM

The cerebellum may be viewed as a machine that processes information from many sources (sensory receptors, vestibular nuclei, reticular formation, and cerebral cortex) and then acts to smooth out the resultant movements or postures. Sudden displacements or lurches are prevented. The large number of inhibitory feedback circuits in the cerebellum (the major influence of Purkinje cells on deep cerebellar nuclei being inhibitory) qualifies the cerebellum for this role. Lesions may then result in undamped oscillation. As a result, tremor perpendicular to the line of movement may occur, called intention or action tremor. Lesions may also impair the ability to respond to sudden displacements, resulting in instability of posture and gait (ataxia). Release of function of ventral lateral nucleus of thalamus may also occur.

The cerebellum is not designed for the direct, fast-conduction control of movements. Thus, it is not surprising that, in the monkey, total ablation may produce little effect, although some deficit in contact placing may be evident. In humans, extensive destruction of cerebellum may be present with little obvious deficit. Moreover, cerebellar symptoms, if present in a "static" disease process (such as cerebrovascular accidents), often disappear with time. However, more specific tests may still reveal a minor deficit in speed and coordination.

More recent studies suggest a role for the cerebellum in classical conditioning and in motor learning, particularly as regards the memory aspect for the timing of movements (Raymond et al., 1996). In addition, a role of the cerebellum in higher order cognitive and emotional functions has been suggested by the studies of Schmahmann and Sherman (1998), Levinsohn et al. (2000), and Riva and Giogi (2000). In patients with lesions of the posterior lobe and vermis, there was an impairment of executive functions such as planning, set shifting, verbal fluency, abstract reasoning, and working memory, as well as visual spatial organization and memory. Higher language disturbances also occurred. In addition, these patients had a personality change characterized by blunting of affect or disinhibition and inappropriate behavior. This cognitive and affective syndrome suggested a disruption of the modulatory effects of cerebellum on the prefrontal, posterior parietal, and limbic circuits discussed in Chapter 18. These changes did not occur with lesions of the anterior lobe. The effects on cognitive and emotional function in patients with prenatal cerebellar hypoplasia may be even more serious and may include autism (Allin et al., 2001; Courchesne et al., 1994).

MAJOR SYNDROMES

While we will discuss three anatomically distinct syndromes of cerebellar disease (the floccular nodular lobe, the anterior lobe, and the lateral hemisphere), it should be pointed out that these strict anatomic borders do not confine many diseases that affect the cerebellum. Moreover, the cerebellum is positioned in a relatively tight compartment with bony walls and a relatively rigid tentorium cerebelli above. An expanding lesion in the posterior fossa, then, may produce a generalized compression of the cerebellum. In such clinical situations, it may be possible to differentiate only between midline (vermal) involvement and lateral (cerebellar hemisphere) involvement. Midline lesions produce disorders of equilibrium and axial ataxia; lateral and lateralized paramedian lesions produce appendicular ataxia and tremor.

Syndrome of the Floccular Nodular Lobe Other Midline Cerebellar Tumors

The major findings in the human, monkey, cat, and dog are a loss of equilibrium and an ataxia (unsteadiness) of trunk, gait, and station. Thus, the patient, when standing on a narrow base with eyes open, has a tendency to fall forward, backward, or to one side. The patient may be unable to sit or stand. The patient walks on a broad base, often reeling from side to side, and often falling. Despite the loss of equilibrium, the patient usually does not complain of a rotational vertigo. When recumbent in bed, the patient often fails to show any ataxia or tremor of limbs. Thus, the finger-to-nose and heel-to-shin tests are performed without difficulty. With unilateral disease of the floccular nodular lobe, a head tilt may be present. In addition, spontaneous horizontal nystagmus may be present as a transitory phenomenon.

In humans, the most common cause of this syndrome is neoplastic. The type of neoplasm depends on the age of the patient. The most likely cause in an infant or child[2] is a medulloblastoma, a tumor arising in nests of external granular cells in the nodulus forming the roof of the fourth ventricle. In older children and young adults, the ependymoma, a tumor arising from ependymal cells in the floor of the fourth ventricle, may cause this syndrome by pressing upward against the nodulus. In adults it is more appropriate to speak of midline tumors of the vermis, since the tumors do not selectively involve the floccular nodular region. In middle-aged adults, the most common cause is probably the midline hemangioblastoma. In older adults, metastatic tumors may produce this syndrome. At all ages, rare arteriovenous malformations may produce the syndrome.[3]

The course of a medulloblastoma is indicated in the following case history.

CASE HISTORY 20.1

This 27-month-old white female had been unsteady in gait, with poor balance, falling frequently since the age of 13 months, when she began to walk. Three months prior to admission, in relation to a viral infection manifested by fever and diarrhea, the patient developed increasing anorexia and lethargy. One month prior to admission, vomiting increased, and the patient also became more irritable. Perinatal history had been normal, and head circumference had remained normal.

Neurologic Examination

Mental status: The child was irritable but cooperative.

Cranial nerves: The fundi could not be visualized. Bobbing of the head was present in the sitting position.

Motor system: A significant ataxia of the trunk was present when sitting or standing. Gait was broad based and ataxic, requiring assistance. No ataxia or tremor of the extremities was present.

Clinical diagnosis: Probable midline cerebellar tumor; based on age, most likely a medulloblastoma.

Laboratory data: *Air-contrast ventriculogram* demonstrated the fourth ventricle was deformed by a mass arising from the nodulus of the cerebellum. There was secondary enlargement of the lateral and third ventricles and marked forward displacement of the cerebral aqueduct.

Hospital course: Dr. Peter Carney performed a suboccipital craniotomy, which confirmed the presence of a medulloblastoma with many malignant cells present in the cerebrospinal fluid obtained at surgery. Radiation therapy to the entire central nervous axis was begun 1 week after surgery. There was initial improvement, but the patient deteriorated 3 months after the surgery and expired 1 month later despite chemotherapy. The findings at autopsy are demonstrated in Figure 20.4.

At present, recommended therapy includes wide resection followed by radiotherapy to the entire central nervous system axis. Dissemination of tumor cells throughout the cerebrospinal fluid is frequent, because of the friable, cellular, nonstromal nature of the lesion. At present, 5-year survival has been increased to 60%. Recurrences may be treated with chemotherapy, although the combination of radiotherapy and chemotherapy may produce significant pathologic alterations in white matter. Refer to Chapters 13 and 27 for additional discussion.

Midline cerebellar tumor in the adult: The following case presents an example of a midline cerebellar tumor metastatic from breast with primary symptoms of gait ataxia, headache, vertigo, and vomiting.

---

[2] Medulloblastomas may occasionally occur in adolescents and young adults.

[3] Progressive multiple sclerosis may produce in the young or middle-aged adult severe involvement of white matter in the cerebellum and brain stem, resulting in severe truncal ataxia, in which the patient is ataxic in both the sitting and standing positions. Such cases almost always also manifest severe appendicular involvement; that is, the cerebellar syndrome is not selective.

Figure 20.4 Medulloblastoma: syndrome of the floccular nodular lobe: Case 20.1. Vomiting and truncal ataxia were present without tremor or ataxia of the extremities. (Courtesy of Dr. John Hills.) Refer to text.

CASE HISTORY 20.2

This 67-year-old white female 6 weeks prior to admission developed intermittent vertigo and then 2 weeks prior to admission a progressive ataxia of gait followed by headaches and vomiting.

Past history: This patient had a poorly differentiated highly malignant infiltrating ductal adenocarcinoma of the left breast for which she had undergone lumpectomy 6 years prior; and a radical mastectomy followed by radiation therapy, 3 years prior to admission.

Neurological Examination (in the emergency room)

Cranial nerves: There was an absence of venous pulsations on funduscopic examination, suggesting a mild increase in intracranial pressure.

Motor system: She had difficulty standing and tended to fall to the right. She was unable to walk because of severe ataxia. There was no limb dysmetria.

Reflexes: The right plantar response was equivocal.

Clinical diagnosis: Midline cerebellar tumor metastatic from breast.

Laboratory data: Computerized tomography (CT) scan demonstrated a large (3–4 cm) enhancing tumor was present involving the midline vermis and right paramedian cerebellum and compressing the fourth ventricle, subsequently confirmed by magnetic resonance imaging (MRI) scans of the brain (Fig. 20.5). CT scan of abdomen demonstrated two possible metastatic lesions in the liver.

Subsequent course: The patient received dexamethasone with significant improvement within 12 hours. At the insistence of the patient, Dr. Gerald McGuillicuddy resected the solitary central nervous system metastatic lesion. Following surgery she received 3000 cGy (rads) whole-brain radiation and was begun on the antitumor agent tamoxifen. She expired at home, 4 months after surgery, of systemic complications of the malignancy.

Syndrome of the Anterior Lobe

Stimulation or ablation of the anterior lobe in the cat or dog may produce significant changes in muscle tone. Thus, stimulation of the middle anterior lobe results in a decrease in spindle discharge and inhibits gamma rigidity of the decerebrate preparation. Stimulation of the intermediate area of the anterior lobe produces an increased spindle discharge and facilitates gamma rigidity in the decerebrate preparation. Actual ablation of the anterior lobe in these animals or functional ablation (cooling) produces an increase in decerebrate rigidity without a change in the gamma system (alpha rigidity). However, in humans, ablation of

Figure 20.5 Metastatic midline cerebellar tumor: Case 20.2. Magnetic resonance imaging (MRI, T1 weighted) (*A*) sagittal section; (*B*) coronal section. Refer to text.

Figure 20.6 Alcoholic cerebellar degeneration: The anterior lobe syndrome. There is a loss of Purkinje cells with atrophy of the cerebellar folia with relatively selective involvement of the anterior lobe: (*A*) schematic representation of the neuronal loss; (*B*) atrophy of the anterior superior vermis in sagittal section. (From Victor, M., R.D. Adams, and E.L. Mancall: 1959. Arch. Neurol. 1:579, 599, 600, AMA.)

the anterior lobe does not change tone.[4] The major symptoms are an ataxia of gait with a marked side-to-side ataxia of the lower extremities as tested in the heel-to-shin test. The upper extremities, in contrast, are affected to only a minor degree.

This area corresponds to the representation of the lower extremities and to the area of projection of the spinocerebellar pathways.

Typical of this syndrome are cases of alcoholic cerebellar degeneration (Fig. 20.6), where a severe loss of Purkinje cells occurs in the anterior lobe. Although this degeneration occurs primarily in alcoholics, the basic etiology may be a nutritional deficiency (the specific factor is most likely thiamine).

The major findings of a broad-based, staggering gait with truncal ataxia and heel-to-shin ataxia can be related to the anterior lobe of the cerebellum. Since symptoms improve or do not progress after the discontinuation of alcohol, and the administration of multiple B vitamins, a toxic or nutritional factor may be postulated. (The reliability of the history of alcohol intake is always open to question. The amount stated by the patient is usually assumed to be the minimum amount.) Note that a similar acute cerebellar syndrome occurs as one aspect of the Wernicke-Korsakoff's syndrome (refer to Chapter 30). At the present time, the diagnosis of cerebellar atrophy may be confirmed by MRI (midline sagittal section) or by CT scan. As a result, evidence of cerebellar atrophy is now found in many patients presenting with other aspects of chronic alcoholism or other nutritional disease who do not necessarily present with initial symptoms of ataxia.

Case 20.3 presented on the CD-ROM illustrates alcoholic cerebellar degeneration.

In other cases, this syndrome is the result of a chronic degenerative disease with a genetic basis. As in alcoholic cerebellar degeneration, the predominant histologic change is the loss of Purkinje cells in the anterior lobe. In contrast to alcoholic cerebellar degeneration, the pathology is usually more widespread and not strictly limited to the anterior lobe. In the following case history, the major involvement was primarily of the anterior lobe. There was definite family history, including evidence of consanguinity.

CASE HISTORY 20.3

A 45-year-old single white male carpenter presented with a 4-year history of progressive unsteadiness in walking, present during the daytime as well as at night, and a minimal loss of coordinated movements in his hands. He felt that his greatest deficit was unsteadiness. He had some numbness at the toes and minor difficulty in swallowing. His mother and father were second cousins. Several aunts and uncles had "trouble with their legs" in later life, resulting in a difficulty in walking.

Neurologic Examination

Cranial nerves: Intact except for minimal dysarthria. Horizontal nystagmus was present on lateral gaze; vertical nystagmus on upward gaze.

Motor system: The patient walked on a broad base with an ataxia of trunk, as though intoxicated, reeling from side to side, with marked unsteadiness on turns. He was unable to walk a tandem gait with eyes open. A mild intention tremor was present, and there was minimal disorganization of alternating movements. In contrast, a marked ataxia and tremor were evident on heel-to-shin test.

Reflexes: There was a relative decrease in ankle jerks compared to knee jerks.

Sensory system: There was a minimal decrease in vibration sensation at the toes.

Clinical diagnosis: Hereditary cerebellar degeneration involving predominantly anterior lobe.

Laboratory data: *Pneumoencephalogram* performed at the University of Virginia Hospital (Dr. Stewart) confirmed the significant atrophy of cerebellum.

Syndrome of the Lateral Cerebellar Hemispheres (Neocerebellar or Middle-Posterior Lobe Syndrome)

A number of disease entities may produce symptoms that can be related to the lateral hemisphere. Some of these disease

---

[4] In general, chronic lesions of cerebellum in humans do not alter tone or tendon reflexes. Acute lesions of cerebellum resulting from hemorrhage or surgery may produce transient hypotonia (Diener and Dichgans, 1992).

Figure 20.7 Generalized cerebellar atrophy most severe in the anterior superior vermis: computerized tomography (CT) scan. This 48-year-old female, following an acute febrile illness and 3 weeks of coma at age 3 years, developed severe ataxia of stance and gait, with dysmetria on heel-to-shin testing, distal weakness in lower extremities, and bilateral Babinski's signs.

entities are mass lesions such as metastatic tumors (Fig. 20.7) or intrinsic tumors (Fig. 20.8). The diagnostic problem, moreover, is complicated by the fact that involvement of the cerebellar peduncles may produce many of the same symptoms that result from direct involvement of the cerebellar hemisphere. The student will recall that the lateral medullary infarct produces an ipsilateral intention tremor and an impairment of alternating movements of the ipsilateral upper extremity. Occlusion of the posterior inferior cerebellar artery may produce an infarct of the lateral medulla and/or of the posterior inferior cerebellum, as demonstrated in Figure 13.12.

Demyelinating disease, that is, multiple sclerosis, may involve in a specific case both the brain stem and cerebellum in a multifocal manner. Cases presenting relatively pure focal involvement of the lateral hemisphere are those patients surviving after gunshot or shrapnel wounds. Such cases have been studied by Holmes (1939); they are not encountered frequently in civilian practice. Diener and Dichgans (1992) provide a more detailed physiologic analysis of lateral cerebellar lesions affecting the limbs.

The major findings in lateral hemisphere lesions are the following signs and symptoms in the ipsilateral extremities: intention tremor, disorganization of alternating movements (dysdiadochokinesia), dysmetria, ataxia, and overshoot on rebound. The intention tremor may be described as a tremor perpendicular to the line of motion, often becoming more

Figure 20.8 Cerebellar atrophy most prominent in anterior superior vermis with predominant anterior lobe syndrome: magnetic resonance imaging (MRI). This 70-year-old female 23 years previously had prolonged markedly elevated temperature related to meningitis, coma, and convulsions with a residual ataxia of stance and gait.

prominent on slower movements and as the target is approached. This intention tremor may be noted in the finger-to-nose test. One may also demonstrate a similar tremor in the lower extremities as the patient attempts to raise the foot off the bed to touch the examiner's finger or in the heel-to-shin test. As with the other signs of cerebellar disease, intention tremor is usually ipsilateral to the hemisphere involved.

At times, in addition to an intention tremor, a sustained postural "tremor" may be evident, more particularly if the superior cerebellar peduncle or its midbrain connections are involved. Brief jerks at the onset of movement (intention myoclonus) may occur when the dentate nucleus or superior cerebellar peduncle is involved.

The intention tremor represents a defect in the ability to dampen oscillations and to dampen overshoot. In the monkey, cerebellar tremor occurs despite deafferentation (section of the dorsal roots), a finding consistent with the concept that there is a central generator of oscillations. (However, other theories reviewed by Diener and Dichgans [1992] suggest the oscillations arise from dysfunction in long-latency transcortical reflexes.)

Having the patient slap the thigh above the knee with the hand at a particular rhythm tests repetitive movements. One can also test for repetitive movement in the lower extremities by having the patient tap toes or heel on the floor. Alternating movements are tested by having the patient slap the hand on the thigh or on the opposite hand, alternating between the palmar and dorsal surface of the hand. In disease of the cerebellar hemisphere a marked disorganization of repetitive and alternating movement occurs. This is almost always ipsilateral to the hemisphere involved.

These patients are also said to demonstrate dysmetria. This may be defined as a defect in the ability or impaired ability to know the force and rate of movement necessary for one to accurately control the range of movement of an extremity. Intention myoclonus may also occur at the onset of movement and may merge with hemichorea.

The effects of isolated lesions of the middle cerebellar peduncles are not certain. There is some evidence that an incoordination of fine limb movements and an ataxia of gait may result. In experimental lesions, circling may result.

OTHER CAUSES OF CEREBELLAR ATROPHY

Prolonged high fever, meningitis, a postinfectious syndrome, and repeated grand mal seizures may all be associated with the development of an ataxia that suggests major involvement of the anterior superior vermis. In some of these cases, more widespread atrophy is found on CT or MRI. At times, as in the case presented in Figure 20.9, other residual neurologic findings may also be present. The topography of cerebellar atrophy, particularly as regards midline structures, can best be studied with MRI. Figure 20.10 demonstrates the findings in a patient with gait ataxia following high fever and meningitis, in which atrophy, although widespread, was most prominent in the anterior superior vermis.

When the ataxia is of acute or subacute onset in childhood, the possibility of a cerebellitis must be considered.

Figure 20.9 Lateral cerebellar syndrome. This patient with bronchiogenic carcinoma had nystagmus and appendicular ataxia. He had this major tumor in the lateral cerebellum and minor metastatic lesions in the cerebral hemispheres. (Courtesy of Dr. John Hills and Dr. Jose Segarra.)

A varicella or other viral infection often precedes this entity. Mononuclear cells may be present in cerebrospinal fluid. Whether this is a direct viral infection or a postinfectious entity remains unclear. The major involvement is of the trunk, although tremors of the head, trunk, and limbs are also present. Recovery usually occurs over 6 months, but occasionally recovery is incomplete.

Diener and Dichgans (1992) discuss the localization of ataxia of standing body posture. Their conclusions are as follows:

1. Lesions of the spinocerebellar portion of the anterior lobe (mainly observed in chronic alcoholics) result in body sway along the anterior/posterior axis with a frequency of three per second. This sway, or tremor, is provoked by eye

Figure 20.10 Syndrome of the lateral hemisphere: hemangioblastoma of cerebellum. This 72-year-old male had a 2-year history of vertex headache (worse on coughing), blurring of vision, diplopia, papilledema, and a lateralized ipsilateral tremor on finger-to-nose testing. (Courtesy of Doctor Jose Segarra.)

closure. Visual stabilization of posture occurs. Since the direction of sway of the trunk is opposite that of the head and legs, the center of gravity is only minimally shifted and the patient does not fall.

2. In contrast, the lesions of the vestibulocerebellum (flocular nodular lobe and lower vermis), which are primarily mass lesions, produce a postural instability of head and trunk during sitting, standing, and walking. Postural sway occurs in all directions often at a frequency of less than 1 per second. Visual stabilization is limited; falls, therefore, are more frequent.

3. Spinal ataxia (as in tabes dorsalis and combined system disease) results predominantly in lateral body sway. Visual stabilization is prominent (positive Romberg test).

VASCULAR SYNDROMES OF THE CEREBELLUM

The development of CT and MRI scan has resulted in an increased recognition of infarcts, hemorrhages, and arteriovenous malformations involving the cerebellum. Many have been clinically silent or previously attributed to brain stem or labyrinthine pathology. We have already considered the blood supply of the cerebellum in Chapter 13, which covers vascular syndromes of the brain stem. Essentially, three circumferential arteries of the vertebral basilar circulation supply the several surfaces of the cerebellum, the arteries being named for the surface they supply:

1. The posterior inferior cerebellar artery (PICA), usually originating from the vertebral artery: an initial medial branch of this vessel supplies the lateral tegmental area of the medulla, and the medial and lateral branches supply the cerebellum.

2. The anterior inferior cerebellar artery (AICA), originating from the lower third basilar artery: the initial branches of this vessel supply the lateral tegmental area of the lower pons.

3. The superior cerebellar artery, originating from the rostral basilar artery: proximal branches supply the lateral tegmental area of the rostral pons and caudal mesencephalon.

All three vessels have extensive leptomeningeal anastomoses over the surface of the cerebellum that are similar to the leptomeningeal anastomoses of the arteries supplying the cortical surface of the cerebral hemispheres. As a consequence, vertebral artery occlusion may result in a lateral medullary infarct and syndrome, but infarction of cerebellum may be absent or limited. As in the cerebral hemispheres, border zone infarctions may occur. On the other hand, embolic occlusion is frequently implicated in cerebellar vascular syndromes.

SYNDROMES OF OCCLUSION AND INFARCTION

This topic has been well reviewed by Amarenco (1991), in an article that summarizes the detailed studies of his group (Amarenco et al., 1989, 1991; Amarenco and Hauw, 1990a, 1990b). The discussion presented here is in large part based on their studies. Refer also to the detailed reviews of Chaves et al. (1994) and Kase et al. (1993).

Although autopsy series localized only between 1.5% and 4.2% of all infarcts to the cerebellum, in a CT scan series (Shenkin and Zavala, 1982) cerebellar infarcts accounted for 15% of all intracranial infarcts. Cerebellar infarcts account for 85% of all cerebellar strokes and hemorrhages for 15%; therefore, our emphasis will be on infarcts.

The symptoms of infarcts and hemorrhages may be similar, particularly if the infarct is large and associated with considerable edema. The large infarct may have what is referred to as a "pseudotumor" presentation. Essentially, the patient has the acute onset of headaches (usually localized to the occipital or cervical occipital area), severe vertigo, nausea, vomiting, and ataxia of gait (often so severe that the patient is unwilling or unable to sit or stand). On examination, nystagmus and ipsilateral dysmetria on finger-to-nose and heel-to-shin tests will be present. Cerebellar type dysarthria is frequent (particularly when the superior cerebellar artery is involved). Coma at the onset or shortly after onset usually indicates severe edema with probable compromise of the fourth ventricle and/or aqueduct of Sylvius or brain stem. Evolving extraocular palsies are also usually indicative of compromise of the brain stem. MRI scan or CT scan allows the following:

a. Distinction between infarct and hemorrhage

b. Determination of whether hydrocephalus is present

c. Determination of the vascular territory of the cerebellum and brain stem involved

Patients presenting in coma or evolving into coma due to hydrocephalus and/or brain stem compression require immediate shunting to reduce the hydrocephalus and sometimes require evacuation of the hemorrhage or infarct (Heros, 1982; Shenkin and Zavala, 1982).

This acute presentation has long been recognized, although occasional patients are still initially misdiagnosed as suffering from acute labyrinthine vertigo, as in the example presented next. The majority (80% to 90%) of cerebellar infarcts have a more benign course not requiring surgical therapy. Many are recognized only in retrospect when a CT scan or MRI is obtained to analyze another central nervous system event (Fig. 20.11). The superior cerebellar artery territory or the posterior inferior cerebellar artery territory is most frequently involved. In our own experience, the symptomatic cerebellar infarct is often in the territory of the posterior inferior cerebellar artery (see following case history and Caplan [1986] and Chaves et al. [1996]). The anterior inferior cerebellar artery is rarely involved in isolation; the posterior inferior cerebellar territory is often also infarcted. One-third of patients with superior cerebellar artery infarcts also have infarcts within the territory of the posterior inferior cerebellar artery, suggesting a possible embolus from the vertebral artery to the more distal basilar artery branches. Although some patients with infarcts in the distribution of the posterior inferior cerebellar artery will also infarct the associated brain stem territory and present a lateral medullary infarct syndrome, as in case history 13.2, the majority have isolated cerebellar infarcts. In

Figure 20.11 Hemangioblastoma of superficial superior and posterior right cerebellar hemisphere. Computerized tomography (CT) scan indicated a densely enhancing mass (arrow) with considerable surrounding edema and cyst formation extending into the opposite cerebellar hemisphere and hydrocephalus. This 60-year-old white female had a several-month history of increasing headaches, exacerbated by straining at stool, laughing, or any head movement; a sense of dizziness; a sense of instability in walking; and a normal neurologic examination. Angiogram demonstrated a vascular mass supplied by the posterior inferior cerebellar and superior cerebellar arteries, as well as meningeal branches. Dr. Bernard Stone removed the tumor with relief of symptoms.

contrast, most patients with cerebellar infarcts of the anterior cerebellar artery territory also have infarcts of the caudal lateral tegmental pontine territory. Most patients with cerebellar infarcts of the territory of the superior cerebellar artery have associated infarcts in the brain stem territory of the rostral basilar artery. It is therefore easy to see that prior to the era of CT/MRI, the clinical features of the associated brain stem infarction (that included involvement of the cerebellar peduncles) dominated the picture and obscured the infarct of the cerebellum. More limited infarcts of parts of the superior cerebellar (lateral and medial) and posterior inferior cerebellar artery (dorsomedial and lateral) or of the cerebellar border zones are discussed in the various papers of Amarenco. The etiology for most infarcts involving the superior cerebellar artery is embolism of cardiac source. Posterior inferior cerebellar artery infarcts are either embolic of cardiac source or due to atherosclerotic occlusion of the vertebral or (less often) the posterior inferior cerebellar artery.

The following case history presents a typical example of posterior inferior cerebellar artery infarct, the territory most frequently affected selectively.

CASE HISTORY 20.4

This 64-year-old, right-handed, married white male on the morning prior to admission, awoke at 3 a.m. with severe posterior headache and severe vertigo, which was exacerbated by head movement; nausea; and projectile vomiting and slurred speech. Shortly afterward he noted a left facial paresthesias, clumsiness of the left upper extremity, and diplopia. Two weeks previously, the patient had been seen for a transient episode of difficulty controlling the right arm, a hissing sensation, and impairment of speech.

Past history was significant for hypertension and coronary artery bypass surgery; six years previously he had episodes of transient weakness and numbness of the right arm with transient aphasia for which he had been placed on long-term anticoagulants. At that time he had normal aortic arch and carotid angiography, but electroencephalography (EEG) had demonstrated focal left frontal/temporal slow-wave activity.

Neurological Examination

Cranial nerves: Conjugate lateral gaze to the left was impaired.

Motor systems: Lateralized cerebellar findings with marked dysmetria of left upper on finger-to-nose testing and impairment of alternating hand movements. In attempting to stand, the patient was markedly ataxic.

Reflexes: Deep tendon reflexes were decreased in both lower extremities. Plantar response was extensor on the right and flexor on the left.

Clinical diagnosis: The acute onset of headache, vertigo, vomiting, ataxia of gait, and dysmetria of the left arm was consistent with a left cerebellar infarct or hemorrhage with a possible minor involvement of brain stem secondary to mass effect.

Laboratory data: CT scan demonstrated a large left cerebellar infarct pressing the fourth ventricle on the right with no actual infarct in the brain stem (Fig. 20.12).

Subsequent course: The patient was somewhat vague with some difficulty in memory during the subsequent 8-day hospitalization and remained ataxic. He had 3 weeks of intensive rehabilitation with continued improvement. Evaluation 6 months after onset of symptoms revealed a slight slowness of alternating movements of the left hand.

A final note should be made regarding the considerable ability of the human nervous system to recover from extensive cerebellar lesions. Considerable recovery is possible because the cerebellum does not have a direct line role in the control of motor movement but instead acts as a modulator of motor and motor planning.

CEREBELLAR DEGENERATIVE DISEASES

The approach of Wood and Harding (2000) is considered, while adding more recent genetic information of Klockgether et al. (2000) and Fujigasaki et al. (2001).

The first step in classification is to separate all of these ataxic disorders into two main categories:

A. The autosomal recessive cerebellar ataxias are usually of early onset (< 20 years of age).

B. The autosomal dominant cerebellar ataxias (ADCAs) are usually of late onset (>20 years of age).

AUTOSOMAL RECESSIVE DISORDERS

The most common disorder in this category is Friedreich's ataxia, which accounts for at least 50% of all cases of hereditary ataxia reported in a large series from the United States

Figure 20.12 Cerebellar infarct in posterior inferior cerebellar artery territory. Case 20.6. Refer to text. Magnetic resonance imaging (MRI): (*A*) T1-weighted sagittal section 10 mm to left of midline. (*B*) T2-weighted posterior coronal section. (*C*) T2-weighted axial sections at level of upper medulla inferior olive.

and Europe. This disorder, which has a prevalence of 1–2 per 100,000, maps to chromosome 9q13. The mutation involves the trinucleotide repeat GAA. The normal number of repeats is 7–22, but in patients with Friedreich's ataxia there are 100–2000 repeats. The marked multiplication undoubtedly explains the early onset and severity of the disease. The gene product is a protein, frataxin. Refer to Chapter 9 for additional discussion.

Other rare disorders in this category include the following:

a. Cerebellar ataxia with retained deep tendon reflexes, in which a mutation in the frataxin gene also occurs. The cases are less severe than Friedreich's ataxia, but with greater cerebellar atrophy on imaging studies.

b. Cerebellar ataxia with hypogonadism in which there is predominant involvement of cerebellum and inferior olivary nuclei.

c. Cerebellar ataxia with myoclonus (formerly called the Ramsay Hunt syndrome or dyssynergia cerebellaris myoclonica) but now recognized to be a heterogeneous syndrome. Included in this category are such entities as (1) the mitochondrial disorder myoclonus epilepsy with ragged red fibers (MERRF) and (2) myoclonic epilepsy of Unverricht and Lundborg (Baltic myoclonus or EPM1). The gene locus which maps to chromosome 21 encodes a small protein cystatin B whose role in the neurological disease is unclear.

d. Other rare disorders in which cerebellar ataxia is associated in various combinations with deafness, optic atrophy, mental retardation, cataracts, or retinopathy.

e. There are also a whole host of relatively rare inherited, usually autosomal recessive metabolic disorders in which progressive cerebellar ataxia may be a prominent feature. One group of disorders involves deficiencies in vitamin E due to genetic mutations or to malabsorption syndromes such as cystic fibrosis. Some of these disorders might be treatable with administration of vitamin E.

An additional disorder carries the designation *ataxia telangiectasia*. This is an autosomal recessive disorder, with onset of a progressive cerebellar ataxia beginning in the first 1 to 2 years of life followed by the development of choreoathetosis. One in 40,000–100,000 live births is affected. An associated finding in all cases, usually appearing by age 6, is the presence of telangiectasis or capillary dilatation of severe and progressive degree, initially involving the conjunctiva but then appearing over the face and neck and the flexor surfaces of the limbs (antecubital and popliteal areas). The neuropathology primarily affects the Purkinje and granule cells of cerebellar cortex. These patients have severe medical problems related to the immune system, affecting both cellular and humoral immunity. The thymus remains in a fetal state. The patients have a marked sensitivity to ionizing radiation and to radiomimetic chemicals, as studied in cultured fibroblasts. The mutation that has been linked in some cases to chromosome 11q results in a defect in repair of DNA. The defective immune state results in a susceptibility to infectious diseases. There is a marked increase in malignancies, particularly leukemia and lymphomas, with rates which are 61 to 184 times normal. More recently, studies of the heterozygotes (who constitute 1% of the general population but do not have neurologic symptoms) have demonstrated a significant increase in cancer rates, with an overall rate approximately 3.5 times that in the general population and breast cancer rates in females 5 times those in the control population. Diagnostic or occupational exposure to ionizing radiation increases the cancer risk of the heterozygotes compared to the controls (Swift et al., 1991).

AUTOSOMAL DOMINANT DISORDERS

These disorders were a problem in classification. The names of the authors of the various papers describing the clinical features and neuropathology of each of the groups of cases or families were attached as labels and included many of the famous neurologists of the late 1800s and early 1900s such as Holmes, Andre Thomas, Marie, Foix, and Alajounine (Greenfield, 1954). Holmes separated these disorders into spinocerebellar degeneration, relatively pure degeneration of the cerebellar cortex, and olivopontocerebellar degeneration. More recently, Harding (1982) proposed a clinical classification into three major categories, of which the first type is the most common.

ADCA I: cerebellar ataxia is accompanied at some point in evolution by supranuclear ophthalmoplegia, optic atrophy, basal ganglia symptoms, dementia, and amyotrophy.

ADCA II: in addition to the above has retinal degeneration.

ADCA III: presents a relatively pure cerebellar syndrome.

ADCA IV: is a recent addition to the classification; cerebellar ataxia is combined with epilepsy.

The problem with all of these classifications from a clinical diagnostic standpoint is that, early in the disease, all three groups might have predominantly cerebellar features. With the unraveling of the molecular genetic basis of the diseases, the term *ADCA* has been replaced by the term *spinocerebellar ataxia* (SCA). To date, 12 different loci have been identified and in many of these the molecular mechanism has been identified (SCA1–SCA12).[5] The gene products of the SCA genes are termed ataxins and are assigned a similar number. In addition two channelopathies causing episodic ataxias have been identified as EA 1 and 2.

GENE MECHANISMS

1. *CAG trinucleotide expansion:* SCA 1, 2, 3, 6, 7, and 12 all involve an expansion of the CAG trinucleotide repeat as in Huntington disease (chromosome 4p16.3) but the chromosome loci are different (SCA 1 at 6p, SCA 2 at 12q, SCA 3 at 14q, SCA 6 at 19p, SCA 7 at 3p, SCA 12 at 5p). This expansion is translated into proteins with expanded polyglutamine tracts. At the ultrastructural level, these expanded proteins are found in neuronal intranuclear inclusions.

2. *CTG trinucleotide expansion:* SCA 8 is a CTG expansion on 13q, the same type of trinucleotide expansion found in myotonic dystrophy.

3. *Channelopathy:* In EA 1 there is a point mutation in a potassium channel on chromosome 12. In EA 2 there is a point mutation in a calcium channel on chromosome 19q.

Patients with EA 1 have frequent brief attacks of ataxia lasting for minutes plus myokymia (a muscle rippling due to peripheral motor nerve hyperexcitability). The patients are normal between attacks. Some cases benefit from acetazolamide or phenytoin. Patients with EA 2 have longer attacks lasting for hours to days involving severe truncal ataxia plus vertigo and vomiting. The patients respond well to acetazolamide. However, nystagmus is noted between attacks and over the years a slowly progressive ataxia develops. The MRI study at that point will confirm the cerebellar atrophy.

SCA 6 also has features of a channelopathy in that the CAG expansion occurs in a gene that encodes a voltage-dependent calcium channel. The chromosome location 19 is similar to EA 2.

4. *Unknown*: The mechanisms involved in SCA 4, SCA 5, SCA 10,[6] and SCA 11 are at the present time unknown. The chromosome locations are SCA 4 at 16q, SCA 5 at 11 centromere, SCA 10 at 22q, and SCA 11 at 15q.

Relationship to the clinical classification: SCA 1, 2, 3, and 12 correspond in general to ADCA I. Whether SCA 2 or SCA 3 is the most frequent mutation depends on the series reviewed (Giunti et al., 1998).[7]

SCA 7 corresponds to ADCA II.

SCA 5, 6, 8, and 11 correspond to ADCA III. SCA 5, however, has some posterior column features. SCA 6 has some sensory and pyramidal features and thus could be placed in the ADCA I group.

SCA 4 has cerebellar features plus a sensory neuropathy and probably would have been classified as ADCA I.

SCA 10[8] combines cerebellar ataxia with epilepsy (ADCA IV).

Azorean Disease: Machado-Joseph Disease

Refer to the reviews of Rosenberg (1992) and Sudarsky et al. (1992).

This autosomal dominant spinocerebellar degeneration is clustered among families who originated in the Portuguese Azorean Islands. This is the region of origin for many families residing in southeastern Massachusetts and the adjacent area of Rhode Island, and the initial cases were described in this area in 1972. Subsequently, other cases have been described in many areas of the world reached by Portuguese seafarers, explorers, whalers, and fishermen (many of whom were recruited in the Azores). The manifestations depend in part on the age of onset.

1. Early-onset (childhood or young adult) cases have predominantly pyramidal features and basal ganglia dysfunction.

2. Intermediate age of onset (20 to 40 years) cases have cerebellar deficits and extraocular disturbances as well as the pyramidal features and basal ganglia dysfunction.

3. Later onset (50 to 60 years) cases are characterized by cerebellar deficits and peripheral neuropathy.

4. Possible late-onset case may have a peripheral neuropathy plus Parkinsonism.

---

[5] As of April 2002, the number of identified loci has grown to 17. SCA 17 involves a CAG trinucleotide expansion.

[6] SCA 10 has now been associated with a pentaneuclotide expansion.

[7] A recent addition to this CAG expansion group is DRPLA (dentatorubropallidoluysian atrophy), a basal ganglia disorder.

[8] and SCA 17.

Since the molecular basis of the disorder is now clear, the more specific molecular diagnosis should be utilized when possible: most families carry the SCA 3 mutation. Occasionally the SCA 1 or the SCA 2 mutations have been found. In contrast to OPCA to be discussed next, the cerebellar cortex and the inferior olivary nucleus are not involved. The ataxia instead correlates with a degeneration of the afferent and efferent cerebellar systems (spinocerebellar tracts and Clarke's column dorsal nucleus) and the lid retraction and other extraocular features reflect involvement of the periaqueductal and third nerve nuclear areas.

OLIVOPONTOCEREBELLAR ATROPHY

This diagnosis once included many of the cases subsequently described as ADCA or SCA. *When cases of progressive adult onset ataxia are familial, they should be assigned a diagnosis based on the genetic classification described earlier.* This entity also has been considered in Chapter 19 on the basal ganglia and is one of the multisystem atrophies considered in the general category of Parkinsonism plus syndromes. In contrast to the data presented in that chapter, Berciano (1988), when considering both familial and sporadic cases of olivopontocerebellar atrophy (OPCA), found cerebellar symptoms (predominantly gait ataxia) to be the most common initial symptom (73%) and the most frequent symptom throughout the course of the disease (88%–97%). Parkinsonian symptoms occurred as the initial feature in 8% but eventually in 35%–57%. The neuropathology involved in all cases the cerebellar cortex, the pontine nuclei, and the inferior olivary nuclei with associated changes in the white matter of cerebellar peduncles (particularly the middle) and of the cerebellar white matter. The substantia nigra is involved in 50% of cases.

Nonfamilial cases of ADCA: Wood and Harding (2000) estimate that approximately two-thirds of cases of degenerative ataxia beginning after age 20 are single cases without a family history, and they suggest that the term *idiopathic late-onset cerebellar ataxia* be utilized rather than the old term, *OPCA*. The majority of cases do demonstrate the pathological findings of OPCA. Some will go on to develop the autonomic features of multisystem atrophy. Some of the patients with onset after age 55 years will demonstrate a relatively pure midline cerebellar syndrome with primarily gait ataxia related to cerebellar atrophy, which is most marked in the vermis. With tests for the molecular basis of the disease now available (particularly as regards the trinucleotide expansions), the number of such sporadic unclassified cases should be reduced. Note that families have become smaller, and full family historical information is not always available. There are, however, other entities to be considered when faced with a sporadic case.

Alcoholic nutritional cerebellar degeneration: refer to earlier discussion in relation to anterior lobe.

Paraneoplastic subacute cerebellar degeneration: This degeneration is associated particularly with cancer of the ovary, breast, small-cell cancer of the lung, and Hodgkin's disease. The neurologic symptoms may precede the discovery of the primary malignancy in the majority of these patients, except in those with Hodgkin's disease, where the diagnosis of the malignancy usually has already been established. In general, these patients present with subacute onset of cerebellar symptoms affecting stance, gait, limbs, and voice (dysarthria). The neuropathology involves a widespread loss of Purkinje cells and evidence of inflammation. The brain stem and dorsal root ganglia and possibly the limbic system may also show inflammatory changes, as part of a wider "encephalitis." Anti-Purkinje cell antibodies can be identified in many of these patients. Anti-yo antibodies which involve the Purkinje cell cytoplasm are found in patients with ovarian cancer, breast cancer, or other gynecological malignancies. Patients with Hodgkin's disease who develop the cerebellar syndrome may have antibodies to a glutamate receptor (Smitt et al., 2000). The paraneoplastic syndromes may improve with control of the primary malignancy. Note, however, that the late cases have evidence on CT or MRI of cerebellar atrophy (Fig. 20.13).

AN OVERVIEW OF TREMORS

Before concluding our discussion of the cerebellum and basal ganglia, we will briefly outline the various types of tremor. This is necessary because many common postural tremors (physiologic and essential) are mistakenly attributed to more serious disease of the basal ganglia or cerebellum. Tremor is defined as an involuntary movement characterized by rhythmic oscillation of a body part (or parts) that develops when there is a synchronized discharge of many motor units. Many peripheral and central factors enter into this synchronization. Hallett (1998), Elble (1998), and Hua (1998) discuss the physiology of tremor and the role of mechanical factors and central oscillators.

Tremor is best classified on the basis of the behavioral situation in which the tremor is observed (Deuschl, 1998; Findley, 1988; Hallet, 1991): (1) tremor at rest and (2) action tremor. Within this second category, postural, kinetic, or intention, and task-specific tremors are distinguished.

1. *Rest tremor:* This is a tremor that occurs in a body part that is not voluntarily activated and is completely supported against gravity. This tremor, particularly when a pill-rolling component is present, is almost always indicative of Parkinson's disease or of related disease of the basal ganglia.

2. *Action tremor:* This is a tremor that is produced by voluntary contraction of muscle. Within this category several subtypes may be specified:

    a. *Postural tremors:* These are by far the most common types of tremor and include the following:

       1. *Physiologic tremor*—usually fine and rapid (6 to 12 Hz), occurs when attempting to sustain a posture. This tremor is significantly increased or "enhanced" by anxiety, excessive caffeine intake, exercise, fatigue. It is also increased by thyrotoxicosis, hypoglycemia, alcohol withdrawal, and beta adrenergic drugs, such as those used in the treatment of asthma and by drugs commonly employed in psychiatry, such as lithium, neuroleptic, or tricyclic medications. Beta

Figure 20.13 (*A*) Large midline-paramedian cerebellar hemorrhage with rupture into the ventricle. This hypertensive (240/110) 61-year-old male had sudden onset of headache, vomiting, dizziness, ataxia of gait and trunk, nystagmus on left lateral gaze, and minor incoordination of the left hand. (Courtesy of Dr. John Hills and Dr. Jose Segarra.) (*B*) Large hypertensive hemorrhage into right cerebellar hemisphere with hydrocephalus. Computerized tomography (CT) scan (nonenhanced). This 65-year-old white male, who had hypertension, diabetes, congestive heart failure, and alcoholism, developed over 1 hour vomiting and a marked ataxia of gait. Examination indicated severe ataxia of gait, marked horizontal nystagmus on gaze to the right, dysmetria on right finger-to-nose and heel-to-shin tests, plus a mild right Horner's syndrome and a mild dysarthria, and bilateral Babinski signs. Symptoms resolved over several weeks.

adrenergic blockers such as propranolol are often effective against this tremor if specific etiologic factors cannot be corrected (use in asthmatics, however, is contraindicated).

2. *Essential tremor:* also called familial, benign, or senile tremor. Aside from physiologic tremor, essential tremor is the most common tremor encountered by the physician. Prevalence studies suggest a high frequency, particularly in older age groups. In the over-40 age group, 5% of the population may be affected. When familial, the genetic pattern appears to be autosomal dominant. Onset of familial cases may occur in childhood, adolescence, in midlife, or later in life. The hands are most commonly affected, but in some patients, the head is primarily involved (side-to-side movement). Some also have involvement of the voice or lips. The frequency of tremor ranges from 4 to 12 Hz. The tremor may remain stable or may slowly progress. Although in some patients the tremor is of relatively small amplitude, in other patients it may become relatively coarse, significantly interfering with fine motor activities. Orthostatic tremor is a variant in which a tremor of trunk and legs and to a lesser degree of arms occurs on prolonged standing and is associated with a high frequency of contractions alternating between antagonist muscles.

The underlying pathology of essential tremor is unknown. Functional imaging studies at rest and on action suggest an abnormal bilateral overactivity of cerebellar connections. Infarcts (homolateral) of the cerebellum or of contralateral motor cortex or of ventrolateral thalamus may result in the disappearance of the tremor (Dupuis et al., 1989). Typical of essential tremor is the temporary reduction in the tremor by ingestion of alcohol. The tremor usually responds to beta adrenergic blockers, such as propranolol. Note that in essential tremor, Parkinsonian and cerebellar features are absent; thus, the patient is able to walk with a good swing of the arms and does not turn en bloc. No pill-rolling tremor emerges as the patient sits at rest or walks. No ataxia of gait or stance is present. These distinctions are of importance because postural tremors (of the outstretched hands) can also occur in patients with clear-cut evidence of akinetic rigid variants of Parkinson's disease, Wilson's disease, dystonia, and cerebellar disease. A postural tremor may also occur in some forms of peripheral neuropathy or in posttraumatic syndromes.

b. *Kinetic tremors* (usually approximately 5 Hz). These are tremors occurring during any voluntary movement. Several types have been specified:

1. *Tremor during targeted, directed movements: intention tremor.* Amplitude increases during visually guided movements toward a target, particularly at the termination of movement. This tremor usually is characteristic of cerebellar disease and is described in detail earlier. Intention tremor is an oscillation perpendicular to the line of movement. Findley (1988) distinguishes the tremor from dysmetria, defining the latter as "the inability to attain the target or normal performance level in a guided, goal-seeking movement." The more severe and violent kinetic tremors are seen in patients with severe multiple sclerosis involving both the brain stem and cerebellum. In these cases, the head and trunk may have a to-and-fro, anterior-to-posterior sway, or tremor,

to which the term "titubation" has been applied (Findley, 1988). Cerebellar intention tremor may be decreased by lesions of the contralateral ventral lateral thalamic nucleus as discussed in Chapter 19.

2. *Task-specific kinetic tremor*: Kinetic tremor that appears or becomes exacerbated during specific activities related to occupation or writing. It is uncertain whether primary writing tremor and some of the occupational tremors of musicians and so on represent a variant of essential tremor or of dystonia, as discussed by Hallet (1991).

MAJOR FIBER PATHWAYS OF THE CEREBELLUM

CEREBELLAR PEDUNCLES

The cerebellum is interconnected to the brain stem by three major fiber bundles, or brachium: superior cerebellar, middle cerebellar, and inferior cerebellar peduncles (Fig. 11A).

1. Superior cerebellar peduncle (brachium conjunctivum). The axons of this pathway are primarily efferent and ascending axons originating in the deep cerebellar nuclei—dentate, emboliform. These fibers cross in the tegmentum of the lower midbrain (decussation of the superior cerebellar peduncle) with some fibers ending on the red nucleus and oculomotor complex. However, the majority of the fibers in the superior cerebellar peduncle distribute to the motor nuclei of the thalamus-ventral lateral and ventral anterior nuclei. This cerebellar projection to the motor cortex permits the well-controlled volitional acts of the corticospinal and corticobulbar systems. The ventral spinocerebellar fibers enter the cerebellum through the superior cerebellar peduncle.

2. Middle cerebellar peduncle (brachium pontis) is the largest cerebellar peduncle and is purely afferent. The largest group of descending fibers from the cerebral hemispheres is directed upon the pontine gray. These fibers form the bulk of the cerebral peduncle and descend from all cortical lobes and the cingulate and insular gyrus, with the largest group of fibers coming from the somatosensory strip and premotor cortex. These corticopontine fibers synapse upon the pontine gray and then pass into the contralateral cerebellar hemisphere. Lesions in these fibers systems do not cause any clinical deficit, although these fibers must be important in all fine movements. The corticopontine fibers end on the pontine nuclei. The axons from the pontine nuclei are crossed and constitute part of the mossy-fiber input to the granule cells.

3. Inferior cerebellar peduncle (restiform body) connects the brain stem and spinal cord with the cerebellum. The *climbing fibers* from the inferior olive enter this peduncle and extend to the Purkinje cells in the deep cerebellar nuclei (Fig. 20.2A). The fibers from the vestibular nuclei, reticular formation, and trigeminal nuclei, as well as the dorsal spinocerebellar fibers, enter through this peduncle. Many of these fibers contribute to the *mossy-fiber* input to the cerebellum. The aminergic fibers from the raphe and locus ceruleus also enter the cerebellum through the inferior cerebellar peduncle. There is a major cerebellar projection onto the reticular formation of the pons and medulla and onto the vestibular nuclei from the fastigial nucleus, as well as a strong cerebellar input onto the vestibular nuclei from the flocculonodular lobe.

SPINOCEREBELLAR TRACTS

The cerebellar cortex must have proprioceptive information to ensure proper muscle tone and coordination. Fibers carrying this information run to the cerebellum in the following pathways: anterior spinocerebellar, posterior spinocerebellar, and cuneocerebellar.

1. Unconscious proprioception from the lower extremity, thorax, abdomen, and pelvis. This information is carried up to the cerebellum by the anterior and posterior spinocerebellar tracts. These tracts carry information from proprioceptive receptors in the body into the cerebellum with the anterior pathway crossed while the posterior is uncrossed.

   a. Anterior spinocerebellar tract, *crossed* (Fig. 20.14, left side). The primary neuron is in the dorsal root ganglion, while the secondary neuron is in cells at the margin of the dorsal horn that are scattered throughout the spinal cord, especially in the lumbar levels. The secondary axon crosses the midline and ascends anterior to the posterior spinocerebellar tract in the lateral funiculus and medulla; it enters the cerebellum via the superior cerebellar peduncle and terminates in the same parts of the cerebellar vermis as the posterior spinocerebellar tract *except it is located on the contralateral side.* The receptors for both tracts are the neuromuscular spindles and Golgi tendon organs.

   b. Posterior spinocerebellar tract, *uncrossed/ipsilateral* (Fig. 20.14, right side). The primary cell bodies are in the ipsilateral dorsal root ganglion; the secondary neuron is located in Clarke's column in the dorsal horn at levels C8 to L3 of the cord. *The secondary axons ascend uncrossed/ipsilateral in the lateral funiculus, enter the cerebellum via the inferior cerebellar peduncle, and terminate in the ipsilateral vermis (midline portion of the cerebellum).*

   c. Cuneocerebellar tract. Unconscious proprioception from the upper extremity and neck and head. Cuneocerebellar pathway. The primary neurons are found in the dorsal root ganglion at cervical levels and in the trigeminal proprioceptive fibers. Their axons ascend in the dorsal columns and end in the external cuneate nuclei (external to the cuneate nucleus) in the lower medullary levels. The secondary axons ascend bilaterally with the posterior spinocerebellar tract and enter the cerebellum primarily uncrossed.

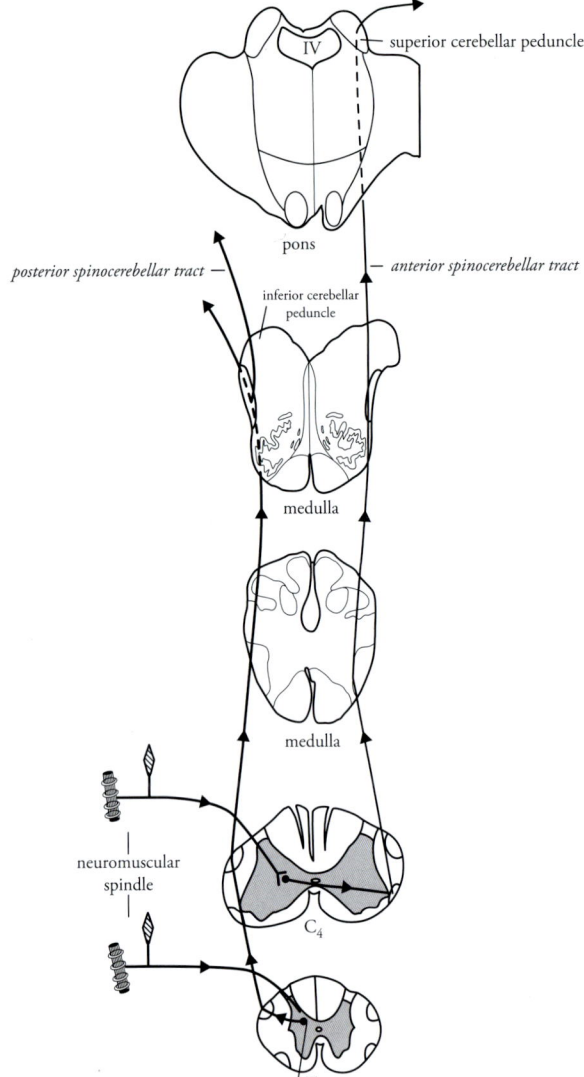

Figure 20.14 Spinocerebellar tracts in spinal cord medulla and pons.

BIBLIOGRAPHY

PART I: GENERAL ANATOMY, PHYSIOLOGY, AND FUNCTIONAL LOCALIZATION

Allin, M., Matsumoto, H., Santhouse, A. M., Nosarti, C., et al. 2001. Cognitive and motor function and the size of the cerebellum in adolescents born very preterm. Brain 124:60–66.

Amarenco, P., Chevrie-Muller, C., Roullet, E., and Bousser, M. G. 1991. Paravennal infarct and isolated cerebellar dysarthria. Ann. Neurol. 30:211–213.

Carrera, R. M. E., and Mettler, F. A. 1947. Physiologic consequences following extensive removals of cerebellar cortex and deep cerebellar nuclei and effect of secondary cerebral ablations in the primate. J. Comp. Neurol. 87:167–288.

Courchesne, E., Townsend, J., and Saitoh, O. 1994. The brain in infantile autism: posterior fossa structures are abnormal. Neurology 44:214–223.

Diener, H. C., and Dichgans, J. 1992. Pathophysiology of cerebellar ataxias. Mov. Disord. 7:95–109.

Dow, R. S., and Moruzzi, G. 1958. The Physiology and Pathology of the Cerebellum. Minneapolis: University of Minnesota Press.

Drepper, J., Timmann, D., Kolb, F. P., and Diener, H. C. 1999. Non-motor associative learning in patients with isolated degenerative cerebellar disease. Brain 122:87–97.

Fiez, J. A., Petersen, S. E., Cheney, M. K., and Raichle, M. E. 1992. Impaired non motor learning and error detection associated with cerebellar damage. A single case study. Brain 115:155–178.

Gilman, S. 1986. Cerebellum and motor function. In A. K. Asbury, G. M. McKhann, and W. I. McDonald.(Eds.) Diseases of the Nervous System Clinical Neurobiology. Vol.1, pp. 401–422. Philadelphia, PA: W. B. Saunders.

Gilman, S., Bloedel, J. R., and Lechtenberg, R. 1981. Disorders of the Cerebellum. Philadelphia, PA: F. A. Davis.

Holmes, G. 1922. Clinical symptoms of cerebellar disease and their interpretation. The Croonian Lectures. Lancet 1:1177–1182, 1231–1237; 2:59–65, 111–115.

Holmes, G. 1939. The cerebellum of man. Brain 62:1–30.

Ito, M. 1984. The Cerebellum and Motor Control. New York, NY: Raven Press.

Lechtenberg, R. 1988. Ataxia and other cerebellar syndromes. In J. Ankovic and E. Tolosa (Eds.) Parkinson's Disease and Movement Disorders, pp. 365–376. Baltimore, MD and Munich, Germany: Urban & Schwarzenberg.

Lechtenberg, R., and Gilman, S. 1978. Speech disorders in cerebellar disease. Ann. Neurol. 3:285–290.

Levinsohn, L., Cronin-Golomb, A., and Schmahmann, J. D. 2000. Neuropsychological consequences of cerebellar tumor resection in children. Brain 123:1041–1050.

Mettler, F. A., and Orioli, F. 1958. Studies on abnormal movement: cerebellar ataxia. Neurology 8:953–961.

Orioli, F. L., and Mettler, F. A. 1958. Consequences of section of the simian restiform body. J. Comp. Neurol. 109:195–204.

Raymond, J. L., Lisberger, S. G., and Mauk, M. D. 1996. The cerebellum: a neurononal learning machine? Science 272:1126–1131.

Riva, D., and Giogi, C. 2000. The cerebellum contributes to higher functions during development. Brain 123:1041–1061.

Sanes, J. N., Dimitrov, B., and Hallett, M. 1990. Motor learning in patients with cerebellar dysfunction. Brain 113:103–120.

Schmahmann, J. D., and Sherman, J. C. 1998. The cerebellar cognitive affective syndrome. Brain 121:561–579.

Thach, W. T. 1987. Cerebellar inputs to motor cortex. In Ciba Foundation Symposium 132. Motor Areas of the Cerebral Cortex, pp. 201–220. Chichester, UK: John Wiley.

Thach, W. T., Goodkin, M., and Keating, J. G. 1992. The cerebellum: the adaptive coordination of movement. Ann. Rev. Neurosci. 15:402–442.

Topka, H., Valls-Sole, J., Massaquoi, S. G., and Hallett, M. 1993. Deficit in classical conditioning in patients with cerebellar degeneration. Brain 116:961–969.

Wood, N. W., and Harding, A. E. 2000. Ataxic disorders. In W. G. Bradley, R. B. Daroff, G. M. Fenichel, and C. D. Marsden (Eds.) Neurology in Clinical Practice. Vol 1., pp. 309–317. Boston, MA: Butterworth Heinemann.

Wood, N. W., and Harding, A. E. 2000. Cerebellar and spinocerebellar disorders. In W. G. Bradley, R. B. Daroff, G. M. Fenichel, and C. D. Marsden (Eds.) Neurology in Clinical practice. Vol. 2, pp. 1931–1951. Boston, MA: Butterworth Heinemann.

PART II: MIDLINE AND LATERAL HEMISPHERE TUMORS (see Chapter 13 AND Chapter 27)

PART III: VASCULAR SYNDROMES OF THE CEREBELLUM (See also Chapters 13 and 26)

Amarenco, P. 1991. The spectrum of cerebellar infarctions. Neurology 41:973–979.

Amarenco, P., and Hauw, J. J. 1990a. Cerebellar infarction in the territory of the superior cerebellar artery: a clinicopathologic study of 33 cases. Neurology 40:1383–1390.

Amarenco, P., and Hauw, J. J. 1990b. Cerebellar infarction in the territory of the anterior and inferior cerebellar artery. Brain 113:139–155.

Amarenco, P., Hauw, J. J., Hinin, D., et al. 1989. Cerebellar infarction in the territory of the posterior inferior cerebellar artery: a clinicopathological study of 28 cases. Rev. Neurol. (Paris) 145:277–286.

Amarenco, P., Kase, C. S., Rosengart, A., et al. 1993. Very small (border zone) cerebellar infarcts. Distribution, causes, mechanisms and clinical features. Brain 116:161–186.

Amarenco, P., Roulellet, E., Goujon, C., et al. 1991. Infarction in the anterior rostral cerebellum (The territory of the lateral branch of the superior cerebellar artery). Neurology 41:253–258.

Caplan, L. R. 1986. Vertebrobasilar occlusive disease. In H. J. M. Barnett, et al. (Eds.) Stroke: Pathophysiology: Diagnosis and Management, pp. 549–619. Elsevier, New York.

Chaves, C. J., Caplan, L. R., Chung, C. S., and Amarenco, P. 1994. Cerebellar infarcts. Curr. Neurol. 14:143–177.

Chaves, C., Pessin, M. S., Caplan, L. R., et al. 1996. Cerebellar hemorrhagic infarction. Neurology 46:346–349.

Greenberg, J., Skubick, D., and Shenkin, H. 1979. Acute hydrocephalus in cerebellar infarct and hemorrhage. Neurology 29:409–413.

Heros, R. 1982. Cerebellar infarction and hemorrhage. Stroke 13:106.

Kase, C. S., and Caplan, L. R. 1986. Hemorrhage affecting the brain stem and cerebellum. In H. J. M. Barnett et al. (Eds.) Stroke: Pathophysiology: Diagnosis and Management, pp. 1015–1020. Elsevier, New York.

Kase, C. S., Norrving, B. O., Levine, S. R., et al. 1993. Cerebellar infarction. Clinical and anatomical observations in 66 patients. Stroke 24:76–83.

Skenkin, H. A., and Zavala, M. 1982. Cerebellar strokes: mortality, surgical indications and results of ventricular drainage. Lancet 11:429–431.

St. Louis, E. K., Wijdicks, E. F., and Li, H. 1998. Predicting neurologic deterioration in patients with cerebellar hematomas. Neurology 51:1364–1369.

Sypert, G. W., and Alvord, E. C. 1975. Cerebellar infarction. A clinicopathological study. Arch. Neurol. 32:357–363.

PART IV: DEGENERATIONS AND SYSTEMIC DISORDERS (See also Chapters 19 and 27)

Baloh, R. W., Yee, R. D., and Honrubia, V. 1986. Late cortical cerebellar atrophy: clinical and oculographic features. Brain 109:159–180.

Berciano, J. 1988. Olivopontocerebellar atrophy. In J. Jankovic and E. Tolosa (Eds.) Parkinson's Disease and Movement Disorders, pp.131–151. Baltimore, MD and Munich, Germany: Urban and Schwarzenberg.

Bhatia, K. P., Griggs, R. C., and Ptacek, L. J. 2000. Episodic movement disorders as channelopathies Mov. Disord. 15:429–433.

Burk, K., Abele, M., Fetter, M., et al. 1996. Autosomal dominant cerebellar ataxia type I clinical features and MRI in families with SCA 1, SCA 2 and SCA 3. Brain 119:1497–1505.

Carbonari, M., Cherchi, M., Pagnelli, R., et al. 1990. Relative increase of T cells expressing the gamma/delta rather than the alpha/beta receptor in ataxia teliangiectasis. N. Engl. J. Med. 322:73–76.

Fujigasaki, H., Verma, I. C., Camuzat, A., et al. 2001. SCA 12 is a rare locus for autosomal dominant cerebellar ataxia: a study of an Indian family. Ann. Neurology. 49:117–121.

Giunti, P., Sabbadini, G., Sweeney, M. G., et al. 1998. The role of the SCA 2 trinucleotide repeat expansion in 89 autosomal dominant cerebellar ataxia. Frequency, clinical and genetic correlates. Brain 121:459–467.

Giunti, P., Sweeney, M. G., and Harding, A. E. 1995. Detection of the Machado-Joseph disease/ spinocerebellar ataxia three trinucleotide repeat expansion in families with autosomal dominant motor disorders including the Drew family of Walworth. Brain 118:1077–1085.

Greenfield, J. G. 1954. The Spinocerebellar Degenerations. Springfield, IL: Charles C. Thomas.

Harding, A. E. 1981. Friedreich's ataxia: a clinical and genetic study of 90 families with an analysis of early diagnostic criteria and intra-familial clustering of clinical features. Brain 104:589–620.

Harding, A. E. 1982. The clinical features and classification of the late onset autosomal dominant cerebellar ataxias. A study of 11 families including descendants of "the Drew family of Walworth." Brain 105:1–28.

Klockgether, T., Ludtke, R., Kramer, B., et al. 1998. The natural history of degenerative ataxia: a retrospective study in 466 patients. Brain 121:589–600.

Klockgether, T., Petersen, D., Gruuddy, W., and Dighans, J. 1991. Early onset cerebellar ataxia with retained tendon reflexes: clinical, electrophysiological and MRI observations in comparison to Friedreich's ataxia. Brain 114:1559–1573.

Klockgether, T., Wullner, U., Spauschus, A., and Evert, B. 2000. The molecular biology of the autosomal- dominant cerebellar ataxias. Mov. Disord. 15:604–612.

Mason, W. P., Graus, F., Lang, B., et al. 1997. Small cell lung cancer, paraneoplastic cerebellar degeneration and the Lambert –Eaton myasthenic syndrome. Brain 120:1279–1300.

Rosen, F. S., and Harris, N. L. 1987. A 30-year-old man with ataxia telangiectasia and dysarthria. Case records of the Massachusetts General Hospital: Case #2–1987. N. Engl. J. Med. 316:91–100.

Rosenberg, R. N. 1992. Machado-Joseph disease: An autosomal dominant motor system degeneration. Mov. Disord. 7:193–203.

Rosenberg, R. N. 1996. DNA-triplet repeats and neurologic disease. N. Engl. J. Med. 335:1222–1224.

Smitt, P. S., Kinoshita, A., De Leeuw, B., et al.2000. Paraneoplastic cerebellar ataxia due to autoantibodies against a glutamate receptor. N. Engl. J. Med. 342:21–27.

Sudarsky, L., Corwin, L., and Dawson, D. M. 1992. Machado-Joseph disease in New England: clinical description and distinction from olivopontocerebellar atrophy. Mov. Disord. 7:204–208.

Swift, M., Morrell, D., Massey, R. B., and Chase, C. L. 1991. Incidence of cancer in 161 families affected by ataxia-telangiectasia. N. Engl. J. Med. 325:1831–1836.

Swift, M., Reitnaver, P. J., Morrell, D., and Chase, C. L. 1987. Breast and other cancers in families with ataxia and telangiectasia. N. Engl. J. Med. 316:1289–1294.

Tolosa, E., and Berciano, J. 1993. Choreas, hereditary and other ataxias and other movement disorders. Curr. Opin. Neurol. and Neurosurg. 6:358–368.

Truman, J. T., Richardson, E. P., Jr., and Dvorak, H. F. 1975. Case records of the Massachusetts General Hospital, Case 22-1975 (ataxia—telangiectasia). N. Engl. J. Med. 292:1231–1237.

Victor, M., Adams, R. D., and Collins, G. H. 1989. The Wernicke Korsakoff Syndrome and Related Neurological Disorders Due to Alcoholism and Malnutrition. 2nd ed. Philadelphia, PA: F. A. Davis.

Victor, M., Adams, R. D., and Mancall, E. L. 1959. A restricted form of cerebellar cortical degeneration occurring in alcoholic patients. Arch. Neurol. 1:579–688.

Yount, W. J. 1981. IgG2 deficiency and ataxia telangiectas (Editorial). N. Engl. J. Med. 306:541–543.

PART V: TREMOR (See also Chapter 19)

Colebatch, J. G., Britton, T., Findley, L. J., et al. 1990. The cerebellum is activated in essential tremor. Lancet 2:1028–1030.

Deuschl, G. 1998. Tremor: basic mechanisms and clinical aspects. Mov. Disord. 3(Suppl. 3):1–149.

Deuschl, G., Wenzelburger, R., Loffler, K., et al. 2000. Essential tremor and cerebellar dysfunction. Clinical and kinematic analysis of intention tremor. Brain 123:1568–1580.

Dupuis, M. J. M., Delwaide, P. J., Boucguey, D., and Gonette, R. E. 1989. Homolateral disappearance of essential tremor after cerebellar stroke. Mov. Disord. 4:183–187.

Elble, R. J. 1998. Animal models of action tremor. Mov. Disord. 13(Suppl. 3): 35–39.

Findley, L. J. 1988. Tremors: differential diagnosis and pharmacology. In J. Jankovic and E. Tolosa (Eds.) Parkinson's Disease and Movement Disorders, pp. 243–261. Baltimore, MD and Munich, Germany: Urban & Schwarzenberg.

Hallett, M. 1991. Classification and treatment of tremor. JAMA. 266:1115–1117.

Hallett, M. 1998. Overview of human tremor physiology. Mov. Disord. 13(Suppl. 3):43–48.

Hua, S., Reich, S. G., Zirh, A. T., et al. 1998. The role of the thalamus and basal ganglia in Parkinsonian tremor. Mov. Disord. 13(Suppl. 3):40–42.

Mc Auley, J. H., and Marsden, C. D. 2000. Physiological and pathological tremors and rhythmic central motor control. Brain 123: 1545–1567.

21.

SOMATOSENSORY FUNCTION AND THE PARIETAL LOBE

The parietal lobe is composed of the postcentral gyrus and superior and inferior parietal lobules. Each area will be considered in terms of cytoarchitecture and functions. For the superior and inferior parietal lobules, the different effects of disease processes in the dominant compared to nondominant hemispheres will be considered. The major sensory pathways have already been covered in Chapters 7 (spinal cord), 11 (brain stem), and 15 (diencephalon). The student may wish to review that material at this time.

POSTCENTRAL GYRUS: SOMATIC SENSORY CORTEX (PRIMARY SENSORY S-I)

The postcentral gyrus is not, from a histological standpoint, homogeneous. Four subtypes may be distinguished:

1. Area 3a at the base of central sulcus

2. Area 3b along the posterior wall of the central sulcus (anterior surface of the gyrus). Both areas are relatively typical granular koniocortex and receive the major projection from the ventral posterior nuclei of the thalamus.

3. Area 1 on the crest of the gyrus

4. Area 2 on the posterior surface of the postcentral gyrus. Both are modified homotypical cortex. While some of the neurons in areas 1 and 2 receive direct input from the ventral posterior thalamic nuclei, other neurons are dependent on collaterals from area 3.

STIMULATION

Stimulation of the postcentral gyrus produces a sensation over the contralateral side of the face, arm, hand, leg, or trunk described by the patient as a tingling or numbness and labeled paresthesias. Less often, a sense of movement is experienced. The patient does not describe the sensation as painful. These various phenomena, occurring at the onset of a focal seizure, may be described as a somatic sensory aura.

There is in the postcentral gyrus a sequence of sensory representation that, in general, is similar to that noted in the precentral gyrus for motor function (Fig. 21.1). The representation of the face occupies the lower 40%; the representation of the hand, the middle upper 40%; and the representation of the foot, the paracentral lobule. As in the precentral gyrus, certain areas of the body have a disproportionate area of representation, that is, the thumb, fingers, lips, and tongue. Those areas of the skin surface that are most sensitive to touch have not only the greatest area of cortical representation but also the greatest number and density of receptors projecting to the postcentral gyrus.[1] The peripheral field of each of these receptors is also very small (e.g., compared to the less sensitive skin areas of the trunk). In addition, at the lower end of the postcentral gyrus, extending into the sylvian fissure (the parietal operculum), there is found a representation of the alimentary tract, including taste. Gustatory hallucinations may arise from seizure foci in this area (Hausser-Hauw and Bancaud, 1987). There is also a representation of the genitalia in the paracentral lobule and the rare patients with seizures beginning in this area have reported paroxysmal sexual emotions, including orgasm and nymphomania.

Microelectrode techniques for recording from single cells in the cerebral cortex of the monkey and cat have allowed a considerable elaboration of the functional localization within the sensory cortex. The studies of Mountcastle (1957) indicated a vertical columnar organization from cortical surface to white matter. While each column is modality specific, each neuron in a particular column is activated by that specific sensory modality, for example, touch, movement of a hair, deep pressure, and joint position. Jones et al. (1982), Jones and Powell (1970), and Killackey and Ebner (1973) discuss the specific thalamocortical relationships. The studies of Kass and his associates (1979, 1981, 1983) provide additional elaboration. Within the postcentral gyrus, four representations of the body and limb surfaces are present in a parallel manner, with each representation relatively modality specific. The cells in area 3a respond primarily to muscle stretch receptors; area 3b to rapidly and slowly adapting skin receptors (as in movement of a hair or skin indentation); area 1 to rapidly adapting skin receptors; and area 2 to deep pressures and joint position.

Within areas 1 and 2, there are additional neurons that do not receive direct thalamic input. These neurons respond instead to more complex properties of the stimulus such as the specific direction of movement and have been labeled complex cells.

Studies of cortical potentials evoked by tactile stimulation in the monkey have suggested that there is a secondary

---

[1] We will discuss in Chapter 30 the more recent observations that indicate a considerable degree of plasticity may be present in sensory cortex. The maps here illustrated then for an individual human or monkey may be subject to some degree of variability. See also Kass et al. (1983).

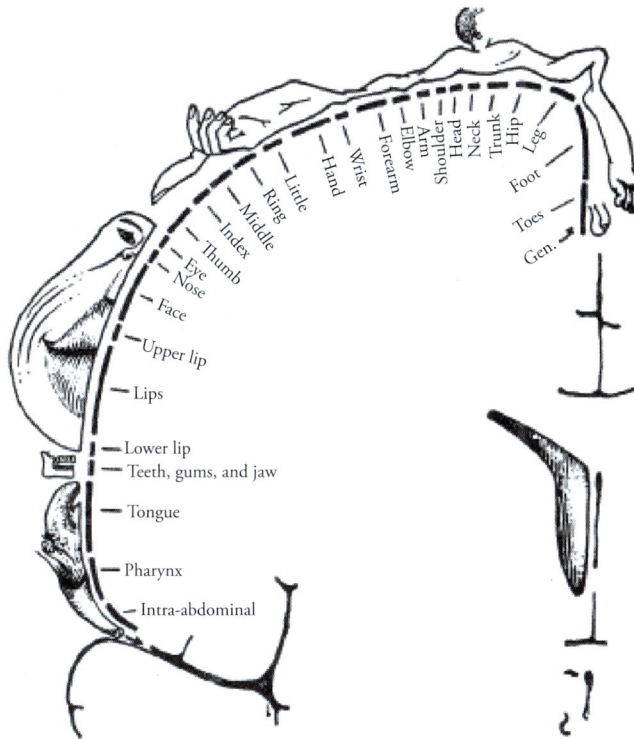

Figure 21.1 Sensory representation as determined by stimulation studies on the human cerebral cortex at surgery. Note the relatively large area devoted to lips, thumb, and fingers. (From Penfield, W., and Rasmussen, T.: The Cerebral Cortex of Man. New York, Macmillan, 1955, p. 214.)

somatic sensory projection area (S-II) in addition to the classic postcentral contralateral projection area. This second area has a bilateral representation and is found partially buried in the sylvian fissure at the lower end of the central sulcus. A similar second area of representation has been reported by Penfield and Jasper (1954), Luders et al. (1985), and Blume et al. (1992) in those seizure patients in whom an abdominal sensation (aura) was followed by a sensation of paresthesias in both sides of the mouth and in both hands (Fig. 18.11). Note also that at times stimulation of the precentral gyrus by the neurosurgeon during surgery has produced contralateral tingling or numbness, in addition to the more frequent motor responses (Penfield and Jasper, 1954). Additional discussion of seizures originating in parietal lobe will be found in Williamson et al. (1992) and Tuxhorn and Kerdar (2001).

ABLATION

Immediately following complete destruction of the postcentral gyrus, there will often be found an almost total loss of awareness of all sensory modalities on the contralateral side of the body. Within a short time there is usually a return of some appreciation of painful stimuli. The patient will, however, often continue to note that the quality of the painful stimulus differs from that on the intact side. An awareness of gross pressure, touch, and temperature also returns. Vibratory sensation may return to a certain degree. Certain modalities of sensation, however, never return or return only to a minor degree. (In partial lesions of the postcentral gyrus, however, these various modalities often return to a variable degree.) *These modalities are often referred to as the cortical modalities of sensation or as discriminative modalities of sensation.* The following types of sensory awareness usually included in this category are summarized in Table 21.1.

In contrast, the sensory modalities of pain, gross touch, pressure, temperature, and vibration are referred to as primary modalities of sensation. Perception of these modalities continues to occur after ablation of the postcentral gyrus, although some alteration in quality of sensation is noted. It has been assumed that the anatomical substrate for such awareness must exist at the thalamic level.

In terms of more specific localization of specific modalities of cortical sensation, the studies of Randolph and Semmes (1974) suggest that in the monkey small lesions restricted to area 3b (hand region) produce deficits in discrimination of

Table 21.1 MODALITIES OF SENSATION LOCATED IN POSTCENTRAL GYRUS

CORTICAL DISCRIMINATIVE SENSORY MODALITIES	TYPE OF STIMULUS
1. Position sense	Ability to perceive movement and the direction of movement when the finger or toe is moved passively at the interphalangeal joint, the hand at the wrist or the foot at the ankle
2. Tactile localization	Ability to accurately localize the specific point on the body or extremity which has been stimulated
3. Two-point discrimination	Ability to perceive that a double stimulus with a small separation in space has touched a given area on the body, limb, or hand
4. Stereognosis	Ability to distinguish the shape of an object and thus to recognize objects based on their three-dimensional tactile form
5. Graphesthesia	Ability to recognize numbers or letters which have been drawn on the fingers, hand, face, or leg
6. Weight discrimination	Ability to recognize differences in weight placed on the hand or foot
7. Perception of simultaneous stimuli	Ability to perceive that both sides of the body have been simultaneously stimulated. When bilateral stimuli are presented but only a unilateral stimulus is perceived, "extinction" is said to have occurred.
8. Perception of texture	Ability to perceive the pattern of surface stimuli encountered by the moving tactile receptors.

texture, size, and shape. Lesions in area 1 interfere with the ability to discriminate texture only; lesions in area 2, size and shape only.

The following case histories demonstrate the type of sensory phenomena found in disease involving the postcentral gyrus.

CASE HISTORY 21.1

One week prior to evaluation, this 40-year-old, right-handed, married white male had the onset of repeated 15- to 21-minute episodes of focal numbness (tingling or paresthesias) involving the left side of the face, head, ear, and posterior neck and occasionally spreading into the left hand and fingers, and rarely subsequently spreading into the left leg. Biting or eating would trigger the episodes. There was no associated pain, headache, weakness, or associated focal motor phenomena.

Initial neurological examination: Totally intact as regards mental status, cranial nerves, motor system, reflexes, and sensory system.

Clinical diagnosis: Focal seizures originating lower third postcentral gyrus, of uncertain etiology.

Laboratory Data

Electroencephalography (EEG): No focal abnormalities were present.

Computerized tomography (CT) scan (Fig. 21.2): The nonenhanced study was normal. The enhanced study demonstrated a small enhancing lesion just above the right sylvian fissure.

Magnetic resonance imaging (MRI) (Fig. 21.3): Demonstrated the more extensive nature of this process involving the operculum—above the right sylvian fissure including the lower end of the postcentral gyrus, the area of representation of the face. A probable infiltrating tumor was suggested as the most likely diagnosis.

Arteriogram demonstrated a tumor blush at the right sylvian area, consistent with a glioblastoma, a rapidly growing infiltrating tumor, originating from astrocytic glia.

Subsequent course: Treatment with an anticonvulsant reduced the frequency of the episodes. Neurosurgical consultation suggested an additional observation period and periodic CT scans. Three months after onset of symptoms, the patient developed a numbness of the left arm and difficulty in coordination of left arm. Exam now demonstrated left central facial weakness, mild weakness of the left hand, and in the left hand a loss of stereognosis and graphesthesia with a relative alteration in pinprick perception. The CT scan showed significant enlargement of the previous lesion. EEG now indicated focal (2–3 Hz delta slow waves) in the right frontal central Rolandic area. Dr. Bernard Stone performed a subtotal resection of a glioblastoma—in the right temporal parietal area. Radiation therapy was administered following surgery, 4000 rads total whole brain and 5210 rad total to the tumor area. Re-evaluation 3 months after surgery indicated only rare focal seizures involving the face. The neurological examination was normal. Repeat CT scans, however, continued to demonstrate a large area of enhancing tumor in the right temporal-frontal-parietal area. Despite the use of dexamethasone and arterial chemotherapy with cis-Platinum, he continued to progress with the development of a left field defect, left hemiparesis, and a loss of all modalities of sensation on the left side. Subsequently he developed significant changes in memory and cognition. CT scan demonstrated progression with extensive involvement of the right side of the brain and spread to the left hemisphere. Death occurred 33 months after onset of symptoms. At postmortem examination of the brain, almost the entire right

Figure 21.2 Glioblastoma somatic sensory cortex: focal sensory seizure with onset in left face. Case 21.1. Computerized tomography (CT) scan with contrast demonstrated a small focal enhancing lesion in the right postcentral gyrus just above the sylvian fissure. (Upper scan) Reference diagram for plane of section. (Lower scan) The enhancing lesion is marked with a white square. See text.

hemisphere was replaced by necrotic infiltrating tumor. The tumor now had spread into the corpus callosum and temporal and occipital lobes. The internal capsule, thalamus, hypothalamus, and basal ganglia were destroyed.

CASE HISTORY 21.2

This 62-year-old white, right-handed housewife, 6 years prior to admission, had undergone a left radical mastectomy for carcinoma of the breast. Five months prior to admission, the patient developed a persistent cough, left pleuritic pain, and a collection of fluid in the left pleural space (pleural effusion). She now had the

Figure 21.3 Glioblastoma, somatosensory cortex focal sensory left facial seizures. Case 21.1. (See text.) Magnetic resonance imaging (MRI) scans demonstrating the more extensive involvement of cortex and white matter: (*A*) coronal section (modified T2); (*B*) horizontal section (T2).

onset of daily headaches in the right orbit, occasionally awakening her from sleep. Four months prior to admission, over a 3- to 4-week period, the patient developed progressive "weakness" and difficulty in control of the right lower extremity. Several weeks later, the patient now experienced aching pain in the right index finger in addition to a progressive deficit in the use of the right hand. This was more a "stiffness and incoordination" than any actual weakness. One month prior to admission the patient noted episodes of pain in the toes of the right foot and numbness of right foot occurred, lasting 2 to 3 days at a time. She subsequently developed difficulty in memory and some minor language deficit, suggesting a nominal aphasia, prompting hospital admission.

Neurological Examination

Mental status: Slowness in naming objects was present, although she missed only one item of six. Delayed recall was slightly reduced to three out of five in 5 minutes.

Cranial nerves: Early papilledema was noted: absence of venous pulsations, indistinctness of disk margins, and minimal elevation of vessels as they passed over the disk margin. A right central facial weakness was present.

Motor system: Mild weakness of the right upper limb was present. A more marked weakness was present in the lower limb (most marked distally). Spasticity was present at the right elbow and knee. In walking, the right leg was circumducted; the right arm was held in a flexed posture.

Reflexes: Deep tendon reflexes were increased on the right. A right Babinski response was present.

Sensation: An ill-defined alteration in pain perception was present in the right arm and leg—more of a relative difference in quality of the pain than any actual deficit. Repeated stimulation of the right lower extremity (pain or touch) produced dysesthesias (painful sensation). Position sense was markedly defective in the right fingers with errors in perception of fine and medium amplitude movement in the right toes.

Simultaneous stimulation resulted in extinction in the right lower extremity.

Graphesthesia (identification of numbers, e.g., 8, 5, 4 drawn on cutaneous surface) was absent in the right hand and fingers and poor in the right leg. Tactile localization and two-point discrimination were decreased on the right side.

Clinical diagnosis: Metastatic tumor to the left postcentral and precentral gyri with a cortical pain syndrome (pseudothalamic pain syndrome).

Laboratory Data

Chest X-ray: Several metastatic nodules were present in the left lung.

EEG: Almost continuous focal 4 to 7 Hz slow-wave activity was present in the posterior frontal central and parietal areas.

Imaging studies were consistent with a focal metastatic lesion in the parasagittal upper left parietal area.

Subsequent course: Because there was evidence in this case that the disease had spread to multiple organs, radiation and hormonal therapy were, therefore, administered rather than any attempt at surgical removal of the left parietal metastatic lesion. Temporary improvement occurred in motor function in the arm, but the patient eventually expired 5 months after admission. Autopsy performed by Dr. Humphrey Lloyd of the Beverly Hospital disclosed extensive metastatic disease in the lungs, liver, and lymph nodes and a single necrotic metastatic brain lesion in the upper postcentral gyrus of the left parietal area, 1.0 cm below the pial surface and measuring 1.2 x 1.0 x 0.6 cm. The occurrence of episodic pain in the involved arms and legs along with the production of an experienced painful sensation on repetitive tactile stimulation (dysesthesias) in patients with sensory pathway lesions is sometimes referred to as a "thalamic" or "pseudothalamic" syndrome. (Refer to discussion of Wilkins and Brody, 1969.) In this case, the anatomical locus for the pseudothalamic syndrome is apparent.

The effects of deficits in cortical sensation on the total sensory motor function of a limb are apparent in this case. The actual disability and disuse of the right arm and leg were far out of proportion to any actual weakness. Such an extremity is often referred to as a "useless limb." The actual weakness that was present undoubtedly reflected pressure effects on the precentral gyrus and the descending motor fibers in adjacent white matter.

Destructive lesions of the postcentral gyrus during infancy or early childhood often produce a retardation of skeletal growth on the contralateral side of the body. Such a patient examined as an adolescent or adult will be found to have not only cortical sensory deficits in the contralateral arm and leg but also a relative smallness of these extremities (shorter arm or leg, smaller hand and glove size, smaller shoe size).

SUPERIOR AND INFERIOR PARIETAL AREAS

In the monkey these areas are collectively designated the posterior parietal cortex. In both the human and the monkey, superior and inferior parietal lobules can be distinguished divided by the intraparietal sulcus. In the human, the superior parietal lobule is composed of Brodmann's cytoarchitectural areas 5 and 7, and the inferior parietal lobule of areas 40 and 39 (the supra marginal and angular gyri). In the monkey, the superior parietal lobule is designated as area 5; the inferior parietal area as primarily area 7. This results in some confusion as correlations are attempted. There is no clear-cut gross homolog of areas 40 and 39 in the monkey cerebral cortex.

All of these areas may be classified as varieties of homotypical cerebral cortex. The major afferent input of the superior parietal lobule area 5 in the monkey is from the primary sensory areas of the postcentral gyrus. Area 7 of the monkey cortex receives indirect cortico-cortical connections. The superior parietal lobule receives projections from the posterior lateral nuclei of the thalamus; the inferior parietal lobule from the pulvinar (see Chapter 15). These secondary sensory areas project to an adjacent tertiary sensory area and then to a multimodal sensory association area at the temporal parietal junctional area. This latter area in the posterior parietal cortex then projects to another multimodal sensory association area in the frontal—periarcuate—principal sulcus area, to the premotor and frontal eye fields (discussed earlier in relationship to premotor and prefrontal motor function). Area 7 has connections to the limbic cortex: cingulate gyrus.

The implications of these connections for the integration of complex movements are clear. It is not surprising then that single-cell studies as reviewed by Darian-Smith et al. (1979) demonstrate responses of neurons in area 5 to manipulation of joints; hand manipulation as in grasping and manipulation objects, or in projecting the hand to obtain a specific object, associate with reward. Neurons in area 7 discharged in relationship to complex eye and limb movements (Lynch et al., 1977). The reviews of Andersen et al. (1997) and Colby and Goldberg (1999) discuss the multiple representations of space in the posterior parietal cortex, particularly the intraparietal sulcus area. When damage to parietal cortex occurs, the patient manifests a variety of spatial deficits. A neglect occurs in relation to multiple sensory modalities but is most prominent with regard to contralateral visual space as we will discuss next. There are corresponding deficits in the generation of spatially directed actions.

STIMULATION

The threshold of the superior and inferior parietal lobules for discharge is relatively high. Although Foerster reported the occurrence of some contralateral paresthesias on stimulation in humans, Penfield did not confirm these results. Stimulation in the inferior parietal areas of the dominant hemisphere did produce arrest of speech, but this is a nonspecific effect, occurring on stimulation of any of the speech areas of the dominant hemisphere. It must, of course, be noted that space-occupying lesions in the parietal lobules may produce sensory or motor seizures by virtue of their pressure effects on the lower threshold postcentral and precentral gyri.

ABLATION

Darian-Smith et al. (1979) have summarized the effects of selective lesions of area 5 and or area 7 in the monkey. The most selective studies were those of Stein (1977) using reversible cooling lesions. Cooling of area 5 resulted in a clumsiness of the contralateral arm and hand so that the animal was unable to search for a small object. Cooling of area 7 produced a much more complex clumsiness which was apparent only when the arm was moved into the contralateral visual field. Movements of the hand to the mouth were intact. (Refer to discussion of Colby and Goldberg [1999] and Wise et al. [1997], for a more recent discussion of the topic.)

Earlier clinical studies in humans had suggested possible sensory deficits in relation to ablation of the inferior or superior parietal areas. The detailed studies of Corkin et al. (1964) on patients subjected to limited cortical ablations of the inferior or superior parietal areas (in the treatment of focal epilepsy) clearly indicated that no significant sensory deficits occurred. The postcentral gyrus rather than the parietal lobules is critical for somatic sensory discrimination. The more recent studies of Pause et al. (1989) confirmed that anterior parietal (postcentral lesions) resulted in somatosensory disturbances, including surface sensibility, two-point discrimination, position sense, and more complex tactile recognition. In contrast, in posterior parietal lesions, there was a preferential impairment of complex somatosensory and motor functions involving exploration and manipulation by the fingers' not explained by any sensory deficit. There was a deficit in the conception and execution in the spatial and temporal patterns of movement. The end result is an impairment of purposive movement, as discussed earlier. The response to visual stimuli in terms of attending to and reaching for objects is impaired (see Baynes et al., 1986; Nagel-Leiby et al., 1990; Perenin et al., 1988; and Pierrott-Deseilligny et al., 1986). Lesions involving the white matter deep to the inferior parietal lobule may damage the superior portion of the optic (geniculocalcarine) radiation, producing a defect in the inferior half of the contralateral visual field, an inferior quadrantanopsia.

PARIETAL LOBE GENERAL FUNCTIONS

DOMINANT HEMISPHERE PARIETAL LOBULES

Destructive lesions of the parietal lobules produce additional effects on more complex cortical functions. Those lesions involving particularly the supramarginal and angular gyri of the dominant (usually the left hemisphere) inferior parietal lobule may produce one or more of a complex of symptoms and signs known as *Gerstmann's syndrome*. These include the following:

a. Dysgraphia (a deficit in writing in the presence of intact motor and sensory function in the upper extremities)

b. Dyscalculia (deficits in the performance of calculations)

c. Left-right confusion

d. Errors in finger recognition, for example, middle finger, index finger, ring finger, in the presence of intact sensation (finger agnosia)

e. In addition, disturbances in the capacity for reading may be present. Some patients may also manifest problems in performing skilled movements on command (an apraxia) at a time when strength, sensation, and coordination are intact.

Usually only partial forms of the syndrome are present. The problem of the dominant parietal lobe in language function will be considered in greater detail and illustrated in the section on language and aphasia. The reader should refer to Chapter 24 for an illustrative case history.

NONDOMINANT HEMISPHERE PARIETAL LOBULES

Patients with involvement of the nondominant parietal lobe, particularly the inferior parietal lobule, often demonstrate additional abnormalities in their concepts of body image, in their perception of external space, and in their capacity to construct drawings.

The disturbance in concept of body image may include the following: (a) a lack of awareness of the left side of the body, with a neglect of the left side of the body in dressing, undressing, and washing. (b) Despite relatively intact cortical and primary sensation, the patient may fail to recognize his arm or leg when this is passively brought into his field of vision. (c) The patient may have a lack of awareness of a hemiparesis despite a relative preservation of cortical sensation (anosognosia) or may have a total denial of illness. At times, this may be carried to the point of attempting to leave the hospital, since, as far as the patient is concerned, there is no justification for hospitalization. The denial of illness undoubtedly involves more than perception of body image.

The disturbance in perception of external space may take several forms: (a) neglect of the left visual field and of objects, writing, or pictures in the left visual field. At times, this is associated with a dense defect in vision in the left visual field; at other times, there may be no definite defect for single objects in the left visual field, but extinction occurs when objects are presented simultaneously in both visual fields. Again, the problem of possible involvement of occipital cortex or of subcortical optic radiation should be considered, as previously noted. (b) An inability to interpret drawings such as a map or to pick out objects from a complex figure. The patient is confused as to figure–background relationship and is disoriented in attempting to locate objects in a room. When asked to locate cities on an outline map of the United States, the patient manifests disorientation as to the west and east coasts and as to the relationship of one city to the next. Chicago and New Orleans may be placed on the Pacific Ocean; Boston on the Florida peninsula; and New York City somewhere west of the Great Lakes.

The disturbance in capacity for the construction of drawings has been termed a constructional apraxia or dyspraxia. An apraxia may be defined as an inability to perform a previously well-performed act at a time when voluntary movement, sensation, coordination, and understanding are otherwise all intact. The following deficits may be present: the patient may be unable to draw a house or the face of a clock; or to copy a complex figure such as a three-dimensional cube, a locomotive, and so forth; in severe disturbances the patient may be unable to copy even a simple square, circle, or triangle. The following case demonstrates many of these features.

CASE HISTORY 21.3 (FIG. 21.4)

This 70-year-old, single, white, female, right-handed, retired candymaker underwent a left radical mastectomy for carcinoma of the breast, 3 years prior to admission. Four months prior to evaluation, the patient became unsteady with a sensation of rocking as though on a boat. She no longer attended to her housekeeping and to dressing.

Figure 21.4 Nondominant parietal constructional apraxia. Case 21.3. The patient's attempts to draw a house are shown on the upper half of the page. Her attempts to copy a drawing of a railroad engine are shown on the lower half of the page (*B* and *C*). The examiner's (Dr. Leon Menzer) original is designated (*A*).

Over a 3-week period, prior to evaluation, a relatively rapid progression occurred with deterioration of recent memory. A perseveration occurred in motor activities and speech. The patient was incontinent but was no longer concerned with urinary and fecal incontinence. For 2 weeks, right temporal headaches had been present. During this time, her sister noted the patient to be neglecting the left side of her body. She would fail to put on the left shoe when dressing. In undressing, the stocking on the left would be only half removed.

Family history: The patient's mother died of metastatic carcinoma of the breast.

Neurological Examination

Mental status: Intact except for the following features: The patient often wandered in her conversation. She often asked irrelevant questions and was often impersistent in motor activities. There was marked disorganization in the drawing of a house or of a clock. A similar marked disorganization was noted in attempts at copying the picture of a railroad engine (Fig. 21.4). There was a marked neglect of the left side of space and of the left side of the body. The patient failed to read the left half of a page. When she put her glasses on, she did not put the left bow over the ear. When getting into bed, she did not move the left leg into bed. She had slipped off her dress on the right side, but was lying in bed with the dress still covering the left side. The patient had been reluctant to come for neurological consultation. Although she complained of headache and nausea, she denied any other deficits. Her relatives provided information concerning these problems. Much additional persuasion over a 2-week period was required before the patient would agree to be hospitalized.

Cranial nerves: A dense left homonymous hemianopsia was present. When reading, the patient left off the left side of a page. She bisected a line markedly off center. Disk margins were blurred and venous pulsations were absent, indicating papilledema. The right pupil was slightly larger than the left. A minimal left central facial weakness was present.

Motor system: Although strength was intact, there was little spontaneous movement of the left arm and leg. The patient was ataxic on a narrow base with eyes open with a tendency to fall to the left, and she was unable to stand with eyes closed even on a broad base.

Sensation: Although pain, touch, and vibration were intact, there was at times a decreased awareness of stimuli on the left side. Errors were made in position sense at toes and fingers on the left. Tactile

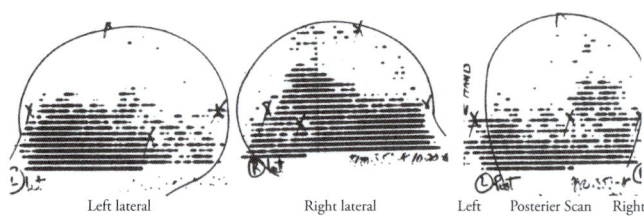

Figure 21.5 Nondominant parietal lesions. Case 21.3. Brain scan Hg[197]. A large uptake of radioisotope is demonstrated in the right parietal and adjacent posterior temporal area. (Courtesy of Dr. Bertram Selverstone.)

localization was poor over the left arm and leg. With double simultaneous stimulation, the patient neglected stimuli on the left face, arm, and leg.

Clinical diagnosis: Metastatic breast tumor to right nondominant parietal cortex.

Laboratory Data

Chest X-ray indicated a possible metastatic lesion at the right hilum.

EEG was abnormal because of frequent focal 3 to 4 cps slow waves in the right temporal and parietal areas, suggesting focal damage in these areas.

Imaging studies (brain scan radioisotope Hg[197] and arteriograms) were consistent with a large well-defined lesion in the posterior section of the right temporal inferior parietal area (Fig. 21.5).

Subsequent course: Treatment with steroids (dexamethasone and estrogens) resulted in temporary improvement. The patient refused surgery. Her condition soon deteriorated with increasing obtundation of consciousness. She expired 2 months following her initial neurological consultation.

A CT scan from a more recent case demonstrating many aspects of this syndrome is illustrated in Figure 21.6. In many cases, the location of lesion may appear to be predominantly posterior temporal. Such large posterior temporal lesions would certainly compromise the cortex and subcortical white matter of the adjacent inferior parietal area.

In this case, marked deficits in perception of the cortical modalities of sensation were present. In other cases, as in the case demonstrated in Figure 21.6, such involvement is much less marked.

In some cases, involvement of the motor cortex is evident with an actual left hemiparesis accompanied by an increase in deep tendon

Figure 21.6 Nondominant parietal lobe syndrome. Computerized tomography (CT) scans. This 68-year-old, left-handed male with diabetes mellitus and hypertension had the sudden onset of left arm paralysis, loss of speech, and loss of ability to read and write, all of which recovered rapidly. On examination 9 months after the acute episode he continued to have the following selective deficits: (1) He was vague in recalling his left hemiparesis. (2) In dressing, he reversed trousers and failed to cover himself on the left side. (3) He had extinction in the left visual field on bilateral simultaneous visual stimulation and over the left arm and leg on bilateral simultaneous tactile stimulation. (4) A left Babinski sign was present. CT scan now demonstrated an old cystic area of infarction in the right posterior temporal-parietal (territory of the inferior division of the right middle cerebral artery).

reflexes and an extensor plantar response. At times in patients with neglect syndromes, there may be several indications in the clinical examination and in the laboratory studies that the involvement of the frontal lobe areas is more prominent than the parietal involvement. We have already indicated that the neglect components of this syndrome may also be noted in lesions of the anterior premotor area (area 8). The prefrontal and premotor areas, as discussed earlier and in Chapter 18, receive projection fibers from the multimodal area of the posterior parietal area. It is possible that in some cases the posterior temporal–inferior parietal location of the lesion may also be critical in interrupting these association fibers. For these several reasons, it is perhaps more appropriate to use the term *syndrome of the nondominant hemisphere*, rather than the more localized designation *nondominant inferior parietal syndrome*. Duffner et al. (1990) have presented the concept of a network for directed attention—with right frontal lesions leading to left hemispatial neglect only for tasks that emphasize exploratory motor components of directed attention, whereas parietal lesions emphasize the perceptual-sensory aspects of neglect.

With lesions of the nondominant hemisphere, there is a significant alteration of the patient's awareness of his environment. The behavior of an individual is in part determined by his own particular perception of the environment. If that perception is altered or disorganized, the behavioral responses of the patient may appear inappropriate to others. Obviously, not all individuals will respond in the same manner to a given environmental situation; part of the response will be determined by the past experience and personality of the individual. Thus, given the same lesion, one individual may be unaware of a hemiparesis, another may deny the hemiparesis but agree an illness is present, a third may claim to be healthy and claim that people are conspiring to keep him in the hospital.

22.

LIMBIC SYSTEM

INTRODUCTION

Cure her of that: Canst though not minister to a mind diseased; pluck from the memory a rooted sorrow; raze out the written troubles of the brain; and with some sweet oblvious antidote clense the stuff'd bosom of that perilous stuff which weighs upon the heart"—Macbeth V;iii.

RHINENCEPHALON

The neurologist Paul Broca in the later half of the 19th century initially designated all of the structures on the medial surface of the cerebral hemisphere the "great limbic lobe." This region, due to its strong olfactory input, was also designated the rhinencephalon.

The olfactory portion of the brain (rhinencephalon, or archipallium) comprises much of the telencephalon in fish, amphibians, and most mammals. In mammals the presence of a large olfactory lobe adjacent to the hippocampus was once considered to be evidence of the important olfactory functions of these regions. However, when a comparative neuroanatomist examined the brains of sea mammals that had rudimentary olfactory apparatus, for example, dolphins and whales, the presence of a large hippocampus suggested other than olfactory functions for this region.

In 1937, Papez proposed that olfactory input was not the prime input for this region, and the experiments of Kluver and Bucy (1937, 1939) and Kluver (1952, 1958) demonstrated the behavioral deficits seen after lesions in this zone. More recently, it has been shown that in primates only a small portion of the limbic lobe is purely olfactory: the olfactory bulb, olfactory tract, olfactory tubercle, pyriform cortex of the uncus, and corticoamygdaloid nuclei (Fig. 22.1). The other portions—hippocampal formation, fornix, parahippocampal gyrus, and cingulate gyrus—are now known to be the cortical regions of the limbic system (Fulton, 1953; Green, 1958; Isaaccson, 1982; Papez, 1958).

EMOTIONAL BRAIN

Since the initial observations of Kluver and Bucy (1937) and Papez (1937), which localized emotions in the telencephalon, many other investigators have added information concerning the localization of behavior. We now know that many cortical and subcortical regions are incorporated in the "emotional brain."

Different investigators have coined different terms to succinctly describe the limbic system, particularly the visceral, vital, or emotional brain. The term "visceral brain" would seem appropriate since much of our emotional response is characterized by specific responses in the viscera (Fulton, 1953). On the other hand, the importance of the emotional response for the self-preservation of the individual and the perpetuation of the species has led other investigators to call this region the "vital brain" (MacLean, 1955). The term used most commonly by investigators and the one used in this chapter is limbic lobe (limbus = margin) because the involved region is located on the medial margin of the cerebrum and surrounds the brain stem as it enters the diencephalon.

We can separate the entire central nervous system into a "somatic brain," which controls the external environment through the skeletal muscles, and a "visceral brain," which controls the internal environment through the control of smooth muscles and glands. Our discussion of this region begins with the olfactory system and continues into the limbic system.

OLFACTORY SYSTEM

The olfactory system must be included in any discussion of the emotional brain as it sends fibers directly into the medial temporal lobe, and this olfactory information is especially important to the emotional brain.

OLFACTORY NERVE

The olfactory nerve (cranial nerve I) originates from the uppermost portions of both nasal fossae, which occupy the mucous membrane covering the superior nasal conchae and adjacent septum. The mucous membrane is attached to the walls of the nasal septum that in this region is formed by the ethmoid bone.

OLFACTORY RECEPTORS

The 100 million or more bipolar receptor cells are embedded in sustentacular cells. The dendrites of the receptor cells are short and ciliated. The cilia are embedded in the odor-absorbing secretion produced by the Bowman glands that forms the mucosa. New cells from the basal layer are constantly replacing the olfactory receptor cells. All of the axons from the olfactory neuroreceptor cells are unmyelinated. They gather together into about 20 bundles (fila olfactoria), which then pass through openings in the cribriform plate of the ethmoid bone to synapse in the olfactory bulb.

OLFACTORY DISCRIMINATION

Vertebrates with a well-developed sense of smell are called macrosmatic, while those with a poorly developed sense of

Figure 22.1 Gross view of ventral surface of the brain, demonstrating the olfactory bulb and the olfactory tract.

smell are called microsmatic. Dogs and cats are macrosmatic animals, while humans and all of the great apes are microsmatic (Fig. 22.2). In the dog, 15% of the brain is devoted to olfactory discrimination, while in the human brain, the portion devoted to olfaction is minute. Most dogs and cats have an olfactory system that is infinitely superior to ours both in sensitivity and the ability to discriminate among odors. Nevertheless, we can still distinguish thousands of different odors, and a multimillion-dollar industry has developed to stimulate our olfactory system. In fact, many people have built careers on their olfactory acuity (wine and coffee sniffers and perfumers). Many blind or deaf people have such a refined sense of smell that they can detect subtle changes in their environment.

Figure 22.2 Diagrammatic representation of the olfactory system and its connections.

The olfactory information is distributed from the olfactory bulb through three olfactory stria:

1. Intermediate stria—olfactory tubercle
2. Medial olfactory stria—septal region and via the anterior commissure into the opposite olfactory bulb
3. Lateral olfactory stria—olfactory cortex of the uncus and corticomedial amygdaloid. The terminations in the amygdala produce a strong response in the emotional brain to substances that stimulate the olfactory systems, especially smoke, food, and pheromones.

LIMBIC REGIONS IN THE BRAIN

The limbic/emotional brain is divided into cortical and subcortical regions. Cortical areas are located in frontal lobe, temporal lobe, and cingulate gyrus, while subcortical areas are found in the brain stem, diencephalon, and septum. Table 22.1 identifies the cortical and subcortical limbic structures.

SUBCORTICAL LIMBIC REGIONS

Reticular Formation of the Brain Stem and Spinal Cord

The spinal and cranial nerve roots are the first-order neurons for sensory information to reach the somatic and visceral brain. These peripheral nerves send much sensory information via axon collaterals into the reticular formation of the spinal cord, medulla, pons, and midbrain. The reticular formation is organized longitudinally, with the lateral area being the receptor zone and the medial area being the effector. In the medial zone are the ascending and descending multisynaptic fiber tracts of the reticular formation: the central tegmental tract.

Throughout the levels of the brain stem there are also certain important limbic nuclear groupings in the reticular formation.

The mesencephalic portion of the reticular formation seems to be especially important, since this zone provides a direct reciprocal pathway to the hypothalamus, thalamus, and septum.

From the locus ceruleus of the upper pons and the raphe of the midbrain the ascending serotoninergic and adrenergic systems run into the diencephalon and telencephalon and provide direct input into these regions.

Interpeduncular Nucleus

The interpeduncular nucleus (posterior perforated substance) is found on the anterior surface of the midbrain in the interpeduncular fossa extending from the posterior end of the mammillary body to the anterior end of the pons. It receives fibers from the habenular nuclei (habenulopeduncular tract) and has reciprocal connections with the hypothalamus and the midbrain limbic region. Amygdaloid information reaches this region through connections via the stria terminalis to the septum and then from the septum to the interpeduncular

Table 22.1 THE SUBCORTICAL AND CORTICAL NUCLEI OF THE LIMBIC SYSTEM

SUBCORTICAL NUCLEI OF THE LIMBIC SYSTEM	CORTICAL STRUCTURES OF THE LIMBIC SYSTEM
1. Reticular formation of the brain stem and spinal cord — Midbrain limbic nuclei (interpeduncular nucleus, paramedian nucleus, ventral tegmental area, ventral half of the periaqueductal gray)	1. Temporal lobe —Amygdala —Parahippocampal cortex —Hippocampal formation —Rostral portion of temporal lobes 2. Frontal lobe
2. Hypothalamus (preoptic, lateral, lateral mammillary nuclei)	—Frontal association areas —Supracallosal gyrus and longitudinal stria —Subcallosal gyrus —Orbital frontal cortex
3. Thalamus (midline, intralaminar, anterior, and dorsal medial nuclei)	3. Cingulate gyrus and cingulate isthmus
4. Epithalamus	
5. Septum	
6. Nucleus accumbens	

nucleus. Hypothalamic input and septal input are also important parts of the autonomic information to the brain stem passing through this nucleus.

Hypothalamus

The hypothalamus (Figs. 22.3 and 22.4; see Chapter 16) is the highest subcortical center of the visceral brain. The basic function of this region is to maintain internal homeostasis (body temperature, appetite, water balance, and pituitary functions) and to establish emotional content. It is a most potent subcortical center due to its control of the autonomic nervous system.

Figure 22.3 Medial surface of a cerebral hemisphere, including entire brain stem and cerebellum.

Figure 22.4 Medial surface of a cerebral hemisphere with medulla, pons, and cerebellum removed.

The hypothalamus receives input from all portions of the limbic system, as well as from the reticular formation, basal ganglia, and frontal association cortex. The hypothalamus connects to the thalamus, midbrain, pons, and medulla via the medial forebrain bundle and the dorsal longitudinal fasciculus (Nauta, 1963). Autonomic fibers from the hypothalamus run in the lateral portion of the reticular formation and descend to the cranial nerves ADD (parasympathetic) and the thoracolumbar (sympathetic) and sacral levels (parasympathetic). The most potent effects result from hypothalamic control of the pituitary gland and the adrenal medulla. The adrenal medulla releases epinephrine and norepinephrine, which produce a decrease in peripheral blood flow, an increase in central blood flow, and an increase in heart rate and force. These agents also stimulate release of glycogen stores from the liver, providing energy for muscular contractions that accompany the response.

The mammillary nuclei (Figs. 22.3, 22.4, and 22.6) of the hypothalamus connect to the anterior thalamic nuclei and habenula, via the mammillothalamic tract, and to nuclei in the brain stem tegmentum via the mammillotegmental tract. The lateral mammillary nucleus receives axons via the fornix from the hippocampus, axons from other portions of the hypothalamus and septum through the medial forebrain bundle, and input from the midbrain tegmentum and substantia nigra via the mammillary peduncle. Effects of hypothalamic stimulation on the autonomic system are listed in Table 22.2.

Stimulation of the hypothalamus can produce the flight-or-fight response (fear or rage), as well as several visceral responses—sweating, salivation, defecation, and retching. These can be produced in adjacent regions or by moving the electrode site or changing the stimulation parameters (e.g., by varying the current). Another interesting result has been noted in cats made docile with amygdaloid lesions; these animals become savage when a lesion is placed in the ventromedial hypothalamic nuclei. The effects of hypothalamic stimulation and ablation on sleep will be considered in Chapter 29.

Thalamus

The anterior, medial, midline, and intralaminar dorsal thalamic nuclei receive input from the ascending nociceptive

Table 22.2 EFFECTS OF HYPOTHALAMIC STIMULATION ON THE AUTONOMIC NERVOUS SYSTEM

STIMULATION OF ANTERIOR HYPOTHALAMUS = PARASYMPATHETIC RESPONSE	STIMULATION OF POSTERIOR HYPOTHALAMUS = SYMPATHETIC RESPONSE OR ANXIETY RESPONSE
Decrease in heart rate, respiration, and blood pressure; increase in peristalsis and in gastric and duodenal secretions; increased salivation; and depending on the internal milieu, even evacuation of the bowels and bladder. Constriction of the pupils; concomitant with the parasympathetic excitation is sympathetic inhibition.	Increase in heart rate, respiration, blood pressure; decrease in peristalsis and in gastric and duodenal secretions; decreased salivation with sweating, and piloerection. Dilation of pupils; concomitant with sympathetic excitation is parasympathetic inhibition.

pathways, hypothalamus, reticular system (especially the midbrain reticular formation), cingulate, and frontal association cortex (see Figs. 22.3 and 22.4). The intralaminar and midline nuclei connect to the medial and other specific dorsal thalamic nuclei, which then project to the cerebral cortex.

Epithalamus

The habenular nuclei (epithalamus) give origin to the habenulopeduncular tract, which projects to the midbrain tegmentum and interpeduncular nucleus. The habenular nuclei receive afferents from the septum and preoptic region via the stria medullaris and connect to the intralaminar nuclei. (See Chapter 16.)

Septum

The septum (Fig. 22.5) forms the medial wall of the frontal horn of the lateral ventricle. The septum consists of two parts: the septum pellucidum containing the septal nuclei (dorsal, lateral, and medial) and the caudal velum interpositum. The septum pellucidum is rostral to the interventricular foramen. The septum pellucidum consists of glial membrane and some pia arachnoid (velum interpositum). This paired glial membrane, along with the fornix, separates the bodies of the lateral ventricles.

The lower part of the septum pellucidum (septal area) consists of many neurons and glia.

This zone receives strong input from the amygdala via the stria terminalis and hypothalamus. The septum connects with the:

1. hypothalamus, interpeduncular nucleus, and the midbrain tegmentum via the medial forebrain bundle,
2. habenula via the stria medullaris, and
3. basolateral amygdaloid nuclei through the diagonal band.

Destruction of the septum in cats causes docile animals to become fearful or aggressive, but only for a short time. Complete destruction of the septum may produce coma, probably because it destroys the strong connections between the septum and hypothalamus.

Nucleus Acumbens

The nucleus acumbens (see Chapter 19) lies below the caudate and receives fibers from the amygdala via the ventral amygdalofugal pathway and from the basal ganglia; thus, it provides a major link between the limbic and basal nuclei. This nucleus has a high content of acetylcholine. In Alzheimer's disease, there is a significant loss of cholinergic neurons in this nucleus.

ROLE OF TEMPORAL LOBE CORTICAL STRUCTURES IN EMOTIONS

PARAHIPPOCAMPAL GYRUS

The uncus (a hook in Latin) forms the anterior-most region in the parahippocampal gyrus on the medial surface of the temporal lobe. Its surface is the olfactory cortex and the principal nucleus of the amygdala lies internally (Figs. 22.4 and 22.5).

AMYGDALOID NUCLEI

The amygdala is uniquely located to provide the intersection between the primary motivational drives of the hypothalamus and septum and the associative learning that occurs at the hippocampal and neocortical levels (Figs. 22.6–22.8).

The amygdala (Fig. 22.9) consists of three main groupings of nuclei: corticomedial, basolateral, and central. In addition to these principal nuclei, there are extratemporal neurons, including the nucleus of the stria terminalis and the sublenticular substantia innominata.

The amygdala receives extensive projections from many cortical areas and in turn sends projections to these areas. In primates, as one expects in comparison to rodents, there has been a significant increase in the projections from and to

Figure 22.5 Medial surface of a cerebral hemisphere with thalamus removed, demonstrating relationship between fornix and hippocampus.

Figure 22.6 Coronal section through diencephalon at level of massa intermedia showing mammillothalamic tract leaving mammillary body.

Figure 22.8 Coronal section through mammillary bodies and amygdala. Magnetic resonance imaging (MRI, T2 weighted).

isocortex (neocortex) as opposed to allocortex and mesocortex. These projections originate from (1) the multimodality sensory areas in temporal, parietal, occipital, and frontal lobes; (2) tertiary unimodal sensory association areas; (3) visual association areas that are particularly prominent in the primates; (4) first- and second-order central sensory neurons of the olfactory system; and (5) from hypothalamus, septum, and anterior cingulate regions.

From the standpoint of the role of the amygdala in emotion and instinctive behavior, there are important connections with the basal forebrain, medial thalamus (medial dorsal nucleus), hypothalamus (preoptic, anterior, ventromedial, and lateral areas), and the tegmentum of the midbrain, pons, and medulla (to various nuclei concerned with visceral function such as chewing, licking, and the motor components of emotional expression). These connections also form the basis of our responses to what one considers a dangerous situation and also the ability for one to recognize familiar faces and those that are not. The more specific connections of the amygdaloid nuclei are listed as follows:

1. *Olfactory nuclei.* The corticomedial group receives olfactory information from the lateral olfactory stria and interconnects with the contralateral corticomedial nuclei (via anterior commissure) and ipsilateral basolateral nuclei. The primary efferent pathway of the corticomedial nucleus is the stria terminalis, which projects to the septum, medial hypothalamus, including preoptic nucleus of the hypothalamus, and to the corticomedial nucleus in the opposite hemisphere.

2. *Limbic nuclei.* The central and basolateral nuclear grouping is associated with the limbic brain, and it has connections with the parahippocampal cortex, temporal pole, frontal lobe, orbital frontal gyri, cingulate lobe, thalamus (especially dorsomedial nucleus), catecholamine-containing nuclei of the reticular formation, and substantia nigra.

3. The *ventral amygdalofugal pathway* projects from the central nucleus to the brain stem and to the septum, the preoptic, lateral, and ventral hypothalamus, and—in the dorsal thalamus—to the dorsomedial, intralaminar, and midline thalamus.

Stimulation of the Amygdaloid Region

In monkeys, cats, and rats, stimulation produces aggressive behavior. The stimulated cats have a sympathetic response of dilated pupils, increased heartbeat, and extension of claws, piloerection, and attack behavior. When the stimulus stops, they become friendly. Animals will even fight when the amygdala is stimulated and stop fighting if the stimulus is off. Eating, sniffing, licking, biting, chewing, and gagging may also be stimulated here. In contrast, studies in the cat indicate that stimulation of the prefrontal areas will prevent aggressive behavior. In humans, stimulation of the amygdala produces feelings of fear or anger (Cendes et al., 1994). A role in sexual behavior has also been postulated, although this may be more prominent in the female.

Figure 22.7 Coronal section through amygdala and hypothalamus. Magnetic resonance imaging (MRI, T1 weighted). Hippocampal gyrus = parahippocampal gyrus.

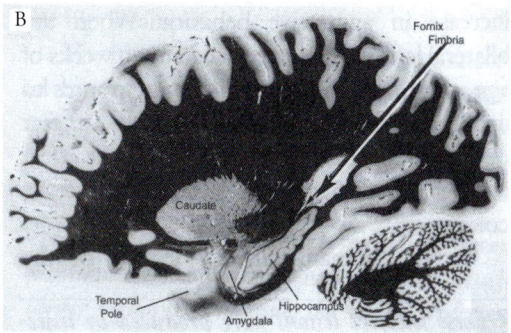

Figure 22.9 (*A*) Sagittal section. Temporal lobe with amygdala and hippocampus. Magnetic resonance imaging (MRI, T1 weighted). (*B*) Sagittal section, Weil myelin stain. Inferior horn LV is the junction of posterior and inferior horns of lateral ventricle.

Ablation of Amygdala

In the studies of Amaral, selective bilateral lesions of the amygdala[1] in the adult monkey significantly decreased the fear response to inanimate objects such as an artificial toy snake. This object was now picked up, whereas previously, such an object had triggered intense fear responses. The social interactions of the lesioned monkey with other members of a colony were significantly altered. The lesioned animals were more sociable with more sexual and nonsexual friendly contacts with other members of the colony. They were described as socially uninhibited. In the male, aggression was decreased, but occasional females had an increase in aggressive behavior. When the bilateral lesions were produced at 2 weeks of age, there was a decrease in fear responses to inanimate objects but an increase in fear responses to other monkeys. This latter effect interfered with their social integration into the colony.

In the human, bilateral lesions of the amygdala have been produced for control of aggression. In patients with bilateral lesions of the amygdala, there is an impairment of the ability to interpret the emotional aspects of facial expression (Adolphs et al., 1996). Patients with high-functioning autism have a similar disorder (Adolphs et al., 1996). On functional magnetic resonance imaging (MRI) studies, these patients failed to activate the left amygdala, as well as the cortical face area or the left cerebellum when implicitly processing facial expressions (Baron-Cohen et al., 2000; Critchley et al., 2000). When quantitative MRI is performed in such autistic patients, there is significant enlargement of the volume of the amygdala. Howard et al. (2000) suggest that these results may indicate that a developmental malformation of the amygdala (possibly an incomplete neuronal pruning) may underlie the social-cognitive impairments of the autistic patient.

THE NEOCORTEX OF THE TEMPORAL LOBE

Lateral Neocortical Areas

As regards the neocortical areas, area 41, the primary auditory projection area, is located on the more anterior of the transverse gyri of Heschl (Fig. 22.13). This area is a primary special sensory region and has a pronounced layer IV (granular or koniocortex) similar to but considerably thicker than areas 17 and 3. Area 41 receives the main projection from the medial geniculate nucleus of the thalamus. Our understanding of the tonal organization in this region comes from studies in the monkey and chimpanzee where the lowest frequencies project to the more rostral areas. Some investigators limit the term "Heschl's gyrus" to the more anterior of the transverse gyri and localize the primary auditory cortex to the posterior aspects of that gyrus (Liegeois-Chauvel et al., 1991).

The remaining neocortical areas of the temporal lobe have a well-defined six cortical layers and are classified as homotypical.

Auditory and Auditory Association

Area 42 surrounds area 41 and receives association fibers from this area. Area 22, in turn, surrounds area 42 and communicates with areas 41 and 42. Both areas 42 and 22 are often designated as auditory association areas, and in the dominant hemisphere they are important in understanding speech as Wernicke's area.

Visual Perceptions

The inferior temporal areas have significant connections with area 18, providing a pathway by which visual perceptions, processed at the cortical level, may then be related to the limbic areas.

HIPPOCAMPAL FORMATION

This region of the limbic system has been of critical importance in our understanding of both the clinical aspects and underlying biological substrate of memory and of complex partial epilepsy.

Anatomical Correlates

From an anatomical standpoint, compared to other lobes of the brain, the temporal lobe is a complex structure. It contains four diverse components:

Neocortex: six layers: superior, middle, and inferior temporal gyri (see Chapter 17)

Allocortex: three layers: the olfactory cortex, hippocampal formation, and subiculum

---
[1] These selective lesions were produced by injection of ibotenic acid, which damages neurons but does not affect fibers of passage.

Mesocortex: a transitional type of six-layer cortex (transitional between neocortex and allocortex): entorhinal/parahippocampal gyrus (the large posterior segment of the pyriform region), presubiculum, and parasubiculum

Cortical nucleus: the amygdala (discussed earlier)

The *hippocampus* is phylogenetically the older part of the cerebral cortex termed *allocortex* and consists of three layers: polymorphic, pyramidal, and molecular. The dentate gyrus fits inside the hippocampus and, like the hippocampus, has three layers: molecular, granular, and polymorphic. The most primitive cortex is the paleocortex of the olfactory bulb.

The fibers of the dentate gyrus,[2] are confined to the hippocampal formation, while the hippocampal fibers leave the hippocampal formation through the fornix and project to either septum or to the mammillary bodies and mesencephalic tegmentum. The cortex adjacent to the hippocampus changes from three layers to six layers and is classified as transitional mesocortex and includes the parahippocampal gyrus (medial to the collateral sulcus), including entorhinal cortex. The pyriform lobe consists of the lateral olfactory stria, uncus, and the anterior part of the parahippocampal gyrus.

Entorhinal Region

The entorhinal/parahippocampal gyrus forms the large posterior segment of the piriform region. This is Brodmann's area 28 and constitutes the bulk of the parahippocampal gyrus. This area has extensive interconnection with the higher association cortex throughout the neocortex and also receives olfactory information from the olfactory stria. This is the major pathway for relating neocortex to the limbic cortex of the hippocampus.[3]

Older classifications have used the terms *archicortex* for the hippocampus, *paleocortex* for the piriform area, and *neocortex* for lateral temporal areas based on presumed phylogenetic considerations. Here we will follow in general the terminology as earlier, employed in the recent monumental work of Gloor (1997). The hippocampus is divided into sectors (referred to as fields) based on cytoarchitectural differences (Fig. 22.10) of CA1–CA4 (or fields of Rose h1–h5). (Note that an older term for the hippocampus is Ammon's [the ram] horn, thus Cornu Ammonis = CA). CA4, the end folium or end blade merges with the hilus of the dentate gyrus. CA1, the sector closest to the subiculum, is referred to as the Sommer's sector. This sector is most severely affected by cell loss following hypoglycemia, anoxia, and status epilepticus (Fig. 22.11). However, this selective vulnerability may also involve CA3 and CA4 with relative sparing of CA2 and the dentate granule cells. The subsequent gliosis (mesial sclerosis) of the hippocampus is the pathology found at surgery or autopsy in 75% of cases of complex partial seizures arising in the hippocampus.

The hippocampal regions are interconnected by a commissure, the hippocampal commissure. In the primate, the dorsal commissure originates in the entorhinal cortex and presubiculum. The ventral commissure originates in the CA3 sector and the dentate hilus primarily in their more rostral areas, for example, in relation to the uncus.

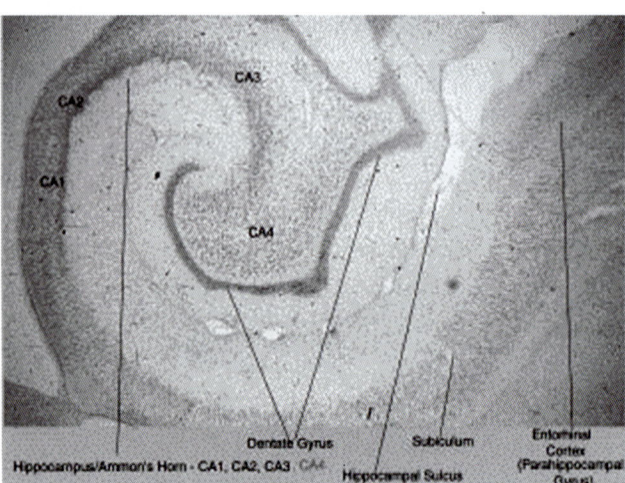

Figure 22.10 The sectors or fields of the hippocampus. The dentate gyrus, subiculum, and related structures are demonstrated. Nissl stain.

Figure 22.11 Selective vulnerability of the hippocampus demonstrated in Nissl stains. (*A*) Normal Ammon's horn with labels for fields h1–h5 of Rose inserted. (*B*) Anesthetic death: recent necrosis in Sommer sector (h1) and partial loss of neurons in h3 and the end plate (h4, h5). (*C*) Hypoglycemic coma: there has been significant loss of pyramidal cells in section h1. (From Meyer, A. in Greenfield, J., et al., Neuropathology 2nd Edition. Baltimore, Williams & Wilkins, 196, p. 256.)

---

[2] In the dentate gyrus in common with the olfactory epithelium and cerebellum, new neurons are formed throughout life. In the vast remainder of the brain there is no differentiation of nerve cells after birth, and when these nerve cells die they are not replaced (Altman, 1962; Gage, 1994). One must expect considerable research in the future to focus on just which genes permit the continued replacement of nerve cells in these regions.

[3] Note that the "entorhinal gyrus" of lower mammals corresponds in humans to a much larger region that includes the middle, inferior, and parahippocampal gyri and the temporal portion of the fusiform gyrus.

Cytoarchitecture of the Hippocampus

In the hippocampus, the three layers are as follows:

1. *Molecular* in which the apical dendrites of the pyramidal cells arborize. This layer is usually divided into a more external stratum lacunosum-moleculare and a more internal stratum radiatum. It is continuous with molecular layer of dentate gyrus and adjacent temporal neocortex.

2. *Pyramidal cell layer* (stratum pyramidalis) contains pyramidal cells that are the principal cells of the hippocampus. Dendrites extend into molecular layer and Schaffer axon collaterals arise from pyramidal neurons and synapse in the molecular layer on dendrites of other pyramidal cells.

3. *Polymorphic layer* (stratum oriens), in which the basilar dendrites of the pyramidal cells are found. Contains axons, dendrites, and interneurons. This layer in CA4 is continuous with the hilus of the dentate gyrus. Only the hippocampus sends axons outside the hippocampal formation.

Cytoarchitecture of the Dentate Gyrus

In the dentate gyrus, the following three layers are found:

1. *Molecular layer* contains dendrites of granule cells.

2. *Granule cell layer.* These small neurons replace the pyramidal cell layer of hippocampus. The granule cells are unipolar; all of the dendrites emerge from the apical end of the cell into the molecular layer. Efferent neurons from the granule cells are mossy fibers that synapse only with cells of hippocampal areas CA2 and CA3.

3. *Polymorphic cell.* Also referred to as the hilus, this layer is continuous with CA4 of hippocampus.

The pyramidal and granule cell neurons are excitatory, utilizing glutamine as the transmitter. In addition, there are inhibitory interneurons (GABA-ergic), basket cells, in the polymorphic layer of both the hippocampus and dentate gyrus. There are also mossy cells in the polymorph layer, probably excitatory interneurons. There are also scattered interneurons in the molecular layers. The connections of the hippocampal formation are summarized in Table 22.3.

The *selective vulnerability of hippocampus* (Fig. 2.11) occurs in diseases such as anoxia and hypoglycemia. In addition, the hippocampus appears to be significantly involved in most seizures of temporal lobe origin.

1. *Why does this selective vulnerability occur?* The CA1 region is rich in NMDA receptors. The dentate hilus and the CA3 sector are rich in kainate receptors. Activation of these receptors by glutamate would allow a considerable entry of calcium ions into the pyramidal neurons, beginning a cascade that could result in cell death. Moreover, the pyramidal neurons of these sectors as compared to CA2 and the granular cells of the dentate gyrus contain very little of the calcium-buffering protein calbinden.

Table 22.3 **CONNECTIONS OF HIPPOCAMPAL FORMATION**

AFFERENT INPUT

1. Perforant pathway from adjacent lateral entorhinal cortex onto granule cells of dentate gyrus and the alvear pathway from the medial entorhinal cortex. The entorhinal areas, in turn, receive their input from many of the highest level of associational cortex in the frontal, orbital, temporal (amygdala), parietal, and cingulate cortex through the cingulum bundle.

2. Septum through the stria terminalis.

3. Contralateral hippocampus via the hippocampal commissure

EFFERENT PROJECTIONS

These fibers, the axons of hippocampal and subiculum pyramidal neurons, form the fornix and have connections with the following structures:

1. Lateral mammillary nuclei, habenulae nuclei, anterior midline, and intralaminar thalamic nuclei, lateral hypothalamic nuclei, midbrain tegmentum, and periaqueductal gray via a column of the fornix

2. Septum, preoptic region, parolfactory and cingulate cortex via the precommissural fornix and supracallosal fornix

---

2. *Seizure activity.* Most seizures beginning after age 15 are classified as partial, and the majority of these are classified as complex partial. Approximately 75% of the complex partial seizures arise in the temporal lobe; the remainder arise in the frontal lobe. While these seizures may arise in temporal neocortex, the majority arise in the mesial temporal structures, particularly the hippocampus. The hippocampus has a low threshold for seizure discharge; consequently, stimulation of any region that supplies hippocampal afferents or stimulation of the hippocampus itself may produce seizures. Hippocampal stimulation produces respiratory and cardiovascular changes, as well as automatisms (stereotyped movements) involving face, limb, and trunk.

3. *Why do not all of the various pathological processes in the hippocampus produce seizures?* There appears to be a critical age during infancy and early childhood for the acquisition of the pathology that is associated with seizures originating in mesial temporal lobe. There may be an age-related remodeling of intrinsic hippocampal connections. Whether a single episode of epileptic status during infancy is sufficient to produce these changes or whether multiple episodes may be required is still under discussion.

4. *Is the hippocampal pathology alone sufficient to explain the complex partial seizures of temporal lobe origin?* As reviewed by Gloor (1997), many of the specimens examined after surgery or at autopsy also demonstrate extensive changes in the amygdala as well as mesial and lateral isocortex. (Overall, however, in the autopsy studies of Margerison and Corsellis [1966] the most frequent site of damage and cell loss was in the hippocampus.) Rather than using the more restrictive term of *hippocampal sclerosis*, it is more appropriate to use the term *mesial temporal*

sclerosis. Even this term fails to include the involvement of more laterally placed neocortex in some of the symptoms in seizures originating in temporal lobe. (See later discussion.)

HIPPOCAMPAL SYSTEM AND MEMORY

The studies of Milner (1972) have shown that bilateral removal or damage of the hippocampus produces great difficulty in learning new information, a condition called anterograde amnesia (see Chapter 30). The excitatory amino acids, L-glutamate and L-aspartate, are important in learning and memory through the mechanism of long-term potentiation. Long-term potentiation is a long-lasting facilitation after repeated activation of excitatory amino acid pathways, is most pronounced in the hippocampus, and may be related to the initiation of the memory trace.

The amygdala and its connections are associated with the conditioning of the emotional response of fear (refer to review of LeDoux, 2000, and earlier discussion).

OTHER CORTICAL REGIONS OF THE LIMBIC SYSTEM

Cingulate Cortex

This region (Fig. 22.5) receives reciprocal innervation from the anterior thalamic nuclei, contralateral and ipsilateral cingulate cortex, and temporal lobe via the cingulum bundle, as well as projecting to the corpus striatum and most of the subcortical limbic nuclei. The cingulate cortex is continuous with the parahippocampal gyrus at the isthmus behind the splenium of the corpus callosum.

Stimulation of cingulate cortex also produces respiratory, vascular, and visceral changes, but these changes are less than those produced by hypothalamic stimulation. Interruption of the cingulum bundle, which lies deep to the cingulate cortex and the parahippocampal gyrus, has been proposed as a less devastating way to produce the effects of prefrontal lobotomy without a major reduction in intellectual capacity. (For additional discussion of the effects of stimulation and of lesions of the anterior cingulate area on autonomic function and behavior, refer to Devinsky et al. [1995].)

PRINCIPAL PATHWAYS OF THE LIMBIC SYSTEM

1. *Entorhinal reverberating circuit* (Fig. 22.12A). This fiber system is an adjunct to the circuit described by Papez (see later). The entorhinal reverberating circuit functions as follows:

    a. Entorhinal cortex receives input from polysensory (multimodal sensory association cortex) cerebral cortex and amygdala.

    b. Entorhinal fibers project via the perforant pathway to the granule cells of the dentate gyrus via the perforant pathway. There are also direct projections to CA1, CA3, and to subiculum.

Figure 22.12 (*A*) The perforant pathway modified. (From Carpenter MB, Core Text of Neuroanatomy. Baltimore, William and Wilkins.) (*B*) The Papez circuit. (*C*) Sagittal section showing medial surface of cerebrum, demonstrating the limbic structures which surround the brain stem and are on the medial surface of the cerebrum. Portions of the Papez circuit are shown, including fornix, anterior nuclei, mammillary bodies, cingulate cortex, and cingulum. Magnetic resonance imaging (MRI), T2 weighted.

c. The major projection of the dentate gyrus is to the proximal dendrites of the CA3 hippocampal pyramidal cells. There are also synapses on the neurons of the polymorphic layer.

d. The CA3 pyramidal cells project via Schaffer collaterals to CA1 pyramidal cells.

e. CA1 pyramidal cell collaterals project to the subiculum and entorhinal cortex.

f. The entorhinal cortex projects back to each of the neocortical polysensory projection areas, completing a reverberating system.

2. *Papez circuit*

   a. Many hippocampal pyramidal cells synapse on the pyramidal cells of the adjacent subiculum. The pyramidal cells of the subiculum constitute the origin of most of the fibers in the fornix.

   b. Fornix projects primarily to the mammillary bodies of the hypothalamus and septum.

   c. Mammillary bodies then project via the mammillothalamic tract to the anterior nuclei of the thalamus.

   d. Anterior thalamic nuclei project to cingulate gyrus.

   e. Cingulate gyrus then projects via the cingulum bundle of fibers to the parahippocampal/entorhinal cortex, which subsequently projects to the hippocampus, as outlined earlier, completing the circuit.

3. *Fornix* (Figs. 22.5, 22.6, and 22.7 and Chapter 16). Note that the fornix is the efferent pathway from the hippocampus and subiculum and is connected to the hypothalamus, septum, and midbrain. This tract takes a rather circuitous pathway to reach the hypothalamus. The fornix originates from the medial surface of the temporal lobe and runs in the medial wall of the inferior horn of the lateral ventricle, passing onto the undersurface of the corpus callosum at the junction of the inferior horn and body of the ventricles, and running in the medial wall of the body of the lateral ventricle suspended from the corpus callosum. The fornix finally enters the substance of the hypothalamus at the level of the interventricular foramen. Different portions of the fornix have specific names:

   a. Portio fimbria (fringe) of the fornix found on the medial surface of the hippocampus and consists of fibers from the fornix and hippocampal commissure.

   b. Portio alveus, band of fornix fibers covering ventricular surface of the hippocampus.

   c. Portio tenia, connecting the hippocampus to the corpus callosum.

   d. Portio corpus, located underneath the corpus callosum and entering the hypothalamus.

   e. Portio columnaris, found in the substance of the hypothalamus.

   The fornix is also divided into a precommissural portion (in front of the anterior commissure), that enters the septum (from the hippocampus), and the postcommissural portion (behind the anterior commissure), that distributes in the mammillary bodies and midbrain (from subiculum). These relationships should be traced out in the atlas section.

4. *Stria terminalis.* The pathway of the stria terminalis (the efferent fiber tract of the amygdala) parallels the fornix, but it is found adjacent to the body and tail of the caudate nucleus on its medial surface (refer to atlas and Chapter 16). The stria terminalis interconnects the medial corticoamygdaloid nuclei, as well as connecting the amygdala to the hypothalamus and septum. There is also a strong termination in the red nucleus of the stria terminalis, which is found above the anterior commissure and lateral to the column of the fornix.

5. *Ventral amygdalofugal pathway.* This fiber pathway originates primarily from the basolateral amygdaloid nuclei and to a lesser degree from the olfactory cortex, spreads beneath the lentiform nuclei, and enters the lateral hypothalamus and preoptic region, the septum, and the diagonal band nucleus. Some of these fibers bypass the hypothalamus and terminate on the magnocellular portions of the dorsomedial thalamic nuclei.

6. *Cingulum.* This fiber bundle is found on the medial surface of the hemisphere and interconnects primarily the medial cortical limbic areas, especially the parahippocampal formation, with one another.

7. *The intracortical association fiber system.* The superior and inferior longitudinal fasciculus and uncinate fasciculus. The limbic regions on the lateral surface of the hemisphere have strong interconnections with polysensory and third-order sensory cortical regions throughout the cerebral cortex through this system.

8. *Limbic system and the corticospinal and corticobulbar pathway.* The bulk of the pyramidal pathway originates in the motor/sensory strip. However, most movements begin with a "thought" in the frontal association areas. A possible example of release of the bulbar areas for emotional expression from frontal-lobe control is seen in pseudobulbar palsy. Such patients exhibit inappropriate response to situations because the interrupted corticonuclear/corticobulbar pathway no longer dampens the strong descending autonomic/limbic input to the brain-stem cranial nuclei. The resultant inappropriate behavior is termed *emotional lability*. A sad story may trigger excessive crying; a funny story, excessive laughter.

SYMPTOMS OF DISEASE INVOLVING THE TEMPORAL LOBE

In considering the functions of the temporal lobe and the effects of temporal lobe lesions, one must bear in mind, as discussed earlier, that the temporal lobe has several structural, phylogenetic, and functional subdivisions (Fig. 22.13). Thus, one may distinguish as follows:

1–the allocortex of the hippocampal formation

2–the transitional mesocortex bordering this area

3–the neocortex that occupies all of the lateral surface and the inferior temporal areas

FIGURE 22.13 The superior and medial surfaces of the temporal lobe. The transverse gyrus of Heschl and the relationships of the temporal lobe to the gyri of other structures surrounding the sylvian fissure are demonstrated. The temporal stem refers to the core of white matter relating the temporal lobe to the remainder of the cerebral hemisphere. The hippocampal gyrus of the figure is now termed the *parahippocampal gyrus*. (From Penfield, W., and Jasper, H.: Epilepsy and the Functional Anatomy of the Human Brain. Boston, Little, Brown & Company, 1954, p. 52.)

4–the amygdala considered previously. When one considers disease processes affecting the temporal lobe, signs and symptoms obviously do not follow the precise subdivisions outlined earlier. There are several reasons for this:

1. The basic lesion (such as a glioma) often involves both neocortical and nonneocortical areas of the temporal lobe.
2. The threshold of the hippocampus for seizure discharge is relatively low, whereas that of the neocortical areas on the lateral surface is relatively high. Since connections from the lateral temporal and inferior temporal area to the hippocampus exist, seizure discharges beginning in the lateral temporal neocortex often activate discharge in the hippocampus.
3. Lesions in the more posterior temporal areas often involve the adjacent posterior parietal areas, that is, the inferior parietal lobule. In contrast, anteriorly placed lesions of the temporal lobe often involve the adjacent inferior frontal gyrus. Lesions spreading into the deeper white matter of the temporal lobe (particularly in its middle and posterior thirds) often involve part or all of the optic radiation.

SYMPTOMS FOLLOWING STIMULATION OF THE TEMPORAL LOBE

Seizures involving the temporal lobe are frequent and produce a variety of symptoms. These may be classified as simple partial if awareness is retained or complex partial if awareness is not retained and the patient is amnestic for the symptoms. A simple partial seizure may progress to a complex partial seizure and may subsequently generalize. These symptoms

Table 22.4 CORRELATION OF TEMPORAL LOBE SEIZURE/LIMITED STIMULATION SYMPTOMS WITH ANATOMY

SYMPTOMS	ANATOMICAL CORRELATION
Autonomic phenomena	Amygdala. Less often cingulate gyrus or orbital frontal
Fear, less often anger or other emotion	Amygdala
Crude auditory sensation: tinnitus	Heschl's transverse gyrus (primary auditory projection)
Visual and auditory illusions: perceptual distortions (22.15)	Higher order visual and auditory association cortex. Superior temporal gyrus in studies of Penfield. For visual predominantly nondominant hemisphere in studies of Penfield
Vestibular sensations: dizziness/vertigo (22.14)	Superior temporal gyrus posterior to auditory cortex
Arrest of speech	Wernicke's area and posterior speech area (posterior temporal/parietal (angular-supramarginal) dominant hemisphere
Olfactory hallucinations	Olfactory cortex of the uncus (termination of lateral olfactory stria). "Uncinate epilepsy of Jackson"
Experiential phenomena/dreamy; more complex illusions such as déjà vu,* déjà vécu,* jamais vu,* other illusions of recognitions, visual and auditory hallucinations (often of past experience) (22.15, 22.16)	Lateral temporal cortex: primarily superior temporal gyru states: controversial. However, ictal phenomena are abolished by ablation limited to lateral temporal neocortex (Blume et al., 1993; Mullan and Penfield, 1959).
Automatisms = repetitive simple or complex often stereotyped motor acts, most commonly involving mouth, lips, etc. Speech or limbs may be involved.	Primary or secondary bilateral involvement of amygdala/hippocampus. Invariably accompanied by confusion and amnesia for the acts.
Defects in memory recording followed by amnesia for the event	Hippocampus

*Déjà vu is a sensation of familiarity, déjà vécu is sensation of strangeness, jamais vu perception is dream-like.

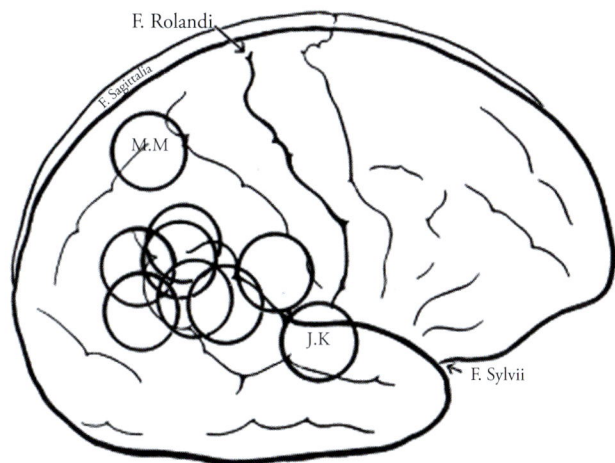

Figure 22.14 Effects of focal discharge in superior temporal gyrus. The location of the discharging lesion at surgery in nine patients with focal seizures beginning with a sensation of vertigo is demonstrated to be primarily superior temporal gyrus. (From Penfield, W., and Kristiansen, K.: Epileptic Seizure Patterns. Springfield, IL, Charles C. Thomas, 1951, p. 49.)

are outlined in Table 22.4 with the most likely anatomical correlate.

In general, as we have indicated, there is mixed symptomatology during partial seizures of temporal lobe origin. The following case history illustrates many of the points just discussed regarding seizures of temporal lobe origin.

CASE HISTORY 22.1

Three months before admission, this 56-year-old, right-handed male baker had the onset of 4-minute episodes of vertigo and tinnitus, unrelated to position, followed by increasing forgetfulness. Later that month he had a generalized convulsive seizure that occurred without any warning. The patient then developed episodes of confusion and unresponsiveness, followed by a left frontal headache. Several studies—electroencephalography (EEG), pneumoencephalogram, and carotid arteriogram—were all negative. One month before admission, the patient began to have minor episodes, characterized by lip smacking and a vertiginous sensation, during which he reported seeing several well-formed, colorful scenes. At times, he had hallucinations of "loaves of bread being laid out on the wall." In addition, he would have a perceptual disturbance (e.g., objects would appear larger than normal). He also had colorful visions and terrifying nightmares "terrifying dreams, crazy things."

Neurological Examination

Seizures observed: The patient had frequent transient episodes of distress characterized by saying, "Oh, oh, oh, my" and at times accompanied by automatisms: fluttering of the eyelids, smacking of the lips, and repetitive picking at bedclothes with his right hand. Consciousness was not completely impaired during these episodes, which lasted from 30 seconds to 3 minutes. The patient reported afterward that at the onset of the seizure he had seen loaves of bread on the wall and smelled a poorly described unpleasant odor. At other times, the olfactory hallucination was described as pleasant, resembling the aroma of freshly baked bread.

Mental status: The patient was disoriented to time, could not recall his street address, and could not pronounce the name of the hospital.

Cranial nerves: A possible deficit in the periphery of the right visual field and a minor right central facial weakness were present.

Reflexes: A right Babinski sign was present.

Clinical diagnosis: Simple and complex partial seizures originating in the left temporal lobe probably involving at various times left lateral superior temporal gyrus, uncus, amygdala, and hippocampus, with tumor the most likely etiology in view of age and the focal neurological findings.

Laboratory Data

EEG: Frequent focal spike discharge was present throughout the left temporal and parietal areas consistent with a focal seizure disorder. A recording 6 days later indicated almost continuous 3 to 5 (Hz) focal slow-wave activity (focal damage) in the left temporal area.

Imaging studies: Left carotid arteriogram indicated a possible avascular mass lesion left posterior lateral frontal.

Subsequent course: These episodes were eventually controlled with anticonvulsant medication. Seizures recurred 7 months after onset of symptoms. An aura of unpleasant odor was followed by a generalized convulsion followed by four or five subsequent seizures of a somewhat different character (deviation of the head and eyes to the right, then tonic and clonic movements of the right hand spreading to

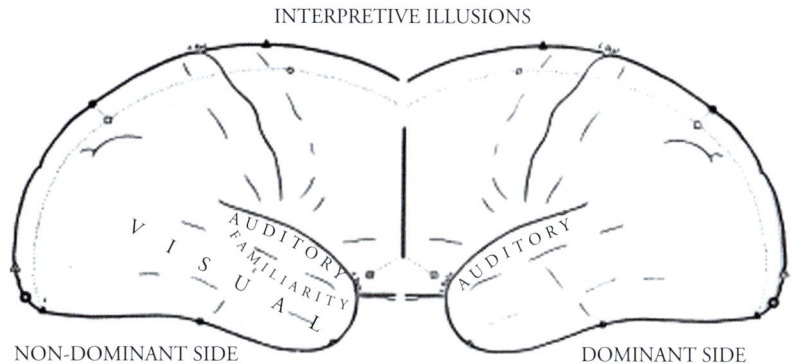

Figure 22.15 Interpretive illusions (disturbances of perception) produced by stimulation at surgery of temporal lobe cortex in patients with temporal lobe seizures. Visual illusions were produced predominantly in the minor (that is, nondominant) hemisphere. Auditory illusions were produced from both sides, chiefly in the superior temporal gyrus. Illusions of familiarity (déjà-vu) were produced predominantly from the nondominant hemisphere. Sensations of fear, unreality, loneliness, or of detachment were produced from stimulation in either temporal region. (From Penfield, W., and Perot, P.: Brain, 86:599, 1963, Oxford University Press. After Mullan and Penfield: Archives of Neurology & Psychiatry, 81:269, 1959.)

EXPERIENTIAL RESPONSES

Figure 22.16 Experimental responses (hallucinations) to stimulation at surgery of temporal lobe and adjacent inferior parietal area in patients with temporal lobe seizures. Auditory responses occur from stimulation in either dominant or nondominant hemisphere (primarily superior temporal gyri). Visual responses occur primarily from stimulation of the nondominant hemisphere. The stippled area within the interrupted lines indicates the posterior speech area of the dominant hemisphere. No experiential responses occur on stimulation of this speech area in the dominant hemisphere. (From Penfield, W., and Perot, P., Brain, 86:676, 1963, Oxford University Press.)

the arm, foot, and leg lasting approximately 1 to 2 minutes, followed by a postictal right hemiparesis). He also experienced minor seizures characterized by sensory phenomena on the right side of the body. Neurologic examination now indicated progression with a marked expressive aphasia, with little spontaneous speech and difficulty in naming objects. There was a dense right homonymous hemianopia, a flattening of the right nasolabial fold, and a right hemiparesis, with a right Babinski sign. The symptoms and findings suggested that the basic disease process might well have spread to involve the adjacent areas across the sylvian fissure—the speech areas of the inferior frontal convolution, premotor areas, and sensory motor cortex. An arteriogram indicated a large space-occupying tumor of the left temporal lobe, and with additional progression, craniotomy was performed by Dr. Robert Yuan 16 months after the onset of symptoms. A necrotic glioblastoma was found involving the superior temporal gyrus, the deeper temporal, and extending superficially under the sylvian fissure to involve the adjacent posterior portion of the inferior frontal gyrus. A temporal lobectomy was performed (from the anterior temporal pole posteriorly for a distance of 6 cm).

Today, CT scan and MRI would be employed for early diagnosis in patients with this type of seizure disorder, as in the following cases, and surgery might be limited to a stereotaxic biopsy.

CASE HISTORY 22.2

This 17-year-old, right-handed male, at age 4 years began to have "staring spells and bizarre behavior." Some episodes had been preceded by the "sound of a musical rhythm." EEG at that time indicated a right temporal spike discharge. Seizures were controlled for 10 years with anticonvulsants but then recurred and were poorly controlled, occurring several times per day.

Neurological Examination

Observed 3-minute seizure: The seizure began with loss of contact and a stare and then automatisms of the hands. He stood up, walked around the room, went to the physician's desk, and attempted to pull open a nonexistent middle drawer. He answered questions vaguely with one- or two-word answers. Confusion was present for 1–2 minutes after the end of the episode.

Cranial nerves: A left central facial weakness was present.

Clinical diagnosis: Focal seizures originating in right temporal lobe. Observed seizure was complex partial. The seizures beginning with the musical sound might be classified as simple partial with secondary complex partial.

Laboratory Data

EEG: Intermittent focal spike discharge anterior-middle temporal area.

CT scan (Fig. 22.17): An area of focal atrophy was present in the right anterior temporal lobe with possible enhancement at the border.

MRI: At the Yale Epilepsy Center it was more consistent with a tumor in the right anterior temporal lobe.

Subsequent course: Dr. Dennis Spencer at the Yale Epilepsy Center performed a temporal lobectomy. This demonstrated a cystic glial tumor with components of astrocytes and oligodendrocytes.

Figure 22.17 Complex and simple partial seizures: cystic-mixed glial tumor and cortical dysplasia right temporal lobe. Case 22.2. Computerized tomography (CT) scan demonstrated an area of atrophy or cyst in the right anterior temporal lobe with possible minimum enhancement at the border. This 17-year-old, right-handed male, at age 4 years began to have "staring spells and bizarre behavior" with some proceeded by the "sound of a musical rhythm." An electroencephalographic (EEG) spike discharge was present in the right anterior-middle temporal area. (Refer to text.)

Figure 22.18 Glioblastoma left temporal lobe. Complex partial seizures with secondary generalization in a 47 year old. Case 22.3. Magnetic resonance imaging (MRI), T2 nonenhanced. (*A*) Horizontal section; (*B*) coronal section. (Refer to text.)

Cerebral cortex also demonstrated abnormal lamination and dysplastic features. Seizures were fully controlled over the next 3 years.

CASE HISTORY 22.3

This 47-year-old ambidextrous male experienced his first seizure 1 month prior to admission. He felt light-headed and warm. Then he was observed to walk 100 feet down a hallway, appearing "dazed" and not recognizing people. He fell to the floor, with a loss of consciousness, bit his tongue, and was confused afterward for several minutes.

Neurological examination: At 2, 16, and 48 hours after the episode a persistent right Babinski sign and slight right hyperreflexia were present.

Clinical diagnosis: Complex partial seizures. In view of age of onset and persistent focal signs, a brain tumor should be suspected as the etiology.

Laboratory Data
Sleep-deprived EEG: Normal.
CT and MRI scans (Fig. 22.18) demonstrated an extensive infiltrating tumor of the left temporal lobe, most likely a glioblastoma.

Subsequent course: Despite anticonvulsant therapy (phenytoin), additional episodes occurred over the next month: loss of train of thought while talking and several minutes of loss of memory. A subtotal resection by Dr. Bernard Stone (St. Vincent Hospital) demonstrated a Grade III–IV astrocytoma (glioblastoma). Despite radiotherapy and chemotherapy, the disease pursued a relentless course, producing early and severe disability prior to death, approximately 1 year after onset of symptoms.

SYMPTOMS FROM ABLATION OF OR DAMAGE TO THE TEMPORAL LOBE

1. *Effects on hearing.* Unilateral lesion of auditory projection area may result in an inability to localize a sound. Bilateral lesions may produce cortical deafness.
2. *Aphasia.* Destruction of area 22 in the dominant hemisphere produces a Wernicke's receptive aphasia. Such a patient not only has difficulty in interpreting speech but also, in a sense, has lost the ability to use previous auditory associations. Lesions that deprive the receptive aphasia area of Wernicke in the dominant temporal lobe (area 22) of information from the auditory projection areas of the right and left hemispheres result in pure word deafness. Such a patient can hear sounds and words but is unable to interpret them.
3. *Visual defects.* Unilateral lesions of the temporal lobe that involve the subcortical white matter often produce damage to the geniculocalcarine radiations. Since the most inferior fibers of the radiation that swing forward around the temporal horn (representing the inferior parts of the retina and referred to as "Meyer's loop") are often the first to be involved, the initial field defect may be a contralateral superior field quadrantanopia.
4. *Klüver-Bucy syndrome.* This syndrome results from bilateral ablation of the temporal pole, amygdaloid nuclei, and hippocampus in the monkey (Klüver and Bucy, 1937). The animals could see and find objects, but they could not identify objects (visual agnosia). The animal showed marked deficits in visual discrimination, particularly in regard to visual stimuli related to various motivations. They also had a release of very strong oral automatisms and compulsively placed objects in their mouths, which, if not edible, were dropped. They had a tendency to mouth and touch all visible objects and manifested indiscriminate sexual practice. They willingly ate food not normally a part of their diet (such as corned beef sandwiches). They showed a lack of response to aversive stimuli and had no recollection or judgment. The animals also lost their fear (release phenomenon) and, in the case of wild monkeys, became tame and docile creatures. They had a marked absence of the fight-or-flight response and also lost fears of unknown objects or objects that previously had frightened them. (See amygdala earlier.) The problems in visual discrimination may reflect a disconnection of the visual association areas from the amygdala/hippocampal areas.
5. *Memory.* Bilateral damage to the hippocampus produces a marked impairment of the ability to form new

associations, an inability to establish new memories at a time when remote memory is well preserved.

6. *Unilateral effects on memory.* Patients with resection of the left temporal lobe may lose the ability to retain verbally related material but gain the ability to retain visually related material relevant to the right hemisphere. The reverse is true for right temporal lobectomy patients.

7. *Psychiatric disturbances.* Waxman and Geschwind (1975) have described an interictal personality disorder characterized by hyposexuality, hyperreligiosity, hypergraphia, and a so-called stickiness or viscosity in interpersonal relationships. In some patients a psychosis may be apparent in periods between seizures (the interictal period) that is often most severe during periods when the seizure disorder is well under control. In other patients a transient psychosis may be related to the actual seizure discharge or the postictal period. There is controversy regarding this issue.

8. *Aggressive behavior.* Aggressive behavior and episodic dyscontrol may be related to dysfunction of the amygdala or to damage to prefrontal areas, which inhibit the amygdala. This remains an area of considerable controversy (Ferguson et al., 1986; Geschwind, 1983; Mark and Ervin, 1970).

9. Complex partial seizures, as discussed earlier, may follow mesial temporal sclerosis.

FRONTAL LOBE: PREFRONTAL CORTEX AND EMOTIONS (AREAS 9, 10, 11, 12, 46, 13, 14)

The term *prefrontal* refers to those portions of the frontal lobe anterior to the agranular motor and premotor areas. The prefrontal region is in a unique position in the brain as it receives a vast stream of information from polysensory, third-order sensory, and from cortical and subcortical limbic areas, including especially dorsomedial nucleus, hypothalamus, and indirectly the amygdala.

In the prefrontal cortex three regions are usually delineated:

1. Lateral-dorsal convexity
2. Medial
3. Orbital

All three are concerned with executive function and relate to the dorsomedial thalamic nuclei. In general, the lateral-dorsal relates to motor association executive function; the orbital-ventral and the medial to the limbic-emotional control executive system. Recent studies have questioned this simplistic approach. Thus, certain functions previously considered to be associated with dorsolateral location have been now localized to a medial location (Stuss et al., 2000). In addition, there is evidence that dorsolateral lesions also alter affect and motivation. Moreover, as the clinical examples will demonstrate, most pathological processes involve the functions associated with more than one division either directly or through pressure effects.

Although the term *prefrontal* traditionally included areas 9, 10, 11, and 12, most studies of stimulation or of ablative lesions involving the prefrontal areas have included, within the general meaning of the term *prefrontal*, areas beyond these Brodmann designations. Thus, the posterior orbital cortex (area 13) and the posteromedial orbital cortex (area 14) have been added to the orbital frontal group (Fig. 18.28). These areas all share a common relationship to the medial dorsal nucleus of the thalamus. Areas 46 and 47, located in humans on the lateral surface of the hemisphere, are also often grouped with areas 9, 10, 11, and 12. Another area, the anterior cingulate gyrus (area 24), is also included in the prefrontal area, although it relates to the anterior thalamic nuclei. Some authors (particularly in discussing frontal epilepsy) also include area 8 and the supplementary motor cortex already discussed earlier in relationship to premotor cortex.

The multiple connections of the prefrontal areas are discussed by Nauta (1964), Pandya et al. (1971). Essentially, all sensory association and polysensory (multimodal) areas and the olfactory cortex project to the prefrontal areas. The prefrontal areas, in turn, have reciprocal connections to the premotor, temporal, inferior parietal, and limbic cortex. The connections to the limbic system include (a) cingulate gyrus and then via cingulum to hippocampus and (b) uncinate fasciculus. Subcortical bidirectional connections are prominent in relationship to the medial dorsal nucleus of the thalamus, amygdala, and hippocampus. Significant projections to the caudate nucleus, putamen, and the premotor areas provide the anatomical substrate for influencing motor function. Projections to the superior colliculus provide the substrate for modifying eye movements—for example, "look to the direction opposite to the target."

Here we will briefly outline the major connections of the major subdivisions

1. *Orbitofrontal cortex.* The orbitofrontal cortex (areas 11 and 12) receives input from the cingulate regions, other sections of the prefrontal cortex, the magnocellular division of the dorsomedial nucleus, the amygdala, and temporal areas. The orbitofrontal cortex, in turn, has strong projections to the autonomic regions of the hypothalamus and magnocellular dorsomedial nucleus of the thalamus in addition to the amygdala and temporal structures. Stimulation of the posterior orbital surface, like stimulation of the cingulate, parahippocampal gyrus, and amygdala, changes the respiration, cardiac rhythm, and visceral contractions. These responses are believed to be the somatic basis of the emotional changes that originate in the limbic cortex.

2. *Frontal association areas/lateral prefrontal granular frontal cortex.* This region that is important in controlling behavior lays rostral to the premotor cortex, areas 6 and 8, and has already been discussed in Chapter 18. The frontal association areas (areas 9, 10, 11, and 12) receive their input from the cingulate regions and cortical association areas in the temporal, parietal, and occipital lobes. They also have a

strong reciprocal connection with the parvicellular portions of the dorsal medial thalamic nucleus via the anterior thalamic radiation. The dorsal medial thalamic nucleus, in turn, receives most of its input from the hypothalamus and the midbrain limbic nuclei. The frontal association region has strong projections to the hypothalamus and thalamus.

Overview of the role of the prefrontal area in motor and cognitive function: this topic has already been discussed in Chapter 18.

STIMULATION COMPLEX PARTIAL SEIZURES

These seizures, partial seizures with impairment of consciousness, were formerly considered to be entirely temporal lobe in origin. It is now recognized that 20%–30% of such seizures are extratemporal in origin—predominantly frontal lobe. Compared to complex partial seizures of temporal lobe origin, complex partial seizures of frontal lobe origin are usually briefer, occur more frequently, and tend to have a much shorter postictal period of confusion. Recent studies of St. Hilaire et al., and Wada and Weiser suggest that these automatisms of orbital or medial parasagittal origin are often complex, involving both arms, both legs, trunk, or pelvis, at times in organized kicking, struggling, running, or screaming. In contrast, automatisms of temporal lobe origin are more often oral or alimentary (licking, chewing, swallowing, etc.). Such frontal lobe seizures must also be differentiated from seizures of psychogenic origin and from the "petit" absence seizures of generalized epilepsy (see Chapter 29). Thus, orbital frontal seizures present many features previously associated with pseudo or psychogenic seizures. Frontal polar seizures or dorsolateral convexity may present as forced thinking or apparent absence seizures. Quesney et al. (1990) make a distinction between discharges originating in the dorsolateral convexity, which are more likely to present with automatisms and affective components compared to parasagittal discharges that are more likely to present with motor or somatosensory components.

The present International Classification provides a summary of the localization types of frontal epilepsy that includes more than the prefrontal areas and is presented in Table 22.5.

PREFRONTAL CORTEX DAMAGE IN HUMANS

In general, most studies of prefrontal function have dealt with bilateral damage or with a unilateral lesion which, because of its parasagittal location in relation to the medial aspect of the prefrontal area, has produced essentially bilateral effects.

The first well-authenticated case of the frontal lobe syndrome is the crowbar case of Mr. Phineas P. Gage reported by Harlow in 1868. In an explosion in 1848, a pointed tamping iron shot through the skull of the patient, an efficient, well-balanced, shrewd, and energetic railroad foreman. The bar, 3.5 feet in length and 1.25 inches in greatest diameter, entered below the left orbit and merged in the midline vertex, anterior to the coronal suture, lacerating the superior sagittal sinus in the process. Following the injury, a marked personality change was noted. The balance "between his intellectual

Table 22.5 SUMMARY OF THE LOCALIZATION TYPES OF FRONTAL EPILEPSY

LOCATION OF SEIZURE	BEHAVIORAL EFFECTS
Supplementary motor	Tonic, postural, and speech arrest
Cingulate	Complex partial
Anterior frontal polar	Forced thinking or initial loss of consciousness plus adversive components
Orbital frontal	Complex partial plus olfactory hallucinations plus illusions
Dorsolateral	Tonic plus or minus aversion
Opercular	Mastication, salivation, swallowing plus speech arrest plus or minus epigastric and gustatory symptoms (see under parietal) plus or minus secondary spread to other simple partial

faculties and animal propensities" had been destroyed. He was "impatient of restraint or advice which conflicts with his desires; at times—obstinate yet capricious and vacillating, devising many plans of future operations which are no sooner arranged than they are abandoned in turn for others appearing more feasible." Additional studies of such patients with bilateral damage to prefrontal areas have been reviewed by Damasio et al. (1994). In humans, gross correlation of location of pathology (trauma and mass lesions) with major behavioral syndromes has been suggested.

1. A *syndrome of "frontal retardation" or "pseudo depression" (abulia)* manifested by apathy, nonconcern, lack of motivational drive, and a lack of emotional reactivity has been associated with lesions involving the *frontal poles and/or the medial aspects of both hemispheres.* In its most severe form a syndrome of akinetic mutism occurs. Some have also noted aspects of this syndrome with dorsolateral frontal lesions.

2. In contrast, the *"pseudopsychopathic" syndrome* is distinguished by a lack of inhibition, including facetiousness ("Witzelsucht"), sexual and personal hedonism, and lack of concern for others has been associated with *orbital frontal* pathology. Some of these patients with ventromedial orbital lesions have been described as manifesting confabulation, a particular disorder of memory found in patients with the Korsakoff syndrome (a syndrome in which lesions of the dorsal medial nucleus of the thalamus have been implicated; Chapter 30). Patients with lesions of lateral orbital and lateral convexity have been described as restless, hyperkinetic, explosive, and impulsive. As indicated earlier, damage in the dorsolateral sector appears to result in impairment of that high-level cognitive ability which allows for abstraction and creative activities. A rigidity or concreteness of response often is present. Additional discussion of the effects of frontal lobe lesions on emotional regulation will be found in Grafman et al. (1986). Most patients do not fall into these discrete groups as regards the effects on emotion and personality, and the

correlation with tumor location is often not precise. Large prefrontal tumors often involve several prefrontal regions.

PREFRONTAL LOBOTOMY

Based on the initial reports of Jacobsen regarding the effects of prefrontal lobotomy on the emotional responses of the chimpanzee, Moniz, a neuropsychiatrist and Lima neurosurgeon, introduced in 1936 the surgical procedures of prefrontal lobotomy to modify the behavior and affect of psychotic patients. Subsequently, Moniz introduced the procedure of prefrontal leukotomy: bilateral disconnection of prefrontal areas from subcortical (thalamic and basal ganglia) and other cortical areas (Fig. 22.19). A more specific approach to problems of severe anxiety, manic behavior, and chronic pain was the procedure of stereotaxic anterior cingulotomy introduced by Ballantine et al. (1967). A number of lobotomies were performed in the 1940s and early 1950s for psychiatric reasons or to modify the emotional response of patient with chronic pain previously requiring large doses of narcotics. Such studies must be interpreted with a certain degree of caution. In the psychiatric patients, the lesions are produced in individuals with preoperative abnormalities of personality function. The effects are not necessarily those that the same lesion would produce in otherwise normal individuals. There is, however, a considerable resemblance in these cases to the effects produced by trauma (to the prefrontal areas) in relatively normal individuals.

The early results did suggest that these procedures did produce an alteration in the emotional response with a reduction of anxiety generated in conflict and painful situations. Emotional response was often detached from the pain and conflicts.

However, these effects on emotion can now be produced by the use of the tranquilizing drugs that were developed beginning in the middle 1950s. The development of these drugs, in addition to the frequent postoperative complications, including seizures and personality alterations, led to the discontinuation of the procedure (Valenstein, 1986). The personality changes are those that have been elaborated earlier. The personality change results from the isolation of the limbic subcortical structures from input provided by the prefrontal areas. Following prefrontal lobotomy or leukotomy, these patients were often impulsive and distractible. Their emotional responses were often uninhibited with an apparent lack of concern over the consequences of their actions. A related finding was an inability to plan ahead for future goals; at times, the patients were unable to postpone gratification, responding to their motivations of the moment. (In a sense, a loss of the reality principle had occurred.) Although distractible, a certain perseveration of response was noted with an inability to shift responses to meet a change in environmental stimuli or cues. A rigidity and concreteness of response was apparent with deficits in abstract reasoning. A somewhat similar but less drastic personality change can be produced by bilateral severance of the anterior thalamic radiation from the dorsomedial nucleus or by direct destruction of the medial nuclei or orbital cortex. This less massive resection of cortex lessens anxiety with fewer personality changes. Destruction of the anterior cingulate regions also produces this less drastic change. Current psychosurgical or functional neurosurgical procedures have been reviewed by Diering and Bell (1991).

The results of partial or complete prefrontal lobotomy have shown that this region is important in motivation, intellect, judgment, abstract reasoning, and emotional control.

Parasagittal Lesions

It must be noted that lesions (e.g., meningiomas) that were initially parasagittal or subfrontal in relation to the prefrontal areas may, as they progress, compromise the function of adjacent premotor areas (8 and 6 and the supplementary motor cortex). The resultant clinical picture may then include not only the changes in personality but also the release of an instinctive tactile grasp and of a suck reflex. An incontinence of urine and feces may be present in addition to an apraxia of gait—an unsteadiness of gait, which is apparent as the patient attempts to stand and begins to walk but clears up once the act has been initiated. The following case histories illustrate many of the features of focal disease involving the prefrontal areas.

CASE HISTORY 22.4 (FIG. 22.20)

Two years before admission, this 69-year-old, right-handed, white housewife visited a relative (a physician) in Israel whom she had not seen in a number of years. He noted a change in the patient's personality. The patient was described as apathetic with silly immature reactions. In retrospect, the patient's husband felt that these alternations had begun insidiously a number of years previously. Her letters became incoherent. Ten months prior to evaluation, a left central facial weakness was first noted followed 2 months later by a decreased left arm swing. Six months prior to evaluation, her husband noted she was purchasing items for which she had no need: 24 pairs of shoes, 15 brassieres. Subsequently she became careless in her housework. On occasions she lost her purse. Her ability to play bridge had decreased over the last year, although her golf game was unchanged.

Neurological Examination

Mental status: There was a marked impersistence in motor activities. She was often inattentive. There was inappropriate joking. Her answers were often irrelevant. (According to her husband, this had been

Figure 22.19 Prefrontal leukotomy. A surgical section has separated the prefrontal connections with the thalamus. (Courtesy of Dr. Thomas Sabin and Dr. Thomas Kemper.)

Left lateral   Right lateral

Right   Anterior   Left   Left   Posterior   Right

Figure 22.20 Frontal parasagittal meningioma. Case 22.4. (Refer to text.) Radioactive brain scan (Hg^{197}) demonstrates dense uptake in right frontal parasagittal area.

present for many years). Digit span was decreased to 5 forward and 3 in reverses. There were marked deficits in serial 7 substractions. At times she began to subtract other numbers; at times she added rather than subtracted. There was a significant spatial disorientation. There was a marked impairment in the ability to copy a cube and deficits in drawing a house. There was disorientation in locating cities on a map.

Cranial nerves: There was a significant neglect of single-stimulus objects in the left visual field and a greater neglect when bilateral simultaneous stimuli were utilized. At times there was a limitation of voluntary gaze to the left. A left central facial weakness was present.

Motor system: There was minimal weakness of the left arm and leg. Variable resistance was present on passive motion at left wrist and elbow, suggesting the "gegenhalten" of frontal lobe disease. There was a decreased swing of the left arm in walking. The gait was initially apraxic but improved as the patient picked up speed.

Reflexes: Deep tendon stretch reflexes were increased on the left, with a left Babinski sign and a bilateral release of the grasp reflex.

Clinical diagnosis: Right frontal lobe tumor: probably a meningioma based on the long history.

Laboratory data: EEG and *imaging studies* (Fig. 22.20) all indicated a right frontal parasagittal lesion. A meningioma was considered most likely since vascular supply was derived from the left and right middle meningeal and left anterior meningeal arteries.

Hospital course: At craniotomy, Dr. Samuel Brendler found a large right posterior parasagittal frontal fibrous, meningothelial meningioma measuring 8 x 8 cm attached to the right side of the superior sagittal sinus.

LIMBIC BRAIN AS A FUNCTIONAL SYSTEM

The emotional brain is organized into a hierarchy of function proceeding from the reticular formation, including mesencephalic midbrain nuclei to the hypothalamus and thalamus to the limbic and neocortical regions.

Reticular Formation

The reticular formation is the site where information is received from the peripheral nerves. This system is so organized that only certain stimuli trigger it to alert the brain. If it were possible for any response to trigger this system, then the individual's survival would be threatened. The response, however, is selective because throughout our lives we have evolved a set of emotional responses that determine whether we will respond to situations calmly or with rage or fear. What happens is that the reticular system, based on the sensory information with probably some subconscious cortical assistance, focuses the attention by sorting out the relevant information, thus enabling the central nervous system to continue functioning efficiently throughout a crisis.

Hypothalamus

By the time the data reach the hypothalamus, there are already distinct, well-organized emotional responses. The hypothalamus, with some assistance from the thalamus, sets the level of arousal needed for the emotional state and organizes and mobilizes the cortical and subcortical centers (especially the autonomic nervous system).

Pleasure/Punishment Areas

Throughout the limbic brain are found pleasure or punishment centers. These were located by implanting electrodes at various subcortical sites in an animal and training it to press a bar that connects the electrode to an electrical current (Olds, 1958). If the electrode is in certain pleasure centers, the animal will self-stimulate until it is exhausted. In fact, the animal would rather press the lever than eat. The pleasure centers are located throughout the limbic system, but especially in the septum and preoptic region of the hypothalamus.

Other brain centers, when stimulated, produce fear responses: pupil dilation, piloerection, and sweating. In these "punishment regions," located in the amygdala, hypothalamus, thalamus, and midbrain tegmentum, the animal quickly stops pressing the bar. If the situation is nonthreatening, the normal operations of the viscera continue. In a mildly stressful situation, such as one involving anger or heavy work, some of the digestive processes slow down, and the heart rate and blood flow increase. If the situation is threatening—triggering the reactions of fear, pain, intense hunger or thirst, or sexual arousal—most of the digestive processes slow down and heart rate, blood flow, and respiration increase. Once the threatening situation passes, conditions quickly return to a normal balance between the sympathetic and parasympathetic nervous systems.

Limbic Cortical Regions

The limbic cortical regions are strongly influenced by the emotional patterns set by the hypothalamus and amygdala, which are then transmitted with only a very few synaptic interruptions into the limbic cortex, where the emotional pattern is elaborated and efficiently organized. The neocortex (prefrontal cortex and, to a lesser degree, the temporal lobe), based on past experience, examines the situation, sorts out the emotional responses from the intellectual, and inhibits or controls

Table 22.6 THE NEUROLOGICAL SUBSTRATES OF PSYCHIATRIC DISORDERS

DISORDER	DEFINING FEATURES	NEUROLOGIC CORRELATE
Schizophrenia	Progressive psychotic* disturbance with deterioration -Positive symptoms: thought disorder: delusions and hallucinations – Negative symptoms: poverty of speech, decreased movements poverty of affect, withdrawal from interpersonal relations Rx: Respond to neuroleptics**	Based on neuropathology, MRI, PET – Decreased gray matter in temporal areas: – left posterior superior temporal and mesial temporal – prefrontal, left parietal and bilateral temporal
Affective disorders	Majority is not psychotic. Disorder is not progressive and no deterioration occurs.-Bipolar – Unipolar-manic – Unipolar depression***	In post-stroke depression, variable location of infarct: left lateral frontal and basal ganglia, or right frontal or right temporal/parietal; metabolites norepinephrine (+) in CSF; norepinephrine and serotonin (–); also hypothalamic with (+) ACTH
Anxiety/panic	Autonomic activation is similar to pattern with fear responses	Brain stem adrenergic and serotonergic centers are implicated in anxiety. In panic attack patient's blood flow to right limbic system is increased between attacks
Obsessive/compulsive	Recurring thoughts trigger repetitive motor acts.	Increased metabolic activity in dorsolateral prefrontal, anterior cingulate, and caudate nucleus
Personality disorders	Various types: hysterical, passive aggressive, antisocial (overlaps with criminal), passive dependent, schizoid, obsessive/compulsive, paranoid	Pseudopsychopathic syndrome may follow prefrontal damage. Studies of violent antisocial individuals indicate smaller prefrontal areas
Autism	Retarded development of social/emotional interactions with development of stereotyped motor automatisms	Cerebellar hypoplasia plus alterations in many limbic structures, including amygdala, hippocampus, entorhinal cortex, septal nuclei, and mammillary
Asperger's	Milder form of autism	Neocortical migration disorders

*Psychosis = gross impairment in reality testing affecting perception, thought, and insight.
**Neuroleptics = dopamine antagonists.
***Antidepressants such as tricyclic agents and monoamine oxidase inhibitors increase norepinephrine and serotonin at selective receptor sites in hypothalamus and the limbic system by inhibition of reuptake of biogenic amines. Selective serotonin reuptake inhibitors (SSRIs) are effective for less severe cases of depression. For mania and bipolar disorder, lithium carbonate is effective. Neuroleptics may decrease manic behavior. For severe affective disorders electroshock therapy may be utilized.
CSF, cerebrospinal fluid; MRI, magnetic resonance imaging; PET, positron emission tomography.

the situation based on what past experience has proven to be expedient for individual survival.

Consider the following examples: a mother responds to her baby's crying, while the father sleeps on; in the middle of the night a jet airplane thundering overhead causes no response, while a whiff of smoke or breaking glass quickly arouses the central nervous system and keeps it focused.

Various types of dysfunction in this system will produce those significant alterations in behavior that represent the spectrum of psychiatric disease, briefly summarized in the next section.

THE ROLE OF THE LIMBIC SYSTEM IN PSYCHIATRIC DISORDERS

The involvement of the limbic system either from a structural or functional standpoint is central to the psychiatric disorders that affect large numbers of patients. These disorders may affect perception, cognition, and affect.

The neurological substrate is presented in Table 22.6. The epidemiology and genetics of the major disorders are presented in Table 22.7.

Table 22.7 EPIDEMIOLOGY AND GENETIC ASPECTS OF THE MAJOR PSYCHIATRIC DISORDERS

DISORDER	POPULATION FREQUENCY (%)	CONCORDANCE IN MONOZYGOTIC TWINS (%)	CONCORDANCE IN DIZYGOTIC TWINS, SIBLINGS, PARENTS (%)
Schizophrenia	0.5–1	68*	11
Affective disorders	10–20	14–25*	
– Unipolar	18–19	40	11
– Bipolar	1–2	72	14

Note. Anxiety disorders and personality disorders affect large numbers of the population.
*Risk is unchanged when adopted at birth and removed from biologic family.

BIBLIOGRAPHY

GENERAL

Adolphs, R., Tranel, D., Damasio, H., and Damasio, A. R. 1995. Fear and the human amygdala. J. Neurosci. 15:5879–5891.

Albert, D. J., Walsh, M. L., and Jonik, R. H. 1993. Aggression in humans: what is its biological foundation? Neurosci. Biobehav. Rev. 17:405–425.

Adrian, E. D. 1950. Sensory discrimination with some recent evidence from the olfactory organ. Brit. Med. Bull. 6:330.

Altman, J. 1962. Are neurons formed in the brains of adult mammals? Science 135:1127–1128.

Anderson, P. 1975. Organization of hippocampal neurons and their interconnections. In R. L. Isaccson and K. H. Pribram (Eds.) The Hippocampus, Vol 1. Structure and Development, pp. 155–173. New York, NY: Plenum.

Bancaud, J. 1987. Semiologie clinique des crises epileptiques d'origine temporale. Rev. Neurol (Paris) 143:392–400.

Bancaud, J. F., and Brunet- Bourgin, P., et al. 1994. Anatomical origin of déjà vu and vivid memories in human temporal lobe epilepsy. Brain 117:71–90.

Blaettner, V., Scherg, M., and VonCramon, D. 1989. Diagnosis of unilateral telencephalic hearing disorders: evaluation of a simple psychoacoustic pattern discrimination test. Brain 112:177–196.

Blume, W. T., Girvin, J. P., and Stenerson, P. 1993. Temporal neocortical role in ictal experiential phenomena. Ann. Neurol. 33:105–107.

Breuer, J., and Freud, S. 1957. (J. Stachey, Trans. and Ed.). Studies of Hysteria. New York, NY: Basic Books.

Burchell, B. 1991. Turning on and turning off the sense of smell. Nature 350:16–18.

Burgerman, R. S., Sperling, M. S., French, J. A., et al. 1995. Comparison of mesial versus neocortical onset of temporal lobe seizures. Epilepsia 36:662–672.

Cendes, F., Andermann, F., Gloor, P., et al. 1994. Relationship between atrophy of the amygdala and ictal fear in temporal lobe epilepsy. Brain 117:739–746.

Crichton, M. 1982. The Terminal Man. New York, NY: Avon Press.

Davidson, R. J., Putnam, K. M., and Larson, C. L. 2000. Dysfunction in the neural circuitry of emotion regulation.- a possible prelude to violence. Science 289:591–594.

Devinsky, O., Morrell, M. J., and Vogt, B. A. 1995. Contribution of anterior cingulate cortex to behavior. Brain 118:279–306.

Delgado-Escueta, A. V., Bascal, F. E., and Treiman, D. M. 1982. Complex partial seizures on closed circuit television and EEG: a study of 691 attacks in 79 patients. Ann. Neurol. 11:292–300.

Diering, S. L., and Bell, W. O. 1991. Functional neurosurgery for psychiatric patients: a historical perspective. Stereotact. Funct. Neurosurg. 57:175–194.

Dionne, V. E. 1988. How do you smell? The principle in question. Trends Neurosci. 11:188–189.

Engel, J., Jr. 1989. Seizures and Epilepsy. Philadelphia, PA: F. A. Davis.

Ferguson, S. M., Rayport, M., and Carrie, W. S. 1986. Brain correlates of aggressive behavior in temporal epilepsy. In B. K. Doane and K. E. Livingstone (Eds.) The Limbic System, pp. 183–193. New York, NY: Raven Press.

Fish, D. R., Gloor, P., Quesney, F. L., and Olivier, A. 1993. A clinical responses to electrical brain stimulation of the temporal and frontal lobes in patients with epilepsy. Pathophysiological implications. Brain 116:397–414.

Fletcher, P. C., and Henson, R. N. A. 2001. Frontal lobes and human memory insight from functional neuroimaging. Brain 124: 849–881.

Foong, J., Symms, M. R., Barker, G. J., et al. 2001. Neuropathological abnormalities in schizophrenia. Brain 124:882–892.

Franceschi, M., Triuizi, F., Ferini-Strombi, L., et al. 1989. Focal cerebral lesions found by MRI in cryptogenic nonrefractory temporal lobe epilepsy patients. Epilepsia 30:540–546.

Freund, F., and Buzsaki, G. 1996. Interneurons of the hippocampus. Hippocampus 6:345–470.

Friberg, L., Olsen, T. S., Roland, P. E., et al. 1985. Focal increase of blood flow in the cerebral cortex of man during vestibular stimulation. Brain 108:609–623.

Fulton, J. F. 1953. The limbic system: a study of the visceral brain in primates and man. Yale J. Biol. 26:107.

Gage, F. H. 1994. Challenging an old dogma; neuronogenesis in the adult hippocampus. J. NIH Res. 6:53–56.

Geschwind, N. 1965. Disconnection syndromes in animals and man. Brain 88:237–294, 585–644.

Geschwind, N. 1983. Interictal behavior changes in epilepsy. Epilepsia 24(Suppl. l):523–530.

Gloor, P. 1990. Experiential phenomena of temporal lobe epilepsy. Facts and hypotheses. Brain 113:1673–1694.

Gloor, P. 1997. The Temporal Lobe and Limbic System. New York, NY: Oxford University Press.

Gloor, P., Olivier, A., Quesney, L. F., Andermann, F., and Horowitz, S. 1982. The role of the limbic system in experiential phenomena of temporal lobe epilepsy. Ann. Neurol. 12:129–144.

Green, J. D. 1958. The rhinencephalon. Aspects of its relation to behavior and the reticular activating system. In H. H. Jasper (Ed.) Reticular Formation of the Brain, p. 607. Boston, MA: Little, Brown and Company.

Halgren, E., Walter, R. D., Cherlow, D. G., and Crandall, P. H. 1978. Mental phenomena evoked by electrical stimulation of the human hippocampal formation and amygdala. Brain 101:83–117.

Honavar, M., and Meldrum, B. S. 1997. Epilepsy. In D. I. Graham and P. L. Lantos (Eds.) Greenfield's Neuropathology. 6th ed., pp 931–971. New York, NY: Oxford University Press.

Horel, J. A., and Misantone, L. G. 1975. Partial Kluver Bucy syndrome produced by destroying temporal neocortex or amygdala. Brain Res. (Amsterdam) 94:347–359.

Isaacson, R. 1982. The Limbic System. 2nd ed. New York, NY: Plenum.

Ishibashi, T., Hori, H., Endo, K., and Sato, T. 1964. Hallucinations produced by electrical stimulation of temporal lobe seizures in schizophrenic patients. Tohoku J. Med. 82:124–139.

Jackson, J. H., and Beevor, C. E. 1889. Case of tumor of the right temporo-sphenoidal lobe, bearing on the localization of the sense of smell and on the interpretation of a particular variety of epilepsy. Brain 12:346–357.

Jackson, J. H., and Colman, W. S. 1898. Case of epilepsy with tasting movements and "dreamy state"-very small patch of softening in the left uncinate gyrus. Brain 21:580–590. (Reprinted In J. Taylor (Ed.). 1958. Selected Writings of John Hughlings Jackson, Vol. 1. On Epilepsy and Epileptiform Convulsions, pp. 458–463. New York, NY: Basic Books)

Jackson, J. H., and Stewart, P. 1899. Epileptic attacks with a warning of crude sensation of smell and with the intellectual aura (dreamy state) in a patient who had symptoms pointing to gross organic disease of the right temporo-sphenoidal lobe. Brain 22:534–549.

Jasper, H. H., and Proctor, L. O. (Eds.). 1958. Reticular Formation of the Brain. Henry Ford Hospital Symposium. Boston, MA: Little, Brown and Company.

Johnston, D., and Amaral, D. G. 1998. Hippocampus. In G. M. Shepherd (Ed.) The Synaptic Organization of the Brain. 4th ed., pp. 417–458. NewYork, NY: Oxford University Press.

Kluver, H. 1952. Brain mechanisms and behavior with special reference to the rhinencephalon. J. Lancet (Minneapolis) 72:567.

Kluver, H. 1958. The "temporal lobe syndrome" produced by bilateral ablations. In E. E. Wolstenhoime and C. M. O'Connor (Eds.) Neurological Bases of Behavior. Ciba Foundation Symposium, p. 175. London, UK: J. A. Churchill.

Kluver, H., and Bucy, P. C. 1937. Psychic blindness and other symptoms following bilateral temporal lobectomy in Rhesus monkeys. Am. J. Physiol. 119:352.

Kluver, H., and Bucy, P. C. 1939. Preliminary analysis of functions of the temporal lobes of monkeys. Arch. Neurol. Psychiatr. 42:979–1000.

Kauer, J. 1988. Real-time imaging of evoked activity in local circuits of the salamander olfactory bulb. Nature 331:166–168.

Kauer, J. 1991. Contributions of topography and parallel processing to odor coding in the vertebrates olfactory pathway. Trends Neurosci. 14:79–85.

Lazard, D., Barak, Y., and Lancet, D. 1989. Bovine olfactory cilia preparation: thiol-modulated odorant-sensitive adenylylcyclase. Biochem. Biophys. Acta 1013:68–72.

Liegeois-Chauvel, C., Musolino, A., and Chauvel, P. 1991. Localization of primary auditory area in man. Brain 114:139–153.

MacLean, P. D. 1955. The limbic system (visceral brain) and emotional behavior. Arch. Neurol. Psychiatr. 73:130.

Margerison, J. H., and Corsellis, J. A. N. 1966. Epilepsy and the temporal lobes. Brain 89:499–530.

Mark, V. P., and Ervin, F. R. 1970. Violence and the Brain. New York, NY: Harper and Row.

Meyer, A. 1963. Intoxications. In J. Greenfield, W. Blackwood, W. H. McMenemy, A. Meyer, and R. M. Norman (Eds.) *Neuropathology*, pp. 235–287. Baltimore, MD: Williamsand Wilkins.

Milner, B. 1972. Disorders of learning and memory after temporal lobe lesions in man. Clin. Neurosurg. 19:421–446.

Mishkin, M. 1972. Cortical visual areas and their interactions. In A. G. Karzmar and J. C. Eccles (Eds.) Brain and Human Behavior, pp. 187–208. Berlin, Germany: Springer Verlag.

Moniz, E. 1936. Tentatives Operatoires dans le Traitement de Certaines Psychoses. Paris, France: Masson et Cie.

Mullan, S., and Penfield, W. 1959. Illusions of comparative interpretation and emotion. Arch. Neurol. Psychiatry 81:269–284.

Nauta, W. J. H. 1963. Central nervous organization and the endocrine motor system. In A. V. Nalbandov (Ed.) Advances in Neuroendocrinology, p. 5. Urbana: University of Illinois Press.

Nauta, W. J. H., and Domesick, V. B. 1981. Ramifications of the limbic system. In S. Matthysse (Ed.) Psychiatry and the Biology of the Human Brain, pp. 43–54. Amsterdam, The Netherlands: Elseveier North Holland Biomedical Press.

Nauta, W. J. H., and Kuypers, H. G. J. M. 1958. Some ascending pathways in brainstem reticular formation. In H. H. Jasper and L. O. Proctor (Eds.) Reticular Formation of the Brain. Henry Ford Hospital Symposium, pp. 3–30. Boston, MA: Little, Brown.

Olds, J. 1958. Self-stimulation experiments and differentiated reward systems. In H. H. Jasper and L. O. Proctor (Eds.) *Reticular Formation of the Brain*, p. 671. Boston, MA: Little, Brown.

Papez, J. W. 1937. A proposed mechanism of emotion. Arch. Neurol. Psychiatry 38:725–743.

Papez, J. W. 1958. The visceral brain, its components and connections. In H. H. Jasper and L. O. Proctor (Eds.) Reticular Formation of the Brain, p. 591. Boston, MA: Little, Brown.

Penfield, W., and Jasper, H. 1954. Epilepsy and the Functional Anatomy of the Human Brain. Boston, MA: Little. Brown.

Penfield, W., and Evans, J. P. 1934. Functional defects produced by cerebral lobotomies. Res. Publ. Assoc. Nerv. Ment. Dis.13:352–377.

Penfield, W., and Perot, P. 1963. The brain's record of auditory and visual experience. Brain 86:595–696.

Penfield, W., and Rasmussen, T. 1950. The Cerebral Cortex of Man: A Clinical Study of Localization of Function. New York, NY MacMillan.

Quesney, L. F., Coustain, M., Fish, D. R., et.al. 1990. Frontal lobe Epilespsyfield of recent emphasis. Am.J. EEG Technology, 30: pp. 177–193.

Reese, T. S., and Shepherd, G. M. 1972. Dendrodenritic synapses in the central nervous system. In G. D. Papas and D. P. Purpura (Eds.) Structure and Function of Synapses, pp. 121–136. New York, NY: Raven Press.

Sachdev, P., Smith, J. S., Matheson, J., et al. 1992. Amygdalohippocampectomy for pathological aggression. Aust. NZ J. Psychiatry 26:671–674.

Seifert, W. (Ed.). 1983. Neurobiology of the Hippocampus. New York, NY: Academic Press.

Sem-Jacobsen, C. W., and Torkildsen, A. 1960. Depth stimulation and electrical stimulation in the human brain. In E. R. Ramey and D. S. O'Doherty (Eds.) Electrical Studies of the Unanesthetized Brain, pp. 275–290. New York, NY: Hoeber.

Sheer, D. E. (Ed.) 1961. Electrical Stimulation of the Brain. Austin University of Texas Press.

So, N. K., Savard, G., Andermann, F.,et al. 1990. Acute postictal psychosis: a stereo EEG study. Epilepsia 31:188–193.

Steinberg, J., Taylor, R., and Haglund, K. 1994. Pheromones: a new term for a class of biologically active substances. J. NIH Res. 6:63–66.

Stevens, J. R. 1975. Interictal clinical manifestations of complex partial seizures. Adv. Neurol. 11:85–112.

Swanson, S. J., Rao, S. M., Grafman, J., et al. 1995. The relationship between seizure subtypes and interictal personality. Results from the Vietnam head injury study. Brain 118:91–103.

Tatnaka, Y., Kamo, T., Yoshide, M., et al. 1991. So-called cortical deafness: clinical, neuropsychological and radiologic observations. Brain 114:238–240.

Taylor, J. (Ed.). 1931. Selected Writing of John Hughlings Jackson, Vol. 1. On Epilepsy and Epileptiform Convulsions, pp. 385–405, 406–411, 458–463. New York, NY: Basic Books. (Reprinted 1958)

Valenstein, E. S. 1986. Great and Desperate Cures: The Rise and Decline of Psychosurgery and Other Radical Treatments for Mental Illness. New York, NY: Basic Books.

Vassar, R., Chao, S. K., Sitcheran, R., et al. 1994. Topographic organization of sensory projections to the olfactory bulb. Cell 79:981–991.

Walczak, T. S. 1995. Neocortical temporal lobe epilepsy. Epilepsia 36:623–635.

Waxman, S. G., and Geschwind, N. 1975. The interictal behavior syndrome of temporal lobe epilepsy. Arch. Gen. Psychiatry 32:1580–1586.

Wieser, H. G. 1988. Selective amygdalo-hippocampectomy for temporal lobe epilepsy. Epilepsia 29(Suppl. 2):100–113.

AMYGDALA, EMOTION, AUTISM, AND PSYCHIATRIC DISORDERS

Adams, R. D., Victor, M., and Ropper, A. H. 1997. Psychiatric disorders. In M. Victor and A. Ropper (Eds.) Principles of Neurology, pp.1501–1562. New York, NY: McGraw Hill.

Adolph, R., Sears, L., and Piven, J. 2001. Abnormal processing of social information from faces in autism. J. Cogn. Neurosci. 13:232–240.

Adolph, R., Tranel, D., and Damasio, A. R. 1998. The human amygdala in social judgment. Nature 393:417–418.

Amaral, D., and LeDoux, J. 2001. Fear and social conditioning in the amygdala. Lectures at the Boston Society of Neurology and Psychiatry, 924th meeting, June 14th 2001. Boston, MA.

Anderson, A. K., and Phelps, E. A. 2000. Expression without recognition: contributions of the human amygdala to motional communication. Psychol. Sci. 11:106–111

Baron-Cohen, S., Ring, H. A., Bullmore, E. T., et al. 2000. The amygdala theory of autism. Neurosci. Biobehav. Rev. 24: 355–364.

Critchley, H. D., Daly, E. M., and Bullmore, E. T. 2000. The functional neuroanatomy of social behaviour. Brain 123:2203–2212.

Foong, J., Symms, M. R., Barker, G. J., et al. 2001. Neuropathological abnormalities in schizophrenia. Brain 124:882–892.

Friston, K. J., Liddle, P. F., Firth, C. D., et al. 1992. The left medial temporal region and schizophrenia. A PET study. Brain 115:367.

Howard, M. A., Cowell, P. E., Boucher, J., et al. Convergent neuroanatomical and behavioural evidence of an amygdala hypothesis of autism. Neuroreport 11:2931–2935.

Kallmann, F. J. 1946. The genetic theory of schizophrenia. An analysis of 691 twin index families. Am. J. Psychiatry 103:309.

Ledoux, J. 2000. Emotion circuits in the brain. Ann. Rev. Neurosci. 23:155–184.

Levine, D. N., and Grek, A. 1984. The anatomic basis of delusionsafter right cerebral infarction. Neurology 34:577–1984.

Robinson, R. G., and Paradiso, S. 1998. Dementia associated with post stroke major depression. ARNMD. 74:141–166.

Schlaepter, T. E., Harris, G. J., Tien, A. Y., et al. 1994. Decreased regional cortical gray matter volumein schizophremia. Am. J. Psychiatry 151:843–848.

Selemon, L. D., and Goldman-Rakic, P. S. 1999. The reduced neuropil hypothesis: a circuit based model of schizophrenia. (Review). Biol. Psychiatry 45:17–25.

Shenton, M. E., Kikinis, R., Jolesz, F. A., et al. 1992. Abnormalities of the left temporal lobe and thought disorder in schizophrenia. A quantitative magnetic resonance imaging study. N. Engl. J. Med. 327:604–612.

Starkstein, S. E., Robinson, R. G., and Price, T. R. 1987. Comparison of cortical and subcortical lesions in the production of post stroke mood disorders. Brain 110:1045–1059.

Stuss, D. T., Gallup, G. G., and Alexander, M. P. 2000. The frontal lobes are necessary for 'theory of mind'. Brain 124:279–286.

23.

VISUAL SYSTEM

Of all our senses, vision is the most important: we perceive the world mostly through our eyes. Even though light intensity varies by a factor of 10 million between the brightest snowy day and a starlit night, our eyes and visual system adapt to these intensity changes. We can discriminate between thousands of hues and shades of color. Our eyes are set in our heads in such a way that each eye sees almost the same visual field, making depth perception possible.

In the visual system the primary, secondary, and tertiary neurons are in the retinae and are all part of the central nervous system. The right field of vision projects to the left cerebral hemisphere; the left field of vision projects to the right cerebral hemisphere.

STRUCTURE OF THE EYE

The anatomy of the receptor organ, the eye, is shown in Figure 23.1A. It has three layers, or tunics:

1. The outer fibrous tunic—cornea and sclera
2. The middle vascular and pigmented tunic—choroid, ciliary body, iris, and pupil
3. The inner neural tunic—retina with pigmented epithelium and neuronal layers

The *outer fibrous tunic* consists of two parts: the anterior transparent cornea and the posterior fibrous white sclera.

The *cornea*, the window to the world, allows light rays to enter the eye. Most of the refraction needed to focus light rays on the retina occurs at the air-cornea junction. The sclera forms the white of the eye and the rest of the outer covering.

The *middle tunic* consists of the choroid, the ciliary body, and the iris. The middle tunic is richly vascular and provides oxygen and nutrients to the inner, photoreceptor layer and the retina.

The choroid is vascular and pigmented and forms the posterior portion of this tunic. Its inner portion is attached to the pigmented layer of the retina. The ciliary body is found in the anterior portion of the middle tunic and consists of a vascular tunic and the ciliary muscle. The ciliary body surrounds the lens and consists of a vascular tunic (the ciliary muscle) and the suspensory ligaments (the zonule), which suspend the lens (Fig. 23.1B). The ciliary muscles consist of meridional and circular fibers. The meridional fibers are external to the circular fibers. The ciliary muscles are the muscles used in accommodation, focusing on near objects.

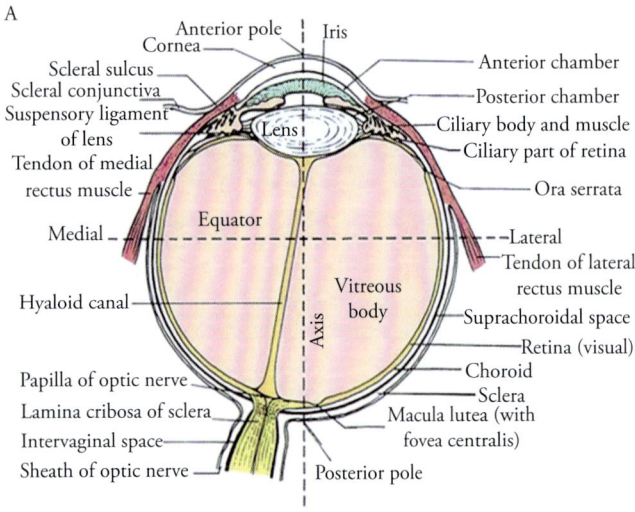

Figure 23.1A Horizontal meridional section of the eye. (From Leeson and Lesson, 1970. Histology, Philadelphia, W.B. Saunders.)

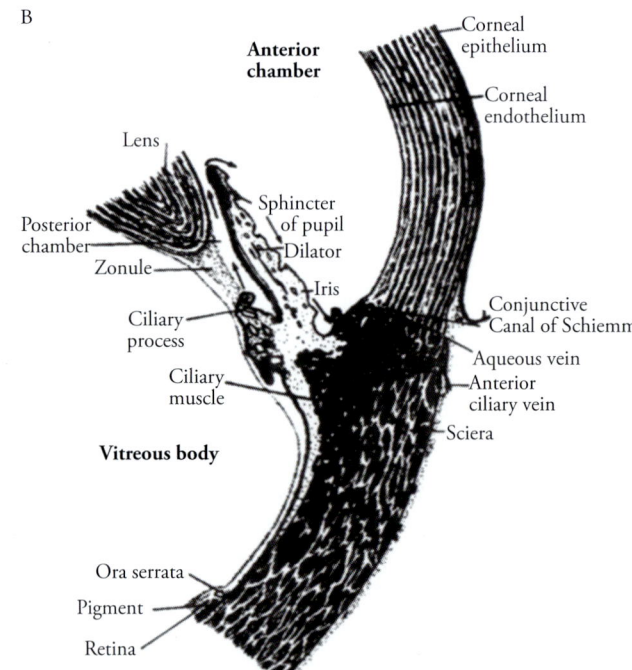

Figure 23.1B Enlargement of a portion of the meridional section to show the angle of the eye. The letter P indicates the pectinate ligament or the trabecular meshwork. The arrows indicate the course of circulation of aqueous fluid. (From Leeson and Leeson, Histology, Philadelphia, WB Saunders, 1970.)

The *lens* separates the anterior chamber from the vitreous body and completes the refraction of the entering light. A fibrous network, the zonule, suspends the lens. For distance vision the fibers are taut and the anterior surface of the lens is pulled flat. For close vision the ciliary muscle contracts, the fibers go slack, and the anterior surface becomes more convex; the eye accommodates. A decreased ability to focus on close objects is a normal consequence of aging. The term "visual acuity" refers to the resolving power of the eye in terms of the ability to focus on near or distant objects. For example, 23/40 means the patient's eye sees at 23 feet what the normal eye sees at 40 feet.

The pigmented iris on the anterior portion of the vascular tunic divides the space between the lens and the cornea into an anterior chamber (between the lens and the cornea) and a narrow posterior chamber (between the suspensory ligaments of the lens and the iris). The iris is a circular structure that acts as a diaphragm to control the amount of light falling on the retina. The opening is analogous to the f-stop of a camera. The eye has a range equivalent to the range from f2 to f22.

PUPILLARY REFLEXES

PUPILLARY MUSCLES

Two sets of muscles in the iris control the size of the pupil, sphincter, and the dilator pupillae. When the circular muscles, the sphincter pupillae, contract, the iris is drawn together and the pupil constricts, such as purse strings close the mouth of the purse. The second set of muscles, the dilator pupillae, are radial and draw the iris back toward the sclera.

The sphincter pupillae are supplied by the parasympathetic nervous system via the ciliary nerves, the fibers of which run together with nerve III. Transmission by this pathway is cholinergic; the dilator pupilla are supplied by the sympathetic nervous system via the superior cervical ganglion. Neurotransmission in this pathway is alpha-adrenergic.

PUPILLARY REFLEXES

When light is flashed into either eye, the pupil constricts; this is the light reflex. When the eye focuses on close objects, accommodation occurs and the pupil constricts.

1. *Light reflex.* In dim light the aperture of the pupil increases (dilator muscle), while in bright light the aperture of the pupil decreases (sphincter muscle). The afferent fibers arise in the retina and travel with the optic nerve and tract; these fibers pass through the lateral geniculate and synapse in the pretectal region of the midbrain. Neurons of the pretectal nuclei project bilaterally to the Edinger-Westphal nucleus.
2. *Accommodation.* This reflex changes the refractive power of the lens by the ciliary muscle contracting and decreasing the force on the suspensory ligament of the lens; the lens assumes a more rounded appearance with a shorter focal length. The neural pathway arises in the occipital lobe and the final efferent fibers run together with nerve III. In looking at distant objects, the pupil dilates while in focusing on nearby objects the pupil constricts.
3. *Fixed pupil.* In the absence of trauma to the eye, a dilated pupil that does not respond to light, fixed, is usually a sign of pressure on the third nerve. This is typically from supratentorial mass lesions that have produced herniation of the mesial segments of the temporal lobe through the tentorium. Compression of the third nerve and of the midbrain occurs. Progressive rostral-caudal damage to the brain stem then evolves. This problem when first detected must be treated as a neurosurgical emergency.

INNER TUNIC (RETINA)

The inner tunic (retina) consists of pars optica, pars ciliaris, and pars iridica. The inner tunic contains photoreceptor cells and nerve cells. They are organized so that photoreceptor cells containing the photopigments are closest to the sclera and the nerve cells are above them. The nerve cells send fibers to the optic nerve through a pigment-free area, the optic disk. Light must traverse the nerve network to reach the photoreceptors.

The pars ciliaris and iridica are primarily a pigmented region on, respectively, the ciliary body and iris. The pars optica contains the photoreceptor cells and will be the focus of our discussion.

The pars optica contains:

- outer pigmented layer,
- inner photoreceptor cells closest to the sclera, and
- nerve cells that are internal to photoreceptors and form the optic nerve that leaves the retinae through a pigment-free area, the optic disk. Light must traverse the nerve network to reach the photoreceptors.

The pars optica of the retina consists of the following layers (Fig. 23.2A):

1. Pigmented epithelium (most external)
2. Receptor cell layer—rods and cones
3. External limiting membrane
4. Outer nuclear layer containing the nuclei of rods and cones
5. Outer plexiform layer containing the synapses of rods and cones with the dendrites of bipolar and horizontal cells, and the cell bodies of horizontal cells
6. Inner nuclear layer containing the cell bodies of bipolar, and amacrine cells
7. Inner plexiform layer containing the synapses of bipolar and amacrine cells with ganglion cells
8. Ganglion cell layer
9. Optic nerve layer
10. Internal limiting membrane

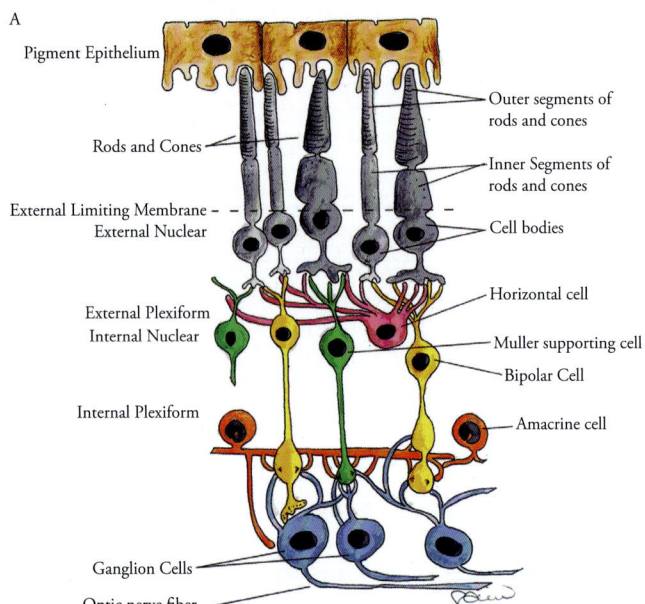

Figure 23.2A Schematic diagram of the ultrastructural organization of the retina. Rods and cones are composed of outer (OS) and inner segments (IS), cell bodies, and synaptic bases. Photopigments are present in laminated disks in the outer segments. The synaptic base of a rod is called a spherule; the synaptic base of a cone is called a pedicle. AM, amacrine cell; DG, diffuse ganglion cell; FB, flat bipolar cell; MB, midget bipolar cell; MG, midget ganglion cell; RB, bipolar cell. (From Carpenter, M.B., A Core Text of Neuroanatomy. Baltimore, Williams and Wilkins.)

PHOTORECEPTORS: RODS AND CONES

There are two types of photoreceptor cells: rods and cones.

The *rods* are sensitive in dim light because they contain more of the photosensitive pigment rhodopsin than the cones. This system has poor resolution; newspaper headlines are the smallest letters that can be recognized.

The *cones* are sensitive to color. There are three separate groups of cones, each of which contains photopigments that are primarily sensitive (1) to blue—short wave lengths, (2) to green—middle wave lengths, or (3) to red—longer wave lengths. Color vision requires light levels greater than bright moonlight and has high resolution; fine detail can be seen. The rods and cones are not uniformly distributed in the retina. Most of the 6 million cone cells are located in an area 2 mm in diameter, the macula lutea (Fig. 23.1A), which can be seen through the ophthalmoscope. In the center of the macula lutea lies a zone of pure cones, the fovea (Fig. 23.2B). The rest of the macula lutea is composed of both rods and cones, and most of the peripheral retina contains only rods. There are about 123 million rods.

BLIND SPOT

The point of entry of the optic nerve and the retinal vessels contains no rod or cone receptors. This area, referred to as the *papilla*, corresponds to the "blind spot" when visual fields are plotted. When swelling of the papilla occurs due to increased intracranial pressures—(*papilledema*)—the blind spot is enlarged.

Rods: Vision in Dim Light and Night Vision

The rods permit vision, *scotopic* (dark vision), in the dark-adapted eye. Rods contain a single pigment, *rhodopsin*, which is related to vitamin A_1 (retinol). The spectral sensitivity of night or scotopic vision is identical to the absorption spectra of rhodopsin (Fig. 23.3). Light that can be absorbed by rhodopsin is seen; light that cannot be absorbed such as red light is not seen at these low light intensities. Scotopic vision has quite poor definition; two light sources must be quite far apart to be distinguished as two sources rather than one. Peripheral vision has progressively poor

Figure 23.2B The densities of cones and rods on or near the horizontal meridian through a human retina. The insert is a schematic map of the retina showing the fovea (F) and the blind spot (B). The striped area represents the regions of the retina, which were sampled in obtaining the counts plotted here. (From Chapanis after Osterberg, Acta Opth, 1935, Suppl. 6, Blackwell.)

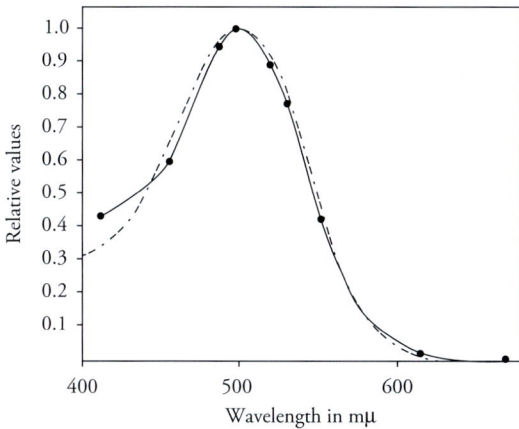

Figure 23.3 Comparison of the absorption curve of pure visual purple (interrupted line) with the intensity of light just visible in a dark-adapted human subject (continuous curve). (Ludwig, Arch. Ophthal. 20:713, 1938, AMA.)

Figure 23.4 The absorption spectra of three types of cones. (Drawn from records in Marks, Dobelle, and MacNichol. 1964. Science 143:1181; and Brown and Wald. 1964. Science 144:45.)

definition. The modern human uses this system very little since we have bright, portable light sources or radar. Several modern inventions, such as night goggles with infrared sensors, are designed to compensate for these limitations.

The visual pigment rhodopsin absorbs photons. Each rhodopsin molecule consists of retinal and opsin. Retinal absorbs the light, while opsin is the protein in the plasma membrane of the rods. The photon converts retinal from the 11-cis form to the all-trans form. The all-trans retinal has to be re-isomerized to 11-cis retinal to reform rhodopsin and to begin the process again. The photons result in hyperpolarization of the plasma membrane that is the light-dependent part of visual excitation. The photoreceptors are depolarized in the dark due to the sodium channels remaining open, called the dark currents. The dark current is turned off in light. Daylight prevents the regeneration of rhodopsin in the rods.

After 5–10 minutes in the dark, scotopic vision begins to return as the rhodopsin is regenerated and reaches maximal sensitivity after 15 to 23 minutes. Since rhodopsin does not absorb red light, using red goggles can preserve night vision.

Cones: Color Vision

Color vision requires much higher light intensities and occurs primarily when the image is focused upon the macula. Each cone contains one of the three color pigments whose absorption spectra are shown in Figure 23.4. The visual pigment of the cones consists of opsin and retinal.

The cones are divided into three separate groups that contain photopigments primarily sensitive to a different part of the visible spectrum as follows:

1. Blue: 423 nanometers (nm) (short wavelengths)
2. Green: 530 nm (middle wave lengths), and
3. Red: 560 nm (longer wavelengths).

Color vision requires light levels greater than bright moonlight and has high resolution so that fine detail can be seen. Any color that does not excite two pigments, such as deep purple (400 nm) and deep red (650 nm), will be hard to discriminate. For this reason, a color of 660 nm in bright light can mimic a color of 640 nm in weaker light. To distinguish the color orange, 600 nm, the visual system compares the relative absorption by two visual pigments, in this case, red and green.

Comparing the absorption by one visual pigment to the overall brightness apparently makes these color discriminations. For this reason a color of 660 nm, in bright light, mimics a color of 640 nm in weaker light. Only when the two types of cones are excited can color and brightness be determined independently.

ELECTROPHYSIOLOGY OF RETINAL PHOTORECEPTORS AND NEURONS

Synaptic Organization of the Rods, Cones, and Neurons in the Retinae (Fig. 23.2A)

1. Rods and cones synapse on the dendrites of bipolar cells and horizontal cells. In the peripheral portion of the retina, 60 degrees from the center, as many as 600 rods may converge on a single bipolar cell, while in the fovea, only one or two cones may do so. In the macula lutea both rods and cones may innervate a single bipolar cell.

2. Axons of bipolar cells and amacrine cells synapse on dendrites of ganglion cells. Once again, the degree of convergence on the ganglion cell depends on the region of the retina. Ganglion cells in the fovea connect with only one bipolar cell.

3. Axons of ganglion cells leave the retina and form the cranial nerve II that synapses in the lateral geniculate, hypothalamus, and midbrain. There are about a million optic nerve fibers. Clearly, considerable data reduction has occurred between the 100 million rods and cones and the 1 million optic nerve fibers.

Two other types of neurons are found in the retina: horizontal and amacrine cells. Horizontal cells are found in the outer plexiform layer (next to the rods and cones); their dendrites make contact with numerous rods and cones over a 230 to 400 μM field. Their axons run transversely along the retina and branch to make contact with many other rods or cones at the bipolar-cell junction. The horizontal cells connect groups of visual receptors in one area with groups in another area. Amacrine cells lie in the inner plexiform layer (next to the ganglion cells). The dendrites form postsynaptic contacts with bipolar cells and presynaptic contacts with ganglion cells; no axon has been described.

RESPONSE OF THE CELLS TO LIGHT

Rods and Cones (Fig. 23.2B). Both rods and cones show a hyperpolarizing response to light. This very surprising result has been obtained in all vertebrate visual receptors studied to date. Contrary to what one would expect, they act as if dark were the stimulus. During darkness, high concentrations of cyclic GMP increase membrane conductance and give rise to a dark current that flows from the outer to inner segment, depolarizing the cell. After absorbing a photon, rhodopsin activates cyclic-GMP-phosphodiesterase, which cleaves cyclic GMP, lowers cyclic GMP levels, and by reducing the membrane conductance, hyperpolarizes the rod. Also contrary to expectation, the rod and cone cells release transmitter when it is dark, but this release ceases when it is light.

Horizontal Cell of Retinae. This hyperpolarizes in response to light, but it has a large receptive field. Even when the light is shining on receptor cells 250μm away, there is a strong hyperpolarizing response. Potential spread through the horizontal layer is by slow potentials; no action potentials have been observed.

Bipolar Cell. Both the direct hyperpolarizing receptor response and the horizontal cell output impinge on the bipolar cell. Here we see the first type of data reduction carried out in the retina: center-surround contrast enhancement. The bipolar cell has one type of output (hyperpolarization) for a bright spot on a dark field and another type of output (depolarization) for a large bright field.

Amacrine Cell. Recordings from the amacrine cell show that it responds primarily to sudden changes in light intensity. Note that it is active primarily when the light turns on or off. This is the second type of processing, or data reduction, that takes place in the retina: dynamic detection.

Ganglion Cells. There are two types of ganglion cell responses: amacrine cell or bipolar cell.

Amacrine Cell Response. This response is primarily a dynamic response to turning the light on or off. Some cells react more strongly to the light coming on than off; others have the opposite response. These cells are inhibited by illumination of both a spot and the surrounding area.

Bipolar Cell Response. The second type of ganglion cell response reflects bipolar cell activity. When only the central portion of its receptive fields is illuminated, the ganglion cell responds with an intense train of action potentials during the illumination that abruptly stops when the light ceases. The frequency of the action potentials during illumination is proportional to the logarithm of the brightness of the light. When both the spot and the surrounding area are illuminated, there is less activity than occurs in the dark (the background level). When only the surround is illuminated, there is no specific response.

A third type of ganglion cell response (not shown in Figure. 23.5) is a center off type. When the center of the receptive field is illuminated, action potential frequency decreases. When the surround is illuminated, activity is greater than the background level but not as intense as in the second type of response to a spot noted earlier.

To summarize, ganglion cells signal the onset and cessation of light flashes and are effectively stimulated only by edges or abrupt transitions between light and darkness in their fields. Diffuse illumination does not stimulate ganglion cells very well.

The axons from the ganglion cells traverse the inner surface of the retina to the optic disk, where they turn and form the optic nerve, which runs for about 1 inch before entering the optic foramen on its way toward the diencephalon.

Optic Nerve. Electrical recordings from optic nerve fibers also show the types of data reduction occurring in the retina. First, there is convergence; many receptors must fire one bipolar cell in the fovea. Consequently the "grain" of the visual image depends on the location on the retinae. Second, brightness can be detected. Third, there is a center-surround contrast enhancement. Lastly, there is a dynamic or motion detection.

Figure 23.5 Responses of the cell types in the Necturus retina. (From F.S. Werblin and J. Dowling. 1969. J. Neurophysiol. 32:339, Amer. Physiol. Soc.)

A spot of light on the retinae will be coded in terms of its brightness and its edges. As it is turned on and off, the dynamic receptors fire to alert higher centers. The spot of light will receive much more attention in the optic nerve bandwidth if it is moved around because each tiny movement will set off a new set of dynamic or movement receptors, and these receptors make up about half the total optic nerve fibers. For example, the rotating flashing lights of emergency vehicles attracts more attention than a fixed light.

VISUAL PATHWAY

Figure 23.6 demonstrates the visual pathway from the eye to the occipital lobe.

1. Origin of cranial nerve II from ganglion cell layer in the retina
2. Optic nerve
3. Optic chiasm
4. Optic tract
5. Synapse in lateral geniculate nucleus of the thalamus
6. Visual radiation from lateral geniculate nucleus to the striate (visual) cortex—area 17 of the occipital lobe
7. Visual association cortex—areas 18 and 19
8. Multimodal associations with cortical regions in the posterior temporal-parietal, and frontal lobes in both hemispheres (Fig. 18.11).

VISUAL FIELDS

RETINA

Each retina is divided into a temporal or nasal half by a vertical line passing through the *fovea centralis*. This also serves to divide the retina of each eye into a left and right half. A horizontal line passing through the fovea would divide each half of the retina and macula into an upper and lower quadrant. Each area of the retina corresponds to a particular sector of the visual fields, which are named as viewed by the patient. For each eye tested alone, there is a left and right visual field corresponding to a nasal and temporal field. Because of the effect of the lens, the patient's left visual field projects onto the nasal retina of the left eye and the temporal retina of the right eye. Similarly, the upper visual quadrants project to the inferior retinal quadrants.

OPTIC NERVE AND OPTIC CHIASM

At the chiasm, the fibers in the optic nerve from the left nasal retina cross the midline and join with the fibers from the right temporal retina to form the right optic tract. This dense bundle of over a million fibers runs across the base of the cerebrum to the lateral geniculate nucleus of the thalamus. Fibers from the inferior nasal retina (the superior, temporal visual field) cross in the inferior portion of the chiasm, which usually lies just above the dorsum sellae.

By this crossing, all the information from the left visual field is brought to the right lateral geniculate nucleus and subsequently to the right calcarine cortex. The fibers of the right nasal retina also cross in the chiasm to join the fibers from the left temporal retina. Thus, the visual pathway repeats the pattern in other sensory systems; the right side of the visual field is represented on the left cerebrum.

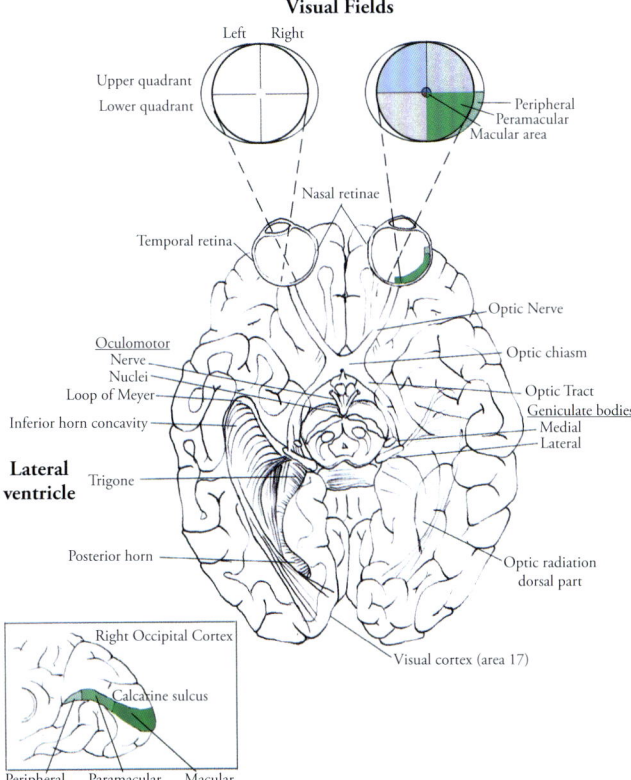

Figure 23.6 The visual pathways viewed from the ventral surface of the brain. Light from the upper half of the visual field falls on the inferior half of the retina. Light from the temporal half of the visual field falls on the nasal half of the retina; light from the nasal half of the visual field falls on the temporal half of the retina. The visual pathways from the retina to the striate cortex are shown. The plane of the visual fields has been rotated 90 degrees toward the reader. The inset (lower left) shows the projection of the quadrants of the right visual field on the left calcarine (striate) cortex. The macular area of the retina is represented nearest the occipital pole. Fibers mediating the pupillary light reflex leave the optic tract and project to the pretectal region; fibers from the pretectal olivary nucleus relay signals bilaterally to the visceral nuclei of the oculomotor complex. (Modified from Carpenter and Sutin. 1983. Human Neuroanatomy. Courtesy of Williams and Wilkins.)

LESIONS IN THE OPTIC PATHWAY

1. In the retina or the optic nerve before the optic chiasm (2 in Fig. 23.7), there is no sight in that eye—monocular blindness. Incomplete lesions produce a monocular scotoma, as in optic neuritis.
2. In the chiasm, the fibers from both temporal visual fields are cut; the result is bitemporal hemianopsia (3 in Fig. 23.7).

Figure 23.7 Common lesions of the optic tract. (1) Normal, (2) optic nerve, (3) optic chiasm, (4) optic tract or complete geniculate or complete geniculocalcarine radiation or complete cortical, (5) temporal segment of geniculocalcarine radiation (Meyer's loop) producing a superior quadrantanopia. If the parietal segment of this radiation were involved, an inferior quadrantanopia would result. (6) Calcarine or posterior cerebral artery occlusion producing a homonymous hemianopia with macular sparing.

3. Lesions behind the optic chiasm produce blindness in one visual field, a homonymous hemianopsia from injury to the optic tract, the lateral geniculate body, or the geniculocalcarine radiation (4 in Fig. 23.7).

4. Partial lesions of the geniculocalcarine radiations produce a quadrantanopsia (5 in Fig. 23.7).

5. Macular sparing is seen with lesions in the visual cortex following calcarine artery infarcts (6 in Fig. 23.7). The macula is represented close to the occipital pole and this area receives anastomotic flow from the middle cerebral artery.

The following case is an example of a lesion in the optic nerve, anterior to the optic chiasm.

CASE HISTORY 23.1

This 53-year-old white right-handed housewife had a progressive 23-year history of right-sided supraorbital headache with decreasing acuity and now almost total blindness in the right eye. During the 3 years before admission, intermittent tingling paresthesia had been noted in the left face, arm, or leg. About 1 year before admission, the patient had a sudden loss of consciousness and was amnestic for the events of the next 48 hours. No explanation for the episode was clearly established. The cerebrospinal fluid protein was reported to be elevated (230 mg/dl). The patient and her family reported some personality changes over a period of several years, including a loss of spontaneity and increasing apathy.

General physical examination: There was a minor degree of proptosis (downward protrusion of the right eye).

Neurologic Examination

Mental status: The patient was, in general, alert but at times would become lethargic. Her affect was flat. At times, she would laugh or joke in an inappropriate manner.

Cranial nerves: There was anosmia for odors, such as cloves, on the right and a reduced sensitivity on the left. Marked papilledema (increased intracranial pressure with elevation of the optic disk and venous engorgement) was present in the left eye. In contrast, there was pallor of the right optic disk, indicating optic atrophy. Visual acuity in the right eye was markedly reduced. This combination of funduscopic findings is termed the Foster Kennedy syndrome. The patient had only a small crescent of vision in the temporal field of the right eye; only vague outlines of objects could be seen. A slight left central facial weakness was present.

Motor system: Movements on the left side were slow.

Reflexes: A release of grasp reflex was present on the left side.

Clinical diagnosis: Subfrontal meningioma rising from the inner third sphenoid wing. Alternative location would be olfactory groove.

Figure 23.8 Sphenoid-wing meningioma producing compression of the right optic and olfactory nerves. Case 23.1 (refer to text). Right carotid arteriogram, venous phase demonstrating tumor blush in the subfrontal area of the anterior fossa, extending into the middle fossa. (Courtesy of Dr. Samuel Wolpert, New England Medical Center Hospitals.)

Figure 23.9 A large pituitary adenoma with secondary hemorrhage has extended upward out of the sella to compress the optic chiasm and optic nerves. This 53-year-old white male 11 months before death experienced difficulty reading small print, with greater involvement of the right eye than the left. This progressed to total blindness in the right eye and shortly thereafter sudden loss of vision in the left eye, an absence of pupillary responses, and a bilateral anosmia. Vision improved after partial surgical removal and irradiation, but fatal meningitis developed. (Courtesy of Drs. John Hills and Jose Segarra.)

Laboratory data: *Imaging studies* demonstrated a tumor blush in the right subfrontal region extending back to the right optic nerve groove, consistent with a meningioma arising from the olfactory groove or inner third sphenoid wing (Fig. 23.8).

Hospital course: A bifrontal craniotomy performed by Dr. Sam Brendler exposed a well-encapsulated smooth tumor, a meningioma attached to the inner third of the sphenoid wing. Approximately 90% to 95% of the tumor was removed, exposing the right optic nerve. Examination 4 months after surgery indicated that right anosmia and right optic atrophy were present.

Optic chiasm: A bitemporal defect results (Figs. 23.9, 23.10, and 23.11). This may be a bitemporal hemianopsia or an incomplete bitemporal field defect. The usual cause is a pituitary adenoma or a suprasellar tumor such as a craniopharyngioma.

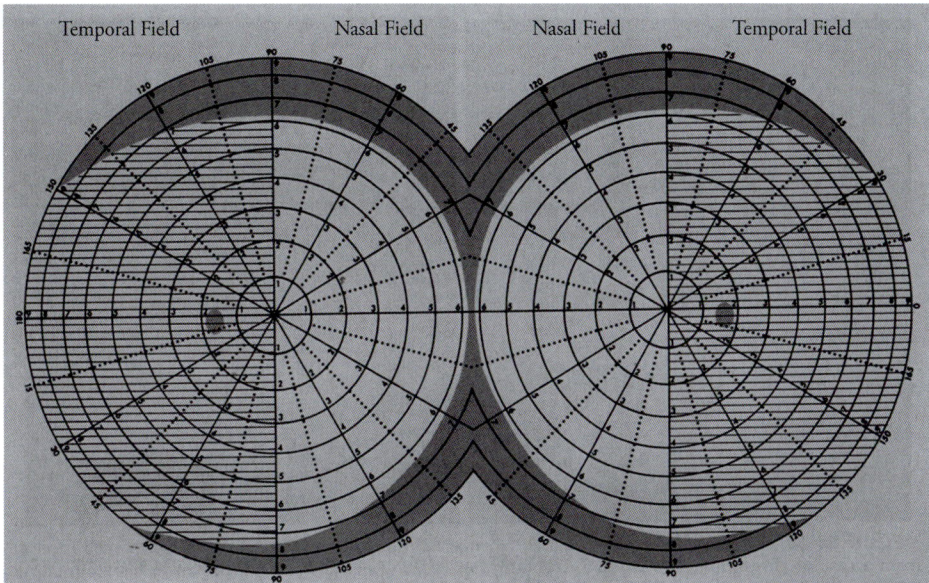

Figure 23.10 Pituitary adenoma. Case 16.2. Visual fields demonstrating a bitemporal hemianopia. O.S. = left eye; O.D. = right eye. This 51-year-old obese male with large puffy hands and a prominent jaw, declining sexual interest for 18 years, an 8-year history of progressive loss of visual acuity, a 6- to 7-month history of diplopia due to a bilateral medial rectus palsy, and headache had stopped driving because he was unable to see the sides of the road. Urinary adrenal and gonadal steroids and thyroid functions were low, with no follicle-stimulating hormone. Imaging studies demonstrated a large pituitary adenoma with significant suprasellar extent.

Figure 23.11 A large pituitary adenoma in a 44-year-old man with a bitemporal hemianopia. Case 23.2. Significant extrasellar extension compresses the optic chiasm. Magnetic resonance imaging (MRI) scans, T1 weighted: (*A*) midline sagittal section; (*B*) coronal section. (T1 with contrast.)

CASE HISTORY 23.2 (PATIENT OF DR. MARTHA FEHR)

This 45-year-old man had an 18-month history of a progressive alteration in vision. He was unable to see objects in the right or left periphery of vision. He was concerned that in the process of driving he might hit pedestrians stepping off the sidewalks in the periphery of vision. He had also experienced, over 6–8 months, progressive headaches, loss of energy, and a lower libido.

Neurologic exam: Normal except for a bitemporal hemianopia.

Clinical diagnosis: Pituitary adenoma compressing the optic chiasm.

Laboratory Data

Endocrine studies: All were normal.

Magnetic resonance imaging (MRI): A large macroadenoma measuring 3 cm in diameter extended outside of the sella turcica to compress the optic chiasm (Fig. 23.11).

Subsequent course: Dr. Gerald McGuillicuddy performed a gross total trans-sphenoidal resection of the tumor, with a significant improvement in vision. Three years later, the patient again had visual symptoms and eye pain. MRI scans indicated regrowth of tumor with possible impression on the right optic nerve. He was treated with radiotherapy.

Note that males are more likely to present with large pituitary adenoma compressing the optic chiasm. Women are more likely to present with microadenomas or small macroadenomas since they are more likely to be seen at an earlier stage due to an initial complaint of amenorrhea.

LATERAL GENICULATE NUCLEUS

The lateral geniculate nucleus (LGN) is primarily a relay station in the visual pathway. The fibers of the optic nerve divide with about half going into the LGN and descend into the pretectal region of the midbrain. Others, for coordinating eye and head or neck movements, descend to the tectum of the superior colliculus. Also some of the retinal fibers synapse in the suprachiasmatic nucleus of the hypothalamus and then project to the pineal by way of the sympathetic fibers, where they influence circadian rhythms and endocrine functions.

The LGN is a six-layer, horseshoe-shaped structure. Visual processing begins in the large and small cells in the LGN. The small cells are in layers 1 to 4, and the large cells in layers 5 and 6. Each LGN cell receives direct input from a specific area of the retina, and each area of the LGN is driven from a specific area of the visual field. Each receptive field has a center that is either on or off and a surround that has the opposite polarity.

The optic nerve fibers from the temporal visual field, the crossed fibers, end in layers 1, 4, and 6. The fibers from the temporal retina (the nasal visual field), the uncrossed fibers, end in layers 2, 3, and 5. Each optic nerve fiber ends in one layer on five or six cells. The total number of cells and fibers is roughly equal. LGN cells respond well to small spots of light and to short, narrow bars of light, as well as to on-off stimuli. Diffuse light is a very poor stimulus.

Cells in the LGN grow rapidly in the first 6 to 12 months after birth, under the influence of visual stimuli. Visual sensory deprivation during this period leads to atrophy and lifelong blindness. Two major streams of visual information leave the retina to the LGN: (1) The magnocellular stream starts in the large cells of the retinal ganglion (Y-cells) that project to the magnocellular layers (layers 1 and 2), which subsequently project to the striate cortex. The cortical neurons of the magnocellular stream respond to movements, orientation, and contrast but respond poorly to color. (2) The parvocellular stream begins with small cells of the retinal ganglion layer (X-cells) that project to parvocellular layer of LGN layers 3 and 6. These cells respond either to shape and orientation or color (red/green and blue/yellow).

OPTIC RADIATION

The fibers to the visual cortex leave the LGN and form the optic radiation, which sweeps around the posterior horn of the lateral ventricle, through the parietal lobe to the occipital lobe and the calcarine cortex (Fig. 23.6). Some fibers from the LGN also enter the inferior pulvinar nucleus.

The visual radiation is so extensive that not all the fibers can pass directly posterior to the calcarine cortex. Only the most dorsally placed fibers pass back deep into the parietal lobe. The more ventrally placed fibers pass forward (Myer's loop) and deep into the temporal lobe, swing posteriorly around the anterior portion of the inferior horn of the lateral ventricle, and continue posteriorly lateral to the ventricle wall to the calcarine cortex. In contrast to the densely packed optic tract, the optic radiation fans out widely on its passage through the parietal and temporal lobes.

OCCIPITAL LOBE

The occipital lobe in Brodmann's numerical scheme consists of areas 17, 18, and 19. From a cytoarchitectural standpoint, area 17 represents a classic example of specialized granular cortex, or koniocortex. Areas 18 and 19 represent progressive modifications from koniocortex toward homotypical cortex (refer to Chapter 17 for a discussion of cytoarchitecture).

Area 17, the striate cortex, the principal visual projection area in humans, is found primarily on the medial surface of the hemisphere, occupying those portions of the cuneus (above) and lingual gyrus (below) that border the calcarine sulcus. For this reason, it is often termed the calcarine cortex. Much of this cortex is located on the walls and in the depths of this sulcus.

The extrastriate visual cortex, including parastriate areas 18 and 19, forms concentric bands about area 17 and is found on both the medial and lateral surfaces. Area 19 in humans extends onto the adjacent mid and inferior temporal gyri.

Most of our understanding of occipital lobe function comes from simian studies. In nonhuman primates five visual areas have been identified: V1, corresponding to area 17 in humans; V2 and V3, corresponding to area 18; and V4 and V5, corresponding to area 19.

Area 17 is the primary visual area and receives the termination of the geniculocalcarine (or optic) radiation. This projection is arranged in a topographic manner, with the superior quadrant of the contralateral visual field represented on the inferior bank of the calcarine fissure, and the inferior quadrant of the contralateral visual field represented on the superior bank. The macula has a large area of representation, which occupies the posterior third of the calcarine cortex and extends onto the occipital pole.

Area 17 receives fibers from and sends fibers to area 18 but does not have any direct callosal or long-association-fiber connections to other cortical areas. The columnar and horizontal organization of the primary visual cortex has been discussed previously in Chapter 17. Area 17 is more mature at birth and has the most precise map. The other visual areas develop through maturation and experience, although experience modifies V1 as well (see Chapter 29).

Area 18 has extensive connections with areas 18 and 19 of the ipsilateral and contralateral hemispheres, which were demonstrated by both the earlier strychnine neuronography studies and the more recent horseradish peroxidase studies.

Callosal fibers enter the opposite hemisphere, and association fibers communicate with the premotor and inferior temporal areas and area 7 of the adjacent parietal cortex.

As discussed in greater detail later, Zeki and associates (1992) studied each of these visual areas to create a map of the retina. Parallel pathways process various aspects of visual information—color (wavelength), motion, stereopsis, and form (line orientation)—and extend from the retina to the LGN, striate cortex, and, finally, extrastriate cortex.

OCULAR DOMINANCE COLUMNS

Ocular dominance columns are seen in the striate cortex. They are seen as an alternating series of parallel stripes that represent a column of neurons in the striate cortex innervated by either the ipsilateral or contralateral eye. Ocular dominance columns extend in alternating bands through all cortical areas and layers, and are absent in only the cortical region representing the blind spot and the cortical area representing the monocular temporal crescent of the visual field. The mosaic appearance of these ocular dominance columns is demonstrated with autoradiography using 2-deoxyglucose and stimulation of only one eye. Simple cells are driven monocularly, while the complex and hypercomplex cells are stimulated from both eyes.

STIMULATION OF AREAS 17, 18, AND 19

Direct electrical stimulation of areas 17, 18, and 19 in conscious people produces visual sensations (Pollen, 1975) (Fig. 23.12).

These images are not elaborate hallucinations (as in complex partial temporal seizures) but rather are described as flickering lights, stars, lines, spots, and so forth. Often the images are described as colored or moving around. The images are usually localized to the contralateral field, at times to the contralateral eye. An illustrative case, 23.4, is presented next.

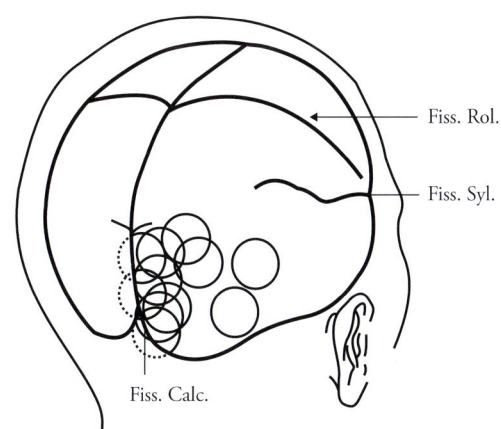

Figure 23.12 Focal discharge in occipital lobe. Location of the lesions at surgery in 11 patients who had focal seizures beginning with visual sensations. (From Penfield, W., and Kristiansen, K.: Epileptic Seizure Patterns, Springfield, IL, Charles C. Thomas, 1951, p. 47.)

At times, the patient cannot determine laterality. In addition, stimulation of areas 18 and 19 (and sometimes 17) produces conjugate deviation of the eyes to the contralateral field and, at times, vertical conjugate movements. Discharge of the occipital cortex may be followed by transient visual defects similar to the transient postictal hemiparesis that may follow focal seizures beginning in the motor cortex (see Aldrich et al., 1989). More complete discussion of seizures beginning in occipital cortex can be found in Salanova et al. (1993) and Williamson et al. (1992).

PHYSIOLOGY

The optic (geniculocalcarine) radiation terminates on the cells in the calcarine cortex, which respond like retinal ganglion cells. Their receptive fields consist of an excitatory region surrounded by an inhibitory region. Fields with the opposite pattern are also seen in higher mammals. These fields are excited by an annulus (donut) of light.

Hubel and Wiesel have described three types of higher order cells in the visual cortex:

1. Simple cell
2. Complex cell
3. Hypercomplex cell

Simple cell. This cell type responds best to a bar of light with a critical orientation and location. The receptive fields of several simple cells are shown in Figure 23.13. The excitatory field of each simple cell is bordered on one or both sides by an inhibitory field as shown for simple cell a. The small portion of the visual field outlined in Figure 23.13 drives thousands of simple cells, each with a discrete location and orientation. Each simple cell appears to receive input from a number of ganglion cells, which have their excitatory and inhibitory fields in a straight line.

Every simple cell can be driven by input from either eye, but they usually show a preference for one eye or the other. For example, a simple cell may be strongly excited by a bar seen with the right eye and only weakly stimulated by the same bar seen with the left eye. This differential sensitivity may form the basis of binocular vision.

Complex cell. A number of simple cells having the same orientation activate a complex cell. The complex cell has a definite orientational preference, but a much larger receptive field. An example of this is complex cell alpha in Figure 23.13. Any horizontal line of any length within the outlined visual field excites complex cell alpha. Lines with different orientations in the same visual field will drive other complex cells.

Hypercomplex cell. The final cell type is a hypercomplex cell. It has characteristics very similar to the complex cell, except it discriminates lines of different lengths. The bottom light bar in Figure 23.13 will inhibit hypercomplex cell 2. If its left-hand border were moved into the visual field, it would strongly excite hypercomplex cell 2. Once again, it is excited by lines of a critical orientation anywhere within a large portion of a visual field, but they must not be too long. Corners and angles also excite these cells.

About half a million optic-tract fibers enter each occipital lobe. It should be clear that there are many more cells processing this information, and indeed, the banks of the calcarine cortex contain many millions of cells.

The response to a large rectangle of light varies with the type of cell. Only if the edge falls on the center of a cell's receptive field will it be excited. Ganglion cells are very sensitive to position, contrast, and dynamics. Ganglion cells, in turn, excite simple cells that outline the edges of the rectangle of light. Simple cells have a larger receptive field than ganglion cells, are less sensitive to position, but are sensitive to the direction of the edge. Simple cells do not respond to continuous light or dark stimuli in their fields or to bars of light with an orientation other than their preferred orientation. Complex cells have much larger receptive fields than simple cells but are heavily influenced by the direction of the edge. Lastly, a hypercomplex cell must have a corner, an angle, or the end of the edge within its field to be activated.

Figure 23.13 Types of visual stimuli that excite each of the four types of cells found in the calcarine cortex. The square represents a box 2 inch by 2 inch, 5 feet away from the monkey's eye. The actual stimuli are bright bars of light on a dark field. (Data from Hubel and Wiesel. 1968. J. Physiol. 195:215.)

When a rectangle of light is flashed upon the retina, the cells described are initially activated but adapt fairly quickly and then are hardly stimulated. However, if the pattern flashes on and off, the cells are repeatedly stimulated. The cortex is also stimulated if the pattern moves a little on the retina. A different group of ganglion and simple cells will react, but because of their larger receptive fields, most of the complex and hypercomplex cells continue to be stimulated. The nervous system has overcome the problem of stationary images by continually producing rapid, saccadic eye movements that constantly shift the image on the retina. Indeed, when the image is stabilized by special contact lenses, it disappears.

In the process of data reduction, the visual system loses the ability to judge absolute light intensity for the most part.

Differences in intensity within a field can be determined easily but not the overall intensity of the field; photographers who estimate exposures usually waste a lot of film. Only the pupillary reflex system retains the ability to measure absolute intensity.

Different calcarine cells within a narrow column perpendicular to the surface repeat this processing for each of the primary-color receptors to give information on form, color, motion, and contrast. Lesions as small as 1 mm result in a detectable loss of all of these modalities in a small area of the visual field.

Zeki and associates (1992) demonstrated how the four identified perceptual pathways (*color, form with color, dynamic form,* and *motion*) relate to the specific visual areas.

The neurons of area V5 (area 19) are responsive to *motion* and are *directionally selective*, but they are nonselective for color. In contrast, the majority of cells in V4 (area 19) are selective for specific wavelengths of light (color sensitive), and many are selective for form (line orientation) as well.

The cells of the adjacent areas V3 and V3A (area 18) are selective for *form (line orientation) but are indifferent to wavelength (color)*. V1 (area 17) and V2 (area 18) distribute information to these specialized fields. V1 has column and intercolumnar areas. The columns stain heavily for the energy-related enzyme cytochrome oxidase. The neurons within the columns are wavelength sensitive, tend to concentrate in layers 2 and 3, and receive input primarily from the parvocellular layers of the LGN. Information concerning color is then projected either directly or through thin-column stripes in area V2 to V4.

By contrast, *form-selective neurons* are located in the intercolumnar areas in V1. Form related to color derives from the parvocellular-neuron layers of the LGN, which project first to the intercolumnar areas of V1 and then to V4.

The second *form system is independent of color* and depends on inputs from the magnocellular layers of the LGN to layer 4B of V1 projecting to V3. Extrastriate areas send projections back to the dorsal LGN and the pulvinar of the thalamus.

The *motion-sensitive system* consists of inputs from the magnocellular layers of LGN to layer 4B of area V1, which then projects to area V5, either directly or through area V2. Each of the prestriate areas, V5, V4, and V3, sends information back to V1 and V2, as well as to the parietal and temporal areas. This provides for more integrated visual perception.

To summarize, let us consider the example of a slowly moving colored ball. Visual information is fractionated into the modalities of form, color, and motion in the calcarine cortex. That information is reassembled elsewhere to give us a unitary view of the ball.

We are just beginning to understand where and how this parallel processing is done.

If the object is the letter A, then further processing takes place in the dominant (usually left) lateral occipital cortex (Brodmann's areas 18 and 19), the visual language association area. Letters seen in the left visual field and represented in the right calcarine cortex must project across the posterior corpus callosum before they can be recognized in the left visual association cortex.

Information needed to reconstruct complex forms flows through the inferior occipital/temporal region, primarily on the nondominant side. Located here are cells that can discriminate between human faces, for example. Similarly, sheep have cells that respond only to the image of a wolf (not of a sheep), and monkeys have cells that respond only to a human face but not to a snake or a banana. Many of these cells are sensitive to gaze, being strongly stimulated by direct eye contact but only weakly stimulated when the eyes are averted.

Extraoccipital higher level visual processing then occurs in area 7 of the parietal lobe, areas 23 and 21 of the temporal lobe, and area 8 of the frontal lobe (see Pandya and Kuypers, 1969).

OCCIPITAL LOBE AND EYE MOVEMENTS

Areas 18 and 19 send fibers to the tectal area of the superior colliculus. Such connections are necessary for visual fixation and accurate following of a moving object. The slow and smooth conjugate eye movements that occur when the eyes are following a moving visual stimulus (pursuit movements) should be distinguished from the independent phenomenon of voluntary (saccadic) conjugate eye movements.

Saccadic movements are rapid and shorter in latency and duration. They do not require a visual stimulus and do not depend on any connections to area 18. Rather, they are dependent on area 8, which sends fibers to the lateral gaze center of the pons.

This discussion of cortical control of eye movements is clearly simplified (see also Chapter 18). Both areas send some fibers to the superior colliculus, and ultimately, both the saccadic and pursuit movements involve the pontine gaze centers. In addition, vestibular and cerebellar influences also determine eye movement.

LESION IN AREA 17

Complete unilateral ablation of area 17 (V1) produces a complete homonymous hemianopia in the contralateral visual field (the same half field in each eye has no conscious visual perception). Such patients may have some crude visual function such as spatial localization, presumably because of optic-tract connections to the superior colliculus. A report by Barbur and colleagues (1993) suggests that conscious perception of the type of visual stimulus and its direction of motion can continue to occur after selective V1 lesions have been made, due to activation of V5 (possibly by subcortical input to V5). Vision is clearly abnormal in this blind field. V1 to V5 input is the dominant input in intact individuals.

With partial lesions, a partial defect results. For example, if only the superior bank of the calcarine fissure is involved, the visual field defect is limited to the inferior quadrant of the contralateral field. A bilateral infarct of either the upper or lower bank of the calcarine fissure may produce a homonymous altitudinal hemianopia in which apparent blindness exists in either the entire lower or upper field of vision (as appropriate).

With such calcarine-cortex lesions, the field defects are usually similar (congruous) in both eyes. By contrast, incomplete optic-tract lesions may produce somewhat unequal (noncongruous) homonymous field defects in both eyes.

Vascular lesions, in particular, occlusion of the posterior cerebral artery, often result in a homonymous hemianopia with macular sparing. That is, vision in the macular area of the involved field remains intact. Such preservation of macular vision probably occurs because the macular area has a large representation in the most posterior third of the calcarine cortex and is the area nearest the occipital pole. This area, then, is best situated to receive leptomeningeal anastomotic blood supply from the middle cerebral and anterior cerebral arteries. Occasionally, with occipital infarcts, there may be preservation of vision in a small peripheral unpaired portion of the visual field, called the temporal crescent (see Benton et al., 1980).

In vascular insufficiency or occlusion of the basilar artery, infarction may occur in the distribution of both posterior cerebral arteries, producing a bilateral homonymous hemianopia and a syndrome of "cortical blindness." Such patients lose all visual sensation, but pupillary constriction in response to light is preserved.

LESIONS OF EXTRASTRIATE AREAS 18 AND 19

Lesions in areas 18 and 19, often referred to as the visual association areas, produce deficits in visual association, including defects in visual recognition and reading. The problem is that in humans with a unilateral lesion, one is almost never dealing with disease limited to areas 18 and 19 (however, see later discussion of more recent studies).

Rather, one finds that adjacent portions of either the inferior temporal areas or of the inferior parietal lobule (the angular and supramarginal gyri) are involved or that the lesion extends into the deeper white matter of the lateral occipital area and involves association and callosal fibers. Such more extensive lesions will, of course, produce the deficits previously noted in the discussion of parietal function. A limited unilateral ablation might produce defects in visual following, as tested by evoking optikokinetic nystagmus (e.g., moving vertical black lines on a white background or looking at telephone poles from a moving train).

Bilateral lesions limited to areas 18 and 19 occur only rarely in humans. In humans such a lesion would deprive the speech areas of the dominant hemispheres of all visual information. The patient would presumably see objects but be unable to recognize them or to place visual sensations in the context of previous experience. The patient would be, moreover, unable to relate these visual stimuli to tactile and auditory stimuli. In monkeys, restricted lesions in the "visual" areas of the temporal and parietal lobes also interfere with pattern discrimination (Mishkin, 1972).

Horton and Hoyt (1991) have reported that unilateral lesions specific to the extrastriate V2/V3 cortex produce quadrantal visual field defects. As discussed by Zeki (1992), rare patients with restricted lesions in V4 present with achromatopia. The patients see the world only in shades of gray but perception of form, depth, and motion are intact. Rare patients with lesions limited to V5 have akinetopia.

Stationary objects are perceived, but if they are in motion, the objects appear to vanish. Plant and coworkers (1993) have reviewed such impaired motion perception. Selective deficits in form perception are even less frequent. Destruction of both form systems and therefore of V3 and V4 (areas 18 and 19) would be required and, as discussed earlier, such a lesion would also destroy V1 (area 17), resulting in total blindness.

The following case illustrates the effects of a space-occupying lesion in the occipital lobe. One should compare these findings to those reported earlier in Case 23.1, a lesion in the visual system anterior to the optic chiasm.

CASE HISTORY 23.3 (FIG. 23.14)

This 47-year-old, white, right-handed, real estate salesman developed a cough with some blood present in the sputum (hemoptysis), 1 month before admission. Five days before admission the patient developed a generalized headache, which was precipitated by coughing or straining and which awakened him or prevented him from sleeping. Two days before admission, the patient noted blurring in the left inferior quadrant of his field of vision. The day before admission, he noted complete loss of vision in this quadrant. On the day of admission, the headache increased, and the patient was unable to see anything in the left visual field. Past history was significant. The patient had multiple pulmonary infections, treated with antibiotics.

Neurologic Examination
Cranial nerves: Early papilledema was present. A noncongruous left homonymous hemianopia was present (Fig. 23.14A).

Clinical diagnosis: Mass lesion in right occipital lobe was suspected, as well as tumor and/or abscess.

Laboratory Data
Imaging demonstrated an enhanced lesion in the posterior and medial aspect of the right hemisphere (occipital and adjacent parietal lobes).

Electroencephalogram (EEG) was abnormal because of frequent focal 3 to 4 cps, slow waves in the right occipital area and, to a lesser degree, the right posterior parietal area.

Cerebrospinal fluid (CSF) pressure was elevated to 210 mm; 97 lymphocytes were present (upper limit is 5 to 7 lymphocytes). Protein was increased to 75 mg/dl. Glucose was 75 mg/dl (normal when compared to blood sugar of 95 mg/dl).

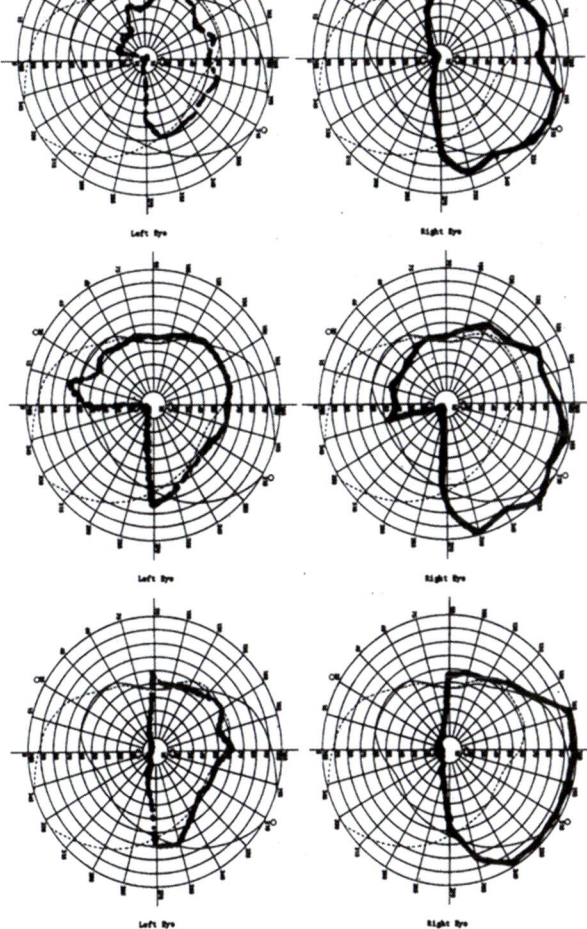

The case that follows is another example of the effects of a lesion in the occipital lobe with very different consequences than those seen in the previous case.

CASE HISTORY 23.4

This 18-year-old, left-handed, single white female restaurant employee had the onset of her seizures at age 14 when she had a sequence of five seizures in less than 12 hours. Each began with flashing lights, "like Christmas tree lights," all over her visual field, plus the sensation "that peoples' faces were moving." She then would have an apparent generalized convulsive seizure. Neurologic examination and computerized tomography (CT) scan were all reported as normal. An EEG reported occasional focal sharp and slow waves in the left hemisphere. The patient was treated with carbamazepine (Tegretol), 400 mg in the morning, and 230 mg at hour of sleep, with no additional.

She apparently had done quite well with no additional grand mal seizures. She had rare episodes of "fear attacks," which would last 23 to 25 minutes. The last attack had occurred 2 years ago, but as recently as 2 months ago, she had had one episode of flashing lights. A recent EEG was normal.

Neurologic examination: Normal.

Clinical diagnosis: Seizures of focal origin, left occipital.

Subsequent course: The patient did well for 3 years, then had a recurrence of a generalized convulsive seizure possibly related to omission of medication. Six weeks later, she reported two additional episodes characterized by flashing lights, then movement of the lights away from a center circle, then dizziness, then a sensation of unreality. She also had other episodes of feeling unreal accompanied by fear.

Figure 23.14 Case history 23.3. Brain abscess, right occipital area: perimetric examination of visual fields. (*A*) Initial examination demonstrated a somewhat asymmetrical (noncongruous) left homonymous hemianopia less in the left eye than the right. The fields are shown from the patient's point of view. (*B*) Sixteen days later, with antibiotic therapy, an improvement had occurred. A noncongruous quadrantanopia is now present. (*C*) Fields after an additional 24 days. A relatively complete homonymous hemianopia, present at the time of readmission, persisted following surgery as shown earlier.

Subsequent course: The patient was treated with antibiotics (cephalothin sodium, penicillin, and streptomycin), and visual fields, EEG, and spinal fluid findings improved. Within 3 weeks the field defect had resolved to a noncongruous left inferior quadrantanopia (Fig. 23.14B).

Ten days later the patient was readmitted to the hospital with a 3-day history of right eye pain, sweats, and chills. Neurologic examination now revealed a recurrence of blurred optic-disk margins, a left homonymous hemianopia, and a slight increase in deep tendon reflexes on the left. Imaging studies now revealed a large space-occupying lesion in the right parietal/occipital region, displacing the right lateral ventricle forward and downward. After 10 days treatment with antibiotics (penicillin and streptomycin), a craniotomy was performed by Dr. Bertram Selverstone, revealing an abscess and a large surrounding area of hard granulomatous cortex and white matter that were removed. The etiologic organism was subsequently found to be a microaerophilic streptococcus. Follow-up examination 6 months after surgery was normal, except for the left homonymous hemianopia (Fig. 23.14C).

Figure 23.15 Case 23.2. Focal visual seizures characterized by "flashing lights" and the sensation of movement of the visual field with secondary generalization beginning at age 14 due to metastatic (thyroid) tumor of the left occipital lobe. Magnetic resonance imaging (MRI), T2-weighted, nonenhanced, demonstrated a small tumor at the left occipital pole with surrounding edema. (See text for details.)

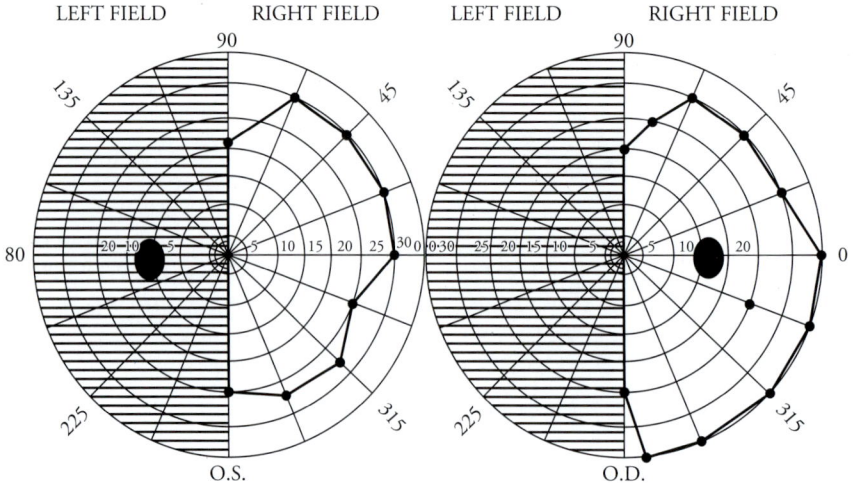

Figure 23.16 Occlusion of right posterior cerebral artery. Case 26.6 on CD-ROM. Tangent screen examination of visual fields, 3 months after the acute event. This 75-year-old woman had the acute onset of headache, bilateral blindness, confusion, vomiting, mild ataxia, and bilateral Babinski signs. All findings cleared except a residual left homonymous hemianopsia with macular sparing. O.S. = left eye; O.D. = right eye.

The neurologic examination demonstrated a minor right central facial weakness not present previously.

Laboratory Data

EEG: Normal.

MRI scan now revealed a small tumor at the left occipital pole (Fig. 23.15).

CT scan: This tumor appeared partially calcified but did show enhancement. Review of the CT scan obtained in Arizona at age 14 indicated similar findings. Angiograms suggested tumor vascularity of a type seen with meningiomas.

Dr. Bernard Stone removed a discrete encapsulated tumor that appeared to be a meningioma. Subsequent microscopic examination, however, indicated a rare type of indolent follicular adenocarcinoma of the thyroid, which sometimes spreads as a single lesion to the brain and remains quiescent for many years. In the postoperative period, a noncongruous right-inferior-field defect was present (partial quadrantanopia). The blood level of thyroid-stimulating hormone (TSH) was elevated. A thyroid nodule was found. A thyroidectomy was performed, and thyroid replacement medication was prescribed. No additional seizures were observed over the next

Figure 23.17 Computerized tomography (CT) scan of a total infarct, presumably embolic in the right posterior cerebral artery cortical territory (occipital and posterior temporal lobes) obtained 5 days after the acute onset of confusion and possible visual hallucinations in an 86-year-old, right-handed male. As confusion cleared, examination indicated a dense left homonymous hemianopia with no evidence of macular sparing. The patient would look to the right and to the midline but would not follow objects to the left beyond the midline. Contrast with Figure 23.18.

Figure 23.18 Computerized tomography (CT) scans of a partial infarct of the left posterior cerebral artery territory (inferior calcarine) with superior quadrantanopia probable basilar vertebral ischemia with artery-to-artery embolic infarction of the occipital (calcarine artery). This 71-year-old, right-handed male with a history of diabetes mellitus and hypertension had acute onset of vomiting, ataxia, minor confusion, and a persistent problem with peripheral vision in the right visual field, followed by episodes of vertical diplopia. Examination the following month demonstrated a homonymous visual field defect involving the right superior field, minor ataxia, and a right Babinski sign. Compare with Figure 23.17.

18 months. The patient subsequently developed a lumbar vertebral metastasis.

Vascular lesions of the calcarine cortex: Various types of visual field defects may occur, including a homonymous hemianopsia, with (Fig. 23.16) or without macular sparing, or a quadrantanopsia. The CT scan correlations are presented in Figures 23.17 and 23.18.

BIBLIOGRAPHY

Aldrich, M. S., Vanderzant, C. W., Alessi, A. C., et al. 1989. Ictal cortical blindness with permanent visual loss. Epilepsia 30:116–120.

Anand, I., and Geller, E. B. 2000. Visual auras. In H. O. Luders and S. Nocachtar (Eds.) Epileptic Seizures: Pathophysiology and Clinical Semiology, pp. 298–303. New York, NY: Churchill Livingstone.

Barbur, J. L., Watson, J. D. G., Frackowiak, R. S. J., and Zeki, S. 1993. Conscious visual perception without V 1. Brain 116:1293–1302.

Benton, S., Levy, I., and Swash, M. 1980. Vision in the temporal crescent in occipital lobe infarction. Brain 103:83–97.

Brindley, G. S., Donaldson, P. E. K., Falconer, M. A., and Rushton, D. N. 1972. The extent of the occipital cortex that when stimulated gives phosphenes fixed in the visual field. J. Physiol. (London) 225:57–58.

Brindley, G. S., and Lewin, W. S. 1968. The sensations produced by electrical stimulation of the visual cortex. J. Physiol. (London) 196:474–493.

Brookhart, J. M. (Ed.). 1984. The Nervous System. In Handbook of Physiology, Vol 3, Pt. 1, Vision. Bethesda, MD: American Physiologic Society.

Geller, E. B., Luders, H. O., Cheek, J. C., and Comair, Y. G. 2000. Electrical stimulation of the visual cortex. In H. O. Luders and S. Noachtar. (Eds.) Epileptic Seizures: Pathophysiology and Clinical Semiology, pp. 219–227. New York, NY: Churchill Livingstone.

Horton, J. C., and Hoyt, W. F. 1991. Quadrontic visual field defects: A hallmark of lesions in extrastriate V2/V3 cortex. Brain 114:1703–1718.

Hubel, D. H., and Wiesel, T. N. 1977. Ferrier Lecture: functional architecture of Macague monkey visual cortex. Proc. R. Soc. London Biol. 198:1–59.

Humphrey, N. K., and Weiskrantz, L. 1967. Vision in monkeys after removal of the striate cortex. Nature 215:595–597.

Kennard, C., and Rose, F. C. 1988. Physiological Aspects of Clinical Neuro-Ophthalmology. Chicago, IL: Year Book Medical Publishers.

Livingstone, M., and Hubel, D. 1988. Segregation of form, color, movement and depth: anatomy, physiology and perception. Science 240:740–749.

Lolley, R. N., and Lee, R. H. 1990. Cyclic GMP and photoreceptor function. FASEB J. 4:3001–3008.

Mishkin, M. 1972. Cortical visual areas and their interactions. In A. G. Karzmar and J. C. Eccles (Eds.) Brain and Human Behavior, pp. 187– 208 Berlin, Germany: Springer.

Moses, W. M. 1987. Adler's Physiology of the Eye: Clinical Application. St.Louis, MO: Mosby.

Pandya, D. N., and Kuypers, H. 1969. Cortico-cortical connections in the rhesus monkey brain. Brain Res. 13:13–16.

Penfield, W., and Jasper, H. 1954. Epilepsy and the Functional Anatomy of the Human Brain. Boston, MA: Little, Brown. (pp. 116–126, 168–173, 401–408)

Plant, G. T., Laxer, K. D., and Barbaro, N. M. 1993. Impaired visual motion perception in the contralateral hemifield following unilateral posterior cerebral lesions in humans. Brain 116:1303–1335.

Pollen, D. A. 1975. Some perceptual effects of electrical stimulation of the visual cortex in man. In T. N. Chase (Ed.) The Nervous System, Vol. 2. The Clinical Neurosciences, pp. 519–528. New York, NY: Raven Press.

Poppel, E., Held, R., and Frost, D. 1973. Residual visual function after brain wounds involving the central visual pathways in man. Nature 243:295–296.

Salanova, V., Andermann, F., and Rasmussen, F. B. 1993. Occipital lobe epilepsy. In E. Wyllie (Ed.) The Treatment of Epilepsy: Principles and Practices, pp. 533–540. Philadelphia, PA: Lea & Febiger.

Stryer, L. 1986. Cyclic GMP cascade in vision. Ann. Rev. Neurosci. 9: 87–119.

VanEssen, D. C. 1979. Visual areas of the mammalian cerebral cortex. Ann. Rev. Neurosci. 2:227–263.

Weiskrantz, L., Warrington, E. K., Sanders, M. D., and Marshall, J. 1974. Visual capacity in the hemianopic field following a restricted occipital ablation. Brain 97:709–728.

Williamson, P. D., Boon, P. A., Thadani, V. M., et al. 1992. Occipital lobe epilepsy. Clinical characteristics, seizure spread patterns and results of surgery. Ann. Neurol. 31:3–13.

Zeki, S. 1992. The visual image in mind and brain. Scientific American 267:69–76.

24.

SPEECH, LANGUAGE, CEREBRAL DOMINANCE, AND THE APHASIAS

In the preceding chapters, we have alluded to various areas in the dominant hemisphere concerned with speech and language. The reader may well have been confused by the introduction of such terms as *aphasia, apraxia, agnosia*, and *dyslexia*. It is well to warn the student beginning the study of language function that prior to the development of modern neuroimaging this was an area of much confusion, with much disagreement and multiple hypotheses. This discussion will be limited to the more practical problems of anatomical localization.

DYSARTHRIA

We should indicate at the onset that we are not concerned here with the problem of dysarthria. Dysarthria refers to a difficulty in articulation of speech from weakness, paralysis, or from mechanical difficulties. Dysarthria may have many causes at many levels of the peripheral or central nervous system, as indicated in Table 24.1.

CEREBRAL CORTEX AND COMPLEX DISTURBANCES OF VERBAL EXPRESSION

There are, however, more complex disturbances regarding verbal expression that occur at a time when the basic motor and sensory systems for articulation are intact. Similarly, there are complex disturbances in language function, as regards comprehension of written and spoken symbolic forms that occur at a time when the basic auditory and visual receptor apparatus is intact. We refer to these more complex acquired disturbances of language function as aphasias. In general, it is possible to relate these language disturbances to disease of the dominant cerebral hemisphere, involving the cerebral cortex or cortical association fiber systems. The term *dysphasia*, which is used in England interchangeably with *aphasia*, is used in the United States in reference to developmental language disorders as opposed to the acquired aphasias.

CEREBRAL DOMINANCE

It is perhaps appropriate at this point to consider the question of cerebral dominance. Most individuals are right-handed (93% of the adult population), and such individuals almost always (>99%) are left-hemisphere dominant for language functions. A minority of individuals (some on a hereditary basis) are left-hand dominant. Baseball appears to have collected a high percentage of these individuals as left-handed pitchers. Some left-handers are right-hemisphere dominant (50%), but a certain proportion is left-hemisphere dominant. It has been estimated that 96% of the adult population are left-hemisphere dominant for speech.

Hand, eye, and foot preference occurs in monkeys, and limb preference occurs in cats (Cole, 1957). One might inquire as to why the majority of humans are right-handed. Although hand preference does not become apparent until 1 year of age, the studies of Yakovlev and Rakic (1966) would suggest that even before this age, there is an underlying anatomical basis for the dominance of the right hand. In the study of the medullae and spinal cords of a large number of human fetuses and neonates, the fibers of the left pyramid were found to cross to the right side in the medullary pyramidal decussation at a higher level in the decussation than fibers of the right pyramid. Moreover, more fibers of the left pyramid crossed to the right side than vice versa. Although the majority of pyramidal fibers decussated, a minority of fibers remained uncrossed. It was more common for fibers from the left pyramid to decussate completely to the right side of the lower medulla (and eventually spinal cord). The minority of fibers that remained uncrossed was more often those descending from the right pyramid into the right side of the lower medulla. The end result, in the cervical region at least, was for the right side of the spinal cord and presumably the anterior horn cells of the right side of the cervical cord to receive the greater corticospinal innervation. There is then an anatomical basis for the preference or dominance of the right hand. Since the majority of fibers supplying the right cervical area have originated in the left hemisphere, on this basis alone one could refer to the dominance of the left hemisphere. Study of the adult brain results in similar conclusions (Kertesz and Geschwind, 1971).

The studies of Geschwind and Levitsky (1968) established that an actual anatomical asymmetry was present in the adult brain between the two hemispheres in an area significant for language function. That area of the auditory association cortex, posterior to Heschl's gyrus on the superior-lateral surface of the temporal lobe (areas 22 and 42) bordering the sylvian fissure and including the speech reception area of Wernicke, was found to be larger in the left hemisphere. Similar differences have been found in the brain of the fetus and newborn infant (Wada et al., 1975). The studies of LeMay and her associates (1972, 1978, and 1978), Galaburda et al. (1978), and Chui and Damasio (1980) elaborated on the asymmetries of the sylvian fissure and occipital lobe demonstrated on arteriography and

Table 24.1 CAUSES OF DYSARTHRIA

LOCATION OF PATHOLOGY	EXAMPLES
Local diseases of the larynx, tongue, or lips	Laryngeal carcinoma
Disease of the muscles affecting the tongue, the lips, or pharynx	Oculopharyngeal dystrophy
Diseases affecting the neuromuscular junction in the muscles of the tongue, lips, and pharynx	Myasthenia gravis, botulinum toxin
Diseases affecting the peripheral nerve supply of the tongue, lips, or pharynx	A) Hypoglossal nerve (carotid endarterectomy) B) Recurrent laryngeal nerve (thyroid surgery) C) Metastatic or regional cancer involving the lymphatics in the neck D) Diphtheritic neuropathy
Diseases of the brain stem motor nuclei, particularly nucleus ambiguus	Lateral medullary infarcts, amyotrophic lateral sclerosis (so-called progressive bulbar palsy), or bulbar poliomyelitis
Bilateral damage to the corticobulbar fibers (cerebral cortex, internal capsule, or upper brain stem)	Bilateral infarcts, multiple sclerosis producing a pseudobulbar palsy

computerized tomography (CT) scan during life. Similar asymmetries were demonstrated in the brains of the great apes, for example, chimpanzee, but not in the Rhesus monkey (LeMay and Geschwind, 1978). LeMay and Culebras (1972) studied the endocranial casts of human fossil skulls in which imprints of the major fissure could be noted and demonstrated similar differences in Neanderthal man. Damasio and Geschwind (1984) provide additional review of this topic.

Development Aspects

It is clear that from a functional standpoint a considerable degree of flexibility exists in the child as regards dominance for language function. Thus, in a child under the age of 5 years, destruction of the speech areas of the dominant left hemisphere during prenatal or postnatal life produces only a minor long-term language disturbance (Vargha-Khadem at al., 1985). If the damage to the speech areas in the dominant hemisphere occurs between the ages of 5 and 12 years, a more severe aphasia occurs; however, some limited recovery of language may occur within a year. These cases suggest an equipotentiality of the two hemispheres for language function during the early years of development. In these cases under the age of 5 years the right hemisphere must assume a dominant role in mediating those learned associations important in language and in the use of symbols either through process compensation and/or reorganization. If total destruction of the speech area of the dominant hemisphere occurs in adult life, only a minor recovery of language functions will occur. Patients with left hemisphere damage sustained under the age of 5 develop a strong left-hand preference. Patients with damage sustained after the age of 5 have only weak left-hand preferences or are ambidextrous. Additional discussion of the role of genetics in dominance and of the effects of early damage to the left hemisphere can be found in Lacaze et al. (2003).

Normal Development of Speech in the Child

There is considerable variability. Milestones may be outlined as follows: At 9–12 months, the child babbles, for example, "mama, dada." At 12 months, the child uses single words and echoes sounds. At 15 months, the child uses several words. At 18 months, the child has a vocabulary of six words and possible hand dominance. At 24 months, the child puts two to three words together into a sentence.

APHASIA

When approaching the patient with aphasia, it is good to keep in mind that textbook discussions of this problem are often artificial, in the sense that such discussions tend to deal with relatively isolated pure types of language disturbance, which have relatively specific localization. The actual patient with aphasia more often presents a mixed disturbance with damage to several areas; some have damage to all major areas in a global aphasia. This is not unexpected when one realizes that all of the major speech areas of the dominant hemisphere are within the cortical vascular territory of the middle cerebral artery. Other areas involved in related disorders are supplied by the anterior cerebral artery (the superior speech area) or by the posterior cerebral artery (those areas involved in pure dyslexia and agnosias). Willmes and Poeck (1993) and Kirshner (2000) provide additional reviews.

Three cortical areas of the dominant hemisphere are of major importance in language disturbances (Fig. 24.1):

1. *Broca's motor aphasia or expressive speech center:* The opercular and triangular portions of the inferior frontal convolution (areas 44 and 45).

2. *Wernicke's receptive aphasia area:* The auditory association area on the superior and lateral surface of the posterior portion of the superior temporal gyrus (area 22 and adjacent parts of area 42).

3. *Inferior parietal lobule:* The angular and supramarginal gyri (areas 39 and 40), at times associated with Gerstmann's syndrome of dysgraphia, dyscalculia, left-right confusion, and finger agnosia.

Other cortical areas: the *supplementary motor cortex (superior speech area)* may also play a role in language function. Stimulation studies by Luders et al. (1988) have also identified a *basal temporal speech area.*

In addition to these cortical areas, the *association fiber systems* relating these areas to each other and to other cortical areas are of considerable importance for certain types of language disturbance, as we will indicate later.

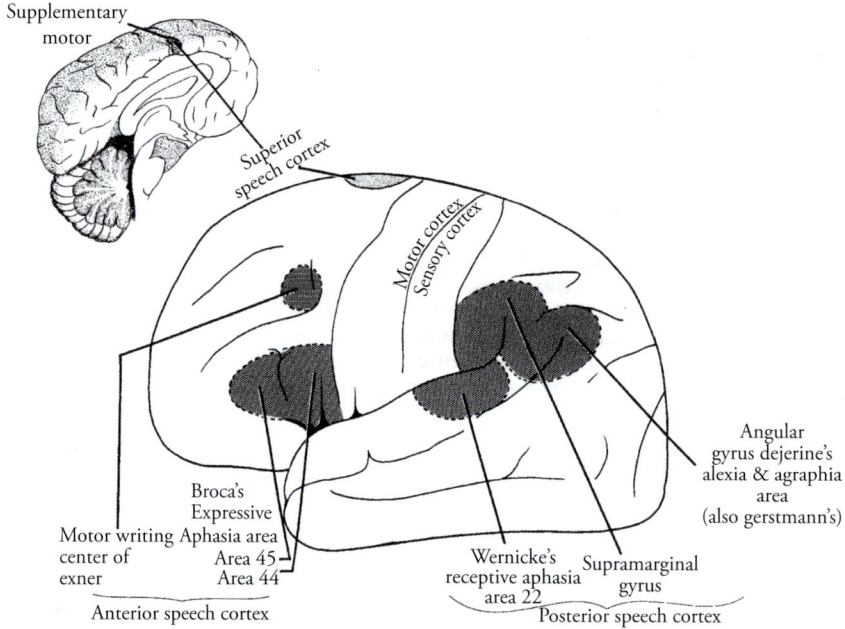

Figure 24.1 Speech areas of the dominant hemisphere; summary diagram combining the data of pathological lesions and stimulation studies. Precise sharp borders are not implied. The designations of Penfield and Roberts (1959), the terms "anterior speech area," "posterior speech area," and "superior speech cortex," are used.

From a practical localization standpoint we can, in a general sense, speak of patients as presenting an anterior or posterior type of aphasia (anterior or posterior to the central sulcus) (Fig. 24.1).

1. The anterior type of aphasia relates to Broca's motor aphasia area. The patient's speech may be generally described as nonfluent with little spontaneous verbalization.
2. The patients with the posterior types of aphasia are fluent and do speak spontaneously. The lesions in such cases involve Wernicke's area in the posterior portion of the superior temporal gyrus or the inferior parietal lobule. However, since the posterior areas are relatively close to one another, it is not unusual for a single disease process to involve both areas. The fluent aphasias include (a) Wernicke's receptive aphasia, (b) disconnection syndromes, (c) Gerstmann's syndrome, (d) dyslexia plus, (e) dyslexia without agraphia, and (f) the agnosias.

Now let us consider in greater detail language functions and the postulated anatomical correlations of these various language centers. In these correlations, it is important to make a distinction between acute and chronic effects.

It is necessary first to review those components of language function that are evaluated in the neurological examination (adapted from Benson, 1985).

1. Conversational speech:
   a. Amount: Nonfluent versus fluent. Mute refers to total absence.
   b. Articulation, rhythm, and melody: Defective in nonfluent, normal in fluent. However, note that the nonverbal aspects of language prosody (the affective, intonation, and melodic aspects of speech) and gesture often involve the right hemisphere (refer to Ross, 1993).
   c. Content:

1. Grammar (referred to as syntax): Nonfluent speech is often telegraphic—lacking the words or word parts and endings needed to express grammatical relations; whereas patients with fluent aphasia can produce long sentences or phrases with a normal grammatical structure.
2. Meaning and substance—(referred to as semantics): Patients with fluent aphasia often demonstrate a number of abnormalities in terms of the choice of words.
   a. The precise word may be replaced by a nonspecific word or phrase.
   b. The correct word or phrase answer may be replaced by a phrase that describes the use of an object (circumlocution). Because such patients are fluent, casual examination may fail to detect such glib features.
   c. The correct word may be replaced by an inappropriate word or phrase substitution (verbal or semantic paraphasias), for example, "clocks for wristwatch."
   d. The correct word may contain replacement sounds or syllables, which are incorrect (literal or phonemic paraphasias), for example, "note for nose."
   e. The correct word may be replaced by a totally new word (neologism), for example, "Zingbam."

2. Repetition: the ability to repeat words or phrases

   a. This may be absent in a mute individual, in a severe nonfluent patient, or in a patient with a severe type of Wernicke's aphasia.

   b. This may be impaired as an isolated symptom (so-called conduction aphasia).

   c. This may be preserved in an individual with otherwise intact language or preserved in isolation (so-called sylvian isolation syndrome).

3. Comprehension of spoken language is tested by providing spoken or written commands that do not require a verbal response, such as "hold up your left hand, close your eyes, and stick out your tongue."

4. Word finding and selection: Naming of objects or selection of the proper name of an object. Defect is defined as anomia or nominal aphasia.

5. Reading: Defect is defined as alexia or dyslexia.

6. Writing: Defect is defined as agraphia or dysgraphia.

7. Related functions:

   a. Calculations: Defect defined as acalculia or dyscalculia.

   b. Perception in visual, auditory, or tactile sphere: Defects in recognition when the sensory modality and naming are otherwise intact are defined as agnosia. The main sensory modality involved is vision and this merges with optic aphasia, dyslexia, and nominal aphasia. The inability to recognize faces (prosopagnosia) and color agnosia are special examples (De Renzi, 2000).

   c. Apraxias: Defects in use of objects when motor and sensory functions are otherwise intact.

STIMULATION OF THE SPEECH AREAS

In general, as demonstrated in Figure 24.2, stimulation of the dominant hemisphere—speech areas—produces arrest of speech ("aphasic arrest" in the terminology of Penfield and Rasmussen). Paroxysmal arrest of speech often occurs as one aspect of seizures involving the dominant hemisphere. More selective aspects of aphasia such as ictal alexia or agraphia or anomia without speech arrest have been reported in rare patients (Ardila and Lopez, 1988; Warner, 1988) with the appropriate localization as noted later. Luders et al. (1988) have recently reviewed this subject with the following conclusions:

1. Speech arrest or interference was elicited in five areas:

   a. Primary motor cortex when stimulating the representation of muscles involved in speech of the dominant or nondominant hemisphere

   b. Negative motor areas (suppressor areas), that is, the supplementary motor areas and inferior frontal gyrus of the dominant hemisphere

   c. Broca's area—dominant hemisphere only (note that Broca's area overlaps the motor suppressor area of the inferior frontal gyrus)

   d. Wernicke's area—dominant hemisphere only

   e. Basal temporal language area—dominant hemisphere only. Dinner and Luders concluded that any effect of stimulating the superior speech area was related to inhibition of motor activity. This area did not appear to have speech function per se. (Ablation-type studies do suggest possible speech functions.)

2. In stimulation of Broca's, Wernicke's, and the basal temporal areas at high stimulus intensities, complete speech arrest occurred with a global receptive and expressive aphasia; however, the patient could still perform nonverbal tasks. At lower intensities of stimulation, the effects were incomplete: speech was slow, and simple but not complex tasks could be performed (both motor sequences and calculations). Simple but not complex material could be repeated. A severe naming defect (anomia) still occurred.

In children some seizures may be associated with long-lasting expressive aphasia (Landau-Kleffner syndrome) (Sawhney et al., 1988).

ABLATION OF SPEECH AREAS: ANATOMICAL CORRELATION OF SPECIFIC SYNDROMES

The Nonfluent Aphasias Involving Broca's Area

In 1861, Broca described patients with nonfluent aphasia: little spontaneous speech with poor repetition but with considerable preservation of auditory comprehension. The spontaneous speech that remained was agrammatic and telegraphic. Based on his examination of the lateral surface of the cerebral hemispheres at autopsy, he emphasized the damage to the third left frontal gyrus, the frontal operculum of the inferior frontal gyrus. Although considerable controversy was generated at the time, Broca's name has continued to be

Figure 24.2 Arrest of speech on stimulation of dominant hemisphere at surgery. (From Penfield, W., and Rasmussen, T.: The Cerebral Cortex of Man. New York, The Macmillan Company, 1955, p. 107.)

associated both with the disorder, nonfluent aphasia, and with the postulated anatomical area. As discussed by Damasio and Geschwind (1984), subsequent CT scans of the museum specimen of Broca's case indicated much more extensive damage than that described by Broca. Damasio (1992), in an extensive recent review of aphasia, discusses in detail the differences between true chronic Broca's aphasia and the more limited and transient effects of lesions restricted to Broca's area alone.

Broca's area is essentially a continuation of premotor cortex and may be considered a specialized motor association area with regard to the tongue, lips, pharynx, and larynx. This area is adjacent to the motor cortex representation of the face, lips, tongue, and pharyngeal muscles. It is not, therefore, unusual for these patients to have also a supranuclear type weakness of the right side of the face and a right hemiparesis. This by itself is not sufficient to explain the problems in speech that these patients manifest, since lesions involving the face area of the nondominant motor cortex do not produce the speech disturbance. Moreover, tongue and pharynx receive a bilateral corticobulbar supply, so that a unilateral cortical lesion involving the motor cortex in this area is not a sufficient explanation. These patients appear to have lost the motor memories for the sequencing of skilled coordinated movements of tongue, lips, and pharynx that are required for the vocalization of understandable single words, phrases, and sentences. They are usually able to vocalize sounds. At times, they may be able to vocalize single words into a proper grammatical sequence for telegraphic sentences.

In the patient with a relatively pure form of Broca's motor aphasia, the capacity to formulate language and to select words in a mental sense is intact. The student might logically inquire as to whether the patient has also lost his motor memories or motor associations for making a nonverbal sequence of movements of the tongue and lips. Frequently, this is the case, as will be demonstrated in the illustrative case history. We may refer to this defect in skilled sequential motor function (at a time when motor, sensory, and cerebellar function are intact, and when the patient is alert and understands what movements are to be performed) as a motor apraxia. There are several types of apraxia with different localization. In general, we may relate the more purely motor forms of apraxia to the motor association areas of the premotor cortex. One could then refer to patients with Broca's motor aphasia as patients with a motor apraxia of speech.

The following presents an example of this type of aphasia. An embolus to the superior division of the left middle cerebral artery produced marked weakness of the face, tongue, and distal right upper extremity and a severe selective nonfluent aphasia. The hand weakness rapidly disappeared; the right central facial weakness, an apraxia of tongue movements, and some expressive difficulties persisted. Most likely, the embolus fragmented and passed into the cortical branches supplying Broca's area.

CASE HISTORY 24.1

This 55-year-old, right-handed white housewife while working in her garden at 10:00 a.m. on the day of admission suddenly developed a weakness of the right side of face and the right arm and was unable to speak. Nine years previously the patient had been hospitalized with a 3-year history of progressive congestive heart failure secondary to rheumatic heart disease (mitral stenosis with atrial fibrillation). An open cardiotomy was performed with a mitral valvuloplasty (the valve opening was enlarged) and removal of a thrombus found in the left atrial appendage. Postoperatively, the patient was given an anticoagulant, bishydroxycoumarin (Dicumarol), to prevent additional emboli since atrial fibrillation continued until the present admission. She had done well in the interim. However, prothrombin at the time of admission was close to normal; that is, the patient was not in a therapeutic range for anticoagulation.

General physical examination: Blood pressure was moderately elevated to 170/80. Pulse was 110 and irregular (atrial fibrillation). Examination of the heart revealed the findings of mitral stenosis: a loud first sound, a diastolic rumble, and an opening snap at the apex as well as the atrial fibrillation.

Neurological Examination

Mental status and language function: She had no spontaneous speech, could not use speech to answer questions, and could not repeat words. She was able to indicate answers to questions by nodding (yes) or shaking her head (no), if questions were presented in a multiple-choice format. In this manner it was possible to determine that she was grossly oriented for time, place, and person. She was able to carry out spoken commands and simple written commands, such as "Hold up your hand, close your eyes." However, she had significant difficulty in performing voluntary tongue moments (such as "wiggle your tongue"; "stick out your tongue") on command.

Cranial nerves: She tended to neglect stimuli in the right visual field and was unable to look to the right on command, although the head and eyes were not grossly deviated to the left at rest. A marked right supranuclear (central) type facial weakness was present. The patient had difficulty in tongue protrusion and was unable to wiggle the tongue. When the tongue was protruded, it deviated to the right.

Motor system: There was a marked weakness without spasticity in the right upper extremity, most prominent distally, and a minor degree of weakness involving the right lower extremity.

Reflexes: Deep tendon stretch reflexes were increased on the right in the arm and leg. Plantar responses were both extensor, more prominent on the right.

Sensory system: Intact within limits of testing.

Clinical diagnosis: Broca's anterior aphasia embolus from heart to left middle cerebral artery, superior division.

Laboratory data: *Electroencephalogram (EEG)* was normal (48 hours after admission). *Electrocardiogram* revealed atrial fibrillation. *Cerebrospinal fluid* was normal.

Subsequent course: Within 24 hours a significant return of strength in the right hand had occurred; independent finger movements could be made. Within 48 hours after admission the patient was able to repeat single words but still had almost no spontaneous speech. She appeared aware of her speech disability and would manifest some frustration. She was able to carry out two- or three-stage commands, although tongue movements and perseveration remained a problem. Within 6 days of admission, the patient used words, phrases, and occasional short sentences spontaneously and was better able to repeat short sentences. At this time strength in the right arm had returned to normal, but a right central facial weakness was still present. Two weeks after admission, she still had expressive disabilities

Figure 24.3 Anterior aphasia: embolic infarct (secondary to rheumatic atrial fibrillation). Case 24.2 (refer to text). Magnetic resonance imaging (MRI): (*A*) T1-weighted, coronal section. (*B*) T2-weighted, horizontal section.

consisting of word-finding and apraxic components in tongue placement and alternating tongue movements. Although complete sentences were used, sentence formulation in spontaneous speech was slow and labored with word-finding difficulties. Repetition was better performed. In reading sentences aloud, substitutions or word omissions were made. The patient did well in naming common pictures and in matching printed words to spoken words or printed words to pictures. She could write from dictation and would often respond preferentially in writing when difficulty in speaking was encountered. A right central facial weakness was still present.

With the passage of time, this type of patient would continue to show some degree of improvement (Mohr, 1973). Improvement could continue to occur over a 2-year period. Although lesions of Broca's area may produce the acute onset of a nonfluent aphasia, rapid amelioration of the deficit occurs even when the acute lesion involves underlying white matter, as well as the superficial cortex.

In order to produce a more persistent severe nonfluent aphasia with good comprehension but poor repetition, more extensive lesions are required. In the CT scan correlation study of Naesar (1983), this larger lesion extended from Broca's area to the anterior parietal lobe, usually including the deep structures such as caudate, putamen, and/or internal capsule. Ludlow et al. (1986) compared persistent versus nonpersistent nonfluent aphasia 15 years after penetrating head injuries of the left hemisphere in the Vietnam War. Both groups had nonfluent aphasia still present at 6 months after injury with equal involvement of Broca's area. The group that failed to recover at 15 years had a more extensive left hemisphere lesion with posterior extension of the CT scan lesion into Wernicke's area and some involvement of the underlying white matter and basal ganglia. The additional study of Naeser et al. (1989) compared severe nonfluency to less severe Broca's aphasia—6 months to 9 years following an infarct of the left cerebral hemisphere. Those patients with severe nonfluency had more extensive lesions of the subcortical white matter involving (a) the subcallosal fasciculus deep to Broca's area containing projections from the cingulate and supplementary motor areas to the caudate nucleus plus (b) the periventricular white matter near the body of the left ventricle deep to the lower motor sensory cortical area for the mouth. The magnetic resonance imaging (MRI) of a case (24.2) with chronic residuals of a more persistent nonfluent aphasia is presented in Figure 24.3.

CASE HISTORY 24.2

On May 30, 1985, at midday, this 37-year-old, right-handed woman with a past history of rheumatic fever, rheumatic heart disease, and "an irregular pulse" (atrial fibrillation) had the sudden onset of loss of speech, central weakness of right face, an inability to protrude the tongue and a right hemiparesis. Although hemiparesis and face and tongue problems disappeared within a week, recovery of speech was slower and limited. At 1 week, she could produce some two-syllable words.

Neurological Examination at 17 Months

Language function: Spontaneous speech was slow and relatively scanty. She could name objects slowly without difficulty, could do some simple repetitions, and could write from dictation. She could carry out two- and three-stage commands. She could read slowly aloud but had little comprehension of what she read.

Reflexes: A residual right Babinski sign and right-sided hyperreflexia were present.

Clinical diagnosis: Anterior aphasia: embolic infarct of superior division of middle cerebral artery.

Laboratory data: Although initial CT scans in May 1985 had been reported as negative, the MRIs in November 1986 and June 1990 demonstrated the infarct, which included Broca's area, as well as adjacent frontal areas with predominant involvement of frontal operculum (inferior frontal gyrus) and adjacent middle frontal gyrus. In addition, a minor independent infarct was present in right occipital area (presumably embolic to the calcarine artery).

Subsequent course: Similar findings were present at 5 years (June 1990).

A brain section from a patient (Case 24.3) with a persistent nonfluent aphasia (is presented in Figure 24.4).

CASE HISTORY 24.3

This 69-year-old, right-handed male expired in 1965. In 1961 and 1963, the patient had experienced transient episodes of right hemiparesis and aphasia, both followed by complete recovery. In 1964, a more persistent right hemiparesis and aphasia had developed.

Figure 24.4 Persistent anterior aphasia after left carotid occlusion with old infarction, predominantly of left middle cerebral territory with lesser involvement of anterior cerebral territory. Case 24.3 (refer to text). (Courtesy of Dr. John Hills and Dr. Jose Segarra.)

General physical examination: No left carotid pulsation was present.

Neurologic Examination (1965)

Language functions: Speech was nonfluent with only a small verbal output. A significant nominal aphasia with paraphasias was present. Reading was limited. Comprehension of spoken language was good. A marked apraxia was present for movements of tongue, lips, and hands.

Motor system: Right hemiparesis with associated reflex findings.

Pathologic diagnosis: Left carotid occlusion with old infarction, predominantly of left middle cerebral territory with lesser involvement of anterior cerebral territory. Note that minor cortical infarcts are also present involving cortex of right hemisphere. (Courtesy of Dr. John Hills and Dr. Jose Segarra.)

THE FLUENT APHASIAS

Wernicke's aphasia and Wernicke's area: In 1874, Wernicke described a type of aphasia that differed significantly from the nonfluent aphasia described by Broca and that had a more posterior localization. This type of patient has fluent spontaneous speech with poor comprehension and poor repetition. The patient has difficulty in understanding symbolic sounds, that is, words that have been heard, and is unable to carry out verbal commands. The patient is unable to use those same auditory associations in the formulation of speech. Moreover, the patient is essentially unable to monitor his own spoken words as he talks, since he lacks the ability to interpret and to compare the sounds, which he himself is producing, to previous auditory associations. The end result is a patient who is fluent but who uses words combined into sentences that lack any meaning to the listeners. Word substitution (paraphasia) is frequent. In severe cases, not only are phrases and words combined into meaningless sentences but also the patient combines syllables into words that have no meaning (jargon aphasia). The patient, however, is usually unaware of his errors. The patient usually fails to show the "rationale" frustration, which is characteristic of patients who have Broca's motor aphasia and who are aware of their errors. At times, the patient shows some awareness that his verbal responses are failing to deal with the environment. At times, the problems in communication are so severe that the patient becomes agitated and is mistaken for psychotic, as demonstrated in the case history that follows. The anatomical localization for Wernicke's aphasia based on early autopsy studies has been confirmed by subsequent CT scan and MRI studies: the posterior temporal parietal area. In the studies of Naeser (1983) the essential lesions involved Brodmann's area 22 (Wernicke area) of the posterior-superior temporal gyrus and the adjacent supramarginal gyrus of the inferior parietal area.

In general, the responsible lesion is usually an infarct within the territory of the inferior division of the left middle cerebral artery, often embolic. There is usually very little evidence of a hemiparesis. In contrast, Broca's aphasia usually reflects infarction within the territory of the superior division of the left middle cerebral artery and a right facial weakness and right hemiparesis are often present. (See Chapter 26 for additional discussion of vascular anatomy.)

Case 24.4 provides an example of a patient with a Wernicke's type aphasia.

CASE HISTORY 24.4

This 40-year-old, right-handed white male had experienced a series of myocardial infarctions beginning 10 months prior to consultation. Angiographic studies indicated occlusion of the right coronary artery and the left anterior descending coronary artery with stenosis of the circumflex artery, and a coronary artery bypass procedure was performed using extracorporeal circulation. The anesthetist noted that the patient was nonreactive 15 minutes after the last administration of halothane anesthesia. When the patient did wake up, he was quite agitated, combative, and in retrospect had transient difficulty using the right arm. Despite medications throughout the postoperative period, he continued to behave in a disoriented and combative manner. Transfer to the psychiatry service was actively planned, but a neurology consultation was obtained.

Neurological Examination

Mental status: He was alert but agitated. Speech was fluent and usually grammatical. He made use of many paraphasias and neologisms (nonsense words). He often appeared unaware of his errors. He was unable to name single objects such as pencil, cup, and spoon, though he could recognize and demonstrate their use. He could read occasional individual words, for example, cat, house. He could not comprehend or carry out either spoken or written commands. His attempts at spontaneous writing produced only a few letters. He was unable to write words or phrases from dictation. He did significantly better when asked to copy a printed sentence or phrase. Repetition of spoken phrases or sentences was poor. Calculations of even a simple nature were poorly performed. *Reflexes:* A minor increase in deep tendon stretch reflexes was present on the right side. The plantar response on the right was equivocal. The left was flexor.

Clinical diagnosis: Wernicke's type of fluent aphasia, probably secondary to an embolus to the inferior division of the middle cerebral artery.

Pure word deafness: We have indicated previously, in discussing the auditory cortex, that this is a related relatively rare problem (Auerbach et al., 1982; Coslett et al., 1984). In cases of pure word deafness, the hypothetical center of auditory word association (Wernicke's area) appears to be intact but auditory information is unable to reach this center from the auditory projection cortex (of either hemisphere); in a sense disconnection has occurred. The auditory word association center is intact. Previous auditory associations may be used in the formulation of the patient's own speech. Input of visual information to the center may also be intact. It should be evident that the distinctions that have been made here between Wernicke's receptive aphasia and word deafness are to some extent artificial. In general, lesions in this area do not respect such artificial distinctions and often destroy not only the center for auditory word associations but also the inputs into this area from the auditory projection areas.

Both Wernicke's receptive aphasia and word deafness are often grouped under the general term *auditory agnosia*.

Conduction or repetition type fluent aphasia: This type of aphasia is characterized by a relatively fluent spontaneous speech but with marked deficits in repetition. Literal paraphasias are present and word-finding problems may be present. The patient is usually aware of the errors made. In contrast to the Wernicke's type of aphasia, auditory comprehension is usually relatively well preserved. The anatomical location of the lesion is somewhat variable (Benson et al., 1973; Damasio and Damasio, 1980; Damasio and Geschwind, 1984; Demasio, 1992; Geschwind, 1965). The lesion essentially serves to disconnect Wernicke's area from Broca's area (the posterior from the anterior speech areas). The essential fiber system is the arcuate fasciculus (Fig. 24.5). This fiber system arches around the posterior end of the sylvian fissure to join the superior longitudinal fasciculus. In the study of Naeser (1983) this system was involved deep to the supramarginal gyrus and/or deep to Wernicke's area. In other cases the white matter deep to insular cortex has been involved (Damasio and Geschwind, 1984). In the resultant conduction aphasia, the patient understands spoken commands and is usually able to carry out complex instructions that do not require a repetition of language. Although able to speak spontaneously with little or no evidence of a Broca's aphasia, the patient is unable to repeat test phrases and sentences, for example, "The rain in Spain falls mainly on the plain" or "no ifs, ands, or buts" and is unable to write from dictation. Often, the syndrome is seen in a less than pure form, as in the case history that accompanies Figure 24.6. This is not surprising since the involved territory is that of the middle cerebral artery, predominantly the inferior division. The essential lesion must spare Broca's and Wernicke's area to a considerable degree but significantly damage the interconnection of these areas. If there is significant damage to either Wernicke's or Broca's areas, repetition will be defective on either the input or output side of the loop. A case demonstrating conduction aphasia will be presented as part of the next section.

Fluent aphasias associated with lesions of the dominant inferior parietal areas: angular and supramarginal gyri: Geschwind (1965) indicated the critical location of the inferior parietal lobule in humans situated between the visual, auditory, and tactile association areas. As such, it may act as a higher association area between these adjacent sensory association areas. In earlier chapters we have already identified this area as the posterior parietal, multimodal sensory association area. Geschwind has suggested that correlated with the development of this area in the human (the angular and supramarginal gyri cannot be recognized as such in the monkey and are present only in rudimentary form in the higher apes), there has developed the capacity for cross modality sensory-sensory associations without reference to the limbic system. He contrasts this situation with that in subhuman forms, where the only readily established sensory-sensory associations are those between a nonlimbic (visual, tactile, or auditory) stimulus and a limbic stimulus: those stimuli related to primary motivations such as hunger, thirst, and sex. (Such considerations, of course, do not rule out the establishment of limbic-nonlimbic stimuli associations in humans, particularly during infancy and childhood.) These theoretical concepts would suggest the underlying basis for human language

Figure 24.5 The arcuate fasciculus: dissection of the long fiber system, the superior longitudinal fasciculus demonstrating the arcuate fasciculus, passing beneath the cortex of inferior parietal, and posterior temporal areas. A small bundle of U fibers are also demonstrated incidentally at posterior, inferior margin of the temporal lobe interconnecting adjacent gyri.

Figure 24.6 Posterior aphasia, infarction left posterior temporal and parietal areas, inferior division, left middle cerebral (probably embolic following left carotid occlusion) computerized tomography (CT) scan. Case 24.6 (refer to text).

functions. It is not surprising then that those aspects of language function that are most dependent on association between auditory and visual stimuli and auditory-visual-tactile stimuli (reading and writing) are most disturbed by lesions of angular and supramarginal gyri. In the words of Geschwind, "It is a region which turns written language into spoken language and vice versa."

The component parts of the resultant syndrome are not constant. The patient will have a varying degree of difficulty in writing (dysgraphia), particularly as regards spontaneous writing. Often the ability to copy letters, words, and sentences will be relatively well preserved. In contrast, the patient will usually have difficulty writing from dictation, although at times, this function may be less affected than spontaneous writing. There is often an associated deficit in reading (dyslexia), although this is not invariable.

Significant defects in spelling and in calculations (dyscalculia) may be present. There may be an associated left-right confusion. Errors may be made in finger identification, with confusion as to index, ring, and middle fingers (finger agnosia). The combination of dysgraphia, dyscalculia, finger agnosia, and left-right confusion is identified as Gerstmann's syndrome.

From the standpoint of localization, several points of caution should be indicated. Dysgraphia may also result from disease involving the premotor cortex anterior to the motor cortex representation of the hand. It is likely that information is conveyed from the inferior parietal area to the premotor motor association cortex and then to the precentral motor cortex. This area of premotor cortex (sometimes termed the writing center of Exner) must function in a manner analogous to Broca's area. It would be reasonable to consider dysgraphia from a lesion in this premotor location as essentially a motor apraxia due to destruction of an area concerned in the motor association memories for writing.

Pure dyslexias may occur without actual involvement of the angular supramarginal areas. The basic lesion, as we will indicate, is a lesion that deprives the inferior parietal cortex of information from the visual association areas.

Many lesions in the inferior parietal area extend into the subcortical white matter involving the long association fiber system, the arcuate fasciculus—as discussed earlier.

Patients with dominant inferior parietal lobule lesions often demonstrate problems in drawing (constructional drawing). Whether this reflects damage to the cortex of the angular and supramarginal gyri or a disconnection of these areas from the more anterior motor areas because of involvement of subcortical association fibers is usually uncertain.

As we have already discussed, many patients have involvement of all of the components of the posterior speech areas, the inferior parietal, the arcuate fasciculus, and Wernicke's area. The following case history demonstrates such a sequence of involvement in a tumor infiltrating this area with greatest difficulty in repetition as the most prominent initial feature.

CASE HISTORY 24.5

This 42-year-old, right-handed truck driver noted fatigue and irritability 6–8 weeks prior to admission. Three to four weeks prior to admission, he noted he was using words which he did not mean to use. Certain words would not come to him. During the week prior to admission, he had two generalized convulsive seizures; each was preceded by a ringing sensation in the ears.

Neurological Examination

Mental status: The patient was alert and oriented to time, place, and person; cooperative; and able to carry out the four-step command: "stick out your tongue, close your eyes, hold up your hand, and touch the thumb to your ear." There was, however, evidence of a significant left-right confusion when laterality was introduced (e.g., "left hand to right ear"). The ability to do even simple calculations was markedly impaired with or without paper (e.g., 100 – 9 = 99). There was little evidence of an expressive aphasia. Flow of speech was slow with only minor mispronunciations. Reading was slow but with few errors. The patient did have minor difficulty in naming objects—a mild nominal aphasia. The patient's greatest difficulty was in repetition of simple test phrases. There were moderate defects in drawings of a house and a clock but few errors in copying simple figures. There was a significant dysgraphia with marked difficulty in writing a simple sentence spontaneously or in writing from dictation. On the other hand, the patient was much better able to copy a simple sentence. Significant errors were made in spelling. Memory was impaired; with immediate object recall limited to 2/5 objects and delayed recall in 5 minutes limited to 0/5. Digit span was limited to 2 forward and 0 in reverse. *Cranial nerves:* A mild right central facial weakness was present.

Sensory system: Tactile localization was impaired on the right side.

Clinical diagnosis: Fluent posterior aphasia, disconnection syndrome plus elements of Gerstmann's syndrome (left-right confusion, dyscalculia, dysgraphia) plus seizures of focal origin (Heschl's gyrus posterior temporal lobe) with secondary generalization. All suggested a lesion in the left posterior temporal-posterior parietal area.

Etiology was uncertain but tumor (glioma) was considered most likely in view of the evolving course.

Laboratory Data

EEG: Focal 4–5 Hz slow-wave activity was present in the left parietal and posterior temporal areas.

Brain scan (radioactive Hg^{197}): Increased uptake of isotope in the left posterior temporal-parietal area measuring 4 x 5 cm.

Left carotid arteriogram: A vascular mass was present in the region of the angular gyrus with tumor stain in the area.

Subsequent course: Papilledema soon developed. Dr. Robert Yuan performed a craniotomy, which revealed a palpable firm mass slightly above and posterior to the angular gyrus. At 2 cm below the surface, firm yellow tumor tissue was encountered. All visible tumor and adjacent cortex of the angular and supramarginal gyri were removed and a partial left temporal lobectomy was performed. Histologic examination indicated a highly malignant glial tumor with active mitosis and necrosis (a glioblastoma). Postoperatively, the patient had a marked expressive and receptive aphasia. By 30 days after surgery, the patient had a significant improvement in fluency; he continued to have a severe posterior type of aphasia. He was unable to carry out simple commands. His speech was incoherent, with nonsense words and neologisms. He appeared unaware of his errors and did not appear frustrated by his failure to follow commands. In addition to this Wernicke's type aphasia, the patient was unable to repeat words of two syllables. He could do no calculations, had severe difficulties in copying drawings, and was unable to even write his name. The patient received radiotherapy, but his condition continued to worsen with the development of a progressive expressive and receptive aphasia and hemiparesis, all suggesting the spread of a rapidly growing glioblastoma. Coma, pupillary changes, and respiratory changes then intervened, suggesting the effects of herniation of the residual temporal lobe. Death occurred 7 months after onset of symptoms and 5 months following surgery.

The neurosurgical approach to the management of a glioblastoma, particularly those involving the speech areas of the dominant hemisphere, has changed in the 35 years since this patient was seen. A limited stereotaxic biopsy under CT scan guidance would be undertaken and the patient would then be treated with dexamethasone and radiotherapy. The end results would have been similar and actually may even have occurred earlier. The postoperative quality of language function may have been transiently better. Unfortunately, this patient had a very malignant and aggressive tumor. The median survival of glioblastomas with surgery alone is 26 weeks; with the addition of radiotherapy, it is 52–60 weeks.

CASE HISTORY 24.6

This 57-year-old female, with a long history of hypertension, in the summer of 1985, had a brief episode of difficulty in word finding and a more prolonged episode in December 1985 with confusion, "visual problems, finding the appropriate words." Following an additional episode in March 1986, she had persistent problems in reading and apraxia of the right hand.

Neurological Examination (May 1986)

Language function: Spontaneous speech was usually quite fluent. She described the room, the environment, and her friend. In contrast, capacity for repetition was very poor both as regards spoken and written speech. Spontaneous writing was very poor except for name and address. Reading to herself aloud was poor with little comprehension. She was able, however, to follow single, one-stage spoken or written commands but unable to do a sequence of commands. Naming of objects was well performed.

Cranial nerves: Extinction occurred in the right visual field for bilateral simultaneous stimuli.

Motor system: No hemiparesis was present.

Reflexes: Right-sided hyperreflexia and a right Babinski sign were present.

Clinical diagnosis: Posterior aphasia, infarction left posterior temporal and parietal areas, probably due to embolic occlusion of inferior division of the left middle cerebral artery.

Laboratory Data

CT scan: Infarct left posterior temporal and parietal areas (Fig. 24.6).

Angiograms: Occlusion of the left internal carotid artery. All left anterior and middle cerebral artery branches filled from the right carotid. An artery-to-artery embolus was presumed.

Global aphasia: These patients have little verbal output either spontaneously or on repetition, no comprehension, and no ability to read or write. CT scans demonstrate massive infarction of the entire middle cerebral artery territory of the dominant hemisphere involving presylvian areas of the frontal, temporal, and parietal areas (see Naeser, 1983).

Anomic, amnesic, or nominal aphasia: There remains a variety of aphasia—nominal aphasia—which is commonly encountered but which is not as readily localized to a particular cortical area. The patient recognizes objects when these are present in the visual or tactile sphere but is unable to name the object or is unable to access the internal dictionary to find the name. Nominal aphasia is often noted as part of other aphasic syndromes. When encountered in relatively pure form, speech output is usually fluent, comprehension is normal, and repetition is normal. The patient will substitute other names but more often will describe the use of the object as a means of naming it, for example, for a light switch—"That's the thing that makes the light go on and off" (circumlocution). At times, associated findings suggest localization to the dominant posterior temporal parietal area; at times, there is some association with a Broca's area motor aphasia.

Mixed transcortical aphasia or isolation of the speech areas: In contrast to the patient with conduction aphasia and to patients with Broca or Wernicke's aphasia, there are patients who have excellent repetition but little spontaneous speech. Broca's area, Wernicke's area, and the arcuate fasciculus are intact. The perisylvian areas supplied by the middle cerebral artery remain intact but are isolated from other cortical areas by infarction at the borders between the middle and anterior cerebral arteries or between the middle and posterior cerebral arteries (see Benson, 1985; Damasio and Geschwind, 1984; Geschwind et al., 1968; Geschwind, 1971). As discussed in greater detail in Chapter 26, carotid artery stenosis may produce a perfusion defect at the border zone of the middle and anterior cerebral artery (watershed infarct). On the other hand, a fall in blood pressure may produce perfusion-related infarction at the border zone between the middle and posterior cerebral artery. The patient can repeat without difficulty (fluent for repetitions) but has little spontaneous speech and little comprehension. At times, the patient echoes (echolalia) everything stated by the examiner.

Transcortical motor aphasia: This relatively rare syndrome reflects isolation of Broca's area from the more anterior frontal areas and from the supplementary motor area. The lesion is within the territory of the anterior cerebral artery. The speech pattern resembles that found in Broca's aphasia except that repetition is intact.

Transcortical sensory aphasia: This relatively rare syndrome reflects isolation of Wernicke's area from more posterior temporal occipital areas. The lesion is within the territory of the posterior cerebral artery. The resultant syndrome resembles Wernicke's aphasia except that repetition is intact.

Damasio and Geschwind (1984), Benson (1985) discuss the different types of transcortical aphasia (motor sensory, mixed) with anatomical correlation.

Visual agnosia and selective dyslexia (alexia without agraphia): Visual agnosia may be defined as a failure to recognize visually presented material. Dyslexia or alexia represents a more selective deficit: a failure to recognize visually presented words (this is sometimes also called word blindness). The student may conceptualize the basic disturbance as a disconnection of the visual areas from the speech areas of the posterior temporal and inferior parietal areas. This disturbance could result from bilateral lesions or from a unilateral lesion. As we have previously indicated, bilateral destruction of the visual association cortex (areas 18 and 19) would theoretically produce this effect. An alternate combination of lesions would involve destruction of the primary visual cortex (area 17) of the dominant left hemisphere and the visual association cortex of the right hemisphere.

A large unilateral lesion producing essentially this same effect has been implicated in dyslexia. This lesion has usually destroyed the visual cortex of the dominant left hemisphere and at the same time damaged the posterior portion or, at least, the splenium of the corpus callosum (or the fibers radiating from the splenium). The fibers conveying visual data from the right hemisphere must presumably reach the speech areas of the dominant hemisphere by passing through the posterior segment of the corpus callosum. The following case would suggest this type of unilateral lesion, producing a transient and partial but selective type of dyslexia.

CASE HISTORY 24.7

Seven days prior to admission, following a period of athletic activity, this 15-year-old, right-handed white male high school student had the onset of a 48-hour period of sharp pain in the left jaw and supraorbital area. The next day the patient noted blurring of vision and the following day had the onset of vomiting. Four days prior to admission, the patient noted that he was unable to read and to translate his Latin lessons. No definite aphasia was apparent. Two days prior to admission, the patient had the sudden onset of severe left facial pain, accompanied by tingling paresthesias of the right leg. The patient became stuporous and then unresponsive for approximately 90 minutes. An examination of spinal fluid at that time revealed pressure elevated to 290 mm of water with 250 fresh blood cells.

Neurological Examination
Mental status and language function: Intact.
Cranial nerves: Small flame-shaped hemorrhages were present on funduscopic examination; slight, right, supranuclear-type (central) facial weakness was present.
Neck: A slight degree of resistance was present on flexion of the neck (nuchal rigidity) consistent with the presence of blood in the subarachnoid space.
Clinical diagnosis: Subarachnoid hemorrhage of uncertain etiology. In view of age and the transient dyslexia, and the transient parerethises of the right leg, an arteriovenous malformation in the left parasagittal parietal-occipital area might be suspected.
Laboratory data: *Arteriograms:* An arteriovenous malformation was present in the left occipital region. The main arterial supply was the posterior temporal branch of the left posterior cerebral artery. The malformation drained into the lateral sinus. The posterior portion of the anterior cerebral artery was shifted across the midline, indicating a hematoma as well as the malformation.
Subsequent course: On the evening after admission, the patient had the sudden onset of a bifrontal headache and was unconscious for a 2- to 3-minute period with deviation (repetitive driving) of both eyes to the right, and with sweating and slowing of the pulse rate. Over the next 2 days an increase in blurring of the optic disk margins was noted (early papilledema). Four days after admission, the patient suddenly complained of being unable to see from his right eye. He became restless and agitated. Additional headache and neck pain with numbness of right arm and leg were reported. Examination now disclosed a dense right visual field defect (homonymous hemianopsia). The deep tendon reflexes were now slightly more active on the right. Funduscopic examination suggested that recent additional subarachnoid bleeding had occurred since new retinal hemorrhages were present. The next day the patient was noted to have a significant reading disability (dyslexia), although other language functions were intact. Because of the progressive evolution of neurological findings due to an expanding intracerebral hematoma, Doctor Robert Yuan performed a craniotomy, which revealed blood present in the subarachnoid space.

The left lateral occipital cortical surface had numerous areas of bluish discoloration, indicating an intracerebral clot. The main arterial vessel was a lateral and inferior branch of the posterior cerebral artery, bearing no relationship to the calcarine region. The draining vein was located in the occipital-temporal area, close to the tentorium. At a depth of 1 cm, a hematoma of 50 cc of clot was found. The clot extended down to the occipital horn of the lateral ventricle but did not enter the ventricle. The malformation, hematoma, and related cerebral tissue of the lateral occipital area were removed. The calcarine area remained intact at the end of the procedure. Over a period of several days, the visual field deficits disappeared.

Detailed language and psychological testing approximately 2 weeks after surgery indicated that language function was intact except for reading. Oral reading was very slow (four times slower than normal for a test paragraph) with halting and stumbling. Comprehension of the material read was good. Minor errors were made in the visual recognition of letters. This was reflected in occasional errors in spelling. Writing and drawing were intact but slow. Visual, auditory, and tactile recognition and naming of objects was intact. Calculations were intact. No right-left confusion or finger agnosia was present. Repetition of speech and spontaneous speech were intact.

Follow-up evaluation at 20 and 30 months indicated that, although the patient was doing well in school, receiving A's and B's with excellent grades in mathematics, he still was described as slow in reading compared to his level prior to illness. No actual errors were made in reading when this was tested.

Geschwind (1965) has reviewed many of the previously reported cases of selective dyslexia. It is uncertain whether the information from area 18 of the nondominant hemisphere passes to the nondominant angular gyrus and then crosses to the dominant temporal parietal areas or whether these fibers pass instead directly to area 18 of the dominant hemisphere with information then conveyed to the dominant temporal parietal areas. He finally concludes that both pathways are probably operative. The relatively minor nature of the final residual deficit in the present case would be consistent with such multiple pathways. It addition, nonfatal hemorrhages always produce less damage than infarcts of comparable size. Finally, Coslett (2000) has reviewed various recovered pure cases of dyslexia where the right hemisphere may have played a role in reading. Such patients do better with concrete nouns than abstract nouns, verbs, and factors (pronouns, prepositions, conjunctions, and interrogatives). It should be noted that a relatively selective dyslexia in the absence of a severe general visual agnosia might occur. Geschwind has suggested that whether a general visual agnosia or dyslexia occurs may depend on the degree of disconnection of the dominant speech areas from the parietal and occipital areas of the nondominant hemisphere. In the patient who already has left occipital cortex damage, dyslexia may require only damage to the splenium, whereas visual agnosia may require more extensive damage to the posterior body of the corpus callosum as well. As noted, bilateral lesions of visual association cortex (areas 18 and 19) would also produce a visual agnosia. (See also Coslett and Saffran [1989] and Friedman and Albert [1985].)

In addition, there are patients who have acquired dyslexia, which is unrelated to the processing of the visual information input. These patients have a central (rather than the peripheral dyslexia of the pure alexia syndrome discussed earlier). The central dyslexic patient has an impairment of the "deeper" or "higher" reading functions by which visual word forms mediate access to meaning or speech production mechanisms. This problem has been reviewed in detail by Coslett (2000). Feinberg and Farah (2000) have reviewed the general topic of agnosia.

APRAXIA

As we have previously indicated, this term may be defined as impairment in motor performance in the absence of a paralysis or sensory receptive deficit and at a time when cerebellar and cognitive functions are otherwise intact. In the carrying out of a skilled movement on command, there are several stages, which are similar to those considered under language function. The command, if auditory, must be received at the cortical sensory projection area of the dominant hemisphere. The information must then be relayed to the auditory association areas for the words of the command to be comprehended, that is, to evoke the appropriate auditory associations. From these areas information must be relayed to the multimodal association area of the dominant inferior parietal association area. Information is then conveyed, as discussed previously, to the premotor and supplementary motor association areas of the dominant hemisphere. Information must then be sent to the dominant motor cortex and via the corpus callosum to the premotor and motor areas of the nondominant hand so that hand can also perform skilled movements on command.

Apraxia then could result from damage at any point in this series of association centers and their interconnections. Depending on the point of disruption in the circuit, the type of impairment will vary. Thus, a lesion of the anterior one-half of the corpus callosum will result in an apraxia limited to the nondominant hand. In contrast, a lesion of the dominant premotor association areas would be more likely to produce a bilateral impairment in certain tongue and hand movements.

The concept that many varieties of apraxia represent a disconnection between various cortical areas, as reintroduced by Geschwind (1965), provides a more anatomically based approach than the use of terms such as *motor or limb kinetic* (motor association areas) or *ideomotor apraxia* (parietal lobe apraxia). Heilman et al. (2000) and Ochipa and Rothi (2000) have provided a more recent analysis of this topic.

The student will also encounter the term *ideational apraxia*. This term, which has received multiple definitions over the years, is now employed to indicate a defect in performing a series of acts in their proper sequence. This problem may occur in diffuse disorders such as Alzheimer's disease or frontal lobe disorders or left parietal disorders. Some would suggest that this type of dysfunction really represents not an apraxia but a deficit in recent memory and would require among the defining conditions of apraxia that dementia not be present. (The topic of apraxia remains an area of controversy.)

NONDOMINANT HEMISPHERE FUNCTIONS

As we have previously indicated, certain symptoms appear to follow damage to the nondominant parietal areas such as lack of awareness of hemiplegia, neglect syndrome, defects in spatial construction, and defects in perception of three-dimensional space. Some have questioned whether a true dominance of these functions actually exists in the hemisphere that is nondominant for speech. Certainly, neglect syndromes may also follow lesions of the dominant parietal area or of either premotor area. As regards concepts of visual space, there is some evidence from the studies of Gazzaniga et al. (1965), on section of the corpus callosum that the dominant left hemisphere is dependent on information that must be conveyed from the right hemisphere. Moreover, the studies of Penfield, which were discussed in Chapter 22, suggest that in patients with temporal lobe seizures, visual hallucinations are more likely to arise from stimulation of the right hemisphere than of the left. The stimulation studies of Fried et al. (1982) suggest short-term memory for visuospatial functions may be localized to the right superior temporal gyrus. Perception for visual spatial material may be localized to the right parietal-occipital and to right frontal operculum. A defect in the recognition of faces (prosopagnosia) has been related to lesions of the right parietal-occipital or inferior temporal-occipital junction (see Fried et al., 1982; Landis et al., 1988; Luders et al., 1988; Sergent and Villemore, 1989).

ROLE OF CORPUS CALLOSUM IN TRANSFER OF INFORMATION

The corpus callosum allows the nondominant hemisphere access to the special language centers of the dominant hemisphere. Thus, the intact right-handed individual can name an object, such as a key, independent of whether the object is placed in the left or right hand. Following section of the corpus callosum, the object can be named when placed in the right hand but not when placed in the left hand. In a similar manner, the corpus callosum allows the dominant hemisphere access to those specialized areas of the nondominant hemisphere concerned with concepts of visual space.

There is also evidence that the corpus callosum is involved in the transfer of information concerned with learned sensory discriminations. Thus, the intact monkey or human, who has been trained to press a key with the right hand only when a particular visual pattern appears in the right visual field, has no difficulty in performing the same discrimination without additional learning when the left visual field and left hand are employed. Section of the corpus callosum interferes with such transfer of learned information. There is evidence, however, that some sensory information and learned sensory discrimination is transferred between hemispheres via noncallosal pathways. (Refer to Ettlinger [1965] and Sergent [1986].)

In considering the functions of the corpus callosum based on studies of patients subjected to callosotomy for control of intractable epilepsy, much caution must be exercised. (1) The patients also have focal multifocal or diffuse cortical damage sustained at variable age. At times, some reorganization of function has occurred. (2) The acute disconnection syndrome which has been described after corpus callosum surgery (see Engel, 1989; Reeves, 1985; Sass et al., 1988) consisting of mutism, agnosia, apraxia of the nondominant limbs, apathy, bilateral grasp release, and gait apraxia may, in part, relate to traction on nondominant parasagittal frontal, supplementary motor, and premotor areas. (3) Ontogenetic effects and effects of staging surgery have been noted. (4) The same deficits do not necessarily occur in patients with agenesis of the corpus callosum.

BIBLIOGRAPHY

APHASIA AND HIGHER CORTICAL DISORDERSR CORICAL DISORDERS

GENERAL OR HISTORICAL REFERENCES

Ajamone-Marsan, C., and Ralston, B. L. 1957. The Epileptic Seizure: Its Functional Morphology and Diagnostic Significance. Springfield, L: Charles C. Thomas.

Alexander, G. E., and DeLong, M. R. 1992. Central mechanisms of initiation and control of movement. In A. K. Asbury, G. M. McKhann, and W. I. McDonald (Eds.) Diseases of the Nervous System: Clinical Neurobiology. 2nd ed., pp. 285–308. Philadelphia, PA: W. B. Saunders.

Brumback, R. A. (Ed.). 1993. Behavioral neurology. Neurol. Clin. 11:1–237.

Coslett, H. B. (Ed.). 2000. Behavioral neurology/higher cortical function. Semin. Neurol. 20:405–515.

Commission on Classification and Terminology of the International League against Epilepsy. 1981. Proposal for re- revised clinical and electroencephalographic classification of epileptic seizures. Epilepsia 22:489–501.

Commission on Classification and Terminology of the International League Against Epilepsy. 1989. Proposal for a revised classification of epilepsies and epileptic syndromes. Epilepsia 30:389–399.

Damasio, H., Damasio, A. R. 1989. Lesion Analysis in Neuropsychology. New York, NY: Oxford University Press.

Engel, J., Jr., 1989. Seizures and Epilepsy. Philadelphia, PA: F.A. Davis.

Ferrier, D. 1873. Experimental researches in cerebral physiology and pathology. Rep. West Riding Lunatic Asylum. 3:30–96.

Foerster, O. 1936. The motor cortex in the light of Hughlings Jackson's doctrines. Brain 59:135–159.

Fulton, J. F. 1949. Physiology of the Nervous System. 3rd ed. New York, NY: Oxford University Press.

Green, J. R. 1987. Sir Victor Horsley: a centennial recognition of his impact on neuroscience and neurological surgery. Barrow Neurol. Inst, Quart. 3:2–16.

Heilman, K. M., and Valenstein, E. D. (Eds.) 1985. Clinical Neuropsychology. 2nd ed. New York, NY: Oxford University Press.

Hitzig, E. 1900. Hughlings Jackson and the cortical motor centres in light of physiological research. Brain 23:545–581.

Kertesz, A. (Ed.) 1983. Localization in Neuropsychology. New York, NY: Academic Press.

Luders, H. O., and Noachtar, S. (Eds.). 2000. Epileptic Seizures: Pathophysiology and Clinical Semiology. New York, NY. Churchill Livingstone.

Martin, J. H., Brust, J. C. M., and Hilal, S. 1991. Imaging the living brain. In E. R. Kandel, J. H. Schwartz and M. Jessell (Eds.) Principles of Neural Science, pp. 309–324. New York, NY: Elsevier.

Meyer, A. 1978. The concept of a sensory motor cortex: its early history with special emphasis on two early experimental contributions by W. Bechterew. Brain 101:673–685.

Palmini, A., and Glood, P. 1992. The localizing value of auras in partial seizures: a prospective and retrospective analysis. Neurology 42:801–808. (In particular: Kertesz, A. Issues in localization. pp.1–20; Galaburda, A. and M.M. Mesulam. Neuroanatomical aspects of cerebral localization. pp. 21–61)

Penfield, W., and Jasper, H. 1954. Epilepsy and the Functional Anatomy of the Human Brain. Boston, MA: Little, Brown. (See pp. 41–154, 350–539)

Penfield, W., and Rasmussen, T. (Eds.). 1957. The Cerebral Cortex of Man: A Clinical Study of Localization. New York, NY: MacMillan.

Reynolds, E. H. 1988. Hughlings Jackson: A Yorkshireman's contributions to epilepsy. Arch. Neurol. 45:675–678.

Schomer, D. L. 1983. Partial epilepsy. N. Engl. J. Med. 309:536–559.

Taylor. J. (Ed.). 1931. Selected Writings of John Hughlings Jackson. New York, NY: Basic Books. (Reprinted 1959, see pp. 1–36, 385–405, 406–411, 458–463)

Wilkins, R. H., and Brody, I. A. 1970. Jacksonian epilepsy. Arch. Neurol. 22:183–188. (see also Taylor above)

SPECIFIC REFERENCES

Amassian, V. E., Cracco, R. Q., and Maccabee, P. J. 1989. Focal stimulation of human cerebral cortex with the magnetic coil: a comparison with electrical stimulation. Electroencephalogr. Clin. Neurophysiol. 74:401–416.

Andrews, R. J. 1991. Transhemispheric diaschisis: review and comment. Stroke 22:943–949.

Ardila, A., and Lopez, M. V. 1988. Paroxysmal aphasias. Epilepsia 29:630–634.

Auerbach, S. H., Allard, T., Naesar, M., et al. 1982. Pure word deafness: analysis of a case with bilateral lesions and a defect at the prephonemic level. Brain 105:271–300.

Ballantine, H. T., Cassidy, W. L., Flanagan, N. B., et al. 1967. Stereotaxic anterior cingulotomy for neuropsychiatric illness and intractable pain. J. Neurosurg. 26:499–495.

Barker, A. T., Jalinous, R., and Freiston, I. L. 1985. Non-invasive magnetic stimulation of human motor cortex. Lancet 1:1106–1107. (See also Amassian, V. E., et al, above.)

Baynes, K., Holtzman, J. D., and Volpe, B. T. 1986. Components of visual attention: alterations in response pattern to visual stimuli following parietal lobe infarction. Brain 109:99–114.

Benson, D. F. 1985. Aphasia. In K. M. Heilman and E. Valenstein (Eds.) Clinical Neuropsychology, pp. 17–47. New York, NY: Oxford University Press.

Benson, D. F., Sheremata, W. A., Bouchard, R., et al. 1973. Conduction aphasia: a clinopathological study. Arch. Neuro. 28:339–346.

Benson, D. F., Metter, E. J., Kuhl, D. E., et al. 1983. Positron computed tomography in neurobehavioral problems. In A. Kertesz (Ed.) Localization in Neuropsychology, pp. 121–139. New York, NY: Academic Press.

Benson, D. F., and Zaidel, E. (Eds.). 1985. The Dual Brain: Hemispheric Specialization in Humans. New York, NY: The Guilford Press.

Black, P., Cianci, S. N., and Markowitz, R. S. 1971. Differential recovery of proximal and distal motor power after cortical lesions. Trans. Amer. Neurol. Assoc. 96:173–177.

Blume, W. T. 1993a. Motor cortex: anatomy, physiology and epileptogenesis. In E. Wyllie (Ed.) The Treatment of Epilepsy: Principles and Practices, pp. 16–25. Philadelphia, PA: Lea & Febiger.

Blume, W. T. 1993b. Focal motor seizures and epilepsia partialis continua. In E. Wyllie (Ed.) The Treatment of Epilepsy: Principles and Practices, pp. 393–399. Philadelphia, PA: Lea Febiger.

Blume, W. T., Jones, D. C., Young, G. B., et al. 1992. Seizures involving secondary sensory and related areas. Brain 115:1509–1520.

Bogousslavsky, J., and Regli, F. 1986. Borderzone infarctions distal to internal carotid artery occlusion: prognostic implications. Ann. Neurol. 20:346–350.

Bottini, G., Corcoran, R., Sterzi, R., et al. 1994. The role of the right hemisphere in the interpretation of figurative aspects of language: a positron emission tomography activation study. Brain 117:1241–1253.

Butter, C. M., Mishkin, K., and Mirsky, A. F. 1968. Emotional response in monkeys with selective frontal lesions. Physiol. Rev. 3:213–215.

Butter, C. M., Snyder, D. R., and McDonald, J. 1970. Effects of orbital frontal lesions on adversive and aggressive behavior in rhesus monkeys. J. Comp. Physiol. Psychol. 72:832–844.

Butters, N., and Pandya, D. 1969. Retention of delayed alternation: effect of selective lesions of sulcus principalis. Science 165:1271–1273.

Calleja, J., Carpizo, R., and Berciano, J. 1988. Organismic epilepsy. Epilepsia 29:635–639.

Cauvel, P., Delgado-Escueta, A. V., Halgren, E., et al. (Eds.). 1992. Frontal lobe seizures and epilepsies. New York, NY: Raven Press. (see also Delgado-Escueta et al. 1988. Epilepsia. 29:204–221 for abstracts)

Chui, H., and Damasio, A. 1980. Human cerebral asymmetries evaluated by computed tomography. J. Neurol. Neurosurg. Psychiatry 43:873–878.

Cole, J. 1957. Laterality in the use of eye, hand and foot in monkeys. J. Comp. Physiol. Psychol. 50:296–299.

Colebatch, J. G., and Gandevia, S. C. 1989. The distribution of muscular weakness in upper motor neuron lesions affecting the arm. Brain 112:749–763.

Corkin, S., Milner, B., and Rasmussen, T. 1964. Effects of different cortical excisions on sensory thresholds in man. Trans. Amer. Neurol. Assoc. 89:112–116.

Coslett, H. B. 2000. Acquired dyslexia. Semin. Neurol. 20:419–426.

Coslett, H. B., Brashear, H. P., and Heilman, K. M. 1984. Pure word deafness after bilateral primary auditory cortex infarcts. Neurology 34:347–352.

Coslett, H. B., and Saffran, E. M. 1989. Evidence for preserved reading in pure alexia. Brain 112:327–359.

Cracco, R. Q., Amassian, V. E., and Maccabee, P. J. 1989. Comparison of human transcallosal responses evoked by magnetic coil and electrical stimulation. Electroencephalograp. Clin. Neurophysiol. 74:417–424.

Cushing, H., and Eisenhardt, L. 1938. Meningiomas: Their Classification, Regional Behavior, Life History and Surgical End Results. Springfield, IL: Charles C. Thomas. (Reprinted 1988, Birmingham, AL: The Classics of Neurology Neurosurgery Library)

Damasio, A. R. 1985. The frontal lobes. In K. M. Heilman and E. Valenstein (Eds.) Clinical Neuropsychology. 2nd ed., pp. 339–375. New York, NY: Oxford University Press.

Damasio, A. R. 1992. Medical progress: aphasia. N. Engl. J. Med. 326:531–539.

Damasio, A. R., and Geschwind, N. 1984. The neural basis of language. Ann. Rev. Neurosci. 7:127–147.

Damasio, H., and Damasio, A. 1980. The anatomical basis of conduction aphasia. Brain 103:337–350.

Damasio, H., Grabowski, T., Frank, R., et al. 1994. The return of Phineas Gage: clues about the brain from the skull of a famous patient. Science 264:1102–1105.

Darian-Smith, I., Johnson, K. O., and Goodwin, A. W. 1979. Posterior parietal cortex relations of unit activity to sensorimotor function. Ann. Rev. Physiol. 41:141–157.

Dellatolas, G., Luciani, S., Castresana, A., et al. 1993. Pathologic left-handed: left-handedness correlatives in adult epileptics. Brain 116:1565–1574.

De Renzi, E. 2000. Disorders of visual recognition. Semin. Neurol. 20:479–486.

DeRenzi, E., and Luchelli, F. 1988. Ideational apraxia. Brain 111:1173–1185.

Duffner, K. R., Ahern, L. L., and Weintraub, S. 1990. Dissociated neglect behavior following sequential strokes in the right hemisphere. Ann. Neurol. 28:97–101.

Duffner, K. R., Mesulam, M. M., Scinto, L. F. M., et al. 2000. The central role of prefrontal cortex in directing attentionto novel eventys. Brain 123:927–939.

Dusser de Barenne, J. G., and McCulloch, W. S. 1941. Suppression of motor response obtained from area 4 by stimulation of area 4S. J. Neurophysiol. 4:311–323.

Ettlinger, F. G. (Ed.). 1965. Function of the Corpus Callosum. Boston, MA: Little, Brown.

Fangel, C., and Kaada, B. R. 1960. Behavior "attention" and fear induced by cortical stimulation in the cat. Electroencephalogr. Clin. Neurophysiol. 12:575–588.

Feinberg, T. E., and Farah, M. J. 2000. Agnosias. In W. G. Bradley, et al. (Eds.) Neurology in Clinical Practice, pp.131–139. Boston, MA: Butterworth Heinemann.

Fletcher, P. C., and Henson, R. N. A. 2001. Frontal lobes and human memory. Insights from functional neuroimaging. Brain 124:849–881.

Freund, H. J. 1987. Differential effects of cortical lesions in humans. In G. Bock, M. O'Connor, and J. Marsh (Eds.) Ciba Foundation Symposium 132. Motor Areas of the Cerebral Cortex, pp. 269–281. Chichester, UK: John Wiley.

Freund, H. J., and Hummelshein, H. 1985. Lesions of the premotor cortex in man. Brain 108:697–733.

Fried, I., Materr, C., Ojemann, G., et al. 1982. Organization of visuospatial functions in human cortex: evidence from electrical stimulation. Brain 105:349–371.

Friedman, R. B., and Albert, M. L. 1985. Alexia. In K. M. Heilman and E. Valenstein (Eds.) Clinical Neuropsychology, pp. 49–73. New York, NY: Oxford University Press.

Fulton, J. F., and Jacobsen, C. F. 1935. The functions of the frontal lobes: a comparative study in monkeys, chimpanzees, and man. Adv. Mod. Biol. (Moscow). 4:113–123.

Galaburda, A. M., LeMay, M., Kemper, T. L., et al. 1978. Right-left asymmetries in the brain. Science 199:852–856.

Gandevia, S. C., Burke, D., and McKeon, B. 1984. The projection of muscle afferents from the hand to cerebral cortex in main. Brain 107:1–13.

Gazzaniga, M. S., Bogen, J. E., and Sperry, R. W. 1965. Observations on visual perception after disconnections of the cerebral hemispheres in man. Brain 88:221–236.

Geier, S., Bancaud, J., Talairach, J., et al. 1977. The seizures of frontal lobe epilepsy: a study of clinical manifestations. Neurology 27:951–958.

Geschwind, N. 1965. Disconnection syndromes in animals and man. Brain 88:237–294, 585–644.

Geschwind, N. 1971. Aphasia. N. Engl. J. Med. 284:654–656.

Geschwind, N., and Levitsky, W. 1968. Human brain: left-right asymmetries in temporal speech region. Science 161:186–187.

Geschwind, N., Quadfasel, F. A., and Segarra, J. 1968. Isolation of the speech area. Neuropsychologia 6:327–340.

Goldman-Rakic, P. S. 1987. Motor control function of the prefrontal cortex. In G. Bock, M. O'Connor, and J. Marsh (Eds.) Ciba Foundation Symposium 132. Motor Areas of the Cerebral Cortex, pp.187–201. Chichester, UK: John Wiley.

Grafman, J., Vance, S. C., Weingartner, H., et al. 1986. The effects of lateralized frontal lesion on mood regulation. Brain 109:1127–1148.

Halsband, U., and Freund, H. J. 1990. Premotor cortex and conditional motor learning in man. Brain 113:207–222.

Halsband, U., Ito, N., Tanji, J., and Freund, H. J. 1993. The role of premotor cortex and the supplementary motor area in the temporal control of movement in man. Brain 116:243–266.

Hausser-Hauw, C., and Bancaud, J. 1987. Gustatory hallucinations in epileptic seizures: electrophysiological, clinical and anatomical correlates. Brain 110:339–360.

Harlow, J. M. 1868. Recovery from the passage of an iron bar through the head. Mass. Med. Soc. Publ. 2:327–346.

Heilman, K. M., and Roth, L. J. G. 1985. Apraxia. In K. M. Heilman and E. Valenstein (Eds.) Clinical Neuropsychology, pp.134–150. New York, NY: Oxford University Press.

Heilman, K. M., Valenstein, E., and Watson, R. T. 2000. Neglect and related disorders. Semin. Neurol. 20:463–470.

Heilman, K. M., Watson, R. T., Valenstein, E., et al. 1983. Localization of lesions in neglect. In A. Kertesz (Ed.) Localization in Neuropsychology, pp. 471–492. New York, NY: Academic Press.

Helmstaedter, C., Kurher, M., Linke, D. B., and Elger, C. E. 1994. Right hemisphere restution of language and memory functions in right hemisphere language dominant patients with left temporal lobe epilepsy. Brain 117:729–737.

Jacobsen, C. F. 1935. Functions of the frontal association area in primates. Arch. Neurol. Psychiat. 33:558–569.

Jacobsen, C. F., and Nissen, H. W. 1937. Studies of cerebral function in primates: IV. The effects of frontal lobe lesion on the delayed alteration habit in monkeys. J. Comp. Physical Psychol. 23:101–112.

Jacobsen, S., and Trojanowski, J. 1977. Prefrontal granular cortex of the rhesus monkey: I. Intrahemispheric cortical afferents. II. Interhemispheric cortical afferents. Brain Res. 132:209–233, 235–246.

Jones, E. G., Friedman, D. P., and Hendra, S. H. C. 1982. Thalamic basis of place and modality specific columns in monkey cerebral cortex: a correlative anatomical and physiological study. J. Neurophysiol. 48:545–568.

Jones, E. G., and Powell, T. P. S. 1970. An anatomic study of converging sensory pathways within the cerebral cortex of the monkey. Brain 93:793–820.

Kass, J. H., Merzenich, M. M., and Killackey, H. P. 1983. The reorganization of somatosensory cortex following peripheral nerve damage in adult and developing mammals. Ann. Rev. Neurosci. 6:325–356.

Kass, J. H., Nelson, R. J., Sur, M., et al. 1979. Multiple representations of the body within somatosensory cortex of primates. Science 204:521–523.

Kass, J. H., Nelson, R. J., Sur, M., et al. 1981. Organization of somatosensory cortex in primates. In F. O. Schmitt et al. (Eds.) The Organization of the Cerebral Cortex, pp. 237–261. Cambridge, MA: MIT Press.

Kertesz, A., and Geschwind, N. 1971. Patterns of pyramidal decussation and their relationship to handedness. Arch. Neurol. 4:326–332.

Killackey, H., and Ebner, F. 1973. Convergent projection of three separate thalamic nuclei into a single cortical area. Science 179:283–285.

Kirsher, H. S. 2000. Aphasia. In W. G. Bradley et al. (Eds.) Neurology in Clinical Practice, pp. 141–159. Boston, MA: Butterworth Heinemann.

Kennard, M. A., and Ectors, L. 1938. Forced circling in monkeys following lesions of the frontal lobes. J. Neurophysiol. 1:45–54.

Lacaze, E., Kieffer, V., Streri, A., et al. 2003. Neuropsychological outcome in children with optic pathway tumours when first-line treatment is chemotherapy. Br J Cancer. 89(11):2038–2044.

Landis, T., Regard, M., Bliestel, A., et al. 1988. Prosopagnosia and agnosia for non-canonical views: an autopsied case. Brain 111:1287–1297.

Legarda, S., Jayakar, P., Duchowny, M., et al. 1994. Benign rolandic epilepsy: high central and low central subgroups. Epilepsia 35:1125–1129.

Lehman, R., Andermann, F., Olivier, A., et al. 1994. Seizures with onset in the sensorimotor face area: clinical patterns and results of surgical treatment in 20 patients. Epilepsia 35:1117–1124.

Leiguarda, R. S., and Marsden, C. D. 2000. Limb apraxias. Higher order disorders of sensori motro integration. Brain 123:860–869.

Leiguarda, R., Starkstein, S., and Berthier, M. 1989. Anterior callosal hemorrhage: a partial interhemispheric disconnection syndrome. Brain 112:1019–1037.

LeMay, M., and Culebras, A. 1972. Human brain morphologic differences in the hemispheres demonstrable by carotid arteriography. N. Engl. J. Med. 287:168–170. (see also N. Geschwind. 1972. Editorial. N. Engl. J. Med. 187:194–195)

LeMay, M., and Kido, D. K. 1978. Asymmetries of the cerebral hemispheres on computed tomograms. J. Computer Assist. Tomography 2:471.

LeMay, M., and Geschwind, N. 1978. Asymmetries of the human cerebral hemispheres. In A. Caramazza and E. B. Zurif (Eds.) Language Acquisition and Breakdown, pp. 311–328. Baltimore, MD: Johns Hopkins.

Luders, H., Lesser, R. P., Dinner, D. S., et al. 1988. Localization of cortical function: new information from extraoperative monitoring of patients with epilepsy. Epilepsia 29(Suppl. 2):56–65.

Luders, H., Lesser, R. P., Dinner, D. S., et al. 1985. The second sensory area in humans: evoked potential and electrical stimulation studies. Ann. Neurol. 17:177–184.

Ludlow, C. L., Rosenberg, J. R., Fair, C., et al. 1986. Brain lesions associated with nonfluent aphasia, fifteen years following penetrating head injury. Brain 109:55–80.

Lynch, J. C., Mountcastle, V. B., Talbot, W. H., et al. 1977. Parietal lobe mechanisms for directed visual attention. J. Neurophysiol. 40:362–389.

Marcus, E. M., Jacobson, S., Watson, C. W., et al. 1970. An experimental model of "petit mal epilepsy" in the monkey: additional studies of the anterior premotor area. Trans. Amer. Neurol. Assoc. 95:279–281.

Marcus, E. M., Watson, C. W., and Simon, S. A. 1968. Behavioral correlates of acute bilateral symmetrical epileptogenic foci in monkey cerebral cortex. Brain Res. 9:370–373.

Meador, K. F., Watson, R. T., Bowers, D., et al. 1986. Hypometria with hemispatial and limb motor neglect. Brain 109:293–305.

Mesulam, M. M., Hoeser, G. W. V., Pandya, D. N., et al. 1977. Limbic and sensory connections of the inferior parietal lobule (area PG) in the rhesus monkey. Brain Res. 136:393–414.

Meyer, B-U., Roricht, S., Gafin von Einsiedel, H., et al. 1995. Inhibitory and excitatory interhemispheric transfers between motor cortical areas in normal humans and patients with abnormalities of the corpus callosum. Brain 118:429–440.

Milner, B., and Teuber, H. L. 1968. Some cognitive effects of frontal lobe lesions in man: reflections on methods. In L. Weiskrantz (Ed.) Analysis of Behavioral Changes, pp. 268–375. New York, NY: Harper and Row.

Mohr, J. P. 1973. Rapid amelioration of motor aphasia. Arch. Neurol. 28:77–82.

Moniz, E. 1936. Tentatives operatories dans le traitement de certaines psychoses. Paris, France: Masson et Cie.

Morris, H. H., III. 1993. Supplementary motor seizures. In E. Wyllie (Ed.) The Treatment of Epilepsy: Principles and Practices, pp. 541–546. Philadelphia, PA: Lea & Febiger.

Morris, H. H., III, Dinner, D. S., Luders, M. D., et al. 1988. Supplementary motor seizures: clinical and electroencephalographic findings. Neurology 38:1075–1082.

Morrow, M. J., and Sharpe, J. A. 1995. Deficits of smooth pursuit eye movement after unilateral frontal lobe lesions. Ann. Neurol. 37:443–451.

Mountcastle, V. B. 1957. Modality and topographic properties of single neurons of cats somatic sensory cortex. J. Neuro-physiol. 20:408–434.

Naeser, M. A. 1983. CT scan lesion size and lesion locus in cortical and subcortical aphasias. In A. Keertesz (Ed.) Localization in Neuropsychology, pp. 63–119. New York, NY: Academic Press.

Naeser, M. A., Palumbo, C. L., Estabrook, N. H., et al. 1989. Severe non-fluency in aphasia: role of the medial subcallosal fasciculus and other white matter pathways in recovery of spontaneous speech. Brain 112:1–38.

Nagel-Leiby, S., Buchtel, H. A., and Welch, K. M. A. 1990. Cerebral control of directed visual attention and orienting saccades. Brain 113:237–276.

Nauta, W. J. H. 1964. Some efferent connections of the prefrontal cortex in the monkey. In J. M. Warren and K. Akert (Eds.) The Frontal Granular Cortex and Behavior, pp. 397–409. New York, NY: McGraw Hill.

Ochipa, C., and Gonzalez Rothi, L. J. 2000. Limb apraxia. Semin. Neurol. 20:471–478.

Ochs, R., Gloor, P., Quesney, F., et al. 1984. Does head turning during seizure have lateralizing or localizing significance? Neurology 34:884–890.

Pandya, D. N., Dye, P., and Butters, N. 1971. Efferent corticocortical projections of the prefrontal cortex in the rhesus monkey. Brain Res. 31:35–46.

Pandya, D. N., and Kuypers, H. 1969. Cortico-cortical connections in the rhesus monkey. Brain Res. 13:13–16.

Pandya, D. N., and Vignolo, L. A. 1971. Intra and inter hemispheric projections of the precentral premotor and arcuate areas in the rhesus monkey. Brain Res. 26:217–233.

Passingham, R. E. 1987. Two cortical systems for directing movement. In G. Bock, M. O'Connor, and J. Marsh (Eds.) Ciba Foundation Symposium 132. Motor Areas of the Cerebral Cortex. pp.151–164. Chichester, UK: John Wiley.

Pause, M., Kunesch, E., Binkofsi, F., et al. 1989. Sensorimotor disturbances in patients with lesions of the parietal cortex. Brain 112:1599–1625.

Perenin, M. T., and Vighetto, A. 1988. Optic ataxia: a specific disruption in visuomotor mechanisms. I. Different aspects of the deficit in reaching for objects. Brain 111:643–674.

Peretz, I., Kolinsky, R., Tramo, M., et al. 1994. Functional dissociations following bilateral lesions of auditory cortex. Brain 117:1283–1301.

Phillips, C. G. 1966. Changing concepts of the precentral motor area. In J. C. Eccles (Ed.) Brain and Conscious Experience, pp. 389–421. New York, NY: Springer Verlag.

Pierrott-Deseilligny, C. H., Cray, F., and Brunot, P. 1986. Infarcts of both inferior parietal lobules with impairment of visually guided eye movement, peripheral visual attention and optic ataxia. Brain 109:81–97.

Pierrott-Deseilligny, C. H., Rivaud, S., Gaymard, B., et al. 1995. Neurological progress—cortical control of saccades. Ann. Neurol. 37:557–567.

Quesney, L. F., Constan, M., Fish, D. R., et al. 1990. The clinical differentiation of seizures arising in the parasagittal and anterolateral dorsal frontal convexities. Arch. Neurol. 47:677–679.

Randolph, M., and Seemes, J. 1974. Behavioral consequences of selective subtotal ablations in the post central gyrus of Macaca mulatta. Brain Res. 70:55–770.

Reeves, A. G. (Ed.). 1985. Epilepsy and the Corpus Callosum. New York, NY: Plenum.

Rizzolatti, G. 1987. Functional organization of inferior area 6. In G. Bock, M. O'Connor, and J. Marsh (Eds.) Ciba foundation Symposium

132. Motor Areas of the Cerebral Cortex, pp. 171–186. Chichester, UK: John Wiley.

Rome, R., and Schultz, W. 1986. Neuronal activity preceding self initiated or externally time arm movements in area 6 of monkey cortex. Exp. Brain Res. 67:656–662.

Saffran, E. 2000. Aphasia and the relationship of Language and brain. Semin. Neurol. 20:409–418.

Sass, K. J., Spencer, D. P., Spencer, S. S., et al. 1988. Corpus callostomy for epilepsy: II. Neurological and neuropsychological outcome. Neurology 38:24–28.

Sawhney, I. M. S., Suresh, N., Dhend, O. K., et al. 1988. Acquired aphasia with epilepsy Landau Kleffner Syndrome. Epilepsia 29:283–287.

Scheffer, I. E., Bhatia, K. B., Lopes-Cendes, I., et al. 1995. Autosomal dominant nocturnal frontal lobe epilepsy. A distinctive clinical disorder. Brain 118:61–73.

Schwartz, B. F., Halgren, E., Delgado-Escueta, A. V., et al. 1989. Neuroimaging in patients with seizures of probable frontal lobe origin. Epilepsia 30:547–558.

Sergent, J. 1986. Subcortical coordination of hemispheric activity in commissurotomized patients. Brain 109:357–369.

Sergent, J., and Villemore, J. G. 1989. Prosopagnosia in a right hemispherectomized patient. Brain 112:975–995.

Shibasaki, H., Sadato, N., Lyshkow, H., et al. 1993. Both primary motor cortex and supplementary motor area play an important role. Brain 116:1387–1398.

Stein, J. F. 1976. The effect of cooling parietal lobe areas 5 and 7 upon voluntary movement in awake rhesus monkeys. J. Physiol. (London) 298:62–63.

Stuss, D. T., and Benson, D. F. 1986. The Frontal Lobes. New York, NY: Raven Press.

Tharp, B. R. 1972. Orbital frontal seizures: a unique electroen-cephalographic and clinical syndrome. Epilepsia 13:627, 642.

Tuxhorn, I., and Kerdar, M. S. 2000. Somatosensory auras. In H. O. Luders and S. Nochtar (Eds.) Epileptic Seizures: Pathophysiology and Clinical Semiology, pp. 286–297. New York, NY: Churchill Livingstone.

Twitchell, T. E. 1951. The restoration of motor function following hemiplegia in man. Brain 74:443–480.

Vargha-Khadem, F., O'Gorman, A. M., and Walters, G. V. 1985. Aphasia and handedness in relation to hemispheric side, age of injury and severity of cerebral lesion during childhood. Brain 108:677–696.

Wada, J. A., Clarke, R., and Hamm, H. 1975. Cerebral hemispheric asymmetry in humans. Arch. Neurol. 32:239–246.

Wada, J., and Rasmussen, T. 1966. Intra-carotid injection of sodium amytal for the lateralization of cerebral speech dominance: experimental and clinical observations. J. Neurosurg. 17:260–282.

Ward, A. A., Pededen, I. K., and Sugar, O. 1946. Cortico-cortical connections in the monkey with special reference to area 6. J. Neurophysiol. 9:453–461.

Warner, J. J. 1988. Ictal alexia, agraphia, anomia without speech arrest. Epilepsia 29:652.

Watson, R. T., Miller, B. D., and Heilman, K. M. 1978. Nonsensory neglect. Ann. Neurol. 3:505–508.

Weiller, C., Isensee, C., Rijntjes, M., et al. 1995. Recovery from Wernicke's aphasia: a positron emmission tomographic study. 37:723–732.

Weiskrantz, L., Liharlovic, L. J., and Gross, G. G. 1962. Effects of stimulation of frontal cortex and hippocampus on behavior in the monkey. Brain 85:487–504.

Welch, K., and Stuteville, P. 1958. Experimental production of unilateral neglect in monkeys. Brain 81:341–347.

Wiesendanger, M., Hummelshein, H., Bianchetti, M., et al. 1987. Input and output organization of the supplementary motor area. In G. Bock, M. O'Connor, and J. Marsh (Eds.) Ciba Foundation Symposium 132. Motor Areas of the Cerebral Cortexm pp. 40–62. Chichester, UK: John Wiley.

Wiesendanger, M., and Wise, S. P. 1992. Current issues concerning the functional organization of motor cortex in non-human primates. In P. Chauvel, A. V. Delgado-Escueta, et al. (Eds.) Frontal Lobe Seizures and Epilepsies, pp. 117–134. New York, NY: Raven Press.

Wilkins, R. H., and Brody, I. J. A. 1969. The thalamic syndrome. Arch. Neurol. 20:550–562.

Williamson, P. D., Boon, P. A., Thadani, V. M., et al. 1992. Parietal lobe epilepsy: diagnostic considerations and results of surgery. Ann. Neurol. 31:193–201.

Williamson, P. D., Spencer, D. D., Spencer, S. S., et al. 1988. Complex partial seizures of frontal lobe origin. Ann. Neurol. 18:497–504.

Willmes, K., and Poeck, K. 1993. To what extent can aphasic syndromes be localized Brain 116:1527–1540.

Wise, S. P. 1985. The primate premotor cortex: past, present and preparatory. Ann. Rev. Neurosci. 8:1–19.

Yakolev, P. I., and Radic, P. 1966. Patterns of decussation of bulbar pyramids and distribution of pyramidal tracts on two sides of the spinal cord. Trans. Amer. Neurol. Assoc. 91:366–367.

25.

CASE HISTORY PROBLEM SOLVING

PART IV: CORTICAL LOCALIZATION

These cases represent the gamut of disease affecting the cerebral cortex. The pathology represented may be tumor, infarction, or hemorrhage. Some of the lesions are intrinsic; others are extrinsic. The nature of the pathology may be uncertain; the location of the pathology, however, should be evident to you.

CASE HISTORY 25.1

Three months prior to admission, this 39-year-old, right-handed, white male had the first of repetitive episodes characterized by "vertical wavy lines" in his left visual field. The initial episode lasted 30 minutes; subsequent episodes, 1 to 2 minutes. The patient had been seen by an ophthalmologist during the first of these episodes, and a left visual field defect, which would disappear at the end of the episode, was detected. An electroencephalogram (EEG) revealed no definite abnormality. Approximately 1 month later, the left visual field defect remained as a permanent deficit. At this time the patient also noted the onset of numbness in his left hand. Two months later the patient noted the onset of bitemporal and bifrontal headaches precipitated by any motion of the head. One week prior to admission there was an onset of vomiting, and these symptoms prompted his admission.

Past history: Not remarkable.
General physical examination: Not remarkable.
Neurological Examination
Mental status: This was intact except for some vagueness in the chronology for events in the present illness. The patient was oriented as to time, place, and person. Delayed recall was intact. No aphasia was present; reading and writing were intact.
Cranial nerves:

a. A complete left homonymous hemianopsia was present.
b. Fundoscopic examination indicated bilateral papilledema with venous engorgement, arteriovenous nicking, and a recent hemorrhage in relation to the right disk. Visual acuity, however, was well preserved.
c. Both pupils demonstrated a sluggish response to light.
d. A left central (supranuclear) type of facial weakness was present with a droop of the left corner of the mouth.

Motor system: Strength was intact and cerebellar tests were negative. However, the patient tended to lean slightly to the left when walking.
Reflexes:

a. Deep tendon reflexes were asymmetrical, being slightly more active on the left than on the right.
b. Plantar responses were flexor. Abdominal reflexes were present bilaterally.
c. No release of grasp and suck reflexes had occurred.

Sensory system:

a. Pain, touch, and vibration were intact.
b. Position sense for fine amplitude movements at the fingers and toes was decreased on the left.
c. On simultaneous tactile stimulation of the left and right side, extinction of stimuli occurred on the left.
d. Errors were made in object identification in the left hand.
e. Occasional errors were made in the identification of numbers drawn on the fingers of the left hand.

Laboratory Data
The electroencephalogram and imaging studies now suggested a single lesion.

Questions

1. Localize the initial symptoms. In your consideration of the location of the lesion, you will wish to consider the localizing significance of the following: (a) the initial episodes of "vertical wavy lines"; and (b) the homonymous hemianopsia.
2. What is the nature of these initial symptoms?
3. Which areas were subsequently involved by the lesion? Take into account the pattern of findings on sensory examination.
4. What is the pathological nature of the lesion? Take into account the short duration of symptoms and the age of the patient.
5. Which diagnostic study would you perform?
6. How would you treat the seizures?
7. How would you manage the basic lesion?
8. Do the fundoscopic findings indicate acute or chronic papilledema?

CASE HISTORY 25.2

This 35-year-old, right-handed, white male had the onset of a sudden pins-and-needles sensation, which began in the left foot and then spread within a few seconds to involve the entire left side of the body, including the arm and the face. The total episode lasted for 8 minutes. Similar episodes then recurred once or twice weekly beginning most frequently on the left side of the face or tongue and less often on the left foot or hand. Four months later, the patient had a similar episode but fell to the floor with a loss of consciousness of several minutes duration during which observers reported some clonic movements of the left arm and leg. Neurological examination, lumbar puncture, and electroencephalogram at that time were reported as normal. The episodes were temporarily controlled with anticonvulsant medication, phenytoin (Dilantin), but then recurred with increasing frequency. At the time of hospital admission, 19 months after onset of symptoms, these episodes of numbness were occurring 3 to 4 times per day.

Past history: There was no history of significant head trauma. There was no family history of seizures.

Neurological Examination

Mental status: Orientation and memory were normal.

Cranial nerves: No abnormalities were present.

Motor system: No relevant findings were present. The patient had fallen during the secondarily generalized seizure, sustaining a fracture of the left humerus and dislocation at the left shoulder. Since that time he had a poor swing of the left arm due to limitation of left shoulder movement. A slight atrophy of the hypothenar eminence with some weakness in the ulnar distribution had also been present since that injury.

Reflexes: Deep tendon reflexes were symmetrical; plantar responses were flexor.

Sensory system: All modalities were intact except for errors in graphesthesia in the left hand.

Laboratory Data

1. *Skull X-rays:* The calcified pineal was shifted 4 to 5 mm compared to a shift of 2 mm in films obtained 1 year previously.
2. *Electroencephalogram:* Focal slow-wave activity of 4 to 6 Hz was present, consistent with focal damage.
3. *Cerebrospinal fluid:* Normal pressure and protein (21 mg/100 ml) were present.
4. The imaging studies were consistent with a single focal lesion.

QUESTIONS

1. Where is the lesion in terms of the origin of the seizure activity?
2. What are the possible pathological diagnoses? In answering this question, you should keep in mind that the patient is of middle age (35), the seizures are clearly focal, and there is a 19-month history. These facts alone, even without the confirmatory laboratory data, should lead to the differential diagnosis.
3. Which diagnostic study would you perform?
4. How would you treat the seizures?
5. How would you treat the basic lesion?

CASE HISTORY 25.3

A 66-year-old, right-handed, white widow developed changes in affect and lack of interest in her surroundings over a 1-month period. Although previously she had

been alert, caring for herself, doing her own shopping, and interested in her relatives, she now took to her bed and became disheveled in appearance. She would talk little if at all. She complained of a vague weakness in her legs, was unwilling to walk, but was able to walk to the bathroom without assistance.

Past history: A myocardial infarct had occurred 10 months previously. There was a 10-year history of Paget's disease involving the bones of the lower extremities.

Neurological Examination

1. *Mental status:*
   a. The patient was apathetic with a dull appearance.
   b. The patient was disoriented for person and time. She knew that she was in a hospital in the state of Massachusetts but did not know the city.
   c. She was unable to recall her birth date or to name any president. She could give no account of her illness.
   d. She was unable to add 5 and 5 and could not do multiplication or subtractions.
   e. She repeated 4 digits forward and none in reverse.
   f. Spontaneous speech was scanty but without a definite dysarthria or aphasia. She could name 3 out of 6 objects, could repeat 6 out of 6, and could read aloud 4 out of 6. She was able to perform slowly a two-step command. She was apparently unable to write.
2. *Cranial nerves:* II–XII were intact except that the left disk margin was blurred on funduscopic examination.
3. *Motor system:*
   a. No focal weakness was present.
   b. There was a variable resistance in both lower extremities described as "gegenhalten."
   c. The patient was very hesitant and very fearful of sitting, standing, or walking. There was some retropulsion (a tendency to fall backward when attempting to sit or walk). When she walked, her right foot appeared to be glued to the floor.
4. *Reflexes:*
   a. Deep tendon reflexes were symmetrical and active.
   b. An equivocal plantar response was present on the right; that on the left was flexor.
   c. Strong grasp reflexes were released at hands and feet. Visual and tactile suck reflexes were also released.
5. *Sensory system:*
   a. Pain, touch, and position sense were intact.
   b. There was a minor decrease in vibratory sensation at the toes, which may well have related to the patient's general nutritional status.

Laboratory Data

1. Sedimentation rate was elevated to 98 mm in 1 hour.
2. Skull X-rays: An osteolytic lesion (area of bone destruction) was present.
3. Lumbar spine X-ray: A suspicious, probably osteolytic lesion was seen in the body of the L1 vertebra.
4. Stool guaiac: A small amount of occult blood was present. Hematocrit and hemoglobin were normal. Rectal and proctoscopic examination revealed a firm mass at approximately 9 cm above the anus.
5. Electroencephalogram indicated a focal lesion having the quality of damage (continuous focal 2 to 4 Hz slow waves).
6. Imaging studies were consistent with a single focal lesion.
7. A lumbar puncture 3 weeks prior to admission had revealed pressure increased to 220 mm of cerebrospinal fluid and protein elevated to 59 mg/100 ml.

QUESTIONS

1. Where is the lesion? (Assume a single central nervous system lesion.)
2. What is the most likely pathology?
3. How would you manage this problem as regards more specific diagnosis and therapy? Which neuroimaging studies would you perform? In considering these questions, you will wish to keep in mind the following points:

   1. As regards the location of the lesion:
      a. The personality change, accompanied by impairment of all areas of mental function

b. The release of strong grasp reflexes in both upper and lower extremities, in addition to suck reflexes
   c. The apparent inconsistent findings as regards resistance to passive motion
   d. The disturbance of sitting posture and of gait.
2. As regards the type of pathology:
   a. The elevation of sedimentation rate
   b. The apparently rapid onset of symptoms
   c. The presence of occult blood in the stool
   d. The presence of osteolytic lesions
   e. The mass noted on examination of the rectum
3. Which diagnostic studies would you perform?

CASE HISTORY 25.4

On the evening prior to admission, his wife noted that this 62-year-old, right-handed, white male had the relatively sudden onset of slurred speech associated with a drooping of the left side of the face. The patient denied that these symptoms were present. The following morning he was examined by his brother, a physician, who confirmed the presence of slurred speech and weakness of the lower one-half of the left side of the face and also noted a weakness of the left arm and leg.

Past history: Gout had been present since age 20. He had sustained an apparent coronary artery occlusion in the past.

Neurological Examination
1. *General*: blood pressure: 130/80; pulse 85 and regular.
2. *Mental status*:
   a. The patient was oriented for time, place, and person.
   b. Memory for recent and remote events was intact. Immediate and delayed recall was intact.
   c. The patient could do simple calculations but had difficulty with more complex problems.
   d. These results may have been influenced by the fact that the patient demonstrated a marked impersistence in following commands. The patient was somewhat apathetic and yawned frequently during the examination. There was a flattening of mood.
   e. The patient denied that he had any particular problems requiring hospitalization. He denied illness and stated he was as healthy now as he had been 1 week prior to hospitalization.
   f. Abstract reasoning was intact, as tested in proverb interpretation (used abstract concepts).
   g. No aphasia was present.
   h. A distinct deficit in the construction of three-dimensional drawings was present.
3. *Cranial nerves*: All were intact except for:
   a. A significant left facial weakness of supranuclear type.
   b. An inconstant neglect of left field on simultaneous stimuli to left and right visual fields.
4. *Motor system*: Strength and gait were intact and cerebellar tests were negative.
5. *Reflexes*: Deep tendon reflexes were symmetrical, plantar responses were flexor, and no pathological grasp reflex was present.
6. *Sensory system*
   a. Pain and touch were intact.
   b. Stereognosis, two-point discrimination, and tactile localization were normal. However, position sense was decreased at toes and fingers on the left. There was a tendency to ignore tactile stimuli on the left face, arm, and leg when simultaneous left and right stimulation was carried out. Graphesthesia was intact in the right hand, but defective on the left.

Laboratory Data
1. Blood serological test for syphilis was negative.
2. Skull X-rays were normal.
3. Electroencephalogram: abnormal because of focal 2–5 Hz slow waves.
4. Brain scan (radioactive Hg^{197}): A diffuse focal uptake was present.

Subsequent course: Over the next 3 months, significant improvement occurred. The patient was able to do complex calculations. He had no difficulty in drawing or in locating points on a map. Sensory examination was normal. The patient still had difficulty in maintaining his concentration. Psychological testing now indicated verbal IQ of 123, performance IQ of 104, with full-scale IQ of 116, compared to much lower scores of 111, 87, and 101, respectively, at the time of his acute illness.

Questions
1. Where is the lesion (be specific)?
2. What is the nature of the lesion? If vascular, discuss the type of lesion and the vascular territory
3. Which studies should be performed (in terms of neuroimaging and nonneurological studies)?

CASE HISTORY 25.5

This 52-year-old housewife was referred for evaluation of episodic "twitching of the left thumb and forefinger" beginning 2 weeks prior to admission. The patient had noted the sudden onset of a numbness of the left thumb, followed in seconds by twitching of the left eyelid and then almost immediately by a twitching of the distal segment of the left thumb. This soon spread to the left forefinger, then to the middle finger, and then involved the hand in repetitive clonic movements. According to observers, the clonic movements then spread into the left arm. The twitching about the eyelid spread to the entire face. This initial episode lasted a total of 15 minutes; there was, however, a residual numbness of the left thumb and index finger: "as though they had fallen asleep." There was also a transient weakness of those areas first involved. Since the first episode, the patient had experienced minor recurrences of "tingling" of the left thumb and index finger.

Past history: Six years prior to admission the patient underwent a right radical mastectomy for carcinoma of the breast. Regional lymph nodes were reported as negative. The patient's mother and sister also had carcinoma of the breast with onset at an age similar to the patient.

Neurological Examination
1. *Mental status*: Intact with no evidence of aphasia. No deficits were noted in drawing.
2. *Cranial nerves*: A minimal left supranuclear central facial weakness was present.

3. *Motor system*: A mild weakness was present in the left upper extremity, and rapid alternating movements of the left hand were slowly performed.
4. *Reflexes*:
   a. Deep tendon stretch reflexes were increased on the left.
   b. An equivocal plantar response was present in the left; that on the right was flexor.
   c. No grasp reflex was present.
5. *Sensory system*:
   a. Pain, light touch, position, and vibration were normal.
   b. There was a slight disturbance in graphesthesia over the left hand and face. There was minor impairment of two-point discrimination over the left thumb and forefinger.

QUESTIONS

1. Indicate the location of the lesion in this case.
2. Indicate the most likely pathology and provide a differential diagnosis.
3. (a) Attach a label to the twitching which begin in the left thumb, then spread to the other fingers, then to left hand, arm, and face.
   (b) Attach a label to the transient weakness, which followed these episodes of twitching.
4. Which diagnostic studies would you perform?
5. Discuss management of this patient.

CASE HISTORY 25.6

This 19-year-old, right-handed, white, male pharmacy student was referred for evaluation of frequent minor seizures. At age 18 months, the patient had fallen and struck his head against a concrete floor; within hours he had lapsed into coma. Later that day he required emergency neurosurgical treatment at the Children's Hospital Medical Center in Boston for a "skull fracture and a bleeding vessel which the neurosurgeon had to tie."

The patient apparently made an excellent recovery. However, from 3 years of age until 5 years of age he experienced "large convulsions" (apparently generalized convulsive seizures). During this time he also experienced minor episodes characterized by the sensation that objects were becoming smaller or larger. The patient recalled that, at times, he had the sensation that bright geometric patterns were present and shrinking in size.

Almost invariably the patient experienced the sensation of fear with these episodes. The patient had no seizures from age 5 years until age 16 years. Since age 16, the patient had frequent minor episodes of several types occurring as frequently as 15 to 30 times a day. One type of episode was accompanied by dreamy sensations lasting a few seconds; at times things looked unreal. At the same time the patient would feel that the whole episode was somehow very familiar, that objects looked very familiar in a manner that could not be described. There was an accompanying sensation of fright. During such an episode the patient would be able to continue driving or walking.

A second type of episode, lasting 30 to 120 seconds, was characterized by an inability to talk properly, a babbling of speech, and an inability to understand speech. During this time a sensation of vague familiarity and fatigue and at times a sense of reincarnation would exist.

A third variety was characterized by the visual sensation of looking down a long dark corridor with a light at the other end. There was no concept of time: at times the corridor seemed to move from right to left. At the end of such an episode things would not look as they should; objects appeared distorted and color was altered. Objects were seen as black and white. The whole scene would seem unworldly. Sounds would be perceived but would fail to be registered and would not make sense.

Neurological Examination

Mental status, cranial nerves, motor-system reflexes, and sensory system were all intact except for a minimal lag of the left side of the face in smiling. During the examination, the patient had a minor episode; his head dropped and he appeared out of contact for 20 to 30 seconds. He did not answer questions directly but replied by saying, "What was then, what was that then, what was that then?" He was confused for several minutes, after the episode. He was subsequently amnestic for the events of the episode.

QUESTIONS

1. The electroencephalogram indicated a stable focus of discharge. Indicate the location of that focus.
2. Classify the seizures according to the International Classification of Seizures. Did he have simple partial, complex partial, or idiopathic (primary generalized) seizures/epilepsy?
3. What is the most likely explanation for the acute events, which occurred at age 18 months?
4. Why did seizures recur at age 16 years?

CASE HISTORY 25.7

This 20-year-old white male had been admitted to Boston City Hospital at age 9 months with acute right-sided hemiconvulsions associated with a fever. A right hemiplegia was present for several days and he continued to have a mild right hemiparesis. Several additional seizure episodes occurred between ages 1 and 3 years. No additional episodes occurred until age 17 when the patient had a focal seizure characterized by tonic posture of the right arm—abducted at the shoulder and flexed at the elbow—followed by turning of the head and eyes to the right. Consciousness was impaired but not completely lost. For several minutes the patient was unable to speak. Upon regaining speech, he was able to follow commands.

Treatment with anticonvulsants (Eskabarb, long-release form of phenobarbital) was relatively effective in preventing seizure recurrence.

Once a month the patient did experience a few seconds of "weakness or limpness" of the right hand with a possible small jerk of the right hand. Approximately 2 weeks before his initial office visit in January 1968, the patient discontinued his medications. Four days prior to this visit, at a time of sleep deprivation, the patient had a focal seizure with tonic movement of the right arm and deviation of the head and eyes to the right followed by a generalized convulsive seizure. Since age 9 months, residual weakness of the right arm had been present. However, language functions had developed and he had done well in school.

Neurological Examination

1. *General*: The patient was left-handed with long-standing smallness of the right side of the face, arm, and leg.
2. *Mental status*: All areas were intact with no aphasia.

3. *Cranial nerves:* All were intact except for a slight lag on the right in smiling.
4. *Motor system:*
   a. There was a mild weakness of the right upper extremity, most marked distally and particularly marked in the thumb.
5. *Reflexes:*
   a. Deep tendon reflexes were increased on the right.
   b. Plantar response was equivocal on the right.
6. *Sensory system:* Minor deficits were present in the right upper extremity characterized by errors in fine-movement perception of the right fingers and errors in graphesthesia of the right hand. Pain and touch were intact.

Subsequent course: With adjustment of anticonvulsant medication, excellent seizure control was attained. Only rare limited focal (partial) seizures occurred over the next 30 years.

Questions

1. Locate the lesion in terms of findings on the neurological examination.
2. What is the origin of focal (partial) seizures characterized by tonic posture of the right arm with deviation of the head and eyes to the right and with arrest of speech?
3. The patient has a right hemiplegia and yet he does not have aphasia. Explain.
4. In view of the acute onset of the hemiplegia at age 9 months and the subsequent lack of progression, speculate concerning the etiology.
5. Why was the weakness most prominent in the distal muscles of the upper extremity (particularly the thumb)?
6. Why did seizures recur?
7. Why has the smallness of the right side occurred?
8. What is the nature of the sensory deficit?
9. How would you manage the seizure problem?
10. Does the recurrence of seizures at age 17, after no seizures since age 3, indicate that a progressive pathology is present?

CASE HISTORY 25.8

This 23-year-old, right-handed, white male was admitted with chief complaints of frequent and increasing headaches and "seizures." The problem apparently began 15 months prior to initial evaluation, when several months after their marriage, the patient's wife noted a change in his personality. In particular, the patient no longer had any desire for sexual intercourse. He became more irritable, at times with only minimal provocation, and he was verbally and physically abusive. Eight months later (7 months prior to initial evaluation), he began to awake from sleep with a numb feeling on the right side of the lips, which quickly spread to the right side of face; it would last a few minutes and resolve. When the patient awoke during such episodes, he found himself sitting upright. These would occur weekly and only as the patient was going to sleep or after he had fallen asleep. After a few weeks the seizures changed in character. While sleeping, the patient would suddenly be thrown toward his right side, his head would arch back and he would have difficulty breathing. He would be aware during these episodes and could understand what people said, but he could not speak. Sometimes the patient would not be thrown to the side but would simply have tonic stiffening and claw-like formation of the right hand, lasting 20 to 30 seconds.

Two months later (5 months prior to evaluation) he underwent a right inguinal herniorrhaphy and had several attacks in the recovery room. Since that time, the patient has experienced one or two seizures per day, some of which occurred while awake. Because of these episodes, he was admitted to a local hospital for evaluation. EEG and lumbar puncture were reported to be normal. Following the lumbar puncture he developed a bifrontal headache. While sitting in a wheelchair, he began to complain of headaches. A nurse placed her hand on his forehead, and his wife told the nurse to get her hand off. According to other observers, he ran down the corridor, pushing the nurses aside, and ran into a wall. He had to be restrained by several people and was given some injections. Psychiatric treatment was begun with no significant improvement. Two months prior to evaluation, the patient's wife inquired of him whether the psychiatrist had been able to tell him anything about the cause of his episodes. He threw a jar of mustard at her, then the plates off of the dinner table. He rushed at her. As she retreated, he kept coming after her. He seemed unaware of his actions and did not seem to recognize her. He placed his hands about her throat and began to choke her. With difficulty, she managed to break free. She noted that he appeared dazed and sleepy. At this point, fearing for her life, the wife decided upon a divorce. The patient denied any memory for this episode. Intermittent bitemporal and bifrontal headaches began to increase in frequency. Occasionally, he had incontinence of urine and tongue biting during his severe nocturnal seizures, which now were occurring, on a daily basis.

Fifteen days prior to admission, the patient became angry at a dog that was barking outside the house. He ran outside to chase the dog, but he could not catch the dog and kicked the fence gate. This is the last he remembers. His girlfriend relates that the patient began punching the brick wall of the house and then began to bang his head forcibly against the wall, stopped, and fell on his back staring, whereupon his girlfriend helped him walk into the house. The patient next recollects the trip to the hospital, where lacerations of his hands were sutured and he was released.

Neurological Examination

On admission evaluation, this was entirely normal. Bilateral paresthesias of the hands were reproduced by hyperventilation.

Subsequent course: Eight months later, minor findings were present:

1. Mental status: He was anxious but affect was indifferent and passive.
2. Cranial nerves: A slight right central facial weakness was present
3. *Reflexes:* Deep tendon reflexes were slightly increased at right biceps, patellar, and Achilles. The right plantar response was equivocal.

Questions

1. What is the most likely explanation and anatomical basis for the episodes of directed aggression in this case?
2. How often does directed aggression occur as an ictal event as opposed to nondirected aggressive behavior during ictal (seizure) or postictal (altered consciousness after seizure) confusional states?
3. From the anatomical standpoint, what is the explanation for the change in personality?

4. What is the localization for the episodes of seizures while sleeping characterized by the following description: "the patient would suddenly be thrown toward his right side, his head would arch back, and he would note difficulty in breathing"?
5. What is the anatomical localization for the episodes of tonic stiffening and claw-like formation of the right hand?
6. What is the explanation for the initial episodes of tingling of the right side of face and lips?
7. How can you tie all of this together into a comprehensive diagnosis?
8. Discuss the possible underlying pathology and your diagnostic and therapeutic management.

26.

CEREBRAL HEMISPHERES

NEUROPATHOLOGY AND CLINICAL CORRELATION I. VASCULAR SYNDROMES

The course and nature of some of the more common diseases affecting the cerebral hemispheres are already familiar to the student on the basis of those case histories presented in the previous chapter on cortical localization. We will refer back to some of those case histories. However, we will not limit our discussion simply to the neocortex but will discuss the cerebral hemispheres in a more general sense. It will also be convenient at this point to consider several broad categories of diseases, not previously discussed, that do not necessarily restrict themselves to the cerebral hemispheres.

Diseases affecting the cerebral hemispheres account for the largest proportion of central nervous system diseases encountered in medical practice. These diseases may be focal or diffuse in nature. There is also a third or intermediate category of multifocal (that is, comprised of many focal events). Our major concern in this chapter will be with focal vascular disease.

VASCULAR SYNDROMES

VASCULAR DISEASES OF THE CEREBRAL HEMISPHERES

Vascular problems account for the largest category of diseases affecting the cerebral hemispheres. Cerebrovascular disease remains the third leading cause of death in the United States. The annual incidence is close to 300,000. Approximately 261,000 fall into the ischemic/occlusive/category and 36,000 into the category of intracerebral and subarachnoid hemorrhage. The overall mortality due to this cause has been falling due to (1) better control of hypertension, (2) better control of cardiac arrhythmias, (3) decreased incidence of rheumatic heart disease, (4) widespread use of statin drugs, and (5) decreased incidence of meningovascular syphilis. Several types must be considered: (1) atherosclerosis with ischemia due to stenosis and occlusion, (2) small infarcts (lacunar infarcts) due to hypertension, (3) embolism, (4) intracerebral hemorrhage, and (5) subarachnoid hemorrhage. These various categories are not mutually exclusive. Thus, occlusive vascular disease usually occurs in relation to the process of atherosclerosis—the deposition of fatty material (cholesterol) in the walls of arteries. However, emboli produce their effect essentially by sudden occlusion of cerebral arteries. Such emboli generally originate from clots within the chambers of the heart. At times, however, such embolic material has originated at an area of occlusive disease when atheromatous material or an overlying thrombus (clot) has broken loose to be carried into the more distal circulation. There is, on the other hand, an overlap between ischemic occlusive disease and intracerebral hemorrhage. Thus, certain areas of tissue damage resulting from ischemia may become hemorrhagic secondarily. The symptoms and signs, which then evolve, may resemble those of intracerebral hemorrhage. The use of angiography, computerized tomography (CT) scan, and magnetic resonance imaging (MRI) has allowed a more precise delineation of infarct versus hemorrhage but has left a group of patients for whom a specific cause of the infarct remains uncertain.

ISCHEMIC-OCCLUSIVE DISEASE

Within this category the subtypes indicated in Table 26.1 may be specified.

Earlier clinical and autopsy studies suggested a higher incidence of large or small vessel disease compared to embolic disease (see Adams et al., 1997).

Atherosclerosis involves the large- and medium-sized extracranial and intracranial portions of the cerebral arteries. With increasing deposition of fatty material at points of bifurcation or angulation, a progressive narrowing (stenosis) of the lumen occurs (Fig. 26.1). Eventually, at approximately 70%–75% stenosis, a decrease in cerebral blood flow through this point of narrowing in the vessel will occur (the actual relationship may be calculated according to Bernoulli's principle). The area supplied by this vessel may then at some point receive less than the required amount of blood (oxygen, glucose, and so forth). When this occurs, we may speak of cerebral ischemia. Kalamo (2005) outline the effects of decreased perfusion as follows: with a blood flow >40% of the normal value, normal spontaneous and evoked activities of nerve cells are still present. Between 30% and 40% of normal flow, neurons

Table 26.1 **TYPES OF ISCHEMIC-OCCLUSIVE DISEASE**

CAUSE OF ISCHEMIC-OCCLUSIVE DISEASE	PERCENT OF TOTAL CASES
1. Large vessel atherosclerosis	15% (internal carotid artery constitutes 9% of all ischemic)
2. Small vessel (lacunar)	9%
3. Embolic	Overall 60% (secondary to atrial fibrillation constitutes 15% of all ischemic)
4. Dissection and other causes	3%

Figure 26.1 Atherosclerosis of arteries in the circle of Willis at the base of the brain. (Courtesy of Drs. John Hills and Jose Segarra.)

are unable to produce sufficient energy to continue transmission of impulses. At <30 % of perfusion, transmission by the neuron no longer occurs, although the neuron is still viable. When perfusion falls below 15% of normal, membrane failure begins to occur. The transmembrane ion gradients are no longer maintained and extracellular potassium rises. Unless perfusion and energy production are restored, irreversible nerve cell damage will occur. Note that there is a zone adjacent to this focal area of damage referred to as the penumbra, where total failure has not yet occurred. This area represents tissue that could be saved by therapeutic measures.

The clinical correlates of this sequence of focal ischemia are as follows. A dysfunction of the involved ischemic area occurs with focal symptoms of weakness, numbness, and the like. This dysfunction may be only temporary in nature, or it may be prolonged with actual tissue death (infarction) and residual neurological deficit.

As progressive narrowing of the lumen occurs, eventually a point of total occlusion is reached. The narrowing of the lumen is, moreover, accentuated by several additional processes: (a) thrombus formation—the formation of a clot of platelets, fibrin, and blood cells due to stasis, change in intimal surface, and so forth; (b) ulceration of the intimal surface at the locus of the atherosclerotic surface at the locus of the atherosclerotic plaque; and (c) subintimal hemorrhage in relation to this area of deposition. The process of ulceration of the intimal wall may produce an originating site for emboli composed of the atheromatous material. Such an ulcerated intimal wall is a likely site of thrombus formation, producing additional stenosis. The study of Eliasziw et al. (1994) confirmed that plaque ulceration more than doubles the risk of stroke at higher degrees of stenosis. Fragments of the clot may also travel as emboli into the distal circulation.

We have used the joint term, *atherosclerotic ischemic occlusive vascular disease*, since there is no one-to-one relationship between actual occlusion of a vessel and tissue death (infarction or encephalomalacia) in the region supplied by that artery. Thus, total occlusion of a vessel may occur with or without the development of significant neurological symptoms and signs. There may be at times persistent symptoms and signs correlated with significant tissue destruction. At other times, with stenosis, there may be only episodes of transient symptomatology without actual tissue destruction. *These transient episodes, related to vascular insufficiency, are referred to as transient ischemic attacks.*

The several factors that account for this lack of close correspondence between the state of a particular artery and the vascular status of the region supplied by that vessel have already been covered in the earlier discussion of basilar vertebral ischemic/occlusive disease. (Refer also to Fig. 26.7.)

1. There are significant variations in the capacity of the circle of Willis to provide collateral circulation.

2. There are significant leptomeningeal anastomoses over the surface of the cerebral cortex between the anterior, middle, and posterior cerebral arteries of a given hemisphere. With regard to each cerebral artery, one may then speak of its area of central supply and its area of peripheral supply. This latter peripheral area usually receives also the peripheral supply of adjacent vessels and is in a sense a border zone or watershed.

3. To a variable degree, anastomoses are present between the external and internal carotid arteries.

4. Finally, a considerable variability occurs because of certain general systemic and metabolic factors. Thus, a narrowed vessel may still deliver sufficient blood when the systemic blood pressure is 190/100 but fails to do so when the blood pressure falls to 120/70 during sleep, on sudden standing after a long period of recumbency, and in relation to antihypertensive medications. Similarly, stenotic blood vessels may deliver a sufficient blood flow when metabolic conditions such as temperature, serum sodium, and glucose are normal, but this blood flow may fail to meet essential requirements when metabolic conditions have changed.

Infarction (Encephalomalacia)

It is appropriate at this point to briefly summarize the gross and microscopic changes, which occur when ischemia has been of a sufficient degree to produce tissue death. The neuropathologist generally distinguishes between pale and hemorrhagic infarction. Most infarcts following ischemia are "pale" and are not complicated by hemorrhage at a gross level. During the first 4 to 6 hours, no gross or microscopic changes are apparent. Between 8 and 48 hours, swelling of gray and white matter is noted; the white matter may appear somewhat granular.

After 48 hours the infarcted area feels soft and mushy; the descriptive term *necrosis* may be used. This state may be generally recognized by visual inspection. Over the next 10 days a decrease in swelling occurs. Through enzymatic processes, liquefaction occurs. By 3 weeks, in larger lesions a gross cavity begins to appear. Within a period of several months, all of the necrotic tissue is replaced by a fluid-filled cavity.

Advances in imaging studies have allowed for earlier detection of ischemia and infarction. (Refer to Shaeblitz and Fisher, 1999.) Perfusion imaging magnetic resonance imaging (MRI) studies will demonstrate decreased perfusion and presumably ischemia within 15 seconds. This ischemia may be reversible. This discrepancy between perfusion imaging and diffusion-weighted imaging allows the identification of tissue which is ischemic but is not yet infarcted, that is, the penumbra of potentially salvageable tissue around the infarct. This information is invaluable for assessing the patient for possible intra-arterial treatment either by intra-arterial administration of thrombolytics or using the ever-increasing number of cleverly designed devices to remove the clot (Ciccone et al., 2013).

This is similar to the older neurophysiologic test, the electroencephalogram, which when employed in the operating room during carotid endarterectomy will begin to detect the changes of ischemia within 10–15 seconds. Diffusion-weighted MRI studies may demonstrate differences between normal and ischemic presumably infarcted tissue within minutes to 1 hour. Standard MRI will detect the increased water content of infarcted tissue at 6–12 hours. Computerized tomography (CT) scans may also begin to detect early subtle changes related to changes in water content (some effacement of sulci and gyri) at 3–4 hours, although the clear-cut appearance of infarction is usually delayed until 18–24 hours (Kalamo 2005).

From the microscopic standpoint, indistinct staining of the neurons (which are more sensitive to anoxia than other elements, e.g., capillaries and glia) may be noted as early as 12 hours. Within 1 to 3 days, swelling, shrinkage, or alteration in the distribution of Nissl substance (chromatolysis) may be noted. Within 2 to 4 days disintegration of cells occurs. As these neuronal changes are developing, alterations are also occurring in the appearance of axons (swelling of myelin sheaths, poor staining, and disintegration) and of glial cells (swelling of astrocytes with fragmentation of processes).

While this process of necrosis is under way, various histological responses to the infarction are also taking place. Within 24 to 36 hours, the area of infarction is infiltrated by neutrophilic polymorphic leukocytes (the acute response cells). Within 24 hours of infarction, phagocytic cells (macrophages) begin to appear. These macrophages arise from various sources: microglia, blood vessel walls, and circulating blood cells. By 48 hours of infarction, macrophages, filled with fatty debris (from myelin and cell breakdown), are noted. These cells remain the predominant repair cell from the period 5 days to 30 days (Fig. 26.2). Some of these cells may be found years later at the edge of the infarct. If some hemorrhagic component has also been present, products from the breakdown of the blood may also be present in these cells. This removal of debris by the macrophages will eventually result in the appearance of the cavity that may be seen grossly.

Figure 26.2 Macrophage stage of reaction in an area of necrosis. Approximately 28 days after a hemorrhagic infarct of the brain stem. Many macrophages are filled with heme pigment. (H&E, 400×). (Courtesy of Dr. John Hills.)

At the same time that macrophages are removing the debris, the capillaries and astrocytes are beginning to engage in repair processes. Within several days to weeks after the infarct, new capillaries are noted at the edge of the lesion. There is also a thickening of the capillary walls with increased cellularity and the appearance of mesodermal fibrils in the adjacent tissue. There also occurs in this adjacent tissue a proliferation of astrocytes (first noted at 3 days) with the formation of reaction astrocytes containing large amounts of pink cytoplasm in H&E stains. There is a correlated proliferation of astroglial fibers. By 4 to 5 weeks a meshwork wall has been formed about the cavity by these mesodermal and glial fibers.

Hemorrhagic infarcts occur in 18%–48% of autopsy studies. Infarcts due to emboli are more likely to be hemorrhagic (51%–71% compared to nonembolic infarcts, 2%–21%). Venous infarcts are often hemorrhagic.

The syndromes associated with ischemic-occlusive disease of each of the arteries supplying the cerebral hemispheres will now be considered in greater detail.[1] The student, however, should interpret this material, keeping in mind those limitations of correlation that have been indicated earlier.

SYNDROMES OF THE MAJOR ARTERIES

Internal Carotid Artery

The carotid artery may be involved by atherosclerosis in its extracranial or intracranial portions. The most common location for stenosis in this system is at the origin of the vessel at

---

[1] At present, most cerebral vascular disease involves the arterial circulation. Disease of the venous circulation is now less common. In the preantibiotic era, infectious processes involving the face, paranasal sinuses, the mastoid, and middle ear could secondarily involve the venous sinuses and cortical veins.

the bifurcation of the common carotid artery into the internal and external carotid branches (Fig. 2.25). Another favorite location is at the carotid siphon. The branches of the internal carotid artery are in order as follows: the ophthalmic, posterior communicating, anterior choroidal, anterior cerebral, and middle cerebral. With stenosis of the internal carotid artery, a variable symptomatology and anatomical pattern of ischemia and infarction may develop (Fig. 26.3). The pattern and time course of the syndrome are dependent on the availability of collateral circulation. One may distinguish among transient ischemic attacks (TIAs), which last less than 24 hours with total recovery,[2] progressing strokes, incomplete or partial strokes, and completed total territory strokes. Transient ischemic attacks may be retinal or hemispheric and may be related to alteration in perfusion or to microemboli originating at the carotid bifurcation. This discussion will emphasize the perfusion etiology.

One syndrome involves the occurrence of repeated episodes of monocular blindness on the side of the involved carotid artery with or without the later development of hemispheric symptoms, for example, motor and sensory symptoms involving the contralateral extremities. The patient may describe a curtain descending over the field of vision of the involved eye. The episodes of monocular blindness are referred to as *amaurosis fugax*. In such cases, when symptoms are limited to monocular blindness, we may presume that there is ischemia predominantly in the ophthalmic artery distribution with the more distal carotid branches temporarily receiving adequate collateral supply from the posterior communicating and anterior communicating arteries and via leptomeningeal anastomoses over the cortical surface. With progression of the occlusive process, even this collateral supply may become inadequate and additional symptoms develop.

One of the common patterns of carotid artery insufficiency is the carotid border zone syndrome (Figs. 26.3 and 26.4). With decreased perfusion by the carotid artery, symptoms will initially develop in the upper extremity, which corresponds to the cortical border zone between the middle and anterior cerebral arteries.[3] As such, it receives some overlap supply from both the anterior and middle cerebral arteries. As perfusion pressure drops in the carotid artery due to severe stenosis, this border zone will be first affected and the patient will experience numbness and weakness involving the arm and hand.

With increasing stenosis and increasing ischemia, there will be involvement of the face with numbness and a supranuclear type weakness. If the ischemia involves the dominant hemisphere, an expressive aphasia will develop due to involvement of Broca's motor speech area. These symptoms indicate the progression to involvement of the more central cortical supply area of the middle cerebral artery. As a general rule, one may assume that carotid ischemia and infarction will occur predominantly over the areas of cerebral cortex within the peripheral and central supply area of the middle cerebral artery (Fig. 26.5). Involvement of the area supplied by the anterior cerebral artery is usually less marked since the anterior cerebral artery is more likely to receive a collateral supply via the anterior communicating artery and via leptomeningeal anastomoses over the corpus callosum from the opposite anterior cerebral artery. At times, however, both the middle and anterior cerebral areas will be involved and infarcted as in case 26.1. At times artery-to-artery embolization will occur involving primarily the middle cerebral artery.

Figure 26.3 Various types of the 40 infarcts in 52 cases of occlusion of carotid artery at autopsy. (*A*) Combined MCA and ACA territories: 37.5%. (*B*) Total MCA: 13%. (*B′*) Proximal MCA: –21%. (*C*) Watershed: 19%. (*D*) Terminal or deep border zone MCA/ACA: 5%. (Modified from Torvik, A., and Jorgensen, L.: J. Neurol. Sci., 3:415, 1966). ACA, anterior cerebral artery; MCA, middle cerebral artery.

Figure 26.4 Left carotid stenosis with old infarction predominantly within the border zone between anterior and middle cerebral arteries. This 72-year-old male had a persistent paralysis of the right upper extremity with defective position sense at fingers. (Courtesy of Drs. John Hills and Jose Segarra.)

---

[2] In reality, most TIAs are minutes in duration and rarely greater than 1 hour in duration. This has significance when the use of the thrombolytic agent recombinant tissue type plasminogen activator (t-PA) is considered, requiring a more realistic definition (see later). This agent must be administered within 3 to 4.5 hours of stroke onset.

[3] For additional discussion, refer to Bogousslavsky and Regli (1986). Note also that although the carotid anterior border zone syndrome may be relatively common as an insufficiency syndrome, actual infarction limited to the border zone alone is less frequent (Mounier-Vehier, 1995).

Figure 26.5 Total middle cerebral artery territory infarct after left carotid clamping and excision 8 months prior to death in a 62-year-old, left-handed male during a radical neck dissection. Patient progressed from a weakness of right hand grip, 8 hours after surgery, to a complete right hemiparesis with right central facial weakness and a mixed aphasia. Subsequently, recovery occurred in the lower extremity. He wrote jargon with his left hand and could copy but was unable to comprehend. (Courtesy of Drs. John Hills and Dr. Jose Segarra.)

Figure 26.6 Combined infarction anterior cerebral artery and middle cerebral artery territories related to severe stenosis of supraclinoid, internal carotid artery, and proximal (M1) segment of middle cerebral artery, with infarction territories of right anterior and middle cerebral arteries. Computerized tomography (CT) scan. Case 26.1. Refer to text.

CASE HISTORY 26.1

This 23-year-old, right-handed female on birth control pills, smoking one pack of cigarettes per day, on June 15, 1985, shortly after intranasal "snorting" of cocaine, complained of gradually increasing right-sided headache and then fell to the floor with a flaccid left hemiplegia with the head and eyes deviated to the right.

Neurological Examination

Mental status: The patient denied any illness and could not explain why she was in the hospital.

Cranial nerves: There was a left homonymous hemianopsia, deviation of head and eyes to the left, and a left central facial weakness.

Motor system: A flaccid left hemiparesis was present.

Reflexes: Deep tendon reflexes were initially depressed on the left side. Plantar responses were extensor bilaterally.

Sensory system: A severe left hemisensory deficit, with a neglect of the left side of space and body was present.

Initial clinical diagnosis: Total right middle cerebral artery territory infarct.

Laboratory Data

Initial CT scan demonstrated hypodensity (infarction in right frontal and parietal areas). *Right carotid angiogram* demonstrated severe stenosis of the supraclinoid segment of the right internal carotid artery with severe stenosis of the M-1 segment of the right middle cerebral artery and multiple areas of narrowing of the remainder of the right MCA. *Left carotid angiogram* indicated only limited cross filling of the distal right middle and anterior cerebral arteries.

On June 21, 1985, 6 days after admission, the previously alert patient suddenly developed a decreased level of consciousness and a fixed, dilated right pupil, suggesting that tentorial herniation had been produced by severe edema or hemorrhagic transformation of the infarct. CT scan now demonstrated massive infarction and edema of the right anterior and middle cerebral artery territories plus transtentorial and sub falx herniation (Fig. 26.6). With emergency management of the increased intracranial pressure (monitor and osmotic agents), the patient became more alert and was transferred to a rehabilitation facility.

The following case histories indicate additional patterns of disease in patients with stenotic-occlusive disease of the carotid artery. In both cases the disease was in the extracranial portion of the vessel; thus, an opportunity for surgical correction of the stenotic lesion was presented. Of course, similar symptoms could have occurred with disease of the intracranial portion of the carotid artery, for example, with stenosis at the siphon. However, in evaluating patients presenting these symptoms, the student should remain alert to the possibility that surgically remedial disease is present. The aim should be recognition of such disease when insufficiency symptoms alone are present, that is, prior to the development of actual infarction. It also should be noted that in some cases no premonitory symptoms will be present, but the patient will present with a completed stroke instead of a transient ischemic attack. A patient with carotid TIAs is presented in Case 26.2.

CASE HISTORY 26.2

This 54-year-old, right-handed, white male for 7 years had experienced twice per month, intermittent, 30- to 60-second episodes of blurring and blacking out of vision in the left eye. Ten days prior to admission, the patient had a 45-minute episode of minor weakness of the right face, arm, and leg plus numbness of the right side of the face accompanied by a transient difficulty in speech (possibly dysarthria, possibly difficulty in word finding). The patient's mother died of a "stroke" at age 66 years, and his father, of heart disease at age 57.

General physical examination: Blood pressure elevated to 160/100 in both arms. Bruits (murmurs) were present over each carotid artery. The retinal artery pulsation was easily obliterated by pressure on the globe of the left eye. Peripheral pulses in the lower extremities were poor.

Neurological examination: Intact except for a minor right central facial weakness.

Clinical diagnosis: Left carotid transient ischemic attacks.

Laboratory data: Cholesterol was elevated to 284 mg%. *Arteriography (aortic arch study)* demonstrated a complete occlusion at the origin of the left internal carotid artery. A *right brachial arteriogram* demonstrated excellent collateral circulation with filling of the left anterior and middle cerebral arteries by cross flow through the anterior communicating artery from the right side. The intracranial portion of the left internal carotid artery filled from the left posterior communicating artery.

Subsequent course: A left carotid endarterectomy performed by Dr. Allan Callow restored blood flow following removal of the occlusive lesion (atherosclerosis with recent thrombosis) at the carotid bifurcation.

In general, carotid TIAs are more likely than vertebral basilar TIAs to proceed to completed strokes. Patients with hemispheric attacks that present with hemiplegia are more likely to proceed to completed strokes than those patients with transient monocular blindness. Cumulative risk for infarct after hemispheric carotid TIAs was 27% compared to 14% for monocular blindness-carotid TIAs. In general, most patients will experience the stroke after one or two transient ischemic attacks. Multiple TIAs over a long period of time are much less likely to result in completed strokes.

Not all patients with carotid TIAs are found to have significant (>75%) stenosis or occlusion of the internal carotid artery. Pessin et al. (1977) found that only 52% of 95 patients with carotid TIAs had significant stenosis (42% if hemispheric, 58% if transient monocular blindness, and 80% if both types). The explanation for TIAs in patients with less than significant stenosis of the carotid artery is not certain. Emboli from ulcerated plaques; emboli from other sources such as the heart (or aortic arch) or micro platelet; and fibrin emboli have all been suggested as possible explanations (see also Amarenco et al., 1992).

The use of the antiplatelet agent aspirin has been effective in reducing both strokes and myocardial infarctions in patients with TIAs by 22%.

A current approach to the management of carotid TIAs is to promptly image the extracranial carotid arteries with ultrasound-Doppler (Duplex scan),[4] magnetic resonance angiography (MRA), or CT angiography to assess the anatomical and flow status within the vessel. If significant stenosis (>70%–75%) is found at the carotid bifurcation in the neck, then MRA or classical angiography followed by endarterectomy is undertaken. In many centers, the initial noninvasive study is the MRA, eliminating the need for both the duplex scan and the angiography. The role of carotid endarterectomy in patients with severe carotid stenosis of 70%–99% and TIAs or non-disabling strokes was clearly established by the randomized North American Symptomatic Carotid Endarterectomy Trial, Moore et al. (1995) and emphasized by the long-term follow-up of these patients (Barnett et al., 1998).

If significant stenosis is not present, then the patient is often treated with both aspirin and clopidogrel for 3 weeks and then aspirin alone. Recent evidence shows that short term use of both antiplatelet agents in small strokes (The SPS3 Investigators, 2012) is associated with a better outcome following a stroke but their long-term use is no better than aspirin alone; indeed, there were more deaths in the group on long-term treatment with both drugs. Many centers are following this protocol in TIA patients as well while awaiting definitive data. Most centers would also place such a patient on statin treatment. Statins appear to improve the outcome in acute stroke as well as reduce the occurrence of stroke and other vascular events over the long term (Flint et al., 2012). Very rarely if the patient remains symptomatic, is not a candidate for surgery, and has trickle flow in the vessel, then anticoagulation with Warfarin derivatives may be considered (see Whisnant and Wieber, 1987). Such therapy, however, is not without risks. The risk of bleeding complications with anticoagulation is greater than with the use of antiplatelet agents.

Since the nineties there has been increasing interest in treating carotid disease by stenting, and this work is continuing but at the present time stenting is associated with an increased frequency of strokes. Stent treatment at this time is usually reserved for people with severe carotid disease who are unable to undergo surgery.

In Caucasians,[5] most symptomatic lesions of the carotid artery occur at the bifurcation of the carotid artery in the neck. In non-Caucasians, intracranial lesions increase in frequency. If attacks persist, angiography may be undertaken to document intracranial lesions before embarking on long-term anticoagulation.

In addition, the absence of a significant extracranial lesion should raise the possibility of a source of multiple emboli from cardiac or other sources (see later).

If total occlusion of the artery is demonstrated, several courses of action have been suggested:

a. Emergency removal of an acute thrombus; for example, if progression is occurring. This may be complicated by intracerebral hemorrhage, particularly if infarction has already occurred and blood flow is restored into infarcted tissue (Piepgras et al., 1988).
b. External carotid to internal carotid artery bypass. This has been found to be of little value (EC-IC Bypass Study Group, 1985).

Controversy exists as to the management of the patient with the asymptomatic carotid artery bruit or with asymptomatic carotid artery stenosis. In the past, many of these patients with no neurological symptoms or with symptoms unrelated to the specific carotid artery were unnecessarily subjected to carotid artery surgery with accompanying morbidity and mortality of that procedure (see Norris and Zhu, 1990). The study of Freischlag et al. (1992) does suggest a definite role for the procedure where the degree of stenosis is over 75% and where perioperative morbidity and mortality are low (<3%). The study of Chambers and Norris (1986) had previously demonstrated that asymptomatic patients with a stenosis of >75% had an ipsilateral stroke rate of more than 10% per year. The editorial of Kistler and Furie (2000) discusses the effects on both low flow and the formation of thrombus leading to embolic phenomena that follow upon stenosis. The results of randomized trials of patients with asymptomatic carotid artery stenosis suggest that severe stenosis (>90%) may benefit from surgery

---

[4] Refer to Hennerici et al. (1992) for a discussion of the technique.

[5] The effects of race and ethnicity on ischemic stroke are discussed by Ethnic Disparities in Stroke. Stroke. 2005. 36:374–386.

but leave unsettled the question of whether lesser degrees of stenosis (50%–90%) may benefit (Barnett, 1993; Barnett & Haines 1993; The CASANOVA Study Group, 1991; Mayberg and Winn, 1995).

The following demonstrates a case in which the patient began with carotid TIAs, progressed to a carotid border zone syndrome of infarction, and then involved additionally all of the middle cerebral artery territory.

CASE HISTORY 26.3 (PATIENT OF DR. THOMAS MULLINS)

This 72-year-old, right-handed white male had two episodes of right upper extremity weakness, each of 2 hours duration, beginning 2 days prior to admission. Following the first episode, the patient had transient slurring of speech, persistent left-right disorientation, dysgraphia, and could not understand what he had read.

Neurological examination: *The only findings related to language function:* Speech was fluent with intact repetition and object naming; however, reading comprehension, writing, and left-right orientation were all impaired. *Carotids:* A bruit was present on the left.

Clinical diagnosis: Carotid artery stenosis with TIA reflecting decreased perfusion in the border zone followed by thrombosis and passage of emboli to the inferior division of the middle cerebral artery.

Laboratory data: *Arteriograms:* (a) the left internal carotid artery was completely occluded just above the bifurcation (Fig. 26.7A). (b) The left external carotid artery filled the left internal carotid artery at the siphon through anastomoses about the orbit (Fig. 26.7B). However, there was a cutoff just below the siphon, suggesting that the thrombus (clot) at the bifurcation had extended to this level. Moreover, the left middle and anterior cerebral arteries failed to fill in this manner. (c) The left posterior cerebral artery did originate from this segment of the otherwise occluded carotid siphon segment but with no retrograde filling into the basilar artery (Fig. 26.7B). (d) The right carotid artery filled not only the right middle cerebral and anterior cerebral artery but also was the source of the right posterior cerebral artery (Fig. 26.7C). (e) The right carotid system also supplied the left anterior cerebral artery and to a limited extent the left middle cerebral artery (Fig. 26.7D).

Subsequent course: On the day following admission, weakness in the right hand at wrist and finger extensors recurred. During the arteriogram, the patient was noted to have additional problems with speech. Weakness in the right upper extremity increased. Despite subsequent anticoagulation, additional progression occurred with total paralysis of the right upper extremity, aphasia, and a right homonymous hemianopsia. The CT scan, which had been normal on admission now, 72 hours after these events, demonstrated acute infarction with severe edema involving the entire cortical and deep territory of the middle cerebral artery and the cortical territory of the posterior cerebral artery but with relative sparing of the anterior cerebral artery territory and most of the thalamic territory of the posterior cerebral artery (Fig. 26.8). Coma developed secondary to the herniation effects on the brain stem and the patient expired 8 days after admission.

Such massive swelling with herniation of temporal lobe through tentorium and secondary brainstem compression is the major acute cause of death in patients dying after acute carotid artery or massive middle cerebral artery infarctions (31%). Other causes of death are pneumonia (29%), cardiac arrest (17%), and pulmonary embolus (13%).

Not all patients with acute carotid infarcts continue to progress. In the series of Jones and Milliken (1976), 39% of patients remained stable. Thirty-five percent had gradual improvement and 19% had a progressing deficit over 48 hours.

Middle Cerebral Artery

The middle cerebral artery is the final branch and, in a sense, the direct continuation of the internal carotid artery. One of

Figure 26.7 Internal carotid artery occlusion at the bifurcation. Transient ischemic attacks with subsequent infarction of middle and posterior cerebral artery territories. Case 26.3 (refer to text.) (*A* and *B*) Left carotid injection (*A*) occlusion of left internal carotid just above the bifurcation. (*B*) External carotid anastomotic branches (periorbital, etc.) allow late filling of the left internal carotid artery at the siphon and its branches. (*C* and *D*) Right carotid injection. (*C*) Lateral view: posterior cerebral artery originates from carotid artery; (*D*) anteroposterior view: cross filling of the left anterior cerebral artery and limited filling of the left middle cerebral artery (arrow).

Figure 26.8 Case 26.3 as in Figure 26.7. Computerized tomography (CT) scan obtained 72 hours after acute massive progression 9B demonstrating infarction and massive edema of the left middle cerebral artery territory and the cortical territory of the posterior cerebral artery, with sparing of the anterior cerebral artery.

the classic internal carotid artery syndromes is essentially a syndrome of the cortical branches of the middle cerebral artery.

Depending on the point of occlusion of the middle cerebral artery and its branches, several syndromes are possible. Essentially these syndromes reflect disease of the lenticulostriate penetrating branches or the cortical branches. In some cases, the clinical picture reflects involvement of the territory of both penetrating and cortical branches due to occlusion at the stem or main trunk of the artery.

Syndrome of the Lenticulostriate Penetrating Branches

The lenticulostriate penetrating branches supply the putamen, most of the caudate nucleus, the outer segments of the globus, pallidus, and most of the adjacent internal capsule (particularly the anterior half of the posterior limb). These vessels ascend with no anastomotic loops between adjacent branches. The classic clinical picture associated with occlusion of these branches is that of the pure motor syndrome, relatively rapid in onset, involving equally the face, arm, and leg in a spastic hemiplegia (so-called capsular hemiplegia). As discussed by Fisher and Curry (1965), there are often no sensory symptoms and no aphasia. These hemiplegic symptoms, reflecting capsular damage, tend to predominate initially over any symptoms related to the basal ganglia, although portions of the basal ganglia may also be infarcted. If the lesion is small (<1.5 cm) termed a *lacune*, the patient may demonstrate a rapid improvement, so that within weeks or months, there is little if any residual motor disability. However, with multiple lacunes, deficits may persist (Fig. 26.9). As indicated in Figure 26.10, however, larger infarcts involving the lenticulostriate territory may result in a

Figure 26.9 Lacunar Infarcts in middle cerebral artery penetrating branch territories. (*A*) Multiple small infarctions in a 71-year-old hypertensive (210/116) who after multiple episodes of right hemiparesis and dysarthria and "dizzy spells" became wheelchair bound, with apraxia of lips, limbs, and gait; and pseudobulbar, bilateral pyramidal and frontal release signs. (*B*) Detail of a small lacunae from a 48-year-old white male, with severe hypertension (250/140). (Courtesy of Drs. John Hills and Dr. Jose Segarra.)

persistent spastic hemiplegia with considerable motor deficits, and symptoms may include sensory and other features.

The basic pathological process has been termed *segmental fibrinoid arterial degeneration* (Fisher, 1969). The walls of these small vessels become thickened and converted into a hyalinized material. Usually but not invariably, this occurs on a background of long-standing hypertension. At times, diabetes mellitus is present. The lenticulostriate branches rising as the initial branches of the middle cerebral artery are under relatively high pressure; not only may these vessels become occluded, they may be the site of small or large intracerebral hemorrhages, also complicating the process of hypertension. We shall have cause to discuss these vessels again later in this chapter. However, not all patients with lacunar infarcts have hypertension, atherosclerosis, or diabetes mellitus, and at autopsy not all patients demonstrate the specific changes in penetrating vessels noted by Fisher (1969). Other disease processes may certainly affect the penetrating vessels and

Figure 26.10 Lenticulostriate penetrating branches of the middle cerebral artery. This 73-year-old hypertensive had at age 53 sustained a right hemiplegia with persistent and dense motor deficits involving the right central face, arm, and leg. (*A*) Coronal section; (*B*) close-up of the cavity. (Courtesy of Drs. John Hills and Jose Segarra.)

Table 26.2 SYNDROMES OF PENETRATING BRANCHES OF CEREBRAL VESSELS

PENETRATING ARTERY SYNDROME	LOCATION OF OCCLUSION
Pure motor syndrome of hemiplegia	Penetrating middle cerebral artery supply to internal capsule, less often basilar pontine paramedian arteries
Pure hemisensory	Posterior cerebral penetrating branches to ventral posterior lateral nucleus of thalamus or penetrating middle cerebral arteries to medial border of the posterior limb of the internal capsule
Dysarthria and clumsy hand syndrome	Paramedian penetrating branches supplying the pons
Ataxic hemiparesis	Infarcts of the corona radiata and less often the posterior limb of the internal capsule-posterior limb (both middle cerebral artery penetrators) and to a minor degree, the pons (basilar-paramedian-penetrating)
Hypesthetic-ataxic hemiparesis	Infarction of the posterior limb (posterior medial segment) of the internal capsule and lateral thalamus (anterior choroidal artery). Less often the posterior cerebral artery penetrating branches are involved.
Hemichorea-hemiballism	Infarction of the subthalamus or thalamus penetrating branches of postcerebral artery or lateral putamen of the striatum (penetrating branches of the middle cerebral artery (see Chapter 19)
"Silent strokes" to clinical history.	Found on computerized tomography or magnetic resonance imaging scan unrelated
Caudate infarcts producing slow state or hyperactive restless state	Lesion in caudate with extension to anterior limb internal capsule perforators proximal anterior or apathetic (abulic) middle cerebral artery

these include the following: (a) small emboli originating in the heart or arteries; (b) the arteritis of meningovascular syphilis (Johns et al., 1987); (c) the arteritis of tuberculous meningitis; (d) the vasculitis of autoimmune diseases such as polyarteritis and lupus erythematosus. Suggest that hypertension and diabetes are more related to multiple as opposed to single lacunar infarcts.

Other Types of Penetrating Branch Infarct, So-Called Lacunar Syndromes

A number of additional syndromes have been identified in the subsequent studies of Fisher and other investigators (Fisher, 1982; Mohr, 1982). These syndromes of penetrating branches of various blood vessels are outlined in Table 26.2.

Although many of these aforementioned lesions can be demonstrated on CT scans, MRI is the most effective technique for confirming localization (Fig. 26.11) (see Larson et al., 1988; Rothcock et al., 1987).

Lacunar State: Over time, some patients have multiple infarcts involving multiple penetrating branches. The patient then begins to manifest a typical clinical syndrome that has been assigned the diagnosis of "lacunar state," based on the findings at the time of pathological examination of multiple small cavities (Figs. 26.9 and 26.11). The patient begins to manifest an apraxia of gait, and a release of grasp reflex occurs as a result of damage to the descending fibers from the premotor areas. Clinical findings associated with disease of the basal ganglia may develop: rigidity and a slowness of movement and, rarely, a minor degree of tremor. These symptoms may reflect the damage to the putamen and globus pallidus or, perhaps, damage to the descending fibers from the premotor areas. This aspect of the syndrome has sometimes been designated as "arteriosclerotic Parkinson's disease" and can usually be distinguished from the classical Parkinson's disease (refer to Chapters 18 and 19). There may be a variable degree of cognitive dysfunction with considerable rigidity in problem solving, a loss of inhibition of emotional responses, and impairment of executive function. Often the patients appear apathetic and are misdiagnosed as manifesting dementia or depression. Subcortical infarcts involving descending frontal systems are responsible.

Syndromes of the Cortical Branches

After providing a series of lenticulostriate branches, the main stem of the middle cerebral artery divides into two main

Figure 26.11 Multiple lacunar infarcts most prominent in penetrating branches of left posterior cerebral artery: thalamus, posterior one-third corpus callosum, and adjacent white matter of left posterior cerebral hemisphere in a 70-year-old, right-handed hypertensive male with multiple episodes of "collapse," possibly related to severe orthostatic changes. (*A*) Magnetic resonance imaging (MRI), T1-weighted sagittal section 12.6 mm left of midline. (*B*) MRI, horizontal section.

cortical divisions: a superior division and an inferior division. At the point of division, the smaller lateral orbital frontal and temporal polar arteries originate. The superior division has pre-rolandic branches (to inferior frontal gyrus and premotor area including Broca's area in dominant hemisphere), Rolandic branches (to pre- and postcentral gyri), and anterior parietal branches (to postcentral gyrus). The inferior division includes anterior temporal, posterior parietal, angular, and posterior temporal branches, named after the areas supplied. The syndrome that results from occlusion will depend on whether the main cortical stem, the superior or inferior division, or the branches thereof have been involved (see Figs. 26.12 and 26.13). In general, the MCA cortical syndromes are assumed to be embolic in origin, particularly in the Caucasian population. The stem, divisions, and the cortical branches of the left middle cerebral artery are a frequent site for the lodgment of embolic material because there is a relatively direct vertical takeoff of the left common carotid artery from the arch of the aorta compared to the right carotid artery. In addition, the middle cerebral artery is the direct continuation of the internal carotid artery; the cortical branches are the direct continuation of the main middle cerebral trunk.

As noted earlier, infarcts may occur due to carotid disease often due to artery-to-artery emboli.

Occlusion of the main cortical stem produces a mixed cortical motor-sensory syndrome involving the contralateral face (supranuclear) and arm; this is termed a *faciobrachial paralysis*. If this occurred in the dominant hemisphere, a mixed type of aphasia would also be present with anterior (nonfluent) and posterior (fluent) components. Face and language involvement would be greater than hand involvement. The degree to which the hand is involved would depend on the degree of collateral circulation. Thus, only the central cortical territory or the entire cortical territory of the middle cerebral artery could be involved.

Occlusion of the superior division in the dominant hemisphere would produce a mixed cortical motor-sensory syndrome involving again predominantly the face and hand plus an expressive Broca's type aphasia. This syndrome has already been illustrated in Chapter 24.

The less frequently encountered occlusion of the inferior division branches produces dominant or nondominant inferior parietal-posttemporal syndromes, including the syndromes of posterior type aphasias and parietal neglect, already discussed in Chapter 24. Refer also to Marler et al., 1986.

Figure 26.12 Acute hemorrhagic infarction of the central cortical territory of the middle cerebral artery: calcific embolus occluded middle cerebral artery following atheromatous occlusion of the carotid artery at the bifurcation. This 74-year-old, right-handed, white male, 5 days prior to death, had the sudden onset of pain in the left supraorbital region and lost consciousness. Upon regaining consciousness, the patient had a right central facial weakness, a right hemiparesis, and was mute but was transiently able to follow commands. (Courtesy of Drs. John Hills and Jose Segarra.)

Figure 26.13 Cortical branches of the middle cerebral artery. Old infarcts involving much of the total cortical territory of the right middle cerebral artery. This 72-year-old, right-handed male with severe hypertension and auricular fibrillation expired after a 3-year history of at least four episodes of left central facial weakness and left hemiplegia involving primarily the arm and a focal seizure involving the left arm. (Courtesy of Drs. John Hills and Jose Segarra.)

Combined Syndrome: Total Occlusion of Initial Segment of Middle Cerebral Artery (Fig. 26.5). The resultant syndrome in this case will be the summation of the lenticulostriate and cortical branches syndrome. The following case history illustrates such an occlusion with massive infarction of the entire territory of the middle cerebral artery.

CASE HISTORY 26.4

This 61-year-old, right-handed, hypertensive black housewife 1 week prior to admission suddenly fell to the floor while taking a bath and lost consciousness. She was found by her son, who noted that she was unable to move her left arm and leg. Her speech had been thick, but no aphasia had been present. No headache had been noted. Both parents had died of heart disease and hypertension.

Physical examination: Blood pressure was 150/100 and pulse was regular at 84.

Neurological Examination

Mental status: The patient was obtunded and slow to respond but grossly oriented to time, place, and person.

Cranial nerves: Papilledema was present bilaterally, particularly in the right fundus, where a recent hemorrhage was present. The head and eyes were deviated to the right. The eyes did not move to the left on command but did move to the left on vestibular stimulation. The patient neglected stimuli in the left visual field. Pain sensation was decreased or neglected on the left side of the face. A marked left central facial weakness was present.

Motor system: A complete flaccid paralysis of the left arm and leg was present.

Reflexes: Deep tendon reflexes were increased on the left compared to the right. The left plantar response was extensor.

Sensory system: All modalities of sensation were decreased on the left side of the body.

Clinical diagnosis: Acute occlusion of the stem of the middle cerebral artery, possibly embolic, although primary occlusions of intracranial arteries may occur in the non-Caucasian population. Hypertensive intracerebral hemorrhage was also possible.

Laboratory data: The electroencephalogram (EEG) indicated severe focal damage with a relative absence of electrical activity in the right temporal area and focal 3 to 5 Hz slow waves most prominent in the right frontal area (Fig. 2.21 and CD EEG atlas). Radioactive brain scan demonstrated a marked right hemisphere uptake of isotope (Hg^{197}) measuring 11 x 6 x 6 cm, extending from the right frontal area to the posterior parietal area that extended from the surface to the deep midline. Right brachial arteriogram revealed a complete occlusion of the right middle cerebral artery at its origin. Cerebrospinal fluid contained no significant cells.

Hospital course: The patient showed no significant improvement during a 4-week hospital course. Prognosis for survival during the acute state of the first week depends on the degree of edema. In patients with massive middle cerebral artery territory infarcts due to MCA occlusion who already had early CT scan evidence of brain swelling within 24 hours of the ictus, 55% of these patients expired, overwhelmingly of herniation effects. Patients older than 45 years had a poorer prognosis than younger patients. Infection of the lungs is a serious complication of large infarcts and a major cause of death during the second week. If the patient survives, prognosis for recovery is related to the size of infarct. Less than 3 cm infarcts may be associated with a good recovery, and greater than 3 cm, with severe disability (Jorgensen et al., 1995).

Anterior Cerebral Artery

In our clinical experience, occlusive disease of the anterior cerebral artery is much less common than that involving the internal carotid or middle cerebral arteries, which account for approximately 1.8% of all ischemic infarcts (Bogousslavsky and Regli, 1990). The anatomical explanation for this is evident. Each anterior cerebral artery receives collateral circulation from several possible sources: (a) leptomeningeal anastomotic end-to-end loops from the middle cerebral artery of the same side, (b) leptomeningeal anastomotic loops from the contralateral anterior cerebral artery over the corpus callosum, and (c) anterior communicating artery from the contralateral anterior cerebral artery. Finally, at postmortem examination atherosclerotic plaques are found less frequently in the anterior cerebral than in the larger internal carotid, middle cerebral, basilar, and vertebral arteries. In the series of Bogousslavsky and Regli (1990), 63% of the 27 patients had infarcts secondary to an embolus from the heart or carotid artery.

Penetrating and cortical branches may be distinguished. *The penetrating branches*, including a larger vessel, the recurrent artery of Heubner, supply the anterior limb of the internal capsule and the anterior head of the caudate nucleus. *The cortical branches*—orbital frontal, frontal polar, callosal marginal, and pericallosal—supply much of the corpus callosum (genu and body), the orbital frontal cortex, and the medial aspects of the frontal and parietal lobes, including the sensory motor areas of the paracentral lobule and the supplementary motor cortex. Symptoms then when they occur will be most severe in the contralateral lower extremity with minor involvement of the contralateral supper extremity and minor or no involvement of the face. Most patients will have involvement of both the cortical and penetrating branch-subcortical territories. Infarcts limited to the penetrating branch territories may occur (Caplan et al., 1990). Note that not all vascular syndromes with predominant leg involvement are due to occlusion of the anterior cerebral artery. Occlusion of the superior sagittal sinus or basilar-vertebral disease affecting the brain stem may also produce predominant leg weakness (refer to Schneider and Gautier, 1994, for additional discussion).

At times both anterior cerebral arteries may be essentially branches of the same proximal segment. Occlusion of this proximal anterior cerebral artery segment will then result in infarction of the medial frontal-parietal areas of both hemispheres (Fig. 26.14). The resultant syndrome will include a more prolonged change in personality and affect (due to involvement of the prefrontal and anterior cingulate areas), an akinetic and mute state (Freeman, 1971) (due to involvement of the prefrontal and premotor areas), urinary incontinence (due to involvement of the para-central lobule, medial premotor, and supplementary motor areas), and a sensory motor syndrome involving both lower extremities (due to involvement of paracentral lobule). There may also be a significant apraxia of the nondominant hand from damage to the corpus callosum, depriving the premotor and motor areas in the nondominant motor hemisphere of information from the dominant hemisphere. A bilateral release of the grasp reflex is present because of the bilateral involvement of the premotor and supplementary motor areas. Many of these features may follow unilateral infarction to a lesser degree. Transient mutism and transcortical motor aphasia are more prominent with dominant hemisphere infarcts; neglect syndromes, with nondominant infarcts. Release of instinctive grasp is usually contralateral to the infarct. An example of infarction in the distribution of the anterior cerebral arteries complicating aneurysm surgery is provided in case 26.9.

Anterior Communicating Artery

Penetrating branches from this vessel supply the anterior hypothalamus, the optic chiasm, and the suprachiasmatic and paraolfactory areas.

Anterior Choroidal Artery

This is the only branch of the internal carotid artery that has not yet been discussed. This vessel supplies the inner portion of the globus pallidus, a small adjacent section of the posterior limb of the internal capsule (including the area occupied by the ansa and fasciculus lenticularis) and to a variable degree the adjacent sector of the ventral posterior lateral nucleus of the thalamus and of the lateral geniculate or geniculocalcarine tract. Various clinical results may follow occlusion of this vessel. There is no single characteristic syndrome. The initial surgical procedures of Cooper indicated that occlusion of this vessel in the patient with Parkinson's disease as discussed in Chapter 19 resulted in a relief of tremor and rigidity in the contralateral limbs without the development of hemiparesis or other focal deficits. Foix in 1925 first described a triad of hemiplegia, hemianesthesia, and homonymous hemianopsia associated with infarction of the territory of the anterior choroidal artery (Bruno et al., 1989). With the development of CT scan and MRI scan, the syndrome is now more frequently recognized. Essentially this is a variable penetrating or lacunar syndrome ranging from a pure motor syndrome to the full-blown triad.

Posterior Cerebral Artery

The posterior cerebral arteries usually originate as the direct continuation of the basilar artery following its bifurcation (Fig. 26.15). At times, then, occlusive disease of the vertebral or basilar artery will be manifested by the development of symptoms within the posterior cerebral territory. At times, a mixture of brain stem and cerebral hemisphere symptoms will be present. At times, bilateral posterior cerebral artery symptoms will be present. Moreover, since the cortical and penetrating vessels of the posterior cerebral artery are the distal branches of the basilar vertebral circulation, they will at times be subject to embolization from extracerebral sources (cardiac) or from occlusive disease in the more proximal sections of the basilar or vertebral arteries. As demonstrated previously in some patients (25%), the cortical divisions of the posterior

Figure 26.14 Anterior cerebral arteries: old bilateral infarcts due to severe bilateral stenosis anterior cerebral artery (complete occlusion on right). Left hemisphere involvement was marked (*A*), with a lesser involvement of the right hemisphere (*B*). This 61-year-old, right-handed female 16 months prior to death developed difficulty in speech, right-sided weakness, and apraxia of hand movements and progressed 2 days later to an akinetic mute state with urinary incontinence. (Courtesy of Drs. John Hills and Jose Segarra.)

Figure 26.15 Posterior cerebral artery: acute hemorrhagic infarction predominantly within the distribution of the right calcarine branch. This 53-year-old male with a right frontal-anterior temporal glioma had tentorial herniation with compression of the right posterior cerebral artery (in addition to brain stem structures). (Courtesy of Drs. John Hills and Jose Segarra.)

cerebral arteries may originate as a direct continuation of the posterior communicating artery.

Essentially two categories of posterior cerebral symptomatology may be recognized: (a) syndromes of the penetrating branches and (b) syndromes of the cortical branches. With main trunk occlusions, a mixture of these two syndromes may be present.

Overall, posterior cerebral artery cortical infarcts account for 5% of all infarcts (Table 26.3). Usually the infarcts reflect embolic occlusion (see Fisher, 1986; Koroshetz and Ropper, 1987; Pessin et al., 1987). Among the 54 cases presented by Kinkel et al. (1984), 11% demonstrated total involvement of the cortical territory. Most had partial involvement primarily of calcarine and/or the posterior temporal artery territory. Nine percent had bilateral infarcts.

The following case history illustrates many aspects of ischemia within the cortical distribution of the posterior cerebral artery. This patient demonstrates the general rule that posterior cerebral cortical infarcts are usually embolic.

CASE HISTORY 26.5

This 55-year-old, ambidextrous, married white female research coordinator at approximately 11:30 a.m. on the day of admission suddenly developed blurring of vision in her left visual field, possibly in her left eye, and was found to have a left visual field defect. Shortly thereafter, she developed tingling paresthesias of the left face, arm, and leg. Hypertension was under treatment with hydrochlorothiazide and flurosemide.

Physical examination: Blood pressure was elevated to 160/70. Weight was elevated to 264 pounds. A small ecchymosis was present under the toenail of the left second digit.

Neurological examination (3 hours after onset)

Cranial nerves: A noncongruous left homonymous hemianopsia was present, greater in the left temporal field than the right nasal field.

Reflexes: Deep tendon stretch reflexes were decreased in the lower extremities (patellar, 1+ and Achilles, 0). Plantar responses were equivocal, with the left probably extensor.

Sensory system: Pain and graphesthesia were decreased over the left foot.

Clinical diagnosis: Posterior cerebral artery ischemia and possible infarct (possibly embolic), involving the right calcarine cortex and thalamus or a lacunar event involving the right thalamus.

Laboratory data: *MRI*, 4 days after onset (Fig. 26.16) demonstrated a small infarct in the right occipital visual cortex area in the distribution of the calcarine artery. *MRA* (Fig. 26.17) demonstrated decreased flow in the right posterior cerebral artery. There was filling of more distal branches via anastomotic flow. *Holter monitoring* demonstrated multiple brief episodes of paroxysmal atrial fibrillation. The *transesophageal echocardiogram* demonstrated a definite patent foramen ovale with right-to-left shunting.

Subsequent course: Re-evaluation of the patient 22 hours after the onset of symptoms demonstrated clearing of all neurologic findings. When seen 2 weeks after the event, her only complaint related to some problems in reading. This patient had already been receiving aspirin at the time of the event, and this was discontinued. She was begun on lifelong systemic anticoagulation with Coumadin by the consultant cardiologist Dr. Filiberti since she had two conditions associated with embolization: paroxysmal atrial fibrillation and

Table 26.3 COMPARISON OF SYNDROMES FROM PENETRATING VERSUS CORTICAL BRANCHES OF POSTERIOR CEREBRAL ARTERY

VESSEL	SYNDROME
The Penetrating Branches – supply the rostral portion of the midbrain and the thalamus (often involved in lacunar infarcts)	– Occlusion of penetrators to midbrain damages the cerebral peduncle, the third cranial nerve, and the red nucleus (Weber's or Benedikt's syndrome) – Occlusion of penetrators to subthalamus and VL nucleus of thalamus produces contralateral hemichorea or hemiballismus – Damage to VPM/VPL of thalamus produces contralateral loss of sensation and possible pain syndrome (thalamogeniculate artery thalamic syndrome).
The Cortical Branches (Figs. 26.15 and 26.16). – anterior temporal and posterior temporal branches to the inferior and medial surfaces of the temporal lobe, posterior cerebral artery then divides into a parieto-occipital branch and the calcarine artery to the visual (calcarine) cortex.	– In bilateral posterior cerebral disease impairment of recent memory may occur, accompanied by a significant degree of confusion and disorientation ±bilateral blindness – If the dominant temporal lobe is involved, a confusional state may follow unilateral posterior cerebral disease. – Ischemia or infarction within the calcarine artery territory produces a contralateral homonymous hemianopsia, often with sparing of the macular area due to collateral circulation from middle cerebral artery (see above if bilateral) (see Chapter 23).

Figure 26.16 Infarct right occipital area, calcarine artery branch territory (embolus to posterior cerebral artery from heart). Magnetic resonance imaging (MRI). Case 26.5.

Figure 26.17 Occlusion of right posterior cerebral artery (arrow). Magnetic resonance angiography. Case 26.5.

patent foramen ovale with right-to-left shunting. The patient did well over the subsequent 5 years.

CEREBRAL EMBOLISM

This topic has already been discussed and illustrated earlier in cases 26.3, 26.4, and 26.5, and in Chapter 24. The middle cerebral and posterior cerebral artery cortical branches are primary targets.

In general, cerebral embolism is a complication of cardiovascular disease. However, as we have indicated, artery-to-artery (the carotid, vertebral or basilar) embolization of thrombus or atheromatous material is also frequent. Rarely, emboli may be composed of tumor cells or, following trauma, of fat or air (Jacobson et al., 1986). The embolus in most cases is a fragment of thrombus (clot, platelets, fibrin, and blood cells) that has become detached from a larger thrombus within the heart or proximal artery. The causes of such a thrombus within the heart are several:

a. A clot will often form in the left auricular appendage when atrial fibrillation is present. This is often the case when a relative stasis of blood in this area occurs as in mitral stenosis.

b. A "mural thrombus" may form on the endocardium in relation to an area of myocardial infarction.

c. Thrombus may collect on heart valves (so-called valvular vegetations), usually the mitral valve, when these valves are the subject of infection and inflammation as in bacterial endocarditis with embolic material breaking off

and entering into the circulation at times of change in cardiac rhythm (Hart et al., 1990; Jones and Siekert, 1989; Salgado et al., 1989).

d. The aorta may be a source of embolic material (Amarenco et al., 1994; Jones et al., 1995; Kistler, 1994).

e. In patients with a patent foramen ovale, within the heart, embolic material may originate in the veins of the legs or pelvis. Such patients may have both pulmonary and "paradoxical" cerebral emboli (Jones et al., 1983; Lechat et al., 1988).

Multiple small emboli of cardiac origin may occur to many cerebral vessels to produce a syndrome of multiple small vessel occlusions with a resultant clinical picture of dementia, alteration in personality, and so forth. Patients with multiple cerebral emboli also have embolization to extracerebral areas as well, such as the femoral artery, the kidney, the spleen, and the skin. Emboli to the kidney will often be detected following the sudden appearance of red blood cells in the urine (hematuria).

Differentiating Embolic from Nonembolic Ischemic-Occlusive Disease

Several points should be considered (see also Ramirez-Lassepas et al., 1987):

a. Perhaps most important is the fact that embolic occlusion of a vessel is sudden. In general, there are no preceding transient ischemic events. At times, the event may be so sudden that the patient stops speaking in mid sentence with a complete loss of speech. On the other hand, infarction due to ischemic occlusive disease is often preceded by one or more transient episodes of ischemia.

b. Since embolic occlusions are sudden, the event may be accompanied by a focal or generalized seizure.

c. Embolic occlusions may occur during any time of the day and often during periods of activity. Ischemic-occlusive infarctions tend to occur during sleep when blood pressure is relatively lower or shortly after arising in relation perhaps to transient falls in blood pressure.

d. Infarction due to embolic occlusion of a vessel is more likely to be hemorrhagic than a nonembolic infarction. This is related to reperfusion of an area of recent necrosis due to disintegration of the embolus or to the development of collateral (leptomeningeal anastomotic flow) (Fisher and Adams, 1951; Ogata et al., 1989; Okada, 1989). In such an area, the walls of blood vessels have also been ischemic and recently damaged. Such vessels when again perfused under a normal head of pressure will then leak blood into the surrounding tissues. In the study of Honig et al. (1993), MRI at 3 weeks demonstrated hemorrhagic transformation in 68% of cardioembolic infarcts but always without clinical deterioration.

e. Infarctions due to embolic occlusions are also often subject to rapid improvement because with the disintegration of embolic material, blood flow is restored. Treatment is discussed later.

MANAGEMENT OF ISCHEMIC AND OF EMBOLIC DISEASE

As regards management of patients with atherosclerotic ischemic-occlusive disease, the student should consult Brott and Bogousslavsky (2000). For patients seen within 3–4.5 hours of an occlusion usually embolic of the middle cerebral artery, the use of intravenous t-PA may be considered if the CT scan does not demonstrate hemorrhage of more than one-third of the middle cerebral artery territory involved by infarction. There has been an important public education program to alert people with the sudden onset of neurologic symptoms (Brain Attack) to report to a hospital in order to fulfill the time criterion to receive IV thrombolysis. Hospitals have to be prepared to rapidly perform a large number of evaluations for these patients, and at the present time only a small percent of eligible patients are treated (Demers et al., 2012). Studies are ongoing to see whether any of these criteria can be waived, since treating patients who do not have a stroke is not very dangerous as they will not likely develop a cerebral hemorrhage. t-PA may prove useful in patients with a minor deficit, a stroke scale of zero, who are classified as rapidly improving who do not meet current criteria for treatment.

For patients seen within 6 hours, direct intra-arterial thrombolysis may be considered. For most patients who have suffered infarcts, there are no specific curative therapies. Considerable recovery will occur in a supportive setting for many patients. Some patients with transient ischemic episodes or infarcts with minimal residual within the carotid distribution will have treatable extracranial vascular disease, which will benefit from surgical correction of the stenosis or occlusion. In addition to direct surgical carotid endarterectomy, the use of balloon angioplasty with or without stents is being developed as for coronary artery disease. Many patients with transient ischemic attacks or with a prior stroke will have a significant reduction in stroke risk with antiplatelet therapy (aspirin) and statins (Callahan et al., 2011) Anticoagulation has a significant role in the prevention of cerebral emboli in patients with atrial fibrillation of both rheumatic and non-rheumatic origin but has little value in other types of occlusive disease. Newer oral anticoagulation with dabigatran is now available. This is a potent antithrombin agent that averts the frequent blood INR determinations and dietary restrictions required with warfarin. Dabigatran is now approved for patients with nonvalvular atrial fibrillation. In patients where anticoagulation is not possible, closure of the left atrial appendage might be considered. The left atrial appendage is a very common source of cerebral emboli and can be closed by various surgical and percutaneous devices (Singh and Holmes, 2010). Some patients may have paradoxical cerebral emboli because of a patent atrial septal defect. These defects can be seen on cardiac echo studies and closed by a device placed by intra-arterial catheter, but the evidence as to the indications for such procedures is not firmly established (Caroll et al., 2013).

The best treatment is prevention. The major factors that can be controlled are hypertension, the risk factors for cardiac disease including the prevention of rheumatic and coronary artery heart disease, cigarette smoking, diabetes mellitus, dietary factors, daily aspirin, statins, and illicit drug use. A major risk factor that unfortunately cannot be well controlled is the family predisposition for cerebrovascular or coronary artery disease (Graffagnino et al., 1994). For a discussion of ischemic-occlusive disease involving the basilar-vertebral circulation, the student should refer to the chapters 11 and 13 on the brain stem and the chapter 20 on the cerebellum.

INTRACRANIAL HEMORRHAGE

There are two types of intracranial hemorrhage: *intracerebral hemorrhage* and *subarachnoid hemorrhage*. In the Framingham study (Di Tullio et al., 1992), intracerebral hemorrhages constituted 5% of all strokes and subarachnoid hemorrhage 9% of all strokes. Both have a high mortality. The young and middle-aged black population in the United States has an increased risk of both intracranial and subarachnoid hemorrhage compared to the white population (Broderick et al., 1992).

Intracerebral Hemorrhage

Intracerebral hemorrhage is primary in 83% of cases and secondary in the remaining 15%. Hemorrhage into the brain may occur in patients receiving anticoagulants (Franke et al., 1990; Kase et al., 1985) or as a complication of various hematological problems which are characterized by bleeding disorders, for example, leukemia (Figs. 26.18 and 26.19). Bleeding into the brain may also occur in relation to arteriovenous

Figure 26.18 Multiple cerebral hemorrhages secondary to acute thrombocytopenia (platelet count of 17,000) with acute lymphatic leukemia. Computerized tomography (CT) scan without contrast in a 24 year old with headache and acute onset of coma, clinical brain death, and a flat electroencephalogram.

such as the lenticulostriate arteries are also involved in occlusion with lacunar infarction in hypertension has led to several hypotheses concerning the etiology of the hemorrhages:

a. The vessel wall may be weakened by this process and may dilate and rupture (the miliary aneurysm of Bouchard and Charcot).

b. The vessel may occlude with infarction. When collateral flow is then introduced into the acutely necrotic area, hemorrhage occurs.

c. Related to this hypothesis is the concept of fluctuations in blood pressure. Certainly such wide fluctuations may occur in some hypertensive patients. With a fall in blood pressure, infarctions would occur. With restoration of elevated blood pressure, these necrotic vessel walls would be unable to take the stress of the increased pressure and would bleed.

d. Another explanation suggests that in some cases venous occlusion may have occurred. Venous occlusions are usually hemorrhagic.

In both explanations (b) and (c) there is implied a concept of hemorrhagic infarction. In some cases of premonitory ischemia, symptoms will be noted.

malformation or to intracranial tumors (such as glioblastomas or metastatic malignancy; Little et al., 1979) or as the complication of the rupture of a saccular aneurysm where there is extension of blood from the subarachnoid space into the substance of the cerebral hemisphere. In general, however, the term *intracerebral hemorrhage* is applied to those primary massive and medium-sized hemorrhages into the parenchyma of the brain. The major risk factor is hypertension. However, in approximately 40% of patients, blood pressure is normal (Brott et al., 1986). Other risk factors include excessive alcohol intake and cerebral amyloid angiopathy with deposition of beta amyloid in cerebral blood vessels. The latter condition is associated with the presence of the ε-2 and ε-4 alleles of the apolipoprotein E gene. Recurrent hemorrhages may occur at different sites. Patients with intracerebral hemorrhages are seen less commonly on general neurological and neurosurgical services than patients with occlusive vascular disease and those with subarachnoid hemorrhage. Patients with intracerebral hemorrhage are, however, relatively common when acute general medical admissions and autopsies are considered. There is certainly a predilection for certain areas of the brain, as demonstrated in Table 26.4.

The basic pathogenesis involved in intracerebral hemorrhage is not certain. The fact that penetrating arteries

Figure 26.19 Resolving hematoma rt. putamen, hypodensity of a cystic cavity with residual hemosiderin and dystrophic calcification (arrow), on MRI T2, 16 months after the acute hemorrhage. This 61 y.o. rt. handed white male had the acute onset of a left hemiparesis, but had an excellent recovery of leg function but continued to have severe spastic weakness in the left upper extremity with tonic neck effects, a hemiplegic gait, decreased pain sensation in left face and arm and a dressing apraxia of his left arm.

Table 26.4 INTRACEREBRAL HEMORRHAGE

LOCATION	VESSEL	FREQUENCY*/FIGURE	CLINICAL MANIFESTATIONS
Putamen-lateral ganglionic mass-internal capsule	Lenticulostriate penetrators: middle cerebral artery	33%-40% (Figs. 26.19 and 26.20)	Progressive headache, hemiparesis, hemianesthesia, confusion, herniation, and coma
Temporal lobe stem and lobar (lobar often secondary to amyloid angiopathy)	Superficial small and medium arteries	23% (Fig. 2.27)	Progressive temporal lobe or other cortical mass with focal seizures. Recurrent or multiple.
Thalamus	Penetrators: posterior cerebral artery	20% (Fig. 26.21)	Unilateral numbness, hemianesthesia, and vertical gaze impairment
Pons	Paramedian penetrators of the basilar artery	7% (Fig 13.26)	Sudden quadriplegia, coma, respiratory impairment, death. Small lateral tegmental lesions may survive.
Cerebellum	Branches posterior inferior or superior cerebellar arteries	8% (Fig. 20.13)	Sudden headache, vomiting, vertigo, ataxia, then extraocular findings and coma

*Based on series of Hier et al. (1977), Kase et al. (1982), and Kase and Caplan (1986).

e. It has been suggested that in younger patients when hypertension is not present, bleeding has occurred from an arteriovenous malformation, the evidence of which has been destroyed by the massive hemorrhage.

f. The use of sympathomimetic drugs utilized in nasal decongestants and cough syrups in addition to amphetamines and the use of illicit street drugs such as "crack" cocaine have also been implicated in younger adults (Levine et al., 1990).

g. In elderly patients when hypertension may or may not be present and when the location of the hemorrhage is lobar involving the superficial small and medium sized arteries rather than small deep penetrating branch vessel, a process of "amyloid angiopathy" has been identified. Deposits of amyloid occur in the media and adventitia of these vessels without the presence of systemic amyloidosis.

The pathological features to be found with an intracerebral hemorrhage may be briefly summarized. The hematoma may continue to expand during the first 3 hours, resulting in continued deterioration. Within a few hours of cessation of the hemorrhage, clotting occurs. In general with hypertensive hemorrhages, bleeding does not again occur into the same area. The blood is not quickly removed from the brain parenchyma. If this hemorrhage is actually a complication of infarction, then in the early stages, the changes of ischemic infarction will be noted with infiltration of adjacent ischemic tissue by polymorphonuclear leukocytes.

The actual clot of a hemorrhage will remain as a red or reddish black mass for a matter of several weeks. Macrophages that may have been already abundant in adjacent necrotic tissue begin to digest red blood cells at the periphery of the hemorrhage, producing the yellow-brown iron pigment hemosiderin. At 3 weeks, this produces at the periphery a rim of orange. The more central area of hemorrhage never undergoes phagocytosis but is converted to a semiliquid mass after several additional weeks or months.

When the brain is examined many months after a hemorrhage, there will be found a residual cleft or cavity with orange-stained walls. The staining is due to the persistence of hemosiderin-containing macrophages. The wall, in general, is similar to that surrounding the cavity, which results from an ischemic infarct. A proliferation of capillaries has occurred with the formation of connective tissue fibers. In adjacent tissue, proliferation of astrocytes has occurred with the formation of glial fibers.

The gross changes over time may be demonstrated with sequential MRI or CT scans (Figs. 26.20 and 26.21).

The clinical manifestations will depend on the location and size of the hemorrhage and are summarized in Table 26.4. In general with the most common variety—those into the putamen—there is the sudden onset of progressive headache, followed by progressive hemiparesis, and then within minutes to hours by hemianesthesia, confusion, and coma. The progression of symptoms is due to the progressive enlargement of the hematoma and to dissection of the hemorrhage along fiber pathways. Displacement of midline brain stem structures and tentorial herniation often occurs. With these brain stem complications and with extension of the hemorrhage into the ventricular system, a decerebrate state and a compromise of respiratory functions develop. Death occurs in a high percentage of such patients (75%) within hours to days. Overall, 50% of patients with large hemorrhages expire. The prognosis for smaller hemorrhages is more favorable (21%). Prognosis is directly related to (a) size of hematoma on CT scan and (b) level of consciousness (Broderick et al., 1992). Patients with small hemorrhages may have only a minimal degree of disability since the hemorrhage displaces structures rather than destroying structures as in an infarct.

The diagnosis of intracerebral hemorrhage may be made on the basis of the sudden onset of symptoms. The onset occurs during a period of activity as opposed to the pattern for arteriosclerotic ischemic-occlusive disease where onset during sleep or shortly after awakening is more characteristic.

Figure 26.20 (*A*) Acute hemorrhage left thalamus on computerized tomography (CT) scan of a 72-year-old woman with clinical findings of severe hypertension (210/130), dense right sided hemiparesis, and sensory deficits plus fluent aphasia. (*B*) Old cystic cavity (arrow) on CT scan, 2.5 years later. She had significant sensory symptoms and cortical sensory deficits in right arm and leg, ataxia of gait, intention tremor of right hand and leg, and occasional choreiform movements of the right hand.

Figure 26.21 Saccular aneurysm (arrow) arising from junction right internal carotid artery and posterior communicating artery demonstrated by right carotid arteriogram. This 70-year-old widow, 18 months previously, had the sudden onset of severe pain in the right eye and complete third nerve paralysis which had partially improved in the interim. (Courtesy of Dr. Samuel Wolpert.) (Compare to Figs. 26.7C and 2.27 for nonaneurysm reference.)

At the present time, the major aids in diagnosis are the CT scan and the MRI scans. There is then no indication for lumbar puncture; such a procedure in any case may be dangerous when increased intracranial pressure is present.

As regards treatment, the deep location within the putamen, thalamus, and pons means that surgical evacuation of these massive hemorrhages is not feasible. Moreover, with most large pontine hemorrhages, death rapidly ensues. With extension of hemorrhages of the putamen or thalamus into the ventricle, death usually occurs within a short time. However, expanding masses of more superficial lobar hematoma within temporal or parietal lobe offer the possibility of surgical therapy. Cerebellar hematomas when diagnosed prior to brain stem compromise are often evacuated with a high degree of recovery. Qureshi et al. (2005) have reviewed current approaches to management.

Occasionally warning prodromal symptoms are present; such warning symptoms, however, are more characteristic of ischemic-occlusive disease.

In general, the cerebrospinal fluid is under increased pressure and usually but not invariably contains red blood cells. The number of such cells, however, is usually less than that found in subarachnoid hemorrhage.

Subarachnoid Hemorrhage

The diagnosis of primary subarachnoid hemorrhage is made on the basis of gross blood present in the cerebrospinal fluid in the absence of primary intracerebral hemorrhage or trauma. Both of these conditions may have secondary leakage of some blood into the subarachnoid space. In 85% of cases of primary subarachnoid hemorrhage in the adult, the source of bleeding is a ruptured saccular aneurysm. (Refer to Table 26.5.) The basic pathology in the saccular or berry aneurysm is a defect in the media and internal elastic membrane of the vessel wall. Since the media of cerebral arteries develops in a multicentric manner, adjacent sections meet at arterial bifurcations where clefts or gaps in the media are

Table 26.5 SUMMARY OF THE CAUSES OF SUBARACHNOID HEMORRHAGE (SAH), ANEURYSM LOCATION, AND MANIFESTATIONS

LOCATION OR TYPE	FREQUENCY OF ALL ANEURYSMS (FIGURE NO., CASE NO.)	FREQUENCY AS CAUSE OF SAH	EARLY MANIFESTATIONS OR SYMPTOMS OF COMPRESSION PRIOR TO RUPTURE
I. ANEURYSMS		85%	Sudden onset of worst-ever headache plus stiff neck
Junction of postcommunicating and internal carotid	30% (Fig. 26.21, Cases 12.1 and 26.8)		Third nerve paralysis since third cranial nerve runs close to and parallel to the posterior communicating artery
Bifurcation MCA	20% (Fig. 26.22, Case 26.9)		Focal symptoms in MCA territory: focal weakness or seizure face, speech, etc.
Junction anterior communicating-anterior cerebral	30% (Figs. 26.23, 26.24, 26.25; Case 26.10)		Compression optic chiasm, or bilateral prefrontal or bilateral lower extremity or coma or mute state or if giant, dementia. Often nonlocalized SAH
Basilar vertebral system	5%–10%		Variable
Multiple aneurysms	15%		Variable; usually only one is the site of SAH
II. OTHER SAH CAUSES		15%	
Perimesencephalic		10%	Nonlocalized: worst-ever headache, stiff neck, drowsiness (Fig. 26.26)
Other: AVM, mycotic aneurysms		5%	Variable depending on location (often distal cortical branches in mycotic). Seizures are frequent in both.

AVM, Arteriovenous Malformation; MCA, middle cerebral artery.

common. These developmental defects in the media probably occur to some extent in all individuals. When later in life thinning or loss of the internal elastic membrane is superimposed at this point of defect, the thin layer of intima bulges out and is covered only by the loose connective tissue of the adventitia. The ballooned protrusion is referred to as a saccular aneurysm.

The unruptured saccular aneurysm is usually asymptomatic. Unruptured saccular aneurysms occur as an incidental finding in 1%–2% of routine autopsies.[6] Most do not rupture and do not cause symptoms. Occasionally, however, symptoms may be noted prior to rupture. Thus, an enlarging aneurysm of the posterior communicating artery may compress the third nerve. At times an aneurysm of the cavernous portion of the carotid artery may invade the pituitary fossa or compress the optic chiasm (Table 26.5) or rupture into the cavernous sinus. In general, the initial symptoms are those related to rupture. The usual symptoms are those of sudden severe headache (the most severe ever experienced by the patient), vomiting, neck pain, and stiffness. The latter symptoms are due to meningeal irritation. Sudden straining, exercise, or sexual activity often precipitates the headache. In massive rupture, sudden onset of coma may occur. In a less severe bleed, consciousness is sometimes well preserved. Often no specific focal symptoms are present, and it may then be difficult to determine, particularly in the comatose patient, on the basis of the clinical findings alone, the actual site of rupture. At times, the presence of minor focal signs will allow the localization of the aneurysm. Those cases where consciousness has been preserved and where few focal signs

Figure 26.22 Giant aneurysm arising from the bifurcation of the right middle cerebral artery. (Courtesy of Dr. C. W. Watson.)

[6] More recent large autopsy studies suggest an overall frequency of intracranial aneurysms of 5% with a population-based incidence of subarachnoid hemorrhage secondary to aneurysms of 10 per 10,000 per year (see Phillips et al., 1980). Patients with autosomal dominant polycystic kidney disease or a family history are at increased risk for aneurysms and require noninvasive screening (Wiebers and Torres, 1992).

Figure 26.23 Saccular aneurysm at junction of anterior communicating and left anterior cerebral artery situated close to the optic chiasm. This 52-year-old white male had the sudden onset one evening of headache, nausea, and vomiting. On examination, the next morning he was stuporous, inattentive, and disoriented but could move all of his extremities; he had bilateral Babinski sign and release of strong grasp reflexes plus urinary and fecal incontinence. Cerebrospinal fluid had >100,000 red blood cells per cubic millimeter; the supernatant fluid was xanthochromic. (Courtesy of Drs. John Hills and Jose Segarra.)

are present can of course be readily distinguished from cases of primary intracerebral hemorrhage. In intracerebral hemorrhage, secondary leakage of blood into the subarachnoid space may occur, but in the early stages, although consciousness may be preserved or clouded, well-developed focal signs are present, for example, hemiparesis, hemianesthesia, hemianopsia, and quadriparesis.

At times in cases of ruptured aneurysm, significant focal or bilateral signs of cerebral involvement will be present. In some cases coma will be an early sign. In some of these cases extension of the hemorrhage into the substance of the cerebral hemisphere has occurred. At times, rupture from the base of the brain into the third ventricle has occurred. At times, the vessel beyond the point of rupture has been deprived of blood,

Figure 26.25 Aneurysm anterior communicating anterior cerebral junction: subarachnoid and intracerebral hemorrhage with rupture into ventricular system and hydrocephalus. Computerized tomography (CT) scan (nonenhanced). This 51-year-old male was found in a confused state and soon lapsed into unconsciousness with mild nuchal rigidity, miotic pupils, decerebrate movements on the left side, flaccidity on the right side, and bilateral Babinski signs. He improved with osmotic shrinking agents (Mannitol), steroids, ventricular drainage, and subsequent clipping of the aneurysm, evacuation of clot, and eventually a shunt procedure.

and infarction has occurred within its territory. Embolism from clot in the dome of the aneurysm may occur. At times, spasm of the artery distal to the point of aneurysm will occur, related perhaps to the presence of blood in the subarachnoid space. Such arterial spasm may produce sufficient vasoconstriction, apparently via adrenergic mechanisms, to result in ischemia and infarction.

Those red blood cells that have entered the subarachnoid space undergo a series of changes. Within a few hours, disruption of red blood cells has begun with a yellow discoloration (so-called xanthochromia) of the spinal fluid. At this time oxyhemoglobin and methemoglobin may also be detected in the spinal fluid. After 48 hours, increasing amounts of bilirubin pigment may be noted with an increase in the degree of xanthochromia. The red blood cells have usually been completely disrupted by 10 days after the hemorrhage. The bilirubin product of this disruption disappears more slowly. The spinal fluid does not become colorless for 15 to 30 days after the hemorrhage. In tissues adjacent to the subarachnoid blood, hemosiderin-filled macrophages may be seen for several weeks after the acute episode of bleeding. Initially in the spinal fluid obtained by lumbar puncture, the ratio of white blood cells to red blood cells is the same as in the peripheral blood. With the passage of time, after the acute hemorrhage, as red blood cells are disrupted and as meningeal reaction occurs, a relative increase in white blood cells will be noted.

Figure 26.24 Saccular anterior communicating aneurysm with rupture into ventricular system. This 65-year-old white male, 14 days after a confirmed subarachnoid hemorrhage without definite localizing findings, had a generalized seizure followed by quadriplegia and coma. (Courtesy of Drs. John Hills and Jose Segarra.)

Evaluation and Management of the Patient with Subarachnoid Hemorrhage

Early recognition of subarachnoid hemorrhage is important since the overall mortality of ruptured aneurysms is at least 50% and the survivors have a significant morbidity. The recent reviews of Schievink (1997) and van Gijn and Rinkel (2001) are excellent sources of information. Prognostic factors include early recognition at the time of the initial hemorrhage, age, level of consciousness, and neurological condition.

Patients presenting at the emergency room with the sudden onset of the worst headache ever should undergo an immediate CT scan searching for subarachnoid blood (Fig. 26.26). The CT scan will be negative in 5%–10% of patients, usually those with a minor bleed, and these patients should undergo a lumbar puncture searching for subarachnoid blood. If either of these studies demonstrates subarachnoid blood, then immediate angiography should be performed, followed by immediate surgery procedure designed to clip the aneurysm. Surgical therapy has as its primary objective the prevention of additional subarachnoid hemorrhage. Modern advances now under development include the use of spiral CT scan angiography or high-resolution MRA. In some patients the direct clipping procedures are being replaced by endoscopic obliteration of the aneurysm. In patients who survive an initial bleed, a second bleed is associated with a very high mortality of 50%. Complications are summarized in Table 26.6.

In considering the matter of therapy, it is important to examine the mortality of the disease. In the study of Di Tullio

Table 26.6 COMPLICATIONS OF THE INITIAL HEMORRHAGE OR OF A SECOND HEMORRHAGE

COMPLICATION	PREVENTION OR TREATMENT
Recurrence of a subarachnoid hemorrhage (SAH)	Prevent by immediate arteriography and clipping of aneurysm after initial SAH
Rupture into the ventricle with brain stem compression death Massive SAH with tentorial and tonsillar herniation	Prognosis poor, coma then possible; use of ventricular drainage and Mannitol
Dissection into brain with hematoma formation	Evacuate hematoma and clip aneurysm to prevent herniation and rebleeding
Vasospasm secondary to aminergic substances in blood	Calcium channel blockers (Nimodipine) and increase blood pressure after clipping aneurysm to increase perfusion
Acute or chronic hydrocephalus due to blockage of cisterns, ventricles, and subarachnoid space	For acute, shunt after ventricular drainage. For chronic, shunt
Seizures	Treat with anticonvulsants: phenytoin or phenobarbital
Compressive effects of large and giant aneurysms	Clip and decompress aneurysm
Cardiac arrhythmias	Treat with pacemaker or appropriate anti-arrhythmia agents

et al. (1992), one-third of the 36 total cases were in coma at the onset and this group had a 30-day mortality of 83%. Two-thirds were conscious at the onset with a 29% mortality at 30 days. Of this conscious group of 24 patients, 15 developed no deficits and 13 of 15 survived with a 30-day mortality of 13%. Of the 9 conscious patients who developed a delayed deficit, the mortality was 56%. The overall 30-day mortality was 47%.

Many patients (18%) die acutely and may never reach a neurosurgical center. In the Cooperative Study of Subarachnoid Hemorrhage, 27% of patients who reached a neurosurgical center died within the first week. Of patients dying within 72 hours, 90% had an associated intracerebral hemorrhage. Rebleeding is a major cause of morbidity and mortality in these patients. Approximately 33% of patients rebleed in the first 30 days with a mortality of 42%. Most episodes of rebleeding occur within the first 14 days, particularly between day 5 and day 9. However, rebleeding continues to occur even 10–20 years after the initial hemorrhage in patients not subjected to surgical therapy. In the series of rebleeding in such patients was estimated at 3.5% per year during the first 10 years with an associated mortality of 67%.

Although direct intracranial surgery was at one time attended by a considerable mortality and morbidity, major advances, including microsurgery, neuroanesthesia with more effective control of blood pressure, and intracranial pressure plus the use of CT scanning, have resulted in a marked improvement in results (see Ropper and Zervas, 1984). The use of calcium channel blockers has decreased vasospasm-induced infarction.

Figure 26.26 Perimesencephalic, unlocalized subarachnoid hemorrhage. Nonenhanced computerized tomography (CT) scan demonstrating blood in the interpeduncular, prepontine, suprasellar, and ambient cisterns. This 46-year-old woman experienced the acute onset of "the worst headache in her life," lethargy, and nuchal rigidity but had an otherwise normal neurological examination. Two series of angiograms and all hematologic studies were normal. She has done well over the subsequent 7 years.

Table 26.7 **HUNT AND HESS CLASSIFICATION WITH CORRELATIONS**

GRADE DESCRIPTION	PROGNOSIS
1 Asymptomatic or minimal headache and slight nuchal rigidity	Excellent, if early surgery
2 Moderate to severe headache and nuchal rigidity but no neurologic deficit	Excellent, if early surgery
3 Drowsiness, confusion, or mild focal deficit	Excellent, if early surgery
4 Stupor, moderate to severe hemiparesis, early decerebrate rigidity, and vegetative disturbance	Poor unless on computerized tomography, treatable hydrocephalus or hematoma
5 Deep coma; decerebrate rigidity and moribund appearance	Very poor unless as above

Patient selection is of considerable importance and this is dependent on grading of the patient as regards level of consciousness and the presence or absence of focal neurological deficit. The classification of Hunt and Hess (1968) (Table 26.7) utilizes a five-grade scale.

The World Federation of Neurological Surgeons' grading scale is discussed by van Gijn and Rinkel (2001).

The Unruptured Intracranial Aneurysm: These aneurysms may be detected because of (a) compression of cranial nerves, (b) angiogram performed in patients with transient ischemic attacks, or ruptured aneurysm at another site (c) the increasing use of CT and MRI scan (Reck et al., 2005). The most extensive study is the International Study of Unruptured Intracranial Aneurysms (Wiebers et al., 1987) demonstrating a clear-cut relationship of aneurysm size and risk of hemorrhage. Essentially those smaller than 10 mm in diameter on angiographic study at the time of diagnosis are unlikely to subsequently rupture; cumulative rate of rupture was less than 0.05% per year. If the patient already had a repaired aneurysm at another site after subarachnoid hemorrhage, the rate of rupture was 0.5% per year. For aneurysms of 10 mm or more in diameter, the rate of rupture approached 1.0% per year for both types of patient, the previously untreated and the previously treated at another site (about 20×–11× the rate for the smaller aneurysms). The rate of rupture for giant aneurysms (more than 25 mm in diameter) was 6% in the first year. Currently, MRI angiography can reliably detect unruptured aneurysms greater than 2–3 mm in diameter, although many earlier studies have utilized 5 mm in diameter as the sensitivity cutoff (see Torres et al., 1990). When two or more members of the same family have aneurysms, MRA of asymptomatic members should be considered.

NEUROLOGIC COMPLICATIONS OF BACTERIAL ENDOCARDITIS

Osler in 1885 first recognized the neurological complications of endocarditis (association of fever, heart murmur, and hemiplegia). The neurological effects of infections of the heart valves remain a major problem. Patients with rheumatic heart disease were once the major patients at risk. At present, other major etiologic factors have emerged, including intravenous drug addiction, prosthetic valves, and the use of various intravenous and intracardiac lines.

Table 26.8 **NEUROLOGIC COMPLICATIONS OF BACTERIAL ENDOCARDITIS**

COMPLICATION	FREQUENCY	MANIFESTATIONS
Cerebral embolism 1 cortical	7% (6%–31%), 3% of all cerebral emboli	Usually MCA territory or stem (see above)
Multiple micro-emboli	11%	Confusional state or personality change or seizures
Mycotic aneurysm	2%–10% (2.5%–6% of all aneurysms)	Subarachnoid hemorrhage often more distal branches of the MCA
Intracerebral hemorrhage	7%–8%	Usually lenticulostriate
Meningitis	16%	In 50% of purulent usually staphylococcus was identified
Brain abscess	Single large is not common	Usually multiple and microscopic; possible confusional state or seizure
Infection of vertebrae or disk space with compression syndromes	Not a common syndrome, although osteomyelitis may occur	Spinal cord or root compression

MCA, middle cerebral artery.

The streptococcus (particularly viridans) remains the predominant organism, although increasingly Staphylococcus aureus and fungi must also be considered. The overall incidence of neurological complication in a large series from the Massachusetts General Hospital amounts to 39% (Pruitt et al., 1978). In 16% of endocarditis patients, the neurological complication was the initial complaint. The development of neurological complications had a significant effect on prognosis. If neurological complications were present, mortality was 58%; if not present, 20%. The major neurological complications are summarized in Table 26.8.

Wilson et al. (2008) discusses the prevention of infective endocarditis.

ARTERIOVENOUS MALFORMATIONS

Included within this diagnostic category of vascular malformations are a variety of pathological entities (based on frequency) such as (1) arteriovenous anomalies, (2) cavernous angiomas, (3) venous malformation, (4) telangiectasis, (5) arteriovenous fistulas, and (6) dual vascular malformations. All are congenital. (However, arteriovenous fistulas may occur with trauma, e.g., carotid cavernous). In general, these represent developmental (at times on a hereditary basis) tangles of abnormal vessels within the substance of the brain (less often involving meningeal vessels). These abnormal vessels provide arteriovenous shunting of blood. Since the vessels are abnormal with defects in their walls, bleeding into the substance of the brain (producing an intracerebral hematoma) or into the subarachnoid space may occur. Moreover, these abnormal vessels are also prone to occlusion with the development of local infarction of cerebral tissue. In general, these malformations produce symptoms earlier in life than do saccular aneurysms. They are moreover less often fatal. Thus, several episodes of subarachnoid hemorrhage may occur without loss of life. The initial manifestations are as follows: seizures, often focal in 50%, intracerebral hemorrhage in 20%, and subarachnoid hemorrhage in 20%. Although involving primarily the cerebral hemisphere, the brain stem, spinal cord, or cerebellum may be involved.

DISORDERS OF THE VEINS AND SINUSES

Cavernous sinus thrombosis or cortical vein thrombosis may occur in adults due to infection and has already been discussed. Occlusion of the superior sagittal and lateral and straight sinus is primarily a disease of the infant less than 1 month of age and reflects dehydration and other systemic and perinatal factors.

BIBLIOGRAPHY

Brodearick, J. P., Brott, T., and Tomiskc, T. 1992. The risk of subarachnoid and intracraebral stroke in blacks as compared to whtes. *N. Eng. J. Med.* 326:733–736.

Brott, T., and Bogousslavsky, J. 2000. Treatment of Acute Ischemic Stroke. *N Engl J Med.* 343:710–722.

Brott, T. G., Hobson, R. W., Howard, G., et al. 2010. CREST investigators: stenting versus endarterectomy for treatment of carotid-artery stenosis. *N. Engl. J. Med.* 363(1):11–23.

Bruno, A., Graff-Radford, N. R., Biller, J., and Adams, H. P. J. 1989. Anterior choroidal artery territory infarction: a small vessel disease. *Stroke* 20:616–619.

Callahan, A., Amarenco, P., Goldstein, L. B., et al. 2011. Risk of stroke and cardiovascular events after ischemic stroke or transient attack in patients with type 2 diabetes or metabolic syndrome: secondary analysis of the Stroke Prevention by Aggressive Reduction in Cholesterol Levels (SPARCL) trial. *Arch. Neurol.* 68(10):1245–1251.

Caroll, J. D., Saver, J. L., Thaler, D. E., et al. 2013. Closure of the patent foramen ovale versus medical therapy after a cryptogenic stroke. *N. Engl. J. Med.* 368(12):1092–1100.

Ciccone, A., Valvasorri, L., Nicholatti, M., et al. 2013. Endovascular treatment for acute stroke. *N. Engl. J. Med.* 368:904–913.

Di Tullio, M., Sacco, R. L., Gopal, A., Mohr, J. P., and Homma, S. 1992. Patent foramen ovale as a risk factor for Cryptogenic Stroke. *Ann. Intern. Med.* 117(6):461–465.

Freeman, F. R. 1971. Akinetic mutism and bilateral anterior cerebral artery occlusion. *J. Neurosurgery and Psychiatry* 34:693–694.

Jorgensen, H. S., Nakayama, H., Raaschou, H. O., et al., and The Cophenagen Stroke Study. 1995. Outcome and time course of recovery in stroke. Part II: Time course of recovery. *Arch. of Phys. Med. and Rehabilitation.* 76:406–412.

Kalimo, H., and Kalaria, R. N. 2005. Hereditary forms of vascular dementia. In H. Kalimo (Ed.) *Cerebrovascular Diseases, Pathology and Genetics*, Vol. 5, pp. 324–384.

Marler, J. R., Price, T. R., Clark, G. L., et al. 1986. Morning increase in onset of ischemic stroke. *Stroke* 36:374–386.

Mayberg, M. R., and Winn, H. R. 1995. Endarterectomy for asymptomatic carotid artery stenosis. *Resolving the controversy.* JAMA 273:1459–1461.

Millikan, C. H., and Futrell, N. 1990. Vertigo of Vascular Origin. *Arch. Neurol.* 47(1):12–13.

Moore, W. S., Barnett, H. J., Beebe, H. G., et al. 1995. Guidelines for endarterectomy. *Am. Heart Association.* 1:188–201.

Norris, J. W., and Zhu, C. Z. 1990. Stroke risk and critical carotid stenosis. *Neurol. Neurosurg. Psychiatry.* 53:235–237.

Pruitt, A. A. 1978. Current treatment options in neurology. Neurologic complications of infective endocarditis. Springer.

Qureshi, A. I., Mohammed, Y. M., et al. 2005. A prospective multi-center study to evaluate the feasibility and safety of aggressive antihypertensive treatment in patients with acute intracerebral hemorrhage. *J Intensive Care Med.* 20:34–42.

Reck, S. D., Zacks, D. N., and Eibschitz-Tsimhoni, M. 2005. Retinal and intracranial arteriovenous malformations: Wyburn-Mason syndrome. J. Neuroophthalmol. 25(3):205–208.

Torres, V. E., Wiebers, D. O., and Forbes, G. S. 1990. Cranial computed tomography and magnetic resonance imaging in autosomal dominant polycystic kidney disease. *J. Am. Soc. Nephrol.* 1(1):84–90.

Whisnant, J. P., and Wieber, D. O. 1987. Clinical Epidemiology of TIAs in the anterior and posterior circulation. In T. M. Sindt (ed.) *Occlusive Cardiovasscular Disease*, W.B. Saunders Philadelphia, pp 60–65.

Wiebers, D. O., Whisnant, J. P. Sundt, T. M., and O'Fallon, W. M. 1987. The significance of unruptured intracranial saccular aneurysms. J. Neurosurgery. 66:23–29.

Wilson, W., Taubert, K. A., Gewitz, M., et al. Prevention of infective endocarditis: guidelines from the American Heart Association: a guideline from the American Heart Association Rheumatic Fever, Endocarditis and Kawasaki Disease Committee, Council on Cardiovascular Disease in the Young, and the Council on Clinical Cardiology, Council on Cardiovascular Surgery and Anesthesia, and the Quality of Care and Outcomes Research Interdisciplinary Working Group. 2008. American Heart Association. *J Am Dent Assoc.* 139 Suppl:3S–24S.

27.

CEREBRAL HEMISPHERES

NEUROPATHOLOGY AND CLINICAL CORRELATION II. NONVASCULAR SYNDROMES

In the era of the automobile, bicycle, and motorcycle, trauma to the head constitutes one of the most frequent neurological problems presented to emergency room physicians. Not all head injuries involve the brain. Significant scalp lacerations and simple skull fractures may be present without the development of significant neurological deficits. On the other hand, closed head injuries may be present with significant neurological signs but without major external signs of head trauma (i.e., scalp and skull appear intact).

TRAUMA

CONCUSSION

Perhaps the most common neurological syndrome occurring in relation to head trauma is the cerebral concussion, a syndrome characterized by a transient alteration of consciousness and of higher cerebral functions lasting a matter of minutes to hours, following a blow to the head. Consciousness may or may not be transiently lost at the onset. The patient complains of "being in a dazed state" with blurring of vision and a sense of unsteadiness. Memory is often impaired for events during this period following the injury: posttraumatic amnesia. The transient inability to record and recall events that occur after the traumatic event is called anterograde amnesia. In addition, memory for events which occurred minutes, hours, or even several days prior to that injury may be impaired: retrograde amnesia. As recovery occurs, this period of retrograde amnesia may shrink.

No definite pathology has been associated with cerebral concussion; the pathophysiology remains unclear. There is some indication that differential acceleration or deceleration of the brain and skull may force the cerebral cortex against the hard surface of the skull, producing a transient neuronal dysfunction. Rotational forces may also set up stresses that result in the stretching (shearing) of white matter systems at a subcortical and brain stem level.

CONTUSIONS AND LACERATIONS

More serious injuries of the cerebral hemisphere involve contusions, lacerations, intracerebral hemorrhages, and edema (see Fig. 27.1).

Contusions (local areas of swelling and capillary hemorrhage resembling bruises) are found particularly at the anterior temporal poles and the under surfaces of the frontal and temporal lobes. These contusions of the cerebral cortex occur as a result of the sudden impact of the cortex against the bony wall of the skull. The anterior portions of the anterior and middle fossa provide relatively constricting compartments favoring the development of such contusions. Contusions may directly underlie the site of the blow to the skull (so-called coup injuries) or may be across from the site of injury (so-called contra coup injuries). When examined at autopsy years later, the brain may show small orange-yellow colored areas of depression on the orbital-frontal and anterior-temporal areas (plaques jaunes).

Intracerebral hemorrhages may also be present. These are usually multiple and small. Occasionally, a single large hematoma may be present requiring surgical therapy if mass effects are present.

Lacerations of the brain involve actual tears in the cortical surface. Both lacerations and contusions may result in the appearance of some red blood cells in the subarachnoid space. In general, patients with contusion and laceration have a loss of consciousness in relation to the injury. Residual alterations in mental function, memory, and personality are often noted. Such alterations are uncommon with a simple concussion. Focal neurological findings may be present during the acute stage, at times remaining as residual deficits. Severe focal deficits such as hemiparesis or aphasia are, however, usually absent.

Complications of Skull Fractures

Certain types of skull injuries provide serious problems as regards the brain and require surgical attention. Thus, depressed skull fracture may compress the cerebral cortex, with bony splinters lacerating the dura and cortex.

Penetrating head injuries (the object causing trauma has penetrated the skin, bone, and meninges) may introduce contaminated material into the brain, producing abscess formation and meningitis. Fractures involving the cribriform plate with laceration of the overlying dura and arachnoid may result in the loss of olfactory sensation (anosmia) and cerebrospinal rhinorrhea: the drainage of spinal fluid through the nose. The presence of such a pathway, of course, allows for the ready entry of bacteria from the nasopharynx into the cerebrospinal

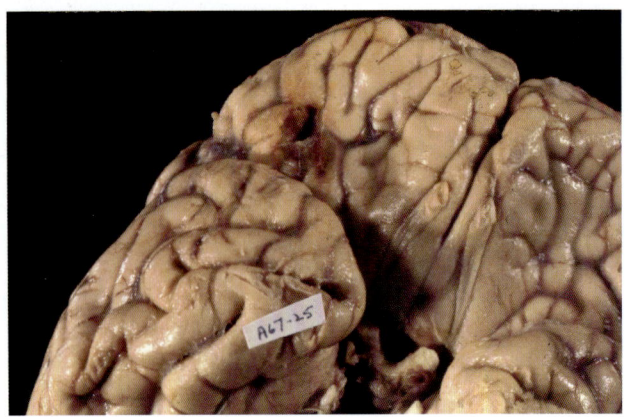

Figure 27.1 Old contusion and laceration of the right orbital frontal area (arrow). This 59-year-old white male had a long history of heavy alcohol intake. In addition to the traumatic lesion shown above, the patient had clinical and pathological evidence of an old Wernicke's encephalopathy involving the mammillary bodies and of alcoholic cerebellar cortical degeneration. (Courtesy of Dr. Jose Segarra.)

fluid spaces, producing recurrent episodes of meningitis. Air may also enter the intracranial cavity through this passageway. Both air and infection may also enter when skull fractures extend into any of the paranasal sinuses or the middle ear. In the latter instance, a cerebrospinal fluid otorrhea may occur: drainage of spinal fluid from the external ear canal. Such basilar skull fractures may extend across the petrous pyramid or tear the tympanic membrane. Blood may be present in the external ear canal or behind the tympanic membrane. If the basilar skull fracture extends into the sigmoid sinus, the tissue over the mastoid may show delayed hematoma with discoloration of the skin and subcutaneous tissue (i.e., "Battle sign").

EXTRADURAL HEMATOMAS AND SUBDURAL HEMATOMAS

Of great importance from the neurological standpoint are these two traumatic conditions in which progressive compression of the cerebral hemispheres occurs. These are conditions where early recognition and treatment will produce excellent results. The failure of recognition will result in progressive deterioration of neurological status with death as the eventual outcome. Note that large traumatic intracerebral hematomas will also produce a progressive course, and these lesions may also benefit from surgical therapy (see also Zervas and Hedley-White, 1972). The use of computerized tomography (CT) scan has revolutionized the diagnostic approach to these problems (see Cordobes et al., 1981; Markwalder, 1981; Masters et al., 1987).

EXTRADURAL HEMATOMA

Extradural hematoma is a complication of skull fractures that extend across a groove containing a meningeal artery, usually the middle meningeal artery. Less often the skull fracture has torn a large venous sinus. Since the bleeding is usually arterial and brisk and the extradural space is narrow (normally the dura is closely applied to the skull), compression of the cerebral hemisphere soon results with the rapid development and progression of neurological symptoms. The classic description is usually that of a short period of unconsciousness related to the acute trauma, then a short lucid interval, which is followed by progressive confusion and coma. A rapidly progressive hemiparesis is often noted with the development of a fixed dilated pupil on the side of the hematoma indicating uncal herniation by the mass that may be placed laterally over the temporal lobe. At other times, as in the following case history, these lateralized findings may be overshadowed by the rapid progression to a stage of functional midbrain transection.

CASE HISTORY 27.1

This 22-year-old, white airman, during a winter storm, was involved in an auto accident at 11:30 p.m., in which he struck his head against the windshield. The patient apparently was dazed, perhaps unconscious, for a matter of seconds to minutes. He was taken by ambulance to the emergency room of the nearby army hospital, where a brief evaluation indicated that the patient was alert, without definite neurological findings, but skull X-rays did indicate a linear fracture over the right temporal area. The patient was apparently alert upon his arrival on the ward. However, by 5 a.m., the patient was reported by the nurses to be agitated and confused.

Neurological Examination (8 a.m.)

Mental status: The patient was agitated and unable to cooperate. He was moving all limbs sitting up in bed, holding his head, which was tender to palpation, moaning and hyperventilating to a marked degree. He answered only occasional questions and then with a yes or no.

Cranial nerves: Pupillary responses were sluggish. The right pupil was perhaps slightly larger and slightly more sluggish than the left.

Reflexes: Deep tendon reflexes were increased bilaterally. Plantar responses were bilaterally equivocal.

Neurological diagnosis: Possible evolving acute bilateral epidural or subdural hematoma.

Subsequent course: Progression occurred. By 4 p.m., the patient was now deeply comatose with little response to stimulation. The pupils were now bilaterally fixed and dilated. The four limbs were extended in a decerebrate posture with significant spasticity on passive motion. The degree of spasticity in the upper limbs could be modified by tonic neck maneuvers. The plantar responses were bilaterally extensor. Spontaneous respirations were now irregular and infrequent, and the patient required the assistance of a mechanical respirator.

Revised neurological diagnosis: Acute tentorial herniation with brain stem compression secondary to epidural hematoma.

Subsequent course: A general surgeon immediately placed burr holes and evacuated an epidural hematoma over the right temporal parietal area. He coagulated and ligated a bleeding middle meningeal artery branch. There was a rapid improvement in the patient's status. The patient returned to active duty but was experiencing some problems related to changes in recent memory, motivation, and personality.

Subdural hematomas: Subdural hematomas (Figs. 27.2 and 27.3) represent the accumulation of blood within the subdural space overlying the cerebral convexities. Such hematomas may be acute, subacute, or chronic. The acute and subacute types are clearly associated with trauma. The acute type is usually associated with other significant

Figure 27.2 Subdural hematoma. This 69-year-old patient with Parkinson's disease had many dizzy spells and had fallen frequently. (Courtesy of Drs. John Hills and Dr. Jose Segarra.)

injuries of the brain such as cerebral contusion, laceration, and intracerebral hematomas. With tears in the arachnoid, blood from the lacerations passes into the subdural space. Moreover, small bridging veins from the pia arachnoid to the superior sagittal sinus are also likely to be torn. The clinical picture of the acute subdural hematoma is often then modified by the clinical manifestations of these associated injuries. At times, however, the typical picture of a rapidly progressive supratentorial space-occupying lesion with progressive obtundation of consciousness and the signs of tentorial herniation will develop in acute (24 to 48 hours) relationship to the head injury. The chronic variety may appear after closed-head trauma, often apparently trivial. At times, there may be no definite history of trauma.

The subacute and chronic subdural hematomas develop after a variable latent period of days, weeks, or months following the injury. The bleeding is venous from small bridging veins passing from the pia arachnoid to the superior sagittal sinus. The resultant accumulation of blood then is relatively slow. Associated injuries to the brain are usually not present. The blood in the subdural space is not readily removed and remains adherent to the dura. Fibroblasts and blood vessels grow from the dura at the edges of the clot, producing a thin membrane that separates the clot from the arachnoid. At the same time, a thicker layer of connective tissue and blood vessels is forming a membrane where the clot is adherent to the inner layer of the dura. The hematoma often continues to increase in size, apparently for several reasons: continued venous oozing may occur; moreover, bleeding may occur from the blood vessels that are growing into the hematoma from the dural surface. Finally, it has been suggested that as some breakdown occurs within the clot, a fluid with high protein content is produced. The resultant fluid of high osmotic pressure then attracts more fluid into the hematoma.

The clinical manifestations are those of a progressive supratentorial mass lesion. At times, progressive focal symptoms and signs are present; for example, hemiparesis, aphasia, and focal seizures. Eventually, alterations in consciousness occur, often of a fluctuating nature. With eventual tentorial herniation, a fixed dilated pupil and the signs of a progressive functional midbrain transection are noted. Often, however, a syndrome is present in which focal symptoms and signs are not prominent, perhaps reflecting the fact that bilateral subdural hematomas are present in a high percentage of cases. The resultant picture then is that of a progressive state of confusion with fluctuating alterations in consciousness. A bilateral grasp reflex is often present. Eventually, if untreated, coma and the signs of tentorial herniation develop. In both types of syndrome, progressive headache may be present, although this complaint as well as the past history of head trauma may be difficult to elicit when the patient is admitted to a hospital in a confused state.

CASE HISTORY 27.2 (PATIENT OF DR. ALEX DANYLEVICH)

This 83-year-old white female struck her head in a motor vehicle accident 2 months prior to admission. She had sustained fractures of her ribs and left clavicle. She had a scalp hematoma in the right frontal area. She was admitted to her local hospital at that time for several days. She was described as having posttraumatic anterograde and retrograde amnesia and obtundation, which cleared over her several-day hospital stay. She returned to her usual activities but then was readmitted with a 3-day history of increasing confusion and lethargy, followed by a mute state.

Neurological Examination
Mental status: The patient was lethargic, mute, and did not follow commands even when relatively alert.
Cranial nerves: Pupils were 2 mm and reactive. There were sudden paroxysmal nystagmoid deviations of the eyes to the right.
Motor system: Tone was increased in the right leg.
Reflexes: Plantar responses were extensor bilaterally.
Clinical diagnosis: Chronic subdural hematomas, probably bilateral.
Laboratory data: The *CT scan* (Fig. 27.3) demonstrated significant bilateral chronic subdural collections much denser on the left

Figure 27.3 Chronic subdural hematoma, bilateral computerized tomography (CT) scans. Case history 27.2. Non–contrast enhanced. This 83-year-old female, 3 months after a motor vehicle accident in which she struck her head, developed fluctuating confusion and lethargy. (See text for details.)

where the lateral ventricle was obscured and shifted to the right. *Serum sodium* was low at 117 mEq/liter.

Hospital course: Serum sodium was corrected. Then, bilateral subdural hematomas were removed via burr holes on the right and a bone flap on the left where substantial chronic membrane and fluid were found. Neurological examination 8 hours after conclusion of the procedure indicated an alert patient who had no apparent language disorder and no weakness. She did develop transient right face and hand focal motor seizures that were treated with anticonvulsants.

There are patients who are at increased risk for subdural hematomas: patients receiving anticoagulant medications or with bleeding disorders (e.g., as in leukemia). The elderly, chronic alcoholics, and patients with Parkinson's disease are also at increased risk, perhaps because such population groups are more prone to unsteadiness and falls (see discussion of Chapter 18). In the patient with cortical atrophy, as in Alzheimer's disease, the bridging veins may be stretched and thus more prone to tear. Because of the atrophy, a large amount of blood may accumulate in the subdural space without producing early symptoms of headache and other symptoms.

The problem also exists in the infant during the first year of life. The picture presented, however, differs significantly from that seen in the adult because in the infant, separation of the sutures may occur, allowing the intracranial cavity to expand. The onset is then often nonspecific and nonfocal: an enlargement of the head, a failure to thrive, a failure to gain weight, and a failure to reach developmental landmarks. At times, generalized seizures, vomiting, and papilledema may be noted. The etiology often relates to presumed birth trauma.

A related problem is the occurrence of subdural effusions in infants following H. influenza meningitis.

MANAGEMENT OF SEVERE HEAD TRAUMA

Severe head injuries represent major problems requiring intensive care. Such patients generally are brought to the emergency room in coma or an obtunded state. As opposed to the patient with a simple concussion (where any loss of consciousness is brief—minutes), these patients continue with an altered level of consciousness for hours, days, weeks, or months. From a pathological standpoint, these patients are found to have contusions, laceration, and multiple hemorrhages within the substance of brain and associated edema and infarction. These findings may be diffuse or concentrated in the diencephalic and midbrain areas involved in maintaining consciousness. At times, the direct effects of trauma have been complicated by cardiopulmonary arrest due to chest injuries or on a central basis producing anoxic encephalopathy. Most do not have epidural or subdural hematomas (epidural in 15%, subdural in 15%). The details of management are considered in Jennett and Teasdale (1981), Bullock and Teasdale (1990), Jaffe and Wesson (1991), White and Likavec (1992), and Ropper et al. (1988). Essentially, the emergency critical care management of the traumatic comatose patient involves the following major steps.

1. ABC: stabilization of vital functions, including Airway, Breathing, and Circulation (control of bleeding and blood pressure).
2. Rapid neurological evaluation with rapid rating of the level of consciousness (see Chapter 29).
3. Emergency CT scan should be obtained. A simple cervical spine series at the same time should serve to rule out cervical fractures and dislocations.
4. Epidural hematomas, significant subdural hematomas, and large focal intracerebral hematomas require emergency neurosurgical intervention.
5. Monitoring and management of increased intracranial pressure are necessary where contusions, edema, small intracerebral hematomas, and small ventricles are present on computerized tomography (CT) scan.
6. Temperature, electrolytes and fluid balance, and nutrition must be maintained to avoid the metabolic causes of coma.
7. Seizures must be treated.
8. Prevention of deep vein thrombosis in the lower extremities and of the subsequent complication of pulmonary embolus (Geerts et al., 1994).

LATE EFFECTS OF HEAD TRAUMA

Posttraumatic Epilepsy

The seizures may be focal or generalized. Penetrating injuries of the head, as in wartime wounds from bullets or shrapnel, are likely to be associated with post-traumatic seizures. In the World War II series of Watson, 41.6% of such patients developed seizures within 3 years of the injury, the majority within 6 to 12 months. There is some evidence that factors such as the location of the wound within the cerebral hemisphere and the complication of abscess may influence the incidence of such post-traumatic seizures. Most head injuries in civilian life, however, are not penetrating missile wounds but rather blunt and nonpenetrating injuries (closed head trauma), and under these circumstances, seizures are much less common. Thus, in the series of Jennett, the overall incidence of seizures in 1000 consecutive blunt head injuries was approximately 5% over a four-year period. In summary, the post-traumatic seizures are more likely to occur in those head injuries where actual structural damage of the cerebral cortex has occurred.

Post-Concussion Syndrome

Another relatively common late complication of head trauma is the posttraumatic or post-concussion syndrome consisting of recurrent episodes of headache and dizziness (vertigo or light-headedness). The episodes often appear to be precipitated by exercise or change in posture from the recumbent to the upright. The severity and duration of the syndrome bear no relationship to the severity of the trauma; the episodes may continue for years after a trivial injury. In a few cases, the vertigo may be related to a traumatic disturbance of the labyrinth. Patients may develop benign positional vertigo. In many cases, the dizziness is actually a light-headedness related to anxiety and hyperventilation. In general, no actual pathology is found.

As a general rule, stable, well-motivated individuals who are anxious to return to their previous occupation or studies do not experience this syndrome in severe degree. On the other hand, individuals with disorders of personality, psychoneurosis, or problems in adjusting to studies or employment appear to be severely affected (Evans, 1992).

In recent years, there has been recognition of possible long duration changes in memory and cognitive function following concussion or other mild head trauma primarily on the basis of neuropsychological testing (see Capruso and Levin, 1992; Packard, 1994 for additional discussion of cognitive effects of head trauma).

PREVENTION

Trauma is the most frequent cause of death and disability in children and young adults. Neurological trauma to brain and spinal cord constitutes the major reason for prolonged costly hospitalizations in young adults since such patients require prolonged intensive critical unit and low-term rehabilitative care. The long-term effects of interruption of what were once hopeful productive careers cannot be calculated simply in terms of the billions of dollars involved but must also take into account the personal and family miseries, which are incurred. Many of the problems are preventable. Table 27.1 summarizes the measures available for prevention of head injuries.

Other traumatic problems include (a) anosmia as in case 30.3 on the CD-ROM (shearing of the olfactory filaments passing through cribriform plate); (b) carotid/cavernous fistula; and (c) dissections of the carotid and vertebral arteries.

NEOPLASMS

Based on the previous chapters, it is evident that particular tumors occur at particular ages. In childhood most intracranial tumors are infratentorial; in adult life, the larger proportion are supratentorial. Meningiomas, glioblastomas, metastatic carcinomas, pituitary adenomas, and vestibular schwannomas (or neurinomas) are tumors of the adult. On the other hand, medulloblastomas and ependymomas are primarily tumors of childhood, while brain stem and spinal cord gliomas are found primarily in older children, adolescents, and adults.

It is also evident that knowledge of the cell type of a tumor taken in isolation does not necessarily enable the observer to predict the future biological and clinical behavior of the tumor. Identity of the cell type and knowledge of the location of the tumor do allow for a higher order of prediction.

Thus, glial tumors may arise in the cerebral hemisphere, the brain stem, and the cerebellum. The biological behavior of the tumor in each location is quite different. Thus, most glial tumors of the cerebral hemispheres in the adult are highly malignant. They are rapidly growing, invasive necrotic tumors with variable cell morphology and frequent nuclear mitotic figures. The brain stem and spinal cord astrocytoma, usually seen in children and young adults, on the other hand, is usually slower growing and has a more constant cellular and nuclear pattern. The cerebellar astrocytoma is a limited cystic and encapsulated tumor of low histological grade, which can be removed in its entirety with essential cure of the patient.

Table 27.1 **PREVENTION OF HEAD INJURIES**

PREVENTATIVE MEASURES	RESULTS OF PREVENTATIVE MEASURE
1. Tricorner seat belts	Mandatory use has been demonstrated to significantly reduce head, face, chest, and spinal cord injuries.
2. Strict enforcement of driving regulations regarding alcohol and drugs	The majority of severe accidents involve the disregard of these regulations. Often the use of these agents is combined with excessive speed.
3. Mandatory use of safety helmets by bicycle and motorcycle riders	Reduces the frequency of: a. Head and neck injury deaths b. Severe head trauma morbidity c. Minor head and neck injuries d. Posttraumatic epilepsy—one of the few preventable causes of one of the major diseases of the nervous system
4. Strict regulation of boxing—professional and amateur with mandatory use of helmets. Compulsory suspensions or revocations after knockouts should be required based on long-term neurological, EEG, and CT scan studies of professional boxers (Ross et al., 1983). Many medical organizations, including the American Medical Association and the American Academy of Neurology, have gone so far as to call for the elimination of all professional boxing.	Reduce the incidence of multiple small contusions and lacerations of the orbital frontal and temporal areas, etc., which result in a chronic frontal lobe syndrome, "the punch drunk" state and possible posttraumatic Parkinsonian state.
5. Effective regulation of sales of arms	Weapons constitute a major cause of injuries and deaths in adolescents and young adults.

CT, computerized tomography; EEG, electroencephalogram.

The clinical manifestations of a particular tumor are determined in part by the cell type of the tumor (astrocytoma, meningioma) and its biological activity (benign meningioma, low-grade astrocytoma, or highly malignant astrocytoma). Much more important in the determination of clinical signs and symptoms is the location of the tumor. This applies to both the local symptoms and signs (focal cortical symptoms and signs or posterior fossa symptoms and signs) and to the general symptoms and signs such as headache, vomiting, drowsiness, and papilledema that reflect the increased intracranial pressure resulting from the tumor mass, cerebral edema, and blockage of the ventricular system. Focal seizures are more likely to occur with low-grade gliomas and meningiomas and less likely to occur with highly malignant gliomas.

HEADACHES

Headache in patients with brain tumors may reflect not only increased intracranial pressure but also the direct or indirect compression of pain-sensitive intracranial structures such as blood vessels, dural sinuses, meninges, or cranial nerves at the base of the brain. At the present time, less than 50% of patients with brain tumors complain of headaches. Headache as an early symptom is more frequent in patients with highly malignant gliomas and less frequent in low-grade gliomas and meningiomas. Supratentorial tumors tend to produce frontal, temporal, orbital, or parietal located headaches. Infratentorial tumors tend to produce occipital or upper cervical located headaches.

In general, patients with headaches alone have another (nontumor) explanation for the headaches. This includes tension headaches; migraine headaches; disease of the nose, nasal sinuses, or orbits; or acute or chronic disease of the cervical spine. Headaches that awaken the patient from sleep or are produced by positional changes or by coughing or similar maneuvers should raise questions about a possible nonbenign pathology. Even under these circumstances, the majority of patients will fall into a benign pathology group. Acute onset of headache, "the worst ever," may indicate a subarachnoid hemorrhage or meningitis.

1. *Migraine headaches.* In general, migraine (vascular headaches) occur intermittently, are throbbing, accompanied by nausea and vomiting, and may be unilateral or bilateral. They are classified as migraine with aura if focal symptoms such as visual phenomena, lateralized tingling, or other cortical phenomena precede the headache. They are classified as migraine without aura if the headache occurs without these phenomena.

2. *Periodic cluster headache.* This variety of unilateral vascular headache often awakens the patient from sleep each night over a period of 1 to 2 weeks. They are throbbing but also involve acute sharp pain localized to the eye. Usually, the headache is accompanied by unilateral tearing of the involved eye and unilateral nasal congestion. They are usually relieved by inhalations of oxygen. Such headaches must be differentiated from the unilateral pain of glaucoma. Acute maxillary sinusitis may also produce unilateral pain in the maxillary and ophthalmic distribution accompanied by nasal congestion, local tenderness, swelling, and erythema.

3. *Muscle tension headaches* tend to occur on a daily basis, and they tend to occur as the problems of the day build up. They are described as a pressure or aching type pain located in the frontal areas but often spreading to the temporal and occipital areas. Often increased tension may be palpated in the temporalis, frontalis, or cervical muscles. Degenerative disease of the cervical spine is frequent and such patients may have chronic muscle tension and aching pain in the cervical and occipital areas.

4. Another common cause of headache is *occipital neuralgia*. This occurs in patients with prior whiplash injuries who have unilateral sharp pains in the distribution of the occipital nerves or the cervical II-nerve root. These patients will have significant local tenderness on palpation of the occipital nerve at the occipital notch. The pain is relieved by cervical traction or local injection of the occipital nerve.

BRAIN TUMOR EPIDEMIOLOGY

The overall relative frequency of the various types of tumors affecting the central nervous system varies from series to series depending on whether a surgical or autopsy series is being reported. In addition, the particular interests of the neurosurgeon have often resulted in a specialized tumor type being referred to a particular neurosurgeon. Table 27.2 presents the data of two neurosurgeons with extensive experience in the surgery of brain tumors. The autopsy data of an earlier period when the postmortem examination was more frequently performed are also presented.

Metastatic tumors are underrepresented in the operative series since patients with multiple metastatic tumors are not considered surgical candidates. Pituitary adenomas were of particular interest to Cushing and, thus, are overrepresented in the operative series. The true clinical frequencies are somewhere between the operative and autopsy incidences. It is important to realize that silent meningiomas may be found on CT scans or magnetic resonance imaging (MRI) scans or at autopsy in older patients. Small pituitary adenomas are found frequently at autopsy.

It is also important to place in perspective the overall frequency of brain tumors.

1. Primary intracranial tumors diagnosed prior to death occur in 11.8 patients per 100,000 per year (Radhakrishman et al., 1995).

2. Asymptomatic tumors. In the same series 7.3 patients per 100,000 per year are found to have asymptomatic tumors.

3. Pediatric age group: Brain tumors are the most frequent form of all solid neoplasm (medulloblastomas, brain stem and cerebellar astrocytomas, ependymomas). Among all malignancies in the pediatric age group, brain tumors are outranked only by leukemia. In the age group 15–34 years, malignant gliomas are the third leading cause of death from cancer.

Table 27.2 RELATIVE FREQUENCY OF VERIFIED INTRACRANIAL TUMORS

TYPE OF TUMOR	COMBINED NEUROSURGICAL SERIES OF 4349 CASES (GRANT AND CUSHING) PERCENT OF TOTAL	AUTOPSY SERIES OF 3010 CASES (COURVILLE) PERCENT OF TOTAL
Gliomas	43.0	41.5
Meningiomas	15.0	11.6
Metastatic tumors	6.5	23.7
Pituitary adenomas	13.0	3.4
Acoustic neuromas	6.5	2.5
Congenital tumors	4.0	3.5
Blood vessel tumors*	7.8	3.0
Miscellaneous: papillomas, granulomas,** and sarcomas	9.0	5.7

*There are very few true tumors of blood vessels (hemangioblastomas and angioblastic meningiomas). Today many of the "tumors" of this group would be considered malformations.
**Today infectious granulomas would not be considered in this series. In some parts of the world tuberculomas and parasitic granulomas still constitute a significant percentage of mass lesions coming to surgery or autopsy.
Source: After Merritt, 1967.

4. Overall, malignant gliomas alone account for 2.5% of deaths due to cancer. Among adults, more die of primary brain tumors than of Hodgkin's disease or of multiple sclerosis.

5. Moreover, 13% of the overall 385,000 cancer deaths per year have some clinical evidence of central nervous system involvement. Autopsy studies suggest that 25% of patients dying of cancer have intracranial metastases. With cancer of the lung, the percentage is even higher.

ETIOLOGY OF PRIMARY BRAIN TUMORS

For the majority of cases, no specific factors can be identified.

1. Radiation of the head early in life for unrelated reasons certainly does significantly increase the risks for all types of tumors involving the nervous system, including gliomas (2.6×), meningiomas (9.5×), and nerve sheath tumors (18.8×), compared to a matched control group. Overall risk for 1.5Gy neural tissue dose was 6.9× control and 20× control for 2.5Gy tissue dosage (Ron et al., 1988).

2. A possible increased risk for the development of gliomas following occupational exposures in the petrochemical, chemical, and rubber industries has been discussed by a number of authors (Selikoff and Hammond, 1982).

3. Head injury of a significant nature, for example, depressed skull fractures, may be associated with meningiomas.

4. In a small number of patients, certain familial syndromes may be present as predisposing factors, for example, *neurofibromatosis* associated with acoustic neuromas, meningiomas and gliomas (of various types—including optic nerve), and *tuberous sclerosis* associated with astrocytomas.

5. Black (1991) and Shapiro and Shapiro (1992) have reviewed concepts of oncogenesis as applied to primary brain tumors. Oncogenes that potentiate or initiate cell mitosis may behave inappropriately or excessively in neoplastic cells. Alternatively, or in addition, neoplastic cells may have lost tumor suppressor sequences. Chromosomal analysis has identified deletion loci on chromosome 22 in meningiomas, chromosome 17 and 22 in acoustic neuromas, and chromosomes 10 and 17 in astrocytomas. Chromosome 7 has been implicated with increased frequency in the cells of malignant gliomas.

5. Other factors: The role of various other growth factors and of immune mechanisms remains to be clarified. Hormonal factors are undoubtedly of importance in meningiomas. These tumors are more common in women than men (2:1 ratio), may undergo growth during pregnancy, and are more common in women with carcinoma of the breast. Estrogen and progesterone receptors have been demonstrated in meningiomas (Lesch et al., 1987).

PRIMARY INTRINSIC TUMORS OF NEUROEPITHELIAL ORIGIN

The most frequent tumors affecting the cerebral hemispheres are those arising from glia. Those of the astrocytic series are by far the most frequent whether operative or autopsy series are considered (Table 27.3). Within this group the glioblastoma is the most frequently encountered, based on autopsy statistics. In the era of Cushing, glioblastomas were often not subjected to surgery. (See later for more recent data and approaches). Oligodendrogliomas are relatively infrequent and ependymomas involving the cerebral hemispheres are rare.

ASTROCYTIC TUMORS

In general, these tumors infiltrate the cerebral hemisphere. The astrocytomas have been subdivided into various types. According to the classification of Kernohan and his associates (1952), these tumors were subdivided into four grades based on their histological degree of malignancy. This classification, to a variable degree, replaced the older nomenclature of Bailey and Cushing (1926), which classified the glial tumors on an embryological basis. (The tumor was classified after the actual or hypothetical embryological cell of closet resemblance.) More recent classifications have utilized features that correlate with prognosis (see Burger and Green, 1985; Burger et al., 1987; Daumais-Duport et al., 1988). Features of importance in grading are degree of (1) hypercellularity; (2) pleomorphism, including nuclear atypia and mitosis; (3) vascular proliferation; and (4) necrosis.

Table 27.3 **THE OVERALL INCIDENCE OF VARIOUS TYPES OF ALL VERIFIED NEUROEPITHELIAL TUMORS***

TYPE OF GLIOMA	NEUROSURGICAL SERIES (CUSHING) TOTAL NO. = 862 PERCENT	AUTOPSY SERIES (COURVILLE) TOTAL NO. = 1259 PERCENT	AVERAGE SURVIVAL: MONTHS AFTER ONSET OF SYMPTOMS**
Astrocytoma grade I	30.0	23.0	76
Astrocytoma grade II	4.0	1.0	28
Glioblastoma (Astrocytoma grades III & IV)	24.0	52.0	12
Polar spongioblastoma	4.0	2.0	46
Ganglioglioma	0.3	2.0	–
Oligodendroglioma	3.0	1.0	66
Ependymoma	3.0	6.5	32
Medulloblastoma	10.0	6.0	17
Pinealoma	2.0	1.0	—
Unclassified	20.0	4.0	—

*The series are not restricted to the cerebral hemisphere but include all gliomas.
**After Merritt, 1967.

In the discussion that follows, we will utilize the several classifications as well as the most recent classification of the World Health Organization.

From a prognostic standpoint, the following grades of astrocytoma are recognized:

The Low-Grade Astrocytoma Tumor (Grade I or II Astrocytoma)

This is a mildly hypercellular tumor with a variable degree of pleomorphism but with no vascular proliferation and no necrosis. There is an increased number of mature astrocytes of relatively normal appearance with no evidence of mitosis. Those arising in the cortex are composed predominantly of protoplasmic astrocytes and were referred to as "gemistocytic"; the cell resembles reactive astrocytes. Those arising in the white matter are composed predominantly of fibrillary astrocytes and sometimes referred to as "piloid or pilocytic." Grossly, the lesion is nonencapsulated, firm, and granular and gray. Cysts may be present. At times, the only hint of the lesion may be a lack of distinction between gray and white matter. On CT the cyst may be evident. The lesion, however, is usually best seen on MRI scan, which initially does not demonstrate tumor enhancement.

Grade I. Mild, hypercellularity, with little pleomorphism or mitosis. The major example is the pilocytic astrocytoma that is predominantly a tumor of children and adolescents. The predominant cell type is usually the fibrillary astrocyte, a relatively uniform elongated mature astrocyte infiltrating along white matter tracts and often found in the pons, optic chiasm, and diencephalon. The term *polar spongioblast* was at one time applied to this type of tumor.

Grade II. The major example in this group is the low-grade fibrillary astrocytoma demonstrating a greater hypercellularity with greater pleomorphism (mitosis present) but with no vascular proliferation or necrosis. Most (65%–95%) present with seizures either focal or secondarily generalized and initially the neurological examination may be without focal features. Most eventually progress to high-grade malignant gliomas. The appearance of progressive neurological findings and of tumor enhancement in the MRI or CT scan may signify such a progression. The median survival despite therapy is 5 years, but some survive for 10–15 years.

Malignant Astrocytoma

These tumors correspond to histologic grades III and IV and unfortunately are the most common glial tumors with an annual incidence of 3 to 4 per 100,000 populations. Two tumors are included: the anaplastic astrocytoma and the very malignant glioblastoma. Both types of tumor have a significant contrast enhancement on CT and MRI scans which is often an irregular ring-like area at the apparent margin. In actuality, the tumor extends beyond this border into the adjacent tissue.

Grade III: The anaplastic astrocytoma tends to begin between the ages of 30 to 50 years. Characteristics include a significant degree of hypercellularity, a significant degree of pleomorphism, and a moderate degree of vascular proliferation (Fig. 27.4). Median survival with aggressive treatment is approximately 3 years. Treatment is similar to that discussed for glioblastoma.

Grade IV. The glioblastoma multiforme accounts for 80% of all malignant gliomas, with the highest frequency of onset of symptoms between the ages of 50 to 70 years. However, there are two categories within this group: primary glioblastomas

Figure 27.4 Gemistocytic astrocytoma, demonstrating a relatively high grade of malignancy: swollen astrocytes, with nuclei often bizarre and multinucleated displaced to the periphery (H&E, 400×). (Courtesy of Dr. David Cowen, Columbia-Presbyterian, Neuropathology.)

that tend to begin in older individuals (mean age: 55years) and secondary glioblastomas, occurring in somewhat younger individuals (mean age: 45 years). These latter tumors have begun as a lower grade of tumor and then have secondarily evolved so that younger patients often appear to have a longer duration of disease. From the histological standpoint, a marked hypercellularity is present with marked variability of cellular and nuclear appearance (Fig. 27.5). Multinucleated cells and mitotic figures are frequent (4–5 per high power field). Hyperplasia of blood vessels is very evident (endothelial proliferation). The additional feature of necrosis serves to distinguish this tumor from the anaplastic astrocytoma. The vascular proliferation often results in hemorrhage into the tumor. The vascular hyperplasia of adventitia and endothelium may be so prominent as to suggest actual sarcomatous alteration. Both the hyperplasia of the blood vessel wall and the rapid growth of the tumor often result in a tumor that outgrows the blood supply with resultant necrosis within the tumor. Grossly, the presence of hemorrhage and necrosis is evident (Fig. 27.6). These features are also evident on CT scans (Fig. 27.7), which will demonstrate area of hemorrhage, necrosis, and edema and, with contrast, a considerable degree of ring enhancement.

Prognosis and Treatment. For malignant astrocytomas, surgery may be employed for purposes of decompression and for debulking the tumor mass so that fewer malignant cells remain to be destroyed by radiotherapy. For the glioblastoma, median survival with surgery only is 6 months; with surgery and radiotherapy, 12 months. The role of chemotherapy is uncertain; the percentage of long-term survivors may be moderately increased. In the study of Shapiro et al. (1989), 29%–37% of patients with glioblastoma receiving radiotherapy survived for 18 months. Chemotherapy produced minor additional survival (approximately 2–3 months).

In general, younger patients with polar lesions who are able to tolerate extensive resection, radiotherapy, and perhaps chemotherapy have the longer survivals (Scott et al., 1999). Why do these patients do poorly? Although at times these tumors may arise superficially in the cerebral cortex, more often they seem to originate in the subcortical white matter. They then appear to infiltrate widely through the cerebral

Figure 27.5 Glioblastoma surgical histological features. Case 27.4. Refer to text and Figure 27.7. (*A*) Low-powered field demonstrating marked cellularity and marked vascular proliferation with areas of micro-hemorrhage (approximately 100× in original). (*B*) High-powered field demonstrating marked pleomorphism, giant cells, and mitotic figures (approximately 400× in original).

Figure 27.6 Glioblastoma multiforme of the left temporal lobe compressing brain stem and ventricular system. This 43-year-old white male had the onset of short "dreamy" states preceded by a distinctive taste and a sensation of familiarity. Despite a craniotomy and radiation therapy, the patient had a 14-month course characterized by a progressive right hemiparesis, a nominal aphasia, a severe receptive aphasia, increasing disorientation, lethargy, headache, vomiting, and papilledema. (Courtesy of Drs. John Hills and Jose Segarra.)

Figure 27.7 Glioblastoma: case 27.4. Refer to text. Computerized tomography (CT) scans. (*A*) Nonenhanced CT scan demonstrated a low-density mass in the left frontal parietal parasagittal region, with areas of hemorrhage. (*B*) CT scan (with contrast) demonstrated an irregular rim of enhancement.

hemisphere, often along white matter systems to involve other areas of the brain (e.g., via the corpus callosum to involve the opposite hemisphere). At times, a multicentric origin may be suspected. Necrosis and hemorrhage are frequent; and progression of neurological deficit is often rapid. At times, the episodes of necrosis and hemorrhage may suggest vascular accidents.

The variable clinical course of a glioblastoma in younger (40-year-old) patients has already been presented in Chapters 21 and 24. Those cases should be reviewed at this time. The clinical course in an older patient with a 4- to 5-day course prior to diagnosis, which initially suggested a possible cerebrovascular event, is presented as case 27.4 and in Figures 27.5 and 27.7. In retrospect, it was evident on the CT scan and at surgery that the acute onset reflected the hemorrhage and necrosis, which had occurred within the tumor.

CASE HISTORY 27.4 (PATIENT OF DR. TOM MULLINS)

This 68-year-old, right-handed white male was admitted to St Vincent Hospital with an apparent 4- to 5-day history of difficulty in doing calculations and in speaking: "he could think of the word, but had difficulty getting it out."

Neurological Examination

Mental status: Speech was limited to short phrases with loss of connectors and sentence structure. Writing was impaired but repetition, comprehension, naming, and reading were intact.

Motor system: Fine motor movements of the right hand were impaired. Tone was increased on the right.

Reflexes: The right patellar reflex was increased. Bilateral Babinski signs were present.

Initial clinical diagnosis: Diagnosis was uncertain. The abrupt onset suggested possible vascular event such as embolus to the middle cerebral artery, but overall pattern including bilateral Babinski sign without significant hemiparesis was unusual.

Laboratory data: *EEG:* Focal left hemisphere delta and theta slow-wave activity. *CT scan* (Fig. 27.7): (a) the *nonenhanced study* demonstrated a low-density mass in the left frontal-parietal parasagittal region with areas of hemorrhage. (b) The *contrast-enhanced study* demonstrated an irregular rim of enhancement. *Angiograms* indicated an avascular mass in the left frontal-parietal area.

Subsequent course: Dr. Alex Danylevich performed a subtotal resection of this tumor that was found to contain blood clot and cystic fluid. The histology of the tumor was glioblastoma multiforme (Fig. 27.5). The patient subsequently received 4000cGy whole-brain radiation and an additional 2000cGy to the tumor site. Three months following surgery, the patient developed increasing obtundation. CT scan revealed a large left frontal necrotic mass. Fever, hypocalcaemia, and hypernatremia developed and he expired 1 month later.

Comments

This patient presented with what appeared to be an abrupt onset of language problems, raising the question of a cerebrovascular accident. In retrospect, it was evident on the CT scan and at surgery that the acute onset reflected the hemorrhage and necrosis that had occurred within the tumor. This was a rapidly growing, extremely malignant tumor, which apparently had outstripped its blood supply despite the neovascularity.

Other types of glial tumors: Oligodendrogliomas: this variety of glioma is found in the cerebral hemisphere of young and middle-aged adults constituting 5%–20% of all glial tumors. The majority is low grade with a long course of 5–15 years; refer to case 18.2. A small percentage are anaplastic or mixed tumors containing anaplastic astrocytoma elements (Fig. 27.8 demonstrates the histology).

Other tumors of neuroepithelial origin: This group contains two very common tumors of the pediatric patient: (1) *primitive neuroectodermal tumor: medulloblastomas* (Fig. 27.9 and case 20.1) and

Figure 27.8 Oligodendroglioma. A relatively uniform mosaic pattern of cells with a small nucleus surrounded by a clear halo of cytoplasm is evident. A small area of calcification is present in this field; much larger areas of calcification were evident in other fields (H&E, 400×) (Courtesy of Dr. David Cowen.)

Figure 27.9 Ependymoma of the fourth ventricle. Clusters of ependymal cells are arranged as rosettes or as perivascular pseudorosettes (H&E, 125×). (Courtesy of Dr. John Hills.)

(2) *ependymomas* (Fig. 27.10). These brain tumors of the posterior fossa constitute the most common solid malignant tumors found in the pediatric population. These tumors have been discussed and illustrated in Chapters 13 and 20.

The other two tumors in this group are rare: (1) *Ganglioglioma or neuroastrocytoma* is now considered to represent the diffuse infiltration by a low-grade astrocytoma among neurons of the cerebral cortex—basal ganglia or diencephalic nuclei. At times, this type of histological picture has been noted in the lesion of tuberous sclerosis. (2) *Pinealomas* figures 27.9 and 27.10: These relatively rare tumors of the pineal have been considered already in relation to the brain stem (Chapter 13). The most common tumor of the pineal region is the germinoma.

OTHER PRIMARY INTRINSIC TUMORS OF THE NONNEUROEPITHELIAL ORIGIN

1. *Primary central nervous system lymphomas:* Prior to 1980, primary intrinsic tumors of the nervous system of non-neuroepithelial origin were considered rare. Primary lymphomas of the central nervous system have now assumed increasing importance and are no longer rare. In general, these malignant tumors have B cell surface markers and are of the diffuse large cell subtype. They were formerly designated reticulum cell sarcoma or microgliomas. As

Figure 27.10 Medulloblastoma. Clusters of small cells with densely staining nuclei are present (H&E, 400×). Refer Chapter 20 for illustration of a gross specimen. (Courtesy of Dr. David Cowen.)

with glioblastomas, the peak incidence occurs in the 50- to 70-year age range. The increased incidence has occurred in both the immune-suppressed (AIDS) and the immune-competent population.

2. *Tumors of blood vessel origin:* Probably the only true vascular neoplasm intrinsic to the central nervous system is the hemangioblastoma of the cerebellum composed of embryonic vascular elements. Giant aneurysms angiomas or arteriovenous malformations of the brain and meninges are composed of adult vascular elements and are not neoplasms but may have mass effect. Hemangioblastomas are discussed in Chapter 20.

EXTRINSIC TUMORS

Meningiomas

The most common extrinsic tumor above the tentorium is the meningioma. Meningiomas constitute 20% of all types of brain tumors. Based on the epidemiological data from Rochester Minnesota (Radhakrishnan et al., 1995), meningiomas have a total annual incidence of 7.8 per 100,000 populations, but the true incidence of symptomatic meningiomas is 2 per 100,000. Most meningiomas (74%) are asymptomatic and are discovered at autopsy or on imaging studies performed for unrelated problems (Fig. 27.11). Meningiomas are tumors of the adult population 30 to 70 years of age. They are more frequent in females due to the fact that many meningiomas contain estrogen receptors. There is an additional increased incidence in patients with breast cancer, at times providing a diagnostic dilemma. Meningiomas arise from arachnoidal cells embedded in the dura. Normally, arachnoidal villi invaginate into the venous sinuses as arachnoidal or pacchionian granulations, but arachnoidal cells may be embedded in the dura. In addition, fibrous and vascular elements are, to a variable degree, also included in these tumors. The variable composition has resulted in a histologic classification according to the following main types:

1. A *syncytial or meningothelial* variety composed of clusters of cells similar to the outer layer of arachnoid arranged in nests or whorls and surrounded by layers of elongated or flattened cells.

2. A *fibrous* variety in which interlacing bundles of fibroblastic elements predominate.

3. A *psammomatous* variety (probably the most common type) consisting of the same type of arachnoidal cells, arranged in a whorl. In the center of the whorl is an area of hyalinization arranged in concentric lamellae and calcified (psammomatous granules). The calcification is often visible on plain X-rays of the skull.

4. A less common *angioblastic* variety, which appears spongy both on gross and microscopic examination, because it contains multiple small vascular channels. (At times, the term *hemangiopericytoma* has been applied to this type of meningioma.)

5. A *mixed or transitional* variety. Considerable overlap is apparent, as demonstrated in Figure 27.12.

Figure 27.11 Meningiomas: incidental discovery multiple asymptomatic in a 71-year-old ambidextrous female with a normal neurological examination. The patient had a history of a transient left posterior thalamic lacunar infarct, which was confirmed on subsequent magnetic resonance imaging (MRI) studies. Those studies also disclosed right prefrontal and right parietal asymptomatic meningiomas (*A*) nonenhanced—T1—right parasagittal section, (*B*) enhanced—T1—frontal coronal section, (*C*) enhanced T1 parietal coronal section. No changes occurred over the next 5 years.

It is unclear that these different histologic types have prognostic significance. However, a small percentage (7%) from a histologic standpoint have atypical or frankly malignant features of a sarcoma. Regardless of the histologic type, all meningiomas on molecular analysis have a loss of chromosome 22q. A similar defect occurs in patients with neurofibromatosis type 2. These latter patients often have multiple meningiomas in addition to bilateral schwannomas of the vestibular nerve.

These tumors are in general benign and slow growing. Almost all occur external to the brain with a dural attachment—compressing, displacing, and at times invaginating into the brain. Rarely, the tumors may be found without a dural attachment within the ventricle or within the sylvian fissure. Although not invading the brain, the otherwise benign meningioma may invade the overlying bone of the skull. Others excite an osteoblastic reaction in the overlying bone with a marked local thickening of the bone (hyperostosis). What is important about meningiomas is not their histological cell type (sarcomatous degeneration is rare) but their location; in general, they are readily amenable to neurosurgical removal. In asymptomatic cases, the risks of surgery may outweigh any conceivable benefit to the patient.

Meningiomas tend to occur in certain specific locations outlined in Table 27.4 (Histological appearance of a mixed meningioma, Fig. 27.12 and Example of meningiomas in sphenoid lesser wing Fig. 27.13).

The course of several meningiomas has been presented already in several of the case histories of Chapters 1, 18, 22, and 23.

Tumors of the Pituitary Gland. See Chapter 16 and later.

Other Extrinsic Tumors Involving the Brain. Refer to Table 27.5.

SECONDARY TUMORS

METASTATIC TUMORS

The greatest number of secondary tumors of the central nervous system spread from a distant site via the bloodstream. The

Figure 27.13 Outer third sphenoid wing meningioma. The dura overlying the sphenoid has been reflected, revealing a large meningioma (arrow) compressing the inferior surface of the anterior temporal lobe and adjacent orbital frontal area. This 73-year-old black male had a 14-year history of complex partial and generalized tonic clonic convulsions. (Courtesy Drs. John Hills and Jose Segarra.)

Figure 27.12 Meningioma. Histological appearance of a mixed or transitional type meningioma. Interlacing fibrous bundles and whorls of meningothelial cells are present in addition to a calcified psammoma body (arrow) (H&E, 100×). (Courtesy of Dr. David Cowen.)

Table 27.4 MENINGIOMAS

LOCATION	FREQUENCY*	MANIFESTATIONS
Parasagittal a) Rolandic b) Prefrontal	21%–23% (or 33%–50%)	a. Focal motor or sensory seizures or leg weakness (cases 1.1, 18.1)
Lateral convexity	17%	Focal motor seizures hand or face
Sphenoid wing	9%–17%	Fig. 27.13.
a) Inner third		Unilateral exophthalmos and optic nerve atrophy + contralateral papilledema**
b) Middle third B		Lateral papilledema, then inner or outer third findings
c) Outer third		Temporal lobe seizures (Fig. 27.13)
Anterior fossa	8%–18%	
a) Olfactory groove		Unilateral anosmia, prefrontal syndrome, dementia (see case 22.5)
b) Tuberculum sellae		May mimic pituitary tumor, with compression of optic chiasm, prefrontal syndrome
Posterior fossa	7%	See Chapter 13, CP angle, foramen magnum, and tentorial syndromes
Other sites		
a) Intraventricular	Not common	Hydrocephalus
b) Spinal cord		Spinal cord compression; see Chapter 9

*Series of Cushing and Eisenhardt (1938), of Courville (1967), and of Taveras and Wood (1964).

**Foster-Kennedy syndrome (see case 23.1).

Table 27.5 OTHER EXTRINSIC TUMORS INVOLVING THE BRAIN

TYPE	LOCATION	STRUCTURES INVOLVED OR MANIFESTATION
Craniopharyngioma	Suprasellar	Pituitary, hypothalamus, optic chiasm (Fig. 27.14)
Epidermoid,	Bone of skull, dura or cisterns C-P	Angle or suprasellar
Dermoids/Teratomas	Usually midline	Pineal, pituitary, 4th ventricle
Chordomas	Clivus	Compression of ventral brain stem, basilar artery
Colloid cysts*	F. Monro of Third ventricle	Acute hydrocephalus with acute headache and coma, often intermittent due to ball valve mechanism (Fig. 27.15, 27.16)
Schwannomas**	Posterior fossa	C-P angle, vestibular nerve most common (see Chap. 12 Fig. 27.17)

*The colloid cyst of the third ventricle although uncommon must be recognized in the emergency room, since death may result.

**Except for Schwannomas at CP angle (Fig. 27.17), which may also arise from cranial nerves (jugular foramen) and from the sensory nerve roots, all of these tumors are relatively rare. Refer to Chapter 13.

majority spread to the cerebral hemisphere or to the cerebellar hemisphere. Metastatic lesions may be solitary or multiple (Figs. 27.18, 27.19, and 27.20). In the series of Delattre et al. (1988), 47% of patients with metastatic lesions to the brain on CT scan had single lesions. These secondary metastatic tumors represent a significant percentage of patients seen with intracranial tumors in a general hospital population. As already noted, 25% of cancer patients have cerebral metastases at autopsy. With increasing length of survival after the diagnosis of cancer, metastatic spread to both brain and leptomeninges has increased in frequency.

1. The most frequent site of primary tumor is the lung, accounting for almost a third of the cases. It has been estimated that almost half of all patients with small cell and nonsquamous, non–small cell carcinoma of the lung, at autopsy will have cerebral metastasis (Cox and Yesner, 1979).

2. The second most frequent site of primary lesion is the breast. Several examples have been presented in Chapter 21.

3. Certain tumors, which have a lower overall frequency of occurrence than carcinoma of the lung and breast, have a particularly high frequency of metastatic spread to the brain: (a) malignant melanoma (usually multiple), (b) hypernephromas (often solitary), and (c) choriocarcinoma. (In the surgical series of Delattre et al. [1988], lung malignancies accounted for 40%, melanoma for 11%, and kidney cancer for 11%.)

Treatment

Solitary metastatic lesions may be subjected to surgical removal, since median survival is significantly improved in series where surgery plus radiation is compared to radiation alone: 40 weeks versus 15 weeks (Patchell et al., 1990) (see Fig. 27.14).

At other times, when multiple metastasis occur, radiation therapy or hormonal therapy may be employed, with a significant reduction in symptoms (for additional discussion, see Posner, 1990, 1992).

Carcinomatous Meningitis: Malignant cells are present in the cerebrospinal fluid implanting on nerve roots, cranial nerves, hemispheres, and meninges (Figs. 27.20 and 27.21). Breast cancer, lymphoma, lung cancer, and melanoma are the most frequent primary lesions. Hydrocephalus is frequent. Additional discussion and illustrative case histories will be found in Hedges et al. (1988), Winkler and DeLaMonte

Figure 27.14 Craniopharyngioma. A 23-year-old female with a 6-year history of headaches and amenorrhea followed by diplopia and papilledema. Contrast enhanced scan demonstrates suprasellar calcification with large cyst, which projects upward into the third ventricle (*A*) thin sections through suprasellar region; (*B*) sagittal and coronal reconstructions.

(1987), Gruber and Sobel (1992), Little et al. (1974), and Olson et al. (1974).

Local Invasive Tumors: Direct extension of tumors to involve the brain is less common than metastatic disease. Common primary sites are carcinomas originating in the nasopharynx and nasal sinuses (Fig. 27.14). These tumors may erode the base of the skull or spread through the foramina at the base of the skull to involve cranial nerves such as nerves V and VI. Treatment involves local radiation; results are dependent on the capacity for response of the primary lesion.

INFECTIONS

The central nervous system may be involved by all of the general types of organisms that infect other systems of the

Figure 27.15 Colloid cyst of the third ventricle. This 20-year-old male had sudden attacks of headache; with the last such attack he presented to the emergency room with rapid onset of coma and death.

body: bacteria, viruses, rickettsiae, fungi, protozoa, and helminths. Certain organisms do have a predilection for the central nervous system and often for particular segments or certain systems of the neuraxis. Thus, we have already seen that the virus of poliomyelitis involves predominantly the motor neurons of the anterior horn and brain stem. Bacteria such as meningococcus and haemophilus influenzae involve predominantly the meninges. In most instances, when infectious agents involve the central nervous system, they also involve to a variable degree other systems of the body in a general or focal manner. The student should bear in mind that the clinical and pathological manifestations of an infectious disease reflect not only the direct effects of the invading organism but also effects that indicate the body's defensive responses to invasion. Moreover, when immune mechanisms have been suppressed, as in AIDS (acquired immune deficiency disease), organisms that do not usually invade the brain or other organs of the adult patient may assume major invasive roles. Examples include toxoplasmosis, fungi, and cytomegalovirus.

Infections involving the nervous system may be considered under two broad categories:

1. Those infections that involve the central nervous system or subdivisions of the central nervous system in a general or diffuse manner
2. Those infections that involve the central nervous system in a focal (or multifocal) manner

FOCAL INFECTIONS OF THE NERVOUS SYSTEM

The problem of focal infections of the nervous system has an importance far out of proportion to the actual frequency of occurrence of such cases. These focal infections represent, in general, rapidly progressive and compressive space-occupying lesions and they often require emergency neurosurgical intervention.

We have already seen that at the level of spinal cord, focal infections are essentially extradural in location. The favorite site of acute focal infection is the fatty tissue of the epidural space. The resultant clinical picture is that of a rapidly progressive extradural compressive lesion of the spinal cord. The symptoms and signs are due both to the direct damage from compression and the indirect destruction of tissue produced by vascular

Figure 27.16 Colloid cyst of third ventricle. This 23-year-old right-handed male had a 4- to 6-week history of generalized throbbing headache and episodic visual obscuration with bilateral papilledema and enlargement of the blind spots. Computerized tomography (CT) scan demonstrated a third ventricular colloid cyst at the level of the foramen of Monro with secondary dilation of the lateral ventricles. (*A*) Contrast-enhanced CT at horizontal level just above foramen of Monro. (*B*) Coronal reconstruction. All symptoms disappeared after Dr. Alex Danylevich drained and removed this cyst and shunted the ventricular system.

Figure 27.17 Vestibular (acoustic) neuroma or schwannoma. Microscopic examination of these tumors usually indicates two tissue types: interwoven bundles of spindle-shaped cells with alignment of nuclei in the form of palisades; and looser, somewhat cystic areas (H&E, 100×). (Courtesy of Dr. David Cowen, Columbia-Presbyterian, Neuropathology.)

compression and occlusion. At the level of the spinal cord also, spinal cord compression may result from the involvement of and collapse of vertebral bodies by chronic tuberculosis.

ACUTE FOCAL INFECTIONS INVOLVING THE BRAIN

Three syndromes should be considered: (1) subdural empyema, (2) purulent brain abscess, and (3) focal viral cerebritis—Herpes simplex.

Figure 27.18 Multiple metastatic tumors to cerebral hemisphere from malignant melanoma, with secondary hemorrhage into several of the pigmented lesions in a 40-year-old white female with excision of primary melanoma of the left knee with dissection of the left groin 5 years prior to death. She had multiple cutaneous metastatic nodules despite chemotherapy and then right temporal headache, nausea and vomiting, sudden coma with papilledema, and sluggish pupils. (Courtesy of Dr. John Hills.)

Figure 27.19 Multiple metastatic tumors to brain. Computerized tomography (CT) scans demonstrate multiple high-density lesions with low-density centers and surrounding areas of edema. Minor enhancement occurred in some of the lesions with contrast. This 43-year-old white male with a 30-pack-year smoking history and a poorly differentiated adenocarcinoma with invasion of peribronchial lymph nodes and of parietal pleura initially presented with hemoptysis. Four months later he presented with a 1-day history of confusion, lethargy, and frontal release signs and died 1 month later.

1. *Subdural empyema:* In general, subdural empyema occurs as a result of the direct extension of purulent infection from an adjacent focus of infection in the nasal sinuses or middle ear or following compound skull fractures. The nasal sinuses are now implicated as the major source of infection. Osteomyelitis of the intervening bone is a frequent finding; thrombophlebitis of the venous sinuses and of the feeding cortical veins is a not unusual complication. The pus is present in a space that offers very little resistance to the expansion of this purulent mass. The mass is apparently never well encapsulated, although in older cases after the removal of the pus, a fibrinous exudate will be found on the inner surface of the dura and the inner surface of the arachnoid. The responsible organism is most commonly the Staphylococcus aureus. A sterile secondary inflammation is usually present in the subarachnoid space. This results in spinal fluid findings on lumbar puncture of moderate increases in cells and protein but a normal sugar and negative culture.

2. *Purulent brain abscess:* A brain abscess (Fig. 27.22) reflects the spread of purulent infection to the brain by several pathways. Direct extension may occur from a nearby focus of infection in the nasal sinuses or mastoid or middle ear. For this reason many solitary brain abscesses tend to be located in the frontal or temporal lobe of the cerebral hemisphere or in the cerebellar hemisphere. Direct introduction of infected material may occur in relation to trauma, for example, compound skull fractures, or in relation to neurosurgical procedures. Finally, hematogenous spread may occur in patients with a primary source in the lung, in patients with bacterial endocarditis, and in

Figure 27.20 Multiple metastatic tumors to brain adjacent to ventricular system and subarachnoid space with carcinomatous meningitis. Which process was the primary one—periventricular solid metastatic lesions or the carcinomatous meningitis—remains uncertain. This 51-year-old white male teamster had progressive headaches for 6–7 weeks and a 2-week history of a progressive third nerve paralysis. Computerized tomography (CT) scans and magnetic resonance imaging (MRI) scans demonstrated at least five distinct areas of contrast-enhancing metastatic tumors. Cerebrospinal fluid contained 90 cells consistent with non–small cell carcinoma. Chest X-ray demonstrated a lesion in the upper lobe of the right lung. He received radiotherapy and dexamethasone with improvement in headache. Three weeks later he developed weakness, tingling, and depression of reflexes in both lower extremities, plus urinary and fecal incontinence. (*A*) T1 horizontal section. (*B*) T1 coronal section.

patients with cyanotic congenital heart disease where the blood may bypass the screening system of the lungs. Patients with pulmonary arteriovenous fistula are also at special risk. Such hematogenous spread is more likely to result in multiple abscesses rather than a solitary abscess.

Since the introduction of antibiotics, there has been a significant decrease in the number of patients presenting with brain abscess, particularly in the number of cases where the abscess is secondary to sinusitis and mastoiditis. Moreover, among the remaining patients there has been a decrease in the percentage of cases with an identifiable primary focus of infection and an increase in cases without an identifiable primary focus. These latter cases may reflect instances where partial

Figure 27.21 "Meningeal carcinomatosis." Five years after a complete remission from diffuse histiocytic lymphoma (Stage III-B non-Hodgkin's lymphoma), which had presented with symptoms of fever, night sweats, abdominal pain, and lymphadenopathy, this 77-year-old female had a biopsy-proven recurrence of disease (lymph nodes and bone marrow). She had drowsiness, poor recall, right eyelid ptosis, and diffuse weakness of the left lower extremity with tenderness over left femoral and sciatic nerves. Over 2 days she progressed to a complete pupil sparing right third nerve paralysis, incomplete left CN III paralysis (downgaze was preserved), left CN VI paralysis, bilateral peripheral facial paralysis, decreased hearing on left, and bilateral toe extensor weakness. Cerebrospinal fluid cytology (approximately 1000×) demonstrated large pleomorphic neoplastic cells. The patient received intrathecal chemotherapy (Methotrexate). (Courtesy of the Pathology Department at St. Vincent Hospital.)

Figure 27.22 Subacute brain abscess with associated ventriculitis. This 41-year-old white male, as a child, had a fibroma of the right maxillary sinus that had been treated with surgery and radon implants. Four months before death he developed the first of four episodes of meningitis with headache, nuchal rigidity, fever, and chills; cerebrospinal fluid contained 495 white blood cells (75% polymorphonuclear) and a cerebrospinal fluid sugar of 40 mg/100 ml. He had chronic sinusitis of right maxillary and ethmoid sinuses on X-rays and defect in the bone and dura in relation to the right ethmoid sinus. (Courtesy of Drs. John Hills and Jose Segarra.)

Figure 27.23 Brain abscess. Computerized tomography (CT) scan: (A) nonenhanced demonstrates an edematous mass in white matter of right posterior temporal parietal-occipital areas with compression of the right lateral ventricle. (B) With contrast a 3–4 cm ring-like enhancement occurs. This 53-year-old, left-handed white male with borderline diabetes mellitus had been treated for an abscess in the muscle of the abdominal wall due to anaerobic Bacteroides with incision drainage and antibiotics. Seven days later he developed severe "blinding" right-sided headaches; confusion; difficulty in reading, word finding, following commands, and repetition of short phrases; plus flat affect, a neglect of the left visual field, and a mild left hemiparesis. All neurological findings resolved over the next 2 days after treatment with antibiotics, dexamethasone, and mannitol (to reduce cerebral edema) and immediate evacuation of the abscess. (Courtesy of Drs. Ralph Sama and Bernard Stone.)

antibiotic therapy has eradicated the primary focus but not the brain abscess.

As might be expected, the most common organism is Staphylococcus aureus. Streptococci and pneumococci are also encountered as responsible organisms. Rarely, under special circumstances, a fungus infection may be implicated, for example, mucormycosis in severely debilitated diabetics and aspergillosis in patients receiving immunosuppressive therapy after renal transplantation or in patients with AIDS.

When the cerebral hemisphere is involved, the clinical symptoms will correspond to the specific area impacted with focal seizures and rapidly evolving focal neurological deficits as the prominent features.

The electroencephalogram is likely to show continuous focal 0.5 to 2 Hz slow-wave activity indicating severe focal damage (refer to Fig. 2.22). The CT scan (Fig. 27.23) will usually demonstrate a contrast ring-enhancing lesion.

In general, the outcome in the untreated brain abscess is fatal. Treatment consists of surgical drainage and total excision of the abscess cavity. In addition, appropriate antibiotic therapy must be administered. In the series of Loeser and Scheinberg (1957), surgical therapy in the period 1940–1944 was associated with a 47% mortality. By the period 1949–1956, an era of specific antibiotics, this mortality had dropped to 19%.

A brain abscess involving the right parietal-occipital area has already been presented in Chapter 23. In reviewing that case, the student should keep in mind that events in a temporal lobe abscess may proceed at a much more rapid pace as regards tentorial herniation with third nerve and brain stem compression.

CHRONIC FOCAL OR MULTIFOCAL INFECTIONS: GRANULOMAS

The following infections may produce granulomas: tuberculosis, cryptococcus, larva of the pork tape worm (cerebral cysticercosis), toxoplasmosis, and schistosomiasis. In some parts of the world these infections are a common cause of mass lesions, seizures, or hydrocephalus. (See also discussion of AIDS.)

GENERAL OR DIFFUSE INFECTIONS

We will consider this section in greater detail on the CD-ROM.

This category of diseases is usually presented in detail in microbiology courses and in the infectious disease sections of internal medicine.

a. Those involving primarily the leptomeninges (pia and arachnoid) producing leptomeningitis. Generalized infection of the dura (pachymeningitis) is uncommon (Figs. 27.24 and 27.25).

b. Those involving primarily the parenchyma of the brain, producing encephalitis (Figs. 27.26, 27.27, and 30.1)

There are some infections, often viral, that involve both structures, producing a meningoencephalitis.

Meningitis (Leptomeningitis)

This is the most common form of infection of the nervous system. The manifestations of meningitis depend on the organism involved, the age of the patient, and the underlying physical status of the patient. Acute, subacute, and chronic forms may be considered.

Acute Purulent (Bacterial or Septic) Meningitis
This is the most common form of infection of the central nervous system among patients requiring hospitalization. In each case, a specific bacterial organism may be isolated from the cerebrospinal fluid in the subarachnoid space. In addition, the

Figure 27.24 Acute meningitis (pneumococcal). This 57-year-old white male had been living in a nursing home with a diagnosis of chronic undifferentiated schizophrenia. Two weeks previously he had become less responsive than usual, then developed a temperature of 104°F for which he received penicillin. On the day of admission, the patient fell out of bed and became comatose. Cerebrospinal fluid was cloudy with 11,861 white blood cells (80% polymorphonuclears) and a sugar of 36 mg/100 ml. Culture of the cerebrospinal fluid subsequently revealed *S. pneumoniae*. A left and then bilateral fixed dilated pupils developed followed by Cheyne-Stokes periodic respirations, decerebrate posture, and death. At autopsy, the brain was swollen with a yellow-green purulent exudate present in the subarachnoid space. (Courtesy of Drs. John Hills and Jose Segarra.)

Figure 27.26 Encephalitis (herpes simplex). A significant collection of mononuclear cells is present in the perivascular space with infiltration of adjacent cerebral cortex. This 32-year-old patient had the acute onset of fever, headache, and generalized convulsions. Over a 30-day period, he developed increasing stupor, bilateral extensor plantar responses, and dilated pupils (H&E, 320×). (Courtesy of Dr. John Hills.)

spinal fluid shows evidence of an acute inflammatory reaction. The fluid is cloudy and under increased pressure with large numbers of white blood cells, predominantly polymorphonuclear leukocytes, for example, 90% to 98% of 500 to 40,000 white blood cells per cubic millimeter. The cerebrospinal fluid sugar content is markedly reduced, relative to the blood sugar. Normal spinal fluid sugar is >50% of the blood sugar. Gram stain of the spinal fluid, latex agglutination tests of cerebrospinal fluid, and cultures will allow identification of the specific organism. The specific organism and the recommended treatment are indicated in Table 27.6.

Clinical Presentation: The clinical picture of acute purulent meningitis depends on the age of the patient. An infant under 6 months of age may be febrile, listless, and drowsy and may vomit and fail to take feedings. The anterior fontanelle of an infant will be under increased pressure and bulging. An older infant or a child is likely to have nuchal rigidity (resistance to passive flexion of the neck), in addition to fever, convulsions, and coma. A posture of opisthotonos may be present (extreme extension of head, neck, trunk, and limbs).

The older child and adult with meningococcal meningitis will usually have a prodromal period characterized by symptoms of an upper respiratory infection, low-grade fever, and various body aches. With septicemia and, then, the subsequent involvement of the meninges, the symptoms of chills, vomiting, severe headache, and nuchal rigidity occur, often followed by an alteration in consciousness. The signs of central nervous system involvement often appear relatively abruptly. A skin rash is common in the stage of bacteremia. Small or large areas of skin hemorrhage (petechiae and purpura) due to involvement and occlusion of the skin capillaries occur during the process of septicemia and are caused either directly by the

Figure 27.25 Acute meningitis (pneumococcal). The subarachnoid space is filled with inflammatory cells, predominantly polymorphonuclear leukocytes. There has been artifactual detachment of the pia from the cortical surface (H&E, 400×). (Courtesy of Pathology Department, Tufts University School of Medicine.)

Figure 27.27 Encephalitis. Rabies. Negri bodies are present as cytoplasmic inclusions in neurons of the hippocampus. Intracellular inclusions are characteristic of viral diseases (H&E, 100×). (Courtesy of Dr. Thomas Smith.)

Table 27.6 ACUTE BACTERIAL MENINGITIS: COMMON ORGANISMS AT SPECIFIC AGES AND RECOMMENDED TREATMENT

AGE OF PATIENT	BACTERIAL ORGANISMS (ON CULTURE)	RECOMMENDED TREATMENT (ALL ARE INTRAVENOUS)
0–1 month	B. streptococcus*	Penicillin G (plus in neonates initially gentamicin for 72 hours)
1–23 months	S. pneumoniae, 45%; N. meningitides, 31%	Vancomycin plus a broad-spectrum cephalosporin for S. pneumonia (see below for N. meningitidis)
2–18 years	N. meningitidis	Penicillin G**
19–59 years	S. pneumoniae, 60%; N. meningitidis, 20%	See above
>60 years	S. pneumoniae	See above

*Prior to introduction in 1990 of H. influenzae conjugate vaccine immunization; most cases were due to this organism. Recommended treatment for H. influenzae is ceftriaxone.
**For epidemics of N. meningitidis in developing countries, a single intramuscular injection of a suspension of chloramphenicol in oil has proven to be effective.
***Less common agents: *L. monocytogenes* ampicillin + gentamicin.
***Enterobacteriaceae-broad spectrum cephalosporin + aminoglycoside.

organism or indirectly as a result of disseminated aggregation of platelets into small thrombi.

The early recognition of acute purulent meningitis is of importance. If it is untreated, serious intracranial complications develop and death is the usual outcome. Prior to the era of specific antimicrobial therapy, the mortality was close to 90%. With specific therapy, this figure has been markedly reduced so that the actual mortality in meningococcal meningitis is now 3%, although the mortality in patients with overwhelming meningococcemia may still approach 40%. For S. pneumoniae the case fatality rate remains high at 21% due to the age of the patients. The case fatality rate for H. influenzae is 6% and for group B streptococcus, 7%. Eleven percent to 19% of survivors of meningococcal disease have sequalae, usually minor if treated early, (peripheral facial weakness, hearing loss), at times major: focal neurological deficit or focal seizures or loss of a limb.

There are several possible complications of meningitis. While these are more likely to occur in delayed or untreated cases, some may occur in those patients receiving adequate treatment. With a marked increase in intracranial pressure (at times, lumbar subarachnoid cerebrospinal fluid pressure at lumbar puncture may be 600 mm of cerebrospinal fluid compared to a normal pressure of 150 mm) herniation of medial temporal areas through the tentorium may occur with compression of the third cranial nerve and midbrain. A vasculitis may involve blood vessel walls, resulting in occlusion of cortical arteries and veins. The occlusion of cortical veins and superior sagittal sinus may lead to hemorrhagic infarction of the parasagittal frontal parietal areas with a resultant weakness of the lower extremities and focal seizures. In addition, a further increase in intracranial pressure may occur.

As we have already indicated, a thick exudate at the base of the brain (somewhat more likely to occur in pneumococcal meningitis) may damage cranial nerves and also obliterate the subarachnoid cisterns. The end result may be a significant degree of hydrocephalus since cerebrospinal fluid will be unable to pass up over the hemispheres to the areas of absorption. In the child, a progressive enlargement of the head occurs.

Overall, in the recent series of Pomeroy et al. (1990), 14% of children had neurological deficits that persisted beyond a year after bacterial meningitis. Of these 10% had only sensory neural hearing deficits and 4% had multiple neurologic deficits. Seven percent had late, nonfebrile seizures (see also Taylor et al., 1990 and Smith, 1990).

Treatment: The present recommendations (Table 27.7; Quagliarello and Scheld, 1997; Rosenstein et al., 2001) as to choice of intravenous antibiotics which are to be started based on the Gram's stain of the cerebrospinal fluid when the patient is first seen but before cerebrospinal fluid or blood cultures are available are presented in Table 27.7.

Once the organism has been identified on cultures or agglutination studies of cerebrospinal fluid or blood, the recommendation of Table 27.6 should be followed.

Acute Aseptic Meningitis

In these cases, the clinical signs and symptoms of meningitis are present in the sense that the patient complains of headache and stiffness of the neck. Vomiting and nuchal rigidity are present. However these findings are usually less fulminating than those in acute purulent meningitis, for example, sudden coma and purpura in the adult is unlikely; consciousness is usually well preserved. The spinal fluid, moreover, is often clear or only minimally cloudy (often described as opalescent). A relatively small number of white blood cells is present (5 to 2000 per cubic millimeter and usually less than 500 per cubic millimeter) in comparison to acute purulent meningitis.

Table 27.7 TREATMENT RECOMMENDATIONS BASED ON CEREBROSPINAL FLUID STAINS PRIOR TO CULTURE RESULTS

IDENTIFICATION OF AGENT IN CEREBROSPINAL FLUID (GRAM STAIN) BEFORE CULTURE	TREATMENT RECOMMENDATIONS (INTRAVENOUS)
COCCI	
Gram-positive cocci	Vancomycin plus a broad spectrum antibiotic
Gram-negative cocci	Penicillin G
BACILLUS	
Gram-positive bacilli	Ampicillin (or penicillin G) plus aminoglycoside
Gram-negative bacillus	Broad spectrum cephalosporin plus aminoglycoside
EMPIRICAL APPROACH	
Children <1 month	Ampicillin plus broad spectrum cephalosporin and vancomycin
Children >1 month	Vancomycin plus cefotaxime or ceftriaxone

Moreover, the white blood cells are predominantly mononuclear (lymphocytes and monocytes). The sugar content of the spinal fluid is normal. Moreover, smears, agglutination studies, and bacteriological cultures of the spinal fluid fail to reveal a responsible organism. In general, the causative organism is a virus: ECHO, Coxsackie, nonparalytic poliomyelitis, mumps, and lymphocytic choriomeningitis.

The student should note, however, that a similar cerebrospinal fluid reaction may also characterize certain diseases where a secondary meningeal reaction occurs: subdural empyema, brain abscess, and venous sinus thrombosis. At times, a similar spinal fluid formula may be noted in a viral encephalitis. The aforementioned viral agents may, of course, at times present a combined syndrome of meningoencephalitis.

Moreover, at times several more significant subacute infections in their early stages may present a predominately mononuclear reaction in the spinal fluid: tuberculous and cryptococcal (fungal) meningitis. Bacterial organisms will be absent on routine smears and cultures of the cerebrospinal fluid. However, both of these infections are characterized by a low spinal fluid sugar, and appropriate stains and cultures (and in the case of cryptococcal infection specific antigen studies) will eventually disclose the organism. These infections, although not common at the present time, in the nonimmunosuppressed population, are of importance because (a) specific therapy is required, and (b) with the increase in cases of acquired immune deficiency syndrome, the incidence of these diseases has increased.

Differentiation of the various types of viral meningitis may be made by specialized immunological techniques for the measurement of neutralizing antibodies. Viral meningitis is a self-limited disease. No specific treatment is available (see later, however, under H. simplex). Recovery is in general complete unless the meningitis is an epiphenomenon in the midst of an encephalitis.

Encephalitis

See also Figures 27.26 and 27.27. A brief introduction is provided here.

The term *encephalitis* refers to a diffuse invasion of the parenchyma of the brain by an infectious agent.

At the present time, clinical presentation of encephalitis is probably less common than those diseases considered under the category of meningitis. During particular epidemics certain infectious agents involving the central nervous system have produced a large number of cases with encephalitis. However, subclinical or minor diffuse involvement of the central nervous system probably occurs in the course of a number of common viral diseases, primarily as a mild aseptic meningitis or meningoencephalitis. Even in epidemics of encephalitis or poliomyelitis, there may be many subclinical cases. For example, for Japanese encephalitis, the ratio of subclinical to overt clinical cases has been estimated at 200 or 300:1 (Monath, 1988).

In general, most cases falling into this category reflect viral infection. Evidence of viral particles will be found as inclusions within the cytoplasm or nuclei of neurons. With the exception of the spirochete, bacteria do not produce a diffuse encephalitis, although bacteria may produce multiple areas of abscess formation. Other infectious agents may produce encephalitic involvement of the nervous system. The rickettsiae, which are intermediate in size between bacteria and viruses, usually produce signs of a meningoencephalitis in addition to a characteristic skin rash. Examples are typhus and Rocky Mountain spotted fever. Moreover, certain protozoal parasites may invade the central nervous system, producing a subacute encephalitis. Examples include toxoplasmosis and trypanosomiasis (African sleeping sickness).

Encephalitis may be acute or chronic. Most cases fall into the acute category; most viral and rickettsial diseases are acute. On the other hand, the spirochetal infection and protozoal infections of the central nervous system are, in general, chronic or subacute processes. Recently, however, several viruses and prions have been implicated in chronic diffuse progressive processes (previously considered to be of an unknown etiology) involving the nervous system.

ACUTE ENCEPHALITIS: ACUTE VIRAL INFECTIONS

The pathology of viral infections of the neural parenchyma involves a viral invasion of neurons with the production of intranuclear or intracytoplasmic inclusions (Fig 27.27) and the acute degeneration and destruction of nerve cells. There is a cellular infiltration of neural tissue and an accumulation of inflammatory cells about the degenerating nerve cells, in a perivascular location (Fig. 27.26). The cells are usually mononuclear, although in some processes (e.g., acute poliomyelitis or in a severe case of encephalitis), there are often noted a significant number of polymorphonuclear leukocytes at times involved in neuronophagia. A microglia proliferation is often noted in the involved neural parenchyma. To a variable degree, adjacent meninges may be infiltrated by inflammatory cells. Depending on the degree of meningeal infiltration and on the severity to which the underlying parenchyma is involved, a variable increase in cells (predominantly lymphocytes) will be noted in the spinal fluid. Occasionally a normal cell count may be present, more often 100 to 500 cells per cubic millimeter are present. The protein content is usually increased; the sugar and chloride content are normal.

The differentiation of the particular virus involved depends on the following:

a. The specific clinical pattern of the disease: some viruses involve particular areas of the central nervous system; some have associated involvement of other organ systems.

b. Virus isolation studies: inoculation of blood, nasal washings, excretions, cerebrospinal fluid, or fresh postmortem brain tissue into susceptible animals. In some specialized centers, tissue culture techniques may be employed.

c. Application of acute and chronic serological tests to measure antibody levels (complement fixation or antibody neutralization tests).

It had been traditional to divide these viral infections into *neurotropic group* (primary involvement of the central nervous system) and a *nonneurotropic group* (involvement of the central

TABLE 27.8 NUTRITIONAL AND RELATED DISORDERS OF THE NERVOUS SYSTEM

STRUCTURES INVOLVED	VITAMIN(S) DEFICENT	MANIFESTATIONS
Cerebral Cortex	Niacin	Pellagra: dementia, dermatitis, diarrhea
	Pyridoxine	Seizures (possibly of hippocampal origin)
	B12	Dementia
Corpus callosum	Specific unknown, possibly toxic, described initially with excess of Italian red wine. Possible role of thiamine.	Marchiafava-Bignami disease: dementia and apraxia. May be seen in patients who also have Wernicke-Korsakoff syndrome.
Diencephalon-thiamine and brain stem and cerebellum-periventricular		Wernicke-Korsakoff syndrome (Chapter 30)
Pons	Specific unclear but does follow too rapid correction of hyponatremia	Central pontine myelinolysis. Patient is mute, spastic, and akinetic (Chapter 13)
Cerebellum	Thiamine or multiple B	Alcoholic cerebellar degeneration (Chapter 20)
Spinal cord	B12	Combined system disease (Chapter 9)
Peripheral nerves	Thiamine, or pyridoxine or B12 or multiple B	Nutritional mixed sensory neuropathy or with thiamine beri-beri.
Optic nerves	Thiamine, B12, riboflavin	Optic neuropathy (retrobulbar neuropathy usually bilateral)

Notes. Muscle may also be involved in an alcoholic myopathy-specific unknown but multiple B suspected.
In infants and children deficiencies of proteins and fat may retard development of nervous system.

nervous system in humans is usually secondary to or less prominent than involvement of other organ systems). As we will discuss with the herpes group of virus infection, the distinction is to some degree artificial. The infections with the neurotropic may be epidemic (the arthropod-borne viruses such as equine encephalitis or West Nile) or nonepidemic such as rabies.

A more modern classification divides viruses into those containing RNA and those containing DNA.

Examples of RNA-containing viruses include the enteroviruses (polio, Coxsackie, ECHO), the arboviruses (Eastern and Western Equine, Japanese, etc.), rubella, mumps and measles, rabies, and HIV.

Examples of DNA containing viruses include Herpes virus, papovavirus, and poxvirus. An overview of viral encephalitis is provided in the review of Whitley (1990).

Neurotropic Group: Epidemic Group

Within the epidemic group several infections may be grouped together because they share common characteristics: (a) equine

Table 27.9 EFFECTS OF HEAVY METALS ON THE NERVOUS SYSTEM

METAL	ACUTE AND HIGH LEVEL	CHRONIC LOW LEVEL
Lead	Encephalopathy: acute cerebral edema	In adults: motor peripheral neuropathy. In children: long-term retardation of cognitive function/intelligence quotient
Inorganic mercury	Acute gastrointestinal, renal and hematologic effects	Cerebellar degeneration and the "mad hatter syndrome": dementia and psychosis
Organic mercury	Blindness, cerebral, cerebellar, pyramidal, and anterior horn cell degeneration primarily affecting fetus infants and children (Minimata Bay in Japan, etc.)	
Arsenic	Acute hemorrhagic encephalopathy	Peripheral neuropathy: sensory/motor
Copper		Hepatolenticular degeneration: Wilson's disease-genetic defect (Chapter 19)
Manganese		Parkinson's disease

encephalomyelitis with eastern United States, western United States, and Venezuelan subtypes (Deresiawicz et al., 1997). (b) Japanese B encephalitis (probably the most common form. Worldwide in recent years). (c) Russian tick encephalitis. (d) St. Louis encephalitis. (e) West Nile encephalitis, a recent problem in the eastern United States (Nash et al., 2001; Tyler, 2001). (f) LaCrosse virus encephalitis, probably the most frequent variety in the United States in recent years (McJunkin et al., 2001).

In each of these infections a relatively diffuse involvement of the cerebral cortex, diencephalon, brain stem, and cerebellum occurs. In each, an arthropod, usually a mosquito, has been implicated as a vector of transmission. A species of bird or mammal has often served as a reservoir of infection. For these reasons, cases have occurred predominantly in a seasonal manner. (In the northeastern United States, for example, most cases of Eastern equine and West Nile encephalitis have occurred in the late summer or early fall months, a time when mosquitoes are frequent.) Vaccines are available for prevention of some of the more common varieties (Hoke et al., 1988).

The clinical syndrome in most cases is characterized by the sudden onset of headache, vomiting, drowsiness, confusion, convulsions, coma, fever, plus or minus stiffness of the neck. Evidence is often present on examination of the patient of diffuse and, at times, multifocal involvement at multiple levels of the neural axis: coma, confusion, myoclonic jerks, status epilepticus, decorticate or decerebrate rigidity, and cerebellar findings. In some cases, cranial nerve findings, aphasia, and hemiplegia will be present. The duration of the disease is a matter of days to several weeks. *The state presented by the patient may be described as an encephalopathy.* The major differential diagnosis is that of toxic metabolic encephalopathy. A variable mortality occurs in part related to the age of the affected patients. The mortality of Eastern equine encephalitis, which has affected children predominantly, has approached 75%, with significant residuals in those recovering. *Encephalitis lethargica (Von Economo's encephalitis)* occurred as an epidemic in the period 1916–1926. More recent cases have been described by Howard and Lees (1987). A viral etiology was suspected but never confirmed: the means of transmission remained uncertain. This infection differed from the previously described varieties of encephalitis in the sense that although diffuse, the pathology tended to be concentrated in a periventricular location with severe involvement of structures bordering the aqueduct and third and fourth ventricles. The periaqueductal region and other structures of the midbrain were particularly affected. Reflecting the significant involvement of the midbrain and of the associated structures of the extrapyramidal system, disorders of eye movement and movement disorders of various types were prominent, in addition to the more general symptoms of lethargy, headache, and fever. Since the involvement of the cortex was less severe, seizures and focal cortical deficits were less frequent. The mortality approached 25%. Among those who survived, postencephalitic residuals were common. In contrast to other forms of encephalitis, Parkinson's disease and other disorders of extrapyramidal function were frequently noted; the Parkinson's disease usually appeared to emerge or evolve as a symptom after the clearing of the acute symptoms (see Chapter 19).

Acute anterior poliomyelitis, the other member of this epidemic group of neurotropic viruses, has already been discussed in relation to the spinal cord. The portal of entry is the gastrointestinal tract. The central nervous system is involved either by spread along the axis cylinders or via a generalized viremia. The virus involves predominantly the large motor neurons of the anterior horn and of the brain stem with lesser involvement of other neurons in the spinal cord.

Nonepidemic Neurotropic Virus Infections

The two most familiar members of this group—Herpes zoster (discussed previously) and rabies—do not have their major effects at the level of cerebral cortex.

Rabies

The virus of rabies is present in the saliva of rabid animals and invades the central nervous system several weeks to months after a bite from an infected animal (dog, cat, wolf, fox, raccoon, squirrel, or bat). The virus travels to the central nervous system along peripheral nerves. The symptoms relate to the characteristic involvement of nuclei of the brain stem, Purkinje cells of the cerebellum, and pyramidal cells of the hippocampus (Ammon's horn). In addition, there is a significant inflammation and necrosis of the spinal cord or brain stem at the segmental site corresponding to the radicular dermatome involved by the bite. The cerebral neocortex is relatively intact and consciousness is preserved.

The initial symptoms consist of numbness and tingling in the distribution of the involved peripheral nerve, followed by headache, vomiting, and a stage of agitation. This latter stage is characterized by restlessness, generalized convulsions, and at times, visual and auditory hallucinations. Marked alteration in emotions occurs: unreasonable fear, rage, and depression. In this stage laryngeal and pharyngeal spasm (with fear of water, "hydrophobia") is prominent. In a later stage of flaccid paralysis, impairment of vocal cords and of respiratory centers develops. In approximately 20% of cases, an ascending flaccid paralysis dominates the acute stage (Plotkin and Koprowski, 1979).

Death occurs within 2 to 5 days of onset of central nervous system symptoms. At autopsy, the diagnosis may be established in humans or other infected animals by the findings of characteristic acidophilic (eosinophilic) inclusions (Negri bodies) within the cytoplasm of hippocampal pyramidal cells (Fig. 27.27).

Because of the long incubation between exposure to the virus and the development of neurological symptoms, prophylactic treatment is possible. Thus, the administration of a vaccine containing the attenuated virus (first introduced by Pasteur) induces the production of antibodies and may prevent the development of neurological symptoms. The combination of this active immunization with passive immunization with antiserum containing antibodies to rabies has been demonstrated to be much more effective. The current vaccine is the human diploid cell vaccine; the current antisera, human rabies immune globulin. Previous treatment protocols involving nervous system derived vaccines resulted in postvaccinal demyelinating reactions. Once neurological symptoms have developed, no effective treatment is available. In underdeveloped areas of the world a high mortality occurs (see Baer and Fishbein, 1987 and Fishbein and Robinson, 1993 for a review of epidemiology and current concepts of treatment).

Nonneurotropic Viral Infections

These viruses were traditionally considered as not producing significant symptoms of central nervous system involvement. Indirect evidence suggests that some of these viruses (mumps, measles, enteroviruses) do invade the central nervous system in a much greater percentage of otherwise asymptomatic cases. In some of these diseases, for example, herpes simplex, there is evidence of direct invasion of the central nervous system when the syndrome of acute encephalitis occurs. In other viral infections, for example, mumps and measles, it is often unclear when central nervous system symptoms develop, whether one is dealing with an actual viral invasion of the central nervous system producing an acute encephalitis (direct invasion of neurons), or whether one is observing an immunological reaction to infection elsewhere, producing an acute allergic postinfectious encephalomyelitis (white matter predominantly involved with perivenous demyelination).

Types of Nonneurotropic Viral Infections

1. *The herpes virus family* includes herpes simplex, herpes zoster/varicella, cytomegalovirus, and Epstein Barr.

   The *herpes simplex virus (HSV)* has two types—*Type 1* associated with the common cold sore of the lip or oral cavity, often activated by fever, and *Type 2*, genital herpes with labial vaginal and penile infection. In both instances, the virus remains in a latent form in neural ganglia (Baringer and Swoveland, 1973), particularly the trigeminal ganglion in the case of Type I HSV and the sacral ganglia in the case of Type 2 HSV.

   Type 1 HSV is the most common cause of nonepidemic, sporadic acute encephalitis in the United States. The early signs of headache and fever are followed by the development of signs that suggest involvement of limbic structures of one or both temporal lobes, and at times orbital frontal (Fig. 30.1). The virus apparently gains access to the central nervous system by infecting structures that are related to the olfactory system, perhaps by axonal transport along the olfactory bulb and its anatomical connections. In some cases spread may be hematogenous (see review of Picard et al., 1993). Personality and behavioral changes may be present for days or a week, followed by seizures, hemiparesis, and aphasia. Rapid or subacute progression to a stage of increasing coma then occurs. In a small number of cases, the patient may present with an overwhelming rapidly fatal state characterized by repeated generalized convulsions, myoclonic jerks of the extremities, decerebrate rigidity, coma, and periodic complexes in the electroencephalogram (EEG). In contrast, in a small number of cases, the clinical picture is that of a progressive subacute dementia and confusional state. The cerebrospinal fluid demonstrates increased pressure, and a variable number of mononuclear cells plus or minus a variable small number of red blood cells. The EEG may provide evidence of focal or bilateral temporal lobe abnormalities, including slow waves. At variable points in the disease course, the radioactive brain scan, contrast enhanced CT scan, or MRI will demonstrate focal or bilateral temporal (and frontal) abnormalities: enhancing necrotic lesions with considerable edema. Sequential serological studies of blood and cerebrospinal fluid may be useful in the diagnosis. The treatment of choice is intravenous acyclovir, which can be administered without serious side effects. The response to treatment is directly related to how long the symptoms have been present and to the level of consciousness. Therefore, if the diagnosis is strongly suspected on clinical grounds, treatment is begun as soon as possible, even though the ancillary laboratory studies are not yet confirmatory. In most instances, a brain biopsy is not obtained unless the patient fails to respond to therapy. Even with acyclovir therapy, 53% of patients will die or will be severely impaired. (See discussions of Hanley, 1990.)

   Type 2 HSV in adults is associated with an aseptic meningitis or with severe radicular symptoms involving the sacral segments. The latter may include urinary retention (Caplan et al., 1977).

   Type 2 HSV infection in the infant or fetus results in severe disseminated disease with multisystem involvement of brain and viscera.

2. *Paramyxovirus* group includes mumps and measles. In the child and adult, mumps encephalitis is rare. In the fetus and neonate, mumps virus infection has been implicated as a possible cause of aqueductal stenosis producing hydrocephalus (see Johnson and Johnson, 1969).

   Measles virus infection may be associated with a variety of central nervous system syndromes, including:

   a. an acute or subacute encephalitis

   b. a postinfectious encephalomyelitis

   c. subacute sclerosing pan-encephalitis (SSPE), a form of progressive chronic encephalitis manifested by dementia, ataxia, seizures, and myoclonus. The disease usually develops in a delayed manner after an early childhood measles infection. There is a reactivation of the measles virus within the central nervous system.

3. *Retrovirus—Human Immunodeficiency Virus (HIV-1)*: This virus infects cells of the immune system (e.g., T helper lymphocytes), producing an

acquired-immune deficiency state (AIDS). Carriers who may be in an early or asymptomatic stage of the disease outnumber actual cases of AIDS or AIDS-related complex (ARC). In the United States during the 1980s, specific groups were at high risk: (a) homosexual or bisexual men (66%); (b) intravenous drug users (17%); (c) heterosexual sexual partners of patients with AIDS (4%); (d) recipients of blood and blood products (3%); and (e) combined risk—homosexual or bisexual male—also drug user (8%).[1] These 1 By the year 2001, Sekowitz quoted figures of 36 million people worldwide infected with HIV, with an additional 21.8 million dead of AIDS. Approximately 70% of cases occur in sub-Saharan Africa, where there are two types of epidemics: (1) a horizontal transmission in adults spread primarily by heterosexual contact and to a lesser degree by shared needles and (2) a vertical transmission, in which infected mothers give birth to infants who have been infected in utero. Significant numbers of cases are also occurring in the Caribbean, Southeast Asia, and South America.

The nervous system is involved in at least 60% of patients with clinical disease. The infections may be generalized or focal due to the immunodeficiency state. Thus, there is an increased incidence of cryptococcal fungal meningitis (10%) and of toxoplasmosis granuloma (5%). A high percentage of patients (>30%) have a direct invasion of the central nervous system by the virus, producing a subacute encephalitis referred to as AIDS dementia or HIV meningitis. In patients with acute HIV-1 infection 24% have an aseptic meningitis.

SYSTEM DISORDERS

1. Degenerations: These disorders are considered in the chapters on muscle, peripheral nerve, spinal cord, basal ganglia, cerebellum, and memory systems.

2. Nutritional disorders: Refer to general medical texts (Table 27.8).

3. Toxic disorders: Various central nervous systems pharmacologic agents taken in excess may all produce effects on central nervous system function (Table 27.9). Some, such as sedatives, anticonvulsants, benzodiazepines, or narcotics, may produce depression of cognitive function and/or ataxia and eventually in severe overdose coma. Neuroleptics may produce extrapyramidal effects. Hallucinogens and amphetamines may produce a psychosis. Use of the latter may be associated with hemorrhagic strokes. Cocaine may produce arrhythmias and stroke. Carbon monoxide may produce headaches or coma.

4. Complications of endocrine disorders: See medical textbooks for discussion on diabetes, thyroid disease, pituitary hormones, and so on.

5. Remote effects of malignancy: see Chapter 21.

DISORDERS OF MYELIN

See also Chapters 9 and 13. Figures 27.28 and 27.29 demonstrate cases with clinical involvement of the cerebral hemispheres.

Figure 27.28 Multiple sclerosis: cerebral involvement. (*A*) Severe involvement of the cerebral white matter has occurred, with multifocal gray sclerotic lesions as well as large confluent lesions in a periventricular location. The large confluent lesions and the relative sparing of the arcuate fibers are reminiscent of Schilder's diffuse sclerosis. Destruction of axons, as well as of myelin, has occurred in the larger lesions. This patient had the onset of multiple sclerosis at age 26 and had a progressive course so that by age 30, the patient was essentially bedridden with paralysis of all four extremities, marked impairment of vision, and marked internuclear ophthalmoplegia, and by age 33 had a severe dementia. (*B*) A more typical area of demyelination in the periventricular subcortical white matter is demonstrated in this coronal section from another case of multiple sclerosis. (Courtesy of Dr. John Hills.)

---

[1] These percentages vary markedly in different geographic areas and in different population groups. Heterosexual cases are increasing significantly among drug users or their contacts and in Africa, South America, and Southeast Asia. New cases among homosexual males are decreasing.

Figure 27.29 Multiple sclerosis. Magnetic resonance imaging (MRI) scans. This 38-year-old white female bank employee had a 15-year history of relapsing-remitting secondarily progressive multiple sclerosis initially affecting spinal cord Lhermitte's sign, then optic nerves, then cerebellum and cognitive function. Cerebrospinal fluid indicated an IgG index of 2.42 (normal 0.45 + 0.1) with 3 oligoclonal bands (normal < 1). In the 5 years following this MRI, she developed dementia and a bedridden state. (*A*) T1 sagittal section. (*B*) T2 horizontal section.

BIBLIOGRAPHY

Bullock, R., and Teasdale, G. 1990. ABC of major trauma: head injuries. BMJ. 300:1515–1518, 1576–1579.

Evans, R. W. (Ed.). 1992. The neurology of trauma. Neurol. Clin. 10:815–1071.

Jaffee, D., and Wesson, D. 1991. Emergency management of blunt trauma in children. N. Engl. J. Med. 324:1477–1482.

Jennett, W. B., and Teasdale, G. 1981. Management of Head Injury. Philadelphia, PA: F. A. Davis.

Plum, F., and Posner, J. B. 1980. The Diagnosis of Stupor and Coma. Philadelphia, PA: F. A. Davis.

Ropper, A. H., Kennedy, S. K., and Zervas, N. T. (Eds.). 1988. Neurologicaland Neurosurgical Intensive Care. Baltimore, MD: University Park Press.

White, R. J., and Likavec, M. J. 1992. The diagnosis and intiial management of head injury. N. Engl. J. Med., 327:1507–1511.

SPECIFIC REFERENCES AND CITATIONS

Annegers, J. F., Hauser, W. A., Coan, S. P., and Rocca, W. A. 1998. A population based study of seizures after traumatic brain injuries. N. Engl. J. Med. 338:20–24.

Capruso, D. X., and Levin, H. S. 1992. Cognitive impairment following closed head injury. Neurol. Clin. 10:879–893.

Cordobes, F., Lobato, R. D., Rivas, J. J., et al. 1981. Observation on 82 patients with extradural hematoma. Comparison of results before and after advent of computerized tomography. Neurosurgery 65:203–210.

Davis, J. M., and Zimmerman, R. A. 1983. Injury to the carotid and vertebral arteries. Neuroradiology 25:55–70.

Duhaime, A. C., Christian, C. W., Rorke, L. B., and Zimmerman, R. 1998. Non accidental head injury in infants. The "shaken- baby syndrome" N. Engl. J. Med. 338:1822–1829.

Evans, R. W. 1992. The Post Concussion Syndrome and the Sequelae of Mild Head Trauma. Neurol. Clin. 10:815–847.

Geerts, W. H., Code, K. I., Jay, R. M., et al. 1994. A prospective study of venous thromboembolism after major trauma. N. Engl. J. Med. 331:1601–1606.

Jennett, W. B. 1962. Epilepsy After Blunt Head Injuries. London, UK: William Heinemann Medical Books.

Jennett, W. B., and Bond, M. 1975. Assessment of outcome after severe brain damage. Lancet 480–484.

PART I: TRAUMA

Jennett, W. B., Teasdale, G., Brachman, R., et al. 1979. Prognosis of patients with severe head injuries. Neurosurg. 4:283–389.

Kellerman, A. L., Rivara, F. P., Lee, R. K., et al. 1996. Injuries due to firearms in three cities. N. Engl. J. Med. 335:1438–1444.

Keane, J. R., and Baloh, R. W. 1992. Post traumatic cranial neuropathies. Neurol. Clin. 10:849–867.

Markwalder, T. M. 1981. Chronic subdural hematomas: a review. J. Neurosurg. 54:637–645.

Marshall, L. F., Smith, R. W., and Shapiro, H. M. 1979. The outcome with aggressive treatment in severe head injuries part I: the significance of intracranial pressure monitoring. J. Neurosurg. 50:20–25.

Masters, S. J., McClean, P. M., Archarese, J. S., et al. 1987. Skull x-ray examination after head trauma: recommendations by a multi-disciplinary panel and validation study. N. Engl. J. Med. 316:84–91.

Packard, R. C. (Ed.). 1994. Mild head injury. Semin. Neurol. 14:1–89.

Rivara, F. P., Grossman, D. C., and Cummings, P. 1997. Injury prevention. N. Engl. J. Med. 337:543–548, 613–618.

Ross, R. J., Cole, M., Thompson, J. S., and Kirn, K. H. 1983. Boxers computerized tomography, EEG and neurological evaluation. JAMA. 249:211–213.

Teasdale, G., and Jennett, B. 1974. Assessment of coma and impaired consciousness: a practical scale. Lancet 2:81.

Thompson, R. S., Rivara, F. P., and Thompson, D. C. 1989. A case control study of the effectiveness of bicycle safety helmets. N. Engl. J. Med. 320:1361–1367.

Walker, A. F., Caveness, W. F., and Critchley, M. (Eds.) 1969. The late effect of head injury. Springfield, IL: Charles C. Thomas.

Watson, C. W. 1952. Incidence of epilepsy following craniocerebral injury II. Three year follow-up study. Arch. Neurol. Psychiatry 68:831–834.

Zervas, N. T., and Hedley-White, J. 1972. Successful treatment of cerebral herniation in five patients. N. Engl. J. Med. 286:1075–1077.

PART II: NEOPLASMS
GENERAL BIBLIOGRAPHY

Black, P. 1991. Medical progress: brain tumors. N. Engl. J. Med. 324:1471–1476, 1555–1564.

Courville, C. B. 1967. Intracranial tumors. Bull. Los Angeles Neurolog. Soc. 2(Suppl.. 2):1–80.

Cushing, H. 1932. Intracranial Tumors: Notes Upon a Series of 2000 Verified Cases with Surgical—Mortality Percentages Pertaining Thereto. Springfield, IL: Charles C. Thomas.

De Angelis, L. M. 2001. Medical progress: brain tumors. N. Engl. J. Med. 344:114–123.

Grant, F. C. 1956. A study of the results of surgical treatment in 2326 consecutive patients with brain tumors. J. Neurosurg. 13:479–488.

Kernohan, J. W., and Sayre, G. P. 1952. Tumors of the Central Nervous System—Fascicle #35. Atlas of Tumor Pathology. Washington, DC: Armed Forces Institute of Pathology.

Osteen, R. T. (Ed.). 1990. Cancer Manual. 8th ed. Boston, MA: American Cancer Society, Massachusetts Division.

Radhakrishnan, K., Mokri, B., Parisi, J. E., et al. 1995. The trends in incidence of primary brain tumors in the population of Rochester Minnesota. Ann. Neurol. 37:67–73.

Rubinstein, L. J. 1992. Tumors of the Central Nervous System Fascicle #6 (2nd series). Atlas of Tumor Pathology. Washington, DC: Armed Forces Institute of Pathology.

Russell, D. S., and Rubinstein, L. J. 1977. Pathology of Tumors of the Nervous System. 4th ed. Baltimore, MD: Williams & Wilkins.

Schmidek, H. H. 1987. The molecular genetics of nervous system tumors. J. Neurosurg. 67:1–16.

Scott, J. N., Rewcastle, N. B., Brasher, P. M. A., et al. 1999. Which glioblastoma multiforme patient will become a long term survivor? A population based study. Ann. Neurol. 46:183–188.

Scott, R. M., Recht, L. D., Linggod, R. M., et al. 1990. Cancer of the central nervous system. In R. T. Osteen (Ed.) Cancer Manual. 8th ed., pp. 394–409. Boston, MA: American Cancer Society, Massachusetts Division.

Shapiro, W. R., and Shapiro, J. R. 1992. Primary brain tumors. In A. K. Asbury, G. M. McKhann, and W. I. McDonald (Eds.) Diseases of the Nervous System. 2nd ed., pp. 1074–1092. Philadelphia, PA: W. B. Saunders

Walker, A. E., Robins, M., and Weinfelder, F. D. 1985. Epidemiology of brain tumors: the national survey of intracranial neoplasms. Neurology 35:219–226.

Zulch, K. J. 1986. Brain Tumors: Their Biology and Pathology. 3rd ed. Berlin, Germany and New York, NY: Springer Verlag.

SPECIFIC REFERENCES AND CITATIONS

Al-Mefty, O. (Ed.). 1991. Meningiomas. New York, NY: Raven Press.

Antunes, J. L., Louis, K. M., and Ganti, S. R. 1980. Colloid cysts of the third ventricle. Neurosurgery 7:450–455.

Asa, S. C., and Kovacs, K. 1983. Histological classification of pituitary disease. Clin. Endocrinol. Metab. 12:567.

Bailey, P., and Cushing, H. 1926. A classification of the tumors of the glioma group on a histogenetic basis with a correlated study of prognosis. Philadelphia, PA: J. B. Lippincott.

Burger, P. C., and Green, S. B. 1987. Patient age, histologic features and length of survival in patients with glioblastoma multiforme. Cancer 59:1617–1625.

Burger, P. C., Vogel, F. S., Green, S. B., et al. 1985. Glioblastoma multiforme and anaplastic astrocytoma: pathologic criteria and prognostic implications. Cancer 56:1106–1011.

Cairncross, J. G., and Laperrier, N. J. 1989. Consensus in neurology low grade glioma. To treat or not to treat. Arch. Neurol. 46:1238–1239. (see also Editorial Comment—Hachinski 46:12–29)

Cairncross, J. G., and MacDonald, D. R. 1991. Consensus in neurology: chemotherapy for oligodendroglioma. Arch. Neurol. 48:225–227. (see also editorial comments of T. L. Casino and V. Hachinski. Arch. Neurol. 48:227)

Carter, J. N., Tyson, J. E., Tolis, G., et al. 1978. Prolactin secreting tumors and hypogonadism in 22 men. N. Engl. J. Med. 299:847–852.

Cooper, P. E., and Martin, J. B. 1992. Hypothalamic—pituitary function and dysfunction. In A. K. Asbury, G. M. McKhann, W. I. MacDonald (Eds.) Diseases of the Nervous System. 2nd ed., pp. 567–583. Philadelphia, PA: W. B. Saunders.

Cox, J. D., and Yesner, R. 1979. Adenocarcinoma of the lung: recent results from the Veterans Administration lung group. Am. Rev. Respir. Dis. 120:1025–1029.

Cushing, H. 1912. The Pituitary Body and Its Diseases. Philadelphia, PA: Lippincott.

Cushing, H. 1932. The basophil adenomas of the pituitary body and their clinical manifestations (pituitary basophilism). Bull. Johns Hopkins Hosp. 50:137–195.

Cushing, H., and Eisenhardt, L. 1938. Meningiomas. Springfield, IL: Charles C. Thomas.

Daumas-Duport, C., Scheithauer, B., O'Fallen, J., and Kelly, P. 1988. Grading of astrocytomas: a simple and reproducible method. Cancer 62:2152–2165.

Dawson, D. M., Hedley-Whyte, T., and Harris, N. 1986. Case records of the Massachusetts General Hospital case #42-1986: a 28-year-old man with renal transplantation and recent disorientation: (malignant lymphoma; diffuse large cell type). N. Engl. J. Med. 315:1079–1081.

DeAngelis, L. M. 1991. Primary central nervous system lymphoma: a new clinical challenge. Neurology 41:619–621.

DeAngelis, L. M., Yahalom, J., Heinemann, M. H., et al. 1990. Primary CNS lymphoma: combined treatment with chemotherapy and radiotherapy. Neurology 40:80–86.

Delattre, J. Y., Krol, G., Thaler, H. T., et al. 1988. Distribution of brain metastases. Arch. Neurol. 45:741–748.

Glasauer, F. F., and Yuan, R. H. P. 1963. Intracranial tumors with extracranial metastases. J. Neurosurg. 20:474–497.

Gruber, M. L., and Sobel, R. A. 1992. A 45-year-old man with confusion, seizures, and few focal findings—metastatic malignant melanoma "encephalitic form in leptomeninges and cerebral cortex. (Case records of the Massachusetts General Hospital—Case 28–1992). N. Engl. J. Med. 327:107–116.

Hall, W. A., and Lunsford, L. D. 1987. Changing concepts in the treatment of colloid cysts—an 11-year experience in the CT era. J. Neurosurg. 66:186–191.

Harding, J. 1973. Transsphenoidal surgery of hypersecreting pituitary tumors. In P. O. Kohler and G. T. Ross (Eds.) Diagnosis and Treatment of Pituitary Tumors, pp.179–198. New York, NY: American Elsevier.

Hedges, T. R., Schoene, W. C., and Albert, D. M. 1988. A 40-year-old man with rapidly progressive blindness and multiple cranial nerve deficits. Case records of the Massachusetts General Hospital Case #14-1988. N. Engl. J. Med. 318:903–915.

Hochberg, F. M., and Miller, D. C. 1988. Primary central nervous system lymphoma. J. Neurosurg. 68:835–853.

Huson, S. M. 1989. Recent developments in the diagnosis and management of neurofibromatosis. Arch. Pis. Childhood 64:745–749.

Jiddene, M., Nicoli, F., Diaz, P., et al. 1986. Intracranial malignant lymphoma. Report of 30 cases and review of the literature. J. Neurosurg. 65:592–599.

Klibanski, A., and Zervas, N. T. 1991. Diagnosis and management of hormone secreting pituitary adenomas. N. Engl. J. Med. 324:822–831.

Kopelson, G., Lingood, R. M., and Kleinmon. 1983. Medulloblastoma the identification of prognostic subgroups and implications for multi-modality management. Cancer 51:312–379.

Kujas, M. 1993. Meningioma. Curr. Opin. Neurol. Neurosurg. 6:882–887.

Kurland, L. T., Schoenberg, B. S., Annergers, J. F., et al. 1982. The incident of primary intracranial neoplasms in Rochester, Minnesota, 1935–1977. Ann. NY Acad. Sci. 381:6–16.

Lesch, K. P., and Gross, S. 1987. Estrogen receptor immunoreactivity in meningiomas: comparison with the binding activity of estrogen progesterone and androgen receptors. J. Neurosurg. 67:237–243.

Levin, V. A., Rodriquez, L. A., Edwards, M. S. B., et al. 1988. Treatment of medulloblastoma with procarbazine, hydroxyurea and reduced radiation doses to the whole brain and spine. J. Neurosurg. 68:383–387.

Little, J. R., Dale, A. J. D., and Okazaki, H. 1974. Meningeal carcinomatosis: clinical manifestations. Arch. Neurol. 30:138–143.

Ludwig, C. L., Smith, M. T., Godfrey, A. D., et al. 1986. A clinicopathologic study of 323 patients with oligodendrogliomas. Ann. Neurol. 19:15–21.

Martuza, R. L., and Roswell, E. 1988. Neurofibromatosis 2-bilateral acoustic neurofibromatosis. N. Engl. J. Med. 318:684–688.

McCormick, W. F., and Halmi, N. S. 1971. Absence of chromophobe adenomas from a large series of pituitary tumors. Arch. Pathol. 92:231–238.

Melmed, S. 1990. Medical progress: acromegaly. N. Engl. J. Med. 322:966–977.

Melmed, S. 1994. Pituitary neoplasia. Endocrinol. Metab Clin. North Am. 23:81–92.

Molitch, M. E., Eiton, R. L., Blackwell, R. E., et al. 1980. Bromocriptine as primary therapy for prolactin secreting macroadenomas results of a prospective multicenter study. J. Clin. Endocrinol. Metab. 60:698–705.

Nelson, J. S., Tsukado, Y., and Schoenfeld, D. 1983. Necrosis as a prognostic criterion in malignant supratentorial astrocytic gliomas. Cancer 52:550–554.

Ojemann, R. G., and Powell, H. C. 1976. Case records of the Massachusetts General Hospital case #36-1976. (Medulloblastoma metastatic to lumbosacral subarachnoid space). N. Engl. J. Med. 295:553–561.

Olson, M. E., Chernick, M. L., and Posner, J. B. 1974. Infiltration of the leptomeninges by systemic cancer. Arch. Neurol. 30:122–137.

Park, T. S., Hoffman, J. H., Henrick, E. B., et al. 1983. Medulloblastoma—clinical presentation and management. Experience at hospital for sick children. J. Neurosurg. 58:543–552.

Patchell, R. A., Tibbs, D. A., Walsh, J. W., et al. 1990. A randomized trial of surgery in the treatment of single metastases to the brain. N. Engl. J. Med. 322:494–500.

Picard, E. H., and Hedley-Whyte, E. T. 1988. Case records of the Massachusetts General Hospital Case #33–1988: a 71-year-old woman with progressive cranial nerve deficits and fever (lymphoma large cell (B Type) of central nervous system involving left temporal and frontal lobes, brain stem and spinal cord meninges and nerve roots). N. Engl. J. Med. 319:426–436.

Pollack, I. F. 1994. Brain tumors in children. N. Engl. J. Med. 331:1500–1507.

Posner, J. B. 1990. Surgery for metastases to the brain (Editorial). N. Engl. J. Med. 322:544–545.

Posner, J. B. 1992. Secondary neoplastic disease. In A. K. Asbury, G. M. McKhann, and W. I. McDonald (Eds.) Diseases of the Nervous System. 2nd ed., pp. 1093–1104. Philadelphia, PA: W. B. Saunders.

Recht, L. D., Lew, R., and Smith, T. W. 1992. Suspected low-grade glioma: is deferring treatment safe? Ann. Neurol. 31:431–436.

Riccardi, V. M. 1981. Von Recklinghausen neurofibromatosis. N. Engl. J. Med. 305:1617–1627.

Riskind, P. N., Richardson, Jr., E. P., and Boroic, G. E. 1986. Case records of the Massachusetts General Hospital—Case #3-1986. (Pituitary adenoma with partial necrosis (pituitary apoplexy). N. Engl. J. Med. 314:229–238.

Ron, E., Modan, B., Boice, J. D., et al. 1988. Tumors of the brain and nervous system after radiotherapy in childhood. N. Engl. J. Med. 319:1033–1039.

Selikoff, I. J., and Hammond, E. C. (Eds.). 1982. Brain tumors in the chemical industry. Ann. NY Acad. Sci. 381:1–364.

Shapiro, W. R. 1998. The therapy of primary nrain tumors. BNI Quart. 14:4–14.

Shapiro, W. R., Green, S. B., Burger, P. C., et al. 1989. Randomized trial of 3 chemotherapy regimens and two radiotherapy regimens in postoperative treatment of malignant glioma brain tumor—cooperative group trial 8001. J. Neurosurg. 71:1–9.

Stakes, J. W., and Sobel, R. A. 1986. Case records of the Massachusetts General Hospital case #22–1986: a 55-year- old woman with a progressive neurological disorder (malignant lymphoma (B cell type) brain right frontal lobe). N. Engl. J. Med. 314:1498–1507.

Stein, B. M., and Fetell, M. R. 1985. Therapeutic modalities for pineal region tumors. Clin. Neurosurg. 32:445–455.

Taveras, J. M., and Wood, E. H. 1964. Diagnostic Neuroradiology. Baltimore, MD: Williams and Wilkins.

Tomita, T., and McLone, D. G. 1986. Medulloblastoma in childhood: results of radical resection and low dose neuro- axis radiation therapy. Neurosurg. 64:239–242.

Tyrrell, J. B., Brooks, R. M., Fitzgerald, P. A., et al. 1978. Cushings disease: selective transsphenoidal resection of pituitary microadenomas. N. Engl. J. Med. 298:753–758.

Walker, M. D., Green, S. B., and Byar, D. P., et al. 1980. Randomized comparisons of radiotherapy and nitrosoureas for the treatment of malignant glioma after surgery. N. Engl. J. Med. 303:1323–1329.

Winkler, G. F., and DeLamonte, S. M. 1987. A 69-year-old woman with multiple cranial nerve abnormalities and inability to walk. Case records of the Massachusetts General Hospital Case #32-1987. N. Engl. J. Med. 317:366–375.

Wood, J. R., Green, S. B., and Shapiro, W. R. 1988. The prognostic importance of tumor size in malignant gliomas: a computed tomographic scan study by the brain tumor cooperative group. J. Clin. Oncol. 6:338–343.

Wood, M. W., White, R. J., and Kernohan, J. W. 1957. One hundred intracranial meningiomas found incidentally at necropsy. J. Neuropathol. Exp. Neurol. 16:337–340.

PART III: INFECTIONS GENERAL

Davis, L. 1992. Spirochetal disease. In A. K. Asbury, G. M. McKhann, and W. I. McDonald (Eds.) Diseases of the Nervous System. 2nd ed., pp. 1359–1370. Philadelphia, PA: W. B. Saunders.

Kennedy, P. G. E., and Johnson, R. T. 1987. Infections of the nervous system. London, UK: Butterworths.

Kocen, R. S. 1992. Tuberculosis of the nervous system. In A. K. Asbury, G. M. McKhann, and W. I. McDonald (Eds.) Diseases of the Nervous System. 2nd ed., pp. 1371–1379. Philadelphia, PA: W. B. Saunders.

Lambert, H. P. 1991. Infections of the Central Nervous System. Philadelphia, PA: B. C. Decker.

McKendall, R. R., and Stroop, W. G. 1994. Handbook of Neurovirology. New York, NY: Marcel Dekker.

Marra, C. (Ed.). 1999. Central nervous system infections. Neurol. Clin. 17(4).

Merritt, H. H., Adams, R. D., and Solomon, H. C. 1946. Neurosyphilis. New York, NY: Oxford University Press.

Newton, B. A. (Ed.). 1985. Trypanosomiasis. Br. Med. Bull. 41:103–199.

Solbrig, M. L. V. (Section Editor). 2000. Infections of the nervous system.. In W. G. Bradley, R. B. Daroff, G. M. Fenichel, and C. D. Marsden (Eds.) Neurology in Clinical Practice. Vol. 2, pp. 1315–1430.

Spach, D. H., Liles, W. C., Campbell, G. L., et al. 1993. Tick borne diseases in the United States. N. Engl. J. Med. 329:936–947.

Tunkel, A. R., and Scheld, W. M. 1992. Bacterial infections in adults. A. K. Asbury, G. M. McKhann, and W. I. McDonald (Eds.) Diseases of the Nervous System. 2nd ed. Philadelphia, PA: W. B. Saunders.

Whitley, R. J. 1990. Medical progress: viral encephalitis. N. Engl. J. Med. 323:1–4.

SPECIFIC REFERENCES AND CITATIONS

Andersson, J., Ehrnst, A., Larson, P. H., et al. 1987. Visualization of defective measles virus particles in cerebrospinal fluid in sub-acute sclerosing panencephalitis. J. Infect. Dis. 156:928–933.

Baer, G. M., and Fishbein, D. B. 1987. Rabies post exposure prophylaxis (Editorial). N. Engl. J. Med. 316:1270–1271.

Baringer, J. J., and Swoveland, P. 1973. Recovery of herpes simplex virus from human trigeminal ganglions. N. Engl. J. Med. 288:638–650.

Basgoz, N., and Frosch, M. P. 1998. Case records of the Massachusetts General Hospital: A 32 year old woman with pharyngeal spasms and parathesias after a dog bite (Rabies). N. Engl. J. Med. 339:105–112.

Bell, B. A., and Britton, J. A. 1991. A brain abscess.. In H. P. Lambert (Ed.) Infection and the Nervous System, pp. 361–373. Philadelphia, PA: B. C. Decker.

Bia, F. J. (Ed.). 1993. Parasitic diseases of the nervous system. Semin. Neurol. 13:131–233.

Bia, F. J., and Barry, M. 1986. Parasitic infections of the nervous system. Neurol. Clin. 4:171–206.

Black, P. H. 1985. HTLV-III, AIDS, and the brain (Editorial). N. Engl. J. Med. 313:1538–1540.

Bousser, M. G., and Barnett, H. J. M. 1992. Cerebral venous thrombosis. In H. J. M. Barnett, J. P. Mohr, B. M. Stein, and F. M. Yatsu. (Eds.)

Stroke Pathophysiology, Diagnosis and Management. 2nd ed., pp. 87–111. New York, NY: Churchill Livingston.

Bromfield, E. B., and Vonsattel, J. P. 2000. Case records of the Massachusetts General Hospital: a 23 year old man with seizures and a lesion in the left temporal lobe.(Neurocysticercosis). N. Engl. J. Med. 343:420–427.

Caplan, L. R., Kleeman, F. J., and Berg, S. 1977. Urinary retention probably secondary to herpes genitalis. N. Engl. J. Med. 297:920–921.

Collinge, J. 1996. New diagnostic tests for prion disease (Editorial). N. Engl. J. Med. 335:963–965.

Daif, B., Awada, A., Al-Rajeh, S., et al. 1995. Cerebral venous thrombosis in adults—a study of 40 cases from Saudi Arabia. Stroke 26:1193–1195.

Dastur, H. M., and Desai, A. D. 1965. Comparative study of brain tuberculomas and gliomas based on 108 case records of each. Brain 88:375–396.

Deresiewicz, R. L., Thaler, S. J., Hsu, L., and Zamani, A. A. 1997. Clinical and neuroradiographic manifestations of eastern equine encephalitis. N. Engl. J. Med. 336:1867–1874.

Durand, M. L., Calderwood, S. B., Webber, D. J., et al. 1993. Acute bacterial meningitis in adults: a review of 493 episodes. N. Engl. J. Med. 328:21–28.

Feigin, R. D., Baker, C. J., Herwaldt, L. A., et al. 1982. Epidemic meningococcal disease in an elementary class room. N. Engl. J. Med. 307:1255–57. (Article concerns use of rifampin and meningococcal polysaccharide vaccine to prevent spread)

Fishbein, D. B., and Robinson, L. L. 1993. Current concepts: rabies. N. Engl. J. Med. 329:1632–1638.

Fowler, K. B., Stagno, S., Nass, R. F., et al. 1992. The outcome of congenital cytomegalovirus infection in relation to maternal antibody status. N. Engl. J. Med. 326:663–667. (See also editorial by M. D. Yow and G. J. Demmler. 1992. N. Engl. J. Med. 326:702–703.)

Gajdusek, D. C. 1967. Slow virus infections of the nervous system. N. Engl. J. Med. 276:392–400.

Galimand, G., Gerbaud, G., Guibourdenche, M., et al. 1998. High level chloramphenicol resistance in Neisseria meningitidis. N. Engl. J. Med. 339:868–874.

Gibbs, C. J., Jr., and Gajdusek, D. C. 1969. Infection as the etiology of spongiform encephalopathy (Creutzfeldt-Jakob disease). Science 165:1023–1025.

Gilden, D. H. 1994. Herpes zoster with postherpetic neuralgia -persisting pain and frustration. N. Engl. J. Med. 330:932–934.

Gilden, D. H., Kleinschmidt-DeMasters, B. K., and La Guardia, J. J. 2000. Medical progress: neurologic complications of the reactivation of varicella-zoster virus. N. Engl. J. Med. 342:635–645.

Gordon, S. M., Eaton, M. E., George, R., et al. 1994. The response of symptomatic neurosyphilis to high-dose intravenous penicillin G in patients with human immunodeficiency virus infection. N. Engl. J. Med. 331:1469–1473.

Gray, F., Gherardi, F., and Scaravilli, F. 1988. The neuropathology of the acquired immune deficiency syndrome (AIDS). Brain 111:245–266.

Griffith, J. F. 1985. Subacute sclerosing panencephalitis and lymphocytes (Editorial). N. Engl. J. Med. 313:952–954.

Hanley, D. 1990. Herpes simplex encephalitis: clinical diagnosis and management. Syllabus Minneapolis annual course 347: infections of the nervous system. Amer. Acad. Neurol. 57:25–37.

Haywood, A. M. 1997. Transmissible spongiform encephalopathies. N. Engl. J. Med. 337:1821–1828.

Henson, J. W., and Ferraro, M. J. 1993. Case records of the Massachusetts General Hospital—a 71-year-old woman with confusion, hemianopia and an occipital mass. N. Engl. J. Med. 329:1335–1341.

Hoban, D. J., Witwick, E., and Hammond, G. W. 1985. Bacterial antigen detection in cerebrospinal fluid of patients with meningitis. Diagn. Microbiol. Infect. Dis. 3:373–379. (Article concerns rapid identification using agglutination for bacterial antigen detection.)

Hoke, C. H., Nisalak, A., and Sangawhipa, N. 1988. Protection against Japanese encephalitis by activated vaccines. N. Engl. J. Med. 319:608–614.

Holman, R. G., Janssen, R. S., Buehler, J. W., et al. 1991. Epidemiology of progressive multifocal leukoencephalopathy in the United States: analysis of national mortality and AIDS surveillance data. Neurology 41:1733–1736.

Holmes, M. D., Brant-Zawodski, M. M., and Simon, R. P. 1984. Clinical manifestations of meningovascular syphilis. Neurology 34:553–556.

Hook, E. W., and Marra, C. M. 1992. Acquired syphilis in adults. N. Engl. J. Med. 326:1060–1068.

Horowitz, S. L., Bentson, J. R., Benson, F., et al. 1983. CNS toxoplasmosis in acquired immunodeficiency syndrome. Arch. Neurol. 40:649–652.

Houff, S. A., Major, E. O., Katz, D. A., et al. 1988. Involvement of J. C. virus-infected mononuclear cells from the bone marrow and spleen in the pathogenesis of progressive multifocal leukoencephalography. N. Engl. J. Med. 318:301–305.

Howard, R. S., and Lees, A. J. 1987. Encephalitis lethargica: a report of four recent cases. Brain 110:35–52.

Johnson, R. T. 1972. Effects of viral infection on the developing nervous system. N. Engl. J. Med. 287:599–604.

Johnson, R. T. 1980. Selective vulnerability of neural cells to viral infections. Brain 103:447–472.

Johnson, R. T. 1982. Current concepts in neurology: the contribution of virologic research to clinical neurology. N. Engl. J. Med. 307:660–662.

Johnson, R. T. 1992. Prion disease. N. Engl. J. Med. 326:486–487.

Johnson, R. T., and Giggs, C. J., Jr. 1998. Medical progress: Creutzfeldt-Jakob disease and related transmissible spongiform encephalopathies. N. Engl. J. Med. 339:1994–2004.

Johnson, R. T., Griffin, D. E., Hirsch, R. L., et al. 1984. Measles encephalomyelitis: clinical and immunologic studies. N. Engl. J. Med. 310:137–141.

Johnson, R. T., and Johnson, K. J. 1968. Hydrocephalus following viral infection: the pathology of aqueductal stenosis developing after experimental mumps virus infection. J. Neuropath. Exp. Neurol. 27:591–606.

Johnson, R. T., and Warren, K. S. 1992. Parasitic infections.. In A. K. Asbury, G. M. McKhann, and W. I. McDonald (Eds.) Diseases of the Nervous System. 2nd ed, pp.130–158. Philadelphia, PA: W. B. Saunders.

Jubelt, B., and Drucker, J. 1993. Post polio syndrome: an update. Semin. Neurol. 13:283–290.

Kahn, J. O., and Walker, B. D. 1998. Current concepts: acute human immunodeficiency virus type I infection. N. Engl. J. Med. 339:33–39.

Lepow, M. L., and Gold, R. 1983. Editorial retrospective: meningococcal A and other polysaccharide vaccines: a 5 year progress report. N. Engl. J. Med. 308:1158–1160.

Lipton, S. A., and Gendelman, H. E. 1995. Seminars in medicine of the Beth Israel Hospital, Boston. Dementia associated with the acquired immunodeficiency syndrome. N. Engl. J. Med. 332:934–940.

Loeser, E., Jr., and Scheinberg, L. 1957. Brain abscesses: a review of ninety-nine cases. Neurology 7:601–609.

Mahalingham, R., Wellish, M., Wolf, W., et al. 1990. Latent varicella zoster viral DNA in human trigeminal and thoracic ganglia. N. Engl. J. Med. 323:627–631.

Marra, C. M. 1995. Neurosyphilis: a guide for clinicians. Neurologist 1:157–166.

Matthews, W. B. 1992. Slow viruses and the central nervous system.. In H. P. Lambert (Ed.) Infections of the Central Nervous System. 2nd ed., pp. 329–342. Philadelphia, PA: B. C. Decker.

McArthur, J. C. 1987. Neurologic complication of AIDS. Medicine 66:407–437.

McArthur, J. C. 1992. Neurologic manifestations of human immunodeficiency virus infection.. In A. K. Asbury, G. M. McKhann and W. I. McDonald (Eds.) Diseases of the Nervous System. 2nd ed, pp. 1312–1330. Philadelphia, PA: W. B. Saunders.

McIntosh, K. 1991. Congenital syphilis: breaking through the safety net (Editorial) N. Engl. J. Med. 316:1569–1572.

McJunkin, J. E., de Los Reyes, E. C., Irazuzta, J. E., et al. 2001: La Crosse encephalitis in America. N. Engl. J. Med. 344:801–807.

Miller, E., Dias, D. S., and Uttlea, D. 1987. Management of subdural empyema: a series of 24 cases. J. Neurol. Neurosurg. Psychiat. 50:1415–1418.

Monath, T. P. 1988. Japanese encephalitis. A plague of the Orient. N. Engl. J. Med. 319:641–643.

Moore, K. A., and Osterholm, M. T. 1998. Meningococcal disease and public health practice (Editorial). JAMA. 279:472–473.

Musher, D. M., and Baughn, R. E. 1994. Editorials—neurosyphilis in HIV-infected persons. N. Engl. J. Med. 331:1517–1518.

Nash, D., Mostashari, F., and Fine, A. 2001. The outbreak of West Nile virus infection in the New York City area in 1999. N. Engl. J. Med. 344:1807–1814.

Padgett, B. L., Walker, D. L., Zurhein, G. M., et al. 1971. Cultivation of papova-like virus from human brain with progressive multi focal leukoencephalopathy. Lancet 1:1257–1260.

Picard, F. J., Poland, S. D., and Rice, G. P. A. 1993. New development with herpes viruses and the nervous system. Curr. Opin. Neurol. Neurosurg. 6:169.

Plotkin, S. A., and Koprowski, H. 1979. Phobia of hydrophobia justified (Editorial). N. Engl. J. Med. 300:620–622.

Pomeroy, S. L., Holmes, S. J., Dodge, P. R., et al. 1990. Seizures and other neurologic sequelae of bacterial meningitis in children. N. Engl. J. Med. 323:1651–1657.

Porter, S. B., and Sande, M. A. 1992. Toxoplasmosis of the central nervous system in the acquired immunodeficiency syndrome. N. Engl. J. Med. 327:1643–1648.

Powderly, W. G., Saag, M. S., Cloud, G. A., et al. 1992. A controlled trial of fluconazole or amphotericin B to prevent relapse of cryptococcal meningitis in patients with the acquired immunodeficiency syndrome. N. Engl. J. Med. 326:793–798. (See also Saag, M. S. et al. 1992. N. Engl. J. Med. 326:83–89)

Prusiner, S. B. 2001. Shattuck lecture-neurodenerative diseases and prions. N. Engl. J. Med. 344:1516–1526.

Quagliarello, V., and Scheld, G. A. 1992. Bacterial meningitis: pathogenesis pathophysiology and progress. N. Engl. J. Med. 327:864–872.

Quagliarello, V., and Scheld, W. M. 1997. Treatment of bacterial meningitis. N. Engl. J. Med. 336:708–716.

Reik, L., Steere, A. C., Bartenhagen, N. H., et al. 1979. Neurologic abnormalities of Lyme disease. Medicine 58:281–294.

Richardson, E. P., Jr. 1988. Progressive multifocal leukoencephalopathy 30 years later. N. Engl. J. Med. 318:315–317.

Rosenstein, N., Levine, O., Taylor, J. P., et al. 1998. Efficacy of meningococcal vaccine and barriers to vaccination. JAMA. 279:435–439.

Rosenstein, N. E., Perkins, B. A., Stephens, D. S., et al. 2001. Meningococcal disease. N. Engl. J. Med. 344:1378–1388.

Sabetta, J. R., and Andriole, V. T. 1985. Cryptococcal infections of the central nervous system. Med. Clin. North Am. 69:333–344.

Salaki, J., Louria, D., and Chmel, H. 1984. Fungal and yeast infections of the central nervous system: a clinical review. Medicine 63:108–132.

Sepkowitz, K. A. 2001. AIDS-the first 20 years. N. Engl. J. Med. 344:1764–1772.

Sharief, M. K., Phil, M., Hentges, R., et al. 1991. Intrathecal immune response in patients with the post polio syndrome. N. Engl. J. Med. 325:751–755.

Schucat, A., Robinson, K., Wenger, J. D., et al. 1997. Bacterial meningitis in the United States in 1995. N. Engl. J. Med. 337:970–976.

Simon, R. P. Neurosyphilis. 1985. Arch. Neurol. 42:606–613.

Simon, R. P. 1990. Neurosyphilis. Syllabus Minneapolis annual course 347: infections of the nervous system. Amer. Acad. Neurol. 12:43–62.

Smith, A. L. 1990. Neurologic sequelae of meningitis. N. Engl. J. Med., 319:141–7.

Steere, A. C. 1989. Medical progress: Lyme disease. N. Engl. J. Med.321: 586–596.

Strauss, S. E. (moderator), Ostrove, J. M., Inchauspe, G., et al. 1988. Varicella zoster virus infections: biology, natural history, treatment and prevention. Ann. Intern. Med. 108:221–227.

Taylor, H. G., Mills, E. L., Ciampi, A., et al. 1990. The sequelae of Haemophilus influenzae meningitis in school age children. N. Engl. J. Med. 323:1657–1667.

Traub, M., Colchester, A. C. F., Kingsley, D. P. C., et al. 1984. Tuberculosis of the central nervous system. Quart. J. Med. 53:81–100.

Tyler, K. L. 2001. West Nile virus encephalitis in America (Editorial). N. Engl. J. Med. 344:1858–1859.

Van Der Horst, C. M., Saag, M. S., Cloud, G. A., et al. 1997. Treatment of cryptococcal meningitis associated with the acquired immunodeficiency syndrome. N. Engl. J. Med. 337:15–21.

Whitley, R. J., Arvin, A., Prober, C., et al. 1991. A controlled trial comparing vidarabine with acyclovir in neonatal herpes simplex virus infection. N. Engl. J. Med. 324:444–449.

Whitley, R. J., and Gnann, J. W., Jr. 1992. Acyclovir: a decade later. N. Engl. J. Med. 327:782–789.

Wood, M. J., Johnson, R. W., McKendrick, M. W., et al. 1994. A randomized trial of acyclovir for 7 days or 21 days with and without prednisolone for treatment of acute herpes zoster. N. Engl. J. Med. 330:896–900.

Wright, P. F., and Karzon, D. T. 1995. Minimizing the risks associated with the prevention of poliomyelitis (Editorial). N. Engl. J. Med. 332:529–530.

ZuRhein, G. M., and Chou, S. M. 1965. Particles resembling papova viruses in human cerebral demyelinating disease. Science 148:1477–1479.

PART IV: NUTRITIONAL, RELATED DISORDERS, AND ALCOHOL EFFECTS (SEE ALSO CHAPTERS 8, 9, AND 20)

Ayus, J. C., Krothanpalli, R. K., and Arieff, A. I. 1987. Treatment of symptomatic hyponatremia and its relation to brain damage. N. Engl. J. Med. 317:1190–1195.

Brody, I. A., and Wilkins, R. H. 1968. Neurological classic IX: Wernicke's encephalopathy. Arch. Neurol. 19:228–232.

Brust, J. C. M. (Ed.). 1993. Neurologic complications of drug and alcohol abuse. Neurol. Clin. 11:503–735.

Charness, M. E., Simon, R. P., and Greenberg, D. A. 1989. Ethanol and the nervous system. N. Engl. J. Med. 321:442–454.

Cuba Neuropathy Field Inveatigation Team. 1995. Epidemic optic neuropathy in Cuba–clinical characterization and risk factors. N. Engl. J. Med. 333:1176–1182.

Czeizel, A. E., and Dudas, I. 1992. Prevention of the first occurrence of neural-tube defects by periconceptional vitamin supplementation. N. Engl. J. Med. 327:1832–1833.

Greenberg, D. A. 1993. Ethanol and sedatives. Neurol. Clin. 11:523–534.

Hauw, J. J., DeBaecque, C., Hausser-Hauw, C., and Serdaru, M. 1988. Chromatolysis in alcoholic encephalopathies. Brain 111:843–857.

Hyvarinen, J., Laakso, M., Roine, R., et al. 1978. Effect of ethanol on neuronal activity in parietal association cortex of alert monkeys. Brain 101:701–715.

Kleinschmidt-DeMasters, B. K., and Norenborg, M. D. 1981. Rapid correction of hyponatremia causes demyelination: relation to central pontine myelinolysis. Science 211:1068–1070.

Lindboe, C. F., and Loberg, E. M. 1989. Wernicke's encephalopathy in non-alcoholics: an autopsy study. N. Engl. J. Med. 90:125–129.

Little, R. E., Anderson, K. W., Ervin, C. H, et al.1989. Maternal alcohol use during breast feeding and infant mental and motor development at one year. N. Engl. J. Med. 321:425–430.

Miller, M. W. 1986. Effects of alcohol on the generation and migration of cerebral cortical neurons. Science 233:1308–1311.

Miller, M. (Ed.) 1991. Development of the Central Nervous System: Effects of Alcohol and Opiates, Vol. 32, pp. 390–402.

Phillips, S. C., Harper, C. G., and Kril, J. 1987. A quantitative histological study of the cerebellar vermis in alcoholic patients. Brain 110:301–314.

Pincus, J. H., Reynolds, E. H., and Glaser, G. H. 1972. Subacute combined system degeneration with folate deficiency. JAMA. 221:496–497.

Porter, R. J., Mattson, R. H., Cramer, J. A., and Diamond, I. (Eds.) 1990. Alcohol and Seizures: Basic Mechanisms and Clinical Concepts. Philadelphia, PA: F. A. Davis.

Rosenberg, I. H. 1992. Folic acid and neural-tube defects—time for action? (Editorial). N. Engl. J. Med. 327:1875–1877.

Serdaru, M., Hausser-Hauw, C., LaPlane, D., et al. 1988. The clinical spectrum of alcoholic pellagra encephalopathy: a retrospective analysis of 22 cases studied pathologically. Brain 111:829–842.

Streissguth, A. P., Aase, J. M., Clarren, S. K., et al. 1991. Fetal alcohol syndrome in adolescents and adults. JAMA. 265:1961–1967.

Toh, B. H., Van Driel, I. R., and Gleeson, P. A. 1997. Pernicious anemia. N. Engl. J. Med. 337:1441–1448.

vanGelder, N. M., Butterworth, R. G., and Drujan, B. D. (Eds.). 1990. (Mal)Nutrition and the infant brain. In Neurology and

Neurobiology—Proceedings of an International Symposium Held in Montreal, Quebec, Canada, May 11–12, 1989.
Victor, M. 1965. The effects of nutritional deficiency on the nervous system. In Brain, Lord, and F. H. Norris (Eds.) The Remote Effects of Cancer on the Nervous System, pp. xx–xx. New York, NY: Grune and Stratton.
Victor, M. 1993. Persistent altered mentation due to ethanol. Neurol. Clin. 11:639–661.
Victor, M., Adams, R. D., and Collins, G. H. 1989. The Wernicke-Korsakoff Syndrome and Related Neurological Disorders due to Alcoholism and Malnutrition. 2nd ed. Philadelphia, PA: F. A. Davis,
Walsh, D. C., Hingson, R. W., Merrigan, D. M., et al. 1991. A randomized trial of treatment options for alcohol abusing workers. N. Engl. J. Med. 325:775–782.

TOXINS GENERAL AND SYMPOSIA

Albers, J. W., and Berent, S. (Eds.). 2000. Clinical neurobehavioral toxicology. Neurol. Clin. 18:517–771.
Brust, J. C. M. (Ed.). 1993. Neurologic complications of drug and alcohol abuse. Neurol. Clin. 11:503–735.
Chang, L. W. (Ed.). 1994. Principles of Neurotoxicology. New York, NY: Marcel Dekker.
Spencer, P. S., and Schumburg, H. H. 1980. Experimental and Clinical Neurotoxicology. Baltimore, MD: Williams & Wilkins.

Heavy Metals: Lead

Baghurst, P. A., McMichael, A. J., Wigg, N. R., et al. 1992. Environmental exposure to lead and children's intelligence at the age of seven years—the Port Pirie Cohort Study. N. Engl. J. Med. 327:1279–1284.
Boothby, J. A., deJesus, P. V., and Rowland, L. P. 1974. Reversible forms of motor neuron disease—lead "neuritis." Arch. Neurol. 31:18–23.
Feldman, R. G. 1978. Massachusetts Department of Public Health -urban lead mining: lead intoxication among deleaders. N. Engl. J. Med. 298:1143–1145.
Goldman, R. H., Baker, E. L., Haman, M., and Kamerow, P. B. 1987. Lead poisoning in automobile radiator mechanics. N. Engl. J. Med. 317:214–218.
Mason, J. O. 1991. U.S. Public Health Service's strategic plan to eliminate child hood lead poisoning. JAMA. 265:2049.
Needleman, H. L., Schell, A., Bellinger, D., Leviton, A., and Allred, E. N. 1990. Exposure to low doses of lead in childhood: an 11-year follow-up report. N. Engl. J. Med. 322:83–88.
Rogan, W. J., Dietrich, K. N., Ware, J. H., et al. 2001. The effect of chelation therapy with succimer on neuropsychological development in children exposed to lead. N. Engl. J. Med. 344:1421–1426.
Rosen, J. F., and Mushak, P. 2001. Primary prevention of childhood lead poisoning- the only solution. 344:1470–1471.

Mercury

Adams, C. R., Ziegler, D. K., and Lin, J. T. 1983. Mercury intoxication simulating amyotrophic lateral sclerosis. JAMA. 250:642–643.
Hammond, A. L. 1971. Mercury in the environment: natural and human factors. Science. 171:778–789.
Hauw, J., Rickards, A. G., McMenemen, W. H., and Cumings, J. N. 1963. Organic mercury encephalopathy. J. Neurol. Neurosurg. Psychiat. 26:199–202.
Kurland, L. T., Faro, S. N., and Siedler, H. 1960. Minimata disease. World Neuro. 11:370–390.
March, D. O., Clarkson, J. W., Cox, C., et al. 1987. Fetal methyl mercury poisoning: relationship between concentration single strands of maternal hair and child effects. Arch. Neurol. 44:1017–1022.
Neal, D. A., and Jones, R. R. 1938. Chronic mercurialism in the hatters' fur-cutting industry. JAMA. 110:337.

Other Agents

Ernst, A., and Zibrak, J. D. 1998. Carbon monoxide poisoning. N. Engl J. Med. 339:1603–1608.

Barbiturates and Benzodiazepines

Busto, U., Sellers, E. M., Naranjo, C. A., et al. 1986. Withdrawal reaction after long term therapeutic use of benzodiazepines. N. Engl. J. Med. 315:854–859.
Farwell, J. R., Lee, Y. J., Hirtz, D. G., et al. 1990. Phenobarbital for febrile seizures—effects on intelligence and on seizure recurrence. N. Engl. J. Med. 322:364–369.

Cocaine and Other Drugs of Abuse: General or Symposia

Ali, S. F. (Ed.). 1998. The neurochemistry of drugs of abuse: cocaine, ibogaine, and substituted amphetamines. Ann. NY Acad. Sci. 844:1–362.
Ali, S. F. (Ed.). 2000. Neurobiologic mechanisms of drugs of abuse: cocaine, ibogaine and substituted amphetamines. Ann. NY Acad. Sci. 914:1–440.
Harvey, J. A., and Kosofsky, B. E. 1998. Cocaine: effets on the developing brain. Ann NY Acad. Sci. 846:1–436.
Richter, R. W. (Ed.). 1975. Medical Aspects of Drug Abuse. Hagerstown, MD: Harper & Row.

Specific References

Altura, B. T., and Altua, B. M. 1981. Phencyclidine, lysergic acid diethylamide and mescaline: cerebral artery spasms an hallucinogenic activity. Science. 212:1051–1052.
Brust, J. C. M. 1993. Other agents: phencyclidine, marijuana, hallucinogens, inhalants and anticholinergics. Neurol. Clin. 11:555–561.
Chiriboga, C. A. 1993. Fetal effects. Neurol. Clin. 11:707–728.
Foley, K. M. 1993. Opioids. Neurol. Clin. 11:503–522.
Freedman, D. X. 1969. The psychopharmacology of hallucinogenic agents. Ann. Rev. Med. 20:409–418.
Cregler, L. L., and Mark, H. 1986. Special report: medical complications of cocaine abuse. N. Engl. J. Med. 315:1495–1499.
Gawin, F. H., and Ellinwood, E. H., Jr. 1988. Cocaine and other stimulants: action, abuse and treatment. N. Engl. J. Med. 318:1173–1182.
Isner, J. H., and Chokshi, S. K. 1989. Cocaine and vasospasms (Editorial). N. Engl. J. Med. 321:1604–1606.
Lange, R. E., Cigarroa, R. A., Yancy, C. W., Jr., et al. 1989. Cocaine-induced coronary artery vasospasm. N. Engl. J. Med. 321:1557–1562.
Leshner, A. I. 1996. Molecular mechanisms of cocaine addiction. N. Engl. J. Med. 335:128–129.
Levine, S. R., Brust, J. C. M., Futrell, N., et al. 1990. Cerebrovascular complications of the use of the "crack" form of alkaloidal cocaine. N. Engl. J. Med. 323:699–704.
Mayes, L. C., Granger, R. H., Bornstein, M. H., and Zuckerman, B. 1992. The problem of prenatal cocaine exposure. JAMA. 267:406–408.
Mendelson, J. H., and Mello, N. K. 1996. Management of cocaine abuse and dependence. N. Engl. J. Med. 334:965–972.
Sanchez-Ramos, J. R. 1993. Psycho stimulants. Neurol. Clin. 11:535–553.
Srnythies, J. R. 1962. Hallucinogenic drugs. In D. Williams (Ed.) Modern Trends in Neurology, pp. 353–366. London, UK: Butterworth & Company.
Volpe, J. J. 1992. Mechanisms of disease—effect of cocaine use on the fetus. N. Engl. J. Med. 327:399–407.
Yul, K., Ikemoto, S., Ishiguro, T., and Goto, K. 1998. Studies of amphetamine or methamphetamine psychosis I japan: relation of metamphetamine psychosis to schizophrenia. Ann. NY Acad Sci. 914:1–12.
Zuckerman, B., Frank, D. A., Hingson, R., et al. 1989. Effects of maternal marijuana and cocaine use on fetal growth. N. Engl. J. Med. 320:762–768.

COMPLICATIONS OF MEDICAL DISORDERS

General Reference

Riggs, J. E. 2002. Neurologic manifestations of systemic disease. Neurol. Clin. 20:1–289.

Diabetes and Thyroid Disease

Alshekhlee, A., Kaminski, H. J., and Ruff, R. 2002. Neuromuscular manifestations of endocrine disorders. Neurol. Clin. 20:35–58.

Boyle, P. J., Schwartz, N. S., Shah, S., et al. 1988. Concentrations at the onset of hypoglycemic symptoms in patients with poorly plasma glucose controlled diabetes and in non-diabetics. N. Engl. J. Med. 318:1487–1492.

Halpern, J. P., Boyages, S. C., Maberly, G. F., Collins, J. K., et al. 1991. The neurology of endemic cretinism: a study of two endemics. Brain 114:825–841.

Ingbar, S. H., and Braverman, L. E. (Eds.). 1986. The Thyroid: A Fundamental and Clinical Text. Philadelphia, PA: J. B. Lippencott.

Sanders, V. 1986. Neurologic manifestations of myxedema. N. Engl. J. Med. 266:547–552, 559.

Swanson, J. W., Kelly, J., Jr., and Mconahey, W. M. 1981. Neurologic aspects of thyroid disease. Mayo Clinic Proc. 56:504–512.

PITUITARY DISORDERS: REFER TO PART II OF THIS CHAPTER ON BRAIN TUMORS.

Renal Disease

Lederman, R. J., and Henry, C. F. 1978. Progressive dialysis encephalopathy. Ann. Neurol. 4:199–204.

Palmer, C. A. 2002. Neurologic manifestations of renal disease. Neurol. Clin. 20:23–34.

Raskin, N. H., and Fishman, R. A. 1976. Neurologic disorders in renal failure. N. Engl. J. Med. 294:143–148, 204–210.

Trompeter, R. S., Polinsky, M. S., Andreoli, S. A., and Fennell, R. S. 1986. Neurological complications of renal failure. Am. J. Kidney Pis. 7:318–323.

IMMUNOLOGIC AND CONNECTIVE TISSUE DISORDERS. LUPUS, VASCULITIS, SARCOID, BECHET'S

Bluestein, H. G. 1987. Neuropsychiatric manifestations of systemic lupus erythematosus (Editorial). N. Engl. J. Med. 317:309–310.

Delaney, P. 1977. Neurologic manifestations in sarcoidosis: review of the literature with a report of 32 cases. Ann. Intern. Med. 87:336–345.

Lim, L., Ron, M. A., Ormerod, I. E. C., David, J., Miller, D. H., et al. 1988. Psychiatric and neurological manifestations in systemic lupus erythematosus. Quart. J. Med. 66:27–38.

McCune, W. J., McGuire, A., Aisen, A., and Gebarski, S. 1988. Identification of brain lesions in neuropsychiatric systemic lupus erythematosus by magnetic resonance scanning. Arthritis Rheum. 31:159–169.

O'Duffy, J. D. 1990. Bechets syndrome. N. Engl. J. Med. 322:326–327.

Nadeau, S. E. 2002a. Neurologic complications of systemic vasculitis. Neurol. Clin. 20:123–150.

Nadeau, S. E. 2002b. Neurologic manifestations of connective tissue disease. Neurol. Clin. 20:151–178.

Sigal, L. H. 1987. The neurological presentation of vasculitic and rheumatologic syndromes. Medicine 66:157–180.

Remote Neurological Manifestations of Malignancy. Paraneoplastic Syndromes (Refer Also to Chapter 20 for Cerebellar Syndrome)

Anderson, N. E., Rosenblum, M. K., Grous, F., Wiley, R. O., and Posner, J. B. 1988. Autoantibodies in paraneoplastic syndromes associated with small cell lung cancer. Neurology 38:1391–1398.

Anderson, N. E., Rosenblum, M. K., and Posner, J. B. 1988. Paraneoplastic cerebellar degeneration: clinical immunological correlations. Ann. Neurol. 24:559–567.

Brain, W. R., and Wilkinson, M. 1965. Subacute cerebellar degeneration associated with neoplasms. Brain 88:465–478.

Clouston, P. D., DeAngelis, L. M., and Posner, J. B. 1992. The spectrum of neurological disease in patients with systemic cancer. Ann. Neurol. 31:268–273.

Dalmau, J., Furneaux, H. M., Rosenblum, M. K., Graus, F., and Posner, J. B. 1991. Detection of the anti hu antibody in specific regions of the nervous system and tumor from patients with paraneoplastic encephalomyelitis/sensory neuronopathy. Neurology 41:1757–1764.

Dropcho, E. J. 2002. Remote neurologic manifestations of cancer. Neurol. Clin. 20:85–122.

Furneaux, H. M., Rosenblum, M. K., Dalmau, J., et al. 1990. Selective expression of purkinje-cell antigens in tumor tissue from patient with paraneoplastic cerebellar degeneration. N. Engl. J. Med. 322:1844–1851.

Henson, R. A., and Urich, H. 1982. Cancer and the Nervous System. London, UK: Blackwell Scientific.

Jones, H. R., Jr., and Richardson, E. P., Jr. 1990. A 45-year-old woman with Hodgkins disease and a neurological disorder. Case records of the Massachusetts General Hospital. Case #8-1990 (acute paraneoplastic sensory ganglionitis). N. Engl. J. Med. 322:531–543.

Koroshetz, W. J., and McKee, A. C. 1988. A 76-year-old woman with confusion, agitation and a gait disorder. Case records of the Massachusetts General Hospital Case #39–1988 (Paraneoplastic Encephalitis Limbic and Brain Stem Encephalitis). N. Engl. J. Med. 319:849–860.

Posner, J. B., and Furneaux, H. M. 1990. Paraneoplastic syndromes. In B. H. Waksman (Ed.) Immunologic Mechanisms in Neurologic and Psychiatric Disease, pp.187–219. New York, NY: Raven Press.

DISORDERS OF MYELIN: LEUKODYTROPHIES

Delong, G. R., Haperin, J. J., and Richardson, E. P., Jr. 1982. A 15-year-old boy with slowly progressive dementia: case records of the Massachusetts General Hospital Case #5-1982, (Adrenoleuko-dystrophy with Peripheral Neuropathy). N. Engl. J. Med. 306:286–293.

Krivit, W., Shapiro, E., Kennedy, W., Lipton, M., et al. 1990. Treatment of late infantile metachromatic leukodystrophy by bone marrow transplantation. N. Engl. J. Med. 322:28–32.

Menkes, J. H. 1990. The leukodystrophies (Editorial). N. Engl. J. Med. 322:54–44.

Sadeghi-Nejad, A., and Senior, B. 1990. Adrenomyeloneuropathy presenting as Addison's disease in childhood. N. Engl. J. Med. 322:13–16.

MULTIPLE SCLEROSIS: SEE ALSO CHAPTERS 9 (SPINAL CORD) AND 13 (BRAIN STEM)

General

Matthews, W. B., Compston, A., Allen, A., and Martyn, C. N. (Eds.). 1991. McAlpine's Multiple Sclerosis. Edinburgh, UK: Churchill Livingstone.

Noseworthy, J. H., and Lucchinetti, C. 2000. Medical progress: multiple sclerosis. 343:938–952.

Paty, D. W., and Ebers, G. C. (Eds.). 1997. Multiple Sclerosis. Philadelphia, PA: F. A. Davis.

Specific

Beck, R. W., Cleary, P. A., Anderson, M. M., Jr., et al. 1992. A randomized. Controlled trial of corticosteroids in the treatment of acute optic neuritis. N. Engl. J. Med. 356:581–588.

Buckley, C., Kennard, C., and Swash, M. 1982. Treatment of acute exacerbations of multiple sclerosis with intravenous methyl-prednisolone. J. Neurol. Neurosurg. Psychiat. 45:179–180.

Confavreux, C., Aimard, G., and Devic, M. 1980. Course and prognosis of multiple sclerosis assessed by the computerized data pro-cessing of 349 patients. Brain 103:281–300.

Dowling, P. C., Bosch, V. V., and Cook, S. D. 1980. Possible beneficial effect of high-dose intravenous steroid therapy in acute demyelinating disease and transverse myelitis. Neurology 30(20):33–36.

Ebers, G. C., Bulman, D. E., Sadovnick, A. D., et al. 1986. A population-based study of multiple sclerosis in twins. N. Engl. J. Med. 315:1638–1642.

IFNB Multiple Sclerosis Study Group. 1993. Interferon beta—1b is effective in relapsing remitting multiple sclerosis. I: clinical results of a multicenter randomized double blind placebo controlled clinical trial. Neurology 43:655–661, 662–667.

Kupersmith, M. J., Kaufman, D., Paty, D. W., et al. 1994. Megadose corticosteroids in multiple sclerosis (Editorial). Neurology 44:1–4.

Lessell, S. 1992. Corticosteroid treatment of acute optic neuritis. N. Engl. J. Med. 326:634–635.

Miller, D., Rudge, P., Johnson, G., et al. 1988. Serial gadolinium enhanced magnetic resonance imaging in multiple sclerosis. Brain 111:927–939.

Morrissey, S. F., Miller, D. H., and Kendall, B. E. 1993. The significance of brain magnetic resonance imaging abnormalities at presentation with clinically isolated syndromes suggestive of multiple sclerosis. A five year follow- up. Brain 116:135–146.

Newcombe, J., Hawkins, C. P., Henderson, C. L., et al. 1991. Histopathology of multiple sclerosis lesions detected by magnetic resonance imaging in unfixed post-mortem central nervous system tissue. Brain114:1013–1024.

Paty, D. W., and Li, D. K. 1993. Interferon beta–1b is effective in relapsing remitting multiple sclerosis. II. MRI analysis results of a multicenter randomized double blind placebo controlled trial. Neurology 43:662–667.

Phadke, J. G. 1990. Clinical aspects of multiple sclerosis in Northeast Scotland with particular reference to its course and prognosis. Brain 113:1597–1628.

Phadke, J., and Best, P. 1983. Atypical and clinically silent multiple sclerosis: a report of 12 cases discovered unexpecpectedly at autopsy. J. Neurol. Neurosurg. Psychiat. 46:414–420.

Phadke, J., and Downie, A. W. 1987. Epidemiology of multiple sclerosis in the northeast (Grampian Region) of Scotland: an update. J. Epidemiol. Community Health. 41:5–13.

Rudick, R. A., Cohen, J. A., Weinstock- Guttman, B., et al. 1997. Management of multiple sclerosis. N. Engl. J. Med. 337:1604–1611.

Runmaker, B., and Andersen, O. 1993. prognostic factors in a multiple sclerosis cohort with twenty-five years of follow-up. Brain 116:117–134.

Weiner, H. L. 1987. COP 1 therapy for multiple sclerosis (Editorial). N. Engl. J. Med. 317:442–443.

Weiner, H. L., and Hafler, D. A. 1988. Immunotherapy of multiple sclerosis—neurological progress. Ann. Neurol. 23:211–222.

Weinshenker, B. C., Bass, B., Rice, G. P. A., et al. 1989. The natural history of multiple sclerosis: a geographically based study. (I.) Clinical course and disability. Brain 112:133–146.

Weinshenker, B. G., Rice, G. P., Noseworthy, J. H., et al. 1991. The natural history of multiple sclerosis: a geographically based study. (3.) Multivariate analysis of predictive factors and models of outcome. Brain 114:1045–1056.

Weinshenker, B. G., Rice, G. P., Noseworthy, J. H., et al. 1991. The natural history of multiple sclerosis: a geographically based study. (4.) Applications to planning and interpretation of clinical therapeutic trials. Brain 114:1057–1068.

Whitaker, J. N. 1998. Effects of pregnancy and delivery on disease activity in multiple sclerosis (Editorial). N. Engl. J. Med. 339:339–340.

POSTINFECTIOUS DEMYELINATION

Arnason, B. G. W. 1987. Neuroimmunology (Editorial). N. Engl. J. Med. 316:406–408.

Hemachudha, T., Griffin, D. E., Giffels, J. J., et al. 1987. Myelin basic protein as an encephalitogen in encephalomyelitis and polyneuritis following rabies vaccination. N. Engl. J. Med. 316:369–374.

Stewart, W. A., Alvord, E. C., Jr., Hruby, S., et al. 1991. Magnetic resonance imaging of experimental allergic encephalomyelitis in primates. Brain 114:1069–1096.

28.

CASE HISTORY PROBLEM SOLVING

PART IV: CEREBRAL HEMISPHERES

A. MATCH THE CASE VIGNETTES, 28.1–28.8 TO THE LESION DIAGRAM FIGS. 28.1 TO 28.8

Case 28.1. A 53-year-old, right-handed housewife with intermittent right-sided headaches and retro-orbital pain for 2 months awoke from sleep with the explosive onset of the "most severe headache" that she had ever experienced (Fig. 28.3).

Case 28.2. This 56-year-old, right-handed white male truck driver had the sudden onset of a transient monocular blindness involving the right eye and the following morning had a transient weak, numb, and useless right arm.

Figure 28.1

Figure 28.3

Figure 28.2

Figure 28.4

Figure 28.5

Figure 28.6

Figure 28.7

Figure 28.8

Case 28.3. A 32-year-old male was admitted to the hospital because of the sudden onset of severe headache, confusion, and aphasia (Fig. 28.4).

Case 28.4. This 73-year-old, right-handed businessman from Maine was involved in an automobile accident in which his auto was struck by a heavy logging truck. Five days later he developed headaches, "fogginess in thinking," and personality change (Fig. 28.6).

Case 28.5. A 62-year-old, right-handed male, 18 months prior to admission, had the onset of focal motor and sensory seizures on the left side of his tongue which spread to the left side of the face and the left arm and hand (Fig. 28.7).

Case 28.6. This 58-year-old right-handed white female with a past history of hypertension and angina pectoris had the acute onset of a right-sided weakness while at work. She had no sensory, visual, or language disturbance (Fig. 28.8).

Case 28.7. This 14-year-old, right-handed female was admitted with a chief complaint of "draining left ear" and left frontal headache followed by a left peripheral facial weakness, and subsequently confusion and language difficulties (Fig. 28.9).

Case 28.8. This 28-year-old, right-handed, school teacher was about to testify in court when she suddenly dropped to the floor with a severe impairment of speech (Fig. 28.10).

B. LESION DIAGRAMS

For each of the preceding figures 28.1 to 28.9 by the cross-hatched lesion. For each structure involved, indicate the expected clinical symptoms or signs with appropriate lateralization. Where appropriate, indicate the vascular territory involved or the designation of the most likely type of pathology.

These cases represent the gamut of disease affecting the cerebral hemispheres. The pathology represented may be tumor, infarction, or hemorrhage. Some of the lesions are intrinsic; others are extrinsic. The nature of the pathology may be uncertain; the location of the pathology, however, should be evident to you.

Diagram each lesion. If the etiology appears to be vascular, attempt to identify the vessel involved.

C. CASE HISTORY

CASE HISTORY 28.1

This 53-year-old, right-handed, white housewife had experienced intermittent right-sided headaches and retro-orbital pain for approximately 2 months. Five days prior to admission to the neurological center, the patient awoke from a sound sleep at 7:00 a.m., complaining of the most severe headache she had ever experienced. "It felt like something bursting inside my head." This was accompanied by nausea and vomiting. Patient was admitted to her local community hospital. Two days prior to transfer to the neurological center, the patient reported ptosis and diplopia. Severe headaches persisted, requiring the administration of meperidine hydrochloride (Demerol hydrochloride).

Neurological Examination

The patient was a well-developed white female with blood pressure of 160/90. Cardiac status was normal.

1. *Mental status:* The patient was lethargic but easily aroused. When aroused, she then responded with alert, appropriate responses.
2. *Cranial nerves:*
   a. The right pupil was dilated and sluggish in response to direct or consensual stimulation with light. The left pupil was of normal size. Ptosis of the right lid was present. There was partial weakness of right medial rectus, inferior rectus, and inferior oblique and superior rectus.
   b. All other cranial nerves were intact.
3. *Motor system:* There was minor weakness of the left arm and left leg with an increase in tone in the left arm and left leg (minor spasticity).
4. *Reflexes:*
   a. Deep tendon reflexes were everywhere increased on the left side.
   b. Plantar responses were extensor bilaterally but much more prominently so on the left.
5. *Sensory system:* No definite abnormalities were present.
6. *Head and neck:*
   a. There was resistance to flexion at neck.
   b. No bruits were present over neck, orbits, and head.

QUESTIONS

1. What is the most likely clinical diagnosis at this point?

Laboratory Data

1. *Skull and chest X-rays* were normal.
2. *Lumbar puncture:*
   a. Opening pressure was 300 mm of cerebrospinal fluid (CSF); closing pressure was 150 mm of CSF.
   b. The fluid was grossly bloody. First tube demonstrated 55,000 red blood cells per cubic millimeter and 60 white blood cells per cubic millimeter. Third tube demonstrated 72,000 red blood cells per cubic millimeter.
   c. The CSF protein was 84 mg/100 ml. The spinal fluid sugar was 60– mg/100 ml with a simultaneous blood sugar of 90 mg/100 ml.

Hospital course: The patient remained relatively stable and alert, and definitive procedures were performed.

QUESTIONS

1. Based on the symptoms and signs in this case, what is your diagnosis?
2. How do you interpret the results of the lumbar puncture?

Figure 28.9

3. If you had seen this patient in the emergency room directly at the onset of symptoms, which study would you have obtained? Would the lumbar puncture have been your initial study?
4. Where is the basic pathologic lesion located? Be specific.
5. Indicate the single most definitive diagnostic procedure that should be performed in this case prior to definitive therapy. When should this be performed?
6. Define definitive therapy in this case. When should this therapeutic procedure be performed?
7. Discuss the complications of this disorder.
8. Discuss prognosis of this clinical problem.

CASE HISTORY 28.2

This 56-year-old, right-handed white male truck driver, on the day prior to admission, had the sudden onset of a transient monocular blindness involving the right eye. On the morning of admission the patient developed a weak, numb, and useless left arm. These symptoms had shown considerable improvement by the time of his initial admission that afternoon.

Past History
1. The patient smoked two packs of cigarettes/day.
2. Occasional symptoms of intermittent claudication had been present.

Physical Examination
1. Blood pressure was 150/80; pulse was 100 and regular.
2. Bruits were present over the right carotid, left subclavian, and both femoral arteries.
3. Posterior tibial pulses were absent.
4. There were no cardiac murmurs.

Neurological Examination
1. *Mental status:* Intact.
2. *Cranial nerves:* Intact.
3. *Motor system:* There was minor weakness and incoordination of the left hand.
4. *Reflexes:* Intact.
5. *Sensory system:* Intact.

Subsequent course: Six days later, the patient had a focal motor seizure involving his left arm. Twenty-three days later, the patient experienced another transient episode of weakness and numbness involving the left arm. Approximately 4 weeks later, definitive diagnostic studies were performed.

Questions

1. What is the most likely diagnosis?
2. Outline your approach to effective management.
3. Which noninvasive studies would you obtain and when would you obtain those studies?
4. You have obtained these studies and the results confirm your clinical diagnosis. Which physician would you now consult?
5. Which surgical procedure would now be appropriate?
6. Indicate the classical definition of a transient ischemic attack (TIA). Now indicate the more modern operational definition that takes account of new developments in the acute treatment of ischemic stroke. What is the definition of the term *reversible ischemic neurological deficit* (RIND)? What is the definition of the term *completed stroke*? What is the meaning of the term *stroke in evolution*?

CASE HISTORY 28.3

This 32-year-old right handed white male was admitted to the hospital because of severe headache, confusion, and aphasia. The patient had been in good health except for frequent headaches for the 10 years prior to admission. Six days prior to admission at approximately 2:00 p.m., the patient returned from a hunting trip and went into the bathroom. His wife heard a noise, a thud, as though the patient had fallen to the floor. She found the patient lying on the floor, moaning and groaning, as if in pain. The patient showed evidence of significant confusion; he was, however, moving all his extremities and she surmised that he had no actual paralysis. The patient was admitted to his local hospital, where a lumbar puncture demonstrated the presence of blood in the spinal fluid. Over the next few days, the patient complained more and more of headaches, became more and more agitated, and was increasingly restless. He was subsequently transferred to a neurosurgical center.

General physical examination: There were no remarkable features. Blood pressure was 125/70.

Neurological Examination
1. *Mental status:*
   a. Patient was oriented for time and place.
   b. The patient was sleepy but agitated when roused from sleep.
   c. The patient had difficulty with word selection and would not cooperate in repeating simple words or identifying simple objects.
   d. The patient often spoke words that were unrelated to questions he had been asked or to the conversation.
2. *Cranial nerves:*
   a. A minor right visual field defect was suggested.
   b. A right central facial weakness was present.
3. *Motor system:* A minor weakness of the right upper extremity was present. When outstretched, the right hand rapidly fell downward.
4. *Reflexes:*
   a. Deep tendon reflexes were symmetric.
   b. Plantar response was extensor on the right and flexor on the left.
5. *Sensory system:* All modalities were intact.
6. *Neck:* Marked nuchal rigidity was present. The patient complained of severe pain on neck motion.

Hospital course: Over the next 4 hospital days, the patient developed increasing expressive aphasia, increasing right central facial weakness, and increasing weakness of right upper extremity. The degree of right upper extremity weakness was now marked, with total paresis of movements of right hand and partial paresis of movement at the shoulder and elbow. The patient continued drowsy and intermittently agitated. Some observers felt that the patient now had a slightly larger pupil on the left side than on the right. Specific diagnostic and therapeutic procedures were performed.

Questions

1. Indicate the original pathology and location of pathology.
2. Indicate the complications of this pathology that occurred prior to surgery and within 2 weeks of the initial episode.

3. Indicate the specific diagnostic procedures that were performed to localize the lesion prior to surgery.
4. What primary indications for surgery were present in this case? When should surgery be undertaken?
5. Which surgical procedure should be performed?

Subsequent course: The patient then underwent a surgical procedure 12 days after the initial episode. Postoperatively the patient had a marked right hemiplegia, with increase in the degree of aphasia. This was a mixed type of aphasia; when the patient did speak, he used jargon and he also appeared unable to understand language.

Eleven days postoperatively, the patient developed a fever of 104°F and a recurrence of nuchal rigidity. Spinal fluid examination now indicated 1200 white blood cells (92% polymorphonuclear); spinal fluid sugar was 50 mg/100 ml with blood sugar of 130 mg/100 ml. Specific treatment was administered.

Questions

1. Indicate the diagnosis that explains this complication of fever and nuchal rigidity. Be as specific as possible in terms of the agent producing fever.
2. How would you treat this complication?

Subsequent course: At the time of discharge, the patient was alert and oriented, but he had a significant expressive aphasia and a moderate hemiparesis (arm greater than leg) in addition to a right central facial weakness. Four months after the initial episode, the patient had a generalized convulsive seizure. Two to three weeks later, he had a focal seizure characterized by clonic movements of right upper extremity. One year after the initial episode, patient had focal seizures consisting of clonic contraction of the right face accompanied by arrest of speech. These seizures were preceded by a sensation of tightness in the face. Twenty-one months later, the patient was reported as having frequent focal seizures characterized by numbness of the right hand and face, followed by transient paralysis of the right lower extremity. Follow-up 33 months after that indicated several minor seizures every day involving numbness of the right hand and perioral area of face. Neurologic examination almost 6 years after the initial episode indicated the following significant residual deficits:

1. Hesitancy in speech with mild expressive aphasia and a more significant nominal aphasia. In addition, left-right confusion was present.
2. Right upper quadrantanopia.
3. Mild right central facial weakness.
4. Minimal weakness, right upper extremity in a right-handed man.
5. Deep tendon reflexes were increased on the right side with a right extensor plantar response.

The patient was treated with specific medications resulting in a reduction of the frequency of his focal seizures.

Questions

1. In the years following surgery, the patient had focal sensory and motor seizures involving hand and face. Indicate the medications to be used in the treatment of these episodes.
2. The patient also had secondarily generalized seizures in the postoperative years. Indicate the recommended medical treatment.

CASE HISTORY 28.4 (PATIENT OF DR. GEORGE ROBERTSON AND DR. HUNTINGTON PORTER)

This 73-year-old, right-handed white businessman from Maine was involved in an auto accident approximately 10 days prior to admission, in which his auto was struck by a heavy logging truck. The patient walked away from his car but was dazed and amnestic for the events of the next 15 minutes. This condition, however, then cleared. At the emergency room of his local hospital, skull X-rays were normal and the patient was found to have no significant injuries except for ecchymosis about the right eye and knee. The patient subsequently, however, did note a steady bilateral frontal temporal headache, which would on occasion awaken him from sleep and which gradually became worse. Five days prior to admission, some fogginess in thinking was noted and the patient's family reported some personality change. The patient reported some weakness of both legs in getting out of a bathtub, perhaps somewhat greater on the right side. Two days prior to admission, the patient was noted to be sleeping longer. On the day of admission, the patient and his physician noted a more persistent left-sided weakness. The patient was admitted to the neurology service.

Past history: Hyperthyroidism had been under treatment for 3 years. Three years prior to admission, the patient had been evaluated for a minor episode of dizziness, which had occurred in relation to bradycardia and a transient fall in blood pressure. The neurological consultant at that time had noted a totally normal examination. The right carotid pulse, however, was noted to be decreased compared to the left.

Neurological Examination (day of admission):

1. *Mental status:* The patient was alert, well oriented in all three spheres, with an excellent knowledge of current events. He could remember 4/5 objects in 5 minutes. His digit span was 8 forward and 5 in reverse.
2. *Cranial nerves:* All were intact except for a questionable left central facial weakness.
3. *Motor system:*
   a. There was a significant decrease in strength predominantly distal in the left leg. To a lesser degree, a mild weakness of the left upper extremity was present.
   b. The patient dragged the left leg in walking.
4. *Reflexes:* Deep tendon stretch reflexes were increased bilaterally in a symmetrical manner. Plantar responses were flexor.
5. *Sensory system:* All modalities were intact.
6. *Carotids:* The right carotid pulse was decreased as previously but no bruits were present.

Questions

1. It is an often quoted axiom in neurology that 75% of neurological diagnosis is based on the history. This patient was seen before the era of the computerized tomography (CT) scan and yet the most likely diagnosis was clear. What is your diagnosis as regards location of the lesion and the nature of the pathology? Be specific.
2. Is the apparent decrease on palpation of the right carotid pulse of any significance?
3. How would you evaluate this patient at this point in time utilizing current technology?

4. An electroencephalogram (EEG) was performed demonstrating focal 3–5 Hz slow-wave activity. Predict the location of that abnormality.
5. The patient had some transient symptoms after the initial trauma; he was dazed and amnestic for a short period of time. What term is applied to those symptoms?

Hospital course: A progressive change in neurological status was soon evident. Twenty-four hours after admission, the patient was found to be intermittently lethargic; if roused, he was able to answer questions, but it was evident that he was disoriented for time. In addition, deep tendon reflexes were now increased on the left side, and a left Babinski sign was now present. Later that day, increasing weakness of the left arm and leg developed. The patient was unable to raise the arm at the shoulder or the leg at the hip. The patient became increasingly more lethargic. Thirty hours after admission, the right pupil was found to be sluggish in response to light. The pupils, which had been previously symmetrical, were now asymmetrical; the right measured 3.5 mm, and the left measured 2.5 mm. An emergency carotid arteriogram was performed. Based on that study, a surgical procedure was immediately undertaken by the neurosurgeon, Dr. Bertram Selverstone.

The patient made a rapid recovery. Examination, 10 hours after surgery, demonstrated an alert and well-oriented patient who was able to lift his leg off the bed and had only a minimal weakness in the left upper extremity. Pupils were now equal. The deep tendon reflexes were now symmetrical and the plantar responses were now flexor. At the time of hospital discharge, 13 days following surgery, the neurological examination was now normal.

Questions

1. What change, if any, would you now make in your diagnosis?
2. Which complication of the original disorder has now occurred?
3. How would you manage that complication?
4. What did the carotid arteriogram demonstrate?
5. Which diagnostic procedure would you perform today? Describe the expected results of that study.
6. Which surgical procedure was performed? Describe the most likely surgical findings.

CASE HISTORY 28.5

This 62-year-old, white, right-handed male, 18 months prior to admission, had the onset of focal motor seizures, which would begin in the left side of the tongue, and then spread to the face, shoulder, arm, and hand.

At the same time, he would note spread of tingling paresthesias over the same parts of the left side of the tongue, face, and hand. Neurological examination at that time was not remarkable.

Anticonvulsant medication produced a significant reduction in focal seizures. However, 1 month prior to admission, the patient had a focal seizure that was followed by transient residual weakness of left face and hand.

Three weeks prior to admission, a minor degree of weakness of the left hand developed. This progressed in degree and also began to involve the left leg and left side of the face as well. Two weeks prior to admission, right-sided headache developed.

Neurological Examination

1. *Mental status:* Intact.
2. *Cranial nerves:* Intact except for a severe left central facial weakness.
3. *Motor system:*
   a. Weakness of the left hand was present, with thumb opposition most severely involved. Minor weakness was present in the left lower extremity.
   b. In walking, the patient dragged the left lower extremity to a minor degree.
4. *Reflexes:*
   a. Deep tendon reflexes were increased on the left.
   b. Instinctive grasp reflex was present on the left.
5. *Sensory system:*
   a. Graphesthesia was decreased over left face and hand.
   b. Tactile localization and two-point discrimination were decreased over the left hand.

Questions

1. Where is the lesion? Be specific.
2. In terms of the pathological diagnosis, list the three most likely possibilities.
3. Indicate the most definitive laboratory test for establishing the diagnosis and the expected findings.
4. Indicate the other studies that would be useful and the expected findings.
5. Indicate a plan of management for each of the possible diagnoses.

CASE HISTORY 28.6

This 58-year-old, white, right-handed female with a past history of hypertension and angina pectoris had the acute onset of a right-sided weakness while at work. She had no change in consciousness, no sensory symptoms, no impairment of language function, and no headache. She had experienced no vertigo, no diplopia, no vomiting, and no visual symptoms. She had no complaints of chest pain or of shortness of breath.

Physical examination: Blood pressure was elevated to 180/120.

Neurological Examination

1. *Mental status:* This was entirely intact, with no evidence of aphasia.
2. *Cranial nerves:* A marked right central facial weakness was present with minimal deviation of the tongue to the right.
3. *Motor system:* A dense right hemiparesis was present.
4. *Reflexes:*
   a. Deep tendon reflexes were increased on the right.
   b. The plantar response was extensor on the right (sign of Babinski).
5. *Sensory system:* All modalities were intact.

Laboratory data: Assume the electrocardiogram (EKG) was not relevant and the cerebrospinal fluid studies were normal.

Hospital course: The patient was stable and alert during the next 2 days and, at her request, was transferred to her local hospital.

Questions

1. What is the most likely diagnosis? How would you confirm the diagnosis?
2. *Contrast with Case 28.1:* Assume that this patient presented with a 1-month history of five transient episodes of numbness

and weakness of the right hand. In addition, the patient had experienced two or three episodes of sudden transient blindness of the left eye. Then on the morning of admission, she awoke with numbness and weakness of the right hand and arm, with increased deep stretch reflexes at the right biceps, triceps, patellar, and Achilles tendons and a right sign of Babinski on plantar stimulation. You also find errors in position sense and in graphesthesia involving the right fingers and hand. The patient has moderate but incomplete recovery over the next week. At no time does the patient complain of headache. What is your conclusion as to the most likely diagnosis? How do you establish the diagnosis and manage the case?

3. *Contrast with Case 28.2:* Assume that this patient has a history of rheumatic heart disease with mitral stenosis and atrial fibrillation. The patient suddenly, while at work at 11:00 a.m., stopped speaking in mid-sentence, fell to the floor with a focal seizure involving the right side, with subsequent generalization. On recovery from the postictal confusion, the patient is found to manifest:
    1. *Mental status:* Patient appears alert but has a dense global aphasia.
    2. *Cranial nerves:*
        a. A dense right homonymous hemianopsia.
        b. Deviation of head and eyes to the left.
        c. A dense right central facial weakness.
    3. *Motor system:* A dense flaccid right hemiparesis.
    4. *Reflexes:*
        a. A depression of the deep tendon reflexes at the right arm and right leg.
        b. A right Babinski sign.
    5. *Sensory system:* Absence of all sensory modalities on the right side. Assume that the initial CT scan at 1 hour after onset of symptoms is interpreted as normal and that the cerebrospinal fluid is clear with no cells.

QUESTIONS

1. After seeing this patient at 12 noon in the emergency room, what conclusions do you reach as to diagnosis and what course of action do you recommend?
2. Unfortunately, the patient is found to have contraindications to the therapy, which you recommended. An alternate course of action is followed. No significant change occurred over the next 10 days except for transient lethargy and the minimal return of deep tendon reflexes. Discuss these issues.
3. Why were the deep tendon reflexes acutely depressed on the side of the hemiparesis?

CASE HISTORY 28.7

This 14-year-old right-handed white female was admitted with a chief complaint of "draining left ear" and left frontal headache. Approximately 4 weeks prior to admission, the patient had the onset of progressive pain in the left ear accompanied by fever up to 104°F. Four days later a discharge from the left ear developed. Three days later a total left-sided facial paralysis developed. The patient was evaluated at the Massachusetts Eye and Ear infirmary, where drainage of the left middle ear was performed, yielding purulent material. Culture of this drainage revealed *Staphylococcus aureus*. The patient was treated with antibiotics with a complete resolution of symptoms. However, 1 week prior to admission, the patient developed a constant severe left frontal headache with swelling about the left eye. There was now a recurrence of discharge of a thick green purulent material from the left ear. Two days prior to admission, the patient developed confusion and delirium. She was also noted to have marked difficulties in language function and in calculations.

General physical examination: Temperature was normal at 98.6°F. The patient appeared chronically ill. Gauze soaked with purulent drainage was present in the left external auditory canal.

Neurological Examination

1. *Mental status:*
    a. The patient was oriented for the day and year but not for the month. There was considerable confusion as to past and recent events.
    b. She had a marked deficit in naming objects. Even when the name of the object was supplied in a multiple-choice scenario, she was unable to recognize the correct name. Paraphasia was evident. She was able to carry out spoken commands. Simple writing and spelling were intact but reading of isolated words was defective. She had no left-right confusion. She was able to identify and to point out the various parts of her body with the exception of the thumb.
    c. At times, the patient acted in a "silly" manner and would giggle inappropriately in response to questions.
2. *Cranial nerves:*
    a. Fundoscopy demonstrated papilledema with elevation of the disk on the right. A recent hemorrhage was present just below the disk of the right eye.
    b. A minor peripheral left facial weakness was present, most prominent in frontalis muscle.
    c. Hearing was decreased on the left.
3. *Motor system:* Strength, gait, and cerebellar functions were intact.
4. *Reflexes:* Deep tendon reflexes were intact. The right plantar response was equivocal; the left was flexor.
5. *Sensory system:* All modalities were intact.

QUESTIONS

1. What is your diagnosis as regards localization and pathology?
2. What laboratory studies would you request?
3. Would you perform a lumbar puncture on this patient? Justify your answer.
4. What is your explanation for the left peripheral facial weakness?

Laboratory Data

1. White blood count and differential were normal.
2. Skull and mastoid X-rays indicated an acute mastoiditis on the left with an increased density throughout the left mastoid extending throughout the medial aspect of the petrous ridge.
3. EEG was abnormal because of focal and hemispheric 2–3 Hz slow-wave activity.

QUESTIONS

1. Do you wish to alter your diagnosis or diagnostic approach?
2. Outline your approach to therapy. Which categories of physicians would you consult?

Subsequent course: Dr. Daniel Miller of the ENT service performed a left mastoidectomy and epidural exploration. Pus was present in the softened mastoid cells. Purulent granulation tissue extended into the adjacent epidural space. Cultures were obtained and antibiotics were reinstituted. Over the next 4 days improvement occurred in the clinical and EEG findings, but then findings worsened. Dr. Sam Brendler of the neurosurgical service then performed more definitive procedures. Following surgery, the patient had a nominal aphasia and a noncongruous right visual field deficit with some sparing of the inferior quadrant. The patient had a single generalized convulsive seizure, 6 years after surgery, and anticonvulsants were instituted. At that point in time, the nominal aphasia had shown marked improvement; she hesitated and stumbled over words. The right visual field defect was unchanged.

Questions

1. Which procedures were performed by the neurosurgeon?
2. Explain the visual field deficits.

CASE HISTORY 28.8

This 29-year-old, right-handed, single white female schoolteacher was about to testify in court in the late afternoon on the day of admission, when she suddenly dropped to the floor. She began to babble but did not lose consciousness. She was taken to the emergency room of the local hospital at 4:15 p.m., where she was initially described as "confused, disoriented, unresponsive to questions, and not verbalizing." At 7:50 p.m., she was subsequently described as agitated with garbled speech. Later that evening, she was transferred to this hospital.

Past history: Patient was receiving birth control pills.

General Physical Examination

1. Blood pressure: 120/70. Pulse: 90 and regular.
2. No heart murmurs were present.
3. No bruits were present over the carotid arteries and carotid pulses were strong.
4. Neck was supple with no nuchal rigidity.

Neurological Examination

1. *Mental status:* The patient was anxious and alert with intermittent agitation. She appeared to understand but only intermittently followed verbal commands. She used only a few words. She attempted to name objects but produced only paraphasia and jargon speech.
2. *Cranial nerves:*
   a. A right homonymous hemianopsia was present.
   b. There was decreased pain and touch over the right side of the face.
   c. A right central facial weakness was present.
3. *Motor system:* A dense right hemiplegia was present.
4. *Reflexes:*
   a. Deep tendon stretch reflexes were increased in the right upper and lower extremities with clonus at the right patellar and Achilles tendon reflexes.
   b. The plantar response was extensor on right and flexor on left.
5. *Sensory system:* An apparent right hemisensory deficit was present to all modalities.

Laboratory Data

1. CSF pressure was normal at 160, with clear fluid (cells = 0, protein = 11mg%, sugar = 75mg% with blood sugar of 104).
2. Skull X-rays were normal.
3. EKG was normal.

Hospital course: By 48 hours after onset, speech had shown some improvement. The patient was using more recognizable words. Occasional appropriate two-word phrases were employed. The dense right hemiparesis had persisted, but the right homonymous field cut and the sensory pain deficit were no longer present. By 72 hours after onset, slight movement was present in the right lower extremity. However, at 5 days after onset, the patient had the sudden development of a cold, pulseless left arm.

Questions

1. Localize the lesion.
2. Characterize the speech deficit at various stages. Did this patient have a dysarthria or aphasia? If aphasia was present, was this primarily fluent or nonfluent?
3. Discuss the use of the term *confusion*. Discuss the use of the term *babbling*.
4. Discuss the pathology and likely etiology and pathophysiology. If vascular, indicate the vascular territory.
5. What other information would you wish to have?
6. This patient was seen before the era of the CT scan. Assume that this patient had arrived in the emergency room today 30 minutes after the acute events, and you are the emergency room physician or the consulting neurologist. How would you manage this problem?

SECTION IV

COMPLEX FUNCTIONS

29.

ALTERATIONS IN CONSCIOUSNESS

SEIZURES, SLEEP, AND COMA

BASIC DEFINITIONS

Consciousness: The waking state in which the individual has awareness, with "the ability to perceive, interact and communicate with the environment and others in the integrated manner which wakefulness normally implies" (Zeman, 2001).

Sleep: A normal periodic alteration in consciousness with various stages. Sleep is an active physiologic process dependent on a complex interaction of cerebral cortex, thalamic, hypothalamic, and brain stem areas. Metabolic activities such as oxygen use remain normal. The level of consciousness may be fully restored by an appropriate stimulus.

Sleep disorders: This term includes such major disorders as insomnia, hyposomnia, narcolepsy, and sleep apnea as well as sleep walking (somnambulism or sleep behavior disorder) and abnormal movements during sleep.

Abnormalities of consciousness: These occur in a brief paroxysmal manner in seizures and syncope and in a more prolonged manner in coma.

Seizure: A sudden (paroxysmal) alteration in behavior due to an excessive discharge of cerebral cortical neurons. The alteration in behavior may be limited or may result in a generalized convulsive seizure. The state of consciousness may be unaffected, may be altered, or may be lost. Seizures represent an alteration in the usual balance between excitation and inhibition. Seizures and epilepsy are most frequent in the infant and in the elderly.

Epilepsy: A chronic condition in which seizures recur at variable frequency over time. The period of seizure activity is termed the *ictus* or *ictal event*. The time between seizures is termed *the interictal period*.

Syncope: A condition in which consciousness and usually posture are briefly impaired in a relatively sudden manner due to a general decrease in cerebral perfusion. This decrease in perfusion may be due to a general peripheral vasodilation (vasovagal reaction), hypotension, or a decrease in cardiac output. The loss of consciousness almost always occurs when the patient is in an upright position. The actual loss of consciousness is preceded by prodromal symptoms that last from seconds to minutes: light-headedness, weakness, "dizziness," sweating, and blurring and dimming of vision. The patient is observed to slump limply to the ground (as opposed to the patient with epilepsy who usually stiffens and then falls violently to the ground). Tonic or clonic movements are rare but may occur. The period of unconsciousness is brief, usually a matter of seconds, and occasionally a minute. During this time, the patient is noted to be pale and sweaty. The pulse is usually weak and the blood pressure often reduced. The return to consciousness is rapid, occurring usually when the patient assumes a recumbent position. There is no significant period of mental confusion following the episode.

Coma: An abnormal state in which various degrees of prolonged alteration of consciousness occur. In contrast to sleep, coma is a passive process in which a loss of function has occurred. Metabolic activities are depressed. Stimulation will not restore a full and persistent state of consciousness. Various gradations of coma exist. In describing the degree of coma, it is best to use operational terms describing brain stem reflexes, response to stimuli, and so on. The Glasgow Coma Scale provides such an approach. Various terms continue in use; in deep coma the responses to stimuli are completely lost. In moderately deep coma, rudimentary responses of a reflex nature only are present (e.g., corneal reflex, withdrawal of a limb to painful stimulus), but psychologically understandable responses to external stimuli and inner need are absent. Various terms have been employed to describe lesser degrees of impairment of consciousness: semicoma, stupor, obtundation, or lethargy.

Confusion: An abnormal state characterized by an impaired capacity to think clearly and with customary speed to perceived stimuli and to remember current stimuli. Confusion includes disorientation and memory impairment. In addition to confusion associated with an altered state of consciousness, confusion may also occur with an alert state in patients with dementia (Chapter 30).

Delirium: An abnormal state in which agitation (of motor activity) is present in addition to confusion.

Akinetic mutism: A state in which the patient lies in bed with eyes open but fails to move or to speak. There are two types. (1) In the mesencephalic/diencephalic variety, usually due to occlusion of a penetrating branch of the posterior cerebral artery or of the proximal/mesencephalic artery segment of the paramedian branch at the top of the basilar artery bifurcation, there is a state of apathetic or somnolent akinetic mutism in which the patient remains in a lethargic state most of the time. The patient may open his eyes in response to strong stimulation but soon closes them and returns to a lethargic state. Paralysis of vertical gaze and of other extraocular movements is usually found. Infarction at the diencephalic-mesencephalic junction is bilateral and includes rostral midbrain tegmentum, the adjacent pretectal area, subthalamus, and periventricular gray matter at the posterior end of the third ventricle. The midline thalamic nuclei: reticular nucleus of the thalamus and intralaminar nuclei of the thalamus (centrum medianum) may also be affected by this lesion. (2) In the bilateral frontal type of hyperalert akinetic mutism (vigilant coma) the patient will follow with intact eye movements and will cycle (alternation periods of agitation). The medial, orbital, and anterior surfaces of the frontal lobes plus adjacent cingulate gyri or the septal area are involved. Although the patient lies immobile in bed, he provides some suggestions of alertness in the sense of appearance. We should distinguish several other conditions. In acute massive infarct of the dominant hemisphere the patient may be mute and hemiparetic. In late Parkinson's disease marked rigidity, akinesia, and mutism may be present but the patient is alert. A similar state may follow bilateral destruction of the putamen or globus pallidus (apallic state). Refer to Segarra (1970).

Locked-in syndrome (pseudo akinetic mutism or pseudocoma): A state in which the patient is aware and conscious but because of paramedian pontine infarction, usually related to thrombosis of the basilar artery, is unable to provide verbal responses. When the midbrain is intact, the patient may provide responses by opening or closing the eyes or by vertical eye movements.

Brain death: Up until the late 1960s, patients were declared dead when cardiac (and respiratory) activity ceased. With the cessation of cardiac respiratory activity, neurological function ceased within 3–4 minutes. With the development of cardiopulmonary resuscitation and of life support equipment, an era dawned in which cardiorespiratory function might be continued or restored but function of the brain could not be restored. Thus, the advance of technology required an expansion of the prior definition of death to include brain death. In most jurisdictions, either by legislative law or by court decision case law, brain death is recognized as legal death.

Brain death is defined by the following criteria:

1. An absence of consciousness.
2. No cerebral responsivity is present.
3. No brain stem reflexes are present.
4. No spontaneous respirations are present.
5. If obtained, the electroencephalogram (EEG) will show no evidence of cortical electrical activity.
6. Spinal cord reflexes may be present.
7. The state is irreversible: reversible metabolic and toxic conditions have been eliminated, a sufficient period of time has elapsed, and appropriate studies have been performed to establish a *diagnosis.*

It is important to note that in those patients who meet the criteria of brain death but where respiratory and blood pressure support is continued, cardiac arrest usually occurs within days, rarely in weeks.

Persistent vegetative state or neocortical death: This term refers to a state in which neocortical death or disconnection has occurred but brain stem reflexes and spontaneous respiration are preserved. Although this condition had long been recognized within the larger group of chronic coma, following cardiac respiratory arrest and trauma, Jennett and Plum popularized the specific term in 1972. Such patients have periods of "wakeful" eye opening and movement. The EEG is usually isoelectric (or occasionally demonstrates a burst suppression pattern). The major cause of the syndrome is cardiac pulmonary arrest with subsequent resuscitation. There is diffuse damage to neocortex and hippocampus. At times, laminar necrosis is present. The patient may live for weeks, months, or years. Such patients never regain consciousness. The management of this state and the ethical dilemmas involved in the continued care of this patient have been a major area of medical and legal controversy. This situation has grown even more complicated by the recent observation that verbally cued tasks produce task-specific activity on functional imaging.

THE BASIS OF THE ELECTROENCEPHALOGRAM: Review Chapter 17 for a discussion of this subject.

ABNORMALITIES OF THE EEG AND CORRELATION WITH SEIZURE DISORDERS: Refer to Chapter 2 for examples of normal and nonseizure abnormalities.

Kershman and Jasper (1941) delineated the two major categories of EEG abnormalities to be found in seizure disorders: (1) those findings which were focal and (2) those findings which were bilateral and relatively symmetrical and synchronous. The international classification of seizures and of the epilepsies has continued to follow this long established distinction.

There are two general rules for the normal electroencephalogram: (1) the left and right hemispheres are relatively similar in appearance (2) for a given age and level of alertness: awake versus drowsy versus asleep, the frequency and rhythm will fall within certain parameters.

All abnormalities of the EEG then will represent deviations from these two general rules.

The first type of abnormality is termed *focal*. The following subtypes may be listed:

a. Focal slow waves correlated with a focal cortical dysfunction with the quality of damage (Fig. 2.22).

b. Focal spikes and sharp waves correlate with a focal dysfunction, having the quality of excessive neuronal discharge, that is, partial epilepsy (Fig. 29.1). Spikes have a duration of less than 75 milliseconds; sharp waves have a duration of greater than 75 milliseconds. Both are named from their contour that shows a rapidly rising slope. These abnormalities are not to be confused with the spike of the short-duration action potential of the axon (a matter of 1–2 msec) for they represent summated postsynaptic potentials. Single focal spikes may occur in interictal (interseizure) periods without the occurrence of the actual focal seizure. In general, the clinical focal seizure is likely to occur when frequent repetitive focal spikes occur or when the focal spike is followed by an afterdischarge. Any focal seizure may secondarily generalize (Fig. 29.2). Additional examples of focal spike discharges with specific correlation have already been presented. Focal (partial) epilepsy is the predominant seizure disorder in those patients with onset of seizures after the age of 15 years and occurs in 45% of patients with seizure onset prior to age 15.

Figure 29.1 (A) Focal spike discharges in the left temporal lobe with phase reversal at the left anterior temporal electrode. Case 22.1. (Refer to text.) Left temporal glioma, with frequent clinical seizures originating in the temporal lobe. ANT.T., anterior temporal; LAT.F., lateral frontal; MID.T., midtemporal; OCC., occipital; PAR., parietal; POST.T., posterior temporal. (B) Focal spike discharge in the right parasagittal Rolandic area (C2–C4) in a 28-year-old woman with focal seizures beginning with clonic movements of the left thigh and numbness of the left leg. Transverse bipolar montage. Case 18.1. (Refer to text.) (C) Focal spike discharges with phase reversal at left mid temporal electrode in a 46-year-old man with subarachnoid hemorrhage secondary to a middle cerebral artery aneurysm. The patient had focal sensory seizures beginning in the right face tongue or thumb.

c. Focal voltage suppression correlates with a reduced electrical activity in the tissue underlying the electrodes, for example, the presence of a subdural or intracerebral hematoma, or massive cerebral infarction (Fig. 2.23).

Figure 29.2 Generalization from an experimental focal spike discharge in the left suprasylvian area (SS) of the cat. After discharge of repetitive spikes occurred at the focus with subsequent spread to other areas of the same and contralateral cerebral hemispheres. P.S., posterior sigmoid gyrus (sensory cortex); V. = visual projection area of marginal gyrus. (Calibrations: 1 second and 100 microvolts). (From Marcus, E.M., Watson, C.W., and Goldman, P.L.: Arch. Neurol. 15:525, 1966, AMA.)

The second type of abnormality is termed *generalized* and the following subtypes are recognized:

a. Continuous generalized slow-wave activity or dominant activity slower than the alpha rhythm correlated with a generalized dysfunction having the quality of damage (Figs. 2.24 and 2.25).

b. Generalized rhythmic paroxysmal electrical discharges correlated with generalized epilepsy: spike–slow wave complexes, polyspike–slow wave complexes, and polyspike (repetitive fast spike discharges). Depending on the clinical findings, and frequency of discharge (e.g., slow 1–2 Hz vs, 2.5–4 Hz vs. >4 Hz spike-wave or polyspike-wave complexes), these EEG findings may be associated with idiopathic (primary) generalized or secondary generalized epilepsy. As explained later, this latter term is to be distinguished from partial epilepsy with secondary generalization.

c. The generalized burst suppression pattern discussed in Chapter 17.

d. Generalized suppression of all electrical activity correlated with neocortical death or with the deepest stage of anesthesia.

UNDERLYING BASIS OF THE FOCAL SEIZURE AND FOCAL SPIKE DISCHARGE

Focal seizures indicate a focal cortical dysfunction and imply an underlying focal cortical pathology. In some cases the actual pathology is in the white matter just below the cortex, and the acute or chronic effects of cortical isolation or deafferentation are being seen. Seizures do not arise from an area of total necrosis since dead neurons do not discharge. Surviving neurons must be present (for example, at the margin of an infarct or hemorrhage).

Table 29.1 CAUSE OF PARTIAL SEIZURES

AGE	CAUSE
Within the first 48 hours of life	Acute birth trauma (poor prognosis)
Within the first 2 years	Birth trauma and congenital malformations (e.g., porencephalic cyst)
From 2 to 10 years	Birth injury and head trauma
From 10 to 20 years	Head trauma and late effects of pathology in infancy and childhood (complex partial seizures)
From 20 to 50 years	Head trauma and neoplasms and late effects of pathology acquired in infancy and childhood (complex partial seizures)
Over 50 years	Tumor and vascular infarcts and degenerations (Alzheimer's disease)

The pathological causes of focal (partial) seizures are variable, dependent in part on the age of the patient and those pathological processes affecting cerebral cortex that are common at that particular age (Table 29.1).

Seizures will occur in approximately 50% of meningiomas, low-grade gliomas, oligodendrogliomas, and brain abscesses involving the cerebral cortex. High-grade gliomas have a lower frequency of approximately 35%. Seizures will occur in 25% of all cerebral infarcts with a higher percentage in embolic middle cerebral artery infarcts of 45%. Cortical migration disorders have a significant association with focal seizure disorders (exact percentage unclear), possibly because of aberrant circuits (Duchowny et al., 2000). Refer to Table 29.2.

REGIONAL CORTICAL VARIATIONS IN THE CAPACITY FOR SEIZURE DISCHARGE

A given pathological process is more likely to cause seizure discharge if it involves an area of low threshold (motor cortex or mesial temporal areas) rather than an area of high relative threshold (prefrontal or occipital areas). (Refer to Chapter 17.)

THE EPILEPTIC FOCUS AND THE EPILEPTIC NEURON

At times, focal seizures may occur in acute or subacute relationship to penetrating head injuries or to the cortical ischemia that follows a cerebral embolus and such patients are more likely to have recurrent seizures. In many cases, however, the spike discharge and the focal seizure begin as a late effect. It is customary to distinguish in all cases between the interictal spike and the ictal discharge. The ictal discharge accompanies the clinical seizure. The spike discharge recorded at the surface represents summated excitatory postsynaptic potentials and therefore are recorded as predominantly surface negative waves. Isolated columns of horizontal layers of rat neocortex in vitro have indicated that the discharges are primarily initiated in the large pyramidal neurons of layer V. Discharges may then propagate both vertically and horizontally. Schmidt

Table 29.2 CAUSES OF NONFOCAL GENERALIZED TONIC CLONIC CONVULSIONS

AGE	ETIOLOGY
Newborn	Metabolic: Na/K, alkalosis, hypoglcemia, hypocalcemia, pyridoxine deficiency, dependency, aminoacidurias (phenylketonuria), respiratory/anoxia, perinatal pathology
Infant	Metabolic disturbance, febrile convulsions,* meningitis/encephalitis, residuals of perinatal pathology
Child	Febrile (<5 years), idiopathic epilepsy, meningitis/encephalitis
Adolescent	Idiopathic epilepsy,** drug use and withdrawal
Young adult	Alcohol/drug withdrawal,*** cocaine use, idiopathic epilepsy
Older adult	Alzheimer's disease and other degenerative disorders, anoxic encephalopathy

*Febrile convulsions are frequent in the age group under 5 years and occur predominantly between 6 months and 3 years of age. It has been estimated that 4% to 7% of all children under the age of 5 years will have at least one generalized convulsive seizure (the majority febrile). Children with febrile seizures have a high familial incidence of seizure disorder, suggesting a factor of genetic predisposition. A significant proportion (but not the majority) of these children will be found later to also have nonfebrile convulsions.
**Note that 86% of juvenile myoclonic epilepsy patients also have generalized convulsive tonic clonic seizures. A related syndrome is that of epilepsy with generalized tonic clonic seizures on awakening, which differs from juvenile myoclonic epilepsy —only in the absence of myoclonic seizures (see Dreifuss, 1989).
***Abrupt withdrawal or reduction of intake after chronic intake of alcohol may trigger seizures within 7–48 hours of the withdrawal. During this period, the electroencephalogram may demonstrate precipitation of myoclonus and of electrical discharges by photic stimulation. There are in these cases of alcohol withdrawal, correlations with low serum magnesium, increased pH, and low pCO_2 levels (see Victor, 1990). More recent cellular studies of sedative drug withdrawal are discussed in Carlen et al. (1990). In these cases the postictal state may then merge into a more prolonged agitated and confusional state of delirium tremens. This same clinical state may also follow withdrawal from short-acting barbiturates, meprobamate, diazepam (Valium), and other benzodiazepines.

and Wilder (1968) define the focus as a group of abnormal cells ("epileptic neurons") with certain unique properties. Engel (1989) has summarized many of the studies utilizing the best-studied acute model of partial epilepsy: topical application of penicillin. Similar changes are observed in chronic models.

1. In the acute and the chronic focus there are bursting units discharging in a paroxysmal manner at high rates of discharge up to 1000 Hz with high-amplitude *paroxysmal depolarization shifts* (PDSs) as the intracellular correlate of the bursting unit discharge. The PDS corresponds to activation of glutamate-mediated synapses.

2. In addition, abnormally hypersynchronous activity of large numbers of adjacent neurons occurs; the PDSs of most of the neurons within the focus summate to produce the interictal spikes recorded at the surface by the EEG. The PDs are followed by prolonged afterhyperpolarizations (AHPs). The AHP reflects activation of calcium and voltage-dependent potassium channels in addition to GABA/A and GABA/B synapses. These AHPs summate to produce the EEG surface

recorded slow wave that follows the EEG spike discharge, as a spike–slow wave complex.

3. Neurons in the cerebral cortex surrounding the focus develop large membrane hyperpolarization. This "inhibitory surround" limits the spread along the surface from the focus but also may interfere with normal activities of those surrounding neurons (Prince and Wilder, 1967). The inhibitory surround is in a sense built into the columnar organization of the neocortex.

As long as the discharge is restricted to the pool of neurons within the seizure focus, in general there are no clinical manifestations. When, however, surround inhibition is surmounted and afterhyperpolarization decreases, propagation to other regions (cortical and subcortical) occurs and clinical seizure phenomena result.

PROPAGATION FROM THE FOCUS

Propagation of discharge from the focus occurs via several pathways: (1) short intracortical pathways involving synapses and neurons within the adjacent neuropil, (2) long fiber systems to other cortical areas within the same cerebral hemisphere, (3) callosal and other commissural pathways to the contralateral cerebral hemisphere, and (4) descending pathways to basal ganglia, thalamus, reticular formation of the brain stem, and to the spinal cord. Obviously, the specific pattern of spread will depend on the location of the focus and on the anatomical connections or projections from the particular cortical area. Refer to Chapter 17 for additional discussion. It is *important to realize that any focal spike discharge may become secondarily generalized* (Fig. 29.2). *From a clinical standpoint, any focal seizure may become a secondarily generalized seizure.*

HISTOLOGICAL CHANGES AT THE FOCUS

There are multiple changes at the chronic focus: damage to capillaries, fibroblastic and capillary invasion from meningeal adhesions (meningocerebral cicatrix), gliosis, mechanical deformation of neuronal processes, a progressive loss of dendritic spines, the development of recurrent collateral excitatory synapses, and partial loss of afferent input (possibly inhibitory) to the neuron (Babb and Pretorius, 1997). Within the hippocampus, neuronal loss and gliosis are accompanied by sprouting of mossy fibers. It is uncertain whether the changes at the chronic focus in the human focus relate to a decrease in the inhibitory transmitter (GABA) or an increase in the excitatory transmitter (glutamate). (See McDonald et al., 1991; Ribak, 1986; Selzer and Richter, 1992.)

SECONDARY EPILEPTOGENESIS

Two experimental models involving the chronic focus suggest that persistent spread of discharge from a focus may produce persistent alterations in excitability in those cortical and subcortical areas that are the targets of the propagated discharge. These projection areas then eventually take on the capacity for independent generation of focal or multifocal discharge.

The first model was described by Morrell (1960, 1991)—*the mirror focus.* The second model was described shortly afterward by Goddard (1967)—*the kindling model.* (Refer also to Mayersdorf and Schmidt, 1982, and to Chapter 30.)

MULTIFOCAL ABNORMALITIES

Many traumatic injuries and other pathologic processes do not produce limited focal damage. Thus, a blow to the occipital area of the skull may not only produce injury to the occipital cortex at the site of the blow but may also produce contusions of the cortex at a distance from the site of injury: the anterior temporal poles and frontal poles and orbital frontal surfaces. The end result may be multifocal slow waves, implying multifocal damage or multifocal spikes, which in turn implies the evolution of multifocal areas of excessive neuronal discharge. Another possible explanation for multifocal spikes when a unilateral pathology may be present is discussed earlier under secondary epileptogenesis. Note also that multiple foci may interact to produce bilateral discharges as discussed next.

GENERALIZED EPILEPSY OR GENERALIZED SEIZURES

In the International Classification of the Epilepsies, this category is defined as those seizures that are generalized from their onset. Other terms that have employed in the past are essential, nonsymptomatic and cryptogenic, or idiopathic—but all of these are now used in a somewhat different context. *The term idiopathic is now used again for this category.*

In this category of epilepsy and seizures, no focal origin is evident for the electrical discharge, and the clinical seizure is characterized from its onset by the loss of consciousness and/or by motor manifestations that are bilateral and symmetrical. In general, these seizures begin in childhood or adolescence.

This type of electrical abnormality and the correlated clinical seizure disorder should be contrasted to the focal spike and the focal (or partial according to the International Classification) seizure disorder, where a focal origin is clearly evident and where total loss of consciousness is usually not the initial sign of the seizure. Such a distinction becomes a little blurry when complex partial seizures, particularly those arising in the frontal lobes, are considered.

Within the overall category of generalized epilepsy or generalized seizures, the classification has two divisions: (A) the major category of primary generalized or idiopathic epilepsy; and (B) secondary or symptomatic generalized epilepsy.

A. Primary generalized or idiopathic epilepsy has the following features:

1. No specific underlying gross neuropathology is present. However, as we will discuss later, there is now evidence that an underlying cortical micro dysgenesis may be present.

2. Neurological and psychological—intellectual status is usually normal.

3. The background EEG activity is relatively normal for the age.

4. A familial genetic background is often present. Early twin studies by Lennox and his associates (1960) indicated a concordance rate for monozygotic twins of 70%–100% and for dizygotic twins of 5%–15%. Seminal studies by Metrakos and Metrakos (1961) demonstrated that the 2.5–3.5 discharge associated with idiopathic epilepsy was inherited as an autosomal dominant. Other studies have suggested a general predisposition gene with other modifying genes determining whether and what type of clinical seizures will occur. The specific altered genetic process is unknown, but studies by Janqua and Andermann (1989) suggested significant abnormalities of amino acids in the serum of both patients and first-degree relatives, particularly increased levels of the excitatory amino acid glutamic acid.

5. The seizures are usually very responsive to medication.

6. The overall course is benign.

Included within this division are the following that shortly will be discussed in greater detail:

1. Childhood absence epilepsy (CA)
2. Juvenile absence epilepsy (JA)
3. Juvenile myoclonic epilepsy (JME)
4. Generalized tonic clonic seizures on awakening
5. Isolated generalized tonic clonic seizure (GTCS)
6. Benign myoclonic epilepsy of childhood

B. Secondary or symptomatic generalized epilepsy has the following features:

1. A diffuse or multifocal pathology is usually present.
2. The neurological examination is abnormal.
3. Mental retardation is present or psychological deterioration develops.
4. The background EEG is abnormal.
5. There is in some cases a progressive course; deterioration may occur.
6. Response to medication is usually poor.
7. A familial genetic background may or may not be present.

Included in this category are the following syndromes:

1. The various progressive myoclonic epilepsies beginning in infancy, childhood, adolescence, and adult life—many due to specific metabolic disorders; lipidosis, lysosomal storage diseases, and mitochondrial disorders

2. Infantile spasms: with the associated EEG pattern of hypsarrhythmia (high-amplitude irregular asynchronous spikes and slow waves) and often as well a decremental pattern resembling burst suppression during sleep (Fig. 29.3)

3. Lennox Gastaut syndrome: childhood encephalopathy with associated EEG pattern of "slow" (1–2 Hz) spike–slow wave complexes. This syndrome may be a residual of infantile spasms. The term "petit mal variant" has been employed in the past. In addition to atypical absence seizures, atonic drop attack seizures, tonic seizures, and generalized tonic/clonic seizures may occur. Multiple foci are often present and section of the corpus callosum may decrease the interaction of these foci (see later).

PRIMARY/IDIOPATHIC GENERALIZED EPILEPSY: MAJOR SYNDROMES

Childhood absence epilepsy (CA) that usually begins between 5 and 10 years of age has the correlated EEG pattern of generalized relatively symmetrical and synchronous bursts of 3 Hz (2.5–4 Hz) spike–slow wave complexes (Fig. 29.4). The spike components of the bursts are most prominent in the frontal-Rolandic parasagittal recording areas. In some cases, the bursts may contain considerable polyspike–slow wave components, particularly during drowsiness and sleep. Short bursts of spike–slow wave complexes (1–2 seconds) in general will have only limited or no definite clinical accompaniment. Bursts of 3–30 seconds duration are in general accompanied by some interruption of consciousness. The absence seizure consists of a short (3–30 seconds) interruption of consciousness in which general postural tone is relatively well preserved. During this brief period, the patient is observed to stare, oblivious to stimuli introduced into the environment. Ongoing activities are interrupted. For example, if in the midst of eating, the patient may stop with his spoon in midair. The interruption is abrupt in onset and relatively abrupt in cessation. The patient's awareness and motor activities return promptly at the

Figure 29.3 Hypsarrhythmia in an infant with myoclonic spasms. Referential (monopolar) recordings from frontal (F), rolandic (C), temporal (T), and occipital (O) areas.

Figure 29.4 Generalized 3 Hz spike wave discharge. This 19-year-old male had a long history of frequent absence seizures characterized by a blank stare, flickering of the eyelids, and a failure to respond to instructions. This accompanying EEG discharge in this episode was of 8 seconds duration. Other episodes were of 20–40 seconds duration.

end of the episode. Memory is defective only for the period of the seizure. It is as though the patient, although physically present, has been absent as regards his higher cortical functions for the brief interval of the seizure. In actuality, the impairment of awareness, the impairment of response capacity, and the impairment of motor activity is a relative phenomenon, occurring in variable degree. Thus, some patients may be unaware of phrases or numbers that are provided as auditory or visual stimuli during the episode. Other patients are aware of these same stimuli and are able to repeat them during questioning at the end of the episode. Some patients are able to continue a familiar recitation during the absence seizure. Whether a response to a stimulus occurs during these brief seizures may, in part, depend on the intensity of the stimulus and the motivation and past experience of the patient. It is the degree of interruption that is variable. There are minor motor phenomena that may often accompany the seizure: eye opening and myoclonus of eyelids and extraocular and facial muscles. Automatisms of mouth, jaw, and hands may also occur. Some minor loss of postural tone in the neck muscles may occur, causing the head to fall onto the chest. Usually many attacks occur per day and interfere with schoolwork. In most patients the attacks may be triggered by hyperventilation.

In many families there is strong evidence of a genetic (autosomal dominant) predisposition to primary generalized epilepsy based on EEG studies. In such families the genetic predisposition is apparently for idiopathic epilepsy and not absence seizures per se. There is a predominance of females affected. For most families a polygenic pattern rather than a monogenic pattern of inheritance is suspected. The high concordance rate in identical twins was noted by Lennox, who was cited earlier. In a minority of cases there is little evidence of a genetic background and the seizures apparently reflect perinatal or other multifocal and diffuse pathological processes beginning in early childhood.

The seizures and the EEG pattern are particularly responsive to medications such as ethosuximide, trimethadione, and valproic acid. Since approximately 50% of these patients will also have generalized convulsive tonic clonic seizures, valproic acid may be the preferred medication since it has significant therapeutic actions against both types of seizures. Note that the terms *pyknolepsy* and *petit mal absence seizure* have been employed in the past.

Juvenile absence epilepsy (JA) has a similar EEG pattern. The attacks are less frequent and there is a higher incidence of generalized tonic clonic seizures. There is no male/female difference.

Juvenile myoclonic epilepsy (JME) was identified in 1957, by Janz and Christian, as a syndrome which incorporated features of juvenile onset, tonic-clonic, and myoclonic seizures with a bilateral symmetrical and synchronous 4–5 Hz polyspike-slow wave pattern (Fig. 29.5). Myoclonus may be defined as a sudden rapid jerk or twitch resulting from the sudden contraction of one or more muscle groups. The jerks may be bilateral and symmetrical or multifocal. Facial muscles, extraocular muscles, and head or limbs or body may be involved. The intensity of the contraction may be strong enough to throw the patient to the floor or isolated and weak enough to result in the twitch of a finger. In 40% of patients, the discharges and often the myoclonus are triggered by intermittent photic stimulation with a stroboscope (Fig. 29.6). In some series, associated with absence seizures the 3–4 Hz spike wave or polyspike slow wave EEG patterns are more common. This syndrome of juvenile myoclonic epilepsy is now recognized as the most common variety of primary generalized epilepsy beginning in the adolescent or young adult years (12–18), accounting for 7%–12% of all seizure patients depending on the series (see Delgado-Escueta et al., 1989; Dreifuss, 1989). Almost all patients have both generalized tonic-clonic and myoclonic seizures, the latter often precipitated by sudden awakening, sleep deprivation, alcohol consumption, or stress. This syndrome has considerable significance.

In the early genetic studies of EEG photosensitivity, this particular trait appeared to be inherited as an autosomal dominant

Figure 29.5 Generalized bursts of polyspikes and slow waves. Juvenile myoclonic epilepsy in a 13 year old who had the onset of sudden single generalized myoclonic jerks, which initially were sufficiently violent to throw the patient to the floor but did not impair consciousness. Neurological examination has remained normal and the patient has never (now age 22 years) experienced generalized convulsive seizures or petit mal absences.

Figure 29.6 Generalized bursts of polyspikes and slow waves triggered by photic stimulation. Juvenile myoclonic epilepsy with photosensitivity. This young woman at age 13 had the onset of generalized convulsive seizures and of frequent myoclonic seizures involving eyelids and arms. The myoclonic seizures involving eyelids, facial muscles, and limbs were clearly triggered by bright flickering light.

(Fig. 29.7), although the majority of affected relatives did not have clinical seizures (Watson and Marcus, 1962). In more recent studies of JME (Delgado-Escueta et al., 1989), 50% of probands had a first- or second-degree relative with epileptic seizures. Among first-degree relatives of the proband, 80% of symptomatic siblings and 6% of asymptomatic siblings had diffuse 4–6 Hz polyspike slow wave discharges. Linkage analysis suggested a relationship to chromosome 6, although subsequent studies have suggested linkage to 15q in other families (Delgado-Escueta et al., 1999). Therapy is very specific: Valproic acid will totally control seizures in 80% of patients but must be continued on a relatively lifelong basis. In the series of Janz (1985), 91% of patients had recurrent seizures when anticonvulsant was discontinued after two seizure-free years.

ANATOMICAL DIFFERENTIAL DIAGNOSIS OF MYOCLONUS

The anatomical substrate for myoclonus is variable. In the monkey, myoclonus may occur as a result of bilateral epileptogenic foci in the motor cortex or the adjacent premotor cortex. A similar cortical onset of discharge has been noted in the light-sensitive baboon (papio, papio). Myoclonus may also occur in various extrapyramidal diseases involving the basal ganglia or ventro-lateral nuclei of the thalamus. In patients with Parkinson's disease, myoclonic jerks may complicate the use of L-Dopa (in addition to the more common choreiform dyskinesia). Segmental myoclonus has been described in viral diseases involving the spinal cord.

In the noncortical varieties of myoclonus, it is possible to have the behavioral phenomenon without the occurrence of accompanying spike or polyspike–slow wave discharges in the electroencephalogram. In the cortical variety of myoclonus, conduction of discharges to the brain stem and spinal cord occurs along both pyramidal and nonpyramidal pathways.

Stimulus-sensitive myoclonus refers to the precipitation of myoclonic jerks by sound, light flash, proprioceptive, or tactile

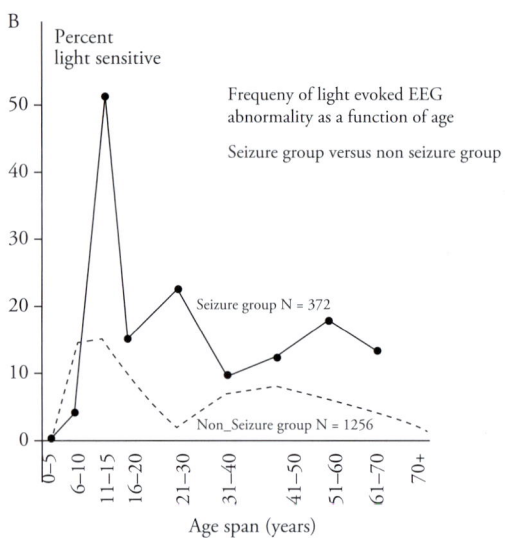

Figure 29.7 (*A*) The electroencephalogram (EEG) trait: photosensitivity as a function of age and sex in 1256 consecutive nonseizure patients. The role of genetics is also demonstrated in the relatives of 60 photosensitive propositi matched for age. Almost all of the propositi had idiopathic epilepsy. Almost all of the photosensitive relatives did not have epilepsy. (*B*) Photosensitivity as a function of age and seizure history. Consecutive seizure and nonseizure patients. The frequency of this trait in those patients with focal (partial) epilepsy did not differ from the nonseizure patients. The excess of photosensitivity in the 10–20 age seizure group reflected the occurrence of idiopathic epilepsy in this age group. The excess in the 50–70 age seizure group may have reflected the occurrence of diffuse disorders in this age group.

stimuli. Usually, the underlying disease is a diffusely distributed process. In some cases, it is primarily cortical; in others it is primarily noncortical. The disease process involves neurons primarily rather than white matter.

ETIOLOGICAL AND PROGNOSTIC CLASSIFICATION OF MYOCLONUS

1. Benign nonprogressive myoclonus: sudden jerks on falling asleep or on awakening are a common normal phenomenon. A familial variety of essential myoclonus may also occur.

2. Nonprogressive myoclonus as a manifestation of idiopathic epilepsy: the JME syndrome.
3. Symptomatic generalized epilepsy, usually with mental retardation
    a. Infantile spasms
    b. Lennox-Gastaut syndrome
4. Progressive myoclonic disorders (Berkovic et al., 1991)
    a. Mitochondrial disorders
    b. Lipidosis-lysosomal storage diseases
    c. Myoclonus epilepsy of Unverricht and Lundborg
    d. Lafora's disease
5. Infectious: viral or prion related
    a. Acute encephalitis, for example, acute herpes simplex
    b. Subacute inclusion body encephalitis: reactivation of the measles virus
    c. Spongiform encephalopathy–Creutzfeldt-Jakob disease–prion disorders
6. Metabolic disorders
    a. Uremia
    b. Hypocalcemia
    c. CO_2 narcosis
    d. Anoxic encephalopathy: acute or chronic effect
    e. Pyridoxine deficiency state of infancy
    f. L-Dopa toxicity
7. Generalized tonic clonic seizures (GTCS): The stereotype of the generalized convulsion, the grand mal seizure, consists of two phases: the tonic and the clonic. Occasionally myoclonic jerks of increasing frequency may precede the actual loss of consciousness and the tonic phase. Unless the tonic-clonic convulsion represents a secondarily generalization of a partial seizure, the onset is abrupt, with loss of consciousness the initial sign. The patient stiffens and, if standing erect, is thrown to the floor. Respiration is arrested and the pupils dilate. After a short but variable period of 10 to 30 seconds, the tonic stage then passes into the clonic stage. The symmetrical jerks of clonus then slow in frequency and cease. The total duration of the actual uncomplicated tonic/clonic phase is usually a matter of 1 minute. This state is followed by a short but variable period of coma, followed by stupor, confusion, and drowsiness. The total duration of confusion and drowsiness is usually less than 30 to 60 minutes. The patient will be amnesic about the onset of the attack, about subsequent events of the seizure, and about the postictal period of confusion. If the bladder has been full, incontinence of urine will have occurred during the seizure. The plantar responses are usually extensor during the attack and will remain extensor during the early part of the postictal period. The following EEG features are correlated with the clinical sequence: fast spike discharge at 8–20 Hz with the tonic phase (Fig. 29.8A), repetitive spike wave or polyspike wave generalized discharge of gradually decreasing frequency with the clonic phase (Fig. 29.8B, C, D), a short period of relative electrical silence in the electroencephalogram (Fig. 29.8E) with the initial postictal stage. Slow-wave activity of 1–3 Hz is then apparent and is correlated with the period of depression of consciousness. With clearing of confusion, the electroencephalogram gradually returns to a normal frequency range. During interictal periods, the electroencephalogram in patients who are subject to generalized convulsive seizures may present a variable appearance. The record often is normal. Generalized bursts of polyspike and slow waves may occur. In some cases, focal or multifocal abnormalities may be present, even though a clinical focus of seizure onset was not apparent. The causes of GTCS at various ages are indicated in Table 29.2. The preferred treatment of idiopathic epilepsy characterized by generalized tonic clonic seizures is valproic acid. For some patients phenytoin may be utilized.

Figure 29.8 Experimental generalized tonic clonic seizure without focal onset in a monkey. The animal was tonic during the fast 8 Hz spike discharge of segment A. The animal had repetitive clonic jerks, during the polyspike–slow wave discharges of segments B, C, and D, gradually decreasing in frequency. The period of relative electrical silence shown at the end of segment E and the subsequent period of 1–2 cps slow-wave activity (not shown) corresponded to the postictal depression of consciousness. Bipolar recordings from left and right premotor-precentral areas.

Several conditions in which a loss of consciousness and postural tone occur must be differentiated from generalized tonic clonic seizures:

1. Syncope (see earlier).

2. Akinetic (atonic) seizures are seizures in which the patient falls suddenly to the floor but then stands up again almost immediately. The loss of consciousness is brief. In some cases, there may be no definite evidence of an actual loss of consciousness. In some cases, the fall represents a sudden loss of postural tone; in other cases, the fall represents a massive myoclonic jerk that throws the patient violently to the floor. Atonic or akinetic seizures are frequently seen in the Lennox Gastaut syndrome in which other seizure types—atypical absence seizures (termed previously petit mal variant), generalized convulsive seizures, and in many cases tonic seizures—are also present.

3. Drop attacks in the adult may occur in relation to ischemia in the paramedian branches of the basilar artery with transient dysfunction in descending motor pathways and of the motor centers of the pontine or medullary reticular formation. In such cases, consciousness is usually preserved but patients often have other symptoms suggesting that basilar vertebral insufficiency may be present (see Chapter 13).

OVERVIEW OF PRIMARY/IDIOPATHIC GENERALIZED EPILEPSY

1. The overlap of syndromes: As demonstrated in Table 29.3 from Genton (1995), although clinical syndromes and their EEG patterns have been delineated, it is important to emphasize the considerable overlap among the various subcategories.

Many of the models to be discussed next illustrate an overlap of syndromes. In addition, both in the human cases and in the experimental models, there is not a 1 to 1 correlation of EEG and behavior.

2. The genetic molecular biology of idiopathic epilepsy: For most cases this has not yet been established. However, a number of specific genetic mutations involving channels and receptors have been identified. Recent papers by McNamara (1999), Prasad et al. (1999), and Steinlein (1999) have reviewed this topic. Specific defects have now been identified in several varieties of presumably monogenic seizure disorders. The genetic studies in epilepsy have defined new, mostly rare seizure types, but the genetic basis for the most common epilepsies requires further research (Sanchez-Carpintero et al., 2007).

a. Partial idiopathic epilepsy: Autosomal dominant nocturnal frontal lobe epilepsy (ADNFLE). This type of nocturnal motor seizure disorder (at times with secondary generalization) was originally misdiagnosed as a sleep disorder. In a large pedigree reported from Australia, linkage to the 20-q 13.3 chromosome site has been established. The α4 subunit of the neuronal acetylcholine nicotinic receptor (CHRNA4) maps to the same region. A missense mutation occurs with the addition of serine to the second transmembrane amino acid sequence. This mutation is present in all affected individuals and in the "carriers" (there is a penetrance of 70%–80%). In a Norwegian family with the same syndrome, an extra leucine was inserted in to the terminal end of the second transmembrane domain on the same receptor subunit.

The overall result of this mutation is a significant reduction of calcium permeability and a hypoactive receptor. The additional step necessary to produce seizures is unclear. However, it is possible that since some acetylcholine receptors are in a presynaptic location a decrease in calcium flux might reduce the release of GABA at this location. More recently a second locus on chromosome 15q24 has been identified; this site also contains multiple subunits of nicotinic cholinergic receptors.

b. Generalized idiopathic epilepsy: Benign, familial neonatal convulsions (BFNCs). This is also a rare autosomal dominant disorder in which partial or generalized clonic convulsions start around the third postnatal day and persist until week 6. Approximately 12% of patients have seizures again later in life. In most families linkage to chromosome site 20q13.3 occurs with a missense mutation in the gene for the voltage-gated potassium channel KCNQ2. There is a loss of amino acids in the sequence at the pore of the channel. *The mutation abolishes the potassium currents that are activated by depolarization. As a result, excitability is increased.* In a few families, the mutation occurs at the KCNQ3 site on chromosome 8 with a similar effect on excitability. Both KCNQ2 and 3 are predominantly expressed in the brain. Neurological development is otherwise normal. A similar mutation in another potassium channel, KCNQ1, produces the cardiac arrhythmia of the long QT syndrome.

c. Generalized idiopathic epilepsy: Generalized epilepsy with febrile seizures plus (GEFS+). In this autosomal dominant syndrome, febrile seizures occur before 3 months or after 3 years of age. In addition, however,

Table 29.3 **SEIZURE TYPES IN IDIOPATHIC EPILEPSY SYNDROMES IN 253 CONSECUTIVE CASES**

MAJOR SYNDROME	NO. OF CASES	SEIZURE TYPE(S)			
		Absences	GTCS	Myoclonic	Other
Childhood absence	73	100%	44%	3%	7%
Juvenile absence	28	100%	75%	11%	11%
Juvenile myoclonic	59	22%	86%	95%	—
GTCS on awakening	30	7%	100%	13%	—
Isolated GTCS	39	—	100%	11%	—

GTCS, generalized tonic clonic seizure.
Source: Modified from Genton (1995).

and this is of particular interest, multiple forms of classical idiopathic seizures occur without fever, including absence, myoclonic, atonic, and generalized tonic-clonic. Different members of the same family may have different types of these seizures despite the presence of the same genetic mutation. The mutant gene maps to chromosome locus 19q13.1. A mutation in the beta subunit of a voltage-gated sodium channel (SCN1B) occurs as a result of amino acid substitution of tryptophan for cysteine.

This is a rapidly evolving area; additional discoveries are to be expected. Note, however, that in most seizure disorders in the human patient, penetrance is often incomplete and transmission may be polygenic.

Later, in our discussion of the idiopathic epilepsies, we will discuss other genetic defects in rodent models.

3. The underlying neuropathology of idiopathic/primary generalized epilepsy: Although a long-standing general criterion cited for this disorder was that no structural neuropathology be present, it is now evident that cortical microdysgenesis is present in those cases that come to autopsy. In most cases, neurons are found in the molecular layer, which is normally relatively devoid of neurons. In the series of Meencke (1996), 100% of 12 patients with childhood absence epilepsy and 100% of 3 patients with JME had significant microdysgenesis; but none had severe migration disorders in the deeper cortical layers. In contrast, 50% of 24 patients with infantile spasms had microdysgenesis and 13% had severe migration disorders. Among 30 patients with the Lennox-Gastaut syndrome, 50% had microdysgenesis and 16% had severe migration disorders. Among 27 patients with temporal lobe epilepsy, only 7% had microdysgenesis but 11% had severe migration disorders. In terms of increased neuron density in the molecular layer (a prominent feature in idiopathic epilepsy), this was most severe in the frontal lobes but also present in other cortical areas. Recent quantitative magnetic resonance imaging (MRI) studies have also raised the question of cerebral gray matter structural changes in all types of patients with idiopathic epilepsy, most prominent in juvenile absence epilepsy (Woermann et al., 1998). In addition, among patients with JME, more specific MRI and positron emission tomography (PET) scan changes have been noted in superior frontal and mesial frontal gyri (Woermann et al., 1999). These patients may also have a correlated deficit in visual working memory.

4. Underlying pathophysiology: A number of models of idiopathic epilepsy are available, which reproduce the behavioral and electrical (EEG), and pharmacologic features of these disorders. If the genetic and biochemical pathophysiology is known in humans, this should be reproduced. Unfortunately, except for a small number of the clinical syndromes that we have earlier reviewed, in relation to genetic disorders of channels, these latter features are often unclear. In general, because of phylogenetic differences in cortical and callosal development, observations in the monkey may be more difficult but have greater validity in terms of generalization to humans. In the models of absence seizures, there is the question of whether the process recorded in the EEG reflects the activity of cerebral cortex alone or of the effects of an interaction of thalamus with cerebral cortex. Studies in the rat are consistent with the thalamo-cortical interaction. Studies in the monkey suggest a cortical basis. As regards the JME syndrome, the baboon with light-induced myoclonus provides a model in which the discharges begin in frontal Rolandic cortex. As regards GTCS, the EEG discharge can be reproduced in a preparation composed of cerebral cortex and corpus callosum. Table 29.4 provides a summary of pathophysiology (Figures 29.9–29.13).

GENETIC MODELS IN THE MOUSE

At present six inbred mouse strains have been reported with spike wave discharges and absence seizures. In each of these strains the bilateral bursts of spike wave discharge are accompanied by behavioral arrest, and the discharges are blocked by drugs that are effective against absence seizures. However, almost all of these strains have other neurological deficits usually related to cerebellar degeneration and the discharge consists of a 6–7 Hz spike and wave. The importance of these strains relates to the monogenic inheritance of actual or presumed ion channel mutations (Ca^{++} or Na^+/H^+). Other genetic seizure disorders in rats are discussed.

CONCLUSIONS REGARDING THE BILATERAL SYNCHRONOUS DISCHARGES OF IDIOPATHIC EPILEPSY

1. All of the models, leaving aside the mouse models, suggest that the basic pathology involves a hyperexcitability of neurons at the cortical level. This is consistent with the now available neuropathological data and MRI data in humans.

2. The bilateral synchrony in the various models in the monkey, baboon, cat, and rat is dependent on the corpus callosum and the related major commissures. There is no direct anatomical substrate in the thalamus of the human providing the basis for the bilateral synchrony found in idiopathic epilepsy.

3. There may be multiple possible mechanisms providing the substrate for the oscillations of excitation and inhibition responsible for the spike–slow wave discharge. The minimal substrate is built into the design of cerebral cortex and of the cortical-callosal circuits. There is little doubt that discharges having begun in cerebral cortex do subsequently spread to the thalamus, basal ganglia, the brain stem, and spinal cord, and these structures do reverberate back to cerebral cortex. However, to what extent the cortico-thalamo-cortical oscillation is necessary to produce and sustain the spike-wave complex in the human

Table 29.4 OUTLINE OF MODELS OF IDIOPATHIC EPILEPSY PATHOPHYSIOLOGY

TYPE OF SEIZURE TYPE OF MODEL	SUBSTRATE OF EEG SEIZURE	MECHANISM FOR BILATERAL SYNCHRONY	BEHAVIOR
Absence			
1. Midline/intralaminar thalamic stimulation; Fig. 29.9	Recruiting response thalamo-cortical Stimulus related 3 Hz SW. Refer to Chapter 17.	Unclear, probably corpus callosum interaction	Arrest of movement
2. Bilateral symmetrical premotor foci (monkey); Figs. 29.10–29.12	Cerebral cortex. Bilateral 2.5–3.5 Hz SW persists in bilateral cortical callosal isolate preparation.	Corpus callosum	Absence: eye opening, staring, arrest of movement, if anterior premotor. Greater myoclonus, if posterior premotor.
3. Feline general penicillin epilepsy (cat); Fig. 29.13	Onset in the cerebral cortex, later in the specific thalamic nuclei, later in nonspecific thalamic nuclei. Thalamic nuclei are recruited into a cortical/thalamic-cortical oscillation. 3.5–6 Hz SW	Corpus callosum	Impairment of responsivity during bursts plus myoclonus of face/ extremities
4. GAERS(rat) (Generalized absence epilepsy of the rat- Strasbuurg)	Discharges are predominant in frontoparietal cortex and posterolateral thalamus, Thalamo-cortical interaction is required. 7–11 Hz SW	Corpus callosum	Animals are immobilized with myoclonus face/ extremities and impairment of responsivity during the bursts.
Myoclonus			
1. Subthreshold pentylene tetrazol (monkey)	Motor cortex: bilateral 3Hz SW	Corpus callosum	Bilateral myoclonic jerks of extremities
2. Bilateral motor cortex foci	Motor cortex: initially bilateral spike discharges	Corpus callosum	Myoclonus of extremities then GTCS**
3. Photosensitive baboon	Origin in frontal/rolandic cortex (areas 4 and 6). Bilateral 4 Hz polyspike slow wave. Blocked by Dopa agonists	Corpus callosum	Bilateral myoclonus of eyelids, face, and limbs. At times, progression to GTCS
Generalized Tonic Clonic Seizure			
Threshold dose of Pentylenetetrazol (monkey/cat). Refer to Chapter 17 for illustrations	Cerebral cortex: onset at low-threshold areas, e.g., motor cortex. Pattern is similar in bilateral cortical callosal isolate	Corpus callosum	GTCS often preceded by bilateral myoclonic jerks

EEG, electroencephalogram; GTCS, generalized tonic clonic seizure.

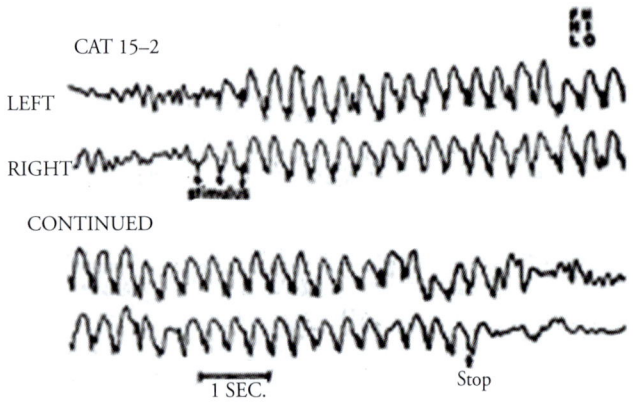

Figure 29.9 Experimental 3 Hz spike wave discharges following midline or intralaminar thalamic stimulation. A stimulus-related bilaterally synchronous spike and wave discharge is produced in cat cerebral cortex by repetitive 3 cps stimulation of the massa intermedia. (From Jasper, H., and Droogleever-Fortuyn, J.: Res. Publ. Ass. Nerv. Ment. Dis. 26:272-298, 1947.)

Figure 29.10 Experimental 3 Hz spike wave discharge following bilateral symmetrical epileptogenic foci in anterior premotor cortex of the monkey. Effects of hyperventilation as in patients with absence seizures. A= just prior to hyperventilation; B, C, D., 2–3 minutes after beginning of hyperventilation. Pre C, precentral gyrus; Pre 0, preoccipital area; SF, superior frontal gyrus. (From Marcus, E.M., and Watson, C.W.: Arch. Neurol. 19:103, 1968, AMA.) Refer also to Chapter 17 for an additional example of a 3–4 Hz spike wave discharge in this preparation.

Figure 29.11 Bilateral symmetrical foci: anterior premotor cortex. Correlation of behavior (absence seizure) with bilateral 3 Hz spike-slow wave discharge. Continuous bipolar recordings: premotor to precentral. Segments A and B are continuous. (1) Head moves to midline and eyes are wide open. (2) Start of testing with pencil moved back and forth across visual fields. The animal failed to follow. (3) Light tap on nose produced only partial blink but no other response of hands or head. (4) Hands were tapped without response, although during nonseizure periods, animal had vigorously grasped the pencil. (5) Animal now blinked fully to approaching object, complete eye closure then opening; no tactile stimulus to nose was required. (6) Animal now followed pencil with head and eye, turning as pencil moved toward the animal's left peripheral field. Licking also occurred (had not occurred during seizure). (Reproduced with permission from Marcus, E.M., et al. Epilepsia, 9:237, 1968b, Blackwell.)

is uncertain. The idiopathic epilepsies and the spike-wave discharge may represent a biological spectrum, rather than a unitary disease, as noted by Berkovic et al. (1988).

4. Behavior is a more complex matter. There is a representation and re-representation of patterns of behavior at various levels of the neuraxis.

WHY ARE AWARENESS AND RESPONSIVITY ALTERED DURING THE ABSENCE SEIZURE?

Several explanations are possible:

1. There is widespread involvement of cerebral cortex in seizure discharge; particularly of the multimodality sensory projection areas and of other frontal and temporal association areas involved in working memory and so on, so that these areas cannot participate in their normal activities.

2. There is impairment in the capacity of the thalamus to transmit information.

3. Both of these explanations are operational in the intact individual since discharge of cerebral cortex secondarily

Figure 29.12 (A) The isolated bilateral cortical callosal preparation in the cat. (B) Prolonged bilateral synchronous 2–3.5 Hz spike-slow wave, polyspike slow wave, and polyspike discharges in the cortical callosal preparation following the production of bilateral epileptogenic foci. (From Marcus, E.M., and Watson, C.W.: Arch. Neurol. 14:632, 1966.) Similar results may be obtained in the monkey. (From Marcus, E.M., Watson, C.W., and Simon, S.A.: Epilepsia, 9:243, 1968, Blackwell.)

Figure 29.13 Generalized penicillin epilepsy in the cat: IM administration. Generalized bursts of polyspike and 3–5 Hz spike-wave discharges occur. (From Gloor, P., Epilepsia 20:571-588, 1979, Blackwell.)

spreading to thalamus via the cortico-thalamic system will also alter the capacity of the thalamus to transmit information.

WHAT ARE THE MECHANISMS FOR ENDING SEIZURE DISCHARGE?

The total explanation for the cessation of the seizures is not entirely clear but presumably could include various inhibitory processes involving the cortex, subcortical nuclei, thalamus, and brain stem. In this regard, we should note that the activity of isolated cerebral cortex is characterized by bursts of activity with intervening periods of relative electrical silence. There are then intrinsic mechanisms within cerebral cortex for cessation of discharge. This is then the most likely overriding consideration. Additional discussion of the role of structures such as the red nucleus, basal forebrain, pontine and medullary reticular formation, and the pars reticularis of the substantia nigra will be found in the cited references (Gale, 1990; Moshe and Sperber, 1990).

GUIDELINES FOR MANAGEMENT OF SEIZURE DISORDERS

EVALUATION

Over 75% of diagnosis in neurology is dependent on the history; this is even more important with regard to seizure disorders. However, in this case, information must be obtained from witnesses regarding events for which the patient may have little recollection. Information from the patient and witnesses regarding focal manifestations, aura, and so on is vital. The neurological examination is critical in terms of the presence or absence of signs suggesting focal cortical pathology. Laboratory studies should include a complete blood count, blood sugar, calcium, electrolytes, and creatinine/BUN. The EEG performed during awake and sleep states may provide information regarding focal or generalized electrical seizure discharges or slow-wave activity. The yield of the EEG may be increased by activation procedures such as sleep deprivation (SD), hyperventilation (HV), and photic stimulation (PS). All patients should have an imaging study. Based on the information considered earlier, whenever possible this should be an MRI with coronal images that allow study of the medial temporal structures. When this is not possible, then a computerized tomography (CT) scan with and without contrast should be obtained.

Specific aspects of seizure management are considered in Table 29.5. The use and properties of anticonvulsants are considered in Tables 29.6, 29.7, and 29.8.

The upper limit of therapeutic range for all of these agents is variable related to protein binding and so on. For valproic acid, the upper limit of therapeutic range is 100–150 μg/ml. The half-life of phenytoin is constant only up to 12 μg/ml above that level the half-life increases with blood level. The time to achieve steady state is approximately 4–5× the half life. Dosing schedule relates to half-life. Note that primidone is in part converted to phenobarbital; both metabolites have anticonvulsant action.

THE MOLECULAR BASIS OF ANTICONVULSANT DRUG ACTION

In general, anticonvulsants that are effective against partial and secondarily generalized seizures are effective in the experimental maximal electroshock test (a model of seizure spread) and produce Na$^+$ channel blockade. In general, those drugs that are effective against spike wave epilepsies, particularly absences: These drugs are also effective against experimental pentylenetetrazol-induced seizures, elevate threshold, and produce T type Ca^{++} channel blockade. However, benzodiazepines and barbiturates are also effective against this type of experimental seizure.

TERATOGENIC AND SIDE EFFECTS OF ANTICONVULSANT MEDICATIONS

1. *Teratogenic effects in the offspring of the pregnant female with seizures.* In general, the nonseizure population has a 2.5% risk of malformation; seizure patients not on anticonvulsants, a 3.5% risk; seizure patients on anticonvulsants, a 5.5% risk. Teratogenic effects occur primarily in the first trimester and consist of cleft lip, neural tube closure defects, and congenital heart disease. The risk of malformation is increased if any of the following factors is present: (1) poor seizure control, (2) polypharmacy, (3) high blood levels, or (4) use of trimethadione. Risk of neural tube defects can be significantly reduced by administration of folic acid.

2. *Other side effects of anticonvulsants fall into three general groups:*

   a. Allergic—dermatological, hepatic, immune, for which the drug must be discontinued

   b. Dose related (ataxia, drowsiness, dizziness, diplopia), for which the dose must be lowered

   c. Chronic—hematological, lymphatic (lymphoma, lupus, etc.), and megodermal.

Since Table 29.6 was created, a number of new anticonvulsant agents have become available. Lacosimide has proven useful in

Table 29.5 MANAGEMENT OF SEIZURE DISORDERS

PROBLEM	MANAGEMENT	EXPECTED RESULTS
Single GTCS	No specific anticonvulsant treatment if: (1) History indicates no focal features, no prior minor seizures, normal growth and development, no mental retardation, and no family history of seizure disorder. (2) Neurological examination is normal. (3) EEG with sleep deprivation, HV, and PS is normal. (4) Imaging studies are normal. (5) Conditions such as fever, sleep deprivation, alcohol and drug withdrawal, or use of drugs such as cocaine, isoniazid, or other agents or metabolic conditions lowering threshold are present.	Annegers et al. (1986) found recurrence rate of 16% at 1 year, 22% at 3 years, 26% at 5 years
Recurrent seizures (epilepsy)	(1) Rule out metabolic abnormality and mass lesion; prevent additional seizures with anticonvulsants. (2) Start with monotherapy push dose to seizure control or toxicity. (3) If still no control, use second or third major agent, then newer add-on agents. (4) Treat for 3–5 years seizure free. If at that point, EEG indicates no seizure discharges, consider gradual withdrawal from medications.	In generalized/idiopathic epilepsy complete control in 63% and significant reduction in an additional 25%. In complex partial, complete control in 20%–35%. If seizure free 5 years and discontinue medication, 30% relapse over 10 years.
Relapses	If on anticonvulsants: (1) Compliance issues, omission of medication. Check levels. (2) Insufficient daily dosage. Check levels and adjust dose. With phenytoin, check the free unbound fraction (usual therapeutic range is 1–2 µg/ml). Alternatively, push dosage until therapeutic effect is attained or dose-related toxicity occurs. (3) Wrong medication for the type of seizure: re-evaluate in terms of history and EEG. Do long-term video-EEG monitoring. Whether on or off medications consider following factors: (1) Sleep deprivation; (2) Alcohol or drug withdrawal; (3) Fever or metabolic abnormalities or use of antihistamines; (4) Falls with frontal or temporal injuries = additional foci; (5) Epileptic status producing hippocampal sclerosis so that additional foci of seizures resulting in complex partial seizures. Re-evaluate in terms of history, EEG, and monitor; (6) Secondary epileptogenesis; (7) Underlying progressive disorder is present; (8) Possible pseudo seizures + actual seizure disorder.	(1) Recurrences are more likely if focal rather than idiopathic, or if long time before initial seizure control or if seizure discharges are still present in EEG. (2) Intensive re-evaluation at an epilepsy center with video EEG monitoring will result in a significant number of patients reclassified with treatment modified. (3) Combination of epilepsy + alcoholism or drug addiction difficult to treat because of compliance issues and withdrawal effects triggering seizures.
Refractory patient despite use of three traditional medications	(1) Consider all factors listed above. (2) If focus is well defined, and psychiatric issues are not present, consider surgery after intensive noninvasive ± invasive monitoring, and determination of dominance. Because of high incidence of complex partial seizures, usual procedure is anterior/mesial temporal resection. Less often, resections in frontal lobe. (3) If poorly controlled secondary generalized epilepsy (e.g., Lennox Gastaut) or multiple foci, consider vagal stimulator or corpus callosotomy.	In patients with complex partial epilepsy due to mesial temporal sclerosis, 78% had complete seizure control at 1 year after anterior medial temporal resection (Doyle and Spencer, 1998) (see also Wiebe et al., 2001). With frontal lobe resections, 68% became seizure free. Vagal stimulator will reduce seizure frequency. Callosotomy will decrease GTCS and drop attacks but focal seizures may increase.
Epileptic status	Discussed	

Note. Refer to CD-ROM for additional discussion.
EEG, electroencephalography; GTCS, generalized tonic clonic seizure.

Table 29.6 PHARMACOLOGIC PROPERTIES OF THE MAJOR ANTICONVULSANT DRUGS

AGENT	USUAL DAILY DOSE CHILDREN (mg/kg)	USUAL DAILY DOSE ADULTS (mg) (TOTAL)	DOSING	HALF-LIFE (HOURS)	BLOOD LEVEL (µg/ml) EFFECTIVE	BLOOD LEVEL (MG/ML) TOXIC
Phenobarbital	3–5	90–180	1×/day	96 ± 12	>15 (4–13)	>40
Phenytoin	4–7	300	Split 2×/day	24 ± 12	>10	>20
Primidone	10–25	750	Split 3×/day	>6	>12	
Ethosuximide	20–30	1000	Split 2×/day	30 ± 6	>40	>100
Carbamazepine	8–20	600–1400	Split 3×/day	12 ± 3	>8 (4–13)	>13
Valproic acid	15 (initial) 15–30 (maintain)	1000–2600	Split 3–4×/day	8	>50	>125

Table 29.7 **MOLECULAR BASIS OF ANTICONVULSANT DRUG ACTION**

TYPE OF ACTION	DRUGS: TRADITIONAL	DRUGS: NEWER AGENTS
Inhibit voltage-gated sodium channel	PHT, CBZ, VPA	FBM, LTG, TPM, ZNA
Enhance GABA/A receptor chlorine channel	PB, BZD	FBM, TPM
Increase brain GABA	VPA	VGB, GBP, TPM, TGB
Inhibits Na$^+$ currents through non-NMDA receptor		TPM
Inhibits Ca^{++} currents through NMDA receptor		FBM
Inhibit slow threshold T-type voltage-gated Ca^{++} channel	ESM (?VPA)	ZNA
Inhibits brain carbonic anhydrase	AZM	

PHT, phenytoin; CBZ, carbamazepine; VPA, valproic acid; PB, phenobarbital; BZD, benzodiazepines; ESM, ethosuximide; AZM, acetazolamide; FBM, felbamate; GBP, gabapentin; LTG, lamotrigine; TPM, topiramate; TGB, tiagabine; VGB, vigabatrin; ZNA, zonisamide.
Source: Modified from Rho and Shankar (1999).

partial seizures and appears to prevent high-frequency neuronal discharges by modifying Na$^+$ channels. It may cause dizziness, diplopia, and prolongation of the PR interval but has minimal interaction with other drugs. An IV preparation is available. Levetiracetam is one of the most widely used of the new-generation anticonvulsants because it is effective in both partial and generalized epilepsy; is well tolerated and has no drug–drug interaction. Pregabalin can be viewed as a more potent form of gabapentin. Rufinamide, which also affects Na$^+$ channels, has been approved for adjunctive treatment of the Lennox-Gastaut syndrome. Oxcarbazepine affects the function of both Na$^+$ and calcium channels with a role in the treatment of partial seizures and can cause severe hyponatremia, ataxia diplopia, gastrointestinal symptoms, and tremor.

Suicide is associated with the anticonvulsant drugs and patients should be warned about this possibility.

Epilepsy surgery is becoming increasingly established for cases with intractable seizures, especially those patients with mesial temporal sclerosis and focal cortical dysgenesis. Radiosurgery and direct open surgery are used. Most of the time this involves referral to one of the National Association of Epilepsy Centers, where a prolonged complex evaluation may be required to succeed in ablation of the seizure foci but not cause damage to normal neural tissue. Prolonged video-EEG telemetry, functional MRI or PET scanning, and placement of electrodes on the cortical surface are examples of techniques that might be required in this setting (Spencer et al., 2005).

Vagal nerve stimulation is an adjunctive treatment that has some use as supplementary therapy in partial seizures for some patients with an inadequate response to good medical therapy. A stimulating device has to be skillfully implanted and follow-up programming is needed. About half of patients so treated will experience significant improvement (Elliott et al., 2011).

A new system of controlling seizures has recently been FDA approved. This system detects the nascent electrical activity of a developing seizure and delivers an electrical stimulus to abort the progress to a full-blown attack (Sohal and Sun, 2011).

Status Epilepticus

This is a frequent major neurological emergency. Overall incidence is at least 41–61 cases per 100,000 population. Less than 1 year of age, the incidence is 156 per 100,000; in the over-65 year group, the incidence is 86 per 100,000 population. Overall 30% of cases are generalized from the onset and 32%–43% are secondarily generalized after focal onset. This acute condition must be recognized and treated as rapidly as possible. The strict terminology of the International Classification of Epileptic Seizures defines epileptic status as any seizure lasting >30 minutes or intermittent seizures lasting >30 minutes without regaining consciousness. Since the usual tonic clonic seizure is usually <1–2 minutes in duration, most experts would now shorten the time before treating as epileptic status to 5–10 minutes. The earlier the treatment, the lower the morbidity and mortality. The epidemiologic data as presented in Table 29.9, indicate a current overall mortality of 22% in cases meeting the 30 minutes criteria. The greatest risk of mortality occurs in those cases that are generalized from the onset or are secondarily generalized after focal onset and in the over-65 age group where mortality is 38%. The causes of morbidity and mortality are cerebral anoxia, cerebral edema, aspiration pneumonitis, hyperthermia, hypotension,

Table 29.8 **SEIZURE TYPES AND DRUG CHOICE**

SEIZURE TYPE	DRUG CHOICE: TRADITIONAL	DRUG CHOICE: NEWER[A,B]
Partial and secondarily generalized	PHT, CBZ, VPA	LTG,[c] TPM, ZNA, GBP, TGB
Absence	ESM, VPA	
Myoclonic	VPA, BZD	
Primary generalized tonic/clonic	VPA, PHT, CBZ	
Infantile spasms	ACTH, BZD	
Status epilepticus: generalized, partial	BZD (intravenous)	

PHT, phenytoin; CBZ, carbamazepine; VPA, valproic acid; PB, phenobarbital; BZD, benzodiazepines; ESM, ethosuximide; AZM, acetazolamide; FBM, felbamate; GBP, gabapentin; LTG, lamotrigine; TPM, topiramate; TGB, tiagabine; VGB, vigabatrin; ZNA, zonisamide; ACTH, adrenocorticotrophic hormone.
[a]With the exception of LTG, all of these newer agents are adjunctive add-on agents.
[b]Additional new agent for partial seizures: levetiracetam.
[c]LTG may also be utilized in the Lennox-Gastaut syndrome.

Table 29.9 EPIDEMIOLOGY OF STATUS EPILEPTICUS

AGE RANGE	INCIDENCE* PER 100,000	MORTALITY (%)	MAJOR ETIOLOGY	PAST HISTORY OF EPILEPSY (%)	TYPE OF SEIZURE IN SE: PARTIAL (%)	TYPE OF SEIZURE IN SE: PARTIAL TO GTCS	TYPE OF SEIZURE IN GTCS(%)
<1 year	156						
1 month–15 year (pediatric)	38	2.5	Non-CNS infection (52%); low levels (21%)	38	28	32	32
16–59 years (adult, nonelderly)	27	14	CVA: acute or remote (>41%); low level (34%)	54	24	43	27
>65–80+	86	38	CVA: acute or remote (61%)	30	Included in adult	Included in adult	Included in adult
Total	41–61	22		42			

*These are minimum figures. Extrapolating from the data for Richmond, Virginia, to the total U.S. population results in an estimate of 152,000 cases and 42,000 deaths per year.

CNS, central nervous system; CVA, cerebrovascular accident; GTCS, generalized tonic clonic seizure; SE, status epilepticus.

and cardiac arrest as possible complications. Due to damage to hippocampal areas, prolonged grand mal status may be followed by prolonged confusion and a residual impairment of recent memory as well as temporal lobe seizures.

The etiology of status epilepticus can be divided into three major groups:

I. Status in patients with prior seizures due to (a) acute withdrawal or omission of medication, and (b) new metabolic factors and fever. (Group I constitutes 42% of all cases.)

II. Status as an acute or remote effect of a focal process, most frequently a cerebrovascular accident (CVA). However, frontal lobe tumor or abscess may also be the underlying focal process.

III. Status as the acute manifestation of systemic disease such as non–central nervous system infection in infants or children (52% of all cases in this age group), and alcohol withdrawal or metabolic factors or hypoxia in the adult.

Treatment has four essential components:

1. Assure stability of vital functions: (a) airway, (b) breathing, and (c) circulation; maintain blood pressure in normal range and maintain temperature in normal range (generalized seizures will produce hyperthermia due to central mechanisms). Draw blood levels and chemistries. Administer intravenous 50% glucose.

2. Stop the seizures: intravenous benzodiazepines: lorazepam (0.1 mg/kg at rate of 1–2 mg/min to maximum dose of 8 mg), diazepam (5–20 mg at rate of 1–2 mg/min), or midazolam. Because of status-induced neuronal changes, the benzodiazepines tend to lose effectiveness as the seizures continue. It is not common practice for EMTs to administer rectal diazepam or sublingual lorazepam prior to reaching the hospital.

3. Prevent additional seizures: load with intravenous phenytoin or fosphenytoin (18–20 mg/kg at rate of 50 mg/min). There has been increasing use of levetiracetam in many in lieu of the phenytoins (Misra et al., 2012).

4. Determine the cause: this will require EEG and CT scan or and/or MRI, blood levels, and so on, as well as neurological examination and observation of the seizures. Must still make distinction: focal versus generalized.

Complicated prolonged status: If status does not end rapidly at the emergency room level, continued intensive care unit monitoring, including continuous EEG, will be required. General anesthesia, including intravenous propofol or pentobarbital, may be required.

Nonconvulsive status: For acute onset of confusional states, consider the diagnosis of complex partial and absence status. The diagnosis will depend on immediate neurological examination and immediate EEG as well as trials of intravenous therapy with benzodiazepines. The availability of EEG monitoring in intensive care units has shown that nonconvulsive status is very common in this setting and managing these seizures is very difficult but crucial to outcomes (Claassen et al., 2004).

This is a skeleton outline of management of status. For greater details, see Delgado-Escueta (1982).

SLEEP STAGES: ANATOMICAL BACKGROUND

Sleep is characterized by a sequence of clinical and EEG stages (Fig. 29.14):

Stage W: Awake. Alpha rhythm of 8–13 Hz with suppression of alpha rhythm and emergence of low-voltage fast activity on eye opening or intense arousal.

Figure 29.14 Polysomnogram. An all-night 7-hour sleep study demonstrating the periodicity of sleep with the rapid eye movement (REM) stage (arrow on interrupted block line), occurring at 60- to 90-minute intervals. Note that in addition to sleep stages, snoring, respiration, electrocardiogram, movements, arousals, and oxygen saturation are all recorded. (Courtesy of Sleep Disorders, Institute of Central New England/Dr. Jay Phadke.) Refer also to Figure 29.16.

Stage 1: Drowsiness. Decrease in alpha amplitude and emergence of intermittent 4–7 Hz theta activity.

Stage 2: Early sleep–high-amplitude diphasic or triphasic sharp waves are present over the vertex areas, termed K complexes, or vertex sharp waves intermixed with 14–15 Hz spindles.

Stages 3 and 4 are characterized by increasing amounts of 0.5–3 Hz delta slow-wave activity (3 = delta 20%–50% of the time; 4 = delta >50% of the time). *Stages 2, 3, and 4 are referred to as slow wave or NREM (non-REM) sleep.*

Stage REM: After 90 minutes in the normal human, there then emerges a different stage of sleep characterized by low-amplitude alpha rhythm and fast activity, rapid eye movement, and a loss of muscle tone. This stage is also called paradoxical sleep since the individual is deeply asleep, but the EEG corresponds to a stage of relative wakefulness. This stage is associated with dreaming.

BRAIN STEM, DIENCEPHALIC, AND CORTICAL STRUCTURES INVOLVED IN CONSCIOUSNESS AND SLEEP

REM SLEEP

Recent studies have indicated an interaction of several areas in the brain stem. *Cholinergic neurons* in two nuclei located in the pontomesencephalic tegmental area of the reticular formation—the pedunculopontine tegmental (PPT) and the lateral dorsal tegmental (LDT)—discharge during REM sleep. These neurons send fibers to the thalamic relay and reticular nuclei. In contrast, during the REM stage of sleep there is an inhibition of activity in the *serotoninergic neurons* in the midline raphe nuclei of the pons and medulla, in the *noradrenergic neurons* of the locus ceruleus in the pontine tegmentum, and in the *histaminergic nuclei* in the hypothalamus. Thus, it is possible to speak of "REM on neurons," as opposed to "REM off neurons" (see reviews of Steriade, 1992, and Chokoverty, 2000, and Table 29.10). Both the cholinergic and the monoamine areas appear to be controlled by the ventrolateral preoptic nuclear complex. Table 29.11 summarizes the relationship between these centers in relation to sleep stages.

Table 29.10 ROLE OF FOREBRAIN, DIENCEPHALIC, AND BRAIN STEM STRUCTURES IN SLEEP AND COMA

STRUCTURE	BEHAVIORAL CHANGE	EEG CHANGE
Basal forebrain, preoptic, orbital frontal: stimulation	Induction of sleep	Slow-wave stage of sleep
Rostral (anterior) hypothalamus: preoptic, suprachiasmatic		
– Lesion*	Insomnia	Desynchronized Aroused
– Stimulation (low frequency)	Decreased spontaneous activity and of muscle tone	
Caudal hypothalamus + upper midbrain – Lesion*	Hypersomnolent	Slow wave pattern
– Stimulation (low frequency)	Behavioral activation	
Lateral hypothalamus-lesion*	Periodic narcolepsy/cataplexy	
Thalamus		
– Anterior/dorsomedial		
– Lesion	Insomnia	
– Stimulation	Sleep induced	Slow wave
-Intralaminar system		
– Lesion	Lethargy	
– Stimulation (high frequency)	Wakefulness	Desynchronized aroused
Mesencephalic reticular formation		
–Lesion	Coma	Slow waves with no arousal
– Stimulation (high frequency)	Shifts animal from sleep to wake	Shifts from slow to low volt fast
Midline raphe nuclei pons and medulla serotonergic neurons: lesion	A marked increase in the total duration of wakefulness. Sleep decreased by 80%–90%	Persistent awake pattern

*Hypothalamic lesions based on neuropathologic correlation studies of Von Economo in encephalitis lethargica or studies of Hess (1949).

Table 29.11 RELATIONSHIP OF BRAIN STEM NEURONS AND SLEEP STAGES

TRANSMITTERS/ NEURONS	AWAKE STAGE	SLOW WAVE STAGES	REM STAGE
Cholinergic	2+	0	2+
Monoamines	2+	1+	0

Source: After Saper et al., 2001.

CIRCADIAN TIMING SYSTEM AND ANATOMICAL BASIS OF SLEEP-WAKE CYCLES

Sleep-wake behavior occurs on an alternating cyclic basis, referred to as *circadian*. Other endocrine and hypothalamic functions also are subject to rhythmic variations over the period of approximately 24 hours, for example. secretion of growth hormone and of cortisol. Most nonprimate mammals sleep during the day and are awake at night. Primates, in general, sleep at night and are awake during the day. It is also evident that, these cyclic rhythms are also altered by the light-dark cycle. Experimental studies reviewed by Moore (1990) indicate that in the presence of constant light (referred to as free running), the cycle still occurs and *that the pacemaker for this rhythmic cycling is located in the suprachiasmatic nucleus of the hypothalamus*. The major projections of the suprachiasmatic nucleus are to other nuclei of the hypothalamus—primarily to the anterior hypothalamus. The hypothalamus has reciprocal connections to the brain stem reticular formation and projects to the nucleus basalis and to the cerebral cortex.

Additional studies have demonstrated a retinal hypothalamic pathway and a lateral geniculate hypothalamic pathway to this nucleus, allowing for the entrainment of this nucleus by visual, light-dark influences. An additional input is also present from the serotonin-secreting neurons of the midbrain raphe nucleus. The secretion of melatonin by the pineal gland is regulated by the suprachiasmatic nucleus. This hormone, in turn, can significantly modify the cyclic activity of neurons within the suprachiasmatic nucleus.

DISORDERS OF SLEEP

INSOMNIA

Insomnia is defined as an inability to enter a state of sleep. *Hyposomnia* is defined as a reduction in sleeping time.

- Both conditions may occur rarely on a neurological basis following lesions of the rostral hypothalamus and preoptic area or anterior or dorsomedial thalamus (Lugaresi, 1992).

- An infrequent cause of fragmented sleep with frequent awakenings is *central sleep apnea*, which may be due to the following conditions: (a) autonomic system lesions; (b) high spinal cord lesions, for example, bilateral cordotomy for control of pain; (c) medullary lesions; (d) abnormalities at the craniocervical junction; (e) muscular disorders; and (f) congestive heart failure. The changes in blood gases may result in significant effects on cardiac rhythm, and sudden death may occur.

- *The most common medical condition associated with insomnia relates to anatomical problems of the airway.* For example, patients with sleep apnea syndrome, particularly obstructive sleep apnea syndrome (who, as discussed later, also manifest excessive daytime sleepiness), will have frequent nocturnal awakenings. These patients who may be obese, have abnormalities of the pharynx, or short, crowded necks may have collapse of the pharynx and cessation of airflow, while diaphragmatic efforts continue, often resulting in snoring. More important from a physiological standpoint, hypoxemia often occurs (arterial pO_2 actually falls as measured by pulse oximetry) and CO_2 retention also occurs. With or without the fall in pO_2, the decrease in airway results in increased diaphragmatic effort and frequent arousals with fragmentation of sleep. As a result, the patient has excessive daytime sleepiness.[2]

- *The most frequent causes of disorders* affecting the initiation and maintenance of sleep (the insomnias) relate to nonneurological factors: (1) poor sleep hygiene, including excessive daytime sleep in elderly patients; (2) underlying psychiatric disorder; (3) pharmacologic factors; and (4) alterations in sleep-wake cycle, jet lag, and so on.

EXCESSIVE DAYTIME SLEEPINESS

As with insomnia, the major causes of excessive somnolence, particularly daytime somnolence, are not associated with specific neuropathological causes.

In most patients, excessive daytime sleepiness is a reflection of poor nighttime sleep. This includes sleep apnea; such cases may be studied with all-night sleep studies utilizing polysomnography.

Specific neuropathological lesions producing somnolence are not common. Tumors or encephalitis or infarcts (Fig. 29.15) involving the areas cited in Table 29.10 may produce somnolence (Culebras, 1992).

Narcolepsy

Narcolepsy is a disorder characterized by paroxysmal attacks of sleep and of a desire to sleep. Following a period of sleep that varies from minutes to hours, the patient awakens refreshed. As in normal sleep, the patient can often be aroused from sleep by strong stimulation. Most cases have no known structural pathology and the neurological examination is normal. At times, a family history of a similar disorder is present. The specific genetic aspects are not clear, whether multifactorial or autosomal dominant remains uncertain. There is

---

[2] The effects of hypoxemia, of CO_2 retention, and of the apneas are much more complex. The responses of the respiratory centers to hypoxia and hypercapnia may be altered (see Grunstein and Sullivan, 1990). Changes in heart rate and rhythms may occur with fatal arrhythmias, resulting in sudden death during sleep (see Krieger, 1990).

Figure 29.15 Excessive daytime sleepiness. Computerized tomography scans, which had been normal 7 years previously, now demonstrated bilateral thalamic paramedian infarcts confirmed on magnetic resonance imaging. Angiograms, echocardiogram, and cerebrospinal fluid were normal and electrocardiogram nonspecific. This 64-year-old, right-handed, usually extroverted male had the acute onset of excessive nocturnal snoring and the following day fell asleep on multiple occasions even while driving. He also had a change in personality, failure to complete his thoughts, and problems in recognition of familiar photographs. Examination, 6 days later, demonstrated only hypertension (180/100), a subdued appearance, a decrease in spontaneous speech, and finger agnosia. He returned to baseline within 3 weeks and had no additional episodes over the next 4 years.

occurrence of periods of desynchronized sleep and rapid eye movements in these patients shortly after onset of sleep (as contrasted to normal where such episodes do not occur for 90 minutes). In the multiple sleep latency tests, five daytime, 20-minute naps are offered at 2-hour intervals. Mean sleep latency and mean REM sleep latency after onset of sleep are calculated. Patients with narcolepsy have daytime sleep latencies of approximately 2–3 minutes; control subjects, 7–12 minutes. Within the 20-minute nap periods, all patients with narcolepsy will have two or more REM periods. (REM within 15 minutes of sleep onset is referred to as REM-onset sleep, as demonstrated in Fig. 29.16.) In the human, the most effective agents in preventing the narcolepsy are those drugs that enhance the presynaptic release of norepinephrine. Agents include methylphenidate and pemoline. The tricyclic antidepressants, such as Protriptyline, are effective in preventing the cataplexy, through blockage of norepinephrine and serotonin reuptake.

COMA IN THE HUMAN

In discussing depression of consciousness in the human, we will consider separately two aspects: (1) the patient who presents at the emergency room or on the general wards of the hospital with acute or subacute onset of coma; and (2) the patient with prolonged depression of consciousness.

EMERGENCY ONSET OF COMA

In the emergency room evaluation of the patient in coma of relatively acute onset, the physician is concerned with the differentiation of three general etiologic categories as presented in Table 29.12.

PROLONGED DISTURBANCES OF CONSCIOUSNESS

There are two major causes: (1) *intrinsic diencephalic and mesencephalic disorders* as in infarcts or infiltrating gliomas (as discussed earlier, von Economo's encephalitis was once included in this category); (2) *disorders producing a diffuse loss of neurons in cerebral cortex* as in cardiac arrest with anoxic encephalopathy and laminar necrosis.

An apathetic-drowsy state may occur in relation to bilateral infraction of the frontal lobe and basal forebrain territory within the distribution of the anterior cerebral arteries, as in anterior communicating-anterior cerebral aneurysms.

It is evident than that from an anatomical standpoint, the conscious state reflects a complex interaction between brain stem structures, diencephalic structures, and the basal forebrain areas, on the one hand, and the cerebral cortex, on the other. *Without functional neocortex, consciousness does not exist. Thus, patients with cerebral anoxia resulting in widespread laminar necrosis of the cerebral cortex are in a state of irreversible coma.*

CARE OF THE COMATOSE PATIENT

Several general rules must be followed if life is to be preserved in the comatose patient until such time as recovery has

a relationship to the HLA (human leukocyte antigen—histocompatibility complex) located on chromosome 6, linked gene—DW-2 (see Honda and Matsuki, 1990). There is no relation to epilepsy.

As regards the underlying basis for narcolepsy, recent studies summarized by Silber and Rye (2001) indicate a marked decrease in the content of a peptide, hypocretin-1 (Hert-1) synthesized by the cells of the ventral and lateral hypothalamus in the brains and cerebrospinal fluid of patients with narcolepsy. These neurons innervate all of the cholinergic and monoaminergic arousal centers discussed earlier.

Many of the patients with narcolepsy manifest other periodic disorders that occur frequently enough to be grouped within the tetrad of the narcolepsy syndrome: cataplexy, sleep paralysis, and hypnogenic hallucinations.

Cataplexy refers to a sudden loss of muscle tone and of postural reflexes, usually occurring in relation to laughter or sudden emotional stimulation. *Sleep paralysis* refers to episodes of inability to move and occurs in relation to the process of falling asleep or awakening. *Hypnogenic hallucinations* are vivid sensory, dream-like experiences that occur upon awakening. Many aspects of the narcolepsy syndrome have been related to the desynchronized, rapid eye movement (REM) stage of sleep. Thus, the multiple sleep latency tests will demonstrate the early

MULTIPLE SLEEP LATENCY TEST
Time of Nap

	Nap 1	Nap 2	Nap 3	Nap 4	Nap 5
Start Time	08:01:02	10:00:34	12:00:16	14:00:14	16:01:12
Stage 1 Latency	1.0	2.5	2.0	1.5	3.0
Stage 2 Latency	3.0	5.0	4.0	4.0	5.0
Stage 3/4 Latency	-	-	-	-	-
REM Latency	4.5	12.5	-	-	-

Mean Sleep Latency (4 naps):
Mean Sleep Latency (5 naps): 2.0 min
Number of REM onsets: 2(Two)

Figure 29.16 Narcolepsy. Multiple sleep latency tests demonstrating mean sleep latency for five naps of 2 minutes with REM onsets in the first two naps at 4.5 and 12.5 minutes. In contrast, the all-night sleep study demonstrated sleep onset at 6.7 minutes and REM onset at 60–90 minutes. This 32-year-old woman had a 7-year history of falling asleep during the day, if sitting at the table or in a car. She also had episodes of sleep paralysis. Her mother had narcolepsy. (Courtesy of Sleep Disorders Institute of Central New England/Dr. Jay Phadke.)

occurred. The ABC (airway, breathing, circulation) approach has already been presented in relation to the management of status epilepticus. The patient must be placed on the side and turned every 2 hours to avoid aspiration and passive congestion of the lungs. This will also serve to avoid decubitus ulcers. Joints must be manipulated passively through their full range of motion several times per day to avoid contractions. The legs should be protected from the weight of bedclothes by cradle. Sandbags should maintain physiological ankle extension. Pressure areas should be protected by foam rubber to avoid decubitus ulcers.

Suctioning is required at periodic intervals to avoid aspiration of nasal and oral secretions. While the intravenous route may provide fluids and glucose temporarily, this will not allow administration of adequate protein, lipids, and carbohydrates. Careful nasogastric feeding will be required to maintain nutritional status, in the short term. After 7–10 days, if swallowing reflexes have not returned, the placement of a percutaneous gastrostomy or jejunostomy should be considered. Nutritional intake and urinary output must be recorded. A condom catheter or indwelling catheter will be required with periodic replacement. Urinary tract and respiratory infections must be treated with antibiotics, but prophylactic antibiotics should not be administered. Constipation and fecal impaction should be avoided by the periodic use of mild cathartics. Enemas may be required. Low-dosage subcutaneous heparin may be administered to prevent thrombophlebitis.

PROGNOSIS IN COMA

Management of the neurological patient includes not only diagnosis of the underlying location of lesion and of the underlying neuropathology but also assessment of the prognostic implications of the diagnosis. From the standpoint of advice to the family of the comatose patient, and from the standpoint of allocation of limited, costly intensive care resources, early assessment must be made as to the likelihood of survival and recovery. This is best done in a uniform, reproducible, and, if possible, quantitative manner. Considering coma in general, prognosis also relates in general to age of patient and etiology.

The prognosis for patients with coma secondary to head injuries or intracranial hemorrhage often is better than for patients with coma secondary to cardiac arrest. For such patients, the standard method utilized is the Glasgow Coma Scale. Values are assigned for (a) degrees of eye opening (E): spontaneous = 4, nil = 1; (b) best motor response (M) obeys = 6, nil = 1; (c) verbal response (V) oriented = 5, nil = 1. The total coma scale is then computed E + M + V and may range from 3 to

Table 29.12 **ETIOLOGY OF COMA OF ACUTE ONSET**

MAJOR CATEGORY	FREQUENCY	MECHANISM	CLINICAL EVALUATION
Toxic/ metabolic/ diffuse	68%	Diffuse biochemical disorder, e.g., alcohol intoxication hypoglycemia, overdoses, ketoacidosis, anoxia, encephalitis	Early depression of consciousness without focal findings
Supratentorial	18%	Herniation due to mass lesions with compression of brain stem, e.g., tumor or abscess of temporal lobe, intracerebral hemorrhage, massive middle cerebral artery infarct	Lateralized hemisphere findings before brain stem findings, then herniation lateral (ipsilateral fixed dilated pupil then bilateral findings) or central (Cheyne Stokes respiration then bilateral midbrain with bilateral fixed pupils) with progressive rostral-caudal deterioration of brain stem function
Infratentorial	10%	Direct damage to brain stem: basilar artery thrombosis, pontine hemorrhage	Onset with brain stem findings usually bilateral, e.g., bilateral pyramidal tract and pontine findings

Source: Adapted from Plum and Posner (1966).

15. There is a clear-cut correlation: patients with a low scale are unlikely to recover; those with a high score are very likely to survive with a good quality of survival.

Essentially, most patients with cardiac arrest outside of the cardiac intensive care unit have a very poor prognosis. For assessing recovery after hypoxic ischemic coma or other forms of nontraumatic coma, Levy et al. (1985) have utilized evaluation of brain stem reflexes (including eye movements, corneal and pupillary responses), motor responses, and verbal responses. Patients who, at first assessment, within the first 24 hours (usually at 6 or 12 hours after onset), had no corneal, pupillary, or oculovestibular (caloric) responses did not recover or remained in a chronic vegetative state, in 97% of cases. Only 1% had a good recovery or moderate disability. By 24 hours, if three of the following (corneal, pupillary or oculovestibular, or motor responses) were not reactive, 98% remained in vegetative state or had no recovery.

Absence of pupillary responses at initial examination was associated with no recovery or vegetative state in 94%, severe disability in 6%. Failure to regain brain stem reflexes by 24 hours is an extremely poor prognostic sign; essentially no patient recovers. At one day, the absence of motor withdrawal and of spontaneous eye movements was associated with no recovery or vegetative state in 95% and severe disability in 4%. If brain stem reflexes have recovered by 24 hours, failure to regain consciousness by day three has a poor prognosis; failure to regain signs of consciousness by day 7, an even bleaker prognosis. At 7 days, absence of motor response to commands and absence of spontaneous eye movements were associated with no recovery or vegetative state outcome in 100% of cases (see Maiese and Caronna, 1988).

The use of the EEG and of evoked potentials may also be of help in assessing prognosis (Marcus and Stone, 1984).

BIBLIOGRAPHY

PART I: SEIZURES AND EPILEPSY

GENERAL CLASSIFICATION AND HISTORICAL

Browne, T. R., and Holmes, G. L. 2001. Epilepsy. N. Engl. J. Med. 344:1145–1151.

Commission on Classification and Terminology International League Against Epilepsy. 1985. Proposal for classification of epilepsies and epileptic syndromes. Epilepsia 26:268–278.

Delgado-Escueta, A. V., Ward, A., Woodbury, D. M., and Porter, R. J. 1986. Advances in Neurology Vol. 44. Basic Mechanisms of the Epilepsies—Molecular and Cellular Approaches. New York, NY: Raven Press.

Delgado-Escueta, A. V., Olsen, R. W., Wilson, W. A., and Porter, R. J. (Eds.). 1999. Advances in Neurology, Vol. 79. Jasper's Basic Mechanisms of the Epilepsies. 3rd ed. Philadelphia: Lippincott Williams and Wilkins.

Dreifuss, F. E. International League Against Epilepsy proposal for revised clinical and electroencephalographic classification of epileptic seizures. 1981. Epilepsia 22:489–501.

Engel, J., Jr., and Pedley, T. A. (Eds.). 1998. Epilepsy: A Comprehensive Textbook, Vols. 1–3. Philadelphia, PA: Lippincott Raven.

Gibbs, F. A., Davis, H., and Lennox, W. G. 1935. The electroencephalogram in epilepsy and in conditions of impaired consciousness. Arch. Neurol. Psychiat. 34:1133–1148.

Gibbs, F. A., and Gibbs, E. L. 1952. Atlas of Electroencephalography, Vol. 2. Epilepsy. Cambridge, MA: Addison Wesley Press.

Gloor, P. (Ed. & Trans.) 1969. Hans Berger: on the electroencepalogram of man. Electroencephalog. Clin. Neurophys. Suppl 28, pp. 1–36.

Jasper, H. H., and Kershman, J. 1941. Electroencephalographic classification of the epilepsies. Arch. Neurol. Psychiat. 45:903.

Luders, H. O., and Nochtar, S. (Eds.). 2000. Epileptic seizures, pathophysiology and clinical semiology. New York, NY: Churchill Livingstone.

Muskens, L. J. J. 1928. Epilepsy: Comparative Pathoqenesis. Symptoms. Treatment. New York, NY: William Wood.

Porter, R. J., and Chadwick, D. (Eds.). 1997. The Epilepsies 2. Boston, MA: Butterworth Heinemann

Prince, D. A.1978. Neurophysiology of epilepsy. Ann. Rev. Neurosci. 1:395–415.

Purpura, D. P., Penry, J. K., Tower, D. B., Woodbury, D. M., and Walter, R. D. (Ed.). 1972. Experimental Models of Epilepsy. New York, NY: Raven Press.

Temkin, O. 1945. The Falling Sickness. Baltimore, MD: Johns Hopkins Press.

Tharp, B. R. 1986. Neonatal and Pediatric Electroencephalography. In M. J. Aminoff (Ed.) Electrodiagnosis in Clinical Neurology. 2nd ed., pp. 77–124. New York, NY: Churchill Livingstone.

Tyner, F. S., Knott, J. R., and Mayer, W. B., Jr. 1983. Fundamentals of EEG Technology, Vol. 1. Basic Concepts and Methods. New York, NY: Raven Press.

Wyllie, E. (Ed.). 1997. The Treatmentof Epilepsy: Principles and Practice. 2nd ed. Baltimore, MD: Williams and Wilkins.

SPECIFIC REFERENCES AND CITATIONS

Ajmone-Marsan, C. 1969. Acute effects of topical epileptogenic agents. In H. H. Jasper, A. A. Ward, and A. Pope (Eds.) Basic Mechanisms of the Epilepsies, pp. 96–110. Boston, MA: Little, Brown.

Andermann, F. 1990. Unanswered clinical questions in generalized epilepsy. In M. Avoli, P. Gloor, G. Kostopoulos, and R. Naquet, (Eds.) Generalized Epilepsy: Neurobiological Approaches, pp.30–35. Boston, MA: Birkhauser.

Annegers, J. F., Shirts, S. B., Hauser, W. A., and Kurland, L. T. 1986. Risk of recurrence after an initial unprovoked seizure. Epilepsia 27:43–50.

Arcelli, P., Frassoni, M. C., Regondi, M. C., De Biasi, S., and Spreafico, R. 1997. GABAergic neurons in mammalian thalamus: a marker of thalamic complexity. Brain Res. Bull. 42:27–37.

Avoli, M., Gloor, P., and Kostopoulos, G. 1990. Focal and generalized epileptiform activity in the cortex: in search of differences in synaptic mechanisms in ionic movements and long-lasting changes in neuronal excitability. In M. Avoli, P. Gloor, G. Kostopoulos, and R. Naquet (Eds.) Generalized Epilepsy: Neurobiological Approaches, pp. 213–231. Boston, MA: Birkhauser.

Babb, T. L., and Pretorius, J. K. 1997. Pathologic substrates of epilepsy. In E. Wyllie (Ed.) The Treatment of Epilepsy: Principles and Practice. 2nd ed., pp. 106–121. Baltimore, MD: Williams &Wilkins.

Barclay, J., and Rees, M. 1999. Mouse models of spike-wave epilepsy. Epilepsia 40(Suppl. 3):17–22.

Berkovic, S. F., Andermann, F., Andermann, E., and Gloor, P. 1987. Concepts of absence epilepsy: discrete syndromes or biological continuum? Neurology 37:993–1000.

Berkovic, S. F., Andermann, F., Carpenter, S., et al. 1986. Progressive myoclonus epilepsies: specific cases and diagnosis. N. Engl. J. Med. 315:296–305.

Berkovic, S. F., So, N. K., and Andermann, F. 1991. Progressive myoclonus epilepsies: clinical and neurophysiological diagnosis. J. Clin. Neurophysiol. 8:261–274.

Buchhalter, J. 1993. The pathophysiology of the genetic epilepsies: what have we learned from animal models? Epilepsia 34:S31–S41.

Carlen, D. L., Daviews, M. F., Rougier-Naquet, I., Reynolds, J. N., and Spigelman, I. 1990. Sedative drug withdrawal seizures: cellular electrophysiological mechanisms. In M. Avoli, P. Gloor, G., Kostopoulos, and R. Naquet (Eds.) Generalized Epilepsy: Neuro-Biological Approaches, pp. 460–470. Boston, MA: Birkhauser.

Caveness, W. F. 1969. Ontogeny of focal seizures. In H. H. Jasper, A. A. Ward, and A. Pope (Eds.) Basic Mechanisms of the Epilepsies, pp. 517–534. Boston, MA: Little, Brown.

Chugani, H. T., Showman, D. A., Sankar, R., Chen, B. C., and Phelps, M. E. 1992. Infantile spasms. II. Lenticular nuclei and brain stem activation on positron emission tomography. Ann. Neurol. 31:212–219.

Duchowny, M., Jayakar, P., and Levin, B. 2000. Aberrant neural circuits in malformations of cortical development and focal epilepsy, Neurology. 55:423–428.

Engel, J. 1989. Seizures and epilepsy. Annals of Neurology. 28(3):398.

Genton, P. 1995. Epilepsy with 3 hz spike and waves without clinically evident absences. In J. S. Duncan and C. P. Panayiotopoulos (Eds.) Typical Absences and Related Epileptic Syndromes, pp. 231–238. Edinburgh, UK: Churchill Livingstone.

Connors, B. W. 1998. Neocortical anatomy and physiology. In J. Engel, Jr. and T. A. Pedley (Eds.) Epilepsy: A Comprehensive Textbook, pp. 307–321. Philadelphia, PA: Lippincott-Raven.

Dam, A. M., Fuglsang-Frederiksen, A., Svarpe-Olsen, U., and Dam, M. 1985. Late onset epilepsy: etiologies, types of seizures, value of clinical investigation, EEG and computerized tomography scan. Epilepsia 26:227–231.

Delgado-Escueta, A. V. 1982. Status epilepticus. N. Engl. J. Med. 306: 1337–1340.

Delgado-Escueta, A. V., Greenberg, D. A., Treiman, L., et al. 1989. Mapping the gene for juvenile myoclonic epilepsy. Epilepsia 30(Suppl. 4):S8–S18.

Delgado-Escueta, A. V., Janz, D., and Beck-Mannagetta, G. 1992. Pregnancy and teratogenesis in epilepsy. Neurology 42(Suppl. 5):1–160.

Delgado-Escueta, A. V., Olsen, R. W., Wilson, W. A., and Porter, R. J. 1999. Introduction to the idiopathic epilepsies. In A. V. Delgado-Escueta, R. W. Olsen, W. A. Wilson, and R. J. Porter (Eds.) Advances in Neurology, Vol. 79. Jasper's Basic Mechanisms of the Epilepsies. 3rd ed, 219–225. Philadelphia, PA: Lippincott Williams and Wilkins.

Delgado-Escueta, A. V., Wasterlain, C. G., Treiman, D. M., and Porter, R. J. (Eds.). 1983. Advances in Neurology, Vol. 34. Status Epilepticus. New York, NY: Raven Press.

Doose, H., and Gerken, H. J. 1973. On the genetics of EEG anomalies in childhood IV. Photoconvulsive reaction. Neuropedia 4:57–75.

Doose, H., Gerken, H. J., and Horstman, T., et al. 1973. Genetic factors in spike wave absences. Epilepsia 14:57–75.

Dreifuss, F. E. 1989. Juvenile myoclonic epilepsy: characteristics of a primary generalized epilepsy. Epilepsia 30(Suppl. 4):S1–7.

Ebersole, J. S. 1987. Physiological substrates of normal and abnormal EEG activity. In O. M. Markand and R. P. Brenner (Eds.) Annual Course Syllabus: State of the Science in Clinical EEG and Electrophysiology. Vol. 1, pp. 101–126. Atlanta, GA: American EEG Society.

Ebersole, J. S., and Chatt, A. B. 1986. Spread and arrest of seizures: the importance of layer 4 in laminar interactions during neocortical epileptogenesis. In A. V. Delgado-Escueta, A. A. Ward, D. M. Woodbury, and R. J. Porter (Eds.) Advances in Neurology, Vol. 44. Basic Mechanisms of the Epilepsies Molecular and Cellular Approaches, pp.545–558. New York, NY: Raven Press.

Engel, J., Jr. 1989. Seizures and Epilepsy. Philadelphia, PA: F. A. Davis (Chapter 4: Basic Mechanisms of Epilepsy, pp.71–111)

Fahn, S., Marsden, C. D., and VanWoert, M. H. (Eds.). 1986. Myoclonus. New York, NY: Raven Press.

Gale, K. 1990. Animal models of generalized convulsive seizures: some neuroanatomical differentiation of seizure types. In M. Avoli, P. Gloor, G. Kostopoulos, and R. Naquet (Eds.) Generalized Epilepsy; Neurobiological Approaches, pp. 329–343. Boston, MA: Birkhauser.

Gastaut, H., Gastaut, Y., Concalves, J. L., et al. 1975. Relative frequency of different types epilepsy: a study employing the classification of the International League Against Epilepsy. Epilepsia 16:457–461.

Gastaut, H., Roger, J., Soulayrol, R., Tassinari, C. A., et al. 1966. Childhood epileptic encephalopathy with diffuse slow spike waves (otherwise known as petit mal variant or Lennox syndrome). Epilepsia 7:139–179.

Genton, P. 1995. Epilepsy with 3 hz spike and waves without clinically evident absences. In J. S. Duncan and C. Panayiotopoulos (Eds.) Typical Absences and Related Epileptic Syndromes, pp. 231–238. Edinburgh, UK: Churchill Livingstone.

Gloor, P., Avoli, M., and Kostopoulos, G. 1990. Thalamocortical relationships in generalized epilepsy with bilateral synchronous spike and wave discharges. In M. Avoli, P. Gloor, G. Kostopoulos, and R. Naquet (Eds.) Generalized Epilepsy: Neurobiological Approaches, pp. 190–212. Boston, MA: Birkhauser.

Gloor, P., Ball, G., and Schul, N. 1977. Brain lesions that produce delta waves in the electroencephalogram. Neurology 27:326–333.

Goddard, G. V. 1967. The development of epileptic seizures through brain stimulation at low intensity. Nature 214:1020–1021.

Hauser, W. A. 1986. Should people be treated after a first seizure? Arch. Neurol. 43:1287–1288.

Hunter, J., and Jasper, H. H. 1949. Effects of thalamic stimulation in unanaesthetised animals. Electroencephalog. Clin. Neurophysiol. 1:305–324.

Ingvar, D. H. 1955. Electrical activity of isolated cortex in the unanesthetized cat with intact brain stem. Acta Physiol. Scand. 33:151–168.

Jacobson, S., and Marcus, E. M. 1970. The laminar distribution of fibers of the corpus callosum: a comparative study in the rat, cat, Rhesus monkey and Chimpanzee. Brain Res. 24:517–520.

Janqua, N. A., and Andermann, E. 1989. Amino acids in the epilepsies. In D. Janz et al. (Eds.) Genetics of the Epilepsies, pp. 1–18. Heidelberg, Germany: Spinger Verlag.

Janqua, N. A., Metrakos, J. D., and VanGelder, N. M. 1982. Plasma amino acids in epilepsy. In V. E. Anderson, W. A. Hauser, J. K. Penry, and C. F. Sing (Eds.) Genetic Basis of the Epilepsies, pp.181–197. New York, NY: Raven Press.

Janz, D., and Christian, W. 1957. Impulsive petit mal. Dtsch. Z. Nervenheilk 176:346–386.

Janz, D., Dam, M., Richens, A., et al. (Eds.). 1982. Epilepsy Pregnancy and the Child. New York, NY: Raven Press. (See in particular Chapters by D. Janz On major malformations and minor anomalies in the offspring of parents with epilepsy. Also, Chapter by E. Andermann)

Jasper, H. H. 1969. Mechanisms of propagation: extracellular studies. In (Ed.) H. H. Jasper, A. A. Ward, Jr., & A. Pope (Eds.) Basic Mechanisms of the Epilepsies, pp. 421–438. Boston, MA: Little, Brown.

Jasper, H. H. 1990. Historical background. In M. Avoili, P. Gloor, G. Kostopoulos, and R. Naquet (Eds.) Generalized Epilepsy: Neuro-Biological Approaches, pp. 1–5. Boston, MA: Birkhauser.

Jasper, H. H., and Droogleever-Fortuyn, J. 1946. Experimental studies on the functional anatomy of petit mal epilepsy. Assoc. Res. Nerv. Dis. Proc. 26:272–298.

Jennett, W. B. 1975. Epilepsy After Blunt Head Injury. 2nd ed. London, UK: Heinemann.

Julien, R. W., Fowler, G. W., and Danielson, M. G. 1975. The effects of antiepileptic drugs on estrogen-induced electrographic spike wave discharge. J. Pharmacol. Exp. Ther. 193:647–656.

Juul-Jensen, P., and Foldspars, A. 1983. Natural history epileptic seizures. Epilepsia 24:297–312.

Killam, K. F., Killam, E. K., and Naquet, R. 1967. An animal model of light sensitive epilepsy, Electroencephalog. Clin. Neurophysiol. 22:497–513.

Killiam, K. F., Naquet, R., and Bert, J. 1966. Paroxysmal responses to intermittent light stimulation in a population of baboons (Papio papio). Epilepsia 7:215–219.

Loiseau, P. 1985. Childhood absence epilepsy. In J. Roger, C. Dravet, M. Bureau, F. E. Dreifuss, and P. Wolf (Eds.) Epileptic Syndromes in Infancy, Childhood and Adolescence, pp.106–120. London, UK: John Libbey.

Luhdorf, K., Jensen, L. K., and Plesner, A. M. 1988. Etiology of epilepsy in the elderly. Epilepsia 27:459–463, 1986.

Magistris, M. R., Mouradian, M. S., and Gloor, P. 1988. Generalized convulsions induced by pentylenetetrazol in the cat: participation of forebrain, brainstem and spinal cord. Epilepsia 29:379–388.

Marcus, E. M. 1972. Experimental models of petit mal epilepsy. In D. P. Purpura, J. K. Penry, D. B. Tower, D. M. Woodbury, and R. D. Walter (Eds.) Experimental Models of Epilepsy, pp. 113–146. New York, NY: Raven Press.

Marcus, E. M. 1985. Generalized seizure models and the corpus callosum. In A. Reeves (Ed.) Epilepsy and the Corpus Callosum, pp.131–206. New York, NY: Plenum Press.

Marcus, E. M., and Watson, C. W. 1966. Bilateral synchronous spike wave patterns in the cat. Arch. Neurol. 14:601–610.

Marcus, E. M., and Watson, C. W. 1968. Bilateral symmetrical epileptogenic foci in monkey cerebral cortex: mechanisms of interaction and regional variations in capacity for synchronous spike slow wave discharges. Arch. Neurol. 19:99–116.

Marcus, E. M., Watson, C. W., and Jacobson, S. 1969. Role of the corpus callosum in bilateral synchronous discharges induced by intravenous pentylenetetrazol. Neurology 19:309.

Marcus, E. M., Watson, C. W., and Simon, S. A. 1968. An experimental model of some varieties of petit mal epilepsy. Epilepsia 9:233–248.

Marseille Consensus Group. 1990. Classification of progressive myo-clonus epilepsies and related disorders. Ann. Neurol. 28:113–116.

Mattson, R. H. 1990. Alcohol related seizures. In Porter et al. (Eds.) Alcohol and Seizures: Basic Mechanisms and Clinical Concepts, pp.143–147. Philadelphia, PA: F. A. Davis.

Mattson, R. H., Cramer, J. A., Collins, J. F., et al. 1985. Comparison of carbamazepine, phenobarbital, phenytoin and primidone in partial and secondarily generalized tonic clonic seizures. N. Engl. J. Med. 313:145–151.

Mattson, R. H., Cramer, J. A., Collins, J. F., and The Department of Veterans Affairs Epilepsy Cooperative Study No. 264 Group. 1992. A comparison of valproate with carbamazepine for the treatment of complex partial seizures and secondarily generalized tonic clonic seizures in adults. N. Engl. J. Med. 327:765–771.

McDonald, J. W., Garofalo, E. A., Hood, T., et al. 1991. Altered excitatory and inhibitory amino acid receptor binding in hippocampus of patients with temporal lobe epilepsy. Ann. Neurol. 29:529–541.

McNamara, J. O. 1999. Emerging insights into the genesis of epilepsy. Nature (Supp.):A15–A22.

McQueen, J. K., Woodbury, D. M. 1975. Attempts to produce spike wave complexes in the electrocorticogram of the rat. Epilepsia 16:295–299.

Mayersdorf, A., and Schmidt, R. P. (Eds.). 1982. Secondary Epileptogenesis. New York, NY: Raven Press.

Meencke, H. J. 1984. Neuron density in the molecular layer of the frontal cortex in primary generalized epilepsy epilepsia. 26:450–454. (See also, Epilepsia 25:8–21, 1985)

Meencke, H. J. 1996. Pathological findings in childhood absence epilepsy. In S. E. Mole, R. E. Weller, H. H. Goebel (Eds.) Typical Absences and Related Epileptic Syndromes, pp. 122–132. Edinburgh, UK: Churchill Livingstone.

Meencke, H. J., and Janz, D. 1985. The significance of microdysgenesis in primary generalized epilepsy: an answer to the considerations of Lyon and Gastaut. Epilepsia 26:368–371.

Metrakos, K., and Metrakos, J. D. 1961. Genetics of convulsive disorders: part 2: genetic and EEG studies in centrencephalic epilepsy. Neurology 11:474–483.

Meyer, J. S., Charney, J. Z., Rivera, V. M., and Mathea, N. J. 1971. Seizures following cerebral embolization. Stroke 2:541–554.

Mirsky, A. F., and Duncan, C. C. 1990. Behavioral and electrophysiological studies of absence epilepsy. In M. Avoli, P. Gloor, G. Kostopoulos, and R. Naquet (Eds.) Generalized Epilepsy: Neurobiological Approaches, pp. 254–269. Boston, MA: Birkhauser.

Morrell, F. 1959/1960. Secondary epileptogenic lesions. Epilepsia 1:538–560.

Morrell, F. 1991. The role of secondary epileptogenesis in human epilepsy (Editorial). Arch. Neurol. 48:1221–1224.

Moshe, S. L., and Sperber, E. F. 1990. Substantia nigra mediated control of generalized seizures. In M. Avoli, P. Gloor, G. Kostopoulos, and R. Naquet (Eds.) Generalized Epilepsy: Neurobiological Approaches, pp. 355–367. Boston, MA: Birkhauser.

Musgrave, J., and Gloor, J. 1980. The role of the corpus callosum in interhemispheric synchrony of spike and wave discharge in feline generalized penicillin epilepsy. Epilepsia 21:369–378.

Mutani, R., Bergamini, L., Fariello, R., and Quattrocolo, G. 1973. Bilateral synchrony of epileptic discharge associated with chronic asymmetrical cortical foci. Electroencephalog. Clin. Neurophysiol. 34:53–59.

Mutani, R., and Fariello, R. 1969. Effeti Enectroencefalografice Comportamental d Foci Epileptogen Sperimentali Cronici Deposti in Modo Bilaerale e Simmetrico Sulla Corteccia del Gatto. Riv. Neurol. 39:521–529.

Naquet, R., and Valin, A. Focal discharges in photosensitive generalized epilepsy. In M. Avoli, P. Gloor, G. Kostopoulos, and R. Naquet (Eds.) Generalized Epilepsy: Neurobiological Approaches, pp. 273–285. Boston, MA: Birkhauser.

Naquet, R., and Wada, J. A. 1992. Role of the corpus callosum in photosensitive seizures of the epileptic baboon. In P. Chauveil, V. Delgado-Escueta, E. Halgren, and J. Bancaud (Eds.) Frontal Lobe Seizures and Epilepsies, pp. 579–587. New York, NY: Raven Press.

Obesco, J. A., Artieda, J., Rothwell, J. C., et al. 1998. Spike-wave complexes and fast components of cortically generated seizures. III. Synchronizing mechanisms. J. Neurophysiol. 80:1480–1494.

Ottino, C. A., Meglio, M., Rossi, G. F., and Tercero, E. 1971. An experimental study of the structures mediating bilateral synchrony of epileptic discharges of cortical origin. Epilepsia 12:299–311.

Pedley, T. A. 1988. Discontinuing anti-epileptic drugs (Editorial). N. Engl. J. Med. 318:982–984.

Pollen, D. A.1964. Intracellular studies of cortical neurons during thalamic induced wave and spike. Electroencephalog. Clin. Neurophysiol. 17:57–67.

Prasad, A. N., Prasad, C., and Stafstrom, C. E. 1999. Recent advances in the genetics of epilepsy: insights from human and animal studies. Epilepsia 40:1329–1352.

Prince, D., and Farrell, D. 1968. "Centrencephalic" spike wave discharges following parenteral penicillin injection in the cat. Neurology 19:309–310.

Quesney, L. F., Andermann, F., and Gloor, P. 1981. Dopaminergic mechanism in generalized photosensitive epilepsy. Neurology 31:1542–1544.

Quesney, L. F., and Reader, T. A. 1990. Role of dopamine in generalized photosensitive epilepsy: electroencephalographic and biochemical aspects. In M. Avoli, P. Gloor, G. Kostopoulos and R. Naquet (Eds.) Generalized Epilepsy Neurobioloqical Approaches, pp. 298–313. Boston, MA: Birkhauser.

Ribak, C. E. 1986. Neurocytology and chemistry of focal epilepsy. In T. A. Pedley and B. S. Meldrum (Eds.) Recent Advances in Epilepsy. Vol. 3, pp. 1–17. Edinburgh, UK: Churchill Livingstone.

Rodin, E., Onuma, T., Wasson, S., Prozak, J., and Rodin, M. 1971. Neuro-physiological mechanisms involved in non-focal grand mal seizures induced by Metrazol and Megimide. Electroencephalog. Clin. Neurophysiol. 30:62–72.

Schmidt, D. 1986. Toxicity of anti-epileptic drugs. In T. A. Pedley and B. S. Meldrum (Eds.) Recent Advances in Epilepsy. Vol. 3, pp. 211–232. Edinburgh, UK: Churchill/Livingstone.

Schmidt, R. P., and Wilder, B. T. 1968. Epilepsy. Volume 2 of Contemporary neurology series. MIT Press.

Selzer, M. E., and Richter, M. A. 1992. Cellular pathophysiology and pharmacology of epilepsy. In A. K. Asbury, G. M. McKhann, and W. I. McDonald (Eds.) Disease of the Nervous System: Clinical Neurobiology. 2nd ed., pp. 916–935. Philadelphia, PA: F. A. Davis.

Shinnar, S., Vining, E. P. A., Mellits, E. D., et al. 1985. Discontinuing anti-epileptic medication in children with epilepsy after 2 years without seizures: a prospective study. N. Engl. J. Med. 313:976–980.

Silva-Barrat, C., and Menini, C. H. 1990. Photosensitive epilepsy of the baboon: a generalized epilepsy with motor cortical origin. In M. Avoli, P. Gloor, G. Kostopoulos, and R. Naquet (Eds.) Generalized Epilepsy: Neurobiological Approaches, pp. 286. Boston, MA: Birkhauser.

Snead, O. C., III. 1994. Pathophysiological mechanisms of experimental generalized absence in rats. In A. Malafosse, P. Genton, E. Hirsh, D. Maresceau, D. Broglin, and R. Bernasconi (Eds.) Idiopathic Generalized Epilepsies: Clinical, Experimental and Genetic Aspects, pp. 133–150. London, UK: John Libbey.

Sourounder, P., and Sjogren, H. 1970. The concept of Alzheimer's disease and its clinical implications. In P. F. W. Wolstenholme and M. O'Connor (Eds.) Alzheimer's Disease and Related Conditions Ciba Foundation Symposium, pp. 11–32. London, UK: J. A. Churchill. (See also in same Symposium: Jacob, H.: Muscular Twitchings in Alzheimer's Disease, pp. 75–93)

Spencer, S. S., Spencer, D. D., Glaser, G. H., Williamson, P. D., and Mattson, R. H. 1984. More intense focal seizure types after callosal section: the role of inhibition. Ann. Neurol. 16:686–693.

Starzl, T. E., Niemer, W. T., Dell, M., and Fosgrave, P. R. 1953. Cortical and subcortical electrical activity in experimental seizures induced by Metrazol. J. Neuropathol. Exp. Neurol. 12:262–276.

Steinlein, O. K. 1999. Idiopathic epilepsies with a monogenic mode of inheritance. Epilepsia 40(Suppl. 3):9–11.

Steriade, M., Amzica, F., Neckelmann, D., and Timofeev, I. 1998. Spike-wave complexes and fastcomponents of cortically generated seizures. II. Extra and intacellular patterns. J. Neurophysiol. 80:1456–1479.

Steriade, M., and Contreras, D. 1998. Spike-wave complexes and fast components of cortically generated seizures. I. Role played by neocortex and thalamus. J. Neurophysiol. 80:1439–1455.

Swann, J. W., and Moshe, S. L. 1998. Developmental issues in animal models. In J. Engel and T. A. Pedley (Eds.) Epilepsy: A Comprehensive Textbook, pp. 467–479. Philadelphia, PA: Lippincott-Raven.

Taylor-Courval, D., and Gloor, P. 1984. Behavioral alteration associated with generalized spike and wave discharges in the EEG of the cat. Exp. Neurol. 83:167–186.

Thurston, J. H., Thurston, D. L., Hixon, B. B., and Keller, A. J. 1982. Prognosis in childhood epilepsy: additional follow-up of 148 children: 15–23 years after withdrawal of anticonvulsant therapy. N. Engl. J. Med. 306:831–836.

Timofeev, I., Grenier, F., and Steriade, M. 1998. Spike-wave complexes and fast components of cortically generated seizures. J. Neurophysiol. 80:1495–1513.

VanWoert, M. H., Rosenbau, D., Howieson, J., and Bowers, M. B., Jr. 1977. Long-term therapy of myoclonus and other neurological disorders with L-5 hydroxytryptophan and carbidopa. N. Engl. J. Med. 296:70–75.

Vas, G. A., and Cracco, J. B. 1990. Diffuse encephalopathies. In D. D. Daly and T. A. Pedley (Eds.) Current Practice of Electroencephalography, pp.371–399. New York, NY: Raven Press.

Velasco, F., and Velasco, M. 1990. Mesencephalic structures and tonic clonic generalized seizures. In M. Avoli, P. Gloor, G. Kostopoulos, et al. (Eds.) Generalized Epilepsy Neurobiological Approaches, pp. 368–384. Boston, MA: Birkhauser.

Vergnes, M., and Marescaux, C. 1994. Pathophysiological mechanisms underlying genetic absence epilepsy in rats. In A. Malafosse, P. Genton, E. Hirsch, C. Marescaux, D. Broglin, and R. Bernasconi (Eds.) Idiopathic Epilepsies: Clinical, Experimental and Genetic Aspects, pp. 151–168. London, UK: John Libbey.

Vergnes, M., Marescaux, C. H., DePaulis, A., Micheletti, G., and Warter, J. M. 1990. Spontaneous spike and wave discharges in Wistar rats: a model of generalized non-convulsive epilepsy. In M. Avoli, P. Gloor, G. Kostopoulos, and R. Naquet (Eds.) Generalized Epilepsy: Neurobiological Approaches, pp. 238–251. Boston, MA: Birkhauser.

Victor, M. 1990. Alcohol withdrawal seizures: an overview. In Porter et al. (Eds.) Alcohol and Seizures: Basic Mechanisms and Clinical Concepts, pp.148–161 Philadelphia, PA: F. A. Davis.

Walker, A. F. 1969. The propagation of epileptic discharge. Mod. Probl. Pharmacopsychiat. 13:13–28. Switzerland, S. Karger).

Ward, A. A., Jr. The epileptic neuron: chronic foci in animals and main. In H. G. Jasper, A. A. Ward, and A. Pope (Eds.) Basic Mechanisms of the Epilepsies, pp. 2630–2288. Boston, MA: Little, Brown.

Watson, C. W., and Marcus, E. M. 1962. The genetics and clinical significance of photogenic cerebral electrical abnormalities, myoclonus, and seizures. Trans. Amer. Neurol. Assoc. 87:251–253.

Westbrook, G. L. 2000. Seizures and epilepsy. In E. R. Kandel, J. H. Schwartz, and T. M. Jessell (Eds.) Principles of Neural Science, pp. 910–935. New York, NY: McGraw Hill.

Wiebe, S., Blume, W. T., Girvin, J. P., et al. 2001. A randomized controlled trial of surgery for temporal lobe epilepsy. N. Engl. J. Med. 341:311–318.

Wilder, B. J., and Morrell, F. 1967. Cellular behavior in secondary epileptic lesions. Neurology 17:1193–1204.

Wilder, B. J., and Schmidt, R. P. 1965. Propagation of epileptic discharge from chronic neocortical foci in monkey. Epilepsia 6:297–309.

Williams, D. 1953. A study of thalamic and cortical rhythms in petit mal. Brain 76:50–69.

Williams, D. 1965. The thalamus and epilepsy. Brain 88:539–556.

Woermann, F. G., Free, S. L., Koepp, M. J., Sisodiya, S. M., and Duncan, J. S. 1999. Abnormal cerebral structure in juvenile myoclonic epilepsy demonstrated with voxel-based analysis of MRI. Brain 122:2101–2107.

Woermann, F. G., Sisodiya, S. M., Free, S. L., and Duncan, J. S. 1998. Quantitative MRI in patients with idiopathic generalized epilepsy Evidence of widespread cerebral structural changes. Brain 121:1661–1667.

Wolf, P. 1985. Juvenile absence epilepsy. In J. Roger, C. Dravet, M. Bureau, F. E. Dreifuss, and P. Wolf (Eds.) Epileptic Syndromes in Infancy, Childhood and Adolescence, pp. 242–246. London, UK: John Libbey.

Woodcock, S., and Cosgrove, J. B. R. 1964. Epilepsy after the age of 50: a 5-year follow-up study. Neurology 14:34–40.

PART II: SLEEP AND COMA

GENERAL REFERENCES

Allredge, B. K., Gelb, A. M., Isaacs, S. M., et al. 2001. A comparison of lorazepam, diazepam and placebo for the treatment of out-of-hospital status epilepticus. N. Engl. J. Med. 345:631–637.

Arana, A., Wentworth, C. E., Ayuso-Mateos, J. L., and Arellano, P. M. 2010. Suicide-related events in patients treated with antiepileptic drugs. N. Engl. J. Med. 363:542–551.

Aldrich, M. S. 1996. Sleep disorders. Neurol. Clin. 14:493–674, 675–855.

Bernat, J. L. (Ed.). 1989. Ethical Issues in Neurologic Practice Neurologic Clinics. Philadelphia, PA: W. B. Saunders. (See in particular: Beresford, H. R.: Legal Aspects of Termination of Treatment Decisions, pp.775–788.)

Allredge, B. K., Gelb, A. M., Isaacs, S. M., et al. 2001. A comparison of lorazepam, diazepam and placebo for the treatment of out-of-hospital status epilepticus. N. Engl. J. Med. 345:631–637.

Arana, A., Wentworth, C. E., Ayuso-Mateos, J. L., and Arellano, P. M. 2010. Suicide-related events in patients treated with antiepileptic drugs. N. Engl. J. Med. 363:542–551.

Bernat, J. L. 1989. Ethical issues in brain death and multiorgan transplantation. Neurol. Clin. 7:715–728.

Cranford, R. E. 1990. The neurologist as ethics consultant and as a member of the institutional ethics committee. Neurol. Clin. 7:697–714.

Gert, B., Nelson, W. A., and Culver, C. M. 1989. Moral theory and neurology. Neurol. Clin. 7:681–696.

Nelson, W. A., Bernat, J. L. 1989. Decisions to withhold or terminate treatment. Neurol. Clin. 7:759–774.

Chokoverty, S. 2000a. Excessive daytime somnolence. In W. G. Bradley et al. (Eds.) Neurology in Clinical Practice, pp. 59–70. Boston, MA: Buttersworth Heiemann.

Chokoverty, S. 2000b. Sleep disorders. In W. G. Bradley et al. (Eds.) Neurology in Clinical Practice, pp. 1781–1828. Boston, MA: Butterworth Heiemann.

Culebras, A. (Ed.). 1992a. The neurology of sleep. Neurology 42: (Suppl. 6):1–94.

Plum, F., and Posner, J. B. 1980. The Diagnosis of Stupor and Coma. 3rd ed. Philadelphia, PA: F. A. Davis.

Thorpy, M. J. (Ed.) 1990. Handbook of Sleep Disorders, pp. 235–258. New York, NY: Marcel Dekker.

SPECIFIC REFERENCES AND CITATIONS

American Academy of Neurology. 1989. Position of the American Academy of Neurology on certain aspects of the care and management of the persistent vegetative state patient. Neurology 38:125–126.

Annas, G. J. 1990. Sounding board—Nancy Cruzan and the right to die case (Editorial). 323: 670–673.

Annas, G. J. 1991. Sounding board—the health care proxy and the living will. N. Engl. J. Med. 324:1210–1213.

Barrett, R., Merritt, H. H., and Wolf, A. 1972. Depression of consciousness as a result of cerebral lesions. Res. Publ. Assoc. Nerv. Ment. Dis. 45:241–272.

Bremer, F. 1935. Cerveau "isole" et physiologie du sommeil. C. R. Soc. Biol. (Paris) 118:1235–1241.

Chatrian, G. E. 1990. Coma, other states of altered responsiveness and brain death. In P. D. Daly and T. A. Pedley (Eds.) Current Practice of Electroencephalography. 2nd ed., pp. 425–487. New York, NY: Raven Press.

Chatrian, G. E. 1986. Electrophysiologic evaluation of brain death: a critical appraisal. In M. J. Aminoff (Ed.) Electrodiagnosis in Clinical Neurology. 2nd ed., pp. 669–736. New York, NY: Churchill Livingstone.

Clemente, C. D., and Sterman, M. B. 1967. Basal forebrain mechanisms for internal inhibition and sleep. Res. Publ. Assoc. Nerv. Ment. Dis. 45:127–147.

Claassen, J., Mayer, S. A., Kowalsky, R. G., et al. 2004. Detection of electrographic seizures with continuous EEG monitoring in critically ill patients. Neurology 62:1743–1748.

Culebras, A. 1992b. Neuroanatomic and neurologic correlates of sleep disturbances. Neurology 42(Suppl.6):19–27.

Grunstein, R. R., and Sullivan, C. E. 1990. Neural control of respiration during sleep. In M. J. Thorpy (Ed.) Handbook of Sleep Disorders, pp. 77–102. New York, NY and Basel, Switzerland: Marcel Dekker.

Elliott, R. E., Morsi, A., Kalhorn, S. P., et al. 2011. Vagus nerve stimulation in 436 consecutive patients with treatment-resistant epilepsy: long term outcomes and predictors of success. Epilepsy Behav 2011:20:57–63.

Honda, Y., and Matsuki, K. 1990. Genetic aspects of narcolepsy. In M. J. Thorpy (Ed.) Handbook of Sleep Disorders, pp. 217–234. New York, NY and Basel, Switzerland: Marcel Dekker.

Jennett, W. B., and Bond, M. 1975. Assessment of outcome after severe brain damage. Lancet 1:470–484.

Jennett, W. B., and Plum, F. 1972. The persistent vegetative state a syndrome in search of a name. Lancet 1:734–737.

Jennett, B., and Teasdale, G.1977. Aspects of Coma After Severe Head Injury. Lancet 1:878–881.

Jouvet, M. 1967. Mechanisms of the state of sleep: a neuropharmacological approach. Res. Publ. Assoc. Nerv. Ment. Dis. 45:86–126.

Kellaway, P., Gol, A., and Proler, M. 1966. Electrical activity of the isolated cerebral hemisphere and isolated thalamus. Exper. Neurol. 14:281–304.

Krieger, J. 1990. Obstructive sleep apnea: clinical manifestations and pathophysiology. In M. J. Thorpy (Ed.) Handbook of Sleep Disorders, pp. 259–284. New York, NY and Basel, Switzerland: Marcel Dekker.

Levy, D. E., Caronna, J. J., Singer, B. H., Lapinski, R. H., Frydman, H., and Plum, F. 1985. Predicting outcome from hypoxic-ischemic coma. JAMA. 253:1420–1426.

Lieberson, A. D. 1992. Advance Medical Directives. Deerfield, IL: Clard, Boardman, Callagher.

Lindsley, D. B., Bowden, J., and Magoun, H. W. 1949. Effect upon the EEG of acute injury to the brain stem activating system. Electroencephalogr. Clin. Neurophysiol. 1:475–486.

Lugaresi, E. 1992. The thalamus and insomnia. Neurology 42:(Suppl. 6):28–33.

Lynn, J. (Chair). 1981. Guidelines for the determination of death. Report of the Medical Consultants on the Diagnosis of Death to the President's Commission for the Study of Ethical Problems in Medicine and Biomedical and Behavioral Research. JAMA. 246: 2184–2186.

Magoun, H. W. 1963. The Waking Brain. Springfield, IL: Charles C. Thomas.

Maiese, K., and Caronna, J. J. 1988. Coma after cardiac arrest: clinical features, prognosis and management. In A. H. Ropper and S. F. Kennedy (Eds.) Neurological and Neurosurgical Intensive Care. 2nd ed., pp. 233–245. Rockville, MD: Aspen Publishers.

Marcus, E., and Stone, B. 1984. Short latency median nerve somatosensory evoked potentials in coma: relationship to BAER, etiology, age and outcome. In R. Nodar & C. Barber (Eds.) Evoked Potentials II, pp. 609–623. Boston, MA: Butterworth,

Marcus, E. M., and Watson, C. W. 1966. Studies of the bilateral cortical callosal preparation. Trans. Am. Neuro. Assoc. 91:291–293.

Misra, U. K., Kalita, J., and Maurya, P. K. 2012. Levitiracetam versus lorazepam in status epilepticus: a randomized open labeled pilot study. J. Neurol. 259(4):645–648.

Moore, R. Y. 1990. The circadian timing system and the organization of sleep-wake behavior. In M. J. Thorpy (Ed.) Handbook of Sleep Disorders, pp. 103–115. New York, NY and Basel, Switzerland: Marcel Dekker.

Moruzzi, G., & Magoun, H. W. 1949. Brain stem reticular formation and activation of the EEG. Electroencephalogr. Clin. Neurophys. 1:455–473.

Munsat, T. L., Stuart, W. H., and Cranford, R. E. 1989. Guidelines in the vegetative state: commentary on the American Academy of Neurology statement. Neurology 38:123–124.

Pallis, C. 1983. ABC of brain stem death. BMJ. 285:1409–1412, 1487–1490, 1558–1560, 1641–1644, 1720–1722, 1983. 286:39, 123–124, 209–210, 284–286.

Sanchez-Carpintero, A. R., Sanmarti Vilaplana, F. X., and Serratosa Fernandez, J. M. 2007. Genetic causes of epilepsy. Neurologist 13(Suppl. 1):S47–51

Saper, C. B., Chou, T. C., and Scammel, T. E. 2001. The sleep switch: hypothalamic control of sleep and wakefulness. Trends Neurosci. 24:726–731.

Scammell, T. E., Nishano, S., Mignot, E., and Saper, C. B. 2001. Narcolepsy and low CSF Orexin (hypocretin) concentration after a diencephalic stroke. Neurology 56:1751–1753.

Segarra, J. M. 1970. Cerebral vascular disease and behavior. Arch. Neurol. 22:408–418.

Shute, C. C. D., and Lewis, P. R. 1967. The ascending cholinergic reticular system: neocortical olfactory and subcortical projections. Brain 90:497–821.

Silber, M. H., and Rye, D. B. 2001. Solving the mystery of narcolepsy. Neurology 56:1616–1618. (Editorial).

Steriade, M. 1992. Basic mechanisms of sleep generation. Neurology 42(Suppl.6):9–18.

Sohal, V. S., and Sun, F. T. 2011. Responsive neurostimulation suppresses synchronized cortical rhythms with epilepsy. Neurosurg. Clin. N. Am. 22(4):481–488.

Villablanca, J., and Salinas-Zeballos, M. E. 1972. Sleep-wakefulness, EEG and behavioral studies of chronic cats without the thalamus the "athalamic" cat. Arch. Ital Biol. 110:383–411.

Walker, A. E. 1985. Cerebral Death. 3rd ed. Baltimore, MD: Urban & Schwarzenberg.

Wijdicks, E. F. M. 2001. Diagnosis of brain death. N. Engl. J. Med. 344:1215–1221.

Zeman, A. 2001. Consciousness. Brain. 124:1263–1289.

30.

LEARNING, MEMORY, AMNESIA, DEMENTIA, INSTINCTIVE BEHAVIOR, AND THE EFFECTS OF EARLY EXPERIENCE

DEFINITIONS

Learning: A relatively permanent change in behavior that results from practice or experience. Learning is the process of acquiring knowledge about the world. This definition implies plasticity in central nervous system function, and it also implies plasticity in the formation of stimulus–response connections. The definition excludes changes in behavior resulting from maturation, sensory adaptation, and fatigue.

Memory: The processes or neural mechanisms involved in the encoding and storage or representation of an experience and the retrieval of that information. At times the definition is restricted to the "read in" consolidation and storage stages, and the terms *remembering* and *retrieval* are defined as the "read out phase" of learning.

Instinctive behavior: Complex behavior occurs on the first presentation of the triggering stimulus. Such behavior occurs in all species, even those raised in isolation. In birds, complex behavior may be triggered by hypothalamic or midbrain stimulation.

Imprinting: Not all behavioral patterns are learned or instinctive. *Certain behavioral patterns require exposure to a specific stimulus at a critical period in development.* The concepts of imprinting evolved from the study of "following" behavior in newly hatched chicks. Thus, chicks will usually follow their natural mother since during the specific critical period after hatching they are usually exposed to the mother. However, if chicks do not encounter the mother but rather encounter a human, they will tend to follow the human. Critical periods in human postnatal development have also been demonstrated.

Disorders of memory: This problem may reflect focal or more generalized disease of the nervous system. The process may be static or progressive. Included in the definition in addition to the focal disorders involving hippocampus and diencephalon are more generalized disorders such as dementia, amentia, and mental retardation.

Dementia: *A progressive impairment* of previously intact mental faculties without loss of consciousness. In general, in the most common type, Alzheimer's disease, the loss involves initially and most severely recent memory and the ability to learn and retain new memories. To some extent, particularly as time passes, other areas of mental capability are also affected: remote memory, abstract reasoning, insight, arithmetic abilities, language function, personality, mood, and social behavior. In other types personality is initially affected, followed later by memory.

Amentia: The term *amentia* implies a *nonprogressive congenital absence or relative deficiency of mental faculties.* At times, in the absence of an adequate history, the distinction from dementia may be difficult to make. The term *mental retardation* is somewhat less specific, referring to retardation in the development of mental abilities or retardation in the development of intelligence.

LEARNING IN HUMANS AND RELEVANT ANATOMICAL SUBSTRATE

Classification of learning and the anatomical substrate can be found in Squire and Zola-Morgan (1991), and Desimone (1992). Essentially, two broad categories are considered: declarative (explicit) learning and nondeclarative (implicit or "reflexive") learning. Declarative learning refers to the conscious recollection of facts or events. This system is rapid; one trial may be sufficient. Nondeclarative learning refers to a nonconscious alteration of behavior by experience. This type of learning is slow and requires multiple trials. Table 30.1 presents the neural substrate for these types of learning.

STAGES OF HUMAN MEMORY: DECLARATIVE LEARNING

The terminology employed has changed with time, particularly as regards the terms short-term and long-term memory. As presented in Table 30.1, there are essentially three major stages.

Immediate or Short-Term Working Memory

This stage has been discussed in Chapter 18. This is a matter of seconds (estimated as <10 seconds. Total capacity has been estimated as less than 12 items. It is best exemplified in simple digit repetition as in digit span testing or the immediate repetition of three or five objects or the *delayed response test* utilized in monkeys and children. Monkeys with prefrontal lesions and infants less than 8 months (presumably with

Table 30.1 TYPES OF LEARNING AND NEURAL SUBSTRATE

TYPE	ANATOMICAL SUBSTRATE
I. Declarative: conscious, facts or events	
Stage 1: short term/ working/immediate memory	Prefrontal
Stage 2: long-term memory: labile stage (transcription/ transduction and consolidation)	Limbic system: hippocampus-thalamus
Stage 3: long-term memory: stage of remote memory	diffuse cerebral cortex
II. Nondeclarative: nonconscious, reflexive	
Motor habit and skill learning	Cerebellum, striatum, and motor cortex
Classical and operant conditioning	Amygdala for emotional responses, cerebellum for motor responses
Nonassociative learning: sensitization*/ habituation**	Reflex mechanisms of spinal cord and brain stem
Priming: recall of words/objects improved by prior exposure to these stimuli	Neocortex

*Sensitization = increased response to nonnoxious stimuli after presentation of noxious stimulus.
**Habituation = decreased response to a benign stimulus when this is presented repeatedly.

immaturity of the frontal function) are unable to consistently perform the task. The neural substrate undoubtedly involves the reception in the appropriate primary sensory projection area with relay to the adjacent sensory association cortex; for example, areas 18, 22, 5/7, then transfer to the multimodal posterior parietal cortex, then relay to prefrontal area for very short-term storage, and then relay to motor association cortex and then to motor cortex if the information is to be recited to the examiner (as in the digit span or immediate recall tests).

Long-Term Memory: Labile Stage

This stage may be considered a transcription and transduction stage. The duration of this intermediate process has been variously estimated in infrahuman species as a matter of 20 to 180 minutes. The time required is probably shorter as one descends the phylogenetic scale. Theoretically, this stage involves the transcription from a relatively localized reverberating neuronal circuit, indicated in the immediate memory stage, into a more permanent macromolecular form of recording. It has been hypothesized that RNA and protein synthesis are involved in this stage. It should be noted that RNA turnover does increase in tissues undergoing learning-like experiences. RNA turnover also increases in areas of neural tissue subjected to repetitive stimulation. It is clear that interference with RNA synthesis or with protein synthesis (by the use of the antibiotic puromycin) interferes with this stage of memory. Presumably, as we will discuss later, an accompanying change in synaptic connection is beginning to occur.

The neural structures involved are the entorhinal cortex, parahippocampal gyri, the hippocampus, the fornix, and the anterior and dorsal medial nuclei of the thalamus (see Zola-Morgan and Squires, 1990, and later). These structures are interrelated as the "limbic system" previously discussed. From a clinical standpoint, we evaluate this stage of memory with a delayed recall test (list of five objects to be remembered for 5 minutes)[1] and by asking the patient to recite a paragraph ("cowboy" or "gilded boy story") that he or she has just read or heard. This ability to learn and to retain new experiences and new material is often referred to as retentive memory. Disturbance of this stage in memory will be considered later under the topic of the amnestic-confabulatory syndrome.

Long-Term Memory: Stage of Remote Memory

This phrase is not discretely localized. Rather, it represents a widespread storage throughout the cerebral cortex and possibly other areas of the central nervous system. Long-term memory would appear to relate more to the actual volume of cortex remaining intact than to any specific localized process (consistent with the concept of Lashley). Although not discretely localized, it must be recalled that the read-out mechanism for such remote memories may be triggered by stimulation of the lateral aspect of temporal lobe in the particular abnormal situation of patients who are subject to complex partial seizures of temporal lobe origin (refer to Chapter 22). In such patients, ablation of the area that on stimulation produces the remote memory does not abolish this remote memory. From a clinical standpoint, we evaluate this stage of memory by asking the patient to indicate long-term knowledge, such as his or her date of birth, date of marriage, dates of World War I and II, and so forth.

FACTORS INFLUENCING LEARNING AND MEMORY

In the consideration of the learning process, it is important to realize the influence of several additional factors.

1. Motivational drives alter the rate of learning. There are primary or instinctive drives such as hunger, thirst, and sex present in all members of a species, irrespective of cultural influences and in general present in the infant. There are learned, secondary drives or motivational forces such as achievement, anxiety, and dependency. These are learned drives in the sense that motivations, such as desire for acquiring money and fame, or particular fears or guilt are not present in the infant and are not present in all members of a species. During the process of development, previously neutral cues may become attached to primary drives and take on the capacity to motivate performance. Some drives such as severe anxiety may trigger responses

---

[1] Other tests utilize three objects for 3 minutes.

that are not goal-directed, thereby interfering with learning. In contrast, lesser degrees of anxiety may motivate performance.

2. Motivation also affects the central process of interpretation of stimuli (perception). In a sense, what we see depends upon what we wish to see and upon our frame of reference, particularly where the stimulus is ambiguous.

3. Whether stimuli are perceived will also depend on the general state of attention or alertness of the individual mediated by the reticular formation and the status of prefrontal and parietal cortex attention influences.

4. At times retention may be intact, but the search and read-out mechanism may be temporarily defective. This may account for the phenomena of shrinking retrograde amnesia following head trauma.

NEUROBIOLOGICAL MECHANISMS IN MEMORY AND LEARNING

The psychologist Hebb, in 1949, had proposed that when in associative learning the axon of neuron A-synapse firing on neuron B in a persistent manner results in a growth process or metabolic change occurring in one or both neurons such that the probability or efficacy of neuron A firing neuron B is significantly increased. Subsequent studies (reviews of Kandel and Hawkins, 1992; Kandel and O'Dell, 1992) have confirmed these observations and demonstrated that the synaptic connection between neuron A and B could be strengthened by a third (modulatory neuron)—acting to enhance release of transmitter from the terminals of the presynaptic neuron. If neuron A and the modulatory neuron discharged simultaneously, then the connection between neuron A and B would also be strengthened. Subsequent studies indicated that eventually the number of presynaptic terminals was increased, providing an anatomical basis for this type of learning.

Long-Term Potentiation

Bliss and Lomo (1973) demonstrated that brief, high-frequency trains of action potentials within each of the three major pathways of the hippocampus would produce a long-lasting increase in synaptic strength in that pathway, lasting for hours in the anesthetized animal but for days and weeks in the alert, freely moving animal. The CA3 to CA1 Shaffer collateral pathway and the perforant-afferent pathway to the dentate gyrus have associative learning properties, and the model of Hebb is followed. The pre- and postsynaptic neurons must fire simultaneously. The transmitter involved is glutamate. Both NMDA and non-NMDA receptors are involved. Similar long-term potentiation has been subsequently demonstrated in other areas of cerebral cortex. The basic point to be made is that long-term potentiation provides a possible mechanism for the labile period of memory—the transition period which maintains memories for hours, days, and weeks, while more permanent transduction is occurring in terms of protein and RNA alterations.

PLASTICITY IN THE NERVOUS SYSTEM

1. Mirror focus: Repeated experimental focal seizure discharge with repeated transcallosal response will produce changes in the excitability of the contralateral hemisphere so that eventually independent focal discharges develop.

2. Kindling: Repeated subthreshold stimulation of the amygdala, hippocampus, or frontal cortex in many species will over time alter the excitability of widespread cortical areas so that eventually spontaneous seizures occur. Both the mirror focus and kindling have been proposed as possible demonstration models of long-term synaptic changes that may be involved in learning, that is, the alteration of neuronal function as a result of experience.

3. Modification of cortical motor and sensory maps. (See Chapter 18.) These maps are not fixed but instead have a plasticity, which can be modified by experience.

4. The corpus callosum also has a role in learning. Thus, a monkey or human trained to carry out a task with one hand, for example, how to follow a maze or somatosensory discrimination, for roughness, and so on, does not have to relearn that task when the other hand is utilized—a rapid transfer of the learned skill or discrimination has occurred.

5. Early experience and postnatal brain development (see Wiesel and Hubel, 1963; Spitz, 1945). A number of studies have demonstrated a significant effect of early environment of the infant animal or human at critical periods on later brain development and function. These observations may be related to the phenomena of imprinting. Beyond a certain critical age of 15 months in the human infant, and 6–12 months in the infant monkey these changes related to environmental deprivation are irreversible. Cultural deprivation at a somewhat later stage of childhood may also produce long-term effects on psychological development. These studies also demonstrate correlated changes in the microscopic structure and biochemistry of the cortex, basal ganglia, or hippocampus. These considerations provide a biological foundation for the use of "headstart" programs in preschool and primary grade students from culturally deprived backgrounds. (Refer to Hellmuth, 1968.)

DISORDERS OF RECENT MEMORY: THE AMNESTIC-CONFABULATORY SYNDROME: WERNICKE-KORSAKOFF ENCEPHALOPATHY

Wernicke, in 1881, described a syndrome that is of relatively acute onset, occurring in alcoholics or nutritionally deficient patients and consisting of a triad: mental disturbance (confusion and drowsiness), paralysis of eye movements, and an ataxia of gait. The basic cause of the syndrome is a dietary deficiency of thiamine. As a deficiency of thiamine and of the other B-complex vitamins also results in a peripheral neuropathy, symptoms relevant to this degeneration of peripheral nerves often will be present as an associated finding.

Table 30.2 WERNICKE'S ENCEPHALOPATHY

SYMPTOM/SIGN	LESION LOCATION	EFFECT OF THIAMINE
Ophthalmoplegia (bilateral)	Predominantly CN VI, less of IIII	Rapid, reversal hours to days
Nystagmus	Vestibular nuclei	Clears over days
Drowsiness	Periaqueductal gray/periventricular diencephalon	Clears over days
Ataxia: gait and heel to shin	Anterior superior vermis cerebellum	If severe, may persist as alcoholic cerebellar degeneration
Confusion/memory deficit	Dorsal medial/anterior thalamic nuclei	If persists: Korsakoff psychosis

The basic pathological process consists of a necrosis of neural parenchyma and a prominence of blood vessels due to a proliferation of adventitial and endothelial cells. Petechial hemorrhages also occur about these vessels. The pathological findings involve the gray matter surrounding the third ventricle, and aqueduct and floor of the fourth ventricle. Lesions in general are usually most prominent in the mammillary bodies and the medial thalamic areas. Table 30.2 correlates the symptoms/signs with lesion location.

The Memory Disturbance

As drowsiness clears it will often be noted that a severe deficit in recent memory is present, particularly if the patient has delayed seeking medical diagnosis and treatment. The patient will be unable to learn new material. He will have little memory of events surrounding his illness but will have little difficulty recalling events in the distant past. The patient may demonstrate confabulation supplying imaginary answers for questions concerning the recent past and for questions involving new material he has been requested to learn by the examiner. A significant disorientation for time is usually present. *The memory disturbance involves both retrograde amnesia (events prior to the illness) and anterograde amnesia (events since the onset of the illness).* The deficit in memory for recent events may be transient, clearing with continued treatment, or it may be more persistent. The persistence of these disorders of recent memory and of the state of confusion as a chronic phenomenon is referred to as Korsakoff's psychosis. In the studies of Victor et al. (1961), pathological examination of the brain in these latter cases revealed persistent lesions in the dorsal medial and anterior nuclei of the thalamus in contrast to cases of Wernicke's encephalopathy without the persistent memory deficits. The following case history illustrates the problem of Wernicke's encephalopathy.

CASE HISTORY 30.1 (PATIENT OF DR. JOHN SULLIVAN AND DR. JOHN HILLS)

This 62-year-old, white, right-handed stonecutter had been a known heavy alcoholic who had engaged in 6- to 8-week drinking sprees for many years. Two years previously, the patient had been admitted to the Boston City Hospital because of delirium tremens (tremor and visual hallucinations). Two months prior to admission, shortly following the death of a brother-in-law, the patient began his most recent drinking spree. Apparently, he had drifted aimlessly for 5 weeks with no definite food intake for a month. He unaccountably found himself in Florida, not knowing where he was and why he was there. The patient was brought back by his family and hospitalized at his local community hospital with diplopia, ataxia, marked impairment of memory, and complaints of numbness of his fingertips and unsteadiness of gait. After beginning treatment, he was transferred to a neurological center.

General physical examination: Enlarged liver with the edge palpated approximately 2-1/2 finger breadths below the costal margin.

Neurological Examination

Mental status: The patient was markedly disoriented for time and place. Confabulation was also evident when it was suggested that he had recently seen various fictitious persons or was in particular locations. The patient was unable to state his age but could provide his birth date. He was confused with little insight as to his disorientation or his condition. At times, the patient often indicated to visitors that his mother and father were still alive, though both parents had been dead for over 20 years. The patient's digit span was normal at 7 forward and 6 in reverse. The patient could name various objects correctly when these were presented to him and yet he was unable to retain any memory of which objects had been presented to him 5 minutes previously. He was unable to retain any information concerning a story that he had been requested to learn. Calculations, reading, and writing were intact.

Cranial nerves: There was horizontal diplopia on right lateral gaze. A minor weakness of the right lateral rectus was suspected. Horizontal nystagmus was present on lateral gaze, bilaterally and vertical nystagmus on vertical gaze.

Motor system: A minor degree of weakness was present in the distal portions of the lower extremities. There was no longer an ataxia of gait but a positive Romberg test was present.

Reflexes: Deep tendon reflexes were absent at patellar and Achilles even with reinforcement.

Sensory system: Pain and touch were decreased in the lower extremities below the mid-calf. Vibratory sensation was absent at the toes and decreased over the tibia to a marked degree and to a lesser degree over the knees and at fingertips and wrists. Position sense was decreased at fingers and toes.

Clinical diagnosis: Wernicke's encephalopathy; nutritional polyneuropathy.

Hospital course: The patient was treated with thiamine. There was a significant improvement in extraocular functions. The patient had no diplopia after the day of admission. There was no significant change in his mental condition or peripheral neuropathy. Evaluation 3 months later indicated persistent disorientation for time and place and severe selective deficits in memory (delayed recall was still grossly defective), suggesting a residual Korsakoff psychosis.

In many cases, the state of confusion in Wernicke's encephalopathy is preceded by or accompanied by a period of delirium tremens, indicating alcohol withdrawal. The use of intravenous glucose feedings without supplemental intravenous thiamine during such a withdrawal state may actually increase the requirements for thiamine, thus exacerbating the thiamine deficiency state. For this reason, all patients under treatment for alcohol withdrawal (or admitted to the hospital with a recent past history of alcoholism) should be treated with high-dosage B vitamins as well, on the presumption that they are candidates for nutritional deficiency.

In general, as we have indicated, the majority of patients with Wernicke's encephalopathy progress to a more persistent memory disturbance. Victor and Adams reported that 75% of their 86 cases progressed to a permanent amnestic confabulatory syndrome. The Korsakoff syndrome with its particular deficits in memory may also occur in other disease states involving the diencephalon:

1. Tumors involving the posterior but not the anterior hypothalamus affect recent memory.

2. Infarcts of the medial or anterior but not the posterior thalamic areas may also produce defects in recent memory. Refer to case 30.7 and Fig. 30.10. In the study of von Cramon et al. (1985) a combined lesion of both the mamillothalamic tract and the ventral portion of the lamina medullaris interna was most effective in producing amnesia. (See also Graff-Radford et al., 1990 and Tatemichi et al., 1992.)

3. Lesions of the fornix may also be associated with significant problems in memory recording. Such damage is likely to occur with colloid cysts or with the surgical procedure necessary to remove this potentially life-threatening nonmalignant tumor (see Fig. 27.11). The effects are most prominent if bilateral but may also occur with unilateral left-sided damage. Recall that the fornix is the major outflow pathway from the hippocampus. Defects in recent memory have also been reported in tumors involving the posterior or anterior portion of the corpus callosum.

4. Lesions of the basal forebrain as in anterior communicating artery rupture (Irle et al., 1992) may produce persistent anterograde and retrograde amnesia.

BILATERAL LESIONS OF HIPPOCAMPUS (BILATER MESIAL TEMPORAL LOBE LESIONS)

The anatomy of the hippocampus and its connections has been considered in detail in Chapter 22 and should be reviewed at this time.

Bilateral Ablation

Scoville and Milner (1957) were the first to observe the effects of bilateral mesial temporal lesions following bilateral ablation of the anterior two-thirds of the hippocampus and the parahippocampal gyrus with removal of the uncus and amygdala. This surgical procedure had been performed for treatment of temporal lobe epilepsy in a patient who had bilateral temporal lobe epileptic spike foci. Following surgery, a gross loss of the ability to retain current experiences and to learn new material was noted, in addition to a significant retrograde amnesia. Remote events were well recalled. It should be noted that a similar defect might follow unilateral ablation of the temporal lobe structures if disease were present in the contralateral temporal lobe (Penfield and Milner, 1958). These observations stimulated considerable clinical and experimental investigation. Extensive studies in the monkey by Squire and Zola-Morgan (1991) have now clarified the relative roles of these structures.

Essentially, monkeys with selective bilateral lesions of the hippocampus are impaired in memory tasks that involve the ability to acquire new information (declarative memory) but are not impaired in their capacity for skill and habit learning (that is, nondeclarative memory). The type of task employed by Squire and Zola-Morgan is the delayed nonmatching to sample: A single object is presented; after a delay, two objects are presented, the original object and a novel object. The animal is rewarded for choosing the novel object and rapidly learns to select the novel object. Monkeys with selective bilateral lesions of hippocampus and parahippocampal and entorhinal cortex were even more impaired than monkeys with a selective hippocampal lesion. The entorhinal/parahippocampal areas receive input from all of the higher sensory association neocortical areas and then project via the perforant and alvear pathways to the hippocampal formation. There are, however, other inputs to the hippocampus. Monkeys with bilateral lesions of the perirhinal cortex and parahippocampal cortex sparing the hippocampus also demonstrated severe impairment on these same memory tasks. Combined bilateral lesions of hippocampus, parahippocampal gyrus, and perirhinal cortex produce greater impairment of memory than the selective lesions of hippocampus and parahippocampal gyrus. Monkeys with selective bilateral lesions of entorhinal cortex demonstrated impairment but recovered when retested at 9–14 months. All of these monkeys had no impairment of remote memory. Monkeys with lesions of the amygdala demonstrated a marked alteration in emotional behavior but had no impairment on memory tests (see Chapter 22 and Zola-Morgan et al., 1991).

While most patients with bilateral medial temporal lesions have both retrograde and anterograde amnesia, several recent studies have allowed a differentiation of these two aspects of amnesia. Zola-Morgan et al. (1986) reported that a patient with selective bilateral lesions of the entire rostral caudal extent of field CA1 of the hippocampus (due to global ischemia) had enduring anterograde amnesia but minimal retrograde amnesia. Rempel-Clower et al. (1996) confirmed this in an additional group of three patients. On the other hand, Kapur et al. (1992) described a patient with a closed head injury who had severe posttraumatic retrograde amnesia (extending back to childhood) but only mild patchy anterograde amnesia. On magnetic resonance imaging (MRI) scan, there was bilateral damage to anterior temporal cortex and to a lesser degree prefrontal areas. There was no damage to hippocampus, thalamus, or other limbic structures of the diencephalon.

Disease involving the medial temporal areas may occur under a variety of circumstances and may result in an inability to retain current experiences and to learn new material. Material learned and already stored in long-term remote memory will be intact. In the clinical discussion that will follow, we will often be considering the medial temporal areas in a more general sense. As already noted, early cases of destruction of medial temporal areas were nonselective. Damage to hippocampus also included damage to amygdala and the adjacent cortex.

Bilateral Infarction

Bilateral infarction of the hippocampal areas may occur with disease of the posterior cerebral artery (De Jong et al., 1969; Victor et al., 1961). Occlusions of the posterior cerebral arteries usually reflect embolic events with the embolus originating in the heart or at a lower level in the vertebral basilar circulation. The ischemia or infarction of the mesial temporal areas may be accompanied by ischemia or infarction of the territories of the calcarine arteries. In other cases, stenosis of the basilar artery may produce decreased blood flow in both posterior cerebral arteries. In still other instances, the ischemia apparently may be limited to the medial temporal area, that is, hippocampal areas, with little involvement of the occipital cortex. In these cases, transient episodes may occur and may be difficult to distinguish from the syndrome of transient global amnesia.

We should note at this point that the posterior cerebral arteries via their penetrating branches also supply the medial diencephalic areas. Such ischemia in the posterior cerebral circulation, then, might well produce ischemia of the dorsal median nucleus, the anterior thalamic nuclei, and the mammillary bodies. Thus, in the case of persistent memory deficit following posterior cerebral artery lesions reported by Victor et al. (1961), the areas of infarction involved not only the hippocampal formation and fornix but also the mammillary bodies. An example of bilateral medial thalamic lesions producing alterations in recent memory has been provided in Chapter 29.

Unilateral Infarcts

The study of Ott and Saver (1993) demonstrated the occurrence of the amnestic syndrome following infarcts within the territory of the posterior cerebral artery involving the hippocampus or the thalamus. In 85% of unilateral infarcts, the lesion was left sided.

Transient Global Amnesia Syndrome

This syndrome involves the sudden onset of a defect in memory. The memory deficit is similar to that which occurs in the amnestic confabulatory syndrome seen in Wernicke's encephalopathy. There is a significant retrograde amnesia for the events of the preceding days, weeks, and months. This retrograde amnesia slowly clears over a period of hours. The patient has a persistent amnesia for the period between the onset of the attack and the point of complete recovery. During the period of the episode, the patient is unable to learn new material, that is, the patient is unable to register new memories. Apart from this defect, the patient usually shows no other abnormality of behavior during the episodes. For some time, a possible vascular etiology involving the posterior cerebral arteries (or basilar vertebral system) has been postulated. Whether the selective transient ischemia involves the hippocampal formation, rather than the diencephalic areas, remains unclear. As discussed, the hippocampus is more likely to manifest a selective vulnerability to anoxia and would be expected to show functional impairment prior to the medial thalamic areas. Mathew and Meyer (1974) demonstrated that elderly patients with transient global amnesia had one or more risk factors for vascular disease, and four-vessel angiography demonstrated significant lesions in the vertebral basilar and posterior cerebral systems. Patients with single episodes had no permanent impairment of memory. Those with recurrent episodes had some degree of permanent memory impairment, as well as mild visual spatial or visual motor dyspraxia. Several recent studies confirm the previously postulated ischemic etiology but leave undecided the location of the ischemia: thalamus versus hippocampus (Goldenberg et al., 1991; Lin et al, 1993; Stillhard et al., 1990). The majority of patients make an apparent total recovery and do not have significant infarcts (see Melo et al., 1992). The following case history illustrates this syndrome. A transient disease process involving the temporal areas is suggested but not proven.

CASE HISTORY 30.2

This 55-year-old, right-handed, white, male college professor awoke at 3:00 a.m. on the morning of admission in an uneasy and restless state. He was confused as to time and kept repeating himself and asking the same questions. His wife arranged for him to be seen early in the morning by his family physician. At approximately 8:00 a.m. he became lost driving a short familiar route to his doctor's office, and when he arrived with the assistance of his wife, he was unable to explain why he had come. He could remember no significant events from the 3-week period prior to the onset of his illness. The patient's more remote recall and other intellectual capacities remained intact.

Neurological examination: When examined in the early afternoon, findings were essentially limited to the mental status examination: the patient was beginning to regain some of his ability to retain new information, but he was still disoriented for the day and month. Store of information was quite intact.

The patient had marked difficulty with delayed recall. He could recall none of the four objects after 5 minutes. He could not remember any of the three test phrases given to him when asked about these 5 minutes later. He did recall in a vague manner that a memory test had been given to him. He was unable to remember his visit to his family physician earlier in the day. Digit retention, however, was relatively well preserved; 6 forward and 5 backward. The patient had no defects in calculation. There was no evidence of a constructional apraxia. Language function was entirely intact.

Clinical diagnosis: Probable transient global amnesia.

Laboratory data: Electroencephalogram (EEG) and cerebrospinal fluid were all within normal limits. The brain scan demonstrated a small area of increased uptake of radioisotope (Hg^{197}) in the left temporal region.

Hospital course: Over the several hours following admission, the patient gradually regained his ability to retain new information and to recall the events of the preceding 3 weeks, the more remote events being recalled first. The memory for the events of the day prior to admission was regained last. This pattern is referred to as a shrinking retrograde amnesia. The specific events that occurred on the morning of admission were never recalled. The following morning delayed recall was four-out-of-four objects after 8 minutes. The patient's mental status and neurological examination were otherwise within normal limits. All brain scan findings had resolved at 5 months. No additional episodes occurred during the 1 year after the acute episode.

EFFECTS FROM STIMULATION OF THE TEMPORAL LOBE

Bilateral stimulation of the temporal lobe or unilateral stimulation with secondary spread to the contralateral hemisphere may occur during limited electric stimulation of the medial temporal structures during epilepsy surgery or unilateral electroshock therapy, during general stimulation of the brain (electrical shock therapy or a spontaneous generalized convulsive seizure), or during a temporal lobe seizure. Thus, it may be demonstrated that electrical stimulation of the depths of the temporal lobe in patients susceptible to temporal lobe seizures can produce a defect in memory for recent events without disturbing the patient's ability to recall remote memories. In general, the longer the stimulation, the longer the duration of retrograde amnesia and the longer the recovery time before the new memories can be recorded. Table 30.3 summarizes the example cited by Doty (1967).

A primary or secondarily generalized convulsive seizure is followed by a period of confusion during which the patient is confused, unable to record new information, and uncertain of memories prior to the seizure. In general, on recovery from this period of confusion, the patient is amnestic for the entire period from the beginning of the seizure until the clearing of the postictal confusion. The patient usually, however, has no impairment of retrograde memories up to the point of the seizure. Thus, any "aura" may be recalled. *The effects produced by electrical stimulation of the hippocampus may also occur as relatively selective ictal and postictal phenomena in a complex partial seizure originating in mesial temporal lobe structures*, as illustrated in the case history 30.3 presented on the CD-ROM. Focal temporal lobe seizure phenomena were followed by a period of impaired recent memory with an inability to record new memories.

SELECTIVE VULNERABILITY OF THE HIPPOCAMPUS TO ANOXIA, HYPOGLYCEMIA, OR STATUS EPILEPTICUS

As discussed in Chapter 22, transient or permanent defects in memory may occur. The effects of repeated seizures on the hippocampus may involve more than simply the effects of hypoxia. Excessive discharge of neurons may also damage the neurons due to excitotoxic effects of the glutamate transmitter.

1. Toxic effects on the hippocampus: An accidental intoxication from consuming contaminated mussels provides additional information about selective damage to the hippocampus resulting in an amnestic syndrome. In 1987, an outbreak characterized by gastrointestinal symptoms and neurological symptoms occurred in Canada in 107 persons who had eaten cultivated mussels from Prince Edward Island. The acute phase symptoms consisted of headaches, seizures, and hemiparesis. Twenty-five percent of patients had persistent severe anterograde amnesia. Positron emission tomography (PET) scanning demonstrated decreased glucose metabolism in the medial temporal areas. In the four patients who died, necrosis and loss of neurons occurred predominantly in the hippocampus and amygdala (Teitelbaum et al., 1990). Two patients also had involvement of the dorsal medial thalamic nucleus. Not all patients with the persistent memory deficits had uncontrolled status epilepticus—which may also produce hippocampal damage. The mussels were found to be contaminated by domoic acid produced by a form of marine vegetation, Nitzchia pungens. Domoic acid has structural similarities to the natural excitatory transmitter glutamic acid and to kainic acid. Both kainic acid and domoic acid bind strongly to the glutamate receptor. Domoic acid is 30–100× more potent than glutamate and 2–3× more potent than kainic acid. Experimental administration of domoic acid or of kainic acid to rats produces limbic seizures, memory disorders, and degeneration of the hippocampus.

2. Herpes simplex encephalitis: As discussed in Chapter 27, the virus herpes simplex type 1, the agent responsible for the common cold sore, may on occasion invade the central nervous system (Fig. 30.1) and produce several syndromes. In addition to the more common acute generalized or focal encephalitis, a third rare syndrome results from a more localized involvement of the medial temporal structures and is characterized by a subacute but progressive dementing process and temporal lobe seizures.

The disturbance of mental status is characterized by confusion and disorientation with a defect in memory for recent events and often for remote events as well. There is a marked inability to form new associations. The selectivity of the memory disturbance is less evident in these cases than in those cases of hippocampal disease previously discussed in detail.

Limbic Encephalitis

This disorder manifests with severe retentive memory loss, florid psychiatric symptoms, seizures, and confusion. If not treated, it may progress to obtundation myoclonus, eye movement abnormalities, and ultimately, respiratory arrest. The MRI often shows T2 and flair hyperintensities in the limbic structures, and there may be a lymphocytic pleocytosis in

Table 30.3 **STIMULATION OF "DEEP" TEMPORAL STRUCTURES**

DURATION OF STIMULATION	LENGTH OF RETROGRADE AMNESIA	LENGTH OF ANTEROGRADE AMNESIA
2 seconds	Just prior to stimulation	1–2 minutes
5 seconds	Current day	5–10 minutes
10 seconds	Previous 3 weeks	1–3 hours

Source: After data of Doty (1967).

Figure 30.1 Herpes simplex encephalitis. Predominant involvement of medial and inferior temporal structures (and of insula) by an acute necrotic process is evident, although a generalized encephalitis was also present. Same case as Figure 27.26. (Courtesy of Dr. John Hills.)

the spinal fluid. This syndrome is associated with identifiable autoantibodies in 40%–60% of cases. These may be paraneoplastic and target cell surface antigens. This permits dramatic responses to immunomodulatory therapy. Limbic encephalitis with anti-NMDA antibodies in women with ovarian dermoids is an excellent example of this situation. Systemic lupus, nervous system Whipple disease, and Sjogren disease may also cause limbic encephalitis. If the antibodies attack intracellular targets, the prognosis is more guarded.

Traumatic Amnesia

Perhaps the most common transient impairment of memory occurs in relation to head injury. When blunt trauma to the head occurs, consciousness is lost. As the individual recovers consciousness, there is a period of confusion before a return to normal behavior. The loss of consciousness and the subsequent period of confusion in such patients are often referred to as concussion. Following this period of confusion, there is often a period during which behavior is otherwise normal, but the ability to form new memories is defective. Examination of the patient at that time will indicate that not only is there no memory of the actual period of unconsciousness and the following confusional state but also that there is defective memory for a period of time preceding the period of injury. The patient has then both an anterograde and retrograde amnesia. In general, the longer the period of retrograde amnesia, the more severe the head injury and, in general, the longer the period of time before memory will be regained. As recovery occurs, the period of retrograde amnesia is gradually reduced. The underlying pathophysiology has been discussed previously in the section on trauma.

PROGRESSIVE DEMENTING PROCESSES

As already defined, dementia refers to a progressive impairment of previously intact mental faculties. In general, in the most common type, Alzheimer's disease, the loss involves initially and most severely recent memory and the ability to learn and retain new memories. To some extent, particularly as time passes, other areas of mental capability are also affected: remote memory, abstract reasoning, insight, and arithmetic abilities, language function, personality, mood, and social behavior. In other types, such as the "frontal temporal dementias," personality and behavior are involved earlier than memory. In still other types, Lewy body dementia, motor function is early involved followed by memory. In general, these processes involve the older adult population. However, certain rare disorders producing a progressive dementia affect infants, children, and adolescents and the young or middle-aged adult. Some of these pediatric disorders reflect known or suspected inborn and genetic errors of metabolism: aminoaciduria, lipidosis, galactosemia, Hurler's disease (accumulation of mucopolysaccharides), and leukodystrophies. Other disorders are placed in the degenerative category because in general the etiology remains unknown, for example, spongy degeneration. A detailed consideration of these various early-onset problems is beyond the scope of this text. Dementia is a major medical problem because of its high frequency in the elderly and because of the significant aging of the population. Life span has been significantly extended, but the capacity to prevent the dementing disorders is limited. The prevalence of dementia and of Alzheimer's disease in the general population is presented in Table 30.4.

Mild cognitive impairment of the elderly is a vague entity that may be a manifestation of normal aging or a bridge between normal aging and Alzheimer's disease (AD). These individuals have difficulty with word retrieval, especially proper nouns, but are not particularly cognitively handicapped in daily life. There is an effort to predict which patients will go on to full-blown dementia. Progress in imaging genetic and biochemical diagnosis of AD will soon clarify this problem. Simple methods of cognitive testing can be used to predict the time of conversion to mild cognitive impairment in the normal elderly. As soon as truly effective treatment for AD is available, early identification will be of paramount importance because AD begins decades before it is clinically evident.

ALZHEIMER'S DISEASE

The most common cause of a progressive impairment of mental faculties in the older adult population is the degenerative disease known as presenile or senile dementia (Alzheimer's

Table 30.4 PREVALENCE OF DEMENTIA AND ALZHEIMER'S DISEASE

Age range (years)	60–64	65–69	70–74	75–79	80–84	85–93[a]
Overall all types/100[b]	0.4	0.9	1.8	3.6	10.5	23.8
Alzheimer's disease/100[c]	0.3[d]		3.2[d]		10.8[d]	

[a] For Alzheimer's disease, age ranges are 60–69, 70–79, and 80–89.
[b] Derived from Bachman et al. 1992 (Framingham).
[c] Derived from Rocca et al., 1991.
[d] Skoog et al., 1993, in 494 patients at age 85 (Sweden); overall prevalence 29.8%: severe 11%, moderate 10%, mild 8%.

Figure 30.2 Cortical atrophy as found in presenile and senile dementia of Alzheimer type. Gross brain: *A* (lateral surface) and *B* (dorsal surface). There is widening of sulci concomitant with narrowing of the gyri especially in this case in the frontal and parietal regions.

disease). Whether the process is called presenile or senile is arbitrary, based on the age of the patient. When the process begins before the age of 65 years, the designation *presenile* is used; when the process begins after the age of 65 years, the designation *senile* is employed. The basic pathological process (Perl, 2000) is, however, the same. Grossly (Fig. 30.2), there is an atrophy of cerebral cortex, involving primarily in a diffuse manner the frontal and temporal areas but sparing the motor cortex, sensory, and visual areas. In some cases (more often presenile) involvement of the parietal association areas is evident as well. There is a thinning of gyri and widening of sulci. There is usually a secondary dilatation of the lateral ventricles. These findings in patients with senile dementia overlap with the patients in the same age group without dementia. In presenile patients, there is less overlap with nondemented patients and the atrophy and the microscopic changes discussed later are also more widespread. There is no one-to-one relationship of the degree of neocortical atrophy with the severity of the dementia. These overall findings are reflected in the neuroimaging studies. Thus, patients with a significant degree of dementia may manifest only a minimal degree of neocortical atrophy, as noted on the computerized tomography (CT) or MRI scan. On the other hand, it is not unusual to find elderly patients with a significant degree of neocortical atrophy on such radiological studies that demonstrate relatively little actual cognitive impairment. There is, however, a significant correlation in Alzheimer's disease between the degree of atrophy of the hippocampus and the presence of dementia. This hippocampal atrophy is evident on the CT scan but is best seen in MRI studies that utilize measurements of hippocampal volume (Fig. 30.3). *It is evident then that the earliest changes occur in the hippocampus and entorhinal cortex.*

The microscopic changes probably have a higher correlation with Alzheimer's disease than the gross changes in brain. Change in the volume of the white matter within the gyri can give the picture of very widened sulci without actual cortical changes. The microscopic changes may be outlined as follows:

1. Loss of neurons in the cerebral cortex (Figs. 30.2A and B and 30.4): the large pyramidal cells of the frontal, temporal,

Figure 30.3 Atrophy of the hippocampus in Alzheimer's disease. Magnetic resonance imaging (MRI): area of hippocampus circled for quantitative analysis. (*A*) Normal hippocampus in a 92-year-old patient with Parkinson's disease but normal cognitive function. (*B*) Severe atrophy of hippocampus in a 72-year-old patient with well-developed Alzheimer's disease. Neocortical atrophy is also present. (Courtesy of Dr. Daniel Sax.)

Table 30.5 CAUSES OF DEMENTIA

NEUROPATHOLOGICAL AND CLINICAL SYNDROME*	PERCENTAGE OF TOTAL
Alzheimer's disease	55%
Dementia with Lewy bodies	15%–20%
Multi-infarct and other vascular dementia**	15%
Combined multi-infarct/vascular plus Alzheimer's disease	12%
Other degenerative causes***	<3%–5%

*Derived from Tomlinson et al., 1970; and other sources.
**Vascular dementia includes a variety of syndromes: (1) A single infarct in areas critical for memory. (2) Infarcts (single or multiple) in which total volume of cortex destroyed is >100 ml. (3) Small vessel disease producing multiple lacunar infarcts. (4) Senile leukoencephalopathy involving periventricular white matter in association with hypertension (Roman et al., 1993).
***Frontal-temporal dementia including Pick's disease, Huntington's disease, and progressive supranuclear palsy (PSP).

Figure 30.4 Alzheimer's disease: microscopic features. This 87-year-old female had a 7-year history of a progressive dementia. This 40× magnification section of the hippocampus CA-1 sector, stained with the Bielschowsky silver stain, demonstrates the following features: (1) loss of neurons, (2) argyrophilic neurofibrillary tangles in surviving pyramidal cells, (3) senile plaques containing fragments of silver staining neuronal and glial processes, (4) dystrophic neurites of silver staining processes surrounding the plaques. (Courtesy Dr. Tom Smith.)

and parietal association areas of the neocortex and particularly the hippocampal and related medial temporal areas. Some loss of neurons occurs in all normal aging individuals, but the degree in Alzheimer's is markedly greater.

2. Loss of neurons in certain subcortical nuclei that project to cerebral cortex: the basal forebrain nucleus of Meynert (cholinergic), the locus ceruleus (noradrenergic), and the amygdala.

3. Loss of dendritic spines and branches affects the pyramidal neurons of the temporal and frontal cortex and the limbic cortex. Normal aging individuals actually have an increase in dendritic trees until the 80s and 90s are attained.

4. Neurofibrillary tangles develop within the cytoplasm of the surviving large pyramidal neurons of these neocortical areas and the hippocampus (Figs. 30.4 and 30.5). These tangles are composed of the spiral (helical) winding of paired protein filaments, probably derived from the protein skeleton of the cytoplasm. They contain tau proteins, a normal constituent of microtubules. Normally these tau proteins are highly soluble. In Alzheimer's disease, the tau protein found in the paired helical filaments is hyperphosphorylated and highly insoluble. These insoluble tau aggregates in the tangles are usually complexed with another protein, ubiquitin. The anterior frontal, temporal neocortex, and particularly the medial temporal area (hippocampus and entorhinal cortex), are primarily affected. The amygdala, basal forebrain, cholinergic nuclei, thalamus, substantia nigra, and locus ceruleus are also affected. Betz cells of the motor cortex and the Purkinje cells of the cerebellum are resistant to the degeneration. Neurofibrillary tangles also occur in a number of other central nervous system diseases that have been grouped together as tauopathies. It is likely that the change in tau protein represents a response of neurons to a variety of pathological insults of a genetic and nongenetic nature. These include such entities as Down's syndrome, postencephalitic Parkinson's disease, amyotrophic lateral sclerosis/Parkinson-dementia complex observed primarily on Guam, progressive supranuclear palsy, corticobasal degeneration, and hereditary frontal temporal dementia (linked to chromosome 17), as well as dementia associated with repeated head trauma in boxers. Some neurofibrillary

Figure 30.5 Neurofibrillary tangles in pyramidal neurons of the hippocampus. Bielschowsky silver stain. 100× magnification. (Courtesy of Dr. Thomas Smith.)

tangles will be found in the brain of intellectually normal individuals, primarily in the anterior medial temporal areas but in comparatively small numbers. In the studies of Tomlinson, 5% of normal patients of 40 years had some minor involvement. By the seventh decade, 50% of patients had some involvement, and all 90-year-old patients were affected to some degree. In Alzheimer's disease not only is the anteromedial temporal lobe affected to a much greater degree but also there is widespread involvement of the remainder of the hippocampus and marked involvement of the neocortex.

In some patients with clinical Alzheimer's disease, an alternate form of neuronal inclusion is found in the cortical pyramidal cells: the Lewy body composed of α-synuclein protein already discussed in relation to Parkinson's disease. These cases are labeled as the Lewy body variant of Alzheimer's disease.

What distinguishes the patient with Alzheimer's disease from the normal elderly patient and from the other tauopathies is the presence of the senile neuritic plaque to be discussed next.

5. Dystrophic neuritis. These are altered neuronal processes (axons, dendrites, and/or synaptic terminals) found free in the neuropil as well as surrounding senile plaques (Fig. 30.4). The study of McKee et al. (1991) noted a significant increase in these dystrophic neurites in Alzheimer's disease and a high correlation of the number of both dystrophic neurites and neurofibrillary tangles with the severity of dementia.

6. Extracellular plaques (senile or neuritic plaques) containing insoluble fibrils of amyloid-beta proteins (Figs. 30.4, 30.6, and 30.7). In Alzheimer's disease fragments of abnormal-appearing neuronal processes (axons and dendrites) surround the amyloid core of these plaques. There is also evidence of surrounding altered astrocytes and microglia. The plaques have a predilection for the frontal temporal and parietal association neocortex and particularly accumulate in the medial temporal areas. A "diffuse" deposit of amyloid in the neuropil, in a nonfibrillar form

Figure 30.6 Senile plaque. Silver stain. 100× magnification. (Courtesy of Dr. Thomas Smith.)

Figure 30.7 Senile plaque. Immunologic stain for beta amyloid. 100× magnification. (Courtesy of Dr. Thomas Smith.)

and without the altered glia and without the surrounding dystrophic neurites may occur in otherwise normal individuals. Similar amyloid may also accumulate in the walls of cerebral blood vessels.

The primary constituent of the amyloid core of the plaque is the B (beta) amyloid peptide of 28–43 amino acids. This peptide is generated by proteolytic cleavage of a larger transmembrane glycoprotein containing 695, 751, or 770 amino-acid residues: the amyloid precursor protein (APP). This cleavage is mediated by a series of proteolytic enzymes, alpha, beta, and gamma secretase. The beta amyloid in the plaque is the internal fragment of the amyloid precursor protein. Selkoe (2001) provides additional discussion of the mechanisms of cleavage.

A secondary area of controversy involves the relationship between the beta amyloid (and the senile plaque) and the neurofibrillary degenerative changes in the neurons and the loss of neurons. One hypothesis suggests that the local microglial activation, reactive astrocytosis, and cytokine release surrounding the plaque may produce a cascade of effects that damage the neuron. An alternative hypothesis is based on the demonstration by Yankner and Mesulam (1991) of a direct toxic effect when beta amyloid is added to tissue cultures of mature neurons. In contrast, a neurotrophic effect is evident when beta amyloid is added to a tissue culture of immature neurons. (For a review of the controversy surrounding these studies and the studies of the effects of direct injection of beta amyloid into the brain, see Marx, 1992.)

That there is some relationship of the senile plaques to the total process is evident, from several standpoints.

a. The plaques tend to be concentrated in those areas with severe neuronal loss and with a high density of neurofibrillary changes.

b. The relationship of Alzheimer's disease to Down's syndrome. Patients with Down's syndrome have trisomy 21. The gene for the amyloid precursor protein localizes to chromosome 21. Patients with Down's syndrome who have in a sense a triple dose of this chromosome develop a severe dementia once they reach age 40–50 (almost 100% after age 50). The dementia from a clinical and neuropathologic standpoint is identical to Alzheimer's disease. Moreover, patients with Down's syndrome dying in their teens, 20s, or 30s before clinical dementia has developed will demonstrate a significant accumulation of plaques and changes surrounding the plaque prior to the development of neurofibrillary changes. Thus, the plaques may be the earliest change.

c. In some families with hereditary Alzheimer's disease of relatively early onset—a linkage to chromosome 21 could be demonstrated. In many of these families, missense mutations in the amyloid protein precursor have been demonstrated. These tend to cluster at the beta secretase cleavage site; others occur just after the gamma secretase cleavage site. All of these various mutations would result in enhanced production of increased amounts of beta amyloid. However, other familial cases have localized to chromosomes 14 or 1. In both of these latter sites, there has been localization to mutations in presenilin 1 or 2. These are membrane proteins that apparently regulate gamma secretase activity. Other late-onset familial cases localize to chromosome 19. Other familial cases, "The Volga Germans," localize to none of these chromosomes. The monograph of Pollen (1993) provides a review of the search for the genetic basis of the disease. Newer advances in genetics have identified that the amyloid precursor protein gene has more than 30 very rare variants associated with early-onset Alzheimer disease (Hooli, 2012). The genetic basis for the common late-onset Alzheimer disease has been more elusive, but recent studies have implicated a TREM2 variant as an important risk factor (Jonsson et al., 2013).

Late-Onset Cases

All of these various mutations do not explain the majority of late-onset nonfamilial Alzheimer's disease cases. Chromosome 19, however, does provide a locus for the apolipoprotein E (ApoE) gene. Three variants (alleles) are found in the general population: E2, E3, and E4. The E3 allele is the most common with a frequency of 0.73. E4 has a frequency of 0.14. In families with late-onset Alzheimer's disease, and individuals with late-onset disease, the frequency of the E4 allele is increased to 0.40. Inheritance of one or two alleles of the E4 variant increases the density of senile plaques and increases the risk and lowers the age of onset of the late-onset disease. Patients with two E4 alleles had an average age of onset 68 years; with one E4 allele, 79 years; and with no E4 allele, 84 years. By age 80, over 90% of patients with two E4 alleles developed Alzheimer's disease, whereas only 50% of patients with no E4 allele developed the disease by this age. ApoE 4 is a risk factor but not an invariant cause of late-onset Alzheimer's disease. The E2 variant may provide some protection from the disease. As regards the mechanism, this is not entirely clear. High concentrations of ApoE are found in liver and brain with production in brain by glial cells. In the Alzheimer brain, ApoE has been localized to the senile plaque and to neurons containing neurofibrillary tangles. The beta-amyloid peptide binds more rapidly to the E4 form than to the E3 form. In contrast, the E3 form binds to tau protein, forming a stable molecular structure, whereas the E4 form does not bind to the tau protein. Additional discussion of this topic will be found in Strittmatter et al. (1993), and Corder et al. (1993). Additional discussion of the molecular biology will be found in Selkoe (2001).

Clinical Findings and Course

The clinical symptomatology in Alzheimer's disease relates to a progressive impairment of mental faculties, usually beginning with recent (retentive) memory. Initially, the social graces, remote memory, and rational reasoning capacities are well preserved. As the disease progresses, these aspects of mental function are also affected. In general, during the early stages, focal motor findings do not develop, deep tendon reflexes remain symmetrical, and plantar responses are flexor. It is not unusual to have a significant degree of nominal aphasia present as the memory impairment becomes more severe. (The patient is unable to recall the names of objects.). Apraxias are also not unusual in these cases. As the disease progresses, a release of a grasp reflex is also often noted. In late stages, frontal lobe gait apraxia becomes prominent, and eventually bilateral Babinski signs emerge. Eventually, the patient becomes bedridden and unable to care for daily needs. A terminal state of paraplegia in flexion or a fetal position may be the final posture. Not all cases have the same initial appearance and not all have the same rate of progression. In some cases, focal aphasia with apparent focal atrophy may be noted as an early presentation (Mesulam, 1982), but these cases are more likely to fall into the diagnostic category of frontal temporal dementia. In a considerable percentage of patients late in the disease course, myoclonus, generalized seizures, or partial seizures may develop and account, along with postinfarct seizures, for a significant increase in the frequency of seizure disorders in the elderly. Criteria for the clinical diagnosis of Alzheimer's disease have been outlined in the report of an NIH work group (McKhann et al., 1984). See also Markesbery (1992) and Katzman (1993).

The following case history presents an example of presenile dementia.

CASE HISTORY 30.4

This 64-year-old, right-handed white male, formerly an administrative assistant for the veteran's administration and newspaper distributor, was evaluated for progressive impairment of recent memory of 10 years' duration. Initially, these problems in memory were attributed to a more "benign" disorder—*mild cognitive impairment of the elderly*. However, such patients, when studied longitudinally, develop Alzheimer's disease at the rate of 12% per year compared to age-matched controls that develop Alzheimer's disease at a rate of 1%–2% per year. At age 60, delayed recall was limited to 0/4, and there was minor time disorientation. During last year there were now personality changes and word-finding difficulties. Family history was negative.

Neurological Examination

Mental status: The mini mental status exam indicated a total score of 19 out of 30. He had particular problems in time orientation. He was able to do the immediate recitation of three objects and of a test phrase but could remember none of these on a delayed recall test. He also had difficulty copying a test figure. The patient was often tangential in his answers and demonstrated inappropriate joking.

Motor system: Premotor/frontal lobe functions were abnormal with a release of the instinctive grasp reflex and impairment of motor sequences.

Clinical diagnosis: Alzheimer's disease.

Laboratory data: All studies were normal, except a CT scan demonstrated significant dilatation of the temporal horns, suggesting hippocampal atrophy, in addition to a general increase in lateral ventricular size with blunting of the angles of the frontal horns. A SPECT scan demonstrated slight decrease in perfusion in the left parietal region.

Subsequent course: After 10 weeks of treatment with 5 mg per day of donepezil (Aricept), a centrally acting acetylcholinesterase inhibitor, and high dosage of vitamin E (a possible antioxidant), the test score had increased to 25 out of 30 with particular improvement in the delayed recall section of the exam. There was, however, no change in personality. Administration of the acetylcholinesterase inhibitor temporarily improved memory function for approximately 18 months. However, by age 67, behavioral disturbance (agitation, aggression, nocturnal wandering, and sexual disinhibition) and urinary incontinence were becoming major problems. He could no longer be managed in his home and day care setting despite the use of haloperidol, and he was placed in a nursing home. At age 69, he was now described as relatively nonfluent, very confused, and restricted to a wheelchair. He was "stiff and afraid" when requested to walk.

The use of the donepezil has been estimated to postpone nursing home placement by approximately 15 months. The rationale for the use of acetylcholinesterase inhibitors is based on the demonstration by Drachman and Leavitt (1974) that administration of scopolamine, an anticholinergic drug that crosses the blood–brain barrier, would produce a transient syndrome similar in many respects to the memory and cognitive changes of Alzheimer's disease. Subsequent studies demonstrated a marked loss of neurons in the basal forebrain nucleus of Meynert, a major source of cholinergic fibers to the cerebral cortex (Growden, 1992; Rogers et al., 1995; Whitehouse et al., 1981). However, a simplistic cholinergic hypothesis is insufficient to explain all of the features of Alzheimer's disease. Administration of acetylcholine esterase inhibitors in mild cases (mini mental status score of 10–25) has only a limited value, as in case 30.4. Other neuronal systems are involved. (Noradrenergic synapses are also involved, and the hippocampal system is severely involved.)

The Evaluation of the Patient with Alzheimer's Disease

The primary purpose of a complete evaluation in these cases is to rule out the treatable causes of dementia. In addition, several less frequent causes of dementia must be differentiated from Alzheimer's disease. The treatable causes of dementia are outlined in Table 30.6. The usual screening tests are the following: thyroid-stimulating hormone (TSH), B12, and folate, relative dose-response (RPR) test or venereal disease research laboratory (VDRL) test, and CT scan. Other causes of progressive dementia are outlined in Table 30.7 and are discussed in greater detail at the end of this chapter. Newer methods of diagnosis are now available but are not in widespread use, often because insurance will not reimburse for expensive testing for an illness with limited treatment. Imaging of the brain beta-amyloid load using the FDA-approved radiopharmaceutical florbetapir F18 is now possible (Yang et al., 2012). The cerebrospinal fluid in Alzheimer disease shows progressive elevation of phosphorylated tau, presumably due to dissolution of neurons while the level beta 1–42 amyloid declines. Ratios of these two substances have diagnostic value and are contained in the new criteria (Honig, 2012).

Table 30.6 **TREATABLE AND RELATED CAUSES OF DEMENTIA**

CATEGORY	SPECIFIC ETIOLOGY	TEST
Infections	Tertiary syphilis (general paresis)*	RPR, or specific FTA or CSF VDRL
	AIDS dementia	If indicated HIV
Nutritional	B12, thiamin, niacin	B12 and folate levels
Intoxications	Various (refer to Chapter 27)	Toxicology screen + if suspected Pb
Endocrine	Hypothyroid	TSH, then if +, T4, T3
Tumors	Frontal meningiomas and gliomas**	CT or MRI scan
Posttraumatic	Chronic subdural hematomas	CT scan
Hydrocephalus	NPH, etc. (ataxia > dementia)	CT scan, improve after CSF removal (30cc)
Vascular	Various types of vascular dementia	Multiple strokes + multifocal signs, CT/MRI
Pseudodementia	Depression > dementia + variability	Trial of antidepressants
Other meningeal	Carcinomatosis of meninges	MRI, CSF cytology

*An example of tertiary syphilis with general paresis; case 30.5 is presented on the CD-ROM.
**See case 30.7 and Figure 30.10. Other progressive disorders producing dementia are summarized in Table 30.7.
CSF, cerebrospinal fluid; CT, computerized tomography; FTA, fluorescent treponemal antibody; MRI, magnetic resonance imaging; RPR, relative dose response test; TSH, thyroid-stimulating hormone; VDRL, venereal disease research laboratory test.

Table 30.7 OTHER PROGRESSIVE CAUSES OF DEMENTIA

DISORDER	DISTINGUISHING CLINICAL	PATHOLOGY
Diffuse Lewy body disease	Parkinsonism and psychotic features with relative sparing of memory at onset	Diffuse Lewy body involvement of cortical and subcortical neurons + senile plaques
Huntington's disease	Chorea and personality changes at onset; autosomal dominant, high penetrance	Atrophy caudate/putamen + cortex, seen CAG trinucleotide repeats
Frontal/temporal dementia (several types)	(1) Personality changes early, memory changes late. (2) Progressive nonfluent aphasia at onset. (3) Semantic dementia in 40% autosomal dominant tauopathies are found linked to chromosome 17.	(1) Bilateral prefrontal atrophy early, hippocampus late. (2) Lobar left temporal-frontal frontal atrophy, (3) Bilateral temporal atrophy with gliosis and/or spongy changes. In some Pick's bodies.
Creutzfeldt-Jakob disease	Rapidly progressive dementia, myoclonus, seizures, pyramidal, basal ganglia signs (+cerebellar in 50%). Familial and new variant (bovine) cases have a younger onset, a slower course, and greater cerebellar involvement.	Transmissible spongiform encephalopathy-Prion disorder (Fig. 30.8). Periodic EEG complexes in sporadic (Fig. 30.9). In new variant, diffuse amyloid plaques + spongiform changes.

CASE HISTORY 30.7 (PATIENT OF DR. THOMAS MULLINS)

This 74-year-old, right-handed widow presented to the emergency room at St Vincent hospital in February with an 8- to 10-week history of worsening memory problems. In the previous December, accompanied by her boyfriend, she made her annual trip to Florida. Although she had been in her usual state of independent living prior to her departure, she was found to have serious problems with memory on arrival. She was unaware as to where she was. In a telephone conversation with her daughter, "she was talking nonsense." During the next 2 months, memory and word finding continued to deteriorate. She was taken to the emergency room of the local hospital in Florida, where a CT scan without contrast on 02/07/02 demonstrated mild cortical atrophy but no acute process. Her son drove to Florida and found that her memory was poor and her conversation did not make sense: "My husband is in the service; my mother died last year." However, she could play cards with her granddaughter. Her gait was slow and stooped. She had urinary incontinence on her way to the bathroom.

She had no history of alcoholism and took various vitamins and herbs.

Family history: Her brother had died of a brain tumor of unknown type.

Neurologic examination: The positive findings were the following:

Mental status: The patient was awake and alert. Overall Mini-Mental Status Score was 19/30. The major problems were in orientation and in delayed recall. She was able to indicate that she was in a hospital in Massachusetts and the date was February. She registered three objects but could not recall any in 3 minutes. She was, however, able to read, name objects, follow instructions, spell "world" backwards, and copy a figure. She was unable to draw a clock with the hands set at 11:10.

Motor system: Although strength and tone were normal, her gait was broad-based and shuffling.

Reflexes: Patellar and Achilles reflexes were absent, but plantar responses were flexor.

Clinical diagnosis: (1) Subacute dementia etiology uncertain, possibly of Alzheimer's or Lewy body dementia. Various entities such as chronic subdurals, tumor, and so on to be ruled out. (2) Peripheral neuropathy; most likely etiology at this age is diabetes mellitus.

Laboratory data: *Basic CBC and chemistries:* Normal except for an elevated fasting glucose. *CT scan* (Fig. 30.10): An enhancing 2.75 cm tumor with a necrotic center was present in the thalamus at the level of the upper third ventricle. There was bilateral involvement of the anterior and medial thalamus but with no involvement of the posterior thalamus or hypothalamus. The study suggested a lymphoma or glioblastoma.

Subsequent course: *Stereotaxic biopsy of the right thalamus:* Frozen section raised the question of a lymphoma or glioblastoma, but special immunological stains were consistent with a glioblastoma. Necrosis and endothelial hyperplasia were present. The patient was treated with dexamethasone and radiotherapy with improvement in gait.

OTHER PROGRESSIVE DISORDERS TO BE DISTINGUISHED FROM ALZHEIMER'S DISEASE

Table 30.8 presents estimates modified from Prusiner (2001) of the prevalence of neurodegenerative disorders in the United States in 2000. Almost all of these disorders have been attributed to the abnormal processing of neuronal proteins.[2]

1. Dementia with Lewy bodies (DLB): Various studies have estimated that 20%–50% of patients with Parkinson's disease will eventually develop dementia that is progressive with changes in memory and other cognitive functions. The prevalence of dementia in this population is higher than in age-matched controls. In some of these patients there is the coincidence of Alzheimer's disease and of Parkinson's disease. More often, however, these patients with both dementia and Parkinson's disease are found to have a significant involvement of cerebral cortical neurons by Lewy bodies and a degeneration of neurons in frontal, anterior cingulate, insular, and temporal areas. Senile plaques are present but neurofibrillary changes are minor. As previously discussed and illustrated in Chapter 19,

---

[2] We have not considered here under the progressive disease rubric, patients with vascular dementia, who develop dementia in relationship to repeated strokes, major or minor (multiinfarct), since such patients from a theoretical standpoint have treatable disease related to stroke prevention: treatment of hypertension, use of statins to reduce atherosclerosis, use of anticoagulants to prevent embolic disease in atrial fibrillation, and so on.

Table 30.8 PREVALENCE OF NEURODEGENERATIVE DISORDERS IN THE UNITED STATES, 2000

DISEASE	NO. PER 100,000 POPULATION
Alzheimer's disease	1450
Dementia with Lewy bodies*	448
Parkinson's disease	360
Frontotemporal dementia + Pick's disease**	14 + 2 = 16
Huntington's disease	11
Amyotrophic lateral sclerosis	7
Progressive supranuclear palsy	5
Spinocerebellar ataxias	4
Prion disease	<1

*This category was not included in Prusiner's original estimates but was probably included as Parkinson's disease or Alzheimer's disease.
**Pick's disease was included as a separate category in Prusiner's Table. If combined with frontotemporal dementia, the overall frequency of frontotemporal dementia would be 16/100,000.

the occurrence of Lewy bodies in the neurons of the substantia nigra is characteristic of patients with Parkinson's disease. This type of dementia syndrome is now estimated to account for 15%–20% of all autopsy confirmed cases of dementia in the elderly. As such, this syndrome is considered the second most common type of degenerative dementia. From the clinical standpoint, in contrast to Alzheimer's disease, these patients are more likely to present with mental slowing, impairment of visual spatial functions, impairment of executive function, a change in personality, depression, and visual hallucinations. Impairment of memory at the onset of the disease is not prominent since there is proportionately less involvement of the hippocampus, entorhinal cortex, and parahippocampal gyrus at this stage. In contrast to Alzheimer's disease, where involvement of these limbic structures is prominent early in the disease and is associated with deficits in memory acquisition and consolidation, these patients develop a deficit in retrieval. In various series, Parkinsonian features are present at onset in 10%–78% of cases. Eventually Parkinsonian features develop in 50%–100% of these cases. In contrast to classical Parkinson's disease, these patients are more likely to have myoclonus, an absence of a resting tremor, and a decreased responsiveness to levodopa.

2. Huntington's chorea occurs on a genetic basis in young and middle-aged adults with an autosomal dominant pattern of inheritance. This not uncommon entity involves progressive degeneration of neurons in the basal ganglia (caudate nucleus and putamen) and to a lesser degree cerebral cortex, predominantly frontal. The resultant clinical syndrome of onset in the middle adult years of a progressive dementia, personality alteration, movement disorder, and gait disturbance has been illustrated in Chapter 19.

The diagnosis is made on the basis of the clinical picture and family history. The diagnosis is confirmed by the laboratory data demonstrating an excessive number of CAG trinucleotide repeats on chromosome 4 and the neuroradiology studies demonstrating atrophy of the caudate nucleus and cerebral cortex.

3. Frontal/temporal dementia (FTD), including Pick's disease and Pick's lobar atrophy.

In this disease, insidious onset and slow progression of behavioral and cognitive changes reflect involvement of the frontal and anterior temporal lobe neocortex in the early stages of the disease. The involvement may be symmetrical or asymmetrical. Depending on the areas involved, aphasia or personality changes may be most prominent. These findings are disproportionate to any degree of memory impairment in the early stages of the disease since hippocampal/limbic involvement is not prominent in the early stages. Three syndromes have been recognized. Involvement of the bilateral prefrontal areas or of the right frontal or right temporal areas produces significant changes in personality. The more selective aspects of the changes in personality are discussed by Rosen et al. (2000). Bilateral prefrontal involvement will also impair executive abilities. Asymmetrical involvement of the left frontal area produces a progressive nonfluent aphasia. Asymmetrical involvement of the left anterior temporal area produces a fluent aphasia characterized by a progressive loss of semantic knowledge about people, facts, and words with an eventual anomia. With progression of the disease, all three variants overlap. A relatively long course of 6 to 8 years may occur. Occasional cases may be difficult to differentiate clinically from Alzheimer's disease or from dementia with Lewy bodies in the early stages. CT scan, MRI, or SPECT scan may be helpful in the diagnosis. At autopsy, the atrophy is more circumscribed than that in Alzheimer's disease. The major distinction occurs at the histological level. All cases have significant pathologic features in the superficial layers of the cerebral cortex of the involved lobes. This is characterized by loss of both large and small neurons, a gliosis which may be marked, and a spongiform appearance. Immunologic staining will demonstrate the presence of tau protein. Neurofibrillary tangles are not present. Some patients also have involvement of the basal ganglia and in these cases Parkinsonian features may be present. In occasional patients frontal temporal dementia is associated with motor neuron disease.

A small subset of patients have additional histologic features that have been described as Pick's disease. Ballooned neurons, referred to as Pick cells, are present; the appearance is similar to neurons undergoing central chromatolysis. These neurons contain silver staining intracytoplasmic inclusions referred to as Pick bodies.[3] These inclusions stain positive for ubiquitin and tau protein.

Frontal temporal dementia then is considered an example of a tauopathy. Approximately 38%–45% of FTD patients have a familial disorder inherited as an autosomal dominant.

---

[3] Both the Pick cells and the Pick bodies were actually first described by Alzheimer.

Figure 30.8 Creutzfeldt-Jakob disease: Histological features. (*A*) Low-power H&E: Diffuse microvacuolization of the neuropil and neuronal cell bodies is present in this biopsy of frontal lobe. (*B*) Higher power, approximately 150×. This 45-year-old female presented in November 1992 with a 3- to 4-week history of progressive ataxia and mental deterioration. EEG evolved into the characteristic periodic pattern. Patient expired after a total course of approximately 5 weeks. See also Figure 3.31 for appearance of cortical tissue from a biopsy of a patient with CJD. (Courtesy of Dr. Tom Mullins and Dr. Tom Smith.)

Genetic studies have linked the disorder to a region of chromosome 17 which codes for tau protein, which binds to microtubules and has a role in maintaining cytoskeletal structure. Subsequent studies have described a variety of mutations in the tau gene. Note that tau protein accumulates as aggregated insoluble fibers in other tauopathies, including Alzheimer's disease, progressive supranuclear palsy, and corticobasal ganglionic degeneration.

Additional discussion will be found in Rosen et al. (2000).

4. Creutzfeldt-Jakob disease[4] (CJD): Spongiform encephalopathy: This is a rare subacute disorder related to an abnormality of prion proteins. An abnormal relatively protease-resistant isoform of the normal cellular glycoprotein prion protein accumulates in the brain. Normal prion proteins are not protease resistant. In addition, diffuse microvacuolation (spongiform changes) of neuropil and cell bodies occurs with cell loss and gliosis involving both cerebral cortex and subcortical nuclei. Eighty-five percent of cases are sporadic. Fifteen percent are familial or related to iatrogenic and infectious causes as discussed later. Sporadic CJD is the major prion disorder in humans. The incidence is approximately 1 case per 1,000,000 population. However, most sporadic cases occur in the 60–74 age group, where there is an incidence of 5 cases per 1,000,000 population in this age group. In combination with rapidly progressive dementia of late adult onset, generalized seizures, myoclonic jerks, fasciculations, rigidity, and ataxia are present. The diagnosis is made on the basis of:

a. The clinical picture with evolution of the process over weeks or a few months.

b. The evolution of a characteristic EEG pattern of generalized periodic spike discharges (Fig. 30.9).

c. Cortical biopsy demonstrating the pathological features of a spongiform encephalopathy (Fig. 30.8).

Figure 30.9 Creutzfeldt-Jakob disease. Biopsy proving spongiform encephalopathy. Electroencephalogram (EEG) features: Frequent periodic discharges of generalized triphasic blunt spikes are present at a late stage of the disease. This 58-year-old male was admitted on January 18, 1993, with a brief subacute onset of ataxia and mild cognitive deficits and a mildly abnormal EEG. He evolved rapidly over a 4-week period (from onset to death), both from the clinical and EEG standpoint. Montage: standard longitudinal. 1-4, left parasagittal; 5-8, right parasagittal; 9-12; left temporal; 13-15, right temporal. (Courtesy of Dr. Tom Mullins and Dr. Sandra Horowitz.)

---

[4] Both authors described similar cases at approximately the same time. Jakob's cases are still recognized as examples of the disease. The cases of Creutzfeldt are not as clearly defined. Both names are still utilized to label human spongiform encephalopathy. The order varies.

d. The presence of a positive immunoassay in cerebrospinal fluid for 14-3-3 proteins (proteins 130–131), which are found in normal brain but not in cerebrospinal fluid. The patient must meet the criteria of a progressive dementia and must not have an acute cerebral infarct or an acute encephalitis. (Refer to Collinge, 1996.)

The usual age range of these sporadic cases overlaps the age range of Alzheimer's disease, which also may manifest in the later stages the combination of dementia and myoclonus.

The following case history presents a typical example.

CASE HISTORY 30.8

Date of admission: April 30, 1984. This 72-year-old, right-handed white housewife, formerly a statistician for a chronic disease hospital in western Massachusetts, was referred for evaluation of progressive problems with gait and balance starting insidiously 2 months prior to admission. The patient and her family had noted a tremor, primarily in the left hand and then involving both hands in July of 1983, but this had developed at a time of great stress when her daughter was hospitalized in an intensive care unit after an accident and the patient had to care for the daughter's twin children between July and December 1983. In February 1984, she began to have significant neurological disability related to difficulty with her balance. This progressed rapidly and was to some degree exacerbated by an elective hysterectomy for benign disease in March 1984. By the time of admission, she was unable to walk even with a cane or a walker and needed assistance.

Initially, her family indicated that her memory was intact, but subsequent history indicated there had been a slow deterioration of memory during this time as well (February to April 1984). She was noted to frequently reminisce about past memories and at times, hallucinate, especially at night. Recently, myoclonic jerks had been noted. She had been incontinent of urine for about a week prior to admission.

Past medical history: Unremarkable.

Family history: The patient's mother developed Parkinson's disease with shaking of the hands and legs beginning at the age of 76. By the time she died at the age of 83 she was bedridden. The patient's brother had been "senile" since open heart surgery several years previously.

Neurologic Examination

Mental status: The patient was alert and sitting in a wheelchair, but she required assistance. She was oriented for place and person but slightly disoriented for time (she gave the date as April 27 or 28, 1984). Speech was fluent with intact naming, repetition, and comprehension, but writing and drawing were impaired by her marked tremor. She was unable to remember any of five objects even with assistance. Formal psychometric examination demonstrated poor attention and considerable apraxia. Full-scale IQ Wechsler Adult Intelligence score (WAIS) was 80 with verbal IQ score of 90 and performance IQ of 69.

Cranial nerves II–XII: Intact.

Motor system: Although no atrophy was present, fasciculations were present in the right calf. Strength was intact. She was unable to stand or walk by herself. She had a marked ataxia and required a broad base when helped to stand or walk. She was ataxic while sitting. Movements were slow. Alternating hand movements were disorganized. An intention tremor was present in hands and to a lesser degree in legs, but this was minor compared to the marked midline ataxia. A minor head tremor was present.

No rigidity was present in the upper extremities but considerable resistance was present in the lower extremities at knees and ankles.

Reflexes: Deep tendon reflexes were symmetrical and physiologic. Plantar responses were flexor. There was no release of the grasp reflexes.

Sensation: Pain sensation was possibly decreased below the knees, but testing was not reliable. Vibration sensation was decreased at toes compared to ankles.

Myoclonus: Loud noises and sudden tactile stimuli would occasionally trigger sudden jerks of the extremities.

Clinical diagnosis: Subacute dementia, most likely spongiform encephalopathy (Creutzfeldt-Jakob disease).

Laboratory data: *Routine CBC* was normal except for a slight increase in white blood cell count to 13,400. B12 and folate levels were normal. Sedimentation rate was 47 mm/hr, but not significantly elevated at age 72. *Complete chemical surveys* were normal as regards electrolytes, glucose, renal and liver function, calcium, and phosphorous. Lead, mercury, arsenic, and manganese levels were normal. Serum copper was slightly elevated but ceruloplasmin was normal. Thyroid functions were normal. *Serum and spinal fluid serological tests for syphilis* were nonreactive, as was the fluorescent treponemal antibody (FTA) test. Antinuclear antibody test for lupus was negative. *Cerebrospinal fluid* was normal as regards cells, protein, sugar, oligoclonal bands, and immunoglobulin G. No tumor cells were present.

Chest X-ray and both enhanced and unenhanced CT scans of head were normal.

Bilateral carotid arteriograms and vertebral arteriograms were normal with no evidence of vasculitis.

Electroencephalograms: A progressive change occurred over a 2-month period with evolution from moderately abnormal to severely abnormal. *April 30, 1984:* occasional multifocal 2–3 Hz slow waves

Figure 30.10 Thalamic dementia secondary to a glioblastoma. Case 30.7: computerized tomography (CT) scan with contrast. An enhancing tumor with a necrotic center involves the anterior and medial thalamus without involvement of the posterior thalamus.

occurred in bursts—left temporal frontal and to a lesser degree independently right temporal. *May 7, 1984*: there were now bilateral frontal and left temporal bursts of 2–3 Hz slow waves. Photic driving response was now marked compared to the previous record. *May 9, 1984*: The bilateral bursts were now more prominent and were now pseudoperiodic. The focal left frontal temporal abnormality was also more prominent. The previous background activity of 10 Hz alpha rhythm was now composed of 5–7 Hz theta rhythm. *May 14, 1984*: The bursts of bilateral slow waves were more periodic and of longer duration. *May 24, 1984*: The background activity was now slower at 5–6 Hz theta waves. Bilateral bursts of paroxysmal triphasic sharp waves now accompanied the 2–3 Hz slow waves. These bursts were again more prominent left frontotemporal and lasted up to 9 seconds. Background activity also was suppressed up to 2 seconds in a periodic manner. *June 1, 1984*: The record was now markedly abnormal, largely consisting of rhythmic triphasic sharp waves and associated slow waves—lasting up to 10 seconds and followed by periods of relative background suppression. The record had a pseudoperiodic appearance.

Evoked potential studies: Brain stem auditory potentials (May 2, 1984, May 24, 1984) were normal.

Somatosensory evoked potentials (May 2, 1984, May 24, 1984). Abnormal: overall conduction times of brachial plexus to cortex were prolonged due to delays at both a cervical spinal cord and cortical level.

Visual evoked potentials: April 30, 1984: Normal. *May 4, 1984*: Abnormal (prolonged) for left eye stimulation. *May 11, 1984*: Abnormal to a greater degree for a left eye stimulation and now abnormal for right eye stimulation.

Nerve conduction studies: Mild axonal neuropathy.

Tremor study: Pattern was consistent with a nonspecific essential tremor.

Biopsy of the left frontal lobe was performed on May 10, 1984: A diffuse spongiform change was present in the cortex (similar to that illustrated in Fig. 30.8). There were numerous round to oval vacuoles, at times confluent within the neuropil. Many were extraneuronal. Some were intracytoplasmic—others indented, the nucleus or cytoplasm of neurons. No definite neuronal loss or gliosis or inflammation was present. The findings were considered pathognomonic of subacute spongiform encephalopathy (Creutzfeldt-Jakob disease). (Note that in patients with a short course, rapid progression of cell loss and gliosis may not be apparent in the biopsy specimen.)

Hospital course: The patient demonstrated a rapid deterioration in cognitive and neurological function. Memory deteriorated; confusion and lethargy developed. She developed marked startle myoclonus and she became more rigid, particularly in the lower extremities. Treatment with phenytoin, and Sinemet and Amantadine had no effect on the disease course. The patient was transferred to a chronic disease hospital, where she expired on June 14, 1984, approximately 11 months after she had first demonstrated a tremor and 4 months after ataxia, memory problems, and neurological disability had developed.

Comments

This unfortunate patient illustrates many of the manifestations of this subacute progressive disease, which involves cerebral cortex, basal ganglia, cerebellum, and brain stem. The exact point of onset was difficult to determine. The tremor, which developed at a time of stress and anxiety, may have been an essential tremor. The onset of rapidly progressive ataxia, dementia, and myoclonus in February of 1984 may then have signified the onset of a rapidly progressive neurological disease which evolved over the subsequent 4–5 months. As noted in the illustrations, other cases may evolve over an even more rapid period of time—a matter of 3–5 weeks. The significance of this disease relates not to its frequency but to the neurobiological studies of the underlying etiology. Questions have been raised as to whether this disease might serve as a model for the study of other "degenerations" affecting the nervous system.

NEUROBIOLOGY OF CREUTZFELDT-JAKOB DISEASE AND OTHER PRION DISORDERS

Creutzfeldt-Jakob disease has been demonstrated to share many characteristics with other subacute progressive neurological diseases: scrapie in sheep, bovine spongiform encephalopathy (mad cow disease) and Kuru in man. Scrapie was recognized as a common disorder over 200 years ago and its infectious nature was first recognized in 1936. The disease scrapie is so named because the affected sheep manifesting irritability and ataxia rubs away its wool against fences, trees, and so on. The disease may be transmitted to other sheep, as well as to goats, mice, hamsters, gerbils, mink, and monkeys (Gilden, 1983). Initially these disorders were classified as "slow virus infections." Studies in the hamster resulted in purification of an insoluble protease-resistant protein PrP27-30, which is a major component of the infectious particle. This class of particles has been assigned the term *prion*. These infectious particles are unique since they do not trigger the usual inflammatory reaction induced by viruses. The infectious particle differs from all other infectious agents in an absence of nucleic acids (DNA and RNA). This particle may polymerize into rods possessing the ultra structure and histochemical characteristics of amyloid. Prusiner and his associates were then able to develop an antiserum to PrP27-30. Purified fractions from the brains of patients with Creutzfeldt-Jakob disease contained protease-resistant proteins of apparent molecular weight 10,000 to 50,000. These fractions cross reacted with the scrapie prion protein PrP27-30. In addition, rod-shaped particles were found in the Creutzfeldt-Jakob brain that were similar to those isolated from the hamster brain infected with scrapie. Bockman et al. (1985) suggested that the amyloid plaques found in the brains of patients with Creutzfeldt-Jakob disease may be composed of these paracrystalline arrays of prion. Normal uninfected cells also contain a cellular prion protein (PrPc). The abnormal prion is termed *PrPsc*. The normal and abnormal prion proteins have an identical chemical composition but differ in their three-dimensional conformation. PrPc has predominantly helical spirals of amino acids (labeled alpha), whereas PrPsc has more flattened sheets of amino acids (labeled beta). Prions reproduce by stimulating the conversion of normal PrPc to Prpsc.

The actual manifestations of the disease differ based on the different conformations of PrPsc, the specific mammal, and the age of the infected host.

Creutzfeldt-Jakob disease can be transmitted to apes and monkeys with inoculation of homogenates of brain, spinal cord, eye, or cerebrospinal fluid. The incubation period is long. Prions from infected animals may infect mice and hamsters, but the incubation period is long and repeated passages are required.

Human-to-human transmission also occurs (Will and Matthews, 1982). The usual route of transmission has been through neurosurgical instruments and depth electrodes used on a suspected or unsuspected patient with the disease and then subsequently employed in a neurosurgical procedure on an uninfected patient. The use of dural grafts has also been associated with transmission of the disease. Rare instances of transmission with corneal transplantation have also occurred. Incubation period after cerebral or ocular inoculations is 15–20 months. Possible transmission through close contact in the house or with a neighbor has also been reported by Will and Matthews. The use of human growth hormone extracted from pituitary glands of cadavers—to treat human congenital dwarfism—has also been associated with the transmission of the disease to children and young adults with cases developing after a 5- to 15-year incubation period (Powell-Jackson et al., 1985). A recent outbreak in France related to the continued use of pooled cadaver pituitaries. A biosynthetic recombinant growth hormone, which eliminates this risk, had been available but had not been utilized in all countries.

Precautions to reduce transmission of disease have been discussed by Behan (1982), Brown et al. (1982), Gajdusek et al. (1977), Greenlee (1982), and Jarvis (1982).

Other Prion Disorders with Human-to-Human Transmission

The first prion disorder in humans with the features of spongiform encephalopathy demonstrated to be transmissible from human to human and to chimpanzees was Kuru. This disorder occurred as an epidemic among the Fore tribal group in the isolated highlands of New Guinea. The disease was acquired through the preparation with bare hands and then the subsequent consumption of the brains of dead relatives. After an incubation period of 4–30 years, cerebellar symptoms of ataxia, tremor, and dysarthria developed and progressed to death over months to a year. Many of the individuals involved in the ritual and in the subsequent disease were children or young adults. With elimination of the ritualistic cannibalism, the disease has disappeared.

Blood or blood products such as intravenous gamma globulin remains a point of concern since prions are present in blood and bone marrow in BSE and in lymphoid tissue in new-variant CJD.

Genetic Aspects of Transmission of Prion Disorders

Of all cases of CJD, 15% of cases occur in families with two or more affected members (Masters et al., 1981). The familial cases in comparison to sporadic cases have an earlier age of onset, a longer duration, and are less likely to have the characteristic EEG pattern. The 14-3-3 protein is present in the cerebrospinal fluid in only 50% of cases. Nevertheless, these cases do have the characteristic pathological picture of spongiform encephalopathy, neuronal loss, and gliosis. Transmission appears to be autosomal dominant with equal involvement of mothers and fathers. Moreover, the familial disease can be transmitted to primates in the same manner as the sporadic cases. A number (20) of different mutations in coding sequence of the gene for the prion protein precursor (PrP) on the short arm of chromosome 20 have been described. The most widely distributed is at codon 200 of the amino acid chain, less often at codon 178 (Brown et al., 1992).

In a related or variant disease, the Gerstmann-Straussler-Scheinker disorder (Masters et al., 1981), an autosomal dominant with prominent cerebellar ataxia, a long course of 5–10 years, and prominent amyloid plaque deposition, the mutation occurs at a different amino acid location, usually codon 102 of the normal prion protein gene.

An even rarer disorder, *fatal familial insomnia*, occurs with some of the mutations at codon location 178. Progressive insomnia, dysautonomia, and dementia occur over 7–15 months. Examination of the brain reveals selective neuronal loss and spongiform changes in the ventral and dorsomedial thalamic nuclei. In other cases with mutations at codon 178, the patients have a typical familial CJD. The difference relates to the amino acid composition at a different site, codon 129. At codon 129, individuals may be homozygous for methionine or valine or heterozygous for methionine/valine. If homozygous for methionine at codon 129, mutations at codon 178 result in fatal familial insomnia. If homozygous for valine at codon 129, mutations at codon 178 result in familial CJD.

The amino acid composition at codon 129 also influences susceptibility to sporadic or acquired CJD, as discussed by Haywood (1997). In healthy controls, 52% are heterozygous at codon 129 (methionine/valine); 37% are homozygous for methionine; and 11% homozygous for valine. In patients with sporadic CJD, 78% are homozygous for methionine; with only 11% heterozygous at codon 129. In patients with iatrogenic CJD, 60% are homozygous at codon 129 with only 11% heterozygous at this location. In patients with new variant CJD to be discussed later, 100% are homozygous for methionine at codon 129 with none heterozygous at this site. Thus, the prion disorders provide an example of the interaction of genetics and environment.

Transmission of Prion Disorders from Animal to Animal, Including Bovine Spongiform Encephalopathy

In addition to scrapie, widespread outbreaks of spongiform encephalopathy have affected domesticated or captive animals. These include transmissible mink encephalopathy, feline spongiform encephalopathy, wasting disease of deer and elk, and bovine spongiform encephalopathy. In almost all of these cases, these outbreaks have been the result of the use of feed contaminated by tissue from infected sheep or cattle secondary to changes in slaughterhouse procedures. The story of bovine spongiform encephalopathy, "mad cow disease," is instructive. In 1985, dairy cows in the United Kingdom were first noted to develop a syndrome of behavioral change (fearful and aggressive) and ataxia. Postmortem examination demonstrated a spongiform encephalopathy similar to scrapie. In 1988, the United Kingdom imposed a ban on feeding cows and other ruminants protein derived from ruminants such as sheep and cattle. Since the incubation period was 4–5 years, cases continued to increase, peaking at 36,000 cases in 1992 and then subsequently declining to 1500 cases in 2000. As of 1998, 170,000 cases of spongiform encephalopathy had been confirmed with severe economic impact on the agriculture industry of the United Kingdom. In the United States, strict bans on importation of ruminants and of ruminant-derived products have been in effect since 1989. A small number of cases have subsequently appeared in other western European countries.

Transmission of Prion Disorders from Animals to Humans (New Variant Creutzfeldt-Jakob Disease)

Until the emergence of "mad cow disease," this remained as an unknown factor. As discussed by Johnson and Gibbs (1998), the incidence of sporadic Creutfeldt-Jakob Disease (CJD) in counties such as Australia and New Zealand without scrapie is no different than in the United Kingdom where scrapie is endemic. Stockyard workers, butchers, chefs, pathologists, and surgeons do not have an increased incidence of the disease. Because of concern that several hundred thousand infected cattle had entered the human food chain, the United Kingdom established a monitoring unit for possible spread to humans. Beginning in 1994, a new type of spongiform encephalopathy began to appear almost entirely in the United Kingdom. As of 2000, 100 cases have been reported. This spongiform encephalopathy differs from the sporadic form of the disease. The patients are younger: mean age of 29 compared to 60 years. The mean duration of disease is longer: 14 months compared to 5 months. The most prominent clinical features at onset consist of psychiatric and sensory symptoms as compared to dementia. Cerebellar signs are present in 100% of the cases compared to 40% in sporadic CJD. Periodic complexes do not occur in the electroencephalogram compared to sporadic cases. The level of 14-3-3 protein in the cerebrospinal fluid is frequently normal. The genetic predisposition to the disease in terms of the homozygosity for methionine at codon 129 has been discussed earlier. At autopsy, the patients have diffuse amyloid plaques as well as spongiform changes. These changes are similar to those found in Kuru and in bovine spongiform encephalopathy. Laboratory transmission studies also demonstrate the relationship to bovine spongiform encephalopathy. Whether new variant disease can be spread by mild cognitive impairment of the elderly is a vague entity that may be a bridge between normal aging and Alzheimer's disease (AD). These individuals have some difficulty with word retrieval, especially proper nouns, but are not particularly cognitively handicapped. This problem is considered a part of normal aging but in some patients does go on to full-blown dementia. Progress in imaging genetic and biochemical diagnosis of AD will soon clarify this problem. Simple methods of cognitive testing can be used to predict the time of conversion to mild cognitive impairment in the normal elderly (Ouhaj et al., 2009). As soon as truly effective treatment for AD is available, early identification will be of paramount importance because AD begins decades before it is clinically evident.

Are prions involved in the more common neurodegenerative disorders? Attempts have been made to transmit the more common Alzheimer's disease to primates using the same methodology. These attempts even in familial cases have not been successful. Disorders such as Alzheimer's disease do not fall into the category of spongiform encephalopathy. While there may be changes in the beta-amyloid protein, apparently infectious particles prions do not result.

BIBLIOGRAPHY

Suggested Readings

Adams, R. D., and Victor, M. 1993. Principles of Neurology. 5th ed. New York, NY: McGraw Hill.

Diamond, A. E. (Ed.) 1990. The development and neural basis of higher cognitive functions. New York: Academy of Sciences.

DeKosky, S. (Ed.). 2000. Dementia. Neurol. Clin. 18:773–1044.

Doty, R. W. 1967. Limbic system. In A. M. Freedman and H. I. Kaplan (Eds.) Comprehensive Textbook of Psychiatry, pp.125–143. Baltimore, MD: Williams & Wilkins.

Gershon, E. S., and Rieder, R. O. 1992. Major disorders of mind and brain. Scientific American 267:126–133.

Harris-Warrick, R. N. 1991. Modulation of neural networks of behavior. Ann. Rev. Neurosci. 14:39–57.

Hebb, D. O. 1949. The Organization of Behavior: A Neuropsycholoqical Theory. New York, NY: John Wiley.

Hubel, D. H. 1988. Eve. Brain and Vision. New York, NY: Scientific American Library.

Jackson, J. H. 1889. On a particular variety of epilepsy ("intellectual aura"), one case with symptoms of organic brain disease. Brain 11:179–207.

Kandel, E. R., and Hawkins, R. D. 1992. The biological basis of learning and individuality. Scientific American 267:79–86.

Kitsch, P. M., Crowden, J. H., Corkin, S., et al. (Eds.) 1992. Alzheime's disease: amyloid precursor proteins, signal transduction and neuronal transplantation. Ann. NY Acad. Sci. 605:1–339.

Kupferman, I. 1991. Learning and memory. In E. R. Kandel, J. H. Schwartz, T. M. Jessell (Eds.) Principles of Neural Science. 3rd ed., pp. 997–1008. New York, NY: Elsevier.

Langston, J. W., and Young, A. (Eds.). 1992. Neurotoxins and neurodegenerative disease. Ann. NY Acad. Med. 648:1–385.

Lashlcy, K. S. 1963. Brain mechanisms and intelligence: a quantitative study of iniurv to the brain. New York, NY: Hafner.

Lynch, G., McGaugh, J. L., and Weinberger, N. M. (Eds.). 1984. The Neurobiolocrv of Learning. New York, NY: Guilford Press.

Mishkin, M., and Appenzeller, T. 1987. The anatomy of memory a scientific American special report. Scientific American l–11.

Olds, J. 1962. Hypothalamic substrates of reward. Physiol. Rev. 42:554–604.

Pavlov, I. P. 1927. Conditioned Reflexes: An Investigation of the Physiological Activity of the Cerebral Cortex (G. U. Anrep Trans.). London, UK: Oxford University Press.

Schatz, C. J. 1992. The developing brain. Scientific American 167:61–76.

Selkoe, D. J. 1992. Aging brain, aging mind. Scientific American 267:134–142.

Squire, L. R., and Lindenlaub, E. (Eds.). 1990. The Biology of Memory. Stuggart, Germany: Schatteuer Verlag.

Tinbergin, N. 1951. The Study of Instinct. London, UK: Oxford University Press.

Tomlinson, B. E., and Corsellis, J. A. N. 1984. Aging and the dementias. In J. Adams, J. A. N. Corsellis, and L. W. Duchen (Eds.) Greenfield's Neuropathology. 4th ed., pp. 951–1025. New York, NY: John Wiley.

Victor, M., Adams, R. D., and Collins, G. H. (Eds.) 1989. The Wernicke-Korsakoff Syndrome and Related Neurologic Disorders due to Alcoholism and Malnutrition. 2nd ed. Philadelphia, PA: F. A. Davis.

Wechsler, D. 1944. The Measurement of Adult Intelligence. Baltimore, MD: Williams and Wilkins.

Weiskrantz, L. 1985. On issues and theories of the human amnesic syndrome In N. M. Weinberger, J. L. McGaugh, and G. Lynch (Eds.) Memory Systems of the Brain: Animal and Human Cognitive Processes, pp. 380–415. New York, NY: Guilford Press.

SPECIFIC REFERENCES (see also chapter 27 for Creuztfeldt-Jakob disease)

Aldhous, P. 1992. French officials panic over rare brain disease outbreak. Science 258:1571–1572.

Bachman, D. L., Wolf, P. A., Linn, R., et al. 1992. Prevalence of dementia and probable senile dementia of the Alzheimer type in the Framingham study. Neurology 42:115–119.

Asztely, F., and Kumlien, E. 2012. The diagnosis and treatment of limbic encephalitis. Acta Neurol. Scand. 126(6):365–375.

Baringa, M. 1992. The brain remaps its own contours. Science 258:216–218.

Bateman, R. J., Xiong, C., Benzinger, T., Fagan, A. M., et al. 2012. Clinical and biomarker changes in dominantly inherited Alzheimer's disease. N. Engl. J. Med. 367(9):795–804.

Baringer, J. R. 1992. Viral infections. In A. K. Asbury, G. M. Mckhann, and W. I. McDonald (Eds.) Diseases of the Nervous System: Clinical Neurobiology. 2nd ed., pp. 1298–1311. Philadelphia, PA: W. B. Saunders.

Behan, P. O. 1982. Creutzfeldt-Jakob disease. BMJ. 284:1658–1659.

Bliss, T. V. P., and Lomo, T. 1973. Long-lasting potentiation of synaptic transmission in dentate area of the anesthetized rabbit following stimulation of the perforant path. J. Physiol. (London) 232:331–356.

Bookman, J. M., Kingsbury, D. T., McKinley, M. P., et al. 1985. Creutzfeldt-Jakob disease prion proteins in human brains. N. Engl. J. Med. 312:73–78.

Boothe, R. G., Dobson, V., Teller, D. Y. 1985. Postnatal development of vision in human and nonhuman primates. Ann. Rev. Neurosci. 8:495–545.

Brown, P., Gajdusek, D. C., Gibbs, C. J., Jr., et al. 1985. Potential epidemic of Creutzfeldt-Jakob disease from human growth hormone therapy. N. Engl. J. Med. 313:728–731.

Brown, P., Goldfarb, L. G., Kovanen, J., et al. 1992. Phenotypic characteristics of familial Creutzfeldt-Jakob disease associated with the Codon 178 Asn PRNP mutation. Ann. Neurol. 31:282–285.

Brown, P., Gibbs, C. J., Amyx, H. L., et al. 1982. Chemical disinfection of Creutzfeldt-Jakob disease virus. N. Engl. J. Med. 306:1279–1282.

Brown, P., Ceruera'kova', L., Goldfarb, L. G., et al. 1994. Iatrogenic Creutzfeldt-Jakob disease: an examples of the interplay between ancient genes and modern medicine. Neurology 44:291–293.

Burkhardt, C. R., Filiey, C. M., Meinschmidt-DeMasters, B. K., et al. 1988. Diffuse Lewy body disease and progressive dementia. Neurology 38:1520–1528.

Calford, M. B., and Tweedale, R. 1990. Interhemispheric transfer of plasticity in the cerebral cortex. Science 249:805–807.

Caplan, L., Chedru, F., Lhermitte, F., et al. 1981. Transient global amnesia and migraine. Neurology 31:1167–1170.

Caplan, L. R., and Schoene, W. C. 1978. Clinical features of subcortical arteriosclerotic encephalopathy (Bunswanger disease). Neurology 28:1206–1215.

Carpenter, W. T., Jr., and Buchanan, R. W. 1994. Schizophrenia. N. Engl. J. Med. 330:681–690.

Corder, E. H., Saunders, A. M., Strittmatter, W. J., et al. 1993. Gene dose of apolipoprotein E type 4 allele and the risk of Alzheimer's disease in late onset families. Science 261:921–923.

Desimone, R. 1992. The physiology of memory: recordings of the past. Science 258:245–246.

Dollard, J., and Miller, N. E. 1950. Personality and Psychotherapy. New York, NY: McGraw Hill.

Drachman, D. A., and Leavitt, J. 1974. Human memory and the cholinergic system—A relationship to aging? Arch. Neurol. 30:113–121.

Drachman, D. A. 1993. New criteria for the diagnosis of vascular dementia: Do we know enough yet? Neurology 43:243–245.

Evans, D. A., Funkenstein, H. H., Albert, M. S., et al. 1989. Prevalence of Alzheimer's disease in a community population of older adults. JAMA. 262:2551–2556.

Friedland, R. P. 1993. Epidemiology, education and the ecology of Alzheimer's disease. Neurology 43:246–249.

Fristoen, K. J., Liddle, P. F., Firth, C. D., et al. 1992. The left medial temporal region and schizophrenia. A PET study. Brain 115:367–382.

Gajdusek, D. C., Gibbs, C. J., Asher, D. M., et al. 1977. Precautions in medical care of, and in handling materials from patients with transmissible virus dementia (Creutzfeldt-Jakob disease). N. Engl. J. Med. 297:1253–1258.

Gallassie, R., Morreale, A., Lorusso, S., et al. 1977. Epilepsy presenting as memory disturbances. Epilepsia 29:624–629.

Gilden, D. H. 1983. Slow virus diseases of the CNA: part II. Scrapie, Kuru, and Jakob-Creutzfeldt disease. Postgrad. Med. 73:113–118.

Goldenberg, G., Podreka, I., Phaffel-Meyer, N., et al. 1991. Thalamic ischemia in transient global amnesia: a SPECT study. Neurology 41:1748–1752.

Graus, F., and Dalmau, J. 2012. Paraneoplastic neurologicl syndromes. Curr Opin Neurol. 25(6):795–801.

Honig, L. S. 2012. Translational research in neurology: dementia. Arch. Neurol. 69(8):969–977.

Hooli, B. V., Mohapatra, G., Mattheisen, M., Parrado, A. R., et. al. 2012. Role of common and rare APP DNA sequence variants in Alzheimer disease. Neurology 78:1250–1257.

Graff-Radford, N. R., Tranel, D., VanHoesen, G. W., et al. 1990. Diencephalic amnesia. Brain 113:1–25.

Greenlee, J. E. 1982. Infection control—containment precautions in hospitals for cases of Creutzfeldt-Jakob disease (Editorial). Infect. Control 3:222–223.

Growdon, J. H. 1992. Treatment for Alzheimer's disease? (Editorial). N. Engl. J. Med. 327:1306–1308. (Ssee also David et al., 1992. N. Engl. J. Med. 327: 1253–1259.)

Grundman, M., and Thal, L. J. 2000. Treatment of Alzheimer's disease. Neurol. Clin. 18:807–828.

Hansen, L., Salmon, D., and Galasko, D. 1990. The lewy body variant of Alzheimer's disease: a clinical and pathologic entity. Neurology 40:1–8.

Harlow, H. 1974. Learning to Love. New York, NY: Jason Aronson.

Heiligenberg, W. 1991. The neural basis of behavior: a neuroethological view. Ann. Rev. Neurosci. 14:247–267.

Hellmuth, J. (Ed.). 1963. Disadvantaged child, Vol. 2. Headstart and Early Intervention. New York, NY: Brunner-Mazel.

Hsiao, K., and Prusiner, S. B. 1990. Inherited human prion diseases. Neurology 40:1820–1827.

Hubel, D. H. 1988. Eve. Brain and Vision. New York, NY: Scientific American Library.

Irle, E., Wowra, B., Kunert, H. J., Hampl, J., and Krunze, S. 1992. Memory disturbances following anterior communicating artery rupture. Ann. Neurol. 31:473–480.

Jarvis, W. R. 1982. Precautions for Creutzfeldt-Jakob disease. Infect. Control 3:238–239.

Jenkins, W. M., Merzenich, M. M., Ochs, M., et al. 1990. Functional reorganization of primary somatosensory motor cortex in adult owl monkeys after behaviorally controlled tactile stimulation. J. Neurophysiol. 63:82–104.

Jonsson, T., Hreinn, S., Steinberg, S., et al. 2013. Variant of TREME associated with risk of Alzheimer's disease. N. Engl. J. Med. 368(2):107–127.

Kaas, J. H., Krubitzer, L. A., Chino, Y. M., et al. 1990. Reorganization of retinotopic cortical maps in adult mammals after lesions of the retina. Science 248:229–231.

Kass, J. 1991. Plasticity of sensory and motor maps in adult mammals. Ann. Rev. Neurosci. 14:137–167.

Kandel, E. R., and Jessell, T. 1991. Early experience and the fine tuning of synaptic connections. In E. R. Kandel, J. H. Schwartz, and T. M. Jessell (Eds.) Principles of Neural Science, pp. 945–958. New York, NY: Elsevier.

Kandel, E. R., and O'Dell, T. J. 1992. Are adult learning mechanisms also used for development? Science 258:243–295.

Kapur, N., Ellison, D., Smith, M. P., et al. 1992. Focal retrograde amnesia following bilateral temporal lobe pathology: a neuropsychological and magnetic resonance study. Brain 115:73–85.

Katzman, R. 1993. Education and the prevalence of Alzheime's disease. Neurology 43:13–20.

Kemper, T. L., and Bauman, M. L. 1993. The contribution of neuropathological studies to the understanding of autism. Neurol. Clin. 11:175–187.

Lin, K. N., Liu, R. S., Yeh, T. P., et al. 1993. Posterior ischemia during an attack of transient global amnesia. Stroke 24:1093–1095.

Madison, D. V., Malenka, R. C., and Nicoll, R. A. 1991. Mechanisms underlying long term potentiation of synaptic transmission. Rev. Neurosci. 14:379–397.

Markesbery, W. R. 1992. Alzheime's disease. In C. M. McKhann and W. McDonald (Eds.) Diseases of the Nervous System: Clinical Neurobiology. 2nd ed., pp. 755–803. Philadelphia: W. B. Saunders.

Marx, J. 1990. Human brain disease recreated in mice. Science 250:1509–1510.

Marx, J. 1992a. A new link in brain's defenses—research news. Science 256:1278–1280.

Marx, J. 1992b. Alzheime's debate boils over—news & comments. Science 257:1336–1338.

Marx, J. 1992c. Familial Alzheimer's linked to chromosome 14 gene—neurobiology. Science 258:550.

Masters, C. L., Gajdusek, D. C., and Gibbs, C. J. 1981. The familial occurrence of Creutzfeldt-Jakob disease and Alzheimer's disease. Brain 104:535–558.

Masters, C. L., Harris, J. O., Gajdusek, D. C., et al. 1979. Creutzfeldt-Jakob disease: patterns of world-wide occurrence and the significance of familial and sporadic clustering. Ann. Neurol. 5:177–187.

Mathew, N. T., and Meyer, J. S. 1974. Pathogenesis and natural history of transient global amnesia. Stroke 5:303–311.

Mayeaux, R., and Sternspanton, S. 1985. Heterogenicity in dementia of the Alzheimer type: evidence of subgroups. Neurology 35:453–461.

Mazzucchi, A., Moretti, G., Caffarra, P., et al. 1980. Neuropsy-chological functions in the follow-up of transient global amnesia. Brain 103:161–178.

McClelland, D. C., and Atkinson, J. W. 1948. The projective expression of needs. J. Psychol. 25:206.

McKee, A. C., Kosik, K. S., and Kowall, N. W. 1991. Neuritic pathology and dementia in Alzheime's Disease. Ann. Neurol. 30:156–165.

Mc Keith, I. G. 2000. Spectrum of Parkinson's disease, Parkinson's dementia and Lewy body dementia. Neurol. Clin. 18:865–884.

McKhann, G., Drachman, D., Folstein, M., et al. 1984. Clinical diagnosis of Alzheimer's disease. Neurology 34:939–944.

Melo, T. P., Ferro, J. M., and Ferro, H. 1992. Transient global amnesia: a case control study. Brain 115: 261–270.

Merzenich, M. M. 1985. Sources of intraspecies and interspecies cortical ap variability in mammals: conclusionsand hypothesis. In J. J. Cohen and A. B. Strumwasser (Eds.) Comparative Neurobiology Modes of Communication in the Nervous System, pp. 105–116. New York, NY: Wiley.

Mesulam, M. M. 1982. Slowly progressive aphasia without generalized dementia. Ann. Neurol. 11:592–598.

Mesulam, M. M. 1990. Schizophrenia and the brain. N. Engl. J. Med. 322:842–844.

Nestor, P. N., and Hodges, J. 2000. Non Alzheimer's dementias. Semin. Neurol. 20:439–446.

Ojemann, G. A., Creutzfeldt, O., Lettich, E., et al. 1988. Neuronal activity in human lateral temporal cortex related to short-term verbal memory, naming and reading. Brain 111:1383–1403.

Ott, B. R., and Saver, J. L. 1993. Unilateral amnesic stroke, six new cases and review of the literature. Stroke 24:1033–1042.

Oulhaj, A., Wilcock, G. K., Smith, A. D., and de Jager, C. A. 2009. Predicting the time of conversion to MCI in the elderly: role of verbal expression and learning. Neurology 73(18):1436–1442.

Penfield, W., and Milner, B. 1958. Memory deficit produced by bilateral lesions in the hippocampal zone. Arch. Neurol. Psychiat. 79:475–497.

Perl, D. P. 2000. Neuropathology of Alzheimer's disease and related disorders. Neurol. Clin. 18:847–864.

Perry, R. H., Irving, D., Blessed, G., et al. 1989. Clinically and neuropathologically distinct form of dementia in the elderly. Lancet 1:166.

Pollen, D. A. 1993. Hannah's Heirs: The Guest for the Genetic Origin of Alzheimer's Disease. New York, NY: Oxford University Press.

Pons, T. P., Garraghty, P. E., Ommaya, A. K., et al. 1991. Massive cortical reorganization after sensory deafferentation in adult macaques. Science 252:1857–1860.

Powell-Jackson, J., Kennedy, P., Whitcomb, E. M., et al. 1985. Creutzfeldt-Jakob disease after administration of human growth hormone. Lancet 2:244–246.

Prusiner, S. B. 1991. The molecular biology of prion diseases. Science 252:1515–1522.

Riesen, A. H. 1966. Sensory deprivation in progress. In E. Stellar and J. M. Sprague (Eds.) Physiological Psychology, Vol. 1, pp.117–147. New York, NY: Academic Press.

Rocca, W. A., Hofman, A., Brayno, C., et al. 1991a. Frequency and distribution of Alzheimer's disease in Europe: a collaborative study of 1980–1990 prevalence findings. Ann. Neurol. 30:381–390.

Rocca, W. A., Hofman, A., Brayne, C., et al. 1991b. The prevalence of vascular dementia in Europe: facts and fragments from 1980–1990 studies. Ann. Neurol. 30:817–824.

Rogers, J. D., Brogan, D., Miran, S. S. 1995. The nucleus basalis of Meynert in neurological disease: a quantitative morphological study. Ann. Neurol. 17:163–170.

Roman, G. C., Tatemich, T. R., Erkinjuntti, T., et al. 1993. Vascular dementia: diagnostic criteria for research studies: report of the NINDS-AIREN International Workshop. Neurology 43:250–260.

Rosen, H. J., Lengenfelder, J., and Miller, B. 2000. Frontotemporal dementia. Neurol. Clin. 18:979–992.

Rosenzweig, M. B., and Leiman, A. L. 1986. Brain functions. Ann. Rev. Psychol. 19:55–98.

Russell, R. W. 1966. Biochemical substrates of behavior. In R. W. Russell (Ed.) Frontiers in Physiological Psychology, pp. 185–246. New York, NY: Academic Press.

Saunders, A. M., Strittmatter, W. J., Schmechel, D., et al. 1993. Association of apolipoprotein E. allele-4 with late onset and sporadic Alzheimer's disease. Neurology 43:1467–1472.

Schatz, C. J. 1992. The developing brain. Scientific American 267:61–76.

Scoville, W. B., and Milner, B. 1957. Loss of recent memory after bilateral hippocampal lesions. J. Neurol. Eurosurg. Psychiatry 20:11–21.

Selkoe, D. J. 2000a. The genetics and molecular pathology of Alzheimer's disease: roles of amyloid and the presenilins. Neurol. Clin. 18:903–922.

Selkoe, D. J. 2000b. Presenilins, B amyloid precursors and the molecular basis of Alzheimer's disease. Clin. Neurosci. Res. 1:91–103.

Shenton, M. E., Kikinis, R., Jolesz, F. A., et al. 1992. Abnormalities of the left temporal lobe and thought disorder in schizophrenia: a quantitative magnetic resonance imaging study. N. Engl. J. Med. 327:604–612.

Silva, A. J., Stevens, C. F., Tonegawa, S., et al. 1992. Deficient hippocampal long term potentiation in B-calcium- calmodulin kinase II mutant mice. Science 257:201–206.

Silva, A. J., Paylor, R., Wehner, J. M., et al. 1992. Impaired spatial learning in B-calcium-calmodulin kinase II mutant mice. Science 257:206–211.

Skoog, L. Nilsson, B., Palmertz, B., et al. 1993. A population-based study on dementia in 85-year-olds. N. Engl. J. Med. 328:153–158.

Sparks, D. L., and Markesbery, W. R. 1991. Altered serotonergic and cholinergic synaptic markers in Pick's disease. Arch. Neurol. 48:796–799.

Spillantini, M. G., and Goedert, M. 2000. Tau mutations in familial frontotemporal dementia. Brain 123:857–859

Spitz, R. 1945. Hospitalism. Psychoanal. Study Child. 1:53.

Squire, L. R., and Zola-Morgan, S. 1991. The medial temporal lobe memory system. Science 253:1380–1386.

Stillhard, G., Landis, T., Schiess, R., et al. 1990. Bitemporal hypoperfusion in transient global amnesia: 99mTC- HM-PAO SPECT and neuropsychological findings during and after an attack. J. Neurol. Neurosurg. Psychiatry 53:339–342.

Strittmatter, W. J., Saunders, A. M., Schmechal, D., et al. 1993. Apolipoprotein E. High avidity binding to B. amyloid and increased frequency of type 4 allele in late onset familial Alzheimer's disease. Proc. Natl. Acad. Sci. USA 90:1977–1981.

Suddath, R. L., Christison, G. W., Torrey, E. F., et al. 1990. Anatomical abnormalities in the brains of monozygotic twins discordant for schizophrenia. N. Engl. J. Med. 322:789–794.

Tassinari, C. A., Ciarmatori, C., Alesi, C., et al. 1991. Transient global amnesia as a postictal state from recurrent partial seizures. Epilepsia 32:882–885.

Tatemichi, T. K., Steinke, W., Duncan, C., et al. 1992. Paramedian thalamopeduncular infarction: Clinical syndromes and magnetic resonance imaging. Ann. Neurol. 32:162–171.

Teitelbaum, J. S., Zatorre, R. J., Carpenter, S., et al. 1990. Neurologic sequelae of domoic acid intoxication due to the ingestion of contaminated mussels. N. Engl. J. Med. 322:1781–1787.

Tomlinson, B. E., Blessed, G., and Roth, M. 1970. Observations on the brains of demented old people. J. Neurol. Sci. 11:205–242.

Tulving, E., and Schacter, D. L. 1990. Priming and human memory systems. Science 247:301–306.

Tuzon, E., and Dalmau, J. 2007. Limbic encephalitis and variants: classification, diagnosis and treatment. Neurologist 13(5):261–271.

Victor, M., Agevine, J. B., Mancall, E. L., et al. 1961. Memory loss with lesions of hippocampal formation. Arch. Neurol. 5:244–263.

von Cramon, D. Y., Hebel, N., and Schuri, V. 1985. A contribution to the anatomical basis of thalamic amnesia. Brain 108:993–1008.

von Cramon, D. Y., Hebel, N., and Schuri, V. 1988. Verbal memory and learning in unilateral posterior cerebral infarction. A report on 30 cases. Brain 111:1061–1078.

Whitehouse, P. J., Price, D. L., Dark, A. W., et al. 1981. Alzheimer's disease: evidence for selective loss of cholinergic neurons in the nucleus basalis. Ann. Neurol. 10:1226.

Wiesel, T. N., and Hubel, D. H. 1963. Efforts of visual deprivation on morphology and physiology of cells in the cat's lateral geniculate lobes. J. Neurophysiol. 26:978–993.

Wiesel, T. N., and Hubel, D. H. 1963. Single cell responses in striate cortex of kittens deprived of vision in one eye. J. Neurophysiol. 26:1003–1007.

Will, R. G., and Matthews, W. B. 1982. Evidence for case-to-case transmission of Creutzfeldt-Jakob disease. Neuro. Neurosurg. Psychiatry 45:235–238.

Williams, M., and Pennybacker, J. 1954. Memory disturbances in third ventricle tumors. J. Neurol. Neurosurg. Psychiatry 17:115–123.

Winker, M. A. 1994. Tacrine for Alzheimer's disease. Which patient, what dose? JAMA. 271:1023–1024. (see also Knapp et al. 1994. JAMA. 271:985–991; and Watkins et al. 1994. JAMA. 271:992–998)

Woods, B. T., and McKee, A. C. 1992. Case records of the Massachusetts General Hospital—a 67-year-old man with aphasia and memory loss followed by progressive dementia. N. Engl. J. Med. 326:397–405.

Yankner, B. A., Dawes, L. F., Fisher, S., et al. 1989. Neuro-toxicity of a fragment of the amyloid precursor associated with Alzheimer's disease. Science 245:117–210.

Yankner, B. A., Duffy, L. K., Kirschner, D. A. 1990. Neurotrophic and neurotoxic effects of amyloid B protein: reversal by tachykinin neuropeptides. Science 250:279–282.

Yang, L., Rieves, D., and Ganley, C. 2012. Brain amyloid imaging-FDA approval of florbetapir F18 injection. N. Engl. J. Med. 367(10): 885–887.

Yankner, B. A., and Mesulam, M. M. 1991. B-amyloid and the pathogenesis of Alzheimer's disease. N. Engl. J. Med. 325:1849–1857.

Zola-Morgan, S., Squire, L. R., and Amaral, D. G. 1986. Human amnesia and the medial temporal region: enduring memory impairment following a bilateral lesion limited to field CA1 of the hippocampus. J. Neurosci. 6:2950–2967.

Zola-Morgan, S. M., and Squire, L. R. 1990. The primate hippocampal formation. Evidence for a time limited role in memory storage. Science 250:288–296.

31.

CASE HISTORY PROBLEM SOLVING

PART V: GENERAL CASES

CASE HISTORY 31.1

This 59-year-old, white, male, married plumbing contractor, approximately 7 years prior to admission, had the onset of a tremor of the right hand occurring mainly at rest. One year prior to admission, the patient had noted progression. The tremor was now present at the wrist and shoulder, in addition to the fingers. During this time, the patient had also noted a stiffness of the right leg when walking. For 1 year prior to admission, since an alleged back injury, he had been unable to straighten up when walking and had to walk in a very stooped position. During the 6 months prior to admission, the patient had experienced short episodes of subjective vertigo, resulting in a tendency to fall forward.

Past History

1. Poliomyelitis at age 2, with residual atrophy of left gastrocnemius muscle.
2. Influenza at age 18.

Neurological Examination

1. *Mental status*:
   a. Patient was depressed and anxious.
   b. There was mild impairment of digit span and of delayed recall, and an inability to retell stories. Some evidence of confabulation was present.
2. *Cranial nerves*: A fixed facies with minor facial asymmetry was present.
3. *Motor system*:
   a. Strength was intact, except for plantar flexion at left ankle, with associated atrophy of gastrocnemius and shortening of the left Achilles tendon.
   b. Gait: The patient walked stooped over, with slow short steps. He turned en bloc. There was a lack of associated movements of the arms, with greater impairment on the right side.
   c. There was a resting tremor of the right upper extremity at the shoulder, wrist, and fingers. The tremor was rhythmical at 3 to 4/second and pill rolling in type.
   d. There was a plastic resistance to passive motion with an intermittent cogwheel component in the right upper extremity at the shoulder, elbow, and wrist. To a lesser degree, rigidity was present in the right lower extremity.
   e. Alternating movements were impaired bilaterally (right more so than left).
4. *Reflexes*:
   a. Deep tendon reflexes: Biceps and triceps were more active on the left; patellar and Achilles were more active on the right.
   b. Plantar responses were extensor bilaterally.
5. *Sensory system*: Intact.

Laboratory Data

1. Thyroid function normal.
2. Cerebrospinal fluid: normal pressure, cells, protein, and Hinton.
3. Electroencephalogram (EEG): Normal.

QUESTIONS

1. Indicate the diagnosis; provide a differential diagnosis.
2. Where is the lesion?
3. What significance do you attach to the bilateral Babinski signs?
4. What significance do you attach to the changes in mental status?
5. Indicate the pathophysiology and etiology.
6. Outline current concepts of diagnostic and therapeutic management.
7. Indicate the prognosis.

CASE HISTORY 31.2

This 42-year-old woman reported to the doctor with a complaint of "trouble with my eyes." At around the age of 20, her menses ceased and never returned. The patient stated she had had an underactive thyroid for 20 years. Her menstrual symptoms did not respond to thyroid medication. During the past few years, the patient had had some automobile accidents and had noted that these accidents occurred when there were objects to her right. During the month before entry, the patient felt excessively tired and was sleeping more than usual but was able to go to work. Her skin had become dry; she had gradually put on weight over the years; her hair was scant with loss of underarm hair and scant pubic hair. A bifrontal dull headache had been present for 1 week.

Physical examination: There was puffiness of hands and face and dryness of the skin. Blood pressure was 108/72; pulse was 82 and regular.

Skin and mucous membranes were pale, and there was bilateral pallor of the optic disks.

Neurological Examination

1. *Mental status:* Intact.
2. *Cranial nerves:* Intact except the visual fields showed a bitemporal upper quadrantic field defect that was almost complete in the right eye and less marked on the left. There was also bilateral pallor of the optic disks. Pupils and ocular movements were normal.
3. *Motor system*: No abnormalities noted.
4. *Reflexes*: Within normal limits.
5. *Sensory system*: Normal.

Subsequent course: Patient returned the next day, having had an emotional upset at work with the onset of a severe pressure headache.

She complained of sudden worsening of vision in the left eye and a film over the temporal fields. On examination, she was pale and sweating. Blood pressure was 100/70; pulse was 100. There was more marked cutting of visual fields, particularly on the left, with a true hemianoptic defect; both eyes now demonstrated a full temporal hemianopia. The patient was drowsy but could provide concise answers. Neurological examination was otherwise normal. The patient was immediately admitted to the hospital. Laboratory studies in the hospital confirmed the clinical impression of hypothyroidism. In addition, there was no follicle-stimulating hormone (FSH) detected on an assay of a 24-hour urine specimen. Plain skull films were positive and bilateral carotid arteriograms were performed. Patient was started on endocrine therapy, and an operation was performed. Three days following surgery, it was noted that the patient was complaining of constant and excessive thirst and was consuming huge quantities of fluids.

Questions

1. In this case, neurological evaluation many years previously would have established the diagnosis. Indicate the location of this lesion. Discuss the differences between this lesion at onset and the lesion at the present time.
2. Indicate the most likely pathology. Speculate as to the other possible causes of this syndrome.
3. What happened the day after the initial office evaluation?
4. Today, which neurodiagnostic study would have best demonstrated the location and nature of the pathology?
5. This patient had 24-hour urine FSH levels performed. Which additional endocrine blood test would be performed today? What are the causes of abnormalities in that additional test?
6. What is the localizing significance of the thyroid dysfunction?
7. What is the localizing significance of the ovarian dysfunction?
8. Why did the patient have excessive thirst and excessive consumption of fluids (polydipsia) after surgery?
9. Why was the patient sleeping more than usual and why was she markedly drowsy at the time of admission? (Several explanations are possible in this case.)

CASE HISTORY 31.3

Three weeks prior to admission, this 60-year-old, right-handed white male had the acute onset of clumsiness of his right hand. Soon thereafter, he noticed weakness and numbness involving the right hand. He then noticed that his right leg was weak, and he fell to the floor. The weakness and numbness of the hand and leg cleared in a matter of minutes. The patient, however, continued to have clumsiness of the right hand. On two subsequent occasions, he had a recurrence of weakness of the right hand.

The patient's history was also of significance in that over a 2-month period, he had had three episodes, each 3 minutes in duration, of a monocular blindness of the left eye. Diabetes mellitus had been present for approximately 20 years.

Six months before admission, the patient had had a sudden onset of weakness and coldness of the right lower extremity, due to sudden occlusion of the right femoral artery.

Cerebellar tests and gait were intact.

Reflexes: Deep tendon reflexes were slightly increased in the right arm compared to the left. The Achilles tendon reflexes were absent bilaterally.

Sensory system:
a. Vibration sensation was decreased bilaterally at the toes.
b. Occasional errors were made in letter and number recognition in the right hand.

Questions

1. What is the diagnosis? Be specific as to the vessel and area involved, if vascular in nature.
2. Outline your diagnostic approach to this problem.
3. Indicate possible therapeutic measures.
4. What is the explanation for the absent Achilles deep tendon reflexes and the decreased perception of vibration at toes?

CASE HISTORY 31.4

The patient was a 20-year-old, right-handed white housewife who was seen initially in the 23rd week of her third pregnancy. The patient presented with a history of generalized convulsive (tonic clonic) seizures beginning at age 7. These apparently would occur once a month without warning. She was begun on treatment with phenytoin and phenobarbital about age 8. She had had recurrences of seizures 2 years prior to the visit and 1 year prior to the visit. On each occasion, these seizures related to her omission of medication for several days. Her medications at the time of the initial visit were phenytoin, 100 mg a day, and phenobarbital, 15 mg a day.

Her symptoms improved when a right femoral endarterectomy with bypass was performed. The patient had had 5- to 10-minute episodes of chest pain (angina pectoris) for a number of years.

Family history was significant in that the patient's mother, father, daughter, and son had all experienced severe diabetes mellitus.

General Physical Examination

1. Blood pressure was 130/80 in both the right and left arms.
2. Light pressure on the left eyeball led to a blackout of vision; similar symptoms were not produced on the right side.

Neurological Examination

1. *Mental status*: The patient was oriented for time, place, and person.
2. *Cranial nerves*: No significant findings.
3. *Motor system*: Strength was intact, except for a minimal drift downward of the outstretched right arm when both arms were outstretched.

Family history: A maternal grandfather had convulsions and staring spells. Two cousins also had a seizure disorder, manifested by staring spells.

Neurological Examination

In detail, the entire examination was normal.

Laboratory Data

1. *Electroencephalogram*: The patient had bilateral, relatively synchronous bursts of polyspike-slow wave complexes most prominent in the frontal recording areas. At times, the bursts would continue for 2 to 3 seconds. No clinical phenomena were noted during the discharges.
2. *Blood levels*: Dilantin blood level was less than 2.5 μg/ml; phenobarbital was 5 μg/ml.

Subsequent course: The patient agreed to increase her intake of Dilantin to 200 mg a day and to increase her intake of phenobarbital to 15 mg two times a day. The blood levels were checked again approximately 3.5 weeks later. Her phenytoin level was still low at 2.8 μg/ml; her phenobarbital was 4.5 μg/ml. The patient did not return again for follow-up until 17 months later. In the interim, she had had no additional seizures of either a major or minor type. Her infant and previous offspring were normal.

Questions

1. Classify these seizures. If possible, be specific.
2. What other types of seizures might be expected in this syndrome?
3. What would be the most appropriate anticonvulsant?
4. What would neuroimaging studies demonstrate?
5. Discuss the relationship between epilepsy and pregnancy.
6. Discuss the relationship between anticonvulsants and pregnancy.
7. Discuss the role of anticonvulsants and related drugs in teratogenesis.
8. Discuss the interaction of anticonvulsants and birth control pills.

CASE HISTORY 31.5

This 23 year-old, white, right-handed army recruit private, on the day prior to admission, was evaluated on sick call for an apparent upper respiratory infection. The patient was given a day of barracks rest. Early on the morning of admission, the patient apparently vomited. At reveille, the patient was found in his bed, unresponsive, and he was found to have been incontinent of urine and feces.

General Physical Examination

1. The patient was febrile with a temperature of 102°F–103°F. Blood pressure was 130/70; pulse was 96.
2. There was a marked degree of nuchal rigidity.
3. Examination of the skin revealed a diffuse petechial rash with a number of ecchymotic areas on the extremities. Some of these areas had apparent necrotic centers.

Neurological Examination

1. *Mental status*: The patient was in a coma; he responded to painful stimuli by withdrawing his extremities.
2. *Cranial nerves*:
   a. The pupils were mid-position and responded very poorly to light.
   b. Funduscopic examination was not remarkable.
3. *Motor system:* There was no definite lateralized weakness. Cerebellar system and gait could not be tested.
4. *Reflexes:*
   a. Deep tendon reflexes were equal but hyperactive throughout.
   b. An extensor plantar response was present on the left side.
5. Sensory system: Could not be adequately tested.

Questions

1. What is your diagnosis?
2. Which studies must be performed and when must they be performed?
3. When must treatment be started? Which treatment would be most appropriate?

Laboratory Data

1. CBC: White blood count was markedly elevated to 42,000, with a differential count of 64% polymorphonuclears, 31% bands, and 5% lymphocytes. Platelets were decreased to 95,000 per mm³. Blood serology was negative.
2. Spinal fluid examination revealed a marked increase in pressure (>600 mm of cerebrospinal fluid). The fluid was grossly cloudy. There were 7250 white blood cells per cubic millimeter; 100% of these were polymorphonuclear leukocytes. Spinal fluid sugar was 6 mg/100 ml (blood sugar was within normal range); spinal fluid protein was increased to 314 mg/100 ml.
3. Smears and eventually cultures of spinal fluid and blood were consistent with the clinical diagnosis.

Subsequent course: The patient was begun on specific therapy. As the patient's level of consciousness began to improve, on the second hospital day it was apparent that a left facial weakness was present. On the fourth hospital day, as the patient began to respond to questions by opening his eyes and moving his right hand, it became apparent that he had a left facial weakness, a weakness of the left arm and leg, and a left Babinski response. On the sixth hospital day, even though the patient was continuing to improve, he had the onset of focal seizures beginning on the left side of the body. Some remained localized to the left side; some became generalized. Following readjustment of therapy, seizures disappeared. With physiotherapy, a significant improvement in function of the left arm and left leg occurred.

Questions (continued)

4. Do you wish to modify your diagnosis and proposed treatment based on the cerebrospinal fluid findings? What do you expect the cultures of blood and cerebrospinal fluid to indicate?
5. Indicate the pathophysiology involved in the complications that developed during the patient's hospitalization.

CASE HISTORY 31.6

This 62-year-old white divorcee was referred for evaluation of memory subsequently of personality change. The patient had a high school education and had been described in the past as a bright, alert, and intelligent lady. The patient was unable to provide a history. She showed little insight into her problem and seemed unaware of any reason for her neurological evaluation. The patient's son indicated that she had begun to show some decline in intellectual capacity as long as 3 or 4 years prior to admission. During the preceding 12 months, a more marked change had occurred, particularly with regard to memory. In more recent months, a lack of concern for her personal appearance and a lack of spontaneity had developed. She had lost interest in her home, friends, and activities.

Past history was unremarkable as regards cardiovascular disease, diabetes, or alcohol or drug and ingestion.

General physical examination: Blood pressure was 140/96; cardiac status was normal.

Neurological Examination

1. *Mental status*:
   a. The patient was pleasant and well mannered.
   b. She was disoriented for the day of the week, for the day of the month, for the month, and for the year.
   c. She was unable to remember any of four test objects after a 5-minute period.
   d. The patient was unable to remember the year she was born.

e. She was unable to recall any president but Kennedy.
  f. She was able to follow very simple directions, but she was unable to remember any instructions beyond these.
  g. She was unable to comprehend subtraction of serial 7s and could not do even simple additions. She was unable to repeat numbers in reverse.
  h. She was unable to draw a triangle but did recognize a circle.
  i. There was a severe dysnomia for even common objects.
2. *Cranial nerves*:
  a. Pupillary reactions were normal.
  b. At times, the patient had extinction of simultaneously presented visual objects in the left or right visual field.
3. *Motor system*:
  a. Strength and gait were intact.
  b. Minor tremulousness was present in the performance of hand and arm movements.
  c. Minor variable resistance on passive motion existed and was described as Gegenhalten.
4. *Reflexes*:
  a. Deep tendon reflexes were symmetric and physiologic.
  b. Plantar responses were flexor bilaterally.
  c. Grasp was absent.
5. *Sensory system*: Normal.

QUESTIONS

1. What cerebrospinal fluid findings are to be expected?
2. What is the natural history and prognosis?
3. What more restricted mental status changes might have been present early in the disease course? What would be a more likely diagnosis if personality changes had been the primary early symptoms? If basal ganglia symptoms had been present early in the course of the disease, which diagnoses might have been considered?

CASE HISTORY 31.7 (PATIENT OF DR. JOHN SULLIVAN AND DR. HUNTINGTON PORTER)

This 67-year-old, white, right-handed retired schoolteacher awoke one morning with numbness over the entire right side of her body. The right corner of her mouth drooped. She was able to go to a family physician but was unsteady on her feet. She had no diplopia or aphasia. Numbness on the right side disappeared gradually over a 2-week period, but then appeared in the left foot. The left hand became restless and would move

1. Does this patient have focal disease or a more generalized disease? If the latter, which areas are predominantly affected? What is the significance of the dysnomia in this case? Which diagnosis would you assign to this case?
2. Describe the most likely pathology in this case. Present a differential diagnosis.
3. What treatable causes of this progressive syndrome must be considered? Discuss in terms of:
  a. Infections
  b. Nutritional diseases
  c. Metabolic diseases
  d. Intoxications
  e. Other treatable etiologies. For each entity indicate the appropriate diagnostic tests.
4. How would you manage this patient as regards diagnosis and treatment?
5. What would an electroencephalogram demonstrate?
6. What would a computerized tomography (CT) scan demonstrate? in a jerky up-and-down movement.

The hand and arm would take on abnormal postures and tend to trail behind her. One week later, this involuntary movement began to affect the left foot, which became restless. Its constant motion seriously interfered with her ability to walk. Over the next several weeks, the movement disorder in the left hand disappeared.

Past history was not remarkable except for menopause at age 30. Family history indicated that her mother died at age 63 of a "heart attack."

Father died at age 72 of a "shock."

General physical examination: Blood pressure was 160/100, with a normal cardiac examination.

Neurological Examination

Mental status: All areas were intact, with no evidence of aphasia.

Cranial nerves:
  a. A slight droop of the left corner of the mouth was present.
  b. There was an unsustained nystagmus on month. Then she began to have sudden "jerky far lateral gaze movements" of the left hand, causing the arm

Motor System: to strike her in the face. The left arm also began to posture in a position of relative flex-

  a. Strength was intact, with good retention of skilled movements of the hands.
  b. In the left leg, there was an almost constant play of movement, smooth and rhythmical, consisting of eversion/inversion of foot and ankle with flexion/extension movements of the toes. In the left arm, the same type of movement was present. This movement was not synchronized with that in the foot and was often absent for periods of time. As the patient used the right arm, the movement disorder became apparent in the left hand. When the patient performed repetitive movements of the left fingers, mirrored movements of the right fingers occurred.
  c. *Gait*: The body was twisted to the left. The left hand trailed behind, with the index finger pointing down and the other fingers clenched. The gait was unsteady. Walking did not dampen the movement in the left leg. At times, the left leg would suddenly buckle.

4. *Reflexes*:
  a. Deep tendon reflexes were symmetric and physiologic.
  b. Plantar responses were flexor bilaterally.
  c. There was no release of the grasp reflex and no repellent apraxia.
5. *Sensory system*: Pain, touch, position, and other discriminative modalities were intact. There was a slight decrease in vibration sensation at the toes.

Laboratory Data

1. *Fasting blood sugar* was elevated to 250 mg/100 ml.
2. *Cerebrospinal fluid*: Opening pressure was 60; no cells; protein was 45 mg/100 ml.

3. *Chest and skull* X-rays were negative, except for calcification of the carotid siphon.
4. *Sedimentation rate* was 17 mm in 1 hour.

Subsequent course: The patient did well for approximately one ion at the elbow, wrist, and fingers. The patient also reported occasional violent flinging movements of the arm. To some extent, numbness had returned to the right upper extremity. When she was re-examined 4 months after the initial episode, certain changes had occurred in the movement disorder. A distal fluid, flowing 2 to 4 Hz movement was still noted at the fingers, toes, hand, and foot, alternating between flexion/supination and extension/pronation. This movement had now appeared at more proximal joints, and some spread of movement into the face was reported. In addition, there were sudden pronation and posterior rotatory movements at the shoulder. At times, this was described as a wild swinging or flinging movement of the left upper extremity. At the time of a visit 5 months later, significant improvement had begun to occur.

By the time of a follow-up 2 months later, approximately 1 year after onset of symptoms, there was little evidence of any movement disorder. Occasional distal movements occurred only when the patient was emotionally excited.

Questions

1. Provide a diagnostic label for the abnormality of movement noted on the initial neurological examination.
2. Provide a diagnostic label for the movement disorder that subsequently evolved.
3. Discuss the neuroanatomic basis of these disorders.
4. Discuss diagnostic and management approaches.

CASE HISTORY 31.8

One week prior to admission, this 51-year-old white housewife developed episodic posterior headaches beginning in the neck and radiating to the vertex of the head. The headaches were usually related to and were definitely exacerbated by straining or coughing. At the same time, the patient noted clumsiness of the left hand and a tendency to fall to the left side.

During the week prior to admission, a progressive gait ataxia also had developed.

Past history: Eight months previously, the patient had been admitted to the gynecology service with a 10-week history of postmenopausal vaginal bleeding. She was found to have an infiltrative anaplastic carcinoma of the uterine cervix. The patient was treated with radiotherapy (4000R to the pelvis), followed by vaginal insertion of radium. Re-evaluation 1 month prior to the present admission had revealed that this anaplastic epidermoid carcinoma of the cervix had spread to the anterior vaginal wall. In addition, metastatic nodules were now present in the lung.

Neurological Examination

1. *Mental status:* The patient was an anxious white female who was cooperative, alert, and well oriented.
2. *Cranial nerves:*
   a. There was coarse nystagmus on gaze to the left.
   b. There was a minor dysarthria for lingual and guttural sounds.
3. *Motor system:*
   a. Strength was intact.
   b. Gait was unsteady, with tendency to fall to the left, especially when turning to the left. On a narrow base, the patient tended to fall backward.
   c. Cerebellar tests revealed no definite truncal ataxia. There was a marked appendicular ataxia on the finger-to-nose test in the left upper extremity and the heel-to-shin test in the left lower extremity.
4. *Reflexes:*
   a. Deep tendon reflexes were active bilaterally. This, however, was felt to be consistent with the patient's degree of anxiety.
   b. Plantar responses were flexor.
5. *Sensory system:* All modalities were intact, except for a minimal decrease in vibratory sensation at the toes.

Laboratory Data

The results of specialized studies were consistent with the clinical diagnosis.

Questions

1. Where is the lesion? Be specific.
2. What pathological process is to be expected?
3. Outline your diagnostic and therapeutic approach for this case.
4. Which is the appropriate neuroimaging study?
5. Should a lumbar puncture be performed? Indicate why or why not.

CASE HISTORY 31.9

A 21-year-old, white, right-handed wife of an air force enlisted man had been married for 2 months and had just moved from her home in the south to an air force base in New Jersey. She had been complaining of increasingly severe right frontal temporal or bifrontal headaches for 3–4 weeks. During the 10 days prior to admission, she had been treated on several occasions at the base dispensary for these headaches, which were relatively constant and were now accompanied by blurring of vision and frequent vomiting.

Various medications had been prescribed for an upper respiratory infection or sinusitis. In the 48 hours prior to admission, the patient had become increasingly confused and ataxic. Her past history was otherwise negative as regards head injury or pulmonary and ear infection.

General Physical Examination

1. The patient was dehydrated and somewhat lethargic.
2. She was complaining of severe headache, particularly on head movement.
3. There was a moderate degree of hyperventilation.
4. No otitis media was present.

Neurological Examination

1. *Mental status:* The patient was disoriented for time and place. She was unable to provide a history and was unable to cooperate for the examination. She was impersistent in fixing gaze or in maintaining eyes in open position.
2. *Cranial nerves:*
   a. On funduscopy, bilateral papilledema was present, with 2 to 3 diopters of disk elevation, accompanied by fresh hemorrhages and venous engorgement.
   b. The right pupil was dilated and fixed in response to light. Extraocular movements were otherwise intact.
   c. A left central facial weakness was present to a marked degree.

3. *Motor system*:
   a. All limbs were moved spontaneously, but there was a downward drift of the outstretched left arm.
   b. The patient was ataxic in a sitting position and in attempting to stand, even on a broad base.
   c. There was a tremor of the outstretched hands, increasing to a minor degree on movement and intention.
4. *Reflexes*:
   a. Deep tendon reflexes were increased on the left in the upper and lower extremities.
   b. Plantar response was extensor on the left and equivocal on the right.
   c. Grasp reflex was present bilaterally.
5. *Sensory system*: Pain sensation was intact; modalities could not be tested.
6. *Neck*: Minor resistance to passive motion.

Laboratory Data

1. Skull and chest X-rays were negative.
2. EEG demonstrated almost continuous focal 1 to 2 Hz slow-wave activity.

Questions

1. This patient was seen relatively late in her disease course. You should be able to localize the primary location of the pathology.
2. Indicate what secondary complications have occurred.
3. The nature of the pathology may be somewhat uncertain to you. However, you should be able to present a differential diagnosis and then to indicate the most likely diagnosis. Keep in mind that the headaches had been present for only 3–4 weeks and the additional symptoms for only 2–10 days.
4. Was the papilledema long-standing?
5. What is the significance of the pupillary findings?
6. Assuming a cerebral hemisphere lesion, why was the patient ataxic in sitting and standing when examined late in her course?
7. Which diagnostic studies would you perform in this case, and when would you perform these?
8. Which diagnostic studies would you not perform? State reasons.
9. How would you manage this problem from a therapeutic standpoint? Indicate when you would institute this therapy.

CASE HISTORY 31.10

This 55-year-old white widow, 6 to 8 years prior to admission, had the onset of a peculiar reeling gait. At the same time, she was noted to be "very nervous," having many peculiar restless movements. At other times, she was described as constantly fidgeting. The patient's children felt that in recent years, she had not been thinking as clearly as she once did. A personality change had also occurred.

Family history: The patient's mother died in her sixties with a disorder that had been labeled as Parkinsonism. From the description of relatives, however, it was evident that the mother had restless movements that were similar to the patient's.

Neurological Examination

1. *Mental status*: The patient was oriented and alert with an intact general store of information. Object recall was three out of four in 10 minutes. Digit span was six forward and three in reverse.
2. *Cranial nerves*: Intact.

3. *Motor system:*
   a. Strength was intact with no significant spasticity or rigidity.
   b. Gait showed a swooping quality of variable degree; there was also a decrease in associated arm movements.
   c. As the patient sat, she would move her head, neck, and feet almost constantly.
   d. The patient was able to walk a tandem gait, and there were no abnormalities of cerebellar function.
4. *Reflexes*: Deep tendon reflexes were symmetric. Plantar responses were flexor. No grasp reflex was present.
5. *Sensory system:* Intact.

Laboratory Data

1. Routine laboratory studies were not remarkable.
2. Specialized neuroradiology studies were consistent with the clinical diagnosis.

Questions

1. Present a differential diagnosis of this problem and indicate the most likely diagnosis.
2. Outline your diagnostic and therapeutic approach to this problem.
3. What did the specialized neuroradiology studies reveal?
4. Which neurodiagnostic study would be most cost-effective and specific in establishing the diagnosis today?
5. Discuss the underlying molecular basis of this disorder.

CASE HISTORY 31.11 (PATIENT OF DR. THOMAS SABIN)

A 50-year-old white man was admitted to the hospital because of drowsiness and confusion of 5 days' duration. His wife stated that he was in good health until that time. For 4 days prior to admission, he merely slept more than usual and napped during the day, but while awake, he was lucid. The day before admission he was confused, and this confusion increased on the day of admission.

Neurological Examination

This was a thin man with normal vital signs who answered questions quickly but often incorrectly. In addition to the confusion, drowsiness, and problems in memory, pertinent findings included the following: Extraocular movements were limited in all directions, and there was horizontal and vertical nystagmus. The gag reflex was diminished bilaterally.

Finger-to-nose and heel-to-shin tests showed a mild deficit. The patient had an unsteady, broad-based gait. No other motor findings were present.

Questions

1. Do you require more historical information? If so, indicate what is required.
2. Present a differential diagnosis.
3. What is the most likely diagnosis?
4. In a general sense, what is the localization of lesions in this disease? What is the localization for each specific symptom or sign (confusion and impairment of new learning, lethargy, impairment of extraocular movement and ataxia)?
5. How could your suspected diagnosis be confirmed?
6. How and when would you treat this patient? Which findings would rapidly resolve over the next 1–2 days?

7. You administer specific treatment but the difficulties with memory fail to clear and 1 year later the patient is still confused and confabulating. How do you modify your diagnosis?
8. You administer specific treatment but 1 year later, the patient is still ataxic. How do you modify your diagnosis?

CASE HISTORY 31.12

This 60-year-old, right-handed, retired priest was referred for evaluation of problems in walking. The history was not precise. Two and a half years previously, he had been admitted to his local hospital, for severe diabetic coma.

Although he recovered, he had some difficulty with memory thereafter. He began to fall. Problems in walking had progressed, particularly in the last 6 to 8 months, so that he was no longer able to walk without assistance. His memory problems had progressed over the last year. He denied numbness in his extremities but was aware of "twitching" of his extremities. He denied any significant family history. He indicated he had been a very heavy drinker and had been hospitalized once in the previous year for treatment of alcoholism. Admitted intake was at least a half liter (500 cc) of gin per day.

Neurological Examination

1. *Mental status*: He was very vague about the date. Delayed recall was limited to two out of five objects in 5 minutes.
2. *Cranial nerves*: All were intact, except for a tremulous voice.
3. *Motor system*:
   a. The patient stood on a broad base and was very unsteady standing on a narrow base, requiring support. This unsteadiness slightly worsened with eye closure.
   b. He had been brought into the office in a wheelchair. He walked with assistance with small steps but was very ataxic.
   c. There was no impairment on finger-to-nose testing, but there was dysmetria on heel-to-shin test.
4. *Reflexes*:
   a. Deep tendon reflexes were everywhere absent.
   b. Plantar responses were not responsive.
5. *Sensory system*:
   a. Pain sensation was absent to the level of the knees.
   b. Position sense was intact.
   c. Vibration sensation was markedly decreased at the toes and moderately decreased at the ankles.

Laboratory Data

1. *Blood studies*: Folic acid, B12 levels, serum and urine immunoelectrophoresis, ESR, and ANA were normal. Serological tests (RPR and FTA) were negative. Liver function studies had been previously elevated but now, except for alkaline phosphatase, were normal.
2. *Electromyogram and nerve conduction* studies indicated a severe sensory-motor peripheral neuropathy, primarily axonal in type, as well as left median nerve (carpal tunnel) and right ulnar nerve (olecranon groove) entrapment neuropathies.
3. *MRI* demonstrated:
   a. Prominence of cerebellar folia, particularly of the superior vermis
   b. Moderate cerebral cortical atrophy
   c. Periventricular white matter involvement (leukoariosis)

Subsequent course: An alcoholism program with discontinuation of all alcohol intake and administration of multiple B vitamins was recommended. When last seen in follow-up, the patient was consuming at least 500 cc of vodka per day. His neurological examination was unchanged except that pain sensation was now intact. He refused additional neurological follow-up.

Questions

This patient had several neurological problems: At least five can be specified, Please list and discuss in terms of:
   a. Ataxia
   b. Memory changes
   c. Peripheral nerve disorders
   d. Toxic and metabolic diseases

32.

CASE HISTORY PROBLEM SOLVING

PART VI: CASE HISTORY REVIEW WITH CORRELATION TO ILLUSTRATIONS

PHOTO SERIES

Each series of photos is derived from a particular case history. Indicate the most likely diagnosis in terms of localization and pathology (see Figs. 32.1–32.12).

CASE HISTORIES 32.1 TO 32.9 FOR PROBLEM SOLVING AND THEN MATCH EACH CASE TO THE CORRECT PHOTO

CASE HISTORY 32.1

This 43-year-old, right-handed, white male, 2 months prior to admission, had the acute onset of blurring of vision and possible diplopia. Two weeks prior to admission, he had the acute onset of ataxia, vomiting, dizziness, and left face numbness. He improved, then developed severe problems with balance, slurring of speech, and difficulty in the use of the left arm, which he labeled as "weakness." The patient was also aware that he had become emotionally labile. Cranial nerve examination demonstrated a paralysis of conjugate lateral gaze to the left. A marked left peripheral facial weakness was present. He had a marked decrease in whisper perception in the left ear. Strength was actually intact. There was a marked dysmetria on the left finger-to-nose and left heel-to-shin tests. The patient was ataxic in walking. Deep tendon reflexes were symmetric; plantar responses were extensor bilaterally. Sensory examination was normal.

QUESTIONS

1. What is the most likely diagnosis in terms of localization and pathology?
2. What study would be most diagnostic or confirmatory of your clinical diagnosis?
3. Select the most appropriate photograph.

Figure 32.1

Figure 32.2

Figure 32.3

Figure 32.4

606 • COMPLEX FUNCTIONS

Figure 32.5

Figure 32.6

32 CASE HISTORY PROBLEM SOLVING: PART VI • 607

Figure 32.7

Figure 32.8

Figure 32.9

Figure 32.10

CASE HISTORY 32.2

This 68-year-old, right-handed, married white female and retired clerical worker was referred for evaluation of "weakness in both lower extremities" of approximately 2 years' duration. She had been falling for at least 1 year. Although the patient and her husband initially denied any bladder symptoms, her daughter, a nurse, was able to indicate that urinary incontinence had occurred on several occasions during the last year. The patient indicated her memory had been "bad" for 1 to 2 years. Her husband minimized this symptom. Her daughter subsequently was able to relate a more significant impairment in mental functions. The patient's mother, age 88, had senile dementia and problems walking.

Neurological Examination

1. *Mental status:* The patient was oriented to time, place, and person. Delayed recall was 0/5 in 5 minutes without assistance: 4/5 with assistance.
2. *Cranial nerves:* The following findings were present:
    a. Tremor of head
    b. Hyperactive jaw jerk
    c. Positive glabellar sign
3. *Motor system:* The following findings were present:
    a. Variable generalized weakness that at times disappeared.
    b. Gait: Small steps, at times waddling, unsteady on the turns.
    c. Sitting: Often tended to fall backward on the examining table.
4. *Reflexes:*
    a. Deep tendon reflexes were everywhere hyperactive.
    b. Plantars responses were equivocally extensor bilaterally.
    c. Grasp reflex was released bilaterally.
    d. Palmomental responses were positive bilaterally.
5. *Sensory system:* Intact.

QUESTIONS

1. Considering the combination of ataxia of gait, impairment of memory, and urinary incontinence, indicate the most likely syndrome.
2. How do you interpret the bilateral release of grasp, the palmomental reflex, the bilateral extensor plantar responses, and the hyperactive jaw jerk?
3. Provide a differential diagnosis of this syndrome.
4. Which study or studies would you obtain to confirm your diagnosis?
5. Select appropriate illustrations (several may be appropriate).
6. If this patient also had severe impairment of upward gaze and headache, what would be the most likely diagnosis and which would be the most appropriate illustration?

Figure 32.11

Figure 32.12

7. If this patient also had a past history of head trauma with resultant coma and recovery 10 years previously, what would be the most likely clinical diagnosis and which illustration would then best correspond?
8. What is the most appropriate therapy?

CASE HISTORY 32.3

This 47-year-old, right-handed, married white female farm manager awoke 1 week before evaluation with numbness and "novocaine-like" sensation involving the entire trigeminal distribution on the right, including the tongue, lip, mucosa, and so on. She had no pain and no other neurological symptoms. Five to six years previously, she had intermittent unsteadiness that was attributed to an "inner ear infection." She also was aware that during the last year, if she sat in a hot tub, she would be totally exhausted.

Neurological Examination

This was entirely within normal limits except for a selective decrease in touch sensation involving the entire distribution of the right trigeminal nerve, including mucous membranes, gums, upper and lower right half of the tongue, and upper and lower lip. Touch sensation was also decreased over the right cornea. In all areas, pain sensation was intact. Graphesthesia over the face was intact.

Subsequent Course

All numbness disappeared approximately 2 months after onset. She returned 5 months later with complaint of 1-week duration of "feeling slightly woozy." Neurological examination was not remarkable. Symptoms were reproduced by rotation.

QUESTIONS

1. What is the location of the lesion corresponding to the sensory symptoms involving the face?
2. What is the appropriate neurodiagnostic study? What other studies might be obtained?
3. Select the appropriate illustration.
4. What is the most likely clinical diagnosis?
5. Which therapy would you recommend?

CASE HISTORY 32.4

This 70-year-old, right-handed, white widow and retired telephone company clerk was referred for evaluation of unsteadiness in walking, which had been present for 23 years. The symptom had begun in relationship to a hospitalization for a myelogram. At that time, the patient had been involved in an automobile accident and had developed lumbar radicular pain. The evening after the myelogram, she had developed "coma, convulsions, and a temperature of 110°F."

The medical records of that hospitalization were not complete but did indicate she had a prolonged, markedly elevated temperature (>104°F) secondary to meningitis.

At that time, the patient also had the onset of episodes of tinnitus, vertigo, olfactory hallucinations of roasting meat, a sense of déjà vu and the sensation of hearing a symphony. She would be observed to be glassy-eyed and inattentive.

Past history indicated the following:

1. Cervical disk surgery at age 30.
2. Lumbar disk surgery at age 38 and age 60.
3. Hyperthyroidism had been treated with radioactive iodine. She was receiving thyroid replacement.
4. Diabetes mellitus had been treated with insulin for 5 years.

Neurological Evaluation

1. *Mental status:* Intact.
2. *Cranial nerves:* Intact.
3. *Motor system:*
   a. Strength intact.
   b. Stance: Unsteady on a narrow base and only slightly worse with eye closure.
   c. Gait: Unable to walk a tandem gait, unsteady on the turns.
   d. Finger-to-nose test and heel-to-shin tests were not remarkable.
4. *Reflexes:*
   a. Deep tendon reflexes: Achilles reflexes were absent bilaterally.
   b. Plantar responses were flexor.
5. *Sensory system:*
   a. Pain sensation was decreased to the knees bilaterally.
   b. Vibration sensation was absent at toes and decreased at ankles.
   c. Position sensation was intact.

Subsequent Course

The neurological examination did not change over the next 2 years.

QUESTIONS

1. As regards the ataxia of stance and gait present since the hospitalization 23 years previously:
   a. Indicate the location of lesion.
   b. Indicate the most likely pathology.
   c. Indicate best study to demonstrate a. and b.
   d. Select the appropriate illustration.

2. As regards the episodes characterized by sensory perception of "roast meat odor," "music of a symphony," tinnitus and vertigo, and so on:
   a. Indicate diagnosis.
   b. Indicate most likely etiology.
   c. Select the best test to support diagnosis.
   d. Indicate the most appropriate treatment.
3. As regards the absent Achilles reflexes, the decreased vibratory sensation, and distal decrease in pain sensation:
   a. Indicate diagnosis.
   b. Indicate the most likely pathology.

CASE HISTORY 32.5

This 70-year-old, single, right-handed, white male priest had been unsteady for at least 1.5 years. He had been stumbling over names for the same period but had no other problems in memory. Urinary symptoms were denied.

Past history indicated atrial fibrillation in the past. Hypertension had been under treatment for 10 to 20 years. There was no definite history of cerebrovascular disease.

Family history: A niece had hydrocephalus that was shunted when she was a child. Two of four sisters had cerebral aneurysms.

Neurological Evaluation

1. *Mental status:* Oriented for time, place, and person. Delayed recall without assistance, 0 out of 5 objects in 5 minutes; with assistance, 3 out of 5 objects.
2. *Cranial nerves:* Intact, including fundi, except for hyperactive jaw jerk.
3. *Motor system:*
   a. Strength intact.
   b. Stance: He was relatively steady until he closed his eyes.
   c. Gait: He walked on a broad base but was able to do tandem gait. He was unsteady on the turns.
   d. Finger-to-nose test demonstrated a slight terminal tremor.
4. *Reflexes:*
   a. Deep tendon stretch reflexes were 2 in the upper extremities, 3 at the patella, and 2–3 at Achilles tendon.
   b. Plantar responses were extensor bilaterally.
   c. There was no release of instinctive grasp.
5. *Sensory system:*
   a. Position sensation was intact at fingers and toes.
   b. Vibration sensation was absent at toes, decreased at ankles, and markedly decreased at fingers compared to wrist, and at wrist compared to elbows.
   c. Pain sensation was decreased at toes to mid arch and over fingers.

Questions

1. As regards ataxia of stance and gait: Localize the lesion. Indicate the pathology.
2. Indicate the best test to support the diagnosis.
3. Select the two best illustrations that would correspond to this case.
4. Does this patient also have another neurological disorder?

Subsequent Course

The patient had periodic neurological follow-up evaluations. He was relatively stable over the next 4 years; then he reported a minor increase in the degree of unsteadiness. Two years later, he developed a sudden onset of diplopia in looking to the left and a minor ptosis of the left lid. Examination now demonstrated:

1. Chronic atrial fibrillation.
2. Moderate ptosis of the left lid.
3. Weakness of the left lateral rectus movements.
4. Decreased hearing in the left ear.
5. Deep tendon reflexes increased on the left.
6. Pain sensation decreased over the entire right side, including the face.
7. Patient stood on broad base and walked with small steps on broad base.

His diplopia cleared, but previous neurological symptoms and signs remained.

Questions (continued)

5. As regards this last sudden episode, localize the pathology. Indicate the nature of the pathology.
6. Indicate the best study to support the clinical diagnosis.
7. Does any illustration correspond to this episode?

CASE HISTORY 32.6

This 36-year-old, right-handed, white male lecturer was referred for evaluation of symptoms related to a motor vehicle accident that occurred 2.5 years earlier. He had initially symptoms in the neck and right arm, but these essentially cleared. A more persistent area of symptomatology related to the lumbar area. Occasional sharp pains extended from the back to the left buttock, the left posterior thigh, the posterior calf, and the ankle. Back pain improved but left leg pain increased. In addition to the shooting pains in the left leg, he complained of intermittent numbness in the left posterior thigh. He denied weakness, bladder problems, or sexual dysfunction. There were no symptoms in the right leg, except for occasional burning in the anterior tibial area.

Neurological Evaluation

Totally intact except for the following:

1. *Reflexes:* Slight decrease in the left patellar reflex and a marked depression of both Achilles deep tendon stretch reflexes.
2. *Back:* The patient could forward flex to 60 degrees to the vertical plane, at which point he complained of pain shooting down the left posterior thigh.
3. *Straight-leg-raising:* This was limited to 50 to 60 degrees on the left, with pain in the left posterior thigh. On the right, straight-leg-raising could be carried out to 90 degrees.
4. *Sciatic nerve:* Tenderness was present on the left.

Questions

1. What is the clinical diagnosis? Be specific as to the localization and pathology.
2. Assuming that this patient had *not* responded to "conservative" measures, which diagnostic study would you obtain? Be specific.
4. Select the illustration corresponding to this case.
5. Define "conservative measures."
6. What therapy would be recommended if these measures had failed and pain progressed?

CASE HISTORY 32.7

This 27-year-old right-handed female college maintenance worker developed progressive numbness in the left arm extending from the elbow to all of the fingers. Initially, this was intermittent, but it soon became constant. She also developed persistent discomfort in the posterior cervical area extending to the left supraclavicular area. There was no history of trauma. Her primary physician obtained initial X-ray studies and, subsequently, referred the patient to a neurosurgeon.

Questions

1. What is the differential diagnosis at this time?
2. What initial study would you, as the primary physician, obtain?
3. Select the appropriate illustration.
4. Based on that illustration, what is the most likely diagnosis?

Subsequent Course

The neurosurgeon found the deep tendon reflexes absent at the left biceps and triceps. He requested a more definitive neuroimaging study. Based on that study, the neurosurgeon performed definitive neurosurgical procedures. The patient had an excellent result, except for residual numbness in the fingers of the left hand and a left Horner's syndrome.

Questions

1. Which definitive study would you, as the neurosurgeon, have requested?
2. Select the appropriate illustration.
3. Based on the illustration, what is the most appropriate diagnosis?
4. Which neurosurgical approaches (procedures) were utilized?
5. Why did the patient have residual sensory deficit in the thumb and index finger?
6. Why did the patient have a residual Horner's syndrome?

Subsequent Course

Six months after her last surgery, she returned to the neurosurgeon, complaining of burning pain in the right scapular area and some intermittent tingling of the fourth and fifth fingers of the right hand. Examination 6 months later demonstrated:

1. *Cranial nerves:*
   a. Mild ptosis of the left eyelid, a smaller pupil on the left, and decreased sweating over the left side of the face.
   b. Whisper perception was decreased bilaterally.
2. *Motor system:* There was mild weakness in the right triceps muscle.
3. *Reflexes:* The triceps and biceps deep tendon reflexes were decreased on the left, but the radial and finger jerks were increased on the left. Plantar responses were flexor.
4. *Sensory system:* Pain sensation was decreased over the thumb and index finger and to a lesser degree over the middle finger of the left hand.
5. *Neck and supraclavicular areas:* She was tender over the right supraclavicular area, with pain extending into the right arm.

Questions (continued)

7. What is the diagnosis of this new problem involving the right arm?
8. Which diagnostic procedure would you request?
9. What is the explanation for the smaller left pupil, mild left lid ptosis, and decreased sweating over the left side of the face?
10. What condition might concern you regarding the bilateral deficit in hearing? How would you evaluate this problem?

CASE HISTORY 32.8

This 20-year-old, left-handed, white male was the product of a prolonged delivery. The mother claimed that "the head was held back." The day after birth, a seizure occurred. At age 10 months, he was noted to have problems in movement of the right arm and leg. He was still unable to stand at 14 months of age. When he was evaluated at the Children's Hospital Medical Center at age 2 years, he was described as having a spastic and dystonic right hemiparesis, with severe delays in expressive speech. At age 4 to 5 years, he began to have frequent seizures, which began with tingling of the right hand and face, and focal movements of the right hand and lips. These would secondarily generalize three to four times per day.

Family history: The mother had a long-standing mild right hemiparesis, with focal sensory seizures involving right face and arm. A brother carried a diagnosis of schizophrenia.

Questions

1. What is your clinical diagnosis (location of lesion, type of pathology) at this point?
2. What study would have best demonstrated the location and nature of the pathology?
3. How would you manage the seizures?
4. How would you manage the spastic dystonic right hemiparesis and expressive speech delay?

Subsequent Course

He had undergone, at age 11, a heel-cord-lengthening and toe-tendon-stretching operation.

At school, he had achieved third-grade proficiency in reading and writing and tenth-grade proficiency in math.

The patient was seen again 10 years later for a second opinion regarding seizure control. Over the intervening years, seizures had occurred at variable frequency. His seizures were primarily focal motor seizures beginning in the right arm. At times, secondary generalization might occur, particularly when flurries of focal seizures occurred. Often a warning occurred, which he could not precisely identify but which had components of a dreamy, strange, or familiar sensation. Over the years, he had been treated with phenytoin, phenobarbital, valproic acid, carbamazepine, and primidone. Despite this, seizures were still occurring in flurries 3 to 4 days per week.

Neurological Evaluation

1. *Mental status:* He was oriented for time, place, and person. Delayed recall was five out of five in 5 minutes. Later, neuropsychological testing indicated that visual nonverbal learning was performed at a much higher level than auditory verbal learning. Reading, spelling, and arithmetic were all severely impaired.
2. *Cranial nerves:* There was smallness of the right side of the face.
3. *Motor system:*
   a. There was smallness of the right hand, thumb, arm, and foot.

b. There was a right-sided weakness of the distal hand muscles, wrist extensor, and triceps.
c. Patient walked with a hemiplegic posture. The right arm was flexed at elbow and there were dystonic movements of the right hand. The leg was extended at hip, with external rotation and circumduction.
d. There was marked resistance to passive motion at the right shoulder and ankle ("tight Achilles tendon"). With rotation of the head, significant alterations occurred in the degree of spasticity in the flexors and extensors at the right elbow.
4. *Reflexes:*
   a. Deep tendon reflexes were increased on the right.
   b. Plantar responses were extensor on the right.
5. *Sensory system:* Intact for all primary and cortical modalities.

QUESTIONS (CONTINUED)

5. Indicate your diagnostic approach.
6. Today, what would be the best study to indicate the location, extent, and nature of the lesion?
7. What would you expect the electroencephalogram to demonstrate?
8. Indicate your therapeutic approach at this point.
9. Discuss the alteration in the spasticity of flexors and extensors at the elbow on rotation of the neck.

CASE HISTORY 32.9

This 18-year-old, right-handed, white male was the product of a prolonged delivery that apparently was complicated by "umbilical cord around the neck." "He did not breathe well at birth and may have aspirated." Three generalized convulsive seizures occurred at birth, and generalized convulsive seizures recurred with vaccination at 9 months of age and then once every 6 to 12 months. No seizures occurred from age 7 to age 15 years. Seizures then recurred in relation to reduction of medication. Warning symptoms preceded most seizures. He would sense a trembling of the extremities, and then vision would black out for 1 to 2 minutes while he was still standing and able to think. Then he would fall down and would be tonic/clonic for 1 to 2 minutes, with greater involvement of the left side. He would be "sleepy and confused afterwards." He was described as having average performance in school but reading had always been slow.

Neurological Evaluation

Intact except for:

1. Slight clumsiness in movements of the left hand.
2. Deep tendon reflexes increased on the left.

Subsequent Course

The patient did well with no seizures for 5 years. Then he had the onset of "trance-like episodes." According to the patient, he would note slurring of speech and then would be unaware of the environment. According to his father, he would appear to stare for 1 minute and would not speak for 1 minute. There would be slight rigidity of both arms, but he would not fall to the ground, and there would not be a generalized convulsive seizure. At the end of the episode, he would be "fully aware of his environment." No automatisms would be noted during or after the episode. With adjustment of medications, the episodes were again controlled. Episodes recurred 7 years later and then, after 8 more years, more frequently (one to three episodes per week).

Several years later, he had a more prolonged episode, beginning with a "seasick sensation and problem with vision of the left eye" and continuing with prolonged confusion. He was "incoherent for 30 minutes and confused for an additional 30 minutes." Eventually, with additional adjustment of medication, control was again eventually achieved.

QUESTIONS

1. What is your diagnosis?
2. Where is the pathology located?
3. What is the nature of the pathology?
4. This patient had multiple electroencephalograms. Indicate the possible findings.
5. Which medication would you utilize in management of this patient?
6. Which neuroimaging study would best demonstrate the location and nature of the pathology?
7. Select the illustration that best correlates with this case.

33.

ATLAS OF THE CEREBRUM

CORONAL AND HORIZONTAL SECTION: GROSS BRAIN SECTIONS

Figure 33.1 *CORONAL SLICE I.* Level: genu of the corpus callosum. In this slice only the cerebral cortex and medullary center of the telencephalon are present.

Gyri. Portions of the frontal and cingulate lobes are present on this slice. The temporal lobe pole is present beneath the inferior surface of the brain.

Arteries. Note that the anterior cerebral arteries are curving around the genu of the corpus callosum. This vessel supplies the medial surface of the hemisphere up to the parieto-occipital fissure.

Figure 33.2 *CORONAL SLICE II.* Level: rostrum of corpus callosum. In this section a portion of the deep telencephalic gray is now seen (caudate and putamen). The temporal lobe is still separated from the remainder of the cerebrum. The corpus callosum is now a thick band of fibers forming the roof of the anterior horn of the lateral ventricle. The olfactory stalk in the olfactory sulcus on the base of the frontal lobe is attached to the inferior surface of the frontal lobe.

Frontal Lobe. The following gyri are present: superior, middle, inferior, orbital, and

rectus. These are the frontal associational areas.

Temporal Lobe. The most anterior tip of the superior, and middle, inferior gyri are present.

Cingulate Lobe. This cortex is found above the corpus callosum in all levels from the genu through the splenium.

White Matter. The anterior limb of the internal capsule separates caudate from putamen.

Arteries. Note that the anterior cerebral arteries are seen in the interhemispheric sulcus above and below the corpus callosum. The middle cerebral arteries are seen entering the lateral fissure.

Frontal Lobe. The same gyri are present as in slice II.

Figure 33.3 *CORONAL SLICE III.* Level: anterior commissure. The temporal lobe is now connected to the remainder of the cerebral hemisphere.

Temporal Lobe. The superior, middle, inferior, occipital-temporal, and parahippocampal gyri are present from the lateral to the medial surface. Note the location of the insular and cingulate cortex.

White Matter. The optic chiasm is seen attached to the base of the brain. The optic recess of the third ventricle is the lumen above the optic chiasm. The septum forms the medial wall separating the body of the lateral ventricles. The anterior limb of the internal capsule is seen between the caudate and putamen.

Arteries. The middle cerebral artery is seen at its point of origin from the internal carotid and in the lateral fissure. Note the anterior cerebrals in the interhemispheric fissure.

Hypophyseal Stalk. This structure is seen medially on the inferior surface of the brain.

Figure 33.4 *CORONAL SLICE IV.* Level: anterior nucleus of the thalamus. This is the first level to include part of the diencephalon.

Frontal Lobe. The superior, middle, inferior, and precentral gyri are present.

Parietal Lobe. This is the first slice to include parietal cortex. The postcentral (sensory) gyrus is seen forming the roof of the lateral fissure.

Temporal Lobe. The superior, middle, inferior, occipito-temporal, and parahippocampal gyri are present. A portion of the transverse temporal gyri (auditory cortex) is found internal to the superior temporal gyri in the depths of the lateral fissure. The hippocampal formation, with the inferior horn of the lateral ventricle at its medial surface, is the most medial portion of the temporal lobe.

Thalamus. The anterior nucleus protrudes into the floor of the lateral ventricle (body). The mammillothalamic tract is seen entering the inferior surface of the anterior nucleus.

Hypothalamus. The mammillary bodies are prominent on the base of the diencephalon. The fornix is seen suspended from the body of the corpus callosum, and the column of the fornix is seen in the hypothalamus. This tract connects the hippocampus to the hypothalamus.

White Matter. The posterior limb of the internal capsule is seen lateral to the thalamus. Many of the fibers of the internal capsule continue to the inferior surface of the brain, where they form the cerebral peduncle.

Figure 33.5 *CORONAL SLICE V.* Level: habenular nucleus. In this section only a small portion of the caudate and putamen remains.

Frontal Lobe. Only the most medial portion of the precentral gyrus (motor cortex) remains.

Parietal Lobe. The postcentral and inferior parietal lobule are present.

Temporal Lobe. The transverse temporal (auditory cortex), superior, middle, inferior, occipitotemporal, and parahippocampal gyrus and hippocampus are found in this level. Cingulate and insular cortex are also evident.

Brain Stem. The bulk of the thalamus at this level consists of the pulvinar nuclei. The laminated lateral geniculate nucleus is found at the inferior, lateral margin of the telencephalon. The fibers of the optic tract synapse in this nucleus. The habenular nucleus of the epithalamus protrudes into the third ventricle. The red nucleus and the pigmented substantia nigra are prominent in the tegmentum of the midbrain. The visual radiation is seen leaving the lateral surface of the geniculate nucleus.

White Matter. The body of the fornix is suspended from the undersurface of the corpus callosum. The visual radiation is seen leaving the lateral surface of the lateral geniculate. The massive brachium pontis forms the base of the brain. The posterior commissure is seen crossing below the habenular nuclei; this fiber bundle interconnects the pretectal, tectal, and posterior portion of the thalamus.

Figure 33.6 *CORONAL SLICE VI.* Level (Fig. 33.6): splenium of the corpus callosum.

Brain Stem. This level is posterior to the thalamus and includes a coronal cut through the inferior colliculus, which receives direct and indirect input from cranial nerve VIII.

One notes in this section the tegmentum and middle cerebellar peduncle of the pons and the upper end of the medullary pyramid.

Frontal and insular cortex are absent from this level.

Cranial Nerves. The rootlets of cranial nerves VII and VIII are seen in the cerebellar pontine angle with the rootlets of cranial nerve XII seen on the lateral surface of the medullary pyramid.

Parietal Lobe. The bulk of the cerebrum temporal gyri are present from the lateral to the medial surface.

Note the location of the insular and cingulate cortex: respectively internal to the lateral fissure and above the corpus callosum.

Occipital Lobe. The deep calcarine fissure marks the location of the primary visual cortex, V1.

The anterior commissure is seen below the lenticular nuclei (globus pallidus and putamen) and above the olfactory area.

White Matter. The optic chiasm is seen attached to the base of the brain. The optic recess of the third ventricle is the lumen above the optic chiasm. The septum forms the medial wall separating the body of the lateral ventricles. The anterior limb of the internal capsule is seen between the caudate and putamen.

Arteries. The middle cerebral artery is seen at its point of origin from the internal carotid and in the lateral fissure. Identify the anterior cerebrals in the interhemispheric fissure.

Hypophyseal Stalk. This structure is seen medially on the inferior surface of the brain.

Figure 33.7. *CORONAL SLICE VII.* Level: calcarine fissure. In this section, parietal, occipital, and temporal gyri are present.

Brain Stem. The medulla is present with the wide fourth ventricle evident below the choroid plexus in the fourth ventricle.

Parietal Lobe. The superior parietal lobule and angular gyrus can be seen.

Occipital Lobe. The lateral occipital gyrus, lingula, and cuneus are present.

Temporal Lobe. The superior, middle, inferior, and occipitotemporal gyri form the main portion of the temporal lobe seen at this level.

Brain Stem. The cerebellar hemispheres and vermis cover the medulla.

Arteries. The posterior cerebral artery is seen adjacent to the calcarine fissure.

Ventricular System. The posterior horn of the lateral ventricles and the fourth ventricle are present. Note the choroid plexus in the fourth ventricle.

Figure 33.8 *HORIZONTAL SLICE IX.* Level: internal capsule. In this slice both hemispheres are present and connected by the corpus callosum.

Gyri. Identify the lateral fissure and the location of the frontal and occipital poles. Note that the interhemispheric fissure is wider in the occipital regions.

White Matter. Identify the anterior limb, genu, and posterior limb of the internal capsule. Note the relationship between the anterior limb, head of the caudate and putamen, posterior limb, thalamus, and globus pallidus. Locate the fornix.

Blood Vessels. Identify the anterior, middle, and posterior cerebrals.

Ventricular System. Locate the third ventricle, anterior horn, body, and inferior horn of the lateral ventricle and note their relationship to the caudate and thalamus.

Figure 33.9 *CORONAL SLICE VIII.* Four levels: sections of cerebrum and diencephalon (upper left), midbrain (lower left), pons (upper right), and medulla (lower right).

Note the presence of the ventricular system in each level: cerebrum and diencephalon, lateral ventricle and third ventricle; midbrain, cerebral aqueduct; pons IV, ventricle; medulla, fourth ventricle. The tectum (roof of the brain stem) in the midbrain (colliculi), pons (cerebellum), and medulla (cerebellum) is labeled.

The tegmentum (floor of the ventricular system) contains the cranial nerves and other nuclei. The basis is labeled in the midbrain, pons, and medulla, and it contains the descending motor pathway to the cerebellum (corticopontines), to brain stem corticobulbars/corticonuclears, and to spinal cord-corticospinals.

For more detail on these levels, read Chapter 6 on the spinal cord, Chapter 8 on the brain stem, Chapter 12 on the cranial nerves, Chapter 15 on the diencephalon, and Chapter 17 on the cerebrum.

INDEX

Note: An italic *t* on a locator indicates a table. An italic *f* on a locator indicates a figure.

A

abdomen, voluntary motor pathways, 366–367, 366*f*
abdominal viscera, autonomic dual innervation, 323
abducens cranial nerve, 79, 227*f*, 232
ablation, 331
abnormal development. *See* neuroembryology of the brain, abnormal development.
abnormalities of consciousness, definition, 549. *See also* coma; seizures; syncope.
accessory cranial nerve, 80
accommodation, pupillary reflex, 445
acetylcholine, 97–98, 98*f*, 99
acetylcholine-activated channels, 98, 98*f*
acoustic neuroma, 246–247, 248*f*, 253*f*
ACTH (adrenocorticotrophic hormone), 315
actin, neuromuscular junction, 93–94
action tremors, 409
activation response, 341
acute anterior poliomyelitis, 176–178, 177*f*, 527
acute inflammatory demyelinating polyneuropathy (AIDP), 148
acute labyrinthitis, 239
acute motor axonal neuropathy (AMAN), 151
acute motor sensory axonal neuropathy (AMSAN), 151
acute progressive motor neuropathy, 148–155
adenomas, 316*f*
adenoma sebaceous, neuroembryology of the brain, 89
ADH (antidiuretic hormone), 318–319
ADNFLE (autosomal dominant nocturnal frontal lobe epilepsy), 558
adrenergic nerve fibers, 320
adrenocorticotrophic hormone (ACTH), 315
afferent nerves, 5
agenesis of the corpus callosum, neuroembryology of the brain, 87–88, 87*f*
aggressive behavior, temporal lobe disease, 436
Agyri-Pachygyri (lissencephaly), neuroembryology of the brain, 86–87
AIDP (acute inflammatory demyelinating polyneuropathy), 148
akathesia, 390
akinesia, 375
akinetic mutism, definition, 549–550
alcoholic cerebellar degeneration of the cerebellum, 402*f*
allocortex, 427

ALS (amyotropic lateral sclerosis)
  case history, 180–181
  correlation of clinical signs and neuropathology, 179*t*
  course of the disease, 180
  degeneration of corticospinal tracts, 180*f*
  differential diagnosis, 179
  laboratory studies, 179
  overview, 178–179
  survival rate, 180–181
Alzheimer's disease, 582–588, 582*t*, 583*f*–584*f*, 584*t*, 585*f*, 587*t*–588*t*
amacrine cells, 448, 448*f*
AMAN (acute motor axonal neuropathy), 151
amaurosis fugax, 485
amentia, definition, 575
amino acids, neurotransmitters, 57
amnesia, 580–582
amnesiac-confabulatory syndrome, 577–579, 578*t*
AMSAN (acute motor sensory axonal neuropathy), 151
amygdala
  ablation, 427
  description, 425–426, 426*f*–427*f*
  stimulation, 426
amygdaloid nuclei, 425–427, 426*f*–427*f*
amyotropic lateral sclerosis (ALS). *See* ALS (amyotropic lateral sclerosis).
anastomotic vessels, 170, 170*f*
anencephaly, neuroembryology of the brain, 86
aneurysms, 257
anosmia, 223
anoxia, memory disorders, 581–582
anterior aphasias, 462
anterior cerebral artery, syndromes of, 492–493, 493*f*
anterior choroidal artery, syndromes of, 493
anterior circulation, 14–15, 257
anterior commissure, 306
anterior communicating artery, syndromes of, 493
anterior horn cells, 113, 113*f*, 176–178
anterior lobe syndrome, in the cerebellum, 401–403, 401*f*–403*f*
anterior nuclei, 291
anterior spinal artery, 170, 170*f*
anterior spinal occlusion, 169–171
anterograde axoplasmic flow, 52
anterolateral pathway, 127*f*, 128
antibiotics, disorders of the neuromuscular junction, 108
anticonvulsant drugs, for epilepsy, 562–565, 563*t*–564*t*
antidiuretic hormone (ADH), 318–319
aphasia, 435, 461–463, 462*f*–463*f*
aphasic arrest, 463
apoptosis, neuroembryology of the brain, 74

apraxia, 471
arachnoid granulations, 16
arachnoid membrane, 18*f*–19
arches, neuroembryology of the brain, 80
archicortex, 428
Arnold-Chiari malformation, 89, 175*f*
arousal response, 341
arterial circle of Willis, 15, 15*f*
arteries, syndromes of. *See also* cerebral hemispheres, vascular diseases; vascular syndromes.
  amaurosis fugax, 485
  anterior cerebral artery, 492–493, 493*f*
  anterior choroidal artery, 493
  anterior communicating artery, 493
  combined syndrome, 492
  faciobrachial paralysis, 491
  internal carotid, 484–488, 485*f*–486*f*
  lacunar syndromes, 489*f*, 490, 490*t*, 491*f*
  lacune, 489
  lenticulostriate penetrating branches, 489–490, 489*f*–490*f*
  middle cerebral, 488–492, 489*f*–490*f*
  monocular blindness, 485
  occlusion of main cortical stem, 491
  occlusion of middle cerebral artery, 486*f*, 492
  occlusion of superior division of dominant hemisphere, 491
  posterior cerebral artery, 493–495, 494*f*, 494*t*, 495*f*
  segmental fibrinoid arterial degeneration, 489–490
  syndromes of cortical branches, 490–492, 491*f*–492*f*
arteries in the brain, illustration, 614*f*–615*f*, 617*f*
arteriovenous malformations, 503*t*
ascending sensory tracts, 127–131
associational fibers, cerebrum, 11
astrocytes, 48*f*, 59–61, 59*t*
astrocytic brain tumors, 512*t*
astrocytoma, 512–515, 513*f*–515*f*
a-synuclein, Parkinson's disease, 377*f*
ataxia telangiectasia of the cerebellum, 407
audition, thalamic nuclei, 292–293
auditory association, 427
auditory division, sensory pathways, 302
augmenting response, 340, 340*f*
autonomic bladder, autonomic dual innervation, 324
autonomic nervous system. *See also* hypothalamus, and the autonomic nervous system.
  adrenergic nerve fibers, 320
  cervical sympathetic ganglia, 321
  cholinenergic nerve fibers, 320
  craniosacral area, 320

description, 319–320
enteric nervous system, 319, 320
facial cranial nerve, 321
glossopharyngeal cranial nerve, 321
illustration, 322*f*
lumbar sympathetic ganglia, 321–322
oculomotor cranial nerve, 321
parasympathetic area, 320
sacral segments, 321
sympathetic area, 320
sympathetic nervous system *vs.* parasympathetic, 320*t*
sympathetic system, 321, 321*f*
thoracic sympathetic ganglia, 321
thoracolumbar area, 320
vagus cranial nerve, 321
autonomic nervous system, autonomic dual innervation
  abdominal viscera, 323
  autonomic bladder, 324
  bladder, 324
  cutaneous vessels, 323, 323*t*
  deep vessels, 323, 323*t*
  eyes, 322
  glands, 323, 323*t*
  hair, 323
  heart, 323
  lacrimal glands, 322
  lungs, 323
  pelvis, 323
  reflex bladder, 324
  salivary glands, 322
  sensory bladder, 324
  summary of structures affected, 320*t*
  uninhibited bladder, 324
autonomic nervous system, disorders of
  blood vessels, 324
  eye, 323–324
  gastrointestinal tract, 324
  heart, 324
autonomic (visceral) division, 5
autosomal dominant disorders of the cerebellum, 407–408
autosomal dominant nocturnal frontal lobe epilepsy (ADNFLE), 558
autosomal recessive disorders of the cerebellum, 406–407
avoiding responses, 352*f*
axonal transport in cellular structures, 48*t*
axon hillock, 53, 53*f*
axoplasmic flow, 51–52
Azorean disease (Machado-Joseph disease), 408–409

B

Babinski response, 130, 130*f*
back pain, 158–160
bacterial endocarditis, 503, 503*t*
BAER (brain stem auditory evoked potentials), 34–35*f*

619

basal ganglia. *See also* movement disorders; tremors.
corpus striatum, 371, 372*t*, 374*t*
description, 8
diagnosing diseases of, 26
extrapyramidal, 371
input nuclei, 371
intrinsic nuclei, 371
lenticular nuclei, 371
major input, 371, 373*t*
outflow pathway, 371–372
output nuclei, 371
transmitter connections, 372*f*, 375*f*
vs. the cerebellum, 374–375
basal ganglia, dopamine
dopaminergic input, 371–373, 374*t*
dopaminergic systems, 374
hypothalamic system, 374
mesocortical system, 374
mesolimbic system, 374
role in movement, 373, 374*t*
basal vein (of Rosenthal), 16
basilar artery, syndromes and diseases, 262–271, 262*f*, 266*f*, 266*f*–268*f*
basilar zone, 6–7
Bassen Kornsweig syndrome, 155
Becker's muscular dystrophy, 100–101
Bell's palsy, 235
bilateral capsular or cortical lesions, 230
bilateral nodular preventricular heterotopia, neuroembryology of the brain, 85
bilateral synchronous discharges, 343–345, 343*f*–344*f*
biogenic amines, neurotransmitters, 57
bipolar cells, 448, 448*f*
bladder, autonomic dual innervation, 324
blood-brain barrier
circum-ventricular organs, 70
definition, 68
extra-cellular space, 70, 70*f*
fluid phase endocytosis, 69
illustration, 69*f*
pinocytosis, 69
receptor-mediated endocytosis, 69
blood supply to the brain
alternate pathways, 18
anterior circulation, 14–15
arachnoid granulations, 16
arterial circle of Willis, 15, 15*f*
basal vein (of Rosenthal), 16
brainstem veins, 16
cavernous sinuses, 17
to the cerebral hemispheres, 15, 15*f*
cerebral veins, 15–18, 16*f*–17*f*
dural sinuses, 17*t*
illustration, 14*f*
inferior cerebellar veins, 16
inferior cerebral veins, 15
inferior sagittal sinus, 17
internal cerebral veins, 16
lateral unpaired sinuses, 17
paired sinuses, 17–18
posterior circulation, 15
sigmoid sinus, 18
sinuses, 16
straight sinus, 17
superficial cerebral veins, 15
superior cerebellar veins, 16
superior cerebral veins, 15
superior sagittal sinus, 17
blood vessel development, neuroembryology of the brain, 75
blood vessels, autonomic nervous system disorders, 324
body temperature, autonomic nervous system, 318

botulism, disorders of the neuromuscular junction, 108
bovine spongiform encephalopathy. *See* prion disease.
brachial neuritis, 140
brachial plexopathy, case history, 141–142
brachial plexus, 138, 141*f*
bradykinesia, 375
brain. *See also* blood supply to the brain; central nervous system; cerebral hemispheres; cranial nerves.
abnormal development. *See* neuroembryology of the brain, abnormal development.
amygdala, 8
basal ganglia, 8
basilar zone, 6–7
brain stem, 6–7*f*
cerebellum, 7–8. *See also* cranial nerves.
claustrum, 8
corpus callosum, 10*f*
corpus striatum, 8
dentatus, 8
development in utero. *See* neuroembryology of the brain.
diencephalon, 8, 8*f*, 8*t*
emboliformus, 8
epiphysis gland, 20
epithalamus, 8, 8*t*
fastigius, 8
four-deep cerebellar nuclei, 8
glands associated with, 20
globosus, 8
gray matter, 6–7
hypothalamus, 8, 8*t*
lesions, 13–14, 13*f*–14*f*
medulla, 6, 9
midbrain, 6
pineal gland, 20
pons, 6
regions, 6. *See also specific regions.*
size of, 9
subthalamus, 8, 8*t*
tectum, 6–7
tegmentum, 6–7
thalamus, 8, 8*t*
ventral horn equivalent, 6–7
white matter, 6–7
brain, cerebral cortex
cingulate gyrus, 9
frontal lobe, 9
functional localization, 9–11
general features, 9
insula, 9
limbic region, 10
occipital lobe, 9
parietal, 9
temporal, 9
brain, cerebral hemispheres. *See also* cerebrum.
corticofugal fibers, 11
corticopetal fibers, 11
dominant functions, 9
illustrations, 9*f*–10*f*, 12*f*
internal capsule, 11
lateral surface of the brain, 12*f*
middle parietal lobe, 9
posterior occipital lobe, 9
rostral frontal lobe, 9
brain, coverings
arachnoid membrane, 18*f* –19
diaphragma sellae, 19
dural compartments, 19*f*
dura mater, 18–19
falx cerebelli, 18
falx cerebri, 18
Meckel's cave, 19

meninges, 17*f*–18*f*
pia mater, 19
tentorium cerebelli, 18
brain death, definition, 550
brain stem
blood supply, 200–201, 204*f*
case histories, problem solving, 281–287
coronal sections, functional localization, 199
cranial nerves, 222*f*
diagnosing diseases of, 26
diagnostic tests, 34–35
dorsal view, 289*f*
glioma, 272*f*
gross appearance, 200*f*
illustration, 616*f*–617*f*
involvement in sleep stages, 566–567, 566*t*–567*t*
medulla, 200–204
overview, 6–7*f*
regions, 199*t*, 200*f*–201*f*
subcortical pathways, 299*t*
transection, 348–349
veins, 16
vertebral arteries, 200–201, 204*f*
vs. spinal cord, 199–200, 202*t*
brain stem, syndromes and diseases
acoustic neuroma, 253*f*
aneurysms, 257
anterior circulation, 257
basilar artery, 15*f*, 262–271, 262*f*, 266*f*, 266*f*–268*f*
brain stem glioma, 272*f*
cerebellar pontine angle syndrome, 34*f*, 253, 253*f*–254*f*
compression of the pretectal area, 255, 255*f*
compression of the superior colliculus, 255–256, 255*f*
degenerative diseases, 277
demyelinating diseases, 274–277, 275*f*, 275*f*–276*f*
developmental and bony abnormalities, 257. *See also* Arnold Chiari malformation.
dorsal-lateral medullary infarct, 259*f*
Duret hemorrhage, 256, 256*f*
ependymoma of the fourth ventricle, 254*f*
extrinsic midbrain syndromes, 255–256
extrinsic tumors and other lesions, 253–257
extrinsic *vs.* intrinsic diseases, 252, 253*f*
flattened base of skull, 257
foramen magnum syndromes, 256–257, 256*f*
hemorrhage, 271–274
hypertensive cerebeller hemorrhage, 257
infections of the brain stem, 277. *See also* Herpes simplex; poliomyelitis.
inferior pontine syndromes, 263–266, 262*f*
intrapontine hemorrhage, 271
intrinsic diseases, 257–262
jugular foramen syndrome, 256
lateral cerebeller hemisphere syndrome, 255, 255*f*
lateral medullary syndrome, 259–261
lateral tegmental superior pontine syndrome, 266–267, 266*f*–267*f*
lateral tegmentum, 263–266
locked-in syndrome, 262*f*
medulloblastoma, 254*f*
meningiomas, 257
midbrain syndromes, 267–271, 268*f*
middle-lower pontine basilar infarct, 262*f*
midline cerebellum syndrome (fourth ventricle), 253–255, 254*f*

multiple sclerosis, 274–277, 275*f*–276*f*
occlusive disease, 258–259
Paget's disease, 257
paramedian lower pontine syndrome, 265
paramedian medullary syndrome, 261, 262*f*
paramedian preventricular mesencephalic-diencephalic junction, 271
paramedian syndrome, upper pons, 262*f*
paramedian syndromes, 267–271, 268*f*
paramedian syndrome with tegmental involvement, 271
paramedian upper pons, 266–267, 266*f*–267*f*
platybasia, 257
pontine glioma, 273*f*
posterior cerebral artery, 263
stenosis of the basilar vertebral arteries, 258
subarachnoid hemorrhage, 271–274
superior pontine syndromes, 266–267, 266*f*–267*f*
syndromes of the cerebellum, 253–255, 254*f*
syndromes of the tentorium, 255*f*–256*f*, 255–256
tentorial meningiomas, 256
Tentorial Notch syndrome, 255*f*–256*f*, 256
total posterior inferior cerebeller artery syndrome, 260*f*
toxic metabolic disorder, 277
vascular syndromes and extrinsic lesions, 257
vertebral arteries, 15, 259
vertibral artery syndrome, 262*f*
vestibular schwannoma, 253*f*
Weber's syndromes, 267–271, 268*f*
brain stem anatomy
basilar zone, 204, 204*f*, 204*t*, 206*f*, 207, 207*t*
central zone, 206, 206*f*
gray matter, 202*t*
inferior colliculus, 208–209, 209*f*
lateral zone, 206, 206*f*
lower pons, facial nerve and facial colliculus, 110*f*, 204*f*, 204*t*, 205–206, 206*f*
medial zone, 206–207
midbrain, 208, 209*f*
motor cranial nerve nuclei, 206, 206*f*
superior colliculus, 209–210, 209*f*
tectum, 207–208, 209*f*
upper pons, motor and main sensory nuclei, 207, 207*t*, 208*f*
ventricular zone, 206–208
white matter, 202*t*, 203, 206*f*
brain stem anatomy, functional centers
cardiovascular, 214
coughing, 215
deglutition, 214
descending reticulospinal system, 212–213, 213*t*
emetic, 214
respiration, 214
reticular formation, 212, 212*t*
vomiting, 214
brain stem anatomy, localization of disease
cerebellar dysfunction, 217–218
corticobulbar pathways, interrupting, 216–217
corticospinal pathways, interrupting, 216–217
cranial nerve dysfunction, 218–219
decerebrate rigidity, 218, 220, 221
guidelines for, 216, 216*f*

lesions in the tegmentum, clinical signs, 219, 219t
long motor pathways, interrupting, 216–217
long sensory systems, interrupting, 218
medial lemniscus, 218
overview, 215–216, 215f–216f
spinothalmics, 218
brain stem anatomy, tegmentum
description, 210, 210f–211f
lesions, clinical signs, 219, 219t
major tracts in tegmental zones, 203t
overview, 199, 200f, 200t
pontine basis tegmentum, 208–209, 209f
zones, 202t, 211t
brain stem auditory evoked potentials (BAER), 34–35f
brain tumors
astrocytic, 512t
astrocytoma, 512–515, 513f–515f
of blood vessel origin, 515
epidemiology, 510–511
etiology, 511t
extrinsic, 515–516, 516f–517f
intrinsic, 511–515
meningeal carcinomatosis, 521f
meningiomas, 515–516, 516f, 517t
metastatic, 516–518, 518f, 520f–521f
neuroepithelials, 511–515
neurofibromatosis, 511
nonneuroepithelials, 515–516
primary central nervous system lymphomas, 515
relative frequency, 511t–512t
secondary, 516–518
tuberous sclerosis, 511
Broca's motor aphasia, 461, 462f
Brown-Sequard hemisection syndrome, 163, 163t

C

CA (childhood absence epilepsy), 554, 554f
CAG trinucleotide expansion, 408
capillary loops, neuroendocrine system, 314
cardiac muscles, 4–5
cardiovascular center, brain stem, 214
carpal tunnel syndrome, case history, 142–144
case histories, problem solving
brain stem, 281–287
cortical localization, 476–481
cranial nerves, 281–287
general cases, 598–604
lesion diagrams, 538–545
muscle diseases, 193–198
nerve root disease, 193–198
peripheral nerve disease, 193–198
photo matching, 605–613
spinal cord disease, 193–198
cataplexy, 568
Ca++ troponin interaction, neuromuscular junction, 94, 96f–97f
cavernous sinuses, 17
cavernous sinus syndrome, 245–246
central lateral premotor area, 359
central nervous system. See also brain; nervous system; neurocytology; neurons; ventricular system.
overview, 5
regeneration, 67, 68
in situ, 6f
spinal cord
cross sections, 6f
description, 5–6
structure, 52–53
ventral horn cells, 5–6
central nervous system, supporting cells

astrocytes, 59–61, 59t
Creutzfeldt-Jakob disease, 62–63
endothelial cells, 61
ependymal cells, 63–64
fibroblasts, 59
functions of, 59t
giant cells, 62
gliotransmitters, 60, 60t
histiocytes, 61
lymphocytes, 61
macroglia, 59
mechanicoreceptor, 58t –59
microglia, 59
microglial cells, 61–62, 61f
monocytes, 61
mononuclear cells, 61–63, 61f
neural crest cells, 64
oligodendrocytes, 48f, 53, 53f, 54–56, 60
pericytes, 61
prion disease, 62–63
prions, 62–63
protoplasmic astrocytes, 59
satellite cells, 59, 63, 63f
Schwann cells, 59, 63, 64f
central nervous system pathways
description, 56
motor-sensory cortex
control of the foot, 12–13
corticospinal pathway, 12
lower motor neuron, 12
lower motor neuron paralysis, 13
overview, 12, 12f
second-order nerve cells, 12
third-order neurons, 12
upper motor neuron, 12, 13t
upper motor neuron paralysis, 13
overview, 11–12
central pattern generators, 347–348
central sleep apnea, 567
centronuclear myopathy, 103
cerebellar agenesis, neuroembryology of the brain, 88
cerebellar atrophy, 403–405, 403f–404
cerebellar dysfunction, localization in brain stem, 217–218
cerebellar peduncles, 411
cerebellar pontine angle syndrome, 253, 253f–254f
cerebellum. See also cranial nerves; tremors.
afferents, 397
cerebellar peduncles, 411
climbing fibers, 396, 396f
cytoarchitecture, 396–397, 396f
description, 7–8
dual motor control, 399
fiber pathways, 411–412f
functions and correlations, 397–399
longitudinal division, 395, 395f, 395t
mossy fibers, 396, 396f
movement, initiation, planning, and timing, 399
parallel fibers, 396, 396f
posture and equilibrium of the trunk, 399
speech/voice control, 399
spinocerebellar tracts, 411–412f
topographic patterns, 397, 398f
transverse division, 395, 395f, 396t
vestibular reflexes and eye movements, 398
vs. basal ganglia, 374–375
cerebellum, effects of disease
alcoholic cerebellar degeneration, 402f
ataxia telangiectasia, 407
autosomal dominant disorders, 407–408
autosomal recessive disorders, 406–407
Azorean disease (Machado-Joseph disease), 408–409

CAG trinucleotide expansion, 408
cerebellar atrophy, 403–405, 403f–404
channelopathy, 408
CTG trinucleotide expansion, 408
degenerative diseases, 406–409, 407f
floccular nodular lobe, 400–401
gene mechanisms, 408–409
hemangioblastoma, 404f, 406f
infarction, 405–406, 407f
lateral cerebellar syndrome, 404f
major syndromes, 400–404, 401f–404f
medulloblastoma, 401f
midline tumors, 400–401, 401f
olivopontocerebellar atrophy, 409, 410f
overview, 399–400
SCA (spinocerebellar ataxia), 408
suns of occlusion, 406f
syndrome of the anterior lobe, 401–403, 401f–403f
syndromes of occlusion, 405–406
vascular syndromes, 405
cerebral aqueduct, 20, 75
cerebral circulation, diagnostic tests, 41, 42f
cerebral cortex
anatomical considerations, 325, 326f
basic design, 327–328
bilateral synchronous discharges, 343–345, 343f–344f
cingulate gyrus, 9
cingulum, 337
complex partial seizures, 330
cortical neuron interaction with thalamic relay neurons, 341–342, 342f
cytology, 325–327, 326f
diagnosing diseases of, 26
epileptic seizures, 330
external granular layer, 328
external pyramidal layer, 328
focal convulsions, 330
focal discharge, 330
focal epilepsy, 330
focal seizure discharge, 342–343, 342f–343f
focal seizures, 330
frontal lobe, 9f, 332, 334f
function, study methods, 330–331, 340–341
functional localization, 9–11
functional organization, 327–328
fusiform layer, 328
ganglionic layer, 328
general features, 9
heterogenetic, 328, 328f
homogenetic, 328, 328f
illustration, 333f
inferior frontal occipital fasciculus, 337
inferior longitudinal fasciculus, 337
insula, 9
internal granular layer, 328
internal layer, 328
large and giant pyramidal cell layer, 328
limbic region, 10
location of pathology, confirming, 331
molecular layer, 328
monitoring activity of. See EEG (electroencephalogram).
motor areas, 332, 332f–334f, 334, 350f, 355f, 362f–363f, 462f–463f
neocortex
afferent inputs, 337–338
cholinenergic pathways, 338
claustrum pathways, 338
dopaminenergic pathways, 338
efferent projections, 338
GABAergic pathways, 338
nonthalamic afferent inputs, 338
noradrenergic pathway, 338

norepinephrine pathway, 338
seritonenergic pathway, 338
thalamic afferent inputs, 337–338
types of, 328–329, 329f–330f
neocortical cytoarchitecture and function, 330f, 332, 332f–333f, 334t
neuroembryology of the brain, 82–83
occipital lobe, 9, 335–336, 335f
ontogenetic factor, 331
parietal, 9
parietal lobe, 334–335, 334t
partial seizures, 330
planum temporale, 330f
plexiform layer, 328
prefrontal-nonmotor areas, 334, 366f
pyramidal cells, 326, 326f
sensory areas, map of, 334f
simple partial seizures, 330
six-layered scheme, 328
smooth stellate cells, 326f, 327, 327f
somatic motor areas, map of, 334f
spindle cell multiform layer, 328
spiny neurons, 326
spiny stellate neurons, 327
subcortical white matter, afferents and efferents, 336–337, 336f–337f
superior longitudinal fasciculus, 337, 467f
temporal, 9
temporal lobe, 330f, 335–336, 335f, 463f
and the thalamus, 295
types of, 328, 328f
uncinate fasciculus, 337, 337f
cerebral cortex, speech and language
ablation of speech areas, 463–466, 465f–466f
anterior aphasias, 462
aphasia, 461–463, 462f–463f
aphasic arrest, 463
apraxia, 471
Broca's motor aphasia, 461, 462f
cerebral dominance, 460–461
components of language function, 462–463
corpus callosum, role of, 471–472
dysarthria, 460–463, 461f
fluent aphasias, 466–471, 467f
inferior parietal lobule, 461, 462f
nondominant hemisphere functions, 471
posterior aphasias, 462
speech arrest, 463
speech development in children, 461
stimulating speech areas, 463, 463f
supplementary motor cortex, 461
Wernicke's receptive aphasia area, 461, 462f
cerebral dominance, 460–461
cerebral embolism, 495–496
cerebral hemispheres
blood flow, 15, 15f
corticofugal fibers, 11
corticopetal fibers, 11
craningiopharyngioma, 518f
diagnostic tests, 35–41
disorders of myelin, 529–530
dominant functions, 9
headaches, 510
heavy metal exposure, 526t
illustrations, 9f–10f, 12f
internal capsule, 11
lateral surface of the brain, 12f
middle parietal lobe, 9
migraine headaches, 510
multiple sclerosis, 529–530, 529f–530f
muscle tension headaches, 510
neoplasms, 509–510
neuroembryology of the brain, 79
nutritional disorders, 526t

cerebral hemispheres (Cont.)
  occipital neuralgia, 510
  periodic cluster headaches, 510
  posterior occipital lobe, 9
  rostral frontal lobe, 9
  system disorders, 529
cerebral hemispheres, brain tumors
  astrocytic, 512t
  astrocytoma, 512–515, 513f–515f
  of blood vessel origin, 515
  epidemiology, 510–511
  etiology, 511t
  extrinsic, 515–516, 516f–517f
  intrinsic, 511–515
  meningeal carcinomatosis, 521f
  meningiomas, 515–516, 516f, 517t
  metastatic, 516–518, 518f, 520f–521f
  neuroepithelials, 511–515
  neurofibromatosis, 511
  nonneuroepithelials, 515–516
  primary central nervous system lymphomas, 515
  relative frequency, 511t–512t
  secondary, 516–518
  tuberous sclerosis, 511
cerebral hemispheres, head trauma
  concussion, 505
  contra coup injuries, 505
  contusions, 505, 506f
  coup injuries, 505
  extradural hematomas, 506–508, 507f
  lacerations, 505, 506f
  late effects of, 508–509
  management of, 508
  post-concussion syndrome, 508–509
  posttraumatic epilepsy, 508
  prevention, 509, 509t
  skull fractures, 505–506
  subdural hematomas, 506–508, 507f
cerebral hemispheres, infections
  acute anterior poliomyelitis, 527
  encephalitis, 523f, 525
  encephalitis lethargica, 527
  encephalopathies, 527
  focal infections of the nervous system, 519–520
  general or diffuse, 522, 523f, 582
  granulomas, 522
  herpes, 582
  HIV - 1, 528–529
  HSV (herpes simplex), 528
  involving the brain, 520–522
  measles, 528
  meningitis, 522–525, 523f, 524t
  mumps, 528
  nonneurotropic, 528–529
  overview, 518–519
  paramyxovirus, 528
  purulent brain abscess, 40, 520–521, 521f–522f
  rabies, 527–528
  retrovirus, 528–529
  subdural empyema, 520
  viral, 523f, 525–529
  Von Economo's encephalitis, 527
cerebral hemispheres, vascular diseases
  arteriovenous malformations, 503, 504t
  bacterial endocarditis, 503, 504t
  cerebral embolism, 495–496
  embolic disease, managing, 496
  encephalomalacia, 483–484, 484f
  infarction, 483–484, 484f
  intracerebral hemorrhage, 496–499, 497f, 498t, 499f
  intracranial hemorrhage, 496–503
  ischemic disease, managing, 496

  ischemic-occlusive disease, 482–484, 482t, 483f, 488f
  necrosis, 484, 484f
  overview, 482
  sinuses, disorders of, 504
  subarachnoid hemorrhage, 499–503, 500t, 502f, 502t–503f
  syndromes of major arteries
    amaurosis fugax, 485
    anterior cerebral artery, 492–493, 493f
    anterior choroidal artery, 493
    anterior communicating artery, 493
    combined syndrome, 492
    faciobrachial paralysis, 491
    internal carotid, 42f, 484–488, 485f–486f
    lacunar syndromes, 489f, 490, 490t, 491f
    lacune, 489
    lenticulostriate penetrating branches, 489–490, 489f–490f
    middle cerebral, 488–492, 489f–490f
    monocular blindness, 485
    occlusion of main cortical stem, 491
    occlusion of middle cerebral artery, 486f, 492
    occlusion of superior division of dominant hemisphere, 491
    posterior cerebral artery, 493–495, 494f, 494t, 495f
    segmental fibrinoid arterial degeneration, 489–490
    syndromes of cortical branches, 490–492, 491f–492f
  TIAs (transient ischemic attacks), 483
  veins, disorders of, 504
cerebral veins, 15–18, 16f–17f
cerebrospinal fluid, 20, 20t
cerebrum
  associational fibers, 11
  commissural fibers, 11
  cortical white matter, 10–11
  functional locations, 10, 11t
  white matter of the cerebrum, 11, 11t
cerebrum, atlas of
  arteries, 614f–615f, 617f
  brain stem, 616f–617f
  cingulate lobe, 615f
  coronal section, 614f
  cranial nerves, 617f
  frontal lobe, 615f–616f
  horizontal section, 614f
  hypophyseal stalk, 615f, 617f
  hypothalamus, 616f
  major gyri, 614f
  occipital lobe, 617f
  parietal lobe, 615f–617f
  temporal lobe, 615f–617f
  thalamus, 616f
  ventricular system, 617f
  white matter, 615f–617f
cervical disk, lateral protrusion, 157f
cervical disk disease, 164–167, 165f–166f
cervical invertebral disks, 155f
cervical spine, 136, 136f, 136f–137f
cervical sympathetic ganglia, 321
channelopathies affecting skeletal muscle, 102, 102t
channelopathy, of the cerebellum, 408
Charcot Marie Tooth (CMT) disease, 153–155
chemical synapses, 56
childhood absence epilepsy (CA), 554, 554f
cholinenergic nerve fibers, 320
cholinergic pathways, to the neocortex, 338
cholinergic neurons, 566

chromatolysis, 64–66
chromosomal trisomy and translocation, neuroembryology of the brain, 88
cingulate cortex, 425f
cingulate gyrus, cerebral cortex, 9
cingulate lobe, illustration, 615f
cingulum, 337, 431
circadian timing cycles, 567
circle of Willis, 15, 15f
circum-ventricular organs, 70
claustrum, 8
claustrum pathways, to the neocortex, 338
climbing fibers, 396, 396f
clinical signs and symptoms, 375–376
CMT (Charcot Marie Tooth) disease, 153–155
cochlear nerve, 236–239, 236f–237f
color sensitivity, eyes, 446–447, 447f
coma
  care of the comatose patient, 568–569
  definition, 549
  emergency onset, 568, 569t
  major causes, 568
  prognosis, 569–570
  prolonged, 568
commissural fibers, cerebrum, 11
commissures, neuroembryology of the brain, 82–83, 83f
complex cells, occipital lobe, 454, 454f
complex partial seizures, 330
compression of
  the pretectal area, 255–256, 255f
  spinal cord
    case histories, 165–167
    consequences of extrinsic compression, 163t
    overview, 162–164
  the superior colliculus, 255, 255f
computerized axial tomography (CT) scan, 31, 33f–34f, 43f
concussion, 505
cones, eyes, 446–448, 446f–448f
confusion, definition, 549
congenital myopathies, 103
congenital neurologic malformations, neuroembryology of the brain, 85t
consciousness, definition, 549
contra coup injuries, 505
contraction, muscles. See neuromuscular junction, contraction.
contusions, 505, 506f
cornea, 444, 444f
corpus callosum
  agenesis of, 87–88, 87f
  illustration, 10f
  memory, 577
  role in speech and language, 471–472
corpus striatum, 8, 371, 372t, 374t
cortical architecture, neuroembryology of the brain, 84
cortical branches, syndromes of, 490–492, 491f–492f
cortical localization; case histories, problem solving, 476–481
cortical microdysgenesias, neuroembryology of the brain, 85–86
cortical neuron interaction with thalamic relay neutrons, 341–342, 342f
cortical nucleus, 428
cortical projections, thalamic nuclei, 295t, 297f
cortical regions, 425f
cortical structures, involvement in sleep stages, 566–567, 566t–567t
cortical structures in emotions
  allocortex, 427
  amygdaloid nuclei, 425–427, 426f–427f

  auditory association, 427
  cingulate cortex, 425f
  cingulum, 431
  cortical nucleus, 428
  cortical regions, 425f
  corticobulbar pathway, 431
  corticospinal pathway, 431
  dentate gyrus, 429, 429t
  entorhinal region, 428, 428f
  entorhinal reverberating circuit, 430, 430f
  fornix, 425f–426f, 431
  hippocampal formation, 427–430
  hippocampus, 428–430, 428f, 429t
  limbic nuclei, 426
  mesocortex, 428
  neocortex, 427, 428
  neocortex of the temporal lobe, 427
  olfactory nuclei, 426
  papez circuit, 431
  parahippocampal gyrus, 424f–425f, 425
  principal pathways, 425f–426f, 430–431, 430f
  stria terminalis, 431
  ventral amygdalofugal pathway, 426, 431
  visual perception, 427
cortical white matter, cerebrum, 10–11
corticobulbar pathways, 216–217, 431
corticofugal fibers, cerebral hemispheres, 11
corticomesencephalic system, 367
corticonuclear system, 367, 367f
corticopetal fibers, cerebral hemispheres, 11
corticorubral spinal system
  central lateral premotor area, 359
  dorsal lateral premotor area, 359
  lateral premotor area, 359
  low-grade glioma, 360
  overview, 358
  premotor cortex, 358–360, 359f
  SMA (supplemental motor area), 359
corticospinal pathway, 12, 431
corticospinal pathways, interrupting, 216–217
corticospinal tracts, 126–127, 129f, 131f, 366–367, 366f
coughing, center in brain stem, 215
coup injuries, 505
cranial bifida, neuroembryology of the brain, 88–89
cranial nerve nuclei, 304
cranial nerves. See also specific nerves.
  in the brain stem, 222f
  brain stem dysfunction, 218–219
  case histories, problem solving, 281–287
  components of, 223, 222f–223f
  illustration, 617f
  localization in the brain stem, 7t
  summary of, 249f
  voluntary control of, 367
cranial nerves, disorders of
  abducens nerve, 227f, 232
  acoustic neuroma, 246–247, 248f
  acute labyrinthitis, 239
  anosmia, 223
  Bell's palsy, 235
  bilateral capsular or cortical lesions, 230
  cavernous sinus syndrome, 245–246
  cochlear nerve, 236–239, 236f–237f
  deafness, 237
  extrinsic lesions, 244–245, 367
  facial diplegia, 235
  facial myokimia, 235
  facial nerve, 233–236, 233f
  glossopharyngeal nerve, 236–240, 240f
  glossopharyngeal neuralgia, 240
  hemofacial spasm, 235
  herpes zoster, 235
  hypoglossal nerve, 244f

jugular foramen syndrome, 247–249
lesions, 240
malformation of base of skull, 250
mandible movements, 230t
mastication muscles, 230t
Meniere's disease, 239
meningiomas, 34
nausea, 238
nystagmus, 239
Paget's disease, 250
parotid gland, tumors of, 235
peripheral autonomic neuropathies, 242–243
pseudobulbar palsy, 245
pterygopalatine ganglia, 234
spinal accessory nerve, 243, 244f
submandibular ganglia, 234
summary of, 245t
taste sensation, 234
tensor vali palatine, 229
tic, douloureux, 230
tinnitus, 237
trigeminal neuralgia, 230
unilateral supranuclear lesions, 230
unsteadiness, 239
vagus nerve, 241–243, 241f
vertigo, 238
vestibular neuropathy, 239
vestibulocochlear nerve, 236–239, 236f
vomiting, 238
cranial nerves, general function
abducens nerve, 227f, 232
cochlear nerve, 236–239, 236f–237f
Edinger-Westphal nucleus, 224
facial nerve, 233–236, 233f
glossopharyngeal nerve, 236–240, 240f
hypoglossal nerve, 244f
mandible movements, 230t
mastication muscles, 230t
oculomotor, 222–224, 227f
olfactory nerve, 223, 226f
optic nerve, 222–224, 226f
pterygopalatine ganglia, 234
spinal accessory nerve, 243, 244f
submandibular ganglia, 234
summary of, 225t
taste sensation, 234
tensor vali palatine, 229
trigeminal nerve, 228f, 228–232
trochlear nerve, 227f, 228
vagus nerve, 241–243, 241f
vestibulocochlear nerve, 236–239, 236f
cranial nerves, neuroembryology
abducens nerve, 79
accessory nerve, 80
facial nerve, 80
glossopharyngeal nerve, 80
hypoglossal nerve, 79
illustration, 81f
innervation, muscles of somite origin, 79
innervation, pharyngeal arches, 79
muscles of somite origin, innervation, 79
oculomotor nerve, 79
olfactory nerve, 81
optic nerve, 81
origins of, 80f
pharyngeal arches, innervation, 79
taste bud nerves, 81
trigeminal nerve, 80
trochlear nerve, 79
types of, 79, 80, 81
vagus nerve, 80
vestibulocochlear nerve, 81
cranigiopharyngioma, 518f
craniosacral area, 320
Creutzfeldt-Jakob disease, 62–63, 292, 590–594, 590f. See also prion disease.

cross-bridges, neuromuscular junction, 95–96, 96f
CT (computerized axial tomography) scan, 31, 33f–34f, 43f
CTG trinucleotide expansion, 408
cutaneous angiomatosis, neuroembryology of the brain, 89
cutaneous vessels, autonomic dual innervation, 323, 323t
cytoplasm organelles, 48

D
dark (scoptic) vision, 446
deafness, 237
decerebrate rigidity, 218, 220.221, 348–349, 349f–350f
decorticate preparation, 350–353, 351f–352f
decorticate rigidity, 350, 351f
deep telencephalic gray, 303–306
deep tendon reflexes, postnatal development, 356
deep tendon stretch reflex, in diagnosis, 27t
deep touch, 300
deep vessels, autonomic dual innervation, 323, 323t
defective fusion of dorsal structures, neuroembryology of the brain, 88–89
degeneration, 64–66
deglutition center in brain stem, 214
delay, spinal cord, 117
delayed response test, 575
delirium, definition, 549
dementia
Alzheimer's disease, 582–588, 582t, 583f–584f, 584t, 585f, 587t–588t
Creutzfeldt-Jakob disease, 590–594, 590f. See also prion disease.
definition, 575
DLB (dementia with Lewy bodies), 588–589, 589t
FTD (frontal/temporary dementia), 589
Huntington's chorea, 589
mild cognitive impairment, 582
neurobiology, 592–594
prion disease, 592–594. See also Creutzfeldt-Jakob disease.
dementia with Lewy bodies (DLB), 588–589, 589f
demyelinating diseases, 186–190, 187f–188f, 274–277, 275f, 275f–276f. See also multiple sclerosis.
dendrites, 45
dendritic spines, 46, 46f, 48, 58
denervation sensitivity, neuromuscular junction, 99
dentate gyrus, 429, 429t
dentatus, 8
dermatome boundaries, 113–114, 113f
dermatome chart, remaining sensibility, 157f
descending reticulospinal system, center in brain stem, 212–213, 213f
descending tracts, 126–127
desynchronization response, 341
developmental and bony abnormalities, of the brain stem, 257
Devic's syndrome, 172f
diabetic mononeuropathy, case history, 145, 150f
diagnosis
deep tendon stretch reflex, 27t
diagrams of the human body, 23f–25f
essential questions, 22
nature of pathology, 28–29
radicular muscle ennervations, 27t
segmental sensory patterns, 27t
superficial reflexes, 27t–28t

symptom categories, 22
diagnosis, diseases of
basal ganglia, 26
brain stem, 26
cerebral cortex, 26
muscle, 22–23
nerve root, 23, 26
neuromuscular junction, 23
peripheral nerve, 23
spinal cord, 26
spinal nerve, 23, 26
diagnosis, history and examination
Mental Status and Language Functions, 29
MMSE (Mini-Mental State Examination), 29–30
diagnosis, studies in neurology
BAER (brain stem auditory evoked potentials), 34–35f
brain stem, 34–35
cerebral circulation, 41, 42f
cerebral hemispheres, 35–41
CT (computerized axial tomography) scan, 31, 33f–34f, 43f
EEG (electroencephalography), 37–40, 38f–39f
electromyography, 30–31
MMPI (Minnesota Multiphasic Personality Index), 41
MRA (magnetic resonance angiography), 41, 42f
MRI (magnetic resonance imaging) scan, 31, 32f, 34f, 36f
muscles, 30–31
nerve, 30–31
nerve conduction velocity test, 30t, 31
nerve root, 31–34
neuropsychological tests, 40–41
PEG (pneumonocephalography), 35, 35f
PET (positron emission tomography), 36, 37f
posterior fossa, 34–35
PSG (polysomnography), 40
skull base, 34–35
sleep disorders, 40
SPECT (single-photon emission computed tomograph), 36, 37f
spinal cord, 31–34, 31f
ventriculography, 35
WAIS (Wechsler Adult Intelligent Score), 40–41
Wechsler Memory Score, 41
Wisconsin Card Sorting Test, 41
diaphragma sellae, 19
diencephalic boundaries, 288, 288f–289f
diencephalic involvement in sleep stages, 566–567, 566t–567t
diencephalon
horizontal section, 294f
major fiber bundles, 294t
neuroembryology of the brain, 79, 79f
subcortical pathways, 299t
subdivisions, 8, 8f, 288. See also specific subdivisions.
white matter, 293–294
disorders of motor development, 365
distal hand movement, postnatal development, 356
DLB (dementia with Lewy bodies), 588–589, 589f
dominant hemisphere parietal lobules, 418–419
dopamine, and the basal ganglia, 371–374, 374t
dopamine-blocking agents, movement disorders, 390–391
dopaminenergic pathways, to the neocortex, 338

dorsal-lateral medullary infarct, 259f
dorsal lateral premotor area, 359
dorsal longitudinal fasciculus, hypothalamus, 313
dorsal root ganglion, 159–160
dorsal thalamus, 337–338
dorsomedial nucleus, 291
double athetosis, 387–388
double cortex, neuroembryology of the brain, 86
Down's syndrome, neuroembryology of the brain, 88
drug-induced Parkinsonian syndrome, 390
dual motor control, 399
Duchenne's muscular dystrophy, 100, 100f
dural compartments, 19f
dural sinuses, 17t
dura mater, 18–19
Duret hemorrhage, 256, 256f
dysarthria, 460–463, 461f
dyskinesia, 375
dysphasia. See aphasia.
dystonia, 375, 389–390
dystonic reactions, 390

E
Eaton-Lambert syndrome, disorders of the neuromuscular junction, 108
ectodermal tissue, neuroembryology of the brain, 89
Edinger-Westphal nucleus, 224
EEG (electroencephalogram)
abnormalities, 40f, 550–551, 551f
activation response, 38f, 341
arousal response, 38f
augmenting response, 340, 340f
bilateral synchronous discharges, 343–345, 343f–344f
cortical neuron interaction with thalamic relay neutrons, 342f
description, 37–40, 38f–39f
desynchronization response, 38f, 341
evoked potentials, 330–331, 340–341, 340f–341f
experimental epilepsy, 343–345, 343f–344f
focal abnormalities, 39–40, 40f, 42f, 550–551, 551f
focal seizure discharge, 342–343, 342f–343f
generalized abnormalities, 39–40, 42f, 551
neurophysiology of the cerebral cortex, 38f–39f, 42f, 338–342, 339f
primary evoked response, 340, 340f
recruiting response, 340–341, 340f–341f
effectors, 58
efferent projections, from the neocortex, 338
electrical synapses, 56
electromyography, 30–31
embolic disease, managing, 496
emboliformus, 8
emetic center in brain stem, 214
emotional brain, 422
emotions, autonomic nervous system, 319
encephalitis, 523f, 525
encephalitis lethargica, 527
encephalomalacia, 483–484, 484f
encephalopathies, 527
endocrine disorders of the muscles, 104
endoneurium, 52
endothelial cells, 61
endplate, neuromuscular junction, 96–98, 97f–98f
enteric nervous system, 319, 320
entorhinal region, 428, 428f
entorhinal reverberating circuit, 430, 430f

ependymal cells, 63–64
ependymoma of the fourth ventricle, 254f
epilepsy. *See also* seizures.
   ADNFLE (autosomal dominant nocturnal frontal lobe epilepsy), 558
   alteration of awareness and responsivity, 561–562
   anticonvulsant drugs, 562–565, 563t–564t
   CA (childhood absence epilepsy), 554, 554f
   definition, 549
   EEG experiment, 343–345, 343f–344f
   ending seizure discharge, 562
   epileptic focus, 552–553
   epileptic neuron, 552–553
   evaluation, 562, 563t–564t
   generalized, 553–556, 555f–556f
   generalized idiopathic, 558–559, 558t
   genetic models in mice, 559
   GTCS (generalized tonic clonic seizures), 552t, 557, 557f
   ictal event, 549
   idiopathic, 553–556, 555f–556f
   infantile spasms, 554, 554f
   interictal period, 549
   JA (juvenile absence), 555
   JME (juvenile myoclonic epilepsy), 555, 555f
   kindling model, 553
   Lennox Gastaut syndrome, 554
   managing seizure disorders, 562–565, 563t–564t
   mirror focus, 553
   multifocal abnormalities, 553
   myoclonus, 555, 556–558
   pathophysiology, 559–561, 560f, 560t, 561f–562f
   PDSs (paroxysmal depolarization shifts), 552
   petit mal seizures, 555
   primary, 558–559, 558t
   pyknolepsy, 555
   secondary epileptogenesis, 553
   status epilepticus, 564–565, 565t
epileptic focus, 552–553
epileptic neuron, 552–553
epileptic seizures, 330
epinephrine, autonomic nervous system, 319
epineurium, 52
epiphysis gland, 20
epithalamus
   afferent inputs to the neocortex, 338
   definition, 8, 8t
   description, 303–304, 306, 319
   limbic regions, 425
essential tremors, 410
evoked potentials, 330–331, 340–341, 340f–341f
excessive daytime sleepiness, 566t, 567–568, 568f, 5689f
excitation contraction coupling, neuromuscular junction, 92
excitatory neurotransmitters, 57
excitatory postsynaptic potential, 116, 116f, 118f
excitatory synapses, 58
exercises. *See* case histories, problem solving.
experimental epilepsy, 343–345, 343f–344f
external granular layer, cerebral cortex, 328
external pyramidal layer, cerebral cortex, 328
extra-cellular space, 70, 70f
extradural hematomas, 506–508, 507f
extrapyramidal, 371
extrinsic, 516f–517f
extrinsic brain tumors, 515–516
extrinsic lesions of the spinal cord, 164–167

extrinsic midbrain syndromes, 255–256
extrinsic *vs.* intrinsic diseases of the brain stem, 252, 253f
eye movements
   central control of saccades, 361–362
   in the cerebellum, 398
   fixation system, 362
   oligodendroglioma, 360, 360f–361f
   saccadic, 360–361
   smooth pursuit, 362
   vergence movements, 362
   vestibulo-ocular movements, 362
eyes. *See also* occipital lobe; vision.
   accommodation, 445
   amacrine cell response, 448
   amacrine cells, 448, 448f
   autonomic dual innervation, 322
   autonomic nervous system disorders, 323–324
   bipolar cell response, 448
   bipolar cells, 448, 448f
   color sensitivity, 446–447, 447f
   cones, 446–448, 446f–448f
   cornea, 444, 444f
   fixed pupil, 445
   ganglion cells, 448, 448f
   horizontal cells, 448, 448f
   inner tunic (retina), 445
   lens, 445
   light reflex, 445
   light sensitivity, 446
   middle tunic, 444f
   movements, occipital lobe, 455
   optic nerve, 448
   optic radiation, 449f, 452–453
   outer fibrous tunic, 444, 444f
   papilla, 446
   papilledema, 446
   pars ciliaris, 445
   pars iridica, 445
   pars optica, 445, 446f
   photoreceptors, 446–448, 446f, 448f
   pupillary muscles, 445
   pupillary reflexes, 445
   rhodopsin, 446
   rods, 446–448, 446f, 448f
   scoptic (dark) vision, 446
   structure of, 444–445, 444f
   visual pathway, 353f, 449, 449f
   voluntary motor pathways, 367
eyes, visual fields
   fovea centralis, 449
   lesions in the optic pathway, 449–452, 450f–452f
   LGN (lateral geniculate nucleus), 452
   optic chiasm, 449
   optic nerve, 449
   retina, 449

F

facial colliculus, 204f, 204t, 205–206, 206f
facial cranial nerve
   anatomy of, 204f, 204t, 205–206, 206f
   enteric nervous system, 321
   general function, 233–236, 233f
   neuroembryology, 80
   taste and general sensation, 302–303
facial diplegia, 235
facial muscles, voluntary motor pathways, 367
facial myokimia, 235
faciobrachial paralysis, 491
facioscapulohumeral (FSH) dystrophy, 101
falx cerebelli, 18
falx cerebri, 18
familial amyloid polyneuropathy autosomal dominant, 155
familial paroxysmal dyskinesia, 391

familial periodic paralysis (periodic paralysis), 102–103
fasciculus cuneatas, 300
fasciculus gracilis, 300
FAS (fetal alcohol syndrome), neuroembryology of the brain, 88
fastigius, 8
fast muscles, neuromuscular junction, 99–100
fatal familial insomnia, 593
fiber bundles, neuromuscular junction, 91–92, 91f
fiber pathways, 411–412f
fibroblasts, 59
filament interaction, neuromuscular junction, 96f–97f
filaments, neuromuscular junction, 91–92
Fisher syndrome, 151–152
five special senses, 3–4
fixation system, 362
fixed pupil, 445
flaccid paralysis, 356
flattened base of skull, 257
flocullar nodular lobe, 400–401
fluent aphasias, 466–471, 467f
fluid phase endocytosis, 69
focal convulsions, 330
focal discharge, 330
focal epilepsy, 330
focal seizure discharge, 342–343, 342f–343f
focal seizures, 330
follicle-stimulating hormone (FSH), 315
food intake, autonomic nervous system, 318
foot control, motor-sensory cortex, 12–13
foramen magnum syndromes, 256–257, 256f
foramen of Monro, neuroembryology of the brain, 75
force-velocity relation, neuromuscular junction, 95–96, 96f
fornix, 83, 83f, 304–305, 425f–426f, 431
four-deep cerebellar nuclei, 8
four general senses, 3–4
fourth ventricle, 20, 75
fovea centralis, 449
fracture dislocations of the spinal cord, 164, 164f
Friedrich's ataxia, 184–186, 185f
frontal association areas, limbic regions, 436–437
frontal epilepsy, limbic regions, 437t
frontal lobe
   description, 332
   illustration, 615f–616f
   limbic regions, 436–437
   major gyri, 9, 334f
frontal retardation, limbic regions, 437
FSH (facioscapulohumeral) dystrophy, 101
FSH (follicle-stimulating hormone), 315
FTD (frontal/temporary dementia), 589
functions and correlations, 397–399
fusiform layer, cerebral cortex, 328

G

GABAergic pathways, to the neocortex, 338
gait disorders of the elderly, 365–366
gamma system, 120–122, 120f–122f
ganglia, 3
ganglion cells, 448, 448f
ganglionic layer, cerebral cortex, 328
gastrointestinal tract, autonomic nervous system disorders, 324
gene mechanisms, of disease in the cerebellum, 408–409
generalized chorea, 384
generalized myasthenia, disorders of the neuromuscular junction, 105
generalized tonic clonic seizures (GTCS), 552t, 557, 557f

genetically linked migration disorders, neuroembryology of the brain, 85–88
giant cells, 62
glands, autonomic dual innervation, 323, 323t
glands associated with, 20
glial response to injury, 68
glioblastoma, parietal lobe, 416f–417f
gliotransmitters, 60, 60t
globosus, 8
glossopharyngeal cranial nerve
   autonomic nervous system, 321
   general function, 236–240, 240f
   general function of, 236–240, 240f
   neuroembryology, 80
   sensory pathways, 302–303
glossopharyngeal neuralgia, 240
glycogen storage diseases, 103–104
Golgi tendon organs, 122
Golgi type II (satellite) cells, 45–46f, 59, 63, 63f
Golgi type I (pyramidal) cells, 45–46f, 47f, 48f, 49f, 50f, 326, 326f
gonadotropin, 315
granulomas, 522
grasp reflex, 351, 352f
gray matter
   brain, 6–7
   brain stem, 202t
   nervous system, 3
   neuroembryology of the brain, 76
growth cone guidance, neuroembryology of the brain, 74
growth hormone (STH), 315–316
GTCS (generalized tonic clonic seizures), 552t, 557, 557f
Guillain Barré syndrome, 148–151

H

hair, autonomic dual innervation, 323
hallucinations, temporal lobe disease, 434f
headaches, 510
head trauma
   concussion, 505
   contra coup injuries, 505
   contusions, 505, 506f
   coup injuries, 505
   extradural hematomas, 506–508, 507f
   lacerations, 505, 506f
   late effects of, 508–509
   management of, 508
   post-concussion syndrome, 508–509
   posttraumatic epilepsy, 508
   prevention, 509, 509t
   skull fractures, 505–506
   subdural hematomas, 506–508, 507f
hearing, temporal lobe disease, 435
heart, 323
heat loss, autonomic nervous system, 318
heat production and conservation, autonomic nervous system, 318
heavy metal exposure, 526t
hemangioblastoma, of the cerebellum, 404f, 406f
hemiballism, 382–383, 382f–383f
hemichorea, 382–383, 382f–383f
hemidystonia, 390
hemofacial spasm, 235
hemorrhage, brain stem, 271–274
hepatolenticular degeneration (Wilson's disease), 388–389
herpes, cerebral hemisphere infections, 582
herpes simplex encephalitis, memory disorders, 581, 582f
herpes simplex (HSV), 528
herpes zoster, cranial nerves, 235

heterogenetic cerebral cortex, 328, 328f
heterotopias, neuroembryology of the brain, 85, 86–87
hippocampal formation, 427–430
hippocampus, 428–430, 428f, 429t, 579–581
histaminergic neurons, 566
histiocytes, 61
histogenesis, neuroembryology of the brain, 73
HIV-1, 528–529
HMSN (hereditary motor and sensory neuropathy). See CMT (Charcot Marie Tooth) disease.
holoprosencephaly, neuroembryology of the brain, 87–88f
homogenetic cerebral cortex, 328, 328f
horizontal cells, 448, 448f
hormones
 ACTH (adrenocorticotrophic hormone), 315
 ADH (antidiuretic hormone), 318–319
 FSH (follicle-stimulating hormone), 315
 lactogenic hormone, 315
 luteinizing, 315
 produced by the hypothalamus, 314–315
 produced in adenohypophysis, 315, 315f, 315t
 prolactin, 315
 somatotropin, 315–316
 STH (growth hormone), 315–316
 TSH (thyrotrophic hormone), 316
Horner's syndrome, case history, 141–142
HSV (herpes simplex), 528
human body, diagrams of, 23f–25f
human embryo, illustration, 73f
Huntington's chorea, 589
Huntington's disease, 373t, 384–387, 385f
hydrocephalus, 20, 90, 90f
hydrophobia. See rabies.
hypercomplex cells, occipital lobe, 454, 454f
hypertensive cerebeller hemorrhage, brain stem, 257
hypnogenic hallucinations, 568
hypoglossal cranial nerve, 79, 244f
hypoglycemia, memory disorders, 581–582
hypophyseal stalk, illustration, 615f, 617f
hypophysiotropic area, neuroendocrine system, 314, 315t
hypophysis cerebri, neuroendocrine system, 312f–313f, 314
hypothalamic-hypophyseal portal system, 313–314, 314f
hypothalamic-hypophyseal tracts, 313, 313f
hypothalamic nuclei
 anterior region, 311, 312f
 functional localization, 312t
 middle region, 311, 312f
 posterior region, 311–312, 312f
 regions, 311–312, 311f–312f
hypothalamus
 afferent pathways, 312–313, 313f
 definition, 8, 8t
 description, 304, 306, 311
 dorsal longitudinal fasciculus, 313
 efferent pathways, 313, 313f
 functional stability, 313–314
 hormones produced by, 314–315
 hypothalamic-hypophyseal portal system, 313
 hypothalamic-hypophyseal tracts, 313, 313f
 illustration, 616f
 light levels, 319
 limbic regions, 424, 424f, 425t, 426f, 440
 mammillotegmental tract, 313
 mammillothalamic tract, 313
 medial forebrain bundle, 313
 melatonin, 319
 neurosecretory system, 313
 oxytocin, 314
 periventricular system, 313
 pineal body, 319
 role in spinal lesions, 349–350
 serotonin, 319
 vasopressin, 314
hypothalamus, and the autonomic nervous system
 ADH (antidiuretic hormone), 318–319
 body temperature, 318
 emotions, 319
 epinephrine, 319
 food intake, 318
 functional localization, 317–318
 heat loss, 318
 heat production and conservation, 318
 neurosecretion, 318–319
 norepinephrine, 319
 overview, 317
 sleep cycle, 318
 water balance, 318–319

I
ictal event, 549
immediate memory, 575–576
imprinting, definition, 575
infantile spasms, epilepsy, 554, 554f
infarction, 483–484, 484f
infections, of the brain stem, 277
infections of the cerebral hemispheres
 acute anterior poliomyelitis, 527
 encephalitis, 523f, 525
 encephalitis lethargica, 527
 encephalopathies, 527
 focal infections of the nervous system, 519–520
 general or diffuse, 522, 523f
 granulomas, 522
 HIV - 1, 528–529
 HSV (herpes simplex), 528
 involving the brain, 520–522
 measles, 528
 meningitis, 522–525, 523f, 524t
 mumps, 528
 nonneurotropic, 528–529
 overview, 518–519
 paramyxovirus, 528
 purulent brain abscess, 520–521, 521f–522f
 rabies, 527–528
 retrovirus, 528–529
 subdural empyema, 520
 viral, 523f, 525–529
 Von Economo's encephalitis, 527
inferior cerebellar veins, 16
inferior cerebral veins, 15
inferior colliculus, 208–209, 209f
inferior frontal occipital fasciculus, 337
inferior hypophyseal arteries, neuroendocrine system, 314
inferior longitudinal fasciculus, 337
inferior parietal area, 418
inferior parietal lobule, 461, 462f
inferior pontine syndromes, 263–266, 262f
inferior sagittal sinus, 17
inflammation, muscle disorders, 104
inhibitory neurotransmitters, 57
inhibitory postsynaptic potential, 116–118, 118f
inhibitory synapses, 58
inner tunic (retina), 445
input nuclei, basal ganglia, 371
insomnia, 567, 593
instinctive grasp, 351, 352f
instinctive tactile avoiding, 352f, 353
instinctive tactile grasp, 352f, 353, 356
insula, cerebral cortex, 9
intentional tremors, 410–411
interictal period, 549
internal capsule, cerebral hemispheres, 11
internal carotid artery, syndromes of, 484–488, 485f–486f
internal cerebral veins, 16
internal granular layer, cerebral cortex, 328
internal layer, cerebral cortex, 328
interneurons, 122–123
interpeduncular nucleus, 423–424
interpretive illusions, temporal lobe disease, 433f
intracerebral hemorrhage, 496–499, 497f, 498t, 499f
intracranial hemorrhage, 496–503
intradural-extramedullary tumors of the spinal cord, 167–169, 167f–168f
intrapontine hemorrhage, 271
intrathecal medications, nerve root disease, 160
intrinsic brain tumors, 511–515
intrinsic diseases, brain stem, 257–262
intrinsic disorders of the spinal cord, 169–176
intrinsic nuclei, basal ganglia, 371
intrinsic vs. extrinsic diseases of the brain stem, 252, 253f
ischemic disease, managing, 496
ischemic-occlusive disease, 482–484, 482t, 483f, 488f
isometric tension, neuromuscular junction, 92f

J
JA (juvenile absence), 555
jaw muscles, voluntary motor pathways, 367
JME (juvenile myoclonic epilepsy), 555, 555f
jugular foramen syndrome, 247–249, 256

K
Kennedy's disease, 178
kindling
 epilepsy, 553
 memory, 577
kinetic tremors, 410–411
Klüver-Bucy syndrome, temporal lobe disease, 435
Kuru. See prion disease.

L
labile memory, 576
lacerations of the head, 505, 506f
lacrimal glands, autonomic dual innervation, 322
lactogenic hormone, 315
lacunar syndromes, 489f, 490, 490t, 491f
lacune, 489
lamina, 3
laminar organization, spinal cord, 123–124, 123f
lamination pattern, tracts, 126, 126f–127f
language. See speech and language.
large and giant pyramidal cell layer, cerebral cortex, 328
lateral cerebellar syndrome, of the cerebellum, 404f
lateral cerebeller hemisphere syndrome, 255, 255f
lateral dorsal nucleus, 291
lateral geniculate nucleus (LGN), 452
lateralized hemichorea, 382
lateral medullary syndrome, 259–261
lateral nuclear mass, 289
lateral prefrontal granular frontal, 436–437
lateral premotor area, 359
lateral surface of the brain, cerebral hemispheres, 12f
lateral tegmental superior pontine syndrome, 266–267, 266f–267f
lateral tegmentum, 263–266
lateral unpaired sinuses, 17
lateral ventricles, 20, 75
learning
 definition, 575
 factors influencing, 576–577
 neurobiological mechanisms, 577
learning, and memory
 immediate, 575–576
 labile, 576
 long term, 576
 remote, 576
 short-term working, 575–576
length-tension relation, neuromuscular junction, 95, 96f
Lennox Gastaut syndrome, 554
lens, eye, 445
lenticular nuclei, basal ganglia, 371
lenticulostriate penetrating branches, 489–490, 489f–490f
lesions
 case histories, problem solving, 538–545
 in occipital lobe, area 17, 455–456
 in occipital lobe, areas 18, 19, 456–459, 457f–459f
 in the optic pathway, 449–452, 450f–452f
 pathology of, Parkinson's disease, 375f, 376–377
lesions, spinal
 brain stem transection, 348–349
 decerebrate rigidity, 348–349, 349f–350f
 decorticate preparation, 350–353, 351f–352f
 decorticate rigidity, 350, 351f
 hypothalamus, role of, 349–350
 midbrain preparation, 349–350, 350f–351f
 noxious stimulus, 349, 350f
 spinal cord transection, 348, 348t, 349f
 tonic labyrinthine reflexes, 349, 350f
 tonic neck reflexes, 349, 349f
Lewy bodies, Parkinson's disease, 377f
LGN (lateral geniculate nucleus), 452
light levels, hypothalamus, 319
light reflex, eyes, 445
light sensitivity, eyes, 446
limb girdle dystrophies, 101
limbic encephalitis, memory disorders, 581–582
limbic nuclei, 426
limbic region, cerebral cortex, 10
limbic regions in the brain
 epithalamus, 425
 frontal association areas, 436–437
 frontal epilepsy, 437t
 frontal lobe, 436–437
 frontal retardation, 437
 hypothalamus, 424, 424f, 425t, 426f, 440
 interpeduncular nucleus, 423–424
 lateral prefrontal granular frontal, 436–437
 nucleus acumbens, 425
 orbital frontal pathology, 437
 orbitofrontal cortex, 436
 parasagittal lesions, 438–439, 439f
 pleasure/punishment areas, 440
 prefrontal cortex and emotions, 436–437
 prefrontal cortex damage, 437–438
 prefrontal lobotomy, 438–439, 438f
 pseudo depression, 437
 pseudopsychopathic syndrome, 437

INDEX • 625

limbic regions in the brain (Cont.)
  reticular formation, 423, 439–440, 440t
  role in psychiatric disorders, 440, 440t
  septum, 425, 425f
  stimulation complex partial seizures, 437, 437t
  subcortical limbic regions, 423–425, 424t
  thalamus, 424–425, 424f
limbic regions in the brain, temporal lobe
  cortical structures in emotions
    allocortex, 427
    amygdaloid nuclei, 425–427, 426f–427f
    auditory association, 427
    cingulate cortex, 425f
    cingulum, 431
    cortical nucleus, 428
    cortical regions, 425f
    corticobulbar pathway, 431
    corticospinal pathway, 431
    dentate gyrus, 429, 429f
    entorhinal region, 428, 428f
    entorhinal reverberating circuit, 430, 430f
    fornix, 425f–426f, 431
    hippocampal formation, 427–430
    hippocampus, 428–430, 428f, 429t
    limbic nuclei, 426
    mesocortex, 428
    neocortex, 427, 428
    neocortex of the temporal lobe, 427
    olfactory nuclei, 426
    papez circuit, 431
    parahippocampal gyrus, 424f–425f, 425
    principal pathways, 425f–426f, 430–431, 430f
    stria terminalis, 431
    ventral amygdalofugal pathway, 426, 431
    visual perception, 427
  disease symptoms
    aggressive behavior, 436
    aphasia, 435
    effects of focal discharge, 433f
    effects on hearing, 435
    following stimulation, 432–435, 432t
    hallucinations, 434f
    interpretive illusions, 433f
    Klüver-Bucy syndrome, 435
    memory, 435–436
    overview, 431–432
    psychiatric disturbances, 436
    seizures, 432–435, 432t, 433f–435f
    from temporal lobe ablation/damage, 435–436
    visual defects, 435
limbic system
  emotional brain, 422
  olfactory system, 422–423, 423f
  rhinencephalon, 422, 423f
limbic thalamic nuclei, 291, 294
limbs, voluntary motor pathways, 366–367, 366f
lissencephaly (Agyri-Pachygyri), neuroembryology of the brain, 86–87
localization of function, cerebral cortex, 9–11
location of pathology, confirming, 331
locked-in syndrome, 262f, 550
longitudinal division, cerebellum, 395, 395f, 395t
long loop reflexes, postnatal development, 353
long motor pathways, interrupting, 216–217
long sensory systems, interrupting, 218

long-term memory, 576
long-term potentiation, 577
Lou Gehrig's disease. See ALS (amyotropic lateral sclerosis).
lower motor neuron, motor-sensory cortex, 12
lower motor neuron paralysis, motor-sensory cortex, 13
lower motor neurons, 129–131, 130t
lower plexus, 141
lower pons, facial nerve and facial colliculus, 204f, 204t, 205–206, 206f
low-grade glioma, 360
Lucy, the mitochondrial Eve, 50
lumbar disk, lateral protrusion, 158f
lumbar plexus, 146f
lumbar puncture, 112, 112f, 160
lumbar sacral plexus, lower extremity, 144, 146f–148f
lumbar spine, 134, 134f, 137f
lumbar sympathetic ganglia, 321–322
lungs, autonomic dual innervation, 323
luteinizing hormone, 315
lymphocytes, 61
lymphomas, primary central nervous system, 515

M
Machado-Joseph disease (Azorean disease), 408–409
macroglia, 59
macrogyria, neuroembryology of the brain, 87
mad cow disease. See prion disease.
magnetic resonance angiography (MRA), 41, 42f
magnetic resonance imaging (MRI) scan, 31, 32f, 34f, 36f
magnocellular portion of the dorsomedial nucleus, 291
mammillotegmental tract, 313
mammillothalamic tract, 313
mandible movements, 230t
mastication muscles, 230t
measles, 528
mechanicoreceptor, 58t–59
Meckel's cave, 19
medial forebrain bundle, 313
medial lemniscus, in the brain stem, 218
medial nuclear complex, 291
medial zone, 206–207
median nerve, 142f, 142f–143f
medulla, 6, 9, 76f, 200–204
medulloblastoma, 254f, 401f
Meige's disease, 389
melatonin, 319
membrane basis of integration, 116–118
memory
  corpus callosum, 577
  cortical motor and sensory maps, 577
  definition, 575
  delayed response test, 575
  early experience, 577
  factors influencing, 576–577
  kindling, 577
  long-term potentiation, 577
  mirror focus, 577
  neurobiological mechanisms, 577
  plasticity in the nervous system, 577
  postnatal brain development, 577
memory, stages
  immediate, 575–576
  labile, 576
  long term, 576
  remote, 576
  short-term working, 575–576
memory disorders

amnesiac-confabulatory syndrome, 516f, 577–579, 578t
anoxia, 581–582
bilateral lesions of the hippocampus, 579–581
bilateral mesial temporal lobe lesions, 579–581
definition, 575
herpes simplex encephalitis, 581, 582f
hypoglycemia, 581–582
limbic encephalitis, 581–582
status epilepticus, 581–582
temporal lobe disease, 435–436
temporal lobe stimulation, 581, 581t
transient global amnesia, 580–581
traumatic amnesia, 582
Wernicke-Korsakoff encephalopathy, 516f, 577–579, 578t
Meniere's disease, 239
meningeal carcinomatosis, 521f
meninges, 17f–18f
meningiomas
  description, 167–168, 167f
  extrinsic brain tumors, 257, 515–516, 516f, 517t
  illustration, 13f
meningitis, 522–525, 523f, 524t
meningomyelocele, neuroembryology of the brain, 88–89f
Mental Status and Language Functions, 29
mesencephalon, neuroembryology of the brain, 78–79
mesial temporal lobe, bilateral lesions and memory disorders, 579–581
mesocortex, 428
mesodermal tissue, neuroembryology of the brain, 89
metabolic myopathies, 103–104
metastatic brain tumors, 516–518, 518f, 520f–521f
metathalamus, 288, 297f–298f
metencephalon (pons and cerebellum), neuroembryology of the brain, 77–78
microencephaly, neuroembryology of the brain, 87
microenvironment, nervous system, 59
microglia, 59
microglial cells, 61–62, 61f
micropolygyria, neuroembryology of the brain, 87, 87f
microtubules, 51–52
midbrain
  extrinsic syndromes, 255–256
  functional anatomy of, 208, 209f
  neuroembryology of the brain, 77f
  preparation, 349–350, 350f–351f
  syndromes, 267–271, 268f
middle cerebral artery, 486f, 488–492, 489f–490f, 492
middle-lower pontine basilar infarct, 262f
middle parietal lobe, cerebral hemispheres, 9
middle tunic, eyes, 444f
midline cerebellum syndrome (fourth ventricle), 253–255, 254f
midline tumors, of the cerebellum, 400–401, 401f
migraine headaches, 510
migration disorders, 85–88
Miller-Dieker syndrome, neuroembryology of the brain, 85
mirror focus
  epilepsy, 553
  memory, 577
mitochondria, 50–51
mitochondrial Eve, 50
mitochondrial myopathies, 103–104

MMPI (Minnesota Multiphasic Personality Index), 41
MMSE (Mini-Mental State Examination), 29–30
modulators of neurotransmitters, 57
molecular architecture, neuromuscular junction, 93–96
molecular layer, cerebral cortex, 328
Mongolism. See Down's syndrome.
monocular blindness, 485
monocytes, 61
mononeuropathies, peripheral nerve disease
  brachial neuritis, 140
  brachial plexopathy, case history, 141–142
  carpal tunnel syndrome, case history, 142–144
  diabetic mononeuropathy, case history, 145, 150f
  Horner's syndrome, case history, 141–142
  of the long thoracic nerve, case history, 142
  lower extremity lumbar sacral plexus, 144, 146f–148f
  lower plexus, 141
  median nerve, anatomy of, 142f–143f
  peroneal nerve, 145, 149f
  sciatic nerve, 144, 146f
  tibial nerve, 145–146
  ulnar nerve dissection, 143f–144f
  upper extremity brachial plexus, 138, 141f
  upper plexus, 140, 141f
mononeuropathy multiplex, 138
mononuclear cells, 61–63, 61f
mossy fibers, 396, 396f
motor areas, cerebral cortex, 332, 332f–334f, 334, 350f, 355f, 362f–363f, 462f–463f
motor/autonomic ganglia, 3
motor center. See also movement disorders.
  avoiding responses, 352f
  central pattern generators, 347–348
  disorders of motor development, 365
  gait disorders of the elderly, 365–366
  grasp reflex, 351, 352f
  instinctive grasp, 351, 352f
  instinctive tactile avoiding, 352f, 353
  instinctive tactile grasp, 352f, 353
  negative motor response, 363–364
  optical righting reflex, 350, 351f
  parieto-occipital eye fields, 333, 333f, 352f, 360–363, 362f–363f
  placing reactions, 350–351
  prefrontal cortex, 364, 364f
  primary motor cortex discharge, 353
  pyramidal tract lesions, 357–358
  reflex activity, 347–348, 347t
  rigidity, 365
  spastic rigidity, 365
  suppressor areas, 363–364
  tactile placing reactions, 351
  visual placing reactions, 350–351
  voluntary motor pathways, corticomesencephalic system, 299t
motor center, corticorubral spinal system
  central lateral premotor area, 359
  dorsal lateral premotor area, 359
  lateral premotor area, 359
  low-grade glioma, 360
  overview, 358
  premotor cortex, 358–360, 359f
  SMA (supplemental motor area), 359
motor center, eye movements
  central control of saccades, 361–362
  fixation system, 362
  oligodendroglioma, 360, 360f–361f
  saccadic, 360–361
  smooth pursuit, 362

vergence movements, 362
vestibulo-ocular movements, 362
motor center, postnatal development
  deep tendon reflexes, 356
  developmental changes in motor responses, 355t
  distal hand movement, 356
  flaccid paralysis, 356
  instinctive tactile grasp, 356
  long loop reflexes, 353
  overview, 353–354, 353f
  prefrontal areas, 353
  premotor cortex, 353
  primary motor cortex, 354–357, 355f, 355t
  primary motor cortex discharge, 353
  projected movement, 356
  selective grasp, 356
  stretch reflexes, 356
  traction response, 356
motor center, primary motor cortex
  focal disease, 357
  postnatal development, 354–357, 355f, 355t
motor center, spinal lesions
  brain stem transection, 348–349
  decerebrate rigidity, 348–349, 349f–350f
  decorticate preparation, 350–353, 351f–352f
  decorticate rigidity, 350, 351f
  hypothalamus, role of, 349–350
  midbrain preparation, 349–350, 350f–351f
  noxious stimulus, 349, 350f
  spinal cord transection, 348, 348t, 349f
  tonic labyrinthine reflexes, 349, 350f
  tonic neck reflexes, 349, 349f
motor center, voluntary motor pathways
  abdomen, 366–367, 366f
  basic principles of motor system, 366
  corticomesencephalic system, 367
  corticonuclear system, 367, 367f
  corticospinal tract, 366–367, 366f
  eye muscles, 367
  facial muscles, 367
  jaw muscles, 367
  limbs, 366–367, 366f
  thorax, 366–367, 366f
  tongue muscles, 367
motor cranial nerve nuclei, 206, 206f
motor nerve, effects on skeletal muscle, 99–100
motor relay thalamic nuclei, 289–291, 294
motor responses, postnatal development, 355f
motor-sensory cortex
  control of the foot, 12–13
  corticospinal pathway, 12
  lower motor neuron, 12
  lower motor neuron paralysis, 13
  overview, 12, 12f
  second-order nerve cells, 12
  third-order neurons, 12
  upper motor neuron, 12, 13t
  upper motor neuron paralysis, 13
motor units, neuromuscular junction, 91
movement; initiation, planning, and timing in the cerebellum, 399. See also motor center.
movement disorders. See also basal ganglia; motor center.
  acute akathesia, 390
  acute drug-induced Parkinsonian syndrome, 390
  acute dystonic reactions, 390
  clinical signs and symptoms, 375–376
  from dopamine-blocking agents, 390–391

double athetosis, 387–388
dystonia, 389–390
familial paroxysmal dyskinesia, 391
generalized chorea, 384
hemiballism, 382–383, 382f–383f
hemichorea, 382–383, 382f–383f
hemidystonia, 390
hepatolenticular degeneration, 388–389
hepatolenticular degeneration (Wilson's disease), 388–389
Huntington's disease, 373t, 384–387, 385f
lateralized hemichorea, 382
Meige's disease, 389
restless leg syndrome, 391
Segawa disease, 390
tardive dyskinesias, 390
tics, 390
movement disorders, clinical signs and symptoms
  akinesia, 375
  bradykinesia, 375
  dyskinesia, 375
  dystonia, 375
  rigidity, 375
  tremor, 375
movement disorders, Parkinson's disease
  a-synuclein, 377f
  case history, 379–380, 380f
  clinical signs, 376, 376t, 377f
  differential diagnosis, 380–382
  etiology, 377–379
  Lewy bodies, 377f
  management, 379
  Parkinsonism plus syndromes, 381–382, 381f
  pathology of lesions, 375f, 376–377
MRA (magnetic resonance angiography), 41, 42f
MRI (magnetic resonance imaging) scan, 31, 32f, 34f, 36f
multiple sclerosis, 186–190, 187f–188f, 274–277, 275f–276f, 529–530, 529f–530f
mumps, 528
muscle proteins, neuromuscular junction, 93–94
muscles
  contraction. See neuromuscular junction, contraction.
  skeletal. See skeletal muscles.
  types of, 4–5
muscles, diseases of. See also neuromuscular junction, disorders of.
  acquired disorders, 104–105
  Becker's muscular dystrophy, 100–101
  centronuclear myopathy, 103
  channelopathies affecting skeletal muscle, 102, 102t
  congenital myopathies, 103
  diagnosing, 22–23
  diagnostic tests, 30–31
  Duchenne's muscular dystrophy, 100, 100f
  endocrine disorders, 104
  FSH (facioscapulohumeral) dystrophy, 101
  glycogen storage diseases, 103–104
  inflammation, 104
  limb girdle dystrophies, 101
  metabolic myopathies, 103–104
  mitochondrial myopathies, 103–104
  muscular dystrophies, 100–104
  muscular dystrophies and the cranial nerves, 101
  myotonic congenita, 102t
  myotonic dystrophy, 101–102
  nemaline myopathy, 103
  overlap polymyositis, 104, 104f

periodic paralysis (familial periodic paralysis), 102–103
problem solving case histories, 193–198
toxic disorders, 104
trauma, 104
muscle spindle, 119–120, 120f
muscle tension headaches, 510
muscular dystrophies, 100–104
muscular dystrophies and the cranial nerves, 101
myasthenia gravis, disorders of the neuromuscular junction, 105–107
myelencephalon (medulla), neuroembryology of the brain, 77–78
myelin, 3
myelin, disorders of, 529–530. See also multiple sclerosis.
myelination, 54–56, 54f, 84t
myoclonus, 555, 556–558
myosin, neuromuscular junction, 93–94
myotonia, 92
myotonic congenita, 102t
myotonic dystrophy, 101–102

N
narcolepsy, 566t, 567–568, 568f, 5689f
nausea, cranial nerve disorder, 238
necrosis, 68, 74, 484, 484f
negative motor response, 363–364
nemaline myopathy, 103
neocortex
  afferent inputs, 337–338
  cholinergic pathways, 338
  claustrum pathways, 338
  dopaminenergic pathways, 338
  efferent projections, 338
  GABAergic pathways, 338
  lateral temporal areas, 427, 428
  limbic system, 427, 428
  nonthalamic afferent inputs, 338
  noradrenergic pathway, 338
  norepinephrine pathway, 338
  seritonenergic pathway, 338
  temporal lobe, 427
  thalamic afferent inputs, 337–338
  types of, 328–329, 329f–330f
neocortical cytoarchitecture and function, 330f, 332, 332f–333f, 334t
neocortical death, definition, 550
neoplasms, 509–510
nerve conduction velocity test, 30t, 31
nerve growth factors (NGF), 68
nerve root
  diagnosing diseases of, 23, 26
  diagnostic tests, 31–34
  problem solving case histories, 193–198
nerve root, peripheral nerve disease
  back pain, 158–160
  cervical disk, lateral protrusion, 157f
  cervical invertebral disks, 155f
  dermatome chart, remaining sensibility, 157f
  dorsal root ganglion, 159–160
  intrathecal medications, 160
  lumbar disk, lateral protrusion, 158f
  lumbar puncture, complications from, 160
  neurofibromas, 159f
  postherpetic neuralgia, 159–160
  radiculopathy, 155–160
  schwannoma, 159–160, 159f
  tabes dorsalis, 159
nerves. See also specific nerves.
  diagnostic tests, 30–31

of right lower leg, 147f, 148f, 149z
of right upper arm, 145f
nervous system, neuroembryology of the brain, 89
nervous system, overview. See also central nervous system.
  afferent nerves, 5
  cardiac muscles, 4–5
  five special senses, 3–4. See also specific senses.
  four general senses, 3–4
  ganglia, 3
  gray matter, 3
  lamina, 3
  motor/autonomic ganglia, 3
  muscles, 4–5
  myelin, 3
  neurons, 3, 4f, 4t
  nuclei, 3
  receptors for general sensation, 4, 5f
  sensory ganglia, 3
  sensory receptors, 4t
  skeletal muscles, 4–5
  smooth muscles, 4–5
  somatic division, 5
  synapse, 3
  visceral (autonomic) division, 5
  white matter, 3
nervous system, response to injury. See also regeneration.
  chromatolysis, 64–66
  degeneration, 64–66
  Wallerian degeneration, 65, 65f–66f
neural crest cells, 64
neuroblasts, neuroembryology of the brain, 73
neurocytology. See also neurons.
  blood-brain barrier, 68–70
  nervous system response to injury, 64–66
  regeneration, 66–68
  supporting cells, 58–64
neuroembryology of the brain
  apoptosis, 74
  blood vessel development, 75
  brain differentiation
    arches, 80
    cerebral cortex, 82–83
    cerebral hemispheres, 79
    commissures, 82–83, 83f
    cortical architecture, changes over time, 84
    diencephalon, 79, 79f
    fornix, 83, 83f
    illustration, 78f
    mesencephalon, 78–79
    metencephalon (pons and cerebellum), 77–78
    myelencephalon (medulla), 77–78
    myelination, 84t
    neuronal maturation, 84t
    neuronal migration, 83–84
    pituitary gland, 79
    primary sulci, 81–82
    prosencephalon (forebrain), 79
    rhombencephalon (hind brain), 77–78
    telencephalon, 79f
  cerebral aqueduct, 75
  cranial nerves
    illustration, 81f
    innervation, muscles of somite origin, 79
    innervation, pharyngeal arches, 79
    origins of, 80f
    types of, 79, 80, 81
  differentiation within the central nervous system, 74
  foramen of Monro, 75

INDEX • 627

neuroembryology of the brain (Cont.)
    fourth ventricle, 75
    gray matter, 76
    growth cone guidance, 74
    histogenesis, 73
    human embryo, illustration, 73f
    illustration, 82f
    lateral ventricles, 75
    layers in the neural tube, 74t
    medulla, 76f
    midbrain, 77f
    necrosis, 74
    neuroblasts, 73
    neuronal death, 74–75
    PCD (programmed cell death), 74
    peripheral nervous system, 75
    pons, 77f
    repair of damaged nervous system, 74
    spinal canal, 75
    spinal cord differentiation, 75–77, 76f
    structure innervated by cranial nerves, 76t
    third ventricle, 75
    by trimester, 72t
    upper spinal nerves, illustration, 81f
    ventricular system, 75
neuroembryology of the brain, abnormal development
    adenoma sebaceous, 89
    agenesis of the corpus callosum, 87–88, 87f
    anencephaly, 86
    Arnold-Chiari malformation, 89
    bilateral nodular preventricular heterotopia, 85
    cerebellar agenesis, 88
    chromosomal trisomy and translocation, 88
    congenital neurologic malformations, 85t
    cortical microdysgenesias, 85–86
    cranial bifida, 88–89
    cutaneous angiomatosis, 89
    defective fusion of dorsal structures, 88–89
    double cortex, 86
    Down's syndrome, 88
    ectodermal tissue, 89
    FAS (fetal alcohol syndrome), 88
    genetically linked migration disorders, 85–88
    in growth, 85
    heterotopias, 85, 86–87
    holoprosencephaly, 87–88f
    hydrocephalus, 90, 90f
    incomplete brain development, 85
    lissencephaly (Agyri-Pachygyri), 86–87
    macrogyria, 87
    meningomyelocele, 88–89f
    mesodermal tissue, 89
    microencephaly, 87
    micropolygyria, 87, 87f
    Miller-Dieker syndrome, 85
    nervous system, 89
    neurofibromatosis (von Recklinghausen's disease), 89
    porencephaly, 87
    Robertsonian translocation, 88
    schizencephaly, 87, 87f
    skin, 89
    Sturge-Weber syndrome, 89
    subcortical band heterotopia, 86
    syringobulbia, 89–90
    syringomyelia, 89
    tuberous sclerosis, 89
    type I X-linked dominant lissencephaly, 85
    in the ventricular system, 89–90
neuroendocrine system

ACTH (adrenocorticotrophic hormone), 315
capillary loops, 314
case histories, 316–317
FSH (follicle-stimulating hormone), 315
gonadotropin, 315
hormones produced in adenohypophysis, 315, 315f, 315t
hypophysiotropic area, 314, 315t
hypophysis cerebri, 312f–313f, 314
hypothalamic-hypophyseal portal system, 314, 314f
inferior hypophyseal arteries, 314
information flow with the brain, 314f
lactogenic hormone, 315
luteinizing hormone, 315
prolactin, 315
somatotropin, 315–316, 451f
STH (growth hormone), 315–316, 451f
TSH (thyrotrophic hormone), 316
neuroepithelial brain tumors, 511–515
neurofibrillar tangles, 53
neurofibromas, 159f
neurofibromatosis, 89, 511
neuromuscular junction
    acetylcholine, 97–98, 98f, 99
    acetylcholine-activated channels, 98, 98f
    denervation sensitivity, 99
    diagnosing diseases of, 23
    drugs acting on, 98–99
    endplate, 96–98, 97f–98f
    fast muscles, 99–100
    fiber bundles, 91–92, 91f
    filaments, 91–92
    isometric tension, 92f
    motor nerve, effects on skeletal muscle, 99–100
    motor units, 91
    muscle speed, 99–100, 99f
    myotonia, 92
    red muscles, 99–100
    reinnervation, 99
    reticular structures, 92, 94f
    sarcomeres, 91–92
    skeletal muscle organization, 93f
    slow muscles, 99–100
    SR (sarcoplasmic reticulum), 92, 94f
    terminal cisternae, 92
    transverse tubules, 92
    T-SR coupling, 92–93, 94f
    T system, 92, 94f
    white muscles, 99–100
neuromuscular junction, contraction
    actin, 93–94
    Ca^{++} troponin interaction, 94, 96f–97f
    cross-bridges, 95–96, 96f
    excitation contraction coupling, 92
    filament interaction, 96f–97f
    force-velocity relation, 95–96, 96f
    length-tension relation, 95, 96f
    molecular architecture, 93–96
    muscle proteins, 93–94
    myosin, 93–94
    overview, 91–92
    SR (sarcoplasmic reticulum), 94f
    tropomyosin, 93–94
    troponin, 93–94
neuromuscular junction, disorders of. See also muscles, diseases of.
    antibiotics, 108
    botulism, 108
    Eaton-Lambert syndrome, 108
    generalized myasthenia, 105
    myasthenia gravis, 105–107
    ocular myasthenia, 105
    postsynaptic disorders, 105–108
    presynaptic disorders, 108

pseudoparalysis, 106
spider venom, 108
neuro myelitis optica (NMO), 172–173
neuronal cytoskeleton, 51, 52f
neuronal death, 74–75. See also nervous system, response to injury.
neuronal maturation, neuroembryology of the brain, 84f
neuronal migration, neuroembryology of the brain, 83–84
neuron doctrine, 45
neurons
    astrocytes, 48f
    axon hillock, 53, 53f
    axoplasmic flow, 51–52
    central nervous system pathways, 56
    central nervous system structure, 52–53
    cytoplasm organelles, 48
    definition, 3
    dendrites, 45
    dendritic spines, 46, 46f, 48
    effectors, 58
    endoneurium, 52
    epineurium, 52
    Golgi type II (satellite) cells, 45–46f
    Golgi type I (pyramidal) cells, 45–46f, 47f, 48f, 49f, 50f
    illustration, 4f, 48f–49f
    microtubules, 51–52
    mitochondria, 50–51
    myelination, 54–56, 54f
    neurofibrillar tangles, 53
    neuronal cytoskeleton, 51, 52f
    neurosecretory granules, 51, 51f
    nodes of Ranvier, 53–54
    nucleus, 48–49
    oligodendrocytes, 48f, 53, 53f, 54–56
    parts of, 45. See also specific parts.
    rates of axonal transport of cellular structures, 48t
    receptors, 58
    regeneration, 67–68
    rough endoplasmic recticulum-nissl body, 459f
    Schwann Cell Cytoplasm, 52
    Schwann cells, 53, 54–56
    soma, 45, 51
    trophic center, 51
    types of, 4t
    ventral horn cell, 459f
neurons, neurotransmitters
    amino acids, 57
    biogenic amines, 57
    description, 57
    excitatory, 57
    inhibitory, 57
    location and function, 57t
    modulators, 57
neurons, peripheral nerves
    classification of axons by function, 55t
    peripheral nerve bundles, 55t
    structures, 52, 55t
neurons, synapses
    chemical, 56
    dendritic spines, 58
    electrical, 56
    excitatory, 58
    excitatory neurotransmitters, 57
    illustration, 56f
    inhibitory, 58
    inhibitory neurotransmitters, 57
    neurotransmitters, 57
    synaptic architecture, 58
    synaptic structure, 56, 56f
    synaptic transmission, 57
    synaptic types, 56, 58
    synaptic vesicles, 57–58, 57t

neuropsychological tests, 40–41
neurosecretory granules, 51, 51f
neurosecretion, autonomic nervous system, 318–319
neurosecretory system, 313
neurotransmitters
    amino acids, 57
    biogenic amines, 57
    description, 57
    excitatory, 57
    inhibitory, 57
    location and function, 57t
    modulators, 57
    synapses, 57
NGF (nerve growth factors), 68
NMO (neuro myelitis optica), 172–173
nociception and pain, 124–126
nociceptive thalamic nuclei, 294
nodes of Ranvier, 53–54
nondominant hemisphere functions, 471
nondominant hemisphere parietal lobules, 419–421, 420f
nonneuroepithelial brain tumors, 515–516
nonspecific associational thalamic nuclei, 289f–290f, 293–294
nonthalamic afferent inputs to the neocortex, 338
noradrenergic neurons, 566
noradrenergic pathway, to the neocortex, 338
norepinephrine, autonomic nervous system, 319
norepinephrine pathway, to the neocortex, 338
noxious stimulus, 349, 350f
nuclei, 3, 288, 290t
nucleus, 48–49
nucleus acumbens, 425
nutritional disorders, 526t
nystagmus, 239

O

object recognition, 300
occipital lobe. See also eyes.
    cerebral cortex, 9
    complex cells, 454, 454f
    description, 335–336
    eye movements, 455
    hypercomplex cells, 454, 454f
    illustration, 617f
    lesions in area 17, 455–456
    lesions of extrastriate areas 18, 19, 456–459, 457f–459f
    major gyri, 335t
    ocular dominance columns, 453
    overview, 453
    physiology, 454, 454f
    saccadic movements, 455
    simple cells, 454, 454f
    stimulation, 453–454, 453f
occipital neuralgia, 510
occlusion
    in the cerebellum, 405–406, 406f
    of main cortical stem, 491
    of middle cerebral artery, 486f, 492
    of superior division of dominant hemisphere, 491
occlusive disease, 258–259
ocular dominance columns, 453
ocular myasthenia, disorders of the neuromuscular junction, 105
oculomotor cranial nerve, 79, 222–224, 227f, 321
olfactory cranial nerve, 81, 223, 226f
olfactory nuclei, 426
olfactory system, 422–423, 423f
oligodendrocytes, 48f, 53, 53f, 54–56, 60

oligodendroglioma, 360, 360f–361f
olivopontocerebellar atrophy, of the cerebellum, 409, 410f
ontogenetic factor, 331
optical righting reflex, 350, 351f
optic chiasm, 449
optic cranial nerve, 81, 302
optic nerve, 222–224, 226f, 448–449
optic radiation, 449f, 452–453
optic thalamus, 303
orbital frontal pathology, 437
orbitofrontal cortex, 436
outer fibrous tunic, 444, 444f
overlap polymyositis, 104, 104f
overview, 358
oxytocin, 314

P

Paget's disease, 250, 257
pain, sensory pathways, 300–301
pain, spinal cord
  modulation of, 125–126
  nociception, 124–126
  presynaptic inhibition, 126
  projection fibers, 126
  receptors, 124–125
  reflexive response to, 115, 116f
  and temperature, 123f, 128–129
  visceral referred, 126
paired sinuses, 17–18
paleocortex, 428
papez circuit, 431
papilla, eyes, 446
papilledema, eyes, 446
parahippocampal gyrus, 424f–425f, 425
parallel fibers, 396, 396f
paramedian lower pontine syndrome, 265
paramedian medullary syndrome, 261, 262f
paramedian preventricular mesencephalic-diencephalic junction, 271
paramedian syndrome
  with tegmental involvement, 271
  upper pons, 262f
  Weber's syndrome, 267–271, 268f
paramedian upper pons, 266–267, 266f–267f
paramyxovirus, 528
parasagittal lesions, 438–439, 439f
parasympathetic area, 320
parasympathetic nervous system, vs. sympathetic, 320t
parietal lobe
  cerebral cortex, 9
  description, 334–335, 334t
  illustration, 615f–617f
parietal lobe, somatosensory functions
  dominant hemisphere parietal lobules, 418–419
  glioblastoma, 416f–417f
  inferior parietal area, 418
  nondominant hemisphere parietal lobules, 419–421, 420f
  postcentral gyrus, 353f, 414–418, 415f, 415t
  superior parietal area, 418
parieto-occipital eye fields, 352f, 360–363, 362f–363f
Parkinson's disease
  a-synuclein, 377f
  case history, 379–380, 380f
  clinical signs, 376, 376t, 377f
  differential diagnosis, 380–382
  etiology, 377–379
  Lewy bodies, 377f
  management, 379
  Parkinsonism plus syndromes, 381–382, 381t
  pathology of lesions, 375f, 376–377

parotid gland, tumors of, 235
pars ciliaris, 445
pars iridica, 445
pars optica, 445, 446f
partial seizures, 330
pathway for inhibition, 116, 116f–117f
PCD (programmed cell death), neuroembryology of the brain, 74
PDSs (paroxysmal depolarization shifts), 552
PEG (pneumonocephalography), 35, 35f
pelvis, autonomic dual innervation, 323
pericytes, 61
periodic cluster headaches, 510
periodic paralysis (familial periodic paralysis), 102–103
peripheral autonomic neuropathies, 242–243
peripheral nerve disease
  brachial plexus, 141f
  histopathology of peripheral nerve I, 150f
  lumbar plexus, 146f
  median nerve, right upper arm, 142f
  median nerve, wrist and hand, 143f
  mononeuropathy multiplex, 138
  nerves of right lower leg, 147f, 148f, 149z
  nerves of right upper arm, 145f
  neuropathological diagnosis at discharge, 150t
  overview, 138
  peripheral nerve innervation, 139f–140f
  posterior tibial nerve, 150f
  problem solving case histories, 193–198
  radicular nerve innervation, 139f–140f
  sacral plexus, 146f
  ulnar nerve dissected, 143f–144f
peripheral nerve disease, mononeuropathies
  brachial neuritis, 140
  brachial plexopathy, case history, 141–142
  carpal tunnel syndrome, case history, 142–144
  diabetic mononeuropathy, case history, 145, 150f
  Horner's syndrome, case history, 141–142
  of the long thoracic nerve, case history, 142
  lower extremity lumbar sacral plexus, 144, 146f–148f
  lower plexus, 141
  median nerve, anatomy of, 142f–143f
  peroneal nerve, 145, 149f
  sciatic nerve, 144, 146f
  tibial nerve, 145–146
  ulnar nerve dissection, 143f–144f
  upper extremity brachial plexus, 138, 141f
  upper plexus, 140, 141f
peripheral nerve disease, nerve root
  back pain, 158–160
  cervical disk, lateral protrusion, 157f
  cervical invertebral disks, 155f
  dermatome chart, remaining sensibility, 157f
  dorsal root ganglion, 159–160
  intrathecal medications, 160
  lumbar disk, lateral protrusion, 158f
  lumbar puncture, complications from, 160
  neurofibromas, 159
  postherpetic neuralgia, 159–160
  radiculopathy, 155–160
  schwannoma, 159–160, 159f
  tabes dorsalis, 159
peripheral nerve disease, polyneuropathies
  acute progressive motor neuropathy, 148–155
  AIDP (acute inflammatory demyelinating polyneuropathy), 148
  AMAN (acute motor axonal neuropathy), 151
  AMSAN (acute motor sensory axonal neuropathy), 151

Bassen Kornsweig syndrome, 155
  chronic common causes, 152–153
  CMT (Charcot Marie Tooth) disease, 153–155
  familial amyloid polyneuropathy autosomal dominant, 155
  Fisher syndrome, 151–152
  Guillain Barré syndrome, 148–151
  hereditary, 153–155
  hereditary peripheral nerve channelopathies, 155
  overview, 146–148
  porphyria, 155
  spino cerebellar degeneration, 155
peripheral nerve I, histopathology of, 150f
peripheral nerves
  classification of axons by function, 55t
  diagnosing diseases of, 23
  innervation, 139f–140f
  peripheral nerve bundles, 55t
  regeneration, 66–67, 66f
  structures, 52, 55t
peripheral nervous system, neuroembryology of the brain, 75
periventricular system, 313
peroneal nerve, 144–145, 149f
persistent vegetative state, definition, 550
petit mal seizures, 555
PET (positron emission tomography), 36, 37f
photoreceptors, 446–448, 446f, 448f
physiologic tremors, 409–410
pia mater, 19
pineal body, 319
pineal gland, 20
pinocytosis, 69
pituitary gland, neuroembryology of the brain, 79
placing reactions, 350–351
planum temporale, 330f
plasma, 20t
platybasia, 257
pleasure/punishment areas, 440
plexiform layer, cerebral cortex, 328
pneumonocephalography (PEG), 35, 35f
poliomyelitis, 176–178, 177f, 527
polyneuropathies, peripheral nerve disease
  acute progressive motor neuropathy, 148–155
  AIDP (acute inflammatory demyelinating polyneuropathy), 148
  AMAN (acute motor axonal neuropathy), 151
  AMSAN (acute motor sensory axonal neuropathy), 151
  Bassen Kornsweig syndrome, 155
  chronic common causes, 152–153
  CMT (Charcot Marie Tooth) disease, 153–155
  familial amyloid polyneuropathy autosomal dominant, 155
  Fisher syndrome, 151–152
  Guillain Barré syndrome, 148–151
  hereditary, 153–155
  hereditary peripheral nerve channelopathies, 155
  overview, 146–148
  porphyria, 155
  spino cerebellar degeneration, 155
polysomnogram, 566f
polysomnography (PSG), 40
pons, 6, 77f
pontine glioma, 273f
porencephaly, neuroembryology of the brain, 87
porphyria, 155
positron emission tomography (PET), 36, 37f

postcentral gyrus, parietal lobe, 414–418, 415f, 415t
post-concussion syndrome, 508–509
posterior aphasias, 462
posterior cerebral artery, 263, 493–495, 494f, 494t, 495f
posterior circulation, 15
posterior columns, 127–128, 127f, 300
posterior fossa, diagnostic tests, 34–35
posterior horn, 123–124
posterior nucleus, 291
posterior occipital lobe, cerebral hemispheres, 9
posterior root fibers, 123f, 124, 130f
posterior spinal artery, 170
posterior tibial nerve, 150f
postherpetic neuralgia, 159–160
postnatal development, motor center
  deep tendon reflexes, 356
  developmental changes in motor responses, 355t
  distal hand movement, 356
  flaccid paralysis, 356
  instinctive tactile grasp, 356
  long loop reflexes, 353
  overview, 353–354, 353f
  prefrontal areas, 353
  premotor cortex, 353
  primary motor cortex, 354–357, 355f, 355t
  primary motor cortex discharge, 353
  projected movement, 356
  selective grasp, 356
  stretch reflexes, 356
  traction response, 356
postsynaptic disorders of the neuromuscular junction, 105–108
posttraumatic epilepsy, 508
postural tremors, 409
posture and equilibrium of the trunk, in the cerebellum, 399
prefrontal areas, postnatal development, 353
prefrontal cortex, 364, 364f
prefrontal cortex and emotions, 436–437
prefrontal cortex damage, 437–438
prefrontal lobotomy, 438–439, 438f
prefrontal-nonmotor areas, cerebral cortex, 334, 366f
premotor cortex, 353, 358–360, 359f
prenatal development. See neuroembryology of the brain.
pressure sense, sensory pathways, 301
presynaptic disorders of the neuromuscular junction, 108
pretectal area, compression, 255–256, 255f
primary evoked response, 340, 340f
primary motor cortex, 354–357, 355f, 355t, 357
primary motor cortex discharge, 353
primary sulci, neuroembryology of the brain, 81–82
principal pathways, 425f–426f, 430–431, 430f
prion disease, 62–63. See also Creutzfeldt-Jakob disease.
prions, 62–63, 592
problem solving. See case histories, problem solving.
programmed cell death (PCD), neuroembryology of the brain, 74
progressive chronic anterior midline compression syndrome, 163–164
progressive subacute anterior midline compression syndrome, 163–164
projected movement, postnatal development, 356
projection fibers, 126

prolactin, 315
proprioception, 300
prosencephalon (forebrain), neuroembryology of the brain, 79
protoplasmic astrocytes, 59
pseudo akinetic mutism. See locked-in syndrome.
pseudobulbar palsy, 245
pseudocoma. See locked-in syndrome.
pseudo depression, 437
pseudoparalysis, disorders of the neuromuscular junction, 106
pseudopsychopathic syndrome, 437
PSG (polysomnography), 40
psychiatric disorders
  epidemiological aspects, 440t
  genetic aspects, 440t
  neurological substrates, 440t
  pseudo depression, 437
  pseudopsychopathic syndrome, 437
  role of the limbic regions, 440, 440t
  role of the limbic system, 440
  temporal lobe disease, 436
pterygopalatine ganglia, 234
pulvinar nuclei, 291–292
pupillary muscles, 445
pupillary reflexes, 445
purulent brain abscess, 520–521, 521f–522f
pyknolepsy, 555
pyramidal (Golgi type I) cells, 45–46f, 47f, 48f, 49f, 50f, 326, 326f
pyramidal tract lesions, 357–358

R

rabies, 527–528
radiation and the internal capsule of the thalamus, 295
radicular muscle ennervations, in diagnosis, 27t
radicular nerve innervation, 139f–140f
radiculopathy, 155–160
receptor-mediated endocytosis, 69
receptors, 58
receptors for general sensation, 4, 5f
reciprocal innervation of a joint, 115–116, 116f
recruiting response, 293, 340–341, 340f–341f
red muscles, 99–100
red nucleus, 303
reflex activity, 347–348, 347t
reflex bladder, autonomic dual innervation, 324
reflexes of a single muscle, 114–115
reflexive response to pain, 115, 116f
regeneration
  in the central nervous system, 67, 68
  of damaged neurons, 67–68
  glial response to injury, 68
  necrosis, 68
  NGF (nerve growth factors), 68
  of peripheral nerves, 66–67, 66f
  scaffolds, 68
  from stem cells, 67–68
reinnervation, neuromuscular junction, 99
remembering, definition, 575
remote memory, 576
REM sleep, 566–567
Renshaw cells, 122–123, 122f–123f
respiration, center in brain stem, 214
restless leg syndrome, 391
rest tremors, 409
reticular formation
  center in brain stem, 212, 212t
  limbic regions, 423, 439–440, 440t
reticular structures, neuromuscular junction, 92, 94f

retina, 449
retrieval (from memory), definition, 575
retrograde axoplasmic flow, 52
retrovirus, 528–529
rhinencephalon, 422, 423f
rhodopsin, 446
rhombencephalon (hind brain), neuroembryology of the brain, 77–78
rigidity
  decerebrate, 348–349, 349f–350f
  decorticate, 350, 351f
  definition, 375
  spastic, 365
Robertsonian translocation, neuroembryology of the brain, 88
rods, eyes, 446–448, 446f, 448f
rostral frontal lobe, cerebral hemispheres, 9
rough endoplasmic recticulum-nissl body, 459f

S

saccades, central control of, 361–362
saccadic movement, 360–361, 455
sacral plexus, 146f
sacral segments, 321
sacral spine, 133–134, 134f, 137f
salivary glands, autonomic dual innervation, 322
sarcomeres, neuromuscular junction, 91–92
sarcoplasmic reticulum (SR), 92, 94f
satellite (Golgi type II) cells, 45–46f, 59, 63, 63f
scaffolds, 68
SCA (spinocerebellar ataxia), 408
schizencephaly, neuroembryology of the brain, 87, 87f
Schwann Cell Cytoplasm, 52
Schwann cells, 53, 54–56, 59, 63, 64f
schwannomas, 159–160, 159f, 168–169, 168f
sciatic nerve, 144, 146f
scoptic (dark) vision, 446
secondary epileptogenesis, 553
second brain. See enteric nervous system.
second-order nerve cells, motor-sensory cortex, 12
Segawa disease, 390
segmental fibrinoid arterial degeneration, 489–490
segmental sensory patterns, in diagnosis, 27t
seizures. See also epilepsy.
  capacity for seizure discharge, 552
  definition, 549
  EEG, focal seizure discharge, 342–343, 342f–343f
  focal, 551–553, 552t
  focal spike discharge, 551–553, 552t
  generalized, 553–556, 555f–556f
  idiopathic, 553–556, 555f–556f
  partial, 330
  simple partial, 330
  stimulation complex partial, 437, 437t
  stimulation complex partial seizures, 437, 437t
  temporal lobe disease, 432–435, 432t, 433f–435f
selective grasp, postnatal development, 356
senses, 3–4. See also specific senses.
sensory areas of cerebral cortex, map of, 334f
sensory bladder, autonomic dual innervation, 324
sensory ganglia, 3
sensory pathways
  auditory division, 302
  clinical lesions, 300
  deep touch, 300
  facial cranial nerve, 302–303
  fasciculus cuneatas, 300

fasciculus gracilis, 300
glossopharyngeal cranial nerve, 302–303
object recognition, 300
optic cranial nerve, 302
pain, 300–301
posterior columns, 300
pressure sense, 301
prioprioception, 300
proprioception, 300
in the secondary trigeminal nuclei, 301
tactile discrimination, 300–301
temperature, 300–301
thalamus, 299–303
in the thalamus, 299–303
touch, 301
two-point discrimination, 300
vagus cranial nerve, 302–303
vestibulocochlear cranial nerve, 302
vibration sensation, 300–301
sensory receptors, 4t
sensory relay thalamic nuclei, 289–291, 294
septum, 425, 425f
seritonenergic pathway, to the neocortex, 338
serotonin, 319
serotoninergic neurons, 566
short-term working memory, 575–576
sigmoid sinus, 18
simple cells, 454, 454f
simple partial seizures, 330
single-photon emission computed tomograph (SPECT), 36, 37f
sinuses, 16
sinuses, disorders of, 504
six-layered scheme, cerebral cortex, 328
skeletal muscles
  description, 4–5
  effects of motor nerve, 99–100
  nerve-muscle junction. See neuromuscular junction.
  organization, 93f
skin, abnormal development, 89
skull
  diagnostic tests, 34–35
  fractures, 505–506
  malformation of base, 250, 257
sleep, definition, 549
sleep cycle, autonomic nervous system, 318
sleep disorders
  cataplexy, 568
  central sleep apnea, 567
  definition, 549
  diagnostic tests, 40
  excessive daytime sleepiness, 566t, 567–568, 568f, 5689f
  fatal familial insomnia, 593
  hypnogenic hallucinations, 568
  insomnia, 567
  narcolepsy, 566t, 567–568, 568f, 5689f
  sleep paralysis, 568
sleep paralysis, 568
sleep stages
  anatomical background, 565–566, 566f
  brain stem involvement, 566–567, 566t–567t
  cholinergic neurons, 566
  circadian timing cycles, 567
  cortical structure involvement, 566–567, 566t–567t
  diencephalic involvement, 566–567, 566t–567t
  histaminergic neurons, 566
  noradrenergic neurons, 566
  polysomnogram, 566f
  REM sleep, 566–567
  serotoninergic neurons, 566
  sleep-wake cycles, 567

sleep-wake cycles, 567
slow muscles, 99–100
slow potentials, 119
SMA (supplemental motor area), 359
smooth muscles, 4–5
smooth pursuit, eye movements, 362
smooth stellate cells, 326f, 327, 327f
soma, 45, 51
somatic division, 5
somatic motor areas of cerebral cortex, map of, 334f
somatosensory functions. See parietal lobe, somatosensory functions.
somatotropin, 315–316
spastic rigidity, 365
specific associational thalamic nuclei, 291–292, 294
SPECT (single-photon emission computed tomograph), 36, 37f
speech and language
  ablation of speech areas, 463–466, 465f–466f
  anterior aphasias, 462
  aphasia, 461–463, 462f–463f
  aphasic arrest, 463
  apraxia, 471
  Broca's motor aphasia, 461, 462f
  cerebral dominance, 460–461
  components of language function, 462–463
  corpus callosum, role of, 471–472
  development in children, 461
  dysarthria, 460–463, 461f
  fluent aphasias, 466–471, 467f
  inferior parietal lobule, 461, 462f
  nondominant hemisphere functions, 471
  posterior aphasias, 462
  speech arrest, 463
  stimulating speech areas, 463, 463f
  supplementary motor cortex, 461
  Wernicke's receptive aphasia area, 461, 462f
speech arrest, 463
speech/voice control, in the cerebellum, 399
spider venom, disorders of the neuromuscular junction, 108
spinal accessory nerve, 243, 244f
spinal canal, 20, 75
spinal cord
  anterior horn cells, 113, 113f
  anterolateral pathway, 127f, 128
  atlas levels, 133–137, 133f–137f
  Babinski response, 130, 130f
  cervical levels, 136, 136f, 136f–137f
  cross sections, 6f, 113–114, 113f
  delay, 117
  dermatome boundaries, 113–114, 113f
  description, 5–6
  diagnosing diseases of, 26
  diagnostic tests, 31–34, 31f
  differentiation, neuroembryology of the brain, 75–77, 76f
  excitatory postsynaptic potential, 116, 116f, 118f
  gamma system, 120–122, 120f–122f
  Golgi tendon organs, 122
  gross anatomy, 111–113, 111f–113f
  inhibitory postsynaptic potential, 116–118, 118f
  interneurons, 122–123
  laminar organization, 123–124, 123f
  lower motor neurons, 129–131, 130t
  lumbar levels, 134, 134f, 137f
  lumbar puncture, 112, 112f
  major pathways, 128t
  membrane basis of integration, 116–118
  muscle spindle, 119–120, 120f

nociception and pain, 124–126
pathway for inhibition, 116, 116f–117f
posterior horn, 123–124
posterior root fibers, 123f, 124, 130f
problem solving case histories, 193–198
reciprocal innervation of a joint, 115–116, 116f
reflexes of a single muscle, 114–115
reflexive response to pain, 115, 116f
Renshaw cells, 122–123, 122f–123f
sacral levels, 133–134, 134f, 137f
slow potentials, 119
stretch receptors, 119–122
stretch reflexes, 115, 115f
synaptic mechanisms, 1189
thoracic levels, 135, 135f, 137f
transection, 348, 348t, 349f
unconscious proprioception, 129–131
upper motor neurons, 129–131, 130t
ventral horn, 123–124, 123f
vs. brain stem, 199–200
spinal cord, diseases
  acute anterior poliomyelitis, 176–178, 177f
  acute compression or transection, 162–164
  ALS (amyotropic lateral sclerosis), 178–181, 179t, 180f, 180t
  anastomotic vessels, 170, 170f
  of the anterior horn cell, 176–178
  anterior spinal artery, 170, 170f
  anterior spinal occlusion, 169–171
  Arnold Chiari malformation, 175f
  Brown-Sequard hemisection sun, 163t
  Brown-Sequard hemisection syndrome, 163
  cervical disk disease, 164–167, 165f–166f
  combined systems disease, 183–185, 183f
  compression, case histories, 165–167
  consequences of extrinsic compression, 163t
  demyelinating diseases, 186–190, 187f–188f
  Devic's syndrome, 172f
  extrinsic lesions, 164–167, 164f–166f
  fracture dislocations, 164, 164f
  Friedrich's ataxia, 184–186, 185f
  intradural-extramedullary tumors, 167–169, 167f–168f
  intrinsic disorders, 169–176
  Kennedy's disease, 178
  meningiomas, 167–168, 167f
  multiple sclerosis, 186–190, 187f–188f
  NMO (neuro myelitis optica), 172–173
  posterior spinal artery, 170
  problem solving case histories, 193–198
  progressive chronic anterior midline compression syndrome, 163–164
  progressive subacute anterior midline compression syndrome, 163–164
  schwannomas, 168–169, 168f
  spinal muscular atrophy, 178
  syringobulbia, 175–176
  syringomyelia, 173–176, 173f–175f
  tabes dorsalis, 181–183, 181f, 182t
  tertiary neurosyphilis syndromes, 182t
  transverse myelitis, 171–174, 172f
  vascular disease, 169–171, 170f
  X-linked Recessive Bulbospinal Neuronopathy, 178
spinal cord, pain
  modulation of, 125–126
  nociception, 124–126
  presynaptic inhibition, 126
  projection fibers, 126
  receptors, 124–125
  and temperature, 123f, 128–129
  visceral referred, 126

spinal cord, tracts
  ascending sensory, 127–131
  corticospinal, 126–127, 129f, 131f
  descending, 126–127
  lamination pattern, 126, 126f–127f
  posterior columns, 127–128, 127f
  spinothalmic, 130f
  tactile discrimination, 127–128
spinal muscular atrophy, 178
spinal nerve, diagnosing diseases of, 23, 26
spindle cell multiform layer, cerebral cortex, 328
spinocerebellar ataxia (SCA), 408
spino cerebellar degeneration, 155
spinocerebellar tracts, 411–412f
spinothalmics, in the brain stem, 218
spinothalmic tracts, 130f
spiny neurons, 326
spiny stellate neurons, 327
SR (sarcoplasmic reticulum), 92, 94f
status epilepticus, 564–565, 565f, 581–582
stem cells, for regeneration, 67–68
stenosis of the basilar vertebral arteries, 258
STH (growth hormone), 315–316
stimulation, as study method, 330–331
straight sinus, 17
stretch receptors, 119–122
stretch reflexes, 115, 115f, 356
stria terminalis, 431
Sturge-Weber syndrome, neuroembryology of the brain, 89
subarachnoid hemorrhage, 271–274, 499–503, 500t, 502f, 502t–503t
subcortical band heterotopia, neuroembryology of the brain, 86
subcortical limbic regions, 423–425, 424t
subcortical white matter, afferents and efferents, 336–337, 336f–337f
subdural empyema, 520
subdural hematomas, 506–508, 507f
submandibular ganglia, 234
substantia negra, 303
subthalamus, 8, 8t, 298–299, 304–306
summary of structures affected, autonomic dual innervation, 320t
superficial cerebral veins, 15
superficial reflexes, in diagnosis, 27t–28t
superior cerebellar veins, 16
superior cerebral veins, 15
superior colliculus, 209–210, 209f, 255–256, 255f
superior longitudinal fasciculus, 337, 467f
superior parietal area, parietal lobe, 418
superior pontine syndromes, 266–267, 266f–267f
superior sagittal sinus, 17
supplemental motor area (SMA), 359
supplementary motor cortex, 461
suppressor areas, 363–364
sympathetic area, 320
sympathetic nervous system vs. parasympathetic, 320t
sympathetic system, 321, 321f
symptom categories, 22
synapses
  architecture, 58
  chemical, 56
  definition, 3
  dendritic spines, 58
  electrical, 56
  excitatory, 58
  illustration, 56f
  inhibitory, 58
  neurotransmitters, 57
  structure, 56, 56f
  transmission, 57

  types, 56, 58
  vesicles, 57–58, 57t
synaptic mechanisms, 1189
syncope, definition, 549
syndromes of the cerebellum, 253–255, 254f
syndromes of the tentorium, 255f–256f, 256
syphilis, tertiary neurosyphilis syndromes, 182t
syringobulbia, 89–90, 175–176
syringomyelia, 89, 173–176, 173f–175f
system disorders, 529

T

tabes dorsalis, 159, 181–183, 181f, 182t
tactile discrimination, 300–301
tactile placing reactions, 351
tardive dyskinesias, 390
task-specific kinetic tremors, 411
taste bud nerves, neuroembryology, 81
taste sensation, 234
tectum, 6–7, 207–208, 209f
tegmentum
  description, 6–7, 210, 210f–211f
  lesions, clinical signs, 219, 219t
  major tracts in tegmental zones, 203t
  overview, 199, 200f, 200t
  pontine basis tegmentum, 208–209, 209f
  zones, 202t, 211f
telencephalic cortex, 307
telencephalon, neuroembryology of the brain, 79f
temperature
  and pain, 123f, 128–129
  sensory pathways, 300–301
temporal lobe. See also limbic regions in the brain, temporal lobe.
  cerebral cortex, 9, 463f
  definition, 305
  description, 335–336, 335f
  illustration, 615f–617f
  neocortex, 330f
  stimulation, memory disorders, 581, 581f
tension headaches, 510
tensor vali palatine, 229
tentorial meningiomas, 256
Tentorial Notch syndrome, 255f–256f, 255–256
tentorium cerebelli, 18
terminal cisternae, 92
tertiary neurosyphilis syndromes, 182t
testing. See diagnosis, studies in neurology.
thalamic afferent inputs to the neocortex, 337–338
thalamic atlas
  anterior commissure, 306
  cerebrum, 307
  cranial nerve nuclei, 304
  deep telencephalic gray, 303–306
  epithalamus, 303–304, 306
  fornix, 304–305
  gross features, 304, 306
  hypothalamus, 304, 306
  illustrations, 304f–306f
  optic thalamus, 303
  red nucleus, 303
  substantia negra, 303
  subthalamus, 304–306
  telencephalic cortex, 307
  temporal lobe, 305
  thalamus, 303–304, 306
  ventricular system, 305–306
thalamic nuclei
  anterior nuclei, 291
  audition, 292–293
  cortical projections, 295t, 297f
  dorsomedial nucleus, 291
  functional groups, 294t. See also specific groups.

  illustration, 290f, 296f
  lateral dorsal nucleus, 291
  lateral nuclear mass, 289
  limbic, 291, 294
  magnocellular portion of the dorsomedial nucleus, 291
  medial nuclear complex, 291
  motor relay, 289–291, 294
  nociceptive, 294
  nonspecific associated, 294
  nonspecific associational, 289f–290f, 293
  posterior nucleus, 291
  pulvinar nuclei, 291–292
  recruiting response, 293
  sensory relay, 289–291, 294
  specific associational, 291–292, 294
  VA (ventral anterior) nucleus, 289, 291
  ventral basal nuclear mass, 289
  ventral lateral nucleus, 291
  ventral posterior nucleus, 291
  ventrobasal complex, lateral posterior, 289–291
  vision, 293, 293f
  VL (ventral lateral) somatic motor thalamus, 291
  VPL (ventral posterior lateral) nucleus, 291
  VPM (ventral posterior medial) nucleus, 291
thalamic relay neutrons, interaction with cortical neurons, 341–342, 342f
thalamus
  afferent inputs to neocortex, 337–338
  afferent pathways to, 297f–298f
  and the cerebral cortex, 295
  clinical considerations, 296–298
  clinical lesions, 300
  Creutzfeldt-Jakob disease, 292
  deep touch, 300
  definition, 8, 8t, 288, 288f
  dorsal, 337–338
  EEG activity, 339–340
  epithalamus
    afferent inputs to the neocortex, 338
    definition, 8, 8t
    description, 303–304, 306, 319
  fasciculus cuneatas, 300
  fasciculus gracilis, 300
  illustration, 616f
  inputs to, 296
  limbic regions, 424–425, 424f
  nuclei, 288, 290t
  object recognition, 300
  posterior columns, 300
  proprioception, 300
  radiation and the internal capsule, 295
  sensory pathways, 299–303
  tactile discrimination, 300
  thalamic syndrome (of Dejerine), 296–298, 297f
  two-point discrimination, 300
  ventral, 338
  vibration sensation, 300
third-order neurons, motor-sensory cortex, 12
third ventricle, 20, 75
thoracic spine, 135, 135f, 137f
thoracic sympathetic ganglia, 321
thoracolumbar area, 320
thorax, voluntary motor pathways, 366–367, 366f
thyrotrophic hormone (TSH), 316
TIAs (transient ischemic attacks), 483
tibial nerve, 145–146
tic, douloureux, 230
tics, 390
tinnitus, 237

tonic labyrinthine reflexes, 349, 350f
tonic neck reflexes, 349, 349f
topographic patterns in the cerebellum, 397, 398f
total posterior inferior cerebeller artery syndrome, 260f
touch, 300–301
toxic disorders of the muscles, 104
toxic metabolic disorder, 277
traction response, postnatal development, 356
tracts, spinal cord
  ascending sensory, 127–131
  corticospinal, 126–127, 129f, 131f
  descending, 126–127
  lamination pattern, 126, 126f–127f
  posterior columns, 127–128, 127f
  spinothalmic, 130f
  tactile discrimination, 127–128
transection of spinal cord, 162–164, 348, 348t, 349f
transient global amnesia, 580–581
transient ischemic attacks (TIAs), 483
transmitter connections, basal ganglia, 372f, 375f
transverse division of the cerebellum, 395, 395f, 396t
transverse myelitis, 171–174, 172f
transverse tubules, 92
trauma, to the muscles, 104
traumatic amnesia, 582
tremors
  action, 409
  essential, 410
  intentional, 410–411
  kinetic, 410–411
  in movement disorders, 375
  physiologic, 409–410
  postural, 409
  rest, 409
  task-specific kinetic, 411
trigeminal cranial nerve, 80, 226f, 228–232
trigeminal neuralgia, 230
trochlear nerve, 79, 227f, 228
trophic center, 51
tropomyosin, neuromuscular junction, 93–94
troponin, neuromuscular junction, 93–94
TSH (thyrotrophic hormone), 316
T-SR coupling, 92–93, 94f
T system, 92, 94f

tuberous sclerosis, 89, 511
two-point discrimination, 300
type I X-linked dominant lissencephaly, neuroembryology of the brain, 85

U

ulnar nerve dissection, 143f–144f
uncinate fasciculus, 337, 337f
unconscious proprioception, 129–131
uninhibited bladder, autonomic dual innervation, 324
unsteadiness, cranial nerve disorder, 239
upper motor neuron, motor-sensory cortex, 12, 13t
upper motor neuron paralysis, motor-sensory cortex, 13
upper motor neurons, 129–131, 130t
upper plexus, 140, 141f
upper pons, motor and main sensory nuclei, 207, 207t, 208f
upper spinal nerves, neuroembryology of the brain, 81f

V

vagus cranial nerve
  autonomic nervous system, 321
  general function, 240–243, 241f
  general function of, 240–243, 241f
  neuroembryology, 80
  sensory pathways, 302–303
vascular disease of the spinal cord, 169–171, 170f
vascular syndromes. See also arteries, syndromes of; cerebral hemispheres, vascular diseases.
  of the cerebellum, 405
  and extrinsic lesions, 257
vasopressin, 314
VA (ventral anterior) nucleus, 289, 291
veins, disorders of, 504
ventral amygdalofugal pathway, 426, 431
ventral basal nuclear mass, 289
ventral horn, 123–124, 123f
ventral horn cells, 5–6, 459f
ventral horn equivalent, 6–7
ventral lateral nucleus, 291
ventral lateral (VL) somatic motor thalamus, 291
ventral posterior lateral (VPL) nucleus, 291
ventral posterior medial (VPM) nucleus, 291
ventral posterior nucleus, 291

ventral thalamus, 338
ventricular system, 305–306. See also central nervous system.
  cerebral aqueduct, 20
  cerebrospinal fluid, 20, 20t
  fourth ventricle, 20
  illustration, 617f
  illustrations, 19f–20f
  lateral ventricles, 20
  neuroembryology of the brain, 75
  overview, 19–20
  plasma, 20t
  spinal canal, 20
  third ventricle, 20
ventricular zone, 206–208
ventriculography, 35
ventrobasal complex, lateral posterior, 289–291
vergence eye movements, 362
vertebral arteries, 200–201, 204f, 259
vertibral artery syndrome, 262f
vertigo, 238
vestibular neuropathy, 239
vestibular reflexes, in the cerebellum, 398
vestibular schwannoma, 253f
vestibulocochlear cranial nerve
  general function, 236–239, 236f
  general function of, 236–239, 236f
  neuroembryology, 81
vestibulocochlear cranial nerve, sensory pathways, 302
vestibulo-ocular movements, 362
vibration sensation, 300–301
visceral (autonomic) division, 5
vision, 293, 293f. See also eye.
visual defects, temporal lobe disease, 435
visual fields
  fovea centralis, 449
  lesions in the optic pathway, 449–452, 450f–452f
  LGN (lateral geniculate nucleus), 452
  optic chiasm, 449
  optic nerve, 449
  retina, 449
visual pathway, 449, 449f
visual perception, 427
visual placing reactions, 350–351
VL (ventral lateral) somatic motor thalamus, 291
voluntary motor pathways
  abdomen, 366–367, 366f

basic principles of motor system, 366
corticomesencephalic system, 367
corticonuclear system, 367, 367f
corticospinal tract, 366–367, 366f
eye muscles, 367
facial muscles, 367
jaw muscles, 367
limbs, 366–367, 366f
thorax, 366–367, 366f
tongue muscles, 367
vomiting, 214, 238
Von Economo's encephalitis, 527
VPL (ventral posterior lateral) nucleus, 291
VPM (ventral posterior medial) nucleus, 291
vs. spinal cord, 202t

W

WAIS (Wechsler Adult Intelligent Score), 40–41
Wallerian degeneration, 65, 65f–66f
water balance, autonomic nervous system, 318–319
Weber's syndromes, 267–271, 268f
Wechsler Adult Intelligent Score (WAIS), 40–41
Wechsler Bellevue Test of Adult Intelligence. See WAIS (Wechsler Adult Intelligent Score).
Wechsler Memory Score, 41
Wernicke-Korsakoff encephalopathy, 577–579, 578t
Wernicke's receptive aphasia area, 461, 462f
white matter
  brain, 6–7
  cerebrum, 10–11, 11t
  cortical, 10–11
  description, 203
  diencephalon, 293–294
  gray matter equivalents, 202t
  illustration, 615f–617f
  nervous system, 3
  ventricular zone, 206, 206f
white muscles, 99–100
Wilson's disease (hepatolenticular degeneration), 388–389
Wisconsin Card Sorting Test, 41

X

X-linked Recessive Bulbospinal Neuronopathy, 178